W9-AWO-093

PLASTIC SURGERY

Editor

JOSEPH G. McCARTHY, M.D.

Lawrence D. Bell Professor of Plastic Surgery and
Director of the Institute of Reconstructive Plastic Surgery
New York University Medical Center
New York, New York

Editors, Hand Surgery Volumes

JAMES W. MAY, JR., M.D.

Director of Plastic Surgery and Hand Surgery Service
Massachusetts General Hospital
Associate Clinical Professor of Surgery
Harvard Medical School
Boston, Massachusetts

J. WILLIAM LITTLER, M.D.

Past Professor of Clinical Surgery
College of Physicians and Surgeons
Columbia University, New York
Senior Attending Surgeon
The St. Luke's–Roosevelt Hospital Center
New York, New York

PLASTIC SURGERY

VOLUME 1

GENERAL PRINCIPLES

W.B. SAUNDERS COMPANY
A Division of Harcourt Brace & Company
Philadelphia • London • Toronto
Montreal • Sydney • Tokyo

W.B. SAUNDERS COMPANY
A Division of
Harcourt Brace & Company

The Curtis Center
Independence Square West
Philadelphia, Pennsylvania 19106

Library of Congress Cataloging-in-Publication Data

Plastic surgery.
Contents: v. 1. General principles—v. 2–3.
The face—v. 4. Cleft lip & palate and craniofacial anomalies—[etc.]
1. Surgery, Plastic. I. McCarthy, Joseph G., 1938–
[DNLM: 1. Surgery, Plastic. WO 600 P7122]

RD118.P536 1990 617′.95 87–9809

ISBN 0–7216–1514–7 (set)

Editor: W. B. Saunders Staff
Designer: W. B. Saunders Staff
Production Manager: Frank Polizzano
Manuscript Editor: David Harvey
Illustration Coordinator: Lisa Lambert
Indexer: Kathleen Garcia
Cover Designer: Ellen Bodner

Volume 1 0–7216–2542–8
Volume 2 0–7216–2543–6
Volume 3 0–7216–2544–4
Volume 4 0–7216–2545–2
Volume 5 0–7216–2546–0
Volume 6 0–7216–2547–9
Volume 7 0–7216–2548–7
Volume 8 0–7216–2549–5
Plastic Surgery 8 Volume Set 0–7216–1514–7

Copyright © 1990 by W. B. Saunders Company.

All rights reserved. No part of this publication may be reproduced or transmitted in any form or by any means, electronic or mechanical, including photocopy, recording, or any information storage and retrieval system, without permission in writing from the publisher.

Printed in the United States of America.

Last digit is the print number: 9 8 7 6 5 4

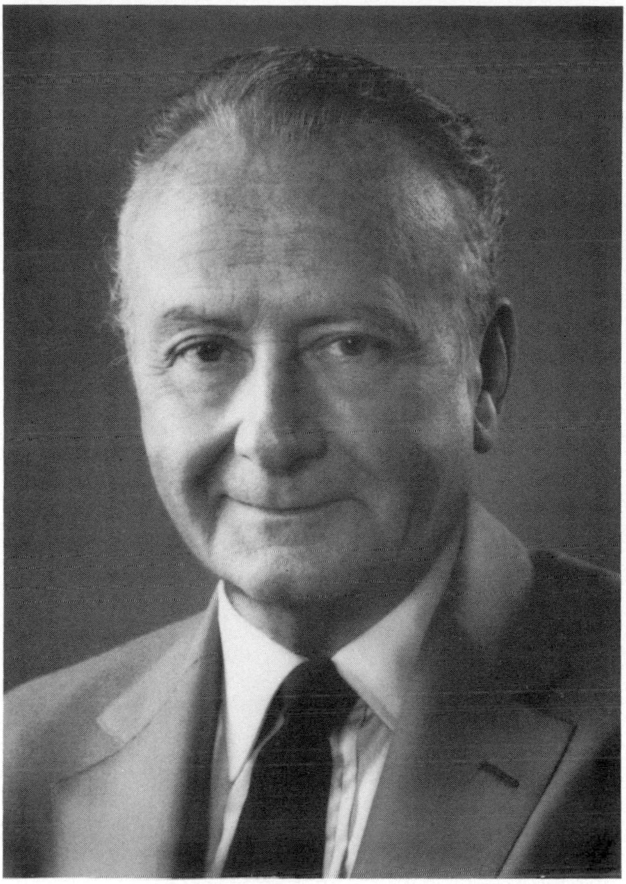

John Marquis Converse

(1909–1981)

This book is dedicated to John Marquis Converse. His enthusiasm for plastic surgery was unrivaled and his contributions to the field were legendary. Through his many writings he not only educated and inspired the plastic surgeon in the era after World War II, but also helped to define modern plastic surgery. This book is a testimony to his professional accomplishments.

Contributors

DAVID B. APFELBERG, M.D.
Assistant Clinical Professor of Plastic Surgery, Stanford University School of Medicine; Director, Comprehensive Laser Center, Palo Alto Medical Foundation, Palo Alto, California.

LOUIS C. ARGENTA, M.D.
Associate Professor of Surgery, University of Michigan School of Medicine; Attending Surgeon, University Hospital, Ann Arbor Veterans Administration Hospital, and St. Joseph Mercy Hospital, Ann Arbor, Michigan.

STEPHAN ARIYAN, M.D.
Professor of Surgery and Chief of Plastic and Reconstructive Surgery, Yale University School of Medicine; Chief of Plastic Surgery, Yale–New Haven Hospital, New Haven; Consultant in Plastic Surgery, Veterans Administration Hospital, West Haven, Connecticut.

SHERRELL J. ASTON, M.D.
Associate Professor of Surgery (Plastic Surgery), New York University School of Medicine; Attending Surgeon, University Hospital and Manhattan Eye, Ear & Throat Hospital, New York, New York.

ERIC D. AUSTAD, M.D.
Clinical Assistant Professor of Surgery, University of Michigan School of Medicine; Attending Surgeon, St. Joseph Mercy Hospital, Ann Arbor, and Chelsea Community Hospital, Chelsea, Michigan.

A. D. BAGNALL, L.C.S.T., M.A.A.S.H.
Speech Pathologist, South Australia Cranio-Facial Unit, Adelaide Children's Hospital, Adelaide, South Australia.

VAHRAM Y. BAKAMJIAN, M.D.
Clinical Associate Professor of Surgery (Plastic Surgery), University of Rochester School of Medicine and Dentistry and Stanford University School of Medicine; Associate Chief, Department of Head and Neck Surgery and Oncology, Roswell Park Memorial Institute, Buffalo, New York.

DANIEL C. BAKER, M.D.
Associate Professor of Surgery (Plastic Surgery), New York University School of Medicine; Attending Surgeon, University Hospital, Bellevue Hospital Center, Manhattan Eye, Ear & Throat Hospital, and Manhattan Veterans Administration Hospital, New York, New York.

THOMAS J. BAKER, M.D.
Assistant Clinical Professor of Surgery (Plastic Surgery), University of Miami School of Medicine; Attending Surgeon, Mercy Hospital and Cedars Medical Center, Miami, Florida.

DONALD L. BALLANTYNE, JR., PH.D.
Professor of Experimental Surgery, New York University School of Medicine; Director of Training and Microsurgical Research Laboratories, Institute of Reconstructive Plastic Surgery, New York University Medical Center, New York, New York.

ALFONSO BARRERA, M.D.
Attending Surgeon, Memorial City Medical Center Hospital and West Houston Medical Center Hospital, Houston, Texas.

FRITZ E. BARTON, JR., M.D.
Professor and Chairman, Division of Plastic Surgery, Department of Surgery, The University of Texas Health Science Center at Dallas; Chief, Plastic Surgery Service, Children's Medical Center; Assistant Chief, Plastic and Reconstructive Surgery Service, Baylor University Medical Center; Attending Surgeon, Parkland Memorial Hospital, Dallas Veterans Administration Hospital, Presbyterian Medical Center, and Gaston Episcopal Hospital, Dallas, Texas.

ROBERT W. BEASLEY, M.D.
Professor of Surgery (Plastic Surgery), New York University School of Medicine; Director of Hand Surgery Services, Institute of Reconstructive Plastic Surgery, New York University Medical Center, New York, New York.

SAMUEL I. BERKOWITZ, D.D.S.
Clinical Professor of Pediatrics, University of Miami School of Medicine; Orthodontist, Dental Clinic, Miami Children's Hospital, Miami, Florida.

PHILIP BONANNO, M.D.
Clinical Professor of Surgery, New York Medical College; Associate Clinical Professor of Plastic Surgery, New York University Medical Center; Attending Surgeon, Bellevue Hospital, New York, Westchester Medical Center, Valhalla, and Northern Westchester Hospital Center, Mount Kisco, New York.

JOHN BOSTWICK III, M.D.
Professor of Surgery, Emory University School of Medicine; Chief of Plastic Surgery, Emory University Hospital, Atlanta, Georgia.

PAUL W. BRAND, C.B.E.-M.B.-B.S., F.R.C.S.
Clinical Professor of Orthopaedics and Surgery, Louisiana State University Medical School; Senior Consultant, Gillis W. Long Hansen's Disease Center, Carville, Louisiana.

BURT BRENT, M.D.
Clinical Associate Professor of Plastic Surgery, Stanford University School of Medicine; Clinical Faculty, Stanford University Hospital; Staff Surgeon, El Camino Hospital, Palo Alto, California.

GARRY S. BRODY, M.D.
Clinical Professor of Surgery (Plastic Surgery), University of Southern California School of Medicine; Chief of Plastic Surgery Research, Rancho Los Amigos Hospital; Attending Surgeon, Downey Community Hospital, Downey, California.

PETER T. BRONSKY, D.M.D., M.S.
Visiting Scientist, Department of Orthodontics and the Dental Research Center, University of North Carolina at Chapel Hill, North Carolina.

EARL Z. BROWNE, JR., M.D.
Chairman, Department of Plastic and Reconstructive Surgery, Cleveland Clinic Foundation, Cleveland, Ohio.

HARRY J. BUNCKE, M.D.
Clinical Professor of Plastic Surgery, University of California, San Francisco, School of Medicine; Director, Department of Microsurgical Transplantation and Replantation, Davies Medical Center, San Francisco; Consultant, San Francisco General Hospital, Fort Miley Veterans Administration Hospital, and Oak Knoll Naval Hospital; Attending Surgeon, Mills Hospital, San Mateo, and Peninsula Hospital, Burlingame, California.

H. STEVE BYRD, M.D.
Associate Professor of Plastic and Reconstructive Surgery, The University of Texas Health Science Center at Dallas; Attending Surgeon, Children's Medical Center, Baylor University Medical Center, Presbyterian Hospital, and St. Paul Hospital, Dallas, Texas.

PHILLIP R. CASSON, M.B., F.R.C.S.
New York University School of Medicine; Attending Surgeon, University Hospital, Bellevue Hospital Center, Manhattan Veterans Administration Hospital, and New York Eye & Ear Infirmary, New York, New York.

ROBERT A. CHASE, M.D.
Emile Holman Professor of Surgery Emeritus, and Chairman, Division of Anatomy, Stanford University Medical Center, Stanford, California.

ZENO N. CHICARILLI, M.D.
Assistant Clinical Professor of Surgery (Plastic Surgery), Yale University School of Medicine; Attending Surgeon, Yale–New Haven Hospital and Hospital of St. Raphael, New Haven, Connecticut.

DAVID T. W. CHIU, M.D.
Assistant Professor of Surgery (Plastic Surgery), New York University School of Medicine; Assistant Attending in Plastic Surgery, New York University Medical Center, Beekman Downtown Hospital, and New York Eye & Ear Infirmary; Attending Surgeon, Cabrini Hospital; Associate Attending Surgeon, Manhattan Eye, Ear & Throat Hospital, New York, New York.

LEO CLODIUS, M.D.
Docent for Plastic Surgery, Zurich University Medical School; Visiting Surgeon, American Medical International Hospital, Zurich, Switzerland.

PETER J. COCCARO, D.D.S.
Formerly Associate Professor of Orthodontics, New York University School of Dentistry, and Research Professor of Clinical Surgery (Orthodontics), New York University School of Medicine, New York, New York.

BENJAMIN E. COHEN, M.D.
Clinical Assistant Professor, Division of Plastic Surgery, Baylor College of Medicine; Academic

Chief and Director, Plastic Surgery Residency Program, and Director, Microsurgical Research and Training Laboratory, St. Joseph Hospital, Houston, Texas.

I. KELMAN COHEN, M.D.
Professor of Surgery and Chairman of Plastic and Reconstructive Surgery, Medical College of Virginia; Attending Surgeon, Medical College of Virginia Hospitals, Richmond Eye & Ear Hospital, St. Mary's Hospital, and McGuire Veterans Administration Hospital, Richmond, Virginia.

M. MICHAEL COHEN, JR., D.M.D., PH.D.
Professor of Oral Pathology, Faculty of Dentistry, and Professor of Pediatrics, Faculty of Medicine, Dalhousie University; Consultant, Izzak Walton Killam Hospital for Children, Halifax, Nova Scotia, Canada.

STEPHEN R. COLEN, M.D., D.D.S.
Assistant Professor of Surgery (Plastic Surgery), New York University School of Medicine; Attending Surgeon, University Hospital, Bellevue Hospital Center, Manhattan Eye, Ear & Throat Hospital, and New York Eye & Ear Infirmary, New York, New York.

ERNEST D. CRONIN, M.D.
Clinical Assistant Professor of Plastic Surgery, Baylor College of Medicine; Chief of Plastic Surgery, St. Joseph Hospital, Houston, Texas.

THOMAS D. CRONIN, M.D.
Clinical Professor of Plastic Surgery, Baylor College of Medicine; Attending Surgeon, St. Joseph Hospital, Houston, Texas.

COURT B. CUTTING, M.D.
Assistant Professor of Surgery (Plastic Surgery), New York University School of Medicine; Attending Surgeon, New York University Medical Center and Bellevue Hospital; Chief of Plastic Surgery, Manhattan Veterans Administration Hospital, New York, New York.

ROLLIN K. DANIEL, M.D.
Attending Staff, Hoag Memorial Hospital Presbyterian, Newport Beach, and Western Medical Center, Santa Ana, California.

DAVID J. DAVID, F.R.C.S., F.R.A.C.S.
Head, South Australian Cranio-Facial Unit, Adelaide Children's Hospital; Head, Department of Plastic and Reconstructive Surgery, Royal Adelaide Hospital, Adelaide, South Australia.

CHARLES J. DEVINE, JR., M.D.
Professor of Urology, The Eastern Virginia Medical School of the Medical College of Hampton Roads, Norfolk, Virginia.

MATTHIAS B. DONELAN, M.D.
Assistant Clinical Professor of Surgery, Harvard Medical School; Chief, Plastic and Reconstructive Surgery, Shriners Burns Institute, Boston; Assistant Surgeon, Massachusetts General Hospital, Boston, Massachusetts.

CRAIG R. DUFRESNE, M.D.
Assistant Professor of Plastic Surgery, Johns Hopkins University School of Medicine; Director, The Facial Rehabilitation Center and Cleft Lip and Palate Clinic, Johns Hopkins Hospital and Children's Hospital; Chief of Plastic Surgery Service, Loch Raven Veterans Administration Medical Center; Attending Physician in Plastic Surgery, The Maryland Institute of Emergency Medical Services Systems, Baltimore, Maryland.

BRADFORD W. EDGERTON, M.D.
Clinical Assistant Professor of Plastic Surgery, University of Southern California, Los Angeles, California; Attending Plastic Surgeon, Southern California Permanente Medical Group, Los Angeles, California

RAY A. ELLIOTT, JR., M.D.
Clinical Professor of Plastic Surgery and Associate Clinical Professor of Orthopedics (Hand), Albany Medical College; Attending Surgeon, Albany Medical Center, Albany Memorial Hospital, and Albany Veterans Administration Hospital, Albany, New York.

DONALD H. ENLOW, PH.D.
Thomas Hill Distinguished Professor of Oral Biology, Case Western Reserve University School of Dentistry, Cleveland, Ohio.

FRED J. EPSTEIN, M.D.
Professor of Neurosurgery, New York University School of Medicine; Attending Surgeon, University Hospital, Bellevue Hospital Center, and St. Vincent's Medical Center, New York, New York.

ISSA ESHIMA, M.D.
Research Fellow, Division of Plastic Surgery, University of California, San Francisco, School of Medicine, San Francisco, California.

MIROSLAV FÁRA, M.D.
Professor of Plastic Surgery, Charles University; Head, Clinic of Plastic Surgery and Burn Unit, Prague, Czechoslovakia.

MICHAEL C. FASCHING, M.D.
Minneapolis, Minnesota.

JOEL J. FELDMAN, M.D.
Associate in Plastic Surgery, Harvard Medical School; Consultant Plastic Surgeon, Shriners Burns Institute and Massachusetts General Hospital, Boston, Massachusetts; Attending Surgeon, Mount Auburn Hospital, Cambridge, Massachusetts.

JOSEPH FISCHER, M.D.
Attending Surgeon, Community General Hospital, Syracuse, New York.

G. GREGORY GALLICO III, M.D.
Assistant Professor of Surgery, Harvard Medical School; Assistant Surgeon, Massachusetts General Hospital, Boston.

GREGORY S. GEORGIADE, M.D.
Associate Professor of Surgery, Division of Plastic, Maxillofacial and Reconstructive Surgery, Duke University School of Medicine, Durham, North Carolina.

NICHOLAS G. GEORGIADE, M.D.
Professor of Surgery, Division of Plastic, Maxillofacial and Reconstructive Surgery, Duke University School of Medicine, Durham, North Carolina.

THOMAS GIBSON, D.Sc., F.R.C.S.
Honorary Clinical Lecturer, Glasgow University Medical School; Emeritus Professor in Bioengineering, University of Strathclyde, Glasgow, Scotland.

BARRY H. GRAYSON, D.D.S.
Associate Professor of Clinical Surgery (Orthodontics), New York University School of Medicine; Associate Professor of Clinical Orthodontics, New York University School of Dentistry, New York, New York.

FREDERICK M. GRAZER, M.D.
Associate Clinical Professor, Division of Plastic Surgery, University of California, Irvine, School of Medicine; Clinical Associate Professor in Plastic and Reconstructive Surgery, Pennsylvania State University School of Medicine; Chairman, Baromedical Committee, Hoag Memorial Hospital Presbyterian, Newport Beach, California.

JAMES C. GROTTING, M.D., F.A.C.S.
Associate Professor of Surgery, Division of Plastic Surgery, University of Alabama Medical School, Birmingham, Alabama.

GRAHAM J. GUMLEY, M.B., B.S., F.R.A.C.S.
Staff Associate, Lahey Clinic Foundation, Burlington, Massachusetts.

VINCENT R. HENTZ, M.D.
Associate Professor of Surgery, Stanford University School of Medicine; Chief, Division of Hand and Upper Extremity Surgery, Stanford University Hospital, Palo Alto, California.

WILLIAM Y. HOFFMAN, M.D.
Assistant Professor of Surgery, Division of Plastic and Reconstructive Surgery, University of California, San Francisco, School of Medicine; Chief, Division of Plastic and Reconstructive Surgery, San Francisco General Hospital, San Francisco, California.

V. MICHAEL HOGAN, M.D.
Clinical Professor of Surgery (Plastic), New York University Medical Center, New York, New York.

RALPH E. HOLMES, M.D.
Associate Professor, Division of Plastic Surgery, University of California, San Diego, School of Medicine; Attending Surgeon, University of California, San Diego, Medical Center, Children's Hospital and Health Center, and Veterans Administration Medical Center, San Diego, California.

CHARLES E. HORTON, M.D.
Professor of Plastic Surgery, The Eastern Virginia Medical School of the Medical College of Hampton Roads, Norfolk, Virginia.

CHARLES E. HORTON, Jr., M.D.
Fellow in Urology, Harvard School of Medicine, Boston, Massachusetts.

SUZANNE B. HOUSMAN, M.D.
Instructor in Psychiatry, New York University School of Medicine, New York, New York.

MICHAEL E. JABALEY, M.D.
Clinical Professor of Plastic Surgery, University of Mississippi School of Medicine; Attending Surgeon, St. Dominic/Jackson Memorial Hospital, Mississippi Baptist Medical Center, River Oaks Hospital, Women's Hospital, and Doctors Hospital; Consultant in Plastic Surgery, Jackson Veterans Administration Hospital, Mississippi Methodist Rehabilitation Center, and University Hospital, Jackson, Mississippi.

IAN T. JACKSON, M.B., CH.B., F.R.C.S., F.A.C.S.
Director, Institute for Craniofacial and Reconstructive Surgery, Providence Hospital, Southfield, Michigan.

GLENN W. JELKS, M.D.
Associate Professor of Surgery (Plastic Surgery), New York University School of Medicine; Attending Surgeon, University Hospital, Bellevue Hospital, Manhattan Eye, Ear & Throat Hospital, Manhattan Veterans Administration Hospital, and New York Eye & Ear Infirmary, New York, New York.

MALCOLM C. JOHNSTON, D.D.S., M.SC.D., PH.D.
Professor of Orthodontics, School of Dentistry; Professor of Cell Biology and Anatomy, School of Medicine, University of North Carolina at Chapel Hill, North Carolina.

GERALD H. JORDAN, M.D.
Assistant Professor of Urology, The Eastern Virginia Medical School of the Medical College of Hampton Roads, Norfolk, Virginia.

HENRY K. KAWAMOTO, JR., M.D., D.D.S.
Associate Clinical Professor, UCLA Division of Plastic Surgery, Los Angeles, California.

PETER P. KAY, M.B., B.CH., F.R.C.S.
Assistant Professor of Plastic and Reconstructive Surgery, Mayo Medical School; Consultant, Division of Plastic and Reconstructive Surgery, and Co-Director, Craniofacial Unit, Mayo Clinic, Rochester, Minnesota.

CAROLYN L. KERRIGAN, M.D.
Assistant Professor of Surgery, McGill University; Acting Surgeon-in-Charge, Division of Plastic Surgery, Royal Victoria Hospital; Consultant, Shriners Hospital for Crippled Children, Quebec, Canada.

LYNN D. KETCHUM, M.D.
Clinical Professor of Surgery, University of Kansas Medical Center, Kansas City; Attending Surgeon, Humana Hospital, Overland Park, Kansas.

DAVID M. KNIZE, M.D.
Assistant Clinical Professor of Surgery, University of Colorado School of Medicine; Attending Surgeon, Swedish Hospital, Porter Memorial Hospital, Denver Children's Hospital, and Colorado General Hospital, Denver, Colorado.

THOMAS J. KRIZEK, M.D.
Professor and Chairman, Department of Surgery, University of Chicago, Chicago, Illinois.

DON LAROSSA, M.D.
Associate Professor of Surgery (Plastic Surgery), University of Pennsylvania School of Medicine; Director, Cleft Palate Program, Children's Hospital of Philadelphia, Philadelphia, Pennsylvania.

R. A. LATHAM, B.D.S., PH.D.
Clinical Instructor in Orthodontics, University of Western Ontario; Assistant Professor of Plastic Surgery, University of Miami School of Medicine; Staff Member, Victoria Hospital Corporation, London, Ontario, Canada.

GOTTFRIED LEMPERLE, M.D.
Professor of Surgery (Plastic Surgery), Johann Wolfgang Goethe University; Chief of the Department of Plastic and Reconstructive Surgery, St. Markus Krankenhaus, Frankfurt-am-Main, Germany.

MALCOLM A. LESAVOY, M.D.
Associate Professor of Surgery, Division of Plastic Surgery, University of California, Los Angeles, School of Medicine; Chief, Plastic & Reconstructive Surgery, Harbor/UCLA Medical Center, Torrance, California.

GRAHAM D. LISTER, M.B., CH.B., F.R.C.S.
Professor of Surgery and Chief, Division of Plastic Surgery, University of Utah School of Medicine; Attending Surgeon, University Hospital, Latter Day Saints Hospital, Primary Children's Hospital, and Shriners Hospital, Salt Lake City, Utah.

J. WILLIAM LITTLER, M.D.
Senior Attending Surgeon, St. Luke's–Roosevelt Hospital Center, New York, New York.

EDWARD A. LUCE, M.D.
Professor and Chief of Plastic Surgery, University of Kentucky College of Medicine; Attending Surgeon, Veterans Administration Hospital and St. Joseph's Hospital; Consultant in Hand Surgery, Shriners Hospital for Crippled Children, Lexington, Kentucky.

JOHN W. MADDEN, M.D., F.A.C.S.
Clinical Professor of Orthopedics, University of New Mexico, Albuquerque; Director, Tucson Hand Rehabilitation Program, Tucson, Arizona.

RALPH T. MANKTELOW, M.D.
Professor and Head, Division of Plastic Surgery, University of Toronto Faculty of Medicine; Head

of the Division of Plastic Surgery, Toronto General Hospital, Toronto, Ontario, Canada.

PAUL N. MANSON, M.D.
Professor of Plastic Surgery, Johns Hopkins University School of Medicine; Director of Plastic Surgery, The Maryland Institute of Emergency Medical Services Systems; Attending Surgeon, Johns Hopkins Hospital, University Hospital, Children's Hospital and Center for Reconstructive Surgery, and Francis Scott Key Medical Center, Baltimore, Maryland.

DANIEL MARCHAC, M.D.
Professor, Collège de Médecine des Hôpitaux de Paris; Director, Center for Cranio-facial Anomalies, Hôpital Necker-Enfants-Malades, Paris, France.

MORTON R. MASER, M.D.
Assistant Clinical Professor of Plastic Surgery, Stanford University Medical Center; Attending Surgeon, Stanford University Hospital, Palo Alto, California.

IVAN MATEV, M.D.
Professor of Orthopaedic Surgery, The Medical Academy; Head, Department of Upper Extremity Surgery, The Institute of Orthopaedics and Traumatology, Sofia, Bulgaria.

STEPHEN J. MATHES, M.D.
Professor of Surgery and Head, Division of Plastic Surgery, University of California, San Francisco, School of Medicine; Professor of Growth and Development, University of California, San Francisco, School of Dentistry; Chief of Plastic Surgery, University of California Medical Center, San Francisco, California.

JAMES W. MAY, JR., M.D.
Chief of Plastic and Reconstructive Surgery and Hand Surgery Service, Department of General Surgery, Massachusetts General Hospital; Associate Clinical Professor, Harvard Medical School, Boston, Massachusetts.

JOSEPH G. MCCARTHY, M.D.
Lawrence D. Bell Professor of Plastic Surgery, New York University School of Medicine; Director, Institute of Reconstructive Plastic Surgery, New York University Medical Center; Attending Surgeon, University Hospital, Bellevue Hospital, Manhattan Eye, Ear and Throat Hospital, and Veterans Administration Hospital, New York, New York.

HAROLD MCCOMB, F.R.A.C.S.
Clinical Lecturer, University of Western Australia; Plastic Surgeon, Princess Margaret Hospital for Children, Perth, Western Australia.

JOHN B. MCCRAW, M.D.
Professor of Plastic Surgery, The Eastern Virginia Medical School of the Medical College of Hampton Roads, Norfolk, Virginia.

ROBERT M. MCFARLANE, M.D.
Professor of Surgery and Head, Division of Plastic Surgery, University of Western Ontario Faculty of Medicine; Head, Division of Plastic Surgery, Victoria Hospital, London, Ontario, Canada.

MARY H. MCGRATH, M.D.
Professor of Surgery and Chief, Division of Plastic and Reconstructive Surgery, George Washington University School of Medicine and Health Sciences; Chief of Service, University Hospital; Attending Surgeon, Children's Hospital National Medical Center, Washington, D.C.

NANCY H. MCKEE, M.D.
Associate Professor of Plastic Surgery, University of Toronto Faculty of Medicine; Attending Surgeon, Mount Sinai Hospital, Toronto General Hospital, and Hospital for Sick Children, Toronto, Ontario, Canada.

DOUGLAS MCMANAMNY, F.R.A.C.S.
Melbourne, Australia.

WYNDELL H. MERRITT, M.D.
Assistant Clinical Professor, Medical College of Virginia, Richmond, Virginia.

D. RALPH MILLARD, JR., M.D.
Light-Millard Professor and Chief of the Division of Plastic Surgery, University of Miami School of Medicine; Attending Surgeon, Jackson Memorial Hospital, Miami Children's Hospital, and Mount Sinai Hospital, Miami, Florida.

TIMOTHY A. MILLER, M.D.
Professor of Surgery (Plastic Surgery), UCLA School of Medicine; Chief of Plastic Surgery, Wadsworth Veterans Hospital, Los Angeles, California.

GUILLERMO MILLICOVSKY, PH.D.
Director of Research, International Craniofacial Institute, Humana Advanced Surgical Institutes, Dallas, Texas.

ERIK MOBERG, M.D., Ph.D.
Professor Emeritus of Hand Surgery and Orthopaedic Surgery, University of Göteborg Medical School, Göteborg, Sweden.

WAYNE A. MORRISON, M.B., B.S., F.R.A.C.S.
Associate, Department of Surgery, University of Melbourne; Assistant Plastic Surgeon and Deputy Director, Microsurgery Research Centre, St. Vincent's Hospital, Melbourne; Plastic Surgeon, Repatriation Hospital, Heidelberg, Melbourne; Consultant Plastic Surgeon, Geelong Hospital, Victoria, Australia.

JOHN B. MULLIKEN, M.D.
Associate Professor of Surgery, Harvard Medical School; Director, Craniofacial Center, Division of Plastic Surgery, Children's Hospital Medical Center and Brigham and Women's Hospital, Boston, Massachusetts.

IAN R. MUNRO, M.D.
Director, Humana International Craniofacial Institute, Humana Hospital, Dallas, Texas.

JAMES F. MURRAY, M.D.
Professor Emeritus, Department of Surgery, University of Toronto Faculty of Medicine; Attending Surgeon, Sunnybrook Medical Center, Toronto, Ontario, Canada.

ALGIMANTAS O. NARAKAS, M.D.
Associate Professor, Medical School of the University of Lausanne; Surgeon-in-Chief and Head of the Longeraie Clinic; Consultant, University Hospital and Children's Hospital, Lausanne, Switzerland.

HENRY W. NEALE, M.D.
Professor of Surgery and Director, Division of Plastic, Reconstructive and Hand Surgery, University of Cincinnati College of Medicine; Attending Surgeon, University Hospital, Children's Hospital Medical Center, and Shriners Burns Hospital, Cincinnati, Ohio.

BERNARD M. O'BRIEN, C.M.G., M.D., M.S., F.R.A.C.S.
Professorial Associate, Department of Anatomy, University of Melbourne; Plastic Surgeon and Director, Microsurgery Research Centre, St. Vincent's Hospital; Consultant Plastic Surgeon, Mercy Maternity Hospital, Melbourne, Australia.

KITARO OHMORI, M.D.
Associate Professor of Plastic Surgery, Juntendo University School of Medicine; Director, Department of Plastic and Reconstructive Surgery, Tokyo Metropolitan Police Hospital, Tokyo, Japan.

MICHAEL G. ORGEL, M.D.
Associate Professor of Surgery (Plastic), University of Massachusetts Medical School at the Berkshire Medical Center; Attending Surgeon, Berkshire Medical Center and Hillcrest Hospital, Pittsfield, Massachusetts.

ANDREW K. PALMER, M.D.
Professor of Orthopedic Surgery, State University of New York Health Center at Syracuse College of Medicine; Coordinator of Hand Service, State University of New York Health Science Center at Syracuse; Consultant and Director of Hand Service, Veterans Administration Hospital, Syracuse, New York.

JOHN H. PALMER, F.R.C.S.
Leeds, United Kingdom.

ERLE E. PEACOCK, Jr., M.D.
Courtesy Staff, North Carolina Memorial Hospital; Attending Staff, Durham County General Hospital, Durham, North Carolina.

IRVING M. POLAYES, M.D., D.D.S.
Clinical Professor of Plastic and Reconstructive Surgery, Yale University School of Medicine; Associate Section Chief, Plastic and Reconstructive Surgery, Yale–New Haven Hospital, New Haven, Connecticut.

GEORGE L. POPKIN, M.D.
Professor of Clinical Dermatology, New York University School of Medicine; Attending Physician, University Hospital, New York, New York.

G. WESLEY PRICE, M.D.
Clinical Assistant Professor of Plastic Surgery, Georgetown University School of Medicine; Clinical Instructor of Plastic Surgery, George Washington University School of Medicine; Attending Surgeon, Sibley Memorial Hospital, Washington, D.C., and Fairfax Hospital, Falls Church, Virginia.

CHARLES L. PUCKETT, M.D.
Professor and Head, Division of Plastic Surgery, University of Missouri–Columbia School of Medi-

cine; Attending Surgeon, University of Missouri–Columbia Hospital and Clinics, Harry S Truman Memorial Veterans Administration Hospital, Boone Hospital Center and Ellis Fischel State Cancer Hospital, Columbia, Missouri.

PETER RANDALL, M.D.
Professor of Plastic Surgery, University of Pennsylvania School of Medicine; Senior Surgeon, Children's Hospital of Philadelphia, Philadelphia, Pennsylvania.

THOMAS D. REES, M.D.
Clinical Professor of Surgery (Plastic Surgery), New York University School of Medicine; Chairman, Department of Plastic Surgery, Manhattan Eye, Ear & Throat Hospital, New York, New York.

RONALD RIEFKOHL, M.D.
Associate Professor of Surgery, Division of Plastic, Maxillofacial and Reconstructive Surgery, Duke University School of Medicine, Durham, North Carolina.

PERRY ROBINS, M.D.
Associate Professor of Clinical Dermatology, New York University School of Medicine; Attending Physician, University Hospital, Bellevue Hospital, and Veterans Administration Hospital, New York, New York.

MARTIN C. ROBSON, M.D.
Truman G. Blocker, Jr. Professor of Surgery and Chief, Division of Plastic Surgery, University of Texas Medical Branch, Galveston, Texas.

PAMELA ROPER, M.D., PH.D.
Attending Staff, St. Joseph Hospital, Women's Hospital of Texas, Park Plaza Hospital, and Hermann Outpatient Surgery Center, Houston, Texas.

R. BRUCE ROSS, D.D.S.
Assistant Professor, Faculty of Dentistry, University of Toronto; Director, Craniofacial Treatment and Research Centre, and Head, Division of Orthodontics, Department of Dentistry, The Hospital for Sick Children, Toronto, Ontario, Canada.

ROSS RUDOLPH, M.D.
Associate Clinical Professor of Plastic Surgery, University of California, San Diego, School of Medicine; Head, Division of Plastic and Reconstructive Surgery, Scripps Clinic and Research Foundation, La Jolla California.

GREGORY L. RUFF, M.D.
Assistant Professor of Plastic Surgery, Duke University School of Medicine, Durham, North Carolina.

ROBERT C. RUSSELL, M.D.
Professor of Surgery, Division of Plastic and Reconstructive Surgery, Southern Illinois University School of Medicine; Chairman of Plastic Surgery, St. John's Hospital, Springfield, Illinois.

RICHARD C. SADOVE, M.D.
Assistant Professor of Plastic Surgery, University of Kentucky Medical Center, Lexington, Kentucky.

ROGER E. SALISBURY, M.D.
Professor of Surgery and Chief of Plastic and Reconstructive Surgery, New York Medical College; Director, Burn Center, Westchester Medical Center, Valhalla; Consultant, Plastic and Reconstructive Surgery, Castle Point Veterans Administration Hospital and Glythedale Children's Hospital; Chief of Plastic and Reconstructive Surgery, Metropolitan Hospital Center, New York, New York.

PAUL F. SAUER, M.D.
Assistant Professor, Department of Plastic Surgery, Medical College of Virginia, Richmond, Virginia.

ROBERT C. SAVAGE, M.D.
Clinical Instructor in Surgery, Division of Plastic Surgery, Harvard Medical School; Associate Surgeon, Massachusetts General Hospital; Attending Surgeon, Faulkner Hospital, Boston, New England Deaconess Hospital, Boston, and Mount Auburn Hospital, Cambridge, Massachusetts.

LEONARD A. SHARZER, M.D.
Clinical Professor of Plastic Surgery, Albert Einstein College of Medicine; Attending Surgeon, Montefiore Medical Center, Bronx, New York.

KEVIN SHAW, M.D.
Head, Section of Plastic Surgery, Mayo Clinic, Jacksonville, Florida.

WILLIAM W. SHAW, M.D.
Associate Professor of Surgery (Plastic Surgery), New York University School of Medicine; Attending Surgeon, Institute of Reconstructive Plastic Surgery, New York University Medical Center; Chief, Plastic Surgery, Bellevue Hospital, New York, New York.

JACK H. SHEEN, M.D.
Associate Clinical Professor of Plastic and Reconstructive Surgery, University of California, Los Angeles, School of Medicine; Attending Surgeon, UCLA Medical Center, Los Angeles, California.

ALAN R. SHONS, M.D., PH.D.
Professor of Surgery, Case Western Reserve University School of Medicine; Director, Division of Plastic Surgery, University Hospitals of Cleveland, Cleveland, Ohio.

JOHN W. SIEBERT, M.D.
Assistant Professor of Surgery, New York University Medical Center; Chief of Plastic Surgery, Bellevue Hospital, New York; Director of Microsurgery, New York University Medical Center and Bellevue Hospital, New York, New York.

NATHANIEL M. SIMS, M.D.
Instructor in Anesthesia, Harvard Medical School; Assistant in Anesthesia, Massachusetts General Hospital, Boston, Massachusetts.

BYRON C. SMITH, M.D.
Consultant in Ophthalmic Plastic Surgery, Manhattan Eye, Ear & Throat Hospital and New York Eye & Ear Infirmary; Attending Surgeon, Mount Sinai Medical Center, New York, New York.

DAVID J. SMITH, JR., M.D.
Professor of Surgery and Section Head for Plastic and Reconstructive Surgery, University of Michigan Medical Center, Ann Arbor, Michigan.

KEVIN L. SMITH, M.D.
Assistant Professor, Department of Plastic Surgery, University of North Carolina School of Medicine, Charlotte Division; Attending Surgeon, Charlotte Memorial Hospital and Presbyterian Hospital, Charlotte, North Carolina.

RICHARD J. SMITH, M.D. (deceased)
Clinical Professor of Orthopaedic Surgery, Harvard Medical School, Boston; Director of Hand Surgical Service, Department of Orthopaedic Surgery, Massachusetts General Hospital, Boston, Massachusetts.

MICHAEL R. SPINDEL, M.D.
Fellow, Reconstructive Urology, The Eastern Virginia Medical School of the Medical College of Hampton Roads, Norfolk, Virginia.

JOHN F. STECKER, M.D.
Professor of Urology, The Eastern Virginia Medical School of the Medical College of Hampton Roads, Norfolk, Virginia.

BRENT V. STROMBERG, M.D.
Assistant Professor of Plastic and Reconstructive Surgery, Creighton University; Attending Surgeon, St. Joseph's Hospital and Omaha Veterans Administration Hospital, Omaha, Nebraska.

JAMES M. STUZIN, M.D.
Attending Surgeon, Mercy Hospital, Cedars Medical Center and Mount Sinai Medical Center, Miami; Clinical Instructor, Department of Plastic Surgery, University of Miami School of Medicine, Miami, Florida.

G. IAN TAYLOR, F.R.A.C.S., F.R.C.S.
Professional Associate, University of Melbourne; Consultant Plastic Surgeon, Royal Melbourne Hospital; Senior Consultant Plastic Surgeon, Preston & Northcote Community Hospital; Honorary Consultant Plastic Surgeon, Royal Children's Hospital, Melbourne, Australia.

JULIA K. TERZIS, M.D., PH.D.
Associate Professor, Department of Plastic and Reconstructive Surgery, and Director, Microsurgical Research Center, Eastern Virginia Medical School; Chief, Microsurgical Service, Norfolk General Hospital, Norfolk, Virginia.

CHARLES H. M. THORNE, M.D.
Assistant Professor of Surgery (Plastic Surgery), New York University School of Medicine; Attending Surgeon, Manhattan Eye, Ear & Throat Hospital, University Hospital, Bellevue Hospital, and Manhattan Veterans Administration Hospital, New York, New York.

JOSEPH UPTON, M.D.
Assistant Professor of Surgery, Harvard Medical School; Active Staff, Division of Plastic Surgery, Department of Surgery, Beth Israel Hospital and Children's Hospital, Boston, Massachusetts.

AUGUSTUS J. VALAURI, D.D.S.
Professor of Surgery (Maxillofacial Prosthetics), New York University School of Medicine; Clinical Professor of Removable Prosthodontics and Occlusion, New York University School of Dentistry; Chief of the Maxillofacial Prosthetics Service, Institute of Reconstructive Plastic Surgery, New York University Medical Center, New York, New York.

CHARLES P. VALLIS, M.D.
Clinical Instructor in Plastic Surgery, Harvard Medical School; Clinical Instructor in Plastic Surgery and Dermatology, Tufts University School of Medicine; Attending Surgeon, Atlanticare Center, Boston, Massachusetts.

ALLEN L. VAN BEEK, M.D.
Clinical Assistant Professor of Surgery, University of Minnesota Medical School; Director of Microsurgery, North Memorial Medical Center, Minneapolis, Minnesota.

LUIS O. VASCONEZ, M.D.
Professor and Chief, Division of Plastic Surgery, University of Alabama at Birmingham, Birmingham, Alabama.

PAUL M. WEEKS, M.D.
Professor of Surgery (Plastic and Reconstructive), Washington University School of Medicine; Chief of Plastic Surgery, Barnes Hospital and St. Louis Children's Hospital, St. Louis, Missouri.

ANDREW J. WEILAND, M.D.
Professor, Department of Orthopaedic Surgery, Division of Plastic Surgery, and Department of Emergency Medicine, Johns Hopkins University School of Medicine, Baltimore, Maryland.

E. F. SHAW WILGIS, M.D.
Associate Professor of Plastic Surgery and of Orthopaedic Surgery, Johns Hopkins University School of Medicine; Chief, Division of Hand Surgery, Union Memorial Hospital, Baltimore, Maryland.

S. ANTHONY WOLFE, M.D.
Clinical Professor of Plastic and Reconstructive Surgery, University of Miami School of Medicine; Chief of Plastic Reconstructive Surgery, Miami Children's Hospital and Victoria Hospital, Miami, Florida.

DONALD WOOD-SMITH, M.D., F.R.C.S.E.
Professor of Surgery (Plastic Surgery), New York University School of Medicine; Chairman, Department of Plastic Surgery, New York Eye & Ear Infirmary; Attending Surgeon (Plastic Surgery), Bellevue Medical Center; Attending Surgeon, New York University Hospital, New York Veterans Administration Hospital, and Manhattan Eye, Ear & Throat Hospital, New York, New York.

R. CHRISTIE WRAY, JR., M.D.
Professor of Surgery, University of Rochester School of Medicine and Dentistry; Plastic Surgeon in Chief, Strong Memorial Hospital, Rochester, New York.

EDUARDO A. ZANCOLLI, M.D.
Professor of Orthopaedics and Traumatology, Medical School of Buenos Aires; Chief of Orthopaedic Surgery of the Rehabilitation Center of Buenos Aires, Buenos Aires, Argentina.

BARRY M. ZIDE, D.M.D., M.D.
Assistant Professor of Surgery (Plastic Surgery), New York University Medical Center; Attending Surgeon, Bellevue Hospital Center, Manhattan Veterans Administration Hospital, and Manhattan Eye, Ear & Throat Hospital, New York, New York.

ELVIN G. ZOOK, M.D.
Professor of Surgery and Chairman of the Division of Plastic Surgery, Southern Illinois University School of Medicine; Attending Surgeon, Memorial Medical Center and St. John's Hospital, Springfield, Illinois.

Preface

Where does a book begin? Initially, I think of a warm September afternoon in a hotel in Madrid when I first organized an outline of the chapters while waiting for an international surgery meeting to begin. However, a scientific book is only an extension of earlier publications. This text is descended from *Reconstructive Plastic Surgery*, edited in 1964 by my predecessor John Marquis Converse, and reedited in 1977. I had been Assistant Editor of the latter. Many of the ideas and principles, if not the exact words, that were integral to the teaching and writing of Dr. Converse live on in the present volumes. *Reconstructive Plastic Surgery* in turn was derived from his earlier collaboration with V. H. Kazanjian, *The Surgical Treament of Facial Injuries*, published in 1949, 1959, and 1974.

Earlier textbooks by Nélaton and Ombrédanne (1904), Davis (1919), Gillies (1920), and Fomon (1939) had played a germinal role in the development of modern plastic surgery. However, even these books represented only a continuum of publications extending back over the centuries to Tagliacozzi and Sushruta. Indeed, there are also the many surgeons who never published but who by their teachings contributed greatly to the body of knowledge that is represented in the present publication. Their concepts, too, have found their way into the plastic surgery literature for the edification of another generation of students.

My own career has been greatly influenced by my teachers, and their spirit has remained an integral part of my personal and professional life. This heritage of the plastic surgeon–teacher represents the spirit of this book.

The title defines the subject—*Plastic Surgery*. Adjectives such as *reconstructive* or *esthetic* are misleading and redundant and represent artificial divisions of this surgical specialty. The parents of the infant undergoing cleft lip repair are more interested in the *esthetic* aspects of the procedure, which traditionally has been regarded as *reconstructive*. The contemporary face lift, long perceived as an *esthetic* operation, represents a surgical reconstruction of the multiple layers of the soft tissues of the face. Plastic surgery, a term first popularized by Zeis in 1838, is preferred.

With the deliberate exception of parts of Chapters 1 and 35, originally written by Dr. Converse and revised through subsequent editions of various books, few paragraphs in these volumes remain unchanged from the 1977 edition. Many of the authors, however, have used material from the previous editions. Line drawings prepared for these editions by Daisy Stillwell have been reproduced again where appropriate. With the death of Ms. Stillwell, I was fortunate to recruit yet another outstanding medical artist, Craig Luce, to draw hundreds of new illustrations to reflect the continuing developments in this specialty.

The purpose of this book is to define the specialty of plastic surgery. To accomplish this goal, contributions have been sought from the acknowledged leaders of this discipline in all of its ramifications. The clinical applications of plastic surgery, practiced over the whole of the human anatomy, range from skin grafting to the management of uncommon craniofacial clefts, to replantation of the lower extremity. Its practice varies from uncomplicated procedures to sophisticated multistage reconstructions that ally the plastic surgeon with other specialists. The chapters that follow vary in the same way from the short and direct to the lengthy and complex. More than any other, this type of surgery strives for the restoration or improvement of form as well as the restoration of function. The teaching of plastic surgery thus lends itself to illustration. The contributors to this book have been encouraged to use drawings and photographs liberally as an enhancement of the principles and techniques described in the text. Special attention has been given to the sizing and placement of more than 5000 illustrations submitted in accordance with this plan. The contributors and publisher have also made every effort to acknowledge and cite the work of other authors. In a text of this magnitude any omission, while understandable, is regrettable.

In Volume 1 will be found discussions of the essential principles basic to all plastic surgery: wound healing, circulation of the skin, microneurovascular repairs, skin expansion, and grafting of tendons, nerves, and bone, as well as their associated methods of repair. This is the largest of the volumes and testifies to the broadening scope of the field. Much of what is now fundamental to the training of a plastic surgeon was only imagined a generation ago.

After the discussion of general principles in Volume 1, the organization of the text is by anatomic regions. Volumes 2 and 3 are devoted to the face; here, as throughout the book, each chapter draws upon the expertise of acknowledged master surgeons particularly experienced in the subjects on which they have written.

Clefts of the lip and palate as well as severe craniofacial anomalies make up Volume 4. In addition to plastic surgery, these chapters incorporate contributions from the allied fields of embryology, craniofacial growth and development, orthodontics, prosthodontics, speech pathology, and neurosurgery.

Volume 5 covers tumors of the skin and head and neck and Volume 6 the trunk, lower extremity, and genitourinary system. Of particular note, the text details recent advances in reconstruction that involve newly developed flaps of ingenious design and considerable sophistication.

The application of plastic surgical principles and techniques of the upper extremity are discussed in Volumes 7 and 8 under the editorship of Drs. James W. May, Jr., and J. William Littler. The latter, one of the most esteemed and influential hand surgeons of the modern era, edited the upper extremity section in 1964 and 1977. He has been joined in this edition by Dr. May, who is qualified in both hand surgery and microsurgical reconstruction. Both, who are my personal friends, brought their usual enthusiasm, experience, and equanimity to bear on this project. Because surgery of the upper extremity is practiced so extensively, ample space has been afforded for the comprehensive description of the reconstructive procedures specifically designed for the restoration of injured parts. Much of the current progress in plastic surgery of the upper extremity has been made possible by the gradual perfection of microvascular techniques, and these newer developments have been incorporated into the text.

Continuing change, the hallmark of all medical and surgical practice, dictates the need for a reference book such as this and makes its accomplishment a challenging task for everyone involved. With the writing of these words the lengthy process of revising, updating, and improving is ended. The book is committed to the press with the promise that it is both complete and current, in the belief that readers will find it an invaluable resource, and with the hope that it makes a contribution to the body of plastic surgery knowledge and to the education of tomorrow's plastic surgeon.

JOSEPH G. MCCARTHY, M.D.

Acknowledgements

The authors or contributors, all with heavy clinical responsibilities and demands, have contributed greatly and are responsible for this text. In addition to outlining their personal views, they have conducted exhaustive literature searches and have organized their illustrative material. They represent the heart and soul of the book.

I wish also to acknowledge my fellow faculty members at the Institute of Reconstructive Plastic Surgery, since their work and concepts, as well as their encouragement, have been so important in the development of this text: Sherrell J. Aston, Donald L. Ballantyne, Robert W. Beasley, Phillip R. Casson, David T.W. Chiu, Peter J. Coccaro, Stephen R. Colen, Court B. Cutting, Barry H. Grayson, V. Michael Hogan, Glenn W. Jelks, Frances C. Macgregor, Thomas D. Rees, Blair O. Rogers, William W. Shaw, John W. Siebert, Charles H. M. Thorne, Augustus J. Valauri, Donald Wood-Smith, and Barry M. Zide. Dr. Frank Cole Spencer, George David Stewart Professor of Surgery and Chairman of the Department of Surgery at the New York University Medical Center, has always championed the goals of the Institute and has especially encouraged development in the newer areas of craniofacial surgery and microsurgery.

I should also pay tribute to Ms. Karen Singer, who did so much of the bibliographic study, and Wayne Pearson and Harry Weissfisch, who provided photographic support. I must also acknowledge my associates at the Institute, Robert E. Bochat, Linda Gerson, Donna O'Brien, Caren Crane, Marilyn Deaton, Margy Maroutsis, Marjorie Huggins, and others for acts of kindness and support during the years of preparation of this book.

Mr. Albert Meier, Senior Editor at Saunders, had a major share in the organization and editing of this book. A friend and colleague since 1974 when we began the Second Edition, I have benefited immensely from his advice and counsel. He has also shown an unusual sense of understanding throughout this project. Special thanks are also due to David Harvey, Frank Polizzano, and Richard Zorab of the W. B. Saunders Company for their support.

I am also grateful to the residents and fellows at the Institute of Reconstructive Plastic Surgery, whose boundless enthusiasm is ever encouraging and who have given generously of their time to proofread manuscripts and galleys: Christopher Attinger, Constance Barone, Richard Bartlett, P. Craig Hobar, William Hoffman, Armen Kasabian, Gregory LaTrenta, George Peck, Rosa Razaboni, Gregory Ruff, John Siebert, R. Kendrick Slate, Henry Spinelli, Michael Stevens, Charles Thorne, and Douglas Wagner.

Special thanks are also due to my colleagues and friends at the National Foundation for Facial Reconstruction, whose support and encouragement have provided a unique environment at the Institute that is conducive to writing and research.

Finally, I want to thank my family, Karlan, Cara, and Stephen, for their love and understanding during the demanding years of this project, especially those times spent at a desk when I may have appeared distracted or lost in thought. They remain my main support and life focus.

I also want to thank my friends, especially Charles and Heather Garbaccio, who had the ability to offer those special moments of lightheartedness, good cheer, and camaraderie.

JGM

Contents

Volume 1
General Principles

Volume 2
The Face (Part 1)

Volume 3

The Face (Part 2)

Volume 4

Cleft Lip & Palate and Craniofacial Anomalies

Volume 5

Tumors of the Head & Neck and Skin

Volume 6

The Trunk and Lower Extremity

Volume 8
The Hand (Part 2)

1

Joseph G. McCarthy

Introduction to Plastic Surgery

Plastic surgery is a specialized branch of surgery concerned with the repair of deformities and the correction of functional deficits.

While the term "plastique" was used by Desault in 1798, it was the publication of Zeis's book *Handbuch der plastischen Chirurgie* in 1838 that popularized the term. Von Graefe was the first to employ the term "plastic" in his monograph entitled *Rhinoplastik* published in Berlin in 1818. It is derived from the Greek word "plastikos," meaning "fit for molding." In most countries, the term "plastic surgery" designates the specialty.

While plastic surgery is largely concerned with form, as is implied in the term "plastic," the functional aspects are also important: for example, reanimating the paralyzed face, restoring the function of the hand, or making possible the healing of a compound fracture of the lower extremity by providing adequate soft tissue coverage.

A sense of form and an innate ability to make an esthetic judgment are critical qualities for the plastic surgeon. Webster in his foreword to the textbook by Gillies and Millard, *The Principles and Art of Plastic Surgery* (1957), quoted from Aristotle's "On the Parts of Animals": "Art, indeed, consists in the conception of the result to be produced before its realization in the material." Perhaps this quality is the most essential requisite for a plastic surgeon; it is the quality that distinguishes him from the technician. For the teacher of plastic surgery it is this artistic quality that is innate (or absent) in the trainee and cannot be formally taught.

It is a rare operation in this discipline that does not involve an esthetic consideration or judgment—the placement of an incision on the dorsum of a hand, the choice of a skin donor site for a lower extremity defect. Because plastic surgery was essentially reconstructive until the turn of this century (congenital and post-traumatic deformities), a distinction arose between *esthetic* and *reconstructive* surgery—a division that is artificial. Tessier always liked to say that the correction of orbital hypertelorism is the ultimate rhinoplasty. Just as most reconstructive surgical procedures have an esthetic component, the opposite is also true—the visual impairment associated with hooding of the upper eyelids, the neck and shoulder pain with massively enlarged breasts. The terms *reconstructive* and *esthetic* also are not helpful in differentiating between the surgery of major and minor defects—witness the modern-day face lift procedure.

Gillies has been widely quoted for his definitions: *reconstructive* surgery is an attempt

---

This chapter incorporates material written by J. M. Converse for the Second Edition of *Reconstructive Plastic Surgery*.

to restore the individual to normal; *esthetic* surgery attempts to surpass the normal.

I suspect that the dilemma will never be resolved and will remain a semantic problem. What is more important is that the surgeon concern himself with those problems that upset his fellow man and affect the quality of his daily life. Some may be predominantly *esthetic* or *reconstructive*; some will be mixed; most, it may be hoped, will lend themselves to surgical correction.

THE AGES OF PLASTIC SURGERY

The philosopher Santayana (1863–1952) has said: "Those who cannot remember the past are condemned to repeat it." The study of surgical history also gives us the perspective to evaluate contemporary surgical practices, and emphasizes the evanescent state of many surgical procedures. Individual surgical techniques may not stand the test of time but the problems remain, awaiting more definitive solutions. In an address to the Royal College of Surgeons, Churchill remarked: "The longer you look back, the further you can look forward."

Ancient Times

The origins of plastic surgery are rooted in ancient history. As emphasized by Majno (1975) in *The Healing Hand*, the history of surgery represents the history of man's struggle to treat wounds and defects inflicted by nature or by other men. Because facial deformities, especially the amputated nose, were so obvious, they received the most attention in ancient records.

Although ancient man practiced trephination of the skull, perhaps as early as 10,000 B.C., specialized surgery appears to have been practiced by the Babylonians during the time of Hammurabi (circa 1950 B.C.) when the operation for cataract was performed as a legitimate surgical procedure.

In India, the famed practitioner Sushruta (circa 600 B.C.) described operations for reconstruction of the nose and the earlobes in the Sushruta Samhita (translated by Bhishagratna, 1916). Since the nose was considered the organ of respect and reputation, amputation of the nose was a common practice to punish criminals and the inhabitants of conquered cities. The operation was performed by members of a caste of potters known as the Koomas. Knowledge of these operations probably filtered to Rome through the Persians; the Greeks; the Arabs; the Nestorian Christian communities in India, Persia, and Iraq; and Jewish scholars (Gnudi and Webster, 1950).

Celsus (25 B.C. to 50 A.D.) used advancement flaps (Fig. 1–1*A* to *C*). It is not clear whether the flaps were raised prior to advancement, as was done in the nineteenth century under the name of "flaps according to the French method" or "gliding flaps" ("lambeaux par glissement"). Celsus was probably the originator of the island flap with a subcutaneous pedicle (Fig. 1–1*D, E*).

Galen (130 to 200 A.D.) did not concern himself with plastic surgery techniques. Progress in surgical techniques during the period of the Roman Empire was epitomized by Paulus Aegineta (625 to 690 A.D.), thought to have been a major link between the medical learning of the Hindu and Arab schools and the increasing number of Western scholars during his lifetime. He may be considered one of the originators of plastic surgery as it is known today (Rogers, 1974). He described procedures varying from the treatment of nasal and jaw fractures to operations for

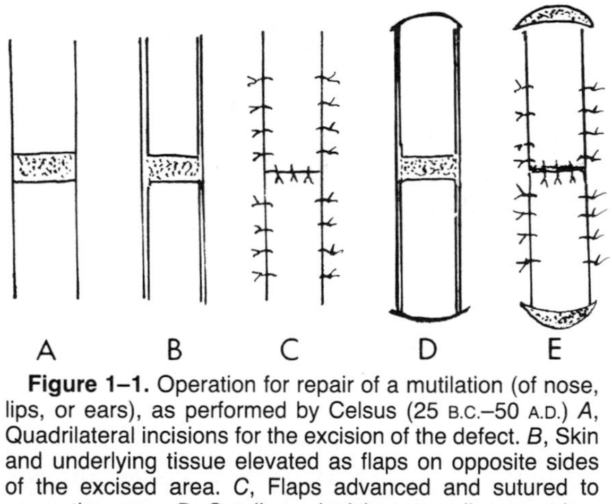

Figure 1–1. Operation for repair of a mutilation (of nose, lips, or ears), as performed by Celsus (25 B.C.–50 A.D.) *A*, Quadrilateral incisions for the excision of the defect. *B*, Skin and underlying tissue elevated as flaps on opposite sides of the excised area. *C*, Flaps advanced and sutured to cover the area. *D*, Semilunar incisions to relieve tension. *E*, Relaxed flaps advanced, leaving two lunate raw areas to heal by secondary intention. (From Spencer, W. G.: Celsus: De medicina; with an English translation. Vol. 3. Cambridge, MA, Harvard University Press, 1938. Redrawn from B. O. Rogers, in Wood-Smith, D., and Porowski, P. C.: Nursing Care of the Plastic Surgery Patient. St. Louis, MO, C. V. Mosby Company, 1967.)

hypospadias. With the death of Paulus Aegineta, the enrichment of medical and surgical knowledge provided by the Greco-Roman period came to an end.

The rise of Islam enhanced the prestige of Arabic medicine. It has been suggested that contacts between the Arabs, the invaders of Sicily, and the local practitioners, such as members of the Branca family, led to the transmission of the art of reconstructive rhinoplasty as practiced in ancient India. Occidental medicine thus is indebted to Arabic medicine. Arabian scholars in the 8th century A.D. provided Arabic translations of the work of Sushruta, which were subsequently translated into Latin (Gnudi and Webster, 1950).

The Renaissance

The period of the Renaissance or rebirth of civilization that marked the transition from the Middle Ages emerged in Italy in the fourteenth century and reached its zenith during the fifteenth and sixteenth centuries. It was during this period that the *Fabrica* of Vesalius was published (1543). The foundations of modern anatomic studies were laid and anatomy changed from a Galenic to a Vesalian discipline.

During the first half of the fifteenth century, plastic surgery came to be practiced in Sicily by members of the Branca family. Sicily was a center of Arabic, Greek, and Occidental learning during the earlier centuries, and it is thought that the elder Branca used the method of repair described by Sushruta. Antonio Branca, the son, abandoned the ancient Indian method and was probably the first surgeon to use a flap from the arm to repair mutilated lips and ears.

During the sixteenth century, the Vianeo family practiced the art of plastic surgery in the region of Calabria in the southwestern part of the Italian peninsula. A number of other practitioners appeared to have repaired mutilated noses. Symonds' observations (1935) on the increase of violence during the period from 1530 to 1600 are of particular interest: "Compared with the Middle Ages, compared with the Renaissance, this period is distinguished by extraordinary ferocity of temper and by an almost unparalleled facility of blood shed."

The need for reconstructive operations during the sixteenth century owing to the frequent duels and clashes of armed men appears to have coincided with an increased interest in this branch of surgery. The renowned surgeon Ambroise Paré (circa 1575) warned, however, of the extreme difficulty and discomfort of the operation for the repair of a mutilated nose:

We have testimony of this from a gentleman named the Cadet of St. Thoan, who, having lost his nose and having long worn one of silver, became angry at the remark that there was never a lack of laughing matter when he was present. And having heard that there was in Italy a master re-maker of lost noses, he went to find him, and he made a new one for him in the way described above as an infinite number of people have since seen him, not without the great marvelling of those who had known him before with a silver nose. Such a thing is not impossible; nevertheless it seems to me very difficult and burdensome to the patient, both because of the trouble of keeping the head down with the arm for so long a time, and because of the pain of the incisions made in healthy parts, cutting and lifting away the part of the flesh of the arm to form the nose; in addition, this flesh is not of the same quality nor similar to that of the nose, and even when agglutinated and reformed it can never be of the same shape and color as that which was former in the place of the lost nose, likewise the openings of the nostrils can never be as they were originally.

Paré apparently shared the common misunderstanding concerning the arm flap technique of nose repair, as he named the biceps muscle as the donor site and specified 40 days as the period requisite for union.

Paré's negative attitude was all the more surprising as he expressed the horror of his contemporaries for facial mutilations in his book published in 1575:

Having arrived in the town, I entered a stable and there I found four soldiers who were dead and three who were leaning against the wall, their faces completely disfigured and they could not see nor could they hear or speak and their clothes were still smoking from the gun powder that had burnt them. As I was looking at them with pity, an old soldier approached me and asked me if there was any way by which I could cure them: I answered that there was no way. Suddenly he approached each one of them and cut his throat, gently and without anger. Seeing this cruel action I told him that he was a bad man to have done this. He answered that he prayed God that if he should be so afflicted there would be someone who would render him the same service rather than allow him to languish miserably.

It would appear that Paré never came to know the work of the man who was to lay the cornerstone of modern plastic surgery, Gaspare Tagliacozzi (1545–1599) of Bologna. The work of Tagliacozzi, particularly in nose reconstruction, was renowned throughout Europe. His treatise "De Curtorum Chirurgia per Insitionem," published in 1597, summarizes his life's work (Fig. 1–2). In describing the technique of preparing the arm flap for transplantation to reconstruct the nose, he specified the details of the delayed flap. In Chapter 10, he stated: "It is not well to implant the flap in its age of infancy because then it is not strong enough, it has suffered the violence of the first operation, and is subject to inflammation or hemorrhage. Nor is its youth the proper time as it is then still not firm enough and is subject to various evils. Nor yet should one await its old age, for by then it has become too wrinkled, blanched, pallid and juiceless." But "when it has reached the age of manhood and has entirely hardened, and now begins to be turned, strong enough and fortified to sustain the force of the operation, it is necessary to take the flap, and to join it with the missing parts in the new union of grafting, for it cannot be done better or more safely. Thus it will satisfy the hopes of ourselves and of the patient abundantly. Between the taking up of the flap and the insertion (about fourteen days) the patient is not limited as to diet and may go about freely" (Gnudi and Webster, 1950).

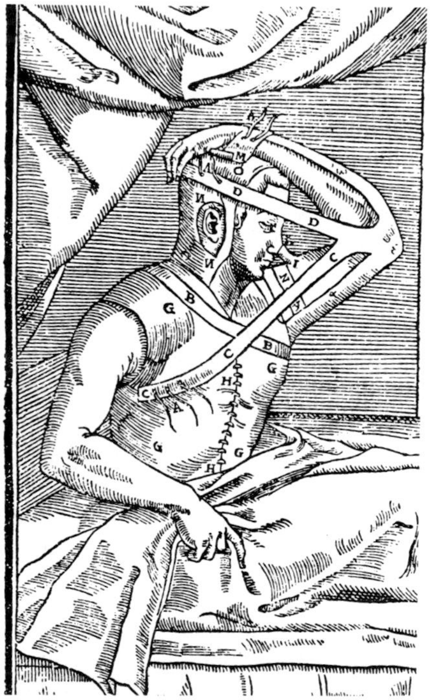

Figure 1–2. Plate VIII illustrating the bandaging. (From Tagliacozzi, G.: De Curtorum Chirurgia per Insitionem. Venice, Gaspare Bindoni, 1597.)

The Seventeenth and Eighteenth Centuries: The Decline

Tagliacozzi's technique was probably little practiced during the seventeenth and eighteenth centuries. The decline of plastic surgery after the death of Tagliacozzi parallels the decline of surgery, which languished throughout all of Europe, particularly in Italy. Indeed, the whole subject, including Tagliacozzi's name, became the object of ridicule from the pens of wits of polite eighteenth century society.

The greatest hindrance to the acceptance and use of plastic surgical operations came from the misconception that reparative tissue could be taken from a slave or person other than the patient and that, under such circumstances, a kind of mystic sympathy existed between the new nose and the person from whom it had been taken, causing the nose to die when the original donor died.

The encyclopedists or "philosophes," a group of scientific determinists (Diderot published the first volume of the "Encyclopédie" in 1751), had great influence during the eighteenth century. One of the encyclopedists, Voltaire, wrote a satirical poem concerning the "sympathetic" slave, the donor tissue having been taken from a slave's buttocks. Ironically, the age of enlightenment was not an age of enlightenment for plastic surgery. Although it has been stated that the Faculty of Medicine of Paris interdicted face repairing during the eighteenth century, there appears to be no truth to the statement. What did happen was that a thesis, "Whether defective noses can be remade from the arm," was rejected by the Faculty. The jokes about "nose and face repairing" during this period, although more cruel, were not unlike the jokes made during the period of development of esthetic surgery in the twentieth century.

The Rebirth

In October, 1794, a letter was written to Mr. Urban, the editor of the Gentleman's

Magazine published in London. The letter stated that a friend in India had communicated to the author the following report on a hitherto unknown operation which had long been practiced successfully in the subcontinent (Fig. 1–3). The letter concerned an incident that had occurred in the Third Mysore War waged by the British East Indian forces against Sultan Tippoo. Since the bullock drivers transported needed grains to the British troops under Cornwallis, the Sultan provided rewards for each nose or ear of the driver or bullock brought back after each attack.

Cowasjee, a bullock driver with the English army in the war of 1792, was made a prisoner by Tippoo, who cut off his nose, and one of his hands. In this state, he joined the Bombay army near Seringapatam, and is now a pensioner of the Honourable East India Company. For about twelve months, he was wholly without a nose; when he had a new one put on, by a Mahratta surgeon. . . . This operation is not uncommon in India, and has been practised from time immemorial.

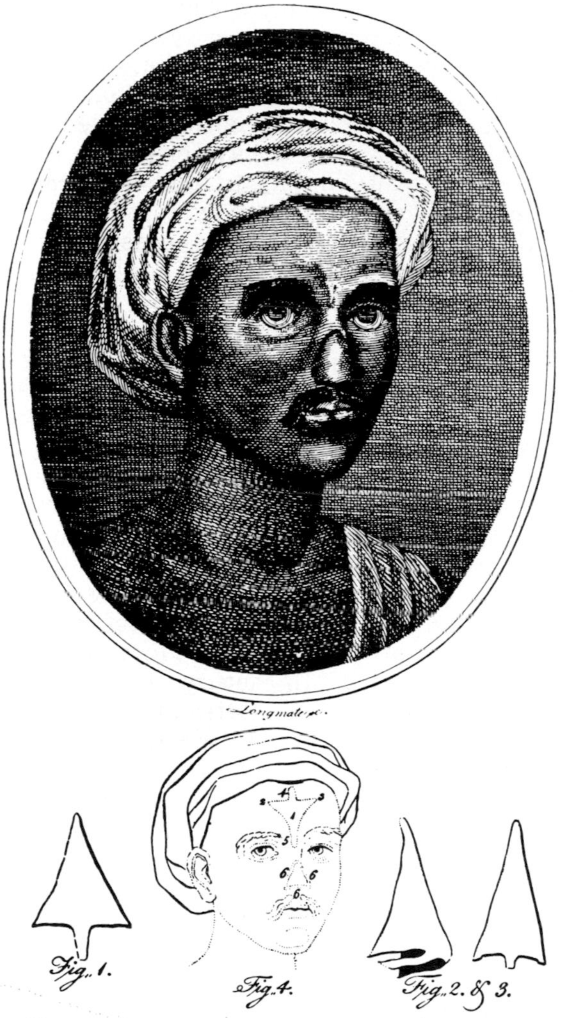

Figure 1–3. Illustration from the celebrated 1794 "Letter to Editor" responsible for the western spread of the "Indian method" for total nasal reconstruction. (From B. L.: Letter to Editor. Gentleman's Magazine, October, 1794, p. 891.)

Two of the medical gentlemen, Mr. Thomas Cruso, and Mr. James Findlay, of Bombay, have seen it performed as follows: a thin plate of wax is fitted to the stump of the nose, so as to make a nose of good appearance; it is then flattened, and laid on the forehead. A line is drawn round the wax, which is then of no further use; and the operator then dissects off as much skin as it covered, leaving undivided a small slip between the eyes. This slip preserves the circulation, till an union has taken place between the new and old parts.

The cicatrix of the stump of the nose is next pared off; and, immediately behind this raw part, an incision is made through the skin, which passes round both alae, and goes along the upper lip. The skin is now brought down from the forehead; and, being twisted half round, its edge is inserted into this incision; so that a nose is formed with a double hold, above, and with its alae and septum below, fixed in the incision.

A little Terra Japonica is softened with water, and, being spread on slips of cloth, five or six of these are placed over each other, to secure the joining. No other dressing than this cement is used for four days; it is then removed, and cloths, dipped in ghee (a kind of butter), are supplied. The connecting slip of skin is divided about the twenty-fifth day, when a little more dissecting is necessary to improve the appearance of the new nose.

For five or six days after the operation, the patient is made to lie on his back; and on the tenth day, bits of soft cloth are put into the nostrils to keep them sufficiently open. This operation is always successful. The artificial nose is secure, and looks nearly as well as the natural one; nor is the scar on the forehead very observable, after a length of time.

Joseph Carpue, who at the time was 30 years old and a surgeon in London, read the story of Cowasjee and reasoned that, if such an operation were possible in India, it should also be possible in Europe. He questioned all the army men and civil servants who returned to London from India, in the hope that they might be able to give him some information. Altogether, he devoted nearly 20 years to investigating this matter.

Carpue located physicians who had witnessed the operation. Barry, who had worked for the East India Company, informed him that the operation had taken 1½ hours and that it had been performed with an old razor, which had to be repeatedly honed in the course of the operation. Carpue obtained another report indicating that the art of nose operations in India was widely practiced by the Koomas, a caste of brickmakers (or potters) in Hindustan. At the beginning of the operation the patient was given betel and arrack. During the operation he had to lie flat on the floor with both hands at the side, and despite the intense pain, the man would unfailingly lie without stirring.

The practice of cutting off noses was common in India to punish thieves, adulterers, and prisoners of war. Only 24 years before the story published in the Gentleman's Magazine, Protwinarajan, the king of Ghorka, captured the city of Kirtipor in Ceylon. The King ordered a census taken by cutting off the noses and lips of all the inhabitants, even the smallest children. The population figure was then to be determined by a count of cut-off noses. Kirtipor was afterwards renamed Naskatapoor, meaning the city of severed noses.

Carpue hesitated to perform the operation until 1814. A man came to him who wore a black patch over his face. The patient told the following story:

In 1801 I entered the Egyptian army as a fledgling officer. There I suffered an attack of jaundice, and the army doctors prescribed mercury. From this you will probably assume that in truth I suffered from a syphilitic disease. I know that syphilis also destroys noses. But I can prove by the testimony of my doctors that I never had any such disease. The mercury which was administered to me in Egypt, then in Malta, then in Ireland, and finally here in London, poisoned me and in the end resulted in the loss of my nose.

Early in October, 1814, Carpue decided to risk the operation. Carpue first made a test to determine whether healing would occur or whether the mercury poisoning had undermined the soundness of the apparently healthy parts of the face. Carpue took a scalpel and made several incisions close to the root of the nose; within a few days the incisions were already beginning to heal. On October 23, the operation took place. Carpue formed the model of the nose out of wax in accordance with the descriptions of the Indian procedure.

Carpue drew lines with the red paint around the stub of the nose, where he would have to make incisions in order to insert the edges of the new nasal skin. The patient did not stir as the knife cut the outlines of the flap on the forehead and freed the skin from the frontal bone. By the end of nine minutes, according to the friend who had accompanied the patient, Carpue was placing the lowest part of the new nose into the incision above the upper lip and suturing it, ligature by ligature, while the blood continued to run from the forehead across the patient's face. After having sutured the two sides of the nose, he cut out the nostril openings and inserted lint to keep them open. Carpue endeavored to bring the edges of the wound on the forehead as much into contact as possible. The patient opened his mouth and said: "It was no child's play—extremely painful—but there was no use complaining." The officer with the watch came up to the foot of the bed and announced 37 minutes, then shook hands heartily with Carpue.

The nose had been covered with a dressing, and the sick room was kept at a torrid temperature in order to simulate the temperature of India. On the third day Carpue removed the dressing in the presence of his assistants and the officer who kept time during the operation. When the dressing was removed, the officer exclaimed: "My God, there is a nose."

Rapid Adoption of Rhinoplasty. Von Graefe, who became Professor of Surgery at the University of Berlin, interrupting his academic career to assume the responsibilities of Surgeon General of the Prussian Army at the end of the Napoleonic Wars (1813 to 1815), reported three cases of reconstructive rhinoplasty in which he had employed the Tagliacotian, the Indian, and a modification of the original Tagliacotian procedure. The reported technique consisted of the immediate application of the flap to the nose without a period of delay. He also shortened to six days, when possible, the period during which the arm was attached to the head. Other than Carpue's report (1816), von Graefe's *Rhinoplastik* (1818) was the first treatise on plastic surgery after Tagliacozzi (1597), and his work, which listed 55 references on the subject, stimulated the development of plastic surgery throughout Europe and the United States.

The recognition of the historical contribution of Tagliacozzi was epitomized by Delpech in his two volumes (1823–1828): "Nothing is more exact than his observations, nothing more wise than his precepts. . . . Tagliacozzi's method was a stroke of genius which can become extremely fruitful in skilled hands. . . ." Delpech wrote not only about his rhinoplastic operations but also about reconstruction of the lips, urethroplasty, and other plastic surgical procedures.

The interest generated in reconstructive rhinoplasty stimulated the development of other plastic surgical procedures. Dieffenbach, a younger contemporary of von Graefe, was especially instrumental in enlarging the scope of plastic surgery. His clinical work was monumental in its variety, inventiveness, and breadth of scope. He should be credited with establishing nasal reconstruction as a feasible technique and he demonstrated the role of secondary operations in refining the shape of the nose (Rogers, 1981). Among his numerous publications, the best known is his *Die operative Chirurgie*, published in 1845 and 1848 in two volumes. John Staige Davis (1941) stated that his "methods and principles have not been improved upon and are still constantly employed."

During the first half of the nineteenth century, Labat (1834) and Blandin (1836) wrote the first treatises on plastic surgery in France.

Serre in 1842 published his "Traité sur l'art de restaurer les déformités de la face" (treatise on the art of repairing facial deformities). Serre was the chief exponent of the sliding (advancement) flap technique, the so-called French method, an adaptation of the technique of Celsus.

The names of two great surgeons of the nineteenth century cannot be omitted: Dupuytren, particularly for his operations for "palmar fibromatosis" described in 1834 and his classification of burns according to their depth, and von Langenbeck, who succeeded Dieffenbach, for his contributions to cleft palate and jaw surgery.

During the remainder of the nineteenth century, hundreds of papers appeared on the subject of plastic surgery. Either surgical treatises devoted entirely to plastic surgery (Zeis's *Handbuch der plastischen Chirurgie*, published in 1838; Jobert's *Traité de Chirurgie Plastique*, published in 1849) or substantive portions of surgical treatises, such as the works of Roux in 1854 and Verneuil in 1877, were published.

A book that also included plastic surgery in its title was published in 1842 by von Ammon and Baumgarten and was translated into French and Italian. In England, Liston devoted a considerable discussion to various plastic surgical procedures in his textbooks published in 1831 and 1837. In France the textbooks of Velpeau (1839) and Malgaigne (1849) also contained sections on plastic surgery. A number of Italian surgeons were performing plastic surgical operations. Sabbatini published a book in 1838 describing the history of plastic surgery and was the first surgeon to describe the "lip switch" operation. The American edition of Velpeau's *Operative Surgery* published in 1851 included, in the first volume under the section "Anaplasty or Autoplasty," a concluding American appendix that described a variety of reconstructive procedures by Pancoast and Mutter of Philadelphia as well as by Mott, Post, and Buck of New York. The publications of Blasius (1839–1843) and a number of other surgeons give an excellent picture of the great advances made during the first half of the nineteenth century. *Surgical Observations*, published in 1867 by Warren of Boston, detailed the surgical treatment of nasal and eyelid defects as well as cleft lip and palate. One of the outstanding works was the *Manual of Operative Surgery* by Szymanowski, published in Russia in 1870.

The Birth of Skin Grafting

In 1804 Baronio of Italy published *Degli Innesti Animali* (On Grafting in Animals) in which he detailed his skin grafting experiments in sheep. Bert's *De la Greffe Animale* (1863) summarized his own animal experiments as well as those of others on transplanting human and animal parts.

The first recorded successful human skin graft was by Sir Astley Cooper, who in 1817 removed the skin from an amputated thumb and used it to cover the stump as a full-thickness skin graft (Balch and Marzoni, 1977). Bünger, a colleague of von Graefe, applied a skin graft from the thigh to the nose in 1823. Warren (1840) in Boston transplanted a full-thickness skin graft to the ala of the nose. Nevertheless, the full clinical import of skin grafting was recognized only near the last quarter of the century, perhaps, in part, because gifted surgeons like Dieffenbach had little success with the technique.

An event took place shortly before the Franco-Prussian War which was to add to the armamentarium of the plastic surgeon: the development of clinical skin grafting. In 1869 Reverdin, a surgical intern in Paris, reported the hastening of the healing of granulating wounds by what he called "epidermic" grafts, which probably contained more dermis than he realized. On December 8, 1869, before the Imperial Society of Surgery of Paris, Reverdin showed a patient on whom he had applied, on a granulating surface, a segment of skin approximately 2 by 3 mm in size excised from the superficial portion of the integument. In the discussion that followed, Guyon stated: "A single experiment is not conclusive. . . . The question of the future of the epidermic graft is today before you. . . . Dr. Reverdin has, on my advice, presented this patient to draw attention to this new method and to receive the recognition which it merits." Claude Bernard, in person, presented Reverdin's work before the Academy of Sciences.

The technique of skin grafting was further developed when Ollier in 1872 described the clinical application of a dermoepidermic graft 4 by 8 cm in size; Thiersch (1874) advocated the use of larger sheets of dermoepidermic grafts to cover wounds and emphasized the importance of the dermal component. The grafts were thin, split-thickness skin grafts often referred to in the English and German literature as "Thiersch" grafts; credit should be given to Ollier and the grafts designated as "Ollier-Thiersch" grafts. Pollock (1870), Lawson (1870), LeFort (1872), and Wolfe (1876) described the use of a full-thickness graft for the treatment of eyelid ectropion; Krause (1893) perfected the technique. The history of skin grafting has been compiled by Klasen (1981).

The nineteenth century literature was compiled and classified by Nélaton and Ombrédanne in two books published in 1904 and 1907. These remained important reference sources until World War II.

It is significant that the early development of plastic surgery appears to have been closely linked to the development of reconstruction of the nose; it was only in the nineteenth century that these principles and techniques were applied to other anatomic areas.

The Early Twentieth Century

The Period of Growth (1914 to 1939). World War I (1914 to 1918), often referred to as the Great War, appears to have been the crucial starting point for the development of what is now considered modern plastic surgery.

Tactical military maneuvering rapidly became limited during the first World War as movement ceased and the conflict became stabilized on the "Western front." Casualties mounted to appalling figures, and trench warfare was responsible for ever-increasing numbers of maxillofacial wounds.

The influx of large numbers of patients with gunshot wounds of the face into military hospitals during World War I required the organization of specialized centers. Few surgeons knew how to cope with the problem. Several treatment centers were established by the French Army, one of which was headed by an outstanding reconstructive surgeon, Morestin, a native of the Caribbean island of Martinique. Well known before World War I for his work in the application of the Z-plasty technique to linear contractures and for developing techniques of cartilage grafting, Morestin conducted an active service at the Val-de-Grâce Military Hospital in Paris. Morestin was one of the first surgeons to show that the skin and subcutaneous tissue could be widely undermined without being subject to necrosis (Converse, 1968).

Morestin died prematurely, a victim of the great influenza epidemic of 1917–1918, and left a void in French plastic surgery. The concept of adapting dental techniques to the treatment of gunshot wounds of the face was foreign to Morestin, who disdained the services of the dental surgeon and claimed: "I can do everything with my scalpel." He rendered an immeasurable service by unwittingly stimulating Sir Harold Gillies' interest in plastic surgery.

Gillies was an otolaryngologist attached to a British general hospital in Rouen, France. A friend of his, an American dentist named Roberts, having returned from a trip to Paris where he had seen Morestin operate, urged Gillies to go to Paris. Gillies was inspired by what he saw and with the help of Sir William Arbuthnot Lane, his army consultant, a unit was established at the Aldershot Military Hospital. This measure was taken as part of the preparation for the Somme offensive (Clarkson, 1966). It is interesting that there appears to have been no further contact between Gillies and Morestin; Morestin even closed the door of his operating room to Gillies (personal communication of J. M. Converse).

A center was subsequently established at the Queen Mary Hospital, Sidcup, Kent. Here Gillies, assisted by Kilner, developed a treatment center for British and allied military casualties. Many allied medical officers came to Sidcup to learn plastic surgery: Ferris

Smith from the United States, Waldron and Risdon from Canada, and Newland and Pickerill from Australia and New Zealand. Gillies was fortunate to have as an associate a dental officer, Kelsey Fry, who applied dental techniques to the many maxillofacial reconstructive problems the surgeons were trying to solve.

Paralleling the development at Sidcup, another center situated not far from the front lines was operational at Etaples, near Boulogne, under the direction of V. H. Kazanjian of Boston. Kazanjian, a dental surgeon, had volunteered to serve in the First Harvard Unit attached to the British Expeditionary Force. Kazanjian applied his knowledge of prosthetic dentistry to the early treatment of gunshot wounds of the face. He perfected methods of fixation of jaw fragments and the use of prosthetic devices prior to delayed primary closure of facial wounds.

At the outbreak of World War I there was no recognized specialty of plastic surgery in the United States. Most general surgeons practiced reconstructive surgery and a few showed interest in this type of work. There were a considerable number of oral surgeons, such as Brophy, Gilmer, Cryer, Marshall, G. V. I. Brown, and Chalmers J. Lyons, who, as a result of their dental training, took a special interest in surgical diseases of the mouth and jaws, particularly cleft lip and palate.

When the United States entered the war in 1917, Surgeon General Gorgas organized, under the Division of Surgery, certain sections, among them a section of head surgery that included subsections of ophthalmology, otolaryngology, brain surgery, and oral and plastic surgery. Vilray P. Blair of Saint Louis headed the last-named section and chose Robert H. Ivy as his assistant. Blair was well known for his work and had written a book, *Surgery and Diseases of the Mouth and Jaws* (1912). As early as 1907 Blair had attempted the surgical correction of mandibular prognathism in collaboration with Edward H. Angle, the orthodontist who is often considered the father of the American school of orthodontics. Blair conceived the idea of setting up teams, each consisting of a general surgeon and a dental surgeon who could pool their respective talents. Officers assigned to these teams were sent to special short courses of instruction in several medical and dental schools. A revised edition of Blair's textbook was prepared and distributed to Army hospitals. A number of officers were sent for short periods of observation and training at British and French hospital centers. Attempts were made to concentrate on patients with face and jaw injuries at Base Hospital 115, Vichy (France).

In the United States, three centers were established where most of the patients with face and jaw injuries were assigned on arrival from Europe: General Hospital No. 11 at Cape May, New Jersey; General Hospital No. 2, Fort McHenry, Baltimore, Maryland; and Walter Reed General Hospital, Washington, D.C. Later, two other centers were established at Columbus Barracks, Ohio and Jefferson Barracks, Missouri (Ivy, 1948).

By the end of the war, names such as Gillies in England, Morestin in France, Lexer, Ganzer, and Lindemann in Germany, Esser and Pichler in Austria, and Burian in Czechoslovakia became widely known, these men being characterized as specialists in plastic surgery or in jaw and face surgery.

One can consider, therefore, that World War I was the beginning of the era during which plastic surgery became a surgical specialty. After World War I, national and international congresses began to include in their scientific programs papers concerned with the methods of treatment of war victims and newly developed plastic surgical procedures for the face.

This was the period when one saw the facially mutilated from the war. Ernest Hemingway (1964), recalling the clients of a particular Parisian Montparnasse café, wrote: "There were other people too who lived in the quarter and came to Lilas, and some of them wore Croix de Guerre ribbons in their lapels and others also had the yellow and green of the Médaille Militaire, and I watched how well they were overcoming the handicap of the loss of limbs, and saw the quality of their artificial eyes and the degree of skill with which their faces had been reconstructed. There was always an almost iridescent shiny cast about the considerably reconstructed face, rather like that of a well-packed ski run and we respected these clients. . . ." There were many others whose faces contained gaping holes, who had no lower jaws; these were the veterans whose faces could not be reconstructed. They formed an organization of mutual aid, "Les Gueules Cassées" ("the broken faces"), which has continued to the present day. In view of the vast number of casualties, the rehabilitation task did not end with the war but continued for many years thereafter.

A number of publications appeared at this time. The first American textbook, *Plastic Surgery—Its Principles and Practice*, was published in 1919 by John Staige Davis of Baltimore. It is ironic that his mentor and chief, the celebrated American surgeon Halsted, refused to write an introduction. Gillies' *Plastic Surgery of the Face* (1920) detailed his war experience and was a landmark publication that influenced several generations of surgeons. The contributions of surgeons and dentists during the war were described in a publication, "La Revue Maxillo-faciale," which appeared in 1919 and 1920. Ivy (1918, 1923) summarized the new knowledge in plastic surgery acquired during the war. A 1922 paper by Blair, "Reconstructive surgery of the face," illustrated the high degree of proficiency achieved in rehabilitating the war disfigured. Other important publications during this period included those of Velter (1917), Steinschneider (1917), Lexer (1919, 1920), Delangenière (1921), and Mauclaire (1922).

With the advent of peace and a period of relative prosperity, a new branch of plastic surgery appeared, designated "esthetic" or "cosmetic." Joseph, an orthopedic surgeon in Berlin who is justly regarded as the founder of modern corrective rhinoplasty, was at the apogee of his career (Natvig, 1982); his classic textbook was published in 1928. He gave courses attended by two pioneers of modern corrective rhinoplasty in the United States, Aufricht and Safian. In France, Passot, Noel, and others were performing surgical procedures to correct the aging face. In the United States C. C. Miller of Chicago was an early advocate of cosmetic surgery of the face and in 1907 published a textbook, *Cosmetic Surgery: The Correction of Featural Imperfections*.

Considerable emphasis was given to the teaching of plastic surgery during this period by the organization of international courses by Lemaitre, an associate professor at the Faculty of Medicine of Paris and chief of an otolaryngologic service in a Paris hospital. Lemaitre had been in charge of a large maxillofacial center at Vichy during the war and had met a number of Allied officers, notably Blair and Ivy. In 1925 he organized an international clinic in his service at l'Hôpital Saint-Louis, which was conducted on a yearly basis until 1928. Gillies also held a series of operative demonstrations, and in the following years Eastman Sheehan, Ferris Smith, Kilner, and Joseph conducted courses that were well attended. There being no other way of learning plastic surgery at this time, a number of surgeons from various parts of Europe and from the United States received their training at these courses. Among these students the most illustrious was Sanvenero-Rosselli of Milan, the president of the Fourth International Congress of Plastic Surgery held in Rome in October, 1967 (Figs. 1–4 and 1–5).

An important contribution to the literature of plastic surgery in the 1920's was Ferris Smith's *Reconstructive Surgery*, which appeared in 1928. Ferris Smith, who had acquired a reputation as a distinguished otolaryngologist, was particularly interested in the technique of repeated partial exicison and the use of local flaps on the face. Many considered him one of the finest technicians of his day. Even in those days he had an appreciation of atraumatic technique, and, above all, he placed emphasis on detail.

In the 1920's and 1930's three personalities—Harold Delf Gillies (Fig. 1–6), John Staige Davis, and Vilray Papin Blair (Fig. 1–7)—helped to shape the present concepts of plastic surgery as it is practiced in the English-speaking world.

Staige Davis was probably the first American surgeon to devote his entire practice to plastic surgery. When there was little recognition for plastic surgery, Davis, working alone and with little encouragement from his own medical school, made many important contributions over the years: "small deep skin" or "pinch" graft, the theory and practice of Z-plasty (1931), serial excision of scars (1929), vascularization of skin grafts (1925), and the delay of skin flaps (German, Finesilver, and Davis, 1933). His textbook *Plastic Surgery*, published in 1919, was the first book of its kind in the English language. This textbook provided the reader with an extensive review of the literature, a critical appraisal by the author of the methods described, and a voluminous description of his personal experience.

Blair and Gillies had a profound influence on the development of plastic surgery, not only in English-speaking countries but also throughout the world at large. Their influence was exerted not only in scientific aspects but also in helping to shape plastic surgery into its present organizational lines.

Each of these men contributed outstandingly to the field of skin transplantation.

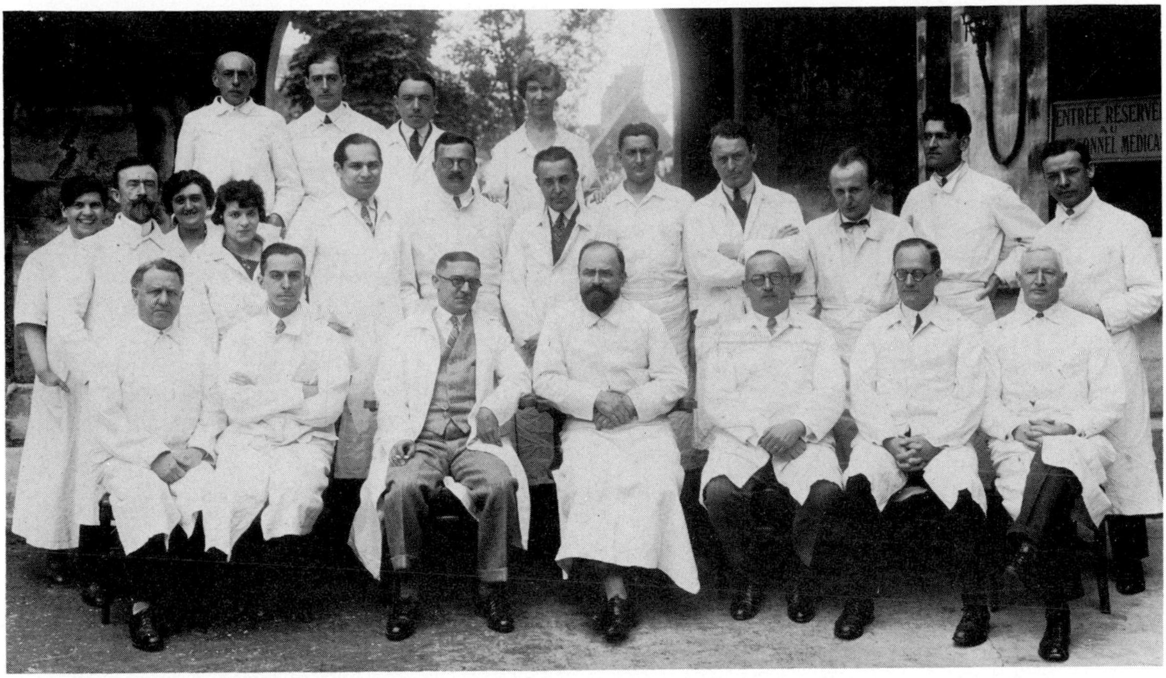

Figure 1–4. A photograph taken at the Hospital Saint-Louis in Paris in 1927 following the International Clinic. From left to right (seated): Myron Metzenbaum (Cleveland), Gustavo Sanvenero-Rosselli (Milan), Ferris Smith (Grand Rapids), Fernand Lemaitre (Paris); the next two are unidentified; extreme right: W. T. Coughlin (New York). Standing behind M. Metzenbaum: M. Roy (Quebec). (From Converse, J. M.: Plastic surgery: The 20th century. The period of growth (1914–1939). Surg. Clin. North Am., *47*:261, 1967.)

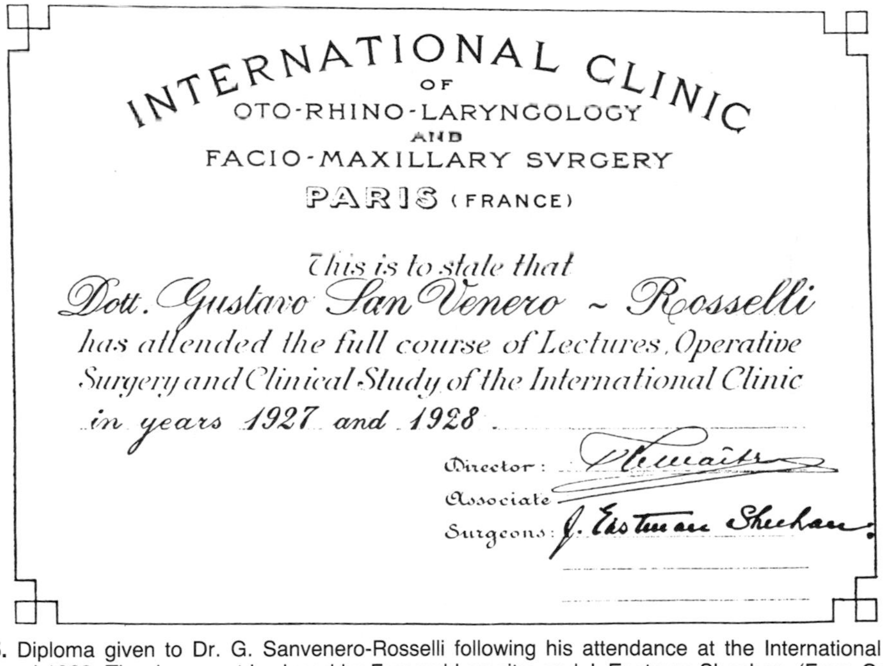

INTERNATIONAL CLINIC
OF
OTO-RHINO-LARYNGOLOGY
AND
FACIO-MAXILLARY SVRGERY
PARIS (FRANCE)

This is to state that
Dott. Gustavo San Venero ~ Rosselli
has attended the full course of Lectures, Operative Surgery and Clinical Study of the International Clinic
in years 1927 and 1928

Director: F. Lemaitre
Associate Surgeons: J. Eastman Sheehan

Figure 1–5. Diploma given to Dr. G. Sanvenero-Rosselli following his attendance at the International Clinic held in Paris in 1927 and 1928. The document is signed by Fernand Lemaitre and J. Eastman Sheehan. (From Converse, J. M.: Plastic surgery: The 20th century. The period of growth (1914–1939). Surg. Clin. North Am., *47*:261, 1967.)

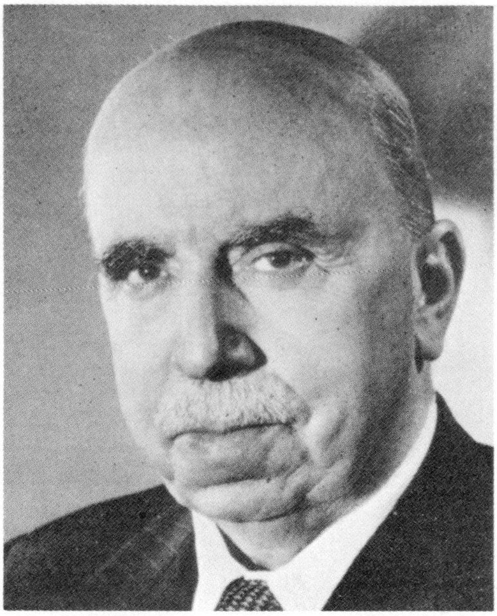

Figure 1–6. Harold Delf Gillies.

Gillies developed the tube flap, coincidentally with Filatov (1917), and showed many applications of the new technique in his book *Plastic Surgery of the Face* (1920). Blair defined the process of delay in nontubulated flaps in his paper, "The delayed transfer of long pedicled flaps in plastic surgery," published in 1921.

The development of the technique of split-thickness skin grafting and the paper on the subject by Blair and his pupil Barrett Brown (1929) constitute a landmark in the history of skin grafting. The thicker split-thickness graft gave a more durable type of repair with less shrinkage and wrinkling than the thin Thiersch graft generally used by surgeons for covering raw surfaces and granulating wounds, or the small, deep, so-called "pinch" grafts, which resulted in even more contraction and scarring.

To facilitate removal of the split-thickness skin graft, Blair developed a special skin-grafting knife and the suction box, which, connected with a negative pressure apparatus, facilitated traction of the skin and flattening of the donor area during the cutting of the graft. In numerous articles written in subsequent years, the St. Louis group advocated early grafting in skin defects resulting from burns and other types of injuries. They espoused the principle that the best dressing for a wound with loss of skin was a skin graft.

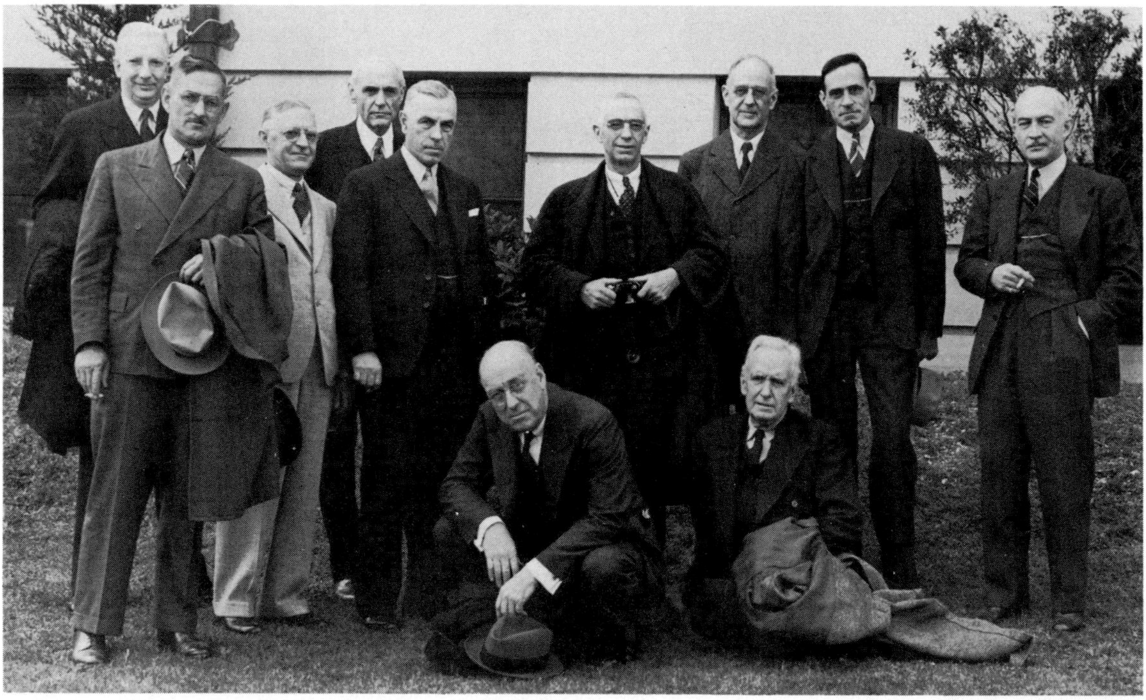

Figure 1–7. First annual meeting of the American Board of Plastic Surgery held in Galveston, Texas, February 2, 1938. From left to right, standing: William S. Kiskadden, George Warren Pierce, Ferris Smith, William E. Ladd, Fulton Risdon, Robert H. Ivy, John Staige Davis, Harold L. D. Kirkham, and Jerome P. Webster. Seated: George M. Dorrance and Vilray Papin Blair. (From Converse, J. M.: Plastic surgery: The 20th century. The period of growth (1914–1939). Surg. Clin. North Am., *47*:261, 1967.)

Skin Grafting by Brown and McDowell (1939) rendered a great service to patients and surgeons during World War II.

Skin grafting was greatly facilitated when Padgett, a plastic surgeon trained by Blair, and Hood, a mechanical engineer, developed the dermatome. Padgett in 1939 described the three-quarter thickness skin graft, which had qualities comparable with those of a full-thickness graft.

The idea of calibration, one of the chief advantages of the dermatome, was not a new one. Finochietto, an Argentine surgeon, had devised a calibrated knife as early as 1920. Humby, while serving as a house surgeon at the Great Ormond Street Hospital for Sick Children in London, added a roller to the Blair knife that permitted calibration of the graft. The Padgett-Hood dermatome, by providing a relatively easy mechanical means for the removal of split-thickness grafts, placed the technique of skin grafting into the hands of all surgeons. Before this development, skin grafting was a specialized technique of the plastic surgeon. The service rendered by the dermatome, an American contribution, in making possible the frequent use of split-thickness grafting during World War II was immeasurable in terms of saving many lives and limbs.

Blair can justly be considered the father of the American Board of Plastic Surgery, established in 1937 (Fig. 1–7). In 1936, in an editorial entitled "Surgery, Specialty Surgery, and 'Plastic Surgery,'" Blair had intimated the need for a Plastic Surgery Board.

It is difficult to realize the precarious status of plastic surgery at that time. To quote Webster: "At that time the public generally considered plastic surgeons as 'face lifters' and 'nose whittlers.' To be sure, a few surgeons throughout the country were known for their capabilities in the special fields of plastic surgery. There were also those who were close to the border of being ethical, if not unethical, in their practice, and some were definitely below that level. Blair felt that those slightly below the ethical line could be raised if given proper recognition, and those with special abilities should be recognized and their qualities brought to bear for the good of the specialty of plastic surgery."

Staige Davis in Baltimore, Ivy and Warren B. Davis in Philadelphia, Kazanjian in Boston, Blair, Brown, Byars, and their associates in St. Louis, Pierce in San Francisco, Peer in Newark, Ferris Smith in Grand Rapids, Webster, Eastman Sheehan, Maliniac, and John M. Wheeler and Wendell L. Hughes, the latter two ophthalmic plastic surgeons in New York, were well known and respected. Safian and Aufricht in New York were perfecting the techniques of corrective rhinoplasty. Many surgeons were practicing corrective rhinoplasty after having taken courses in Europe either with Joseph in Berlin in the 1920's, or in other centers, such as Vienna, where such courses were also available.

Opportunities for learning plastic surgery were few in the 1930's. Preceptorships were not numerous and there were few well-organized plastic surgery services in the hospitals. One of the first active hospital services in the United States was that organized by Eastman Sheehan at the Postgraduate Hospital, the predecessor to the Institute of Reconstructive Plastic Surgery at the New York University Medical Center. Sheehan trained Straatsma, Milton Adams, Peer, and Barsky. Sheehan was a brilliant technician who had a predilection for operating upon members of the European nobility and was not averse to publicity. He wrote a number of books, including *Plastic Surgery of the Orbit* (1927), and did much work on the wounded armies of General Franco during the Spanish Civil War.

By an unusual set of circumstances, Sheehan was responsible for the establishment of the Nuffield Professorship of Plastic Surgery at Oxford University. Through a doctor-patient relationship with Lord and Lady Nuffield, he was offered the Nuffield Chair of Plastic Surgery. Because Sheehan had been regarded as a Fascist following his activities in Spain, Lord Nuffield was obliged to intervene with Prime Minister Churchill in order to obtain a visa permitting him to enter England. The Council of Oxford University, however, disapproved of his appointment. Because of faculty opposition also to Gillies, T. Pomfret Kilner was appointed the first (and unfortunately last) Nuffield Professor of Plastic Surgery.

Before the establishment of approved residencies and with the exception of the few available preceptorships, the only method of learning was observation, and there were well-trodden paths by young surgeons to St. Louis, Baltimore, New York, Boston, and London.

A residency in maxillofacial surgery was

established by Ivy in Philadelphia. Another residency was started at King's County Hospital in Brooklyn by Coakley. For a number of years Ivy's residents spent an additional year in Coakley's service. Webster established his residency program in New York in 1939, which graduated a whole generation of leaders of plastic surgery. This service earned the respect of many influential American surgeons from other disciplines.

A curious phenomenon was the publication in 1939 of a book, *Surgery of Injury and Plastic Repair*, by Fomon. Not a plastic surgeon but a medical writer, Fomon had proposed to Kazanjian that he write a book for him. When Kazanjian declined the offer, Fomon made a similar proposition to Eastman Sheehan, who accepted. Some disagreement occurred subsequently, and Fomon published a book under his own name. Although lacking in many ways, the deficiencies reflecting the author's inexperience, the book rendered a service by collecting the known techniques, some of which were well illustrated, and by assembling an exhaustive and accurate bibliography. It is ironic that a textbook by an author who was not a plastic surgeon was a major reference source in plastic surgery in the mid-twentieth century.

In Great Britain, before World War II, plastic surgery was a monopoly in the hands of Gillies, McIndoe, and Mowlem (all from New Zealand) and Kilner, an Englishman. McIndoe, who had been trained in surgery at the Mayo Clinic, was consultant to the Royal Air Force, and Kilner was in charge of plastic surgery at the Ministry of Pensions. These surgeons were active in a number of London hospitals.

A Swedish surgeon, Ragnell, was trained in England by Gillies and returned to Stockholm in the 1930's, where he later headed a service established at the Karolinska Institute. This was the beginning of the Swedish school of plastic surgery.

Léon Dufourmentel was an otolaryngologist and son-in-law of Sebileau, who was professor of otolaryngology at the University of Paris during World War I and during the immediate postwar period. Unfortunately, he was not appointed head of one of the Paris hospital services and was obliged to restrict his activities to private practice. This fact, in addition to the untimely death of Morestin, was responsible for a long period of stagnation in the development of reconstructive plastic surgery in France. Plastic surgery became commonly known as "chirurgie esthetique," and it was not until after World War II that a new and dynamic generation of plastic surgeons arose. This generation made notable contributions to the specialty of plastic surgery.

Victor Veau, a pediatric surgeon, started making surgical contributions to the treatment of cleft lip and palate in the early 1920's as well as conducting outstanding research in the embryology of the cleft lip in the 1930's (Converse, 1962).

Lexer, a general surgeon in Germany, summarized his own work in reconstructive surgery in his treatise *Die gesamte Wiederherstellungschirurgie*, published in 1931 (May, 1962).

A colorful individualist between the two World Wars was Esser, a Dutch surgeon who had volunteered to work with the Austrian army during World War I. Esser did much of his work in Vienna during the war and made a number of notable contributions, such as the application of the rotation flap to the repair of facial defects, the artery island flap that he termed the "biologic flap," and the important contribution of the "epithelial" or skin graft inlay technique. His textbook *Esser (Epithelial) Inlay* was published in Leiden in 1940.

Following the war, Esser appears to have led the life of a wandering surgeon. For a long time he was established in Munich and then in Monte Carlo. In the late 1930's he conceived the grandiose plan of establishing a world center for plastic surgery. For this purpose he requested an audience with Benito Mussolini. In the Palazzo Venezia in Rome, Mussolini had his desk at the end of an enormous room, and the visitor walked the long distance under the steady gaze of the head of the Fascist state. It is said that Esser picked up a chair and sat down next to Il Duce, much to the latter's amazement. He then requested an island in "Mare Nostrum" (Mussolini's Imperial Roman term for the Mediterranean Sea) in which to establish the world center for plastic surgery! The advent of World War II put an end to this grandiose plan (personal communication of J. M. Converse).

The period between the two wars also saw the birth of the oldest plastic surgery society, the American Association of Oral and Plastic Surgeons, which was established in 1921 by

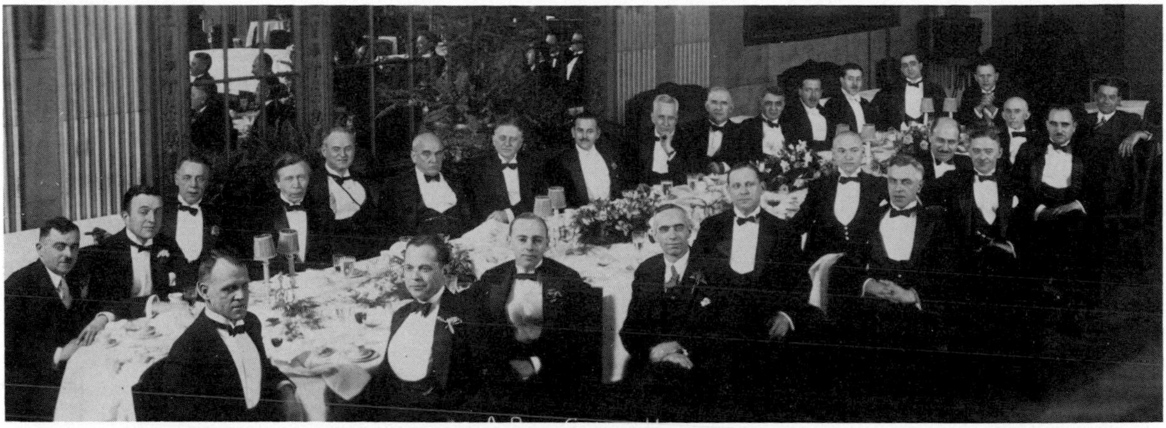

Figure 1–8. Meeting of the American Association of Plastic and Oral Surgeons in New York, 1927. Back row, left to right: Drs. Waldron, Dunning, McCaffrey, Vilmajalmur Stefansson (Arctic explorer), Judge Conboy, Drs. J. Erdman, Sheehan, Blair, Lyons, Kazanjian, Gillies, unidentified, Beck, Straatsma. Front row, left to right: Drs. Lucius Johnson, Stout, Parker, Ivy, Schamberg, Vaughan, Risdon, Douglas Quick, Ferris Smith, McCurdy, unidentified, H. A. Potts. (Courtesy Plastic Surgery Archives, Harvard Medical School Library)

Brophy, Moorehead, and Dunning. The name of the society was changed to the American Association of Plastic Surgeons in 1941; the double-degree requirement had been dropped in 1927 (Fig. 1–8). Annual meetings were held; these were small, intimate gatherings until World War II. The meetings comprised operating room sessions at which members gathered around their host and watched him operate. Under the leadership of Maliniac, Aufricht, Palmer, Wheeler, and Peer, another society, the American Society of Plastic and Reconstructive Surgeons, was established in 1931. The proceedings of the Society were published in a European publication, *Revue de Chirurgie Plastique,* until 1940, after which the Society published its own proceedings.

The first issue of the *Revue de Chirurgie Plastique* was published in 1931 under the editorship of Coelst (Fig. 1–9). Coelst was a practitioner in Brussels, Belgium, who does not appear to have had any official university or hospital appointments. Through his personal initiative and efforts, he assembled a series of papers of good quality for the period. At the suggestion of Esser, the name of the publication was later changed to *Revue de Chirurgie Structive* (Fig. 1–10). Esser pointed out that "plastic" was a poor term that did not define the specialty, and that the term "structive," derived from the Latin *structo* (I build), was more appropriate. Coelst brought together an international editorial board of high quality that included many well-known names (Fig. 1–11). The papers were published in whatever language was preferred by the author and summarized in English, German, and French. By contrast with this early effort, the American journal *Plastic and Reconstructive Surgery* and the *British Journal of Plastic Surgery* commenced publication only after World War II.

In 1931 the first congress of the French Society of Reparative and Esthetic Surgery was held in Paris. This group published in book form the papers read at the congress, edited by Claoué and Dartigues. Participants in the congress and authors of the papers published in the *Revue* comprised, in addition to the few full-time practicing plastic surgeons, general surgeons, otolaryngologists, ophthalmologists, oral and dental surgeons, and orthodontists who were involved either full or part time in the various aspects of plastic surgery.

Of major interest in the history of this period was the establishment in 1936 of a European Society of Structive Surgery, which held its first congress in Brussels in that year (Fig. 1–11). Eminent personalities in the field such as Gillies, Esser, and Kilner participated. The second congress was held the following year in London, and the third in Milan in 1938. At the time of the Milan congress there appeared the first issue of a new international review entitled *Plastica Chirurgica,* edited by Sanvenero-Rosselli, who established a teaching course for the training of plastic surgeons in Italy. The publication of

Année 1931 **Revue trimestrielle** **N° 1, Avril**

REVUE
DE
CHIRURGIE PLASTIQUE

Revue internationale de Chirurgie restauratrice, plastique et esthétique.
International Review for restoring, plastic and esthetical surgery.
Internationale Zeitschrift für wiederherstellende, plastische und ästhetische Chirurgie.

SOMMAIRE :

Figure 1–9. Title page of the first issue of the *Revue de Chirurgie Plastique* (From Converse, J. M.: Plastic surgery: The 20th century. The period of growth (1914–1939). Surg. Clin. North Am., *47*:261, 1967.)

6ᵉ **Année.** **Nos 3 et 4, Décembre 1936.**

REVUE
DE
CHIRURGIE
STRUCTIVE

(Ancienne Revue de Chirurgie Plastique)

Revue Internationale de Chirurgie restauratrice et plastique
International Review for restoring, and plastic Surgery.
Internationale Zeitschrift für wiederherstellende und plastische Chirurgie.

Directeur-Fondateur : Dʳ **M. COELST** (Bruxelles)

Collaborateurs : MM. les Professeurs et Docteurs :

Albee, F.-H. *(New-York)* — Anopol, G. *(New-York)* — Aubert *(Marseille)* — Bames, H.-O. *(Los Angeles)* — Bettman, A.-G. *(Portland)* — Boisson, R. *(Bruxelles)* — Bourguet, J. *(Paris)* — Burian, F. *(Prague)* — Claoué, Ch. *(Paris)* — Corachan, M. *(Barcelona)* — Dantlo, R. *(Moyeuvre)* — Dantrelle *(Paris)* — Darcissac, M. *(Paris)* — Dartigues *(Paris)* — Decoster, L. *(Bruxelles)* — Deselaers, A. *(Barcelona)* — Dieulafé *(Toulouse)* — Dobrzaniecki, W. *(Lwow)* — Dufourmentel, L. *(Paris)* — Eastman-Sheehan *(New-York)* — Esser, J.-F.-S. *(Monaco)* — Ferrari, R.-C. *(Buenos-Aires)* — Ferris Smith *(Grand Rapids)* — Fruhwald *(Wien)* — Gumpert, M. *(New-York)* — Halle, M. *(Berlin)* — Hofer, Otto *(Wien)* — Horno Alcorta *(Zaragoza)* — Ivanissevich, O. *(Buenos-Aires)* — Ivy, R.-H. *(Philadelphia)* — Jiano, J. *(Bucarest)* — Joseph, J. *(Berlin)* † — Karfik *(Prague)* — Kilner, T.-P. *(London)* — Kubertova, E. *(Prague)* — Lapierre, V. *(Lyon)* — Larroudé, C. *(Lisboa)* — Lexer *(München)* — Lumière, A. *(Lyon)* — Lyons, Hunt *(New-York)* — Madureira, A. *(Lisboa)* — Maliniak, J.-W. *(New-York)* — Manna, A. *(Roma)* — Marchal *(Anvers)* — Maurel, Gérard *(Paris)* — Michalek-Grodzki *(Warszawa)* — O' Connor, C.-B. *(San-Francisco)* — Passot, R. *(Paris)* † — Péri, M. *(Alger)* — Pierre-Robin *(Paris)* — Pohl, L. *(Wien)* — Pont, A. *(Lyon)* — Portmann, G. *(Bordeaux)* — Prevot *(Marseille)* — Raul *(Thionville)* — Rebello-Neto *(Sao Paulo)* — Réthi *(Budapest)* — Rocher *(Bordeaux)* — Roy, J.-N. *(Montréal)* — Sanvenero-Rosselli *(Milano)* — Sargnon *(Lyon)* — Schultz, J.-H. *(Berlin)* — Sercer, A. *(Zagreb)* — Simon, Paul-W. *(Berlin)* — Straith, C.-L. *(Detroit)* — Stephan Wahl *(New-York)* — Ulrich *(Paris)* — Wallet *(Paris)* — Warren Pierce, G. *(San Franscisco)* — Wodak, E. *(Prague)* — Gerald Brown O'Connor M. D. *San Francisco)*.

Rédaction : Centre de Chirurgie Structive
3, Boulevard du Centenaire
Administration : 17, Rue de la Longue-Haie, Bruxelles

Abonnement pour quatre numéros :

Belgique, 20 belgas ; Etranger, 25 ou 30 belgas selon les conventions postales.

Figure 1–10. Title page of the first issue of the *Revue de Chirurgie Structive* (From Converse, J. M.: Plastic surgery: The 20th century. The period of growth (1914–1939). Surg. Clin. North Am., *47*:261, 1967.)

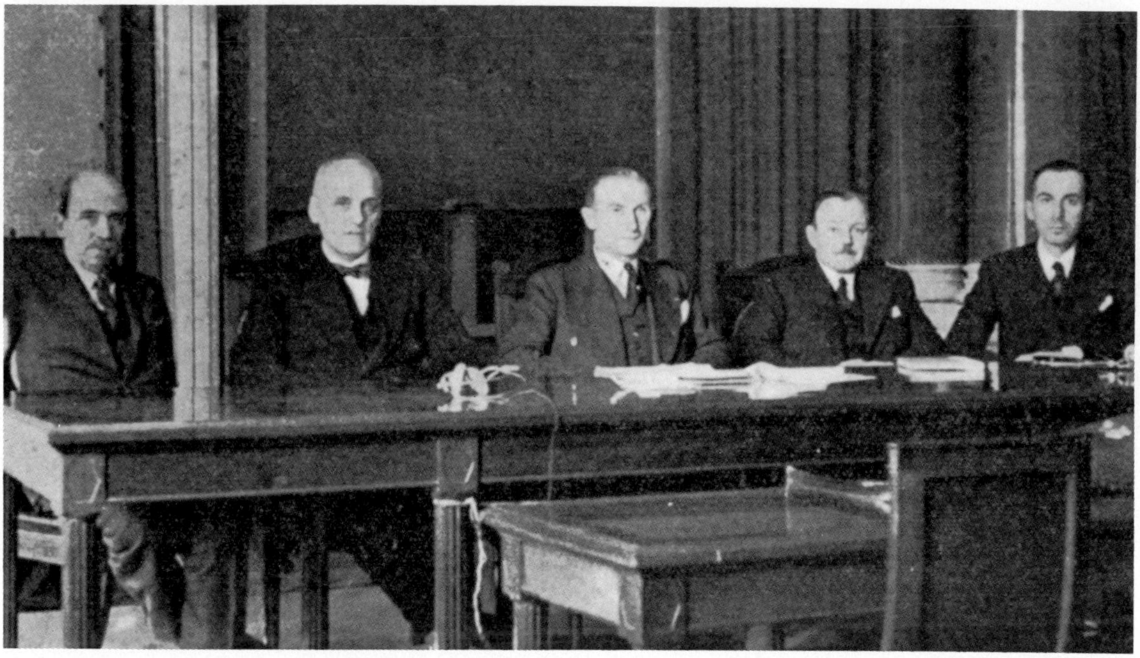

Figure 1–11. Officers of the First European Congress of Structive Surgery held in Brussels in October, 1936. From left to right: Sir Harold Gillies, J. F. S. Esser, M. Coelst. T. Pomfret Kilner, and G. Sanvenero-Rosselli. (From Converse, J. M.: Plastic surgery: The 20th century. The period of growth (1914–1939). Surg. Clin, North Am., *47*:261, 1967.)

subsequent issues was interrupted by World War II. These international congresses of the European Society of Structive Surgery represented the high point of development of plastic surgery before World War II. The contributions to the congresses were of high quality and represented milestones of progress toward recognition, not only by the public at large but also by the academic world, of the existence of this new branch of surgery.

Throughout the period between the wars loomed the towering figure of Sterling Bunnell. Bunnell, along with other pioneers—Kanavel, Koch, Auchincloss, and Cutler in the United States; Wood-Jones in Great Britain; and Iselin in France—originated the anatomic and physiologic concepts of reconstructive hand surgery. This type of reconstructive plastic surgery reached its fruition during World War II with the establishment of specialized hand centers under the consultantship of Bunnell. It was at such a center (Cushing General Hospital) that J. William Littler was introduced to hand surgery as a young physician in 1944.

Plastic surgery had thus passed the stage when it was more or less confined to the correction of nasal deformities or, during World War I, to maxillofacial surgery.

World War II and the Postwar Era: The Growth to Maturity

Since World War II the scope of plastic surgery has changed. During this conflict it was necessary to treat complicated fractures of the extremities and craniofacial skeleton, to replace lost structures, to repair paraplegic pressure sores, frostbite, and burns, and to prepare soft tissues for orthopedic surgery and the repair of peripheral nerves. Impetus was given to the development of surgery of the hand and the treatment of burns. It was also during this wartime period that research in tissue transplantation began (Medawar, 1944). In this way, reconstructive plastic surgery, as it is now known, came into being.

Because of the fear of massive civilian casualties resulting from air raids, special centers were established in strategic locations in Great Britain to treat both civilian and military casualties under the direction of the Emergency Medical Service. Gillies was the leader in insisting on adequate facilities for the treatment of all patients requiring plastic surgery, military or civilian, including those with severe burns. From the beginning of the war it became obvious that tank warfare would cause numerous burns. During the

Battle of Britain the pilots of fighter aircraft were ordered to land their planes in flame in order that they could be repaired and returned to intercept German bombers. As a result many Royal Air Force pilots sustained severe facial and hand burns. McIndoe, a pupil and relative of Gillies, was the first British surgeon to utilize split-thickness skin grafting on a large scale for the early as well as the definitive repair of burns, especially of the periorbital area.

The Plastic Surgery and Jaw Centres in Great Britain became teaching centers for surgeons of the Western Allies, and there was considerable progress in the development of surgical techniques during this period. A young American plastic surgeon, John Marquis Converse of New York, first worked with the Free French Army in North Africa and later with the British at the Churchill Hospital in Oxford. It was at the latter that Converse (1942) devised the technique of the scalping flap for nasal reconstruction.

Similar units were organized in the United States in a certain number of Army and Navy General Hospitals. Hand surgery centers were also established and generally associated with Plastic Surgery Centers under the guidance of Bunnell.

Plastic surgery gained much stature among the medical profession and the public at large as a result of the accomplishments of military surgeons during World War II, many of whom subsequently headed training programs in the specialty in the United States: Blocker, Brown, Cannon, Converse, Conway, Dingman, Lewin, Littler, Robinson, Tanzer, and White.

Unlike the pioneering surgeons in the maxillofacial units of World War I, the plastic surgeons of World War II could return to peacetime and continue their work in their chosen field. Not only had the military surgeons demonstrated the scope and efficacy of plastic surgical reconstruction, but the lay public demand for it had increased dramatically. Until the war the medical profession had essentially dealt only with the critically ill—those with infectious diseases, malignancy and cardiovascular disease. Following the war *elective* surgery became popular. The public was no longer willing to accept the stigmata of club feet, facial scars, and congenital defects. It is significant that pediatricians established "well baby clinics" during this period. For the first time public demand and pressure mounted for surgical procedures that would improve the quality of life and were not necessarily associated with saving a life. It was the development of this concept that contributed so much to the growth of plastic surgery in the last 40 years.

Coupled with these changes in societal attitudes were technical and scientific advances. Cleft palate and burn centers were established, and training in plastic surgery became more formalized in the postwar years. The publication of *Surgical Treatment of Facial Injuries* by Kazanjian and Converse in 1949 was a milestone because it was the first comprehensive discussion of the subject. The American journal *Plastic and Reconstructive Surgery* commenced publication in 1946 under the editorship of W. B. Davis and later of Robert Ivy. This was also the period when the Educational Foundation of the American Society of Plastic and Reconstructive Surgeons was founded under the leadership of Maliniac.

The postwar years were also characterized by an increased emphasis on research in plastic surgery, best illustrated by the studies in transplantation. Gibson and Medawar (1943) had described the events that led to the rejection of allografts and the rejection of second set allografts. In addition to Gibson, other plastic surgeons contributed significantly to research in this area: Converse, who was the first president of the Transplantation Society; Conway, who organized one of the first research laboratories; Rogers; Edgerton; Peer, whose book *Transplantation of Tissues* (1955, 1959) was the first review of the subject; and Murray, who performed the first successful renal allotransplantation in monozygomatic twins (Murray, Merrill, and Harrison, 1955).

The period of the late 1960's and the decade of the 1970's may well be recorded as the Golden Age of Plastic Surgery, characterized by a proliferation of new surgical techniques, a rapid increase in the number of practicing plastic surgeons, and an increased public awareness of the discipline.

At the Fourth International Congress of Plastic and Reconstructive Surgery held in Rome in 1967, Tessier and colleagues presented their concepts of craniofacial surgical techniques and revolutionized the surgical approach to the correction of severe craniofacial deformities. This development was responsible for the organization of multidisciplinary craniofacial surgery teams around the world. Pioneered by plastic surgeons, this discipline grew rapidly, and in 1983 the International Society of Craniomaxillofacial Surgery was founded.* Craniofacial surgery techniques have been employed on patients of all ages including infants for the corrections of congenital and post-traumatic deformities and the eradication of advanced neoplasms.

By the 1960's flap surgery had changed little since the development of the tube flap by Gillies and Filatov during World War I. The introduction of the deltopectoral flap by Bakamjian (1965) focused attention on the vascular basis of flap design and resulted in the development of a large number of axial pattern flaps that obviated the need for multiple-staged procedures.

In their search for new flaps, plastic surgeons turned their attention to muscles, and the result of the clinical studies of Ger, Vasconez and McCraw was a proliferation of flap techniques.

At approximately the same time the era of microsurgery began with the microvascular transfer of omentum by McClean and Buncke (1972) in the United States, scalp by Harii, Ohmori, and Ohmori (1974) in Japan, and groin flaps in Australia by Daniel and Taylor (1973) and O'Brien and associates (1973).

In 1962 Malt of Boston performed the first successful arm replantation (Malt and McKhann, 1964), and by the 1970's replantation of limbs, digits, and other amputated parts had become a clinical reality.

The dramatic increase in the scope of flap surgical technology was also responsible for a host of new breast reconstruction techniques. General surgeons and their patients began to look to the plastic surgeon to reconstruct the postablative breast defect.

The 1960's and 1970's also witnessed an increase in the demand for esthetic surgery of the face. This type of surgery was no longer reserved for a small segment of the population, as patients from all strata of society sought plastic surgery to rejuvenate their faces. The American Society for Aesthetic Plastic Surgery was founded in 1967.

As an example of the growth of the specialty in the United States, one can cite the following statistics. From 1960 to 1969, 458 plastic surgeons were trained and certified by the American Board of Plastic Surgery. Thus, the total number of practicing, board-certified plastic surgeons was 907. However, in the decade after 1969 the total number of board-certified plastic surgeons in the United States had increased to over 2000.

*The founding members were Drs. Caronni, David, Edgerton, Jackson, Johanson, Kawamoto, Marchac, McCarthy, Munro, Murray, Ortiz-Monasterio, Psillakis, Salyer, Stricker, Tessier, van der Meulen, Whitaker, and Wolfe.

THE SCOPE OF PLASTIC SURGERY

I always say to my residents that plastic surgery can be defined as a problem solving surgical discipline. It is unique in that it spans the entire body and does not have a defined anatomic area (such as the genitourinary tract in urologic surgery). It is ironic that the plastic surgeon, operating on all anatomic areas of the body, has evolved into the modern day "general surgeon."

Verdan stated in his opening speech on the occasion of the tenth anniversary of the founding of the Swiss Society of Plastic and Reconstructive Surgery in 1974:

It is true that plastic surgery is a specialty that is difficult to define and that all the other surgical specialties with the exception of pediatric surgery have a regional character which is anatomically defined. The plastic surgeon extends his surgical activities not only to the skin and its adnexa but also to certain subjacent tissues in locations as diverse as the face and hands, the neck and abdominal wall, the extremities and the genitourinary apparatus, the breasts and scalp. To the term plastic surgery is added the adjective "reconstructive" which implies an extension of the plastic surgeon's activities to the most diverse reconstructive procedures such as vascular and microvascular surgery, peripheral nerve surgery, transplantation of muscles and tendons and arthroplasties thus overlapping the specialty of orthopedic surgery.

With the development of craniofacial surgery by Tessier and associates (1967), the plastic surgeon finds himself invading the interior of the cranium, the previously private domain of the neurosurgeon. The wide application of microsurgical techniques has made the plastic surgeon a "general surgeon"—reconstructing a compound fracture of the lower extremity, a postmastectomy chest wall deformity, or a brachial plexus injury.

It is interesting that the development of the modern era of plastic surgery dating from World War I originated from the activities of surgeons of disparate specialties. Morestin and Blair were general surgeons; Ivy and Kazanjian were originally dental surgeons; and Gillies was an otolaryngologist (to name only a few pioneers of the modern era). The founding members of the American Society of Plastic and Reconstructive Surgeons in 1931 included a physiotherapist, a dermatologist, an anesthesiologist, a radiologist, an otolaryngologist, a medicolegal authority, and four plastic surgeons. It is therefore understandable that practitioners of other surgical specialties lay claim to certain plastic surgical procedures that fall into the anatomic domain of their specialty. It is as reasonable for the plastic surgeon to abstain from performing operations for which he has not been trained as for the specialists in allied specialties to refrain from plastic surgery procedures for which they are not qualified. In many cases plastic surgery is competently performed in specialized areas of oral surgery, otolaryngology, ophthalmology, and orthopedic surgery.

J. William Littler, who acquired extensive experience in hand surgery during World War II under the overall guidance of Sterling Bunnell, played a decisive role in bringing hand surgery into the field of plastic surgery in the United States. His influence was preponderant and he trained innumerable plastic surgeons. The development of limb replantation surgery also increased the number of plastic surgeons practicing this special field of surgery.

The fragmentation of plastic surgery occurred early on the European continent, probably because of the emphasis on maxillofacial surgery, which was needed for the large number of facial gunshot wounds inflicted on the thousands of survivors of World War I.

In Vienna, von Eiselsberg, a general surgeon and professor of surgery at the Allgemeines Krankenhaus, sought a close and intimate collaboration with Pichler, a dentist and physician, as early as 1903. Von-Eiselsberg applied for a maxillofacial unit to furnish Pichler with a position. In 1915 the Austrian Imperial Reserve Hospital No. 17 was organized, and Foramitti and Esser from Holland were among its experienced surgeons, capable of performing plastic surgery. In 1917 the outpatient department was also opened to civilians, but the beneficial work of the unit was terminated at the end of the war. It was von Eiselsberg who made every effort to preserve the facilities. He succeeded by applying to the university and the government, stating that "the unit would not only be most beneficial for so many patients and the teaching of students, but also to attract foreign physicians and patients."

Thus, the personal efforts of a general surgeon led to the foundation of one of the schools of maxillofacial surgery in Austria, which subsequently included Trauner, Köle, and Obwegeser.

Wilflingseder, who trained under Gillies, became the head of a division of plastic surgery at the University Hospital in Innsbruck in 1957. In 1966 a chair of Plastic and Reconstructive Surgery was founded for Wilflingseder, and a Department of Plastic Surgery was placed under his direction.

In Germany, departments of maxillofacial surgery were organized early in the 1920's in the military hospitals for the facially disfigured. These were headed by Axhausen in Berlin, Rosenthal in Leipzig, and Lindemann in Düsseldorf. These three men became the founders of German face and jaw surgery and were later joined by the much younger Wassmund, who was in Berlin. The pupils of these men, especially Schuchardt and Schmid, led the transition from maxillofacial to plastic surgery.

In Hamburg the Nordwestdeutschen Kieferklinik was established after World War II, when Schuchardt, a student of Wassmund, was asked to come to Hamburg. He transferred from a hospital in Schleswig-Holstein 200 wounded soldiers whom he managed to bring out of an area occupied by the Russians.

These origins explain why there are two separate German societies of plastic surgeons. The Vereinigung Deutscher Plastischer Chirurgen strives to have plastic surgery considered as a specialty in its own right; the older, dental-oriented group clings to a regional specialty concept (Kiefer und Gesichtschirurgie: jaw and face surgery). There is also the Society of Plastic and Reconstructive Surgery, which developed as a section, later a branch, of the Deutsche Gesellschaft für Chirurgie. Its membership is open to all physicians who are interested in plastic surgery.

Before World War II Burian in Prague established an outstanding plastic surgery service. In 1948 he was appointed the Professor and Chairman of the Department of Plastic Surgery at Charles University.

In France, surgeons who had been trained in Great Britain and the United States after World War II rapidly established the French school under the leadership of Claude Du-

TRANSACTIONS OF
THE INTERNATIONAL SOCIETY OF

Plastic Surgeons

FIRST CONGRESS

Stockholm and Uppsala 1955

Edited by

Tord Skoog, M.D., *General Secretary of the Congress, in cooperation with* Robert H. Ivy, M.D., *and the Editorial Board of Plastic & Reconstructive Surgery.*

Translations of abstracts into

French by Dr. Morel-Fatio, *Paris*
German by Professor Karl Schuchardt, *Hamburg*
Spanish by Dr. Mario Gonzalez Ulloa, *Mexico City*

Figure 1–12. Title page of the Transactions of the First International Society of Plastic Surgeons held in Stockholm in 1955.

fourmentel (the son of Léon Dufourmentel) and Morel-Fatio; they were followed by surgeons in Switzerland and other countries of Europe and throughout the world. The pioneering work of Tessier attracted plastic surgeons from around the world to l'Hôpital Foch in the 1970's and was responsible for the international development of this discipline.

Marino and Malbec provided leadership for the specialty in South America. Today, Brazil has one of the largest groups of plastic surgeons in the world.

The presently thriving specialty of plastic surgery in Australia began under the leadership of Rank and Wakefield after they had acquired additional training in England and experience during World War II. O'Brien of Melbourne was one of the pioneering microsurgeons and trained young surgeons from around the world in this new discipline.

Penn, who had served as chief of a hospital for the wounded requiring plastic surgery during World War II, was the founder of the specialty in South Africa.

As a specialist in dermatology and urology, Ohmori, the founder of the Japanese Society of Plastic and Reconstructive Surgery, treated patients with scar contractures from burns after observing plastic surgical operations in the United States, England, and Scotland. A program started in 1958 at Tokyo University Hospital and the Tokyo Metropolitan Police Hospital was used to train a group of outstanding microsurgeons.

In Peking, Song developed a plastic surgery service after studying under Ivy in Philadelphia. Chang in Shanghai established a comprehensive program at the Ninth People's Hospital. It should be noted that Chen, an orthopedist in Shanghai, was a pioneer in the development of extremity replantation.

Ten years after the end of World War II, in 1955, the International Society of Plastic Surgeons was organized under the aegis of Tord Skoog and held its first International Congress in Stockholm (Fig. 1–12). Subsequent meetings were held in London (1959), Washington (1963), Rome (1967), Melbourne (1971), Paris (1975), Rio de Janeiro (1979), Montreal (1983), and New Delhi (1987). The transactions of each Congress have been published. In addition subsections or chapters were established in esthetic plastic surgery, craniofacial surgery, and microsurgery.

The International Society of Aesthetic Plastic Surgery was established in 1970.

PLASTIC SURGERY AS A SPECIALTY: ITS FUTURE

During the early part of the nineteenth century, before the discovery of general anesthesia and the development of the concepts of antisepsis, the surgeon was mostly concerned with what was referred to as "external pathology." This explains the large number of reconstructive plastic surgical operations performed during this period.

Specialization came much later, especially during the middle of the present century and with increasing impetus. Even the "general" surgeon is becoming a specialist in many respects. Let us read the words of a Professor of Surgery, Francis Moore: "Are we to go along with the concept that those who operate on the face, the neck, the head, the lip, the eye, the hand, and the breast are the *only* persons who should do any of those operations?" A plastic surgeon will reply: "Of course, the answer is 'no,' but in the case of many *particular* operations in those regions, if the plastic surgeon can do these operations not only *better*, but also more *safely* and more efficiently *without increasing the medical cost*, then those operations probably should be done by a plastic surgeon whenever one is available. We must deliver reconstruction not only better, but also more efficiently" (Edgerton, 1974).

The principles of plastic surgical techniques are specialized, and the conceptual application of these principles requires special training. Once indoctrinated, the plastic surgeon can apply these concepts in any area of the body if he has had comprehensive training in "general" surgery. During his early surgical training he must seek training in as many areas of surgical endeavor as possible.

The optimal training for a plastic surgeon poses a dilemma. While a broad-based surgical background remains the ideal for the person entering plastic surgery training, the significant increase of the scope of the discipline has obviously mandated a longer training. At the same time the specialty has become somewhat subdivided and the trainee may wish to spend time in such an area as microsurgery or craniofacial, hand, or esthetic surgery. The training of the plastic surgeon of the future will probably entail three components: (1) broad experience in a variety of surgical disciplines, (2) a formalized plastic surgery residency, and (3) a postresidency fellowship in one of the subspecialties of plastic surgery (McCarthy, 1985).

After completion of training, the education of the plastic surgeon is a continuing obligation during his entire professional career. The widespread availability of symposia and specialty board recertification promote this concept.

The answer to comprehensive and quality coverage of all phases of plastic surgery remains the team approach, whether in a university setting or in large-city private practice. After a broad introductory training in surgery with periods spent in the surgical specialties and in plastic surgery, each plastic surgeon of the team can subspecialize in his area of preference. The team should include not only plastic surgeons but also members of allied specialties in the field of medicine and dentistry. Thus, the various talents are centralized for the benefit of the patient. The multidisciplinary approach has been brought to the foreground in the treatment of craniofacial malformations. Various surgical, medical, and dental specialists and representatives of the basic sciences are members of the team. It is the interdisciplinary interchange that makes for optimal, cost-efficient patient care and should be conducive to teaching and research.

In smaller cities and towns the plastic surgeon will find himself called upon to solve problems that the general surgeon or other specialists think it necessary to refer to him. He will cover the broad field of plastic surgery, seek collaboration with other specialists, and refer to the large centers those patients whom he feels he is not equipped to treat.

Esthetic surgery has become a legitimate and integral component of plastic surgery. Because of the psychologic component in the patient's motivation for this type of corrective surgery, the indications for surgery should be carefully evaluated. The psychologic and, often, vocational gains resulting from esthetic surgery, whether large or small, often have a considerable impact on the patient's life style.

In 1597 Tagliacozzi wrote: "We restore, repair, and make whole those parts . . . which nature has given but which fortune has taken away, not so much that they may delight the eye but that they may buoy up the spirit and help the mind of the afflicted."

Tagliacozzi was damned, exhumed, and buried in unconsecrated ground because of his reconstructive nasal operations, which were then illegal and considered against nature. Only in our time have the problems and purpose of plastic surgery been valued theologically. Pope Pius XII declared on October 14, 1958: "If we consider physical beauty in its Christian light and if we respect the conditions set by our moral teachings, then esthetic surgery is not in contradiction to the will of God, in that it restores the perfection of that greatest work of creation, man" (Wilflingseder, 1975).

FACE TO FACE WITH DEFORMITY

The plastic surgeon must first make an accurate evaluation of the deformity, the degree of displacement of the tissues, the extent of the defect, and the functional disability. Is the deformity apparent or real? What is the extent of the true defect? Having made his appraisal, the surgeon must then consider various methods of treatment in relation to the type of deformity, the age of the patient, and the patient's mental attitude toward the surgery. The methods to be employed are also considered: a simple and rapid technique may give an adequate result; a more complex and multiple-staged type of repair may provide a more optimal result. Which is the best suited to the particular patient? A primary defect may be satisfactorily repaired, but the result may be obtained at the expense of a secondary defect that is a more serious deformity than the original one.

Certainly, complex surgical reconstruction and a superior final result are possible only in the patient who is willing to give the highest degree of cooperation. The demands of the patient stimulate the surgeon toward progress. In developing countries the patient may be satisfied with a type of result that would not satisfy someone in a country where competition for employment and social status necessitate the best result possible in appearance and function. Careful diagnosis for the restoration of function is particularly important in hand surgery.

Planning the Reconstruction

In planning reconstruction, the surgeon must choose from many methods of treatment: grafts of skin or other tissue; transfer of local or distant flaps; restoration of the skeletal framework by bone or cartilage; repair or grafting of nerves; or microsurgical transfers of composite tissue. He must consider the advisability of inorganic implants in certain favorable sites.

The unhurried and deliberate approach to the problem at hand is the key to success in plastic surgery.

THE APPARENT VERSUS THE TRUE DEFECT

In many cases the defect is evident. In a deformity of the mandible, the change in the occlusal relationships of the teeth provides a satisfactory guide to the size of the defect. A retracted, everted lower eyelid may be compared with the contralateral lower eyelid and an accurate estimate of the required amount of skin readily obtained. A missing ala may be compared with the contralateral side and the size of the composite graft to repair the nasal defect readily estimated.

A method of actually mapping the extent of the true defect and comparing it with the apparent defect is illustrated in Figure 1–13. Measurements are made from landmarks such as the acromion and the styloid process,

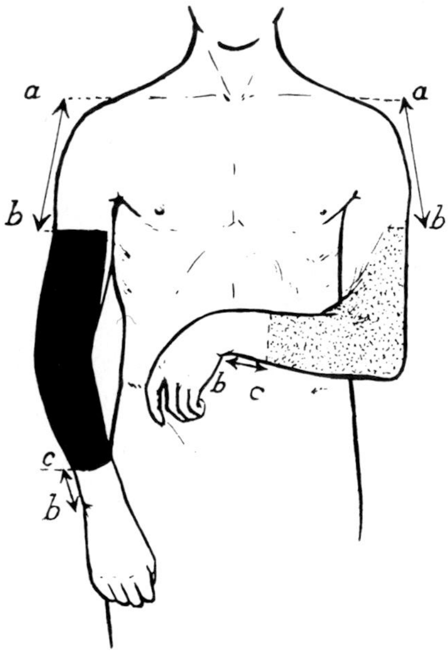

Figure 1–13. True versus apparent defect in a severe burn contracture of the left upper extremity. Because of the contracture, the apparent defect is smaller than the true defect plotted on the right upper extremity. Fixed points, such as the acromion and the styloid process of the ulna, are employed to obtain the distances a-b and c-d, which, when transferred to the unaffected extremity, permit estimation of the upper and lower limits of the true defect.

and in this manner the size of the area to be covered by grafts or a flap can be evaluated with a certain degree of precision. When the defect is bilateral, as in an extensive burn contracture of the neck (Fig. 1–14*A*), fixed points at the mental symphysis and the sternal notch permit one to obtain a fairly accurate evaluation of the amount of missing skin by measuring the distance between these two points in another individual of approximately the same size and comparing this distance with that between similar points in the patient.

The apparent defect is often the result of the loss of tissue followed by the contraction of the scar and contracture of the adjacent parts (Fig. 1–14*B*). The apparent defect may also be a relative one: the chin may appear deviated to one side because of a deviation of the nose; the nose may appear too prominent in the profile because of lack of development of the mental symphysis.

Aids in Planning

There is no substitute for a careful clinical examination of the patient. In deformities of the face, photographs taken in standardized positions according to the Frankfort horizontal and the midsagittal plane of the face help to establish a diagnosis and a plan of treatment. Serial photographs are indispensable for following progress. Facial casts (moulage) aid in planning contour restoration or other changes in form, but usually are not required in the average case. Bony deformities require a careful roentgenographic examination;

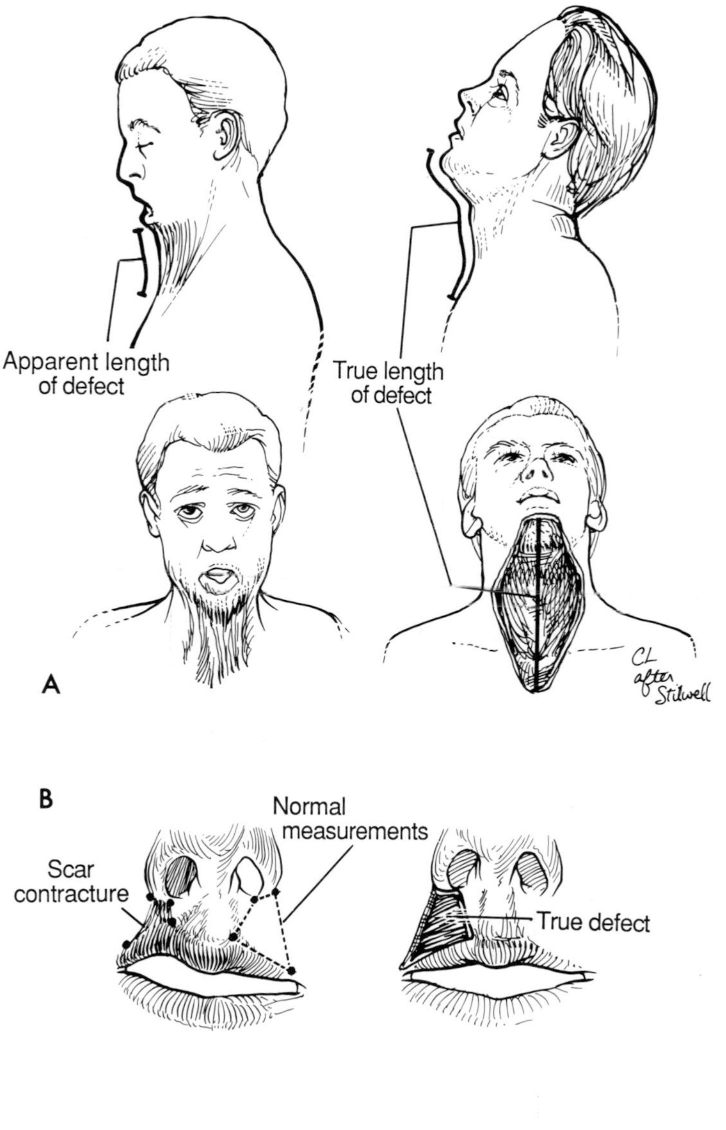

Figure 1–14. True versus apparent defect. *A*, In bilateral involvement, as in neck contractures, a measurement between two fixed points (mental symphysis and sternal notch) in an unaffected individual of the same size gives the length and size of the true defect. *B*, Upper lip scar and contracture. The apparent defect is smaller because of the resulting contracture of the adjacent parts. (From Kazanjian and Converse.)

cephalometric roentgenograms are of invaluable assistance in planning changes in the form of the skeletal facial framework. The more complex craniofacial deformities require a three-dimensional CT analysis.

The team approach is essential for progress. Many problems in plastic surgery require consultation with specialists in other fields. The collaboration of dental specialists is essential to treat such problems as jaw fractures, cleft lip and palate, and other craniofacial malformations and in reconstruction after excisional surgery for malignant disease. Postoperative physiotherapy, guided by the surgeon, is an important part of hand rehabilitation.

Certain intangible qualities make for excellence in plastic surgery: a sense of proportion and contour, esthetic judgment, and attention to minute detail may spell the difference between success and failure. Often these qualities are innate and cannot be taught. An everyday preoccupation with problems that require solution makes for excellence in plastic surgery.

Not the least of the aspects of treatment is the psychologic support provided by the surgeon and his team; psychiatric treatment is obligatory in some cases. The psychologic make-up of the patient often influences the technique or repair; simple methods may be required in problem cases.

A characteristic of plastic surgery is its diversity, both in the problems to be solved and in the methods available to solve them. "There are more ways than one to skin a cat": the simple and effective way, and the complicated way. The beginner often chooses the most devious route when he is blind to the most obviously simple. One of the most vital aspects of residency training is to impart the importance, after the deformity has been diagnosed, of considering in turn all possible methods of treatment, weighing the alternatives, and choosing the most suitable.

Regional Entities of the Face and Neck

In reconstructive procedures involving the face—for example, in skin grafting for burn contractures—it is important to observe the confines of the esthetic units of the face (Fig. 1–15). The first of these is the forehead, extending from the eyebrows to the hairline; for example, a one-piece, split-thickness skin graft will provide a satisfactory esthetic result. Other regional entities are the orbital region, the region of the lips, limited laterally by the nasolabial folds and secondary lines of expression situated laterally to the angle of the mouth, and the labiomental fold. The nasal unit can be divided into subunits: dor-

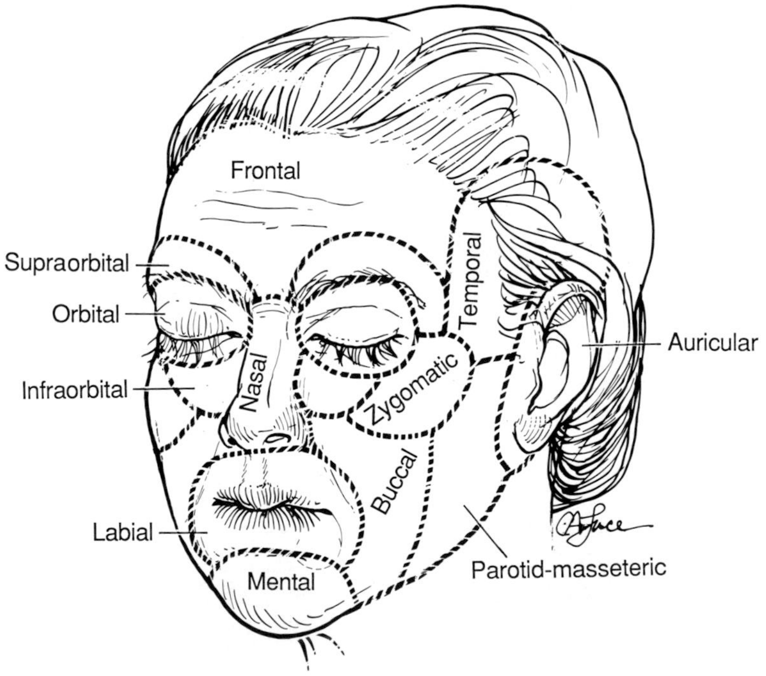

Figure 1–15. Esthetic units of the face.

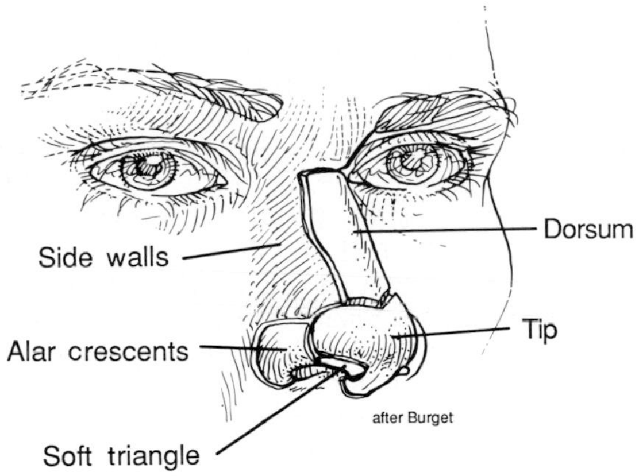

Figure 1–16. Subunits of the nasal esthetic unit.

sum, side walls, tip, soft triangles, and alar wings (Fig. 1–16) (Burget and Menick, 1985). The region of the cheek is subdivided into two entities: an anterior, which is soft, pliable, and mobile; and a posterior, extending over the parotidomasseteric region, which is relatively firm and less mobile.

Interpretation of the Deformity

The deformity may be minor to an impartial observer. To the patient, however, the deformity may assume a magnitude out of all proportion to reality. One of the main purposes of plastic surgery is to restore the mental health of the patient, thus permitting a return to active social participation. The psychologic trauma suffered by the patient may be related to the injury and the circumstances of the accident or may be due to comments of relatives or friends. One distressing aspect of this type of surgery is that the successful repair of even major traumatic deformities is not necessarily followed by a cure. Deep seated psychologic disturbances may persist.

In major deformities, despite the significant progress made in surgery, the improvement achieved does not always restore the physical appearance of the patient. The severity of the psychologic disturbance is not necessarily related to the severity of the deformity, nor is it directly proportional to the degree of improvement accomplished by surgery. Cultural aspects complicate this picture. A classic example is the scar resulting from the student duels in Heidelberg, considered an emblem of manliness rather than a disfigurement.

In civilized man the face alone remains unclothed and exposed. An injury resulting in distortion of the features thus sets the unfortunate individual apart in a highly organized society in which a premium is placed on beauty and facial symmetry. Because disfigurement of the face becomes a serious social handicap, the surgical treatment of facial injuries is of special significance, serving to restore the inner feelings of happiness and well-being in addition to the outer appearance and function.

The need to rehabilitate the facially disfigured is well recognized in the present era. Following World War II a change took place in the treatment of patients requiring massive resection for head and neck cancer. In the past, the disease-oriented surgeon proceeded with the necessary mutilating surgery, following the philosophy that all means are indicated to preserve life, irrespective of the esthetic and functional consequences for the patient. This philosophy no longer prevails: the patient demands more than the preservation of life. The quality of life is important to the patient as is the quantity of life that the ablation is able to achieve. While the anticipation that radical extirpative surgery gives the best chance for a cure is reassuring to the surgeon, the expectation that satisfactory reconstruction is feasible is also comforting to the patient.

Body Image

The body image is a basic component of our self concept and our feeling of personal identity. It includes both the mental picture we have of our physical characteristics and our attitudes toward these characteristics. It stems from both conscious and unconscious sources (Macgregor, 1974).

The body image develops slowly and undergoes many changes in the course of growth and development. The perception of one's physical characteristics begins to take shape probably around the age of 6 months when infants explore and discover their bodies. Later, as they begin to play with other children, they gradually develop a vague idea of what their bodies can or cannot do. This is the beginning of the development of the body concept. As time passes, the attitudes of others play a major role in this self-image.

A patient can incur a deformity or undergo correction of the deformity, but his reactions may well depend on the reactions of others, which may in turn bring about a change in his *body concept.* Some people incorporate defects or corrections in the body image, while others retain a distorted image. By using preoperative photographs of the patient or a mirror to determine how the patient views himself, it is often possible to learn to what extent the patient's perception of himself is realistic or distorted.

ANTHROPOMETRIC POINTS OF THE FACE

Physical anthropologists employ methods of measurement that permit determination of significant likenesses and differences between individuals and races. These standardized measurements can be useful when attempting to restore the structure and contour of the deformed face (Farkas, 1981). Among the commonly employed anthropometric points (Fig. 1–17) are: *trichion*, an imprecise landmark, the midpoint at the hairline on the forehead; *nasion*, the most anterior point of the midline of the frontonasal suture; *subnasale*, the point beneath the nasal spine where the nasal columella merges with the upper lip in the midsagittal plane; *pogonion*, the most anterior point on the contour of the chin; and *menton*, the lowest point on the symphyseal outline. The midsagittal line, a vertical line passing through these points, divides the face into halves. *Tragion* is the notch immediately above the tragus of the ear; *orbitale* is the lowest point on the infraorbital margin; and the *Frankfort horizontal* passes through these points and is a helpful plane in establishing the head of the person being examined in the symmetrical or "neutral" position.

Measurements of facial dimensions are taken according to three planes: vertical (facial length), frontal (facial width), and sagittal (facial depth). Facial width is obtained by measuring the distance between the most prominent points on the zygomatic bones. Facial depth is determined by measuring the distance from the external auditory canal to various points such as nasion, subnasale, and gonion. The distance between pogonion and gonion, the tip of the angle of the jaw, determines the length of the body of the mandible; the distance from the nasion to the tip of the nose equals the length of the nose.

Horizontal lines passing through trichion, nasion, subnasale, and menton divide the physiognomic face into thirds, theoretically of equal height; in practice, however, each third of the face differs in size from the others.

PRINCIPLES OF ARTISTIC ANATOMY

Beauty has no universal criteria and varies from culture to culture and from century to century. Burkhardt (1929) cited the work of Firenzuola (1802) on female beauty written

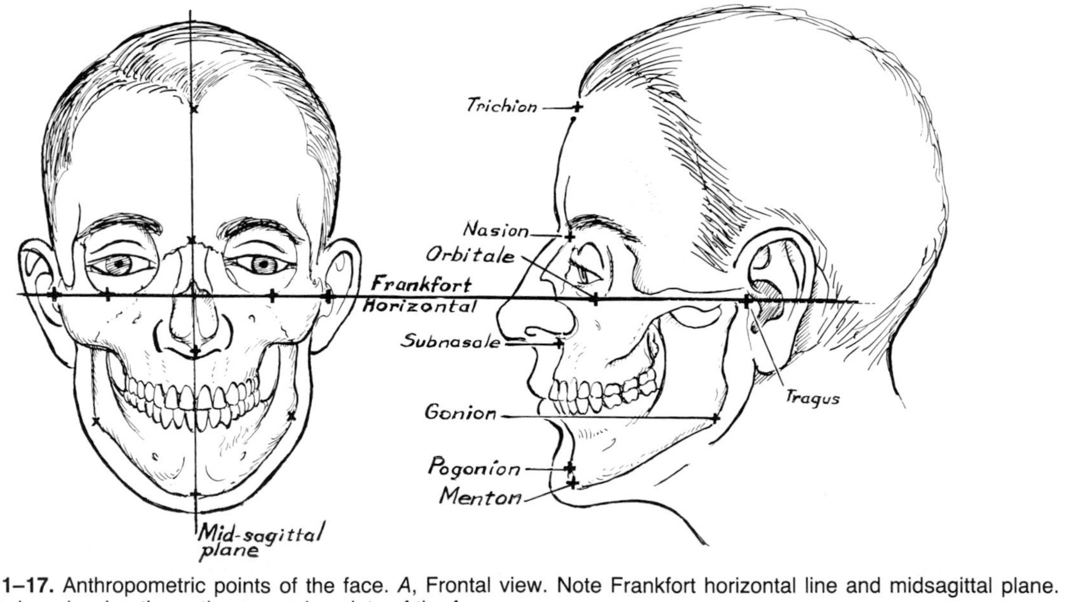

Figure 1–17. Anthropometric points of the face. *A*, Frontal view. Note Frankfort horizontal line and midsagittal plane. *B*, Lateral view showing the anthropometric points of the face.

in the sixteenth century: "The nose, which chiefly determines the value of the profile, must recede gently and uniformly in the direction of the eyes; where the cartilage ceases there may be a slight elevation, but not so marked so as to make the nose aquiline, which is not pleasing in women. . . ." As delicacies of details, he mentions a dimple in the upper lip, a certain fullness of the lower lip, and a tempting smile in the left corner of the mouth. Such a description would imply that the smile of "La Gioconda" (the Mona Lisa) is not necessarily one of mystery but rather a habit induced by what was considered the preferred style of the period. Large hips and a robust body were much admired as recently as the Victorian age; crease lines around the neck were called the "necklace of Venus" (Fig. 1–18).

Contemporary standards of beauty are epitomized in advertisements showing young, slender-bodied models with perfectly proportioned facial features. It is implied that these are the ideals of beauty for all ages. Beauty basically reflects an assemblage of esthetic properties that commands approbation in the specific culture at that point in time.

Today, people turn to plastic surgeons in increasing numbers to give them these valued features, to correct minor defects, and to repair the ravages of age. It is their hope that such surgery will improve their life style in a highly competitive society that places considerable emphasis on youth and accepted standards of beauty.

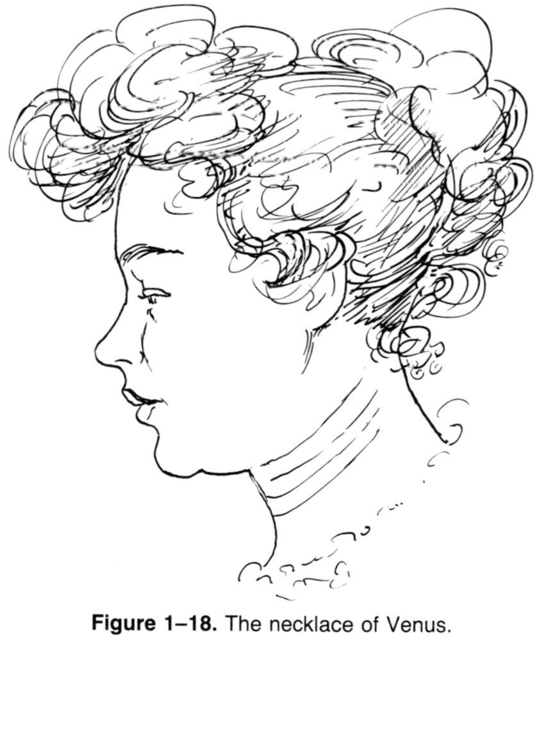

Figure 1–18. The necklace of Venus.

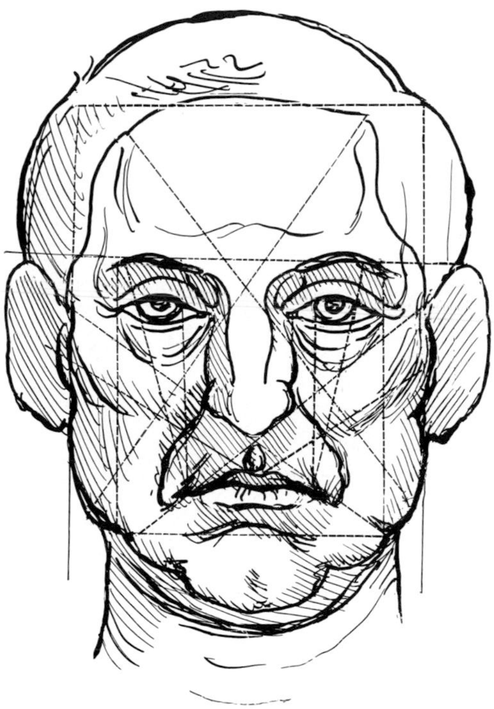

Figure 1–19. Tracing of a sketch by Leonardo da Vinci. An analysis of the relationships of the various facial structures.

Proportions of Human Form. The surgeon, when making his corrections, tries to reform the affected body or face to an acceptable cultural or societal standard. In doing so, he must also be as well acquainted with the accepted proportions of the human form as are the artists who specialize in portraits or nudes.

Leonardo da Vinci, after conducting extensive anatomic studies, sketched and measured many faces and figures to determine geometrically what he called "the divine proportions." Many of his measurements and divisions remain the basic tools in art school for teaching life classes in drawing. Figure 1–19 is a penline copy of a well-known crayon sketch by Leonardo in which he analyzed the shape and relationships of the various features of the face. No descriptive accompanying notes explain his geometric lines. Figure 1–20*A* is also a tracing of a sketch by Leonardo. A translation of his notes reads as follows: "Proportions of the head. From the eyebrow to the junction of the lip with the chin, and from there to the posterior angle of

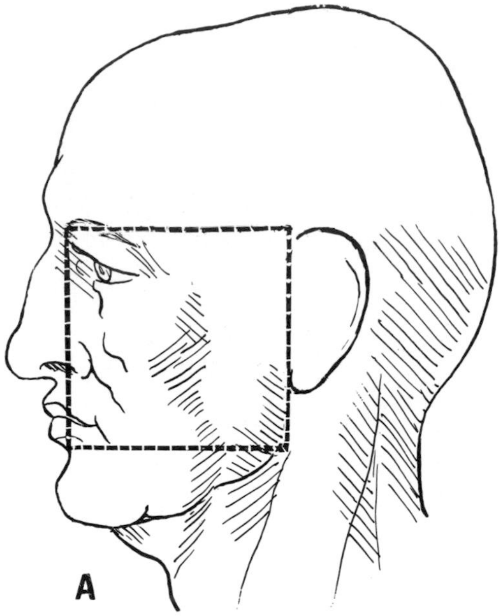

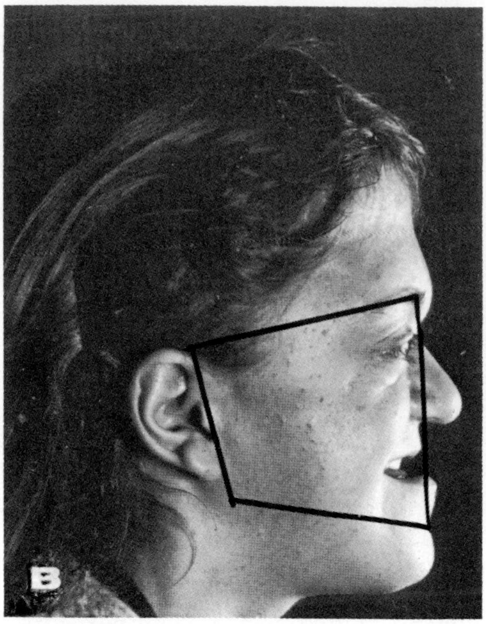

Figure 1–20. *A*, The square in the face described by Leonardo (after Leonardo). *B*, Distortion of the square in Apert's syndrome (acrocephalosyndactyly).

the jaw, and from there to the upper edge of the ear near the temple, there is a perfect square, the side of which measures half a head, and the hollow of the cheek bone is halfway between the tip of the nose and the back portion of the jaw." Figure 1–20*B* shows distortion of the square in a patient with Apert's syndrome.

If one takes the same Leonardo sketch and superimposes the ear (Fig. 1–21), his following note is understood: "From the edge of the orbit to the ear, there is the same distance as the length of the ear, in other words one-third of the head." It would then apparently follow that the distance from the hairline to the chin is three ears long and also three noses long. He wrote: "The distances from the chin to the nose and from the hairline to the eyebrows are equal, each of them to the height of the ear and to one-third of the face."

Other proportions of the face taught in art schools today are still credited to Leonardo. For example, the distance between the eyes is equal to the width of one eye (Fig. 1–22*A*). It is also pointed out that, in the ideal Caucasian form, the nostrils should not flare more laterally than a line dropped vertically from the medial canthus (Fig. 1–22*B*, line *f*). The mouth should extend laterally to a line dropped from the medial margin of the limbus (Fig. 1–22*B*, line *e*). Beyond this point the mouth is too large. Figure 1–22*C* is a tracing of a patient with orbital hypertelorism, showing the wide deviation from normal measurements. The eyes are two lengths apart, and lines *e* and *f* are no longer vertical.

In considering the face in relation to the

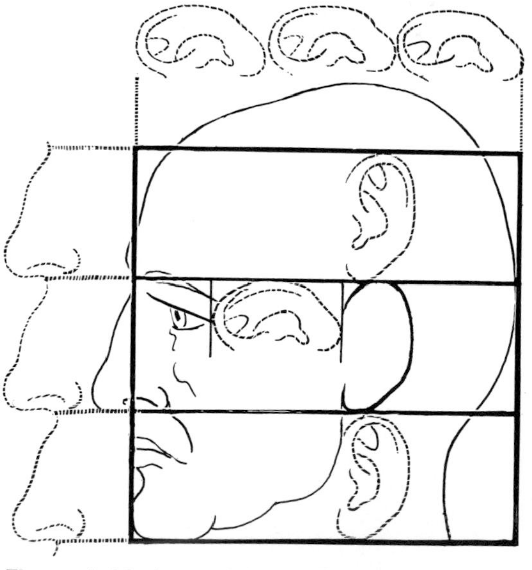

Figure 1–21. Leonardo's measurements of the face superimposed on a tracing of a sketch by him.

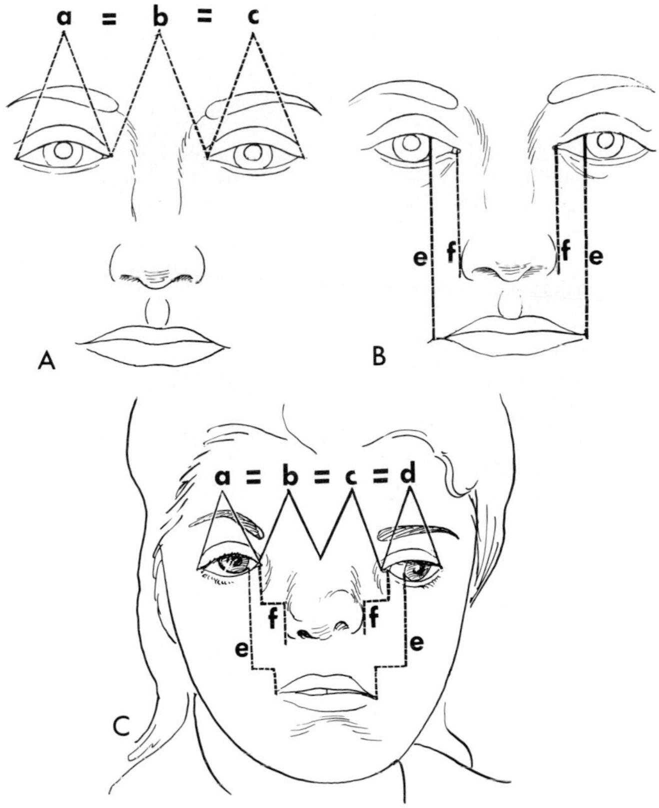

Figure 1–22. Proportions of the face. *A*, Ideal relationships of the eyes and the interorbital space. *B*, Ideal relationships of the nostrils, the corners of the mouth, and the eyes. *C*, Tracing from a photograph of a patient with orbital hypertelorism, showing the distorted relationships.

body, one should remember that the face from chin to hairline is the same length as that of the hand, and the nose is the same length as that of the thumb (Fig. 1–23*A*). The eyes are situated in the exact center of the head, between the top of the skull and the chin (Fig. 1–23*B*). The patient with Apert's syndrome shown in Figure 1–24*A*, if the mouth were closed, would have eyes placed three-fifths of the distance down from the top of the head to the chin. His appearance suggests mental deficiency. This impression is corrected in the sketch (Fig. 1–24*B*) by placing a normal-sized cranium above the same features and closing the mouth so that the chin is shorter and the teeth are in occlusion.

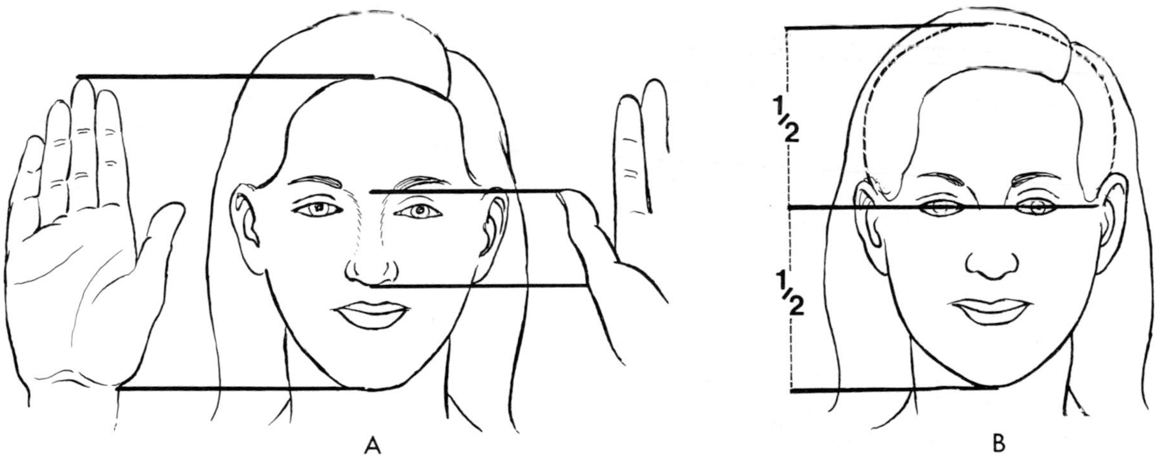

Figure 1–23. *A*, The hand has the same length as the face, and the nose is as long as the thumb. *B*, The eyes are in the exact middle of the head.

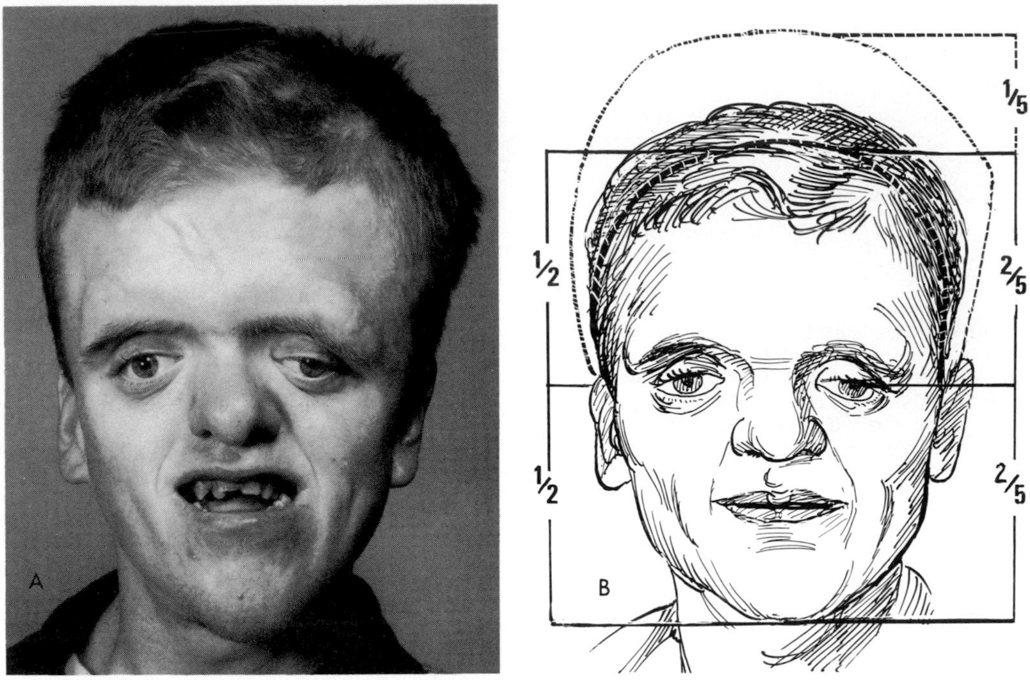

Figure 1–24. A knowledge of the correct proportions of the face can be of a great value in analyzing a deformity. *A*, Photograph of patient with acrocephalosyndactyly (Apert's syndrome). *B*, The tracing of the photograph (dotted) demonstrates the increase in size of the cranial vault.

Figure 1–25 shows a patient with eyes set too high in the face.

Eyebrows should ideally lift as they follow the rim of the orbit laterally, to give a youthful appearance (Fig. 1–26*A*). The brow should never follow the same curvature as the two lines just below it—the line of the superior contour of the globe and the line of the upper

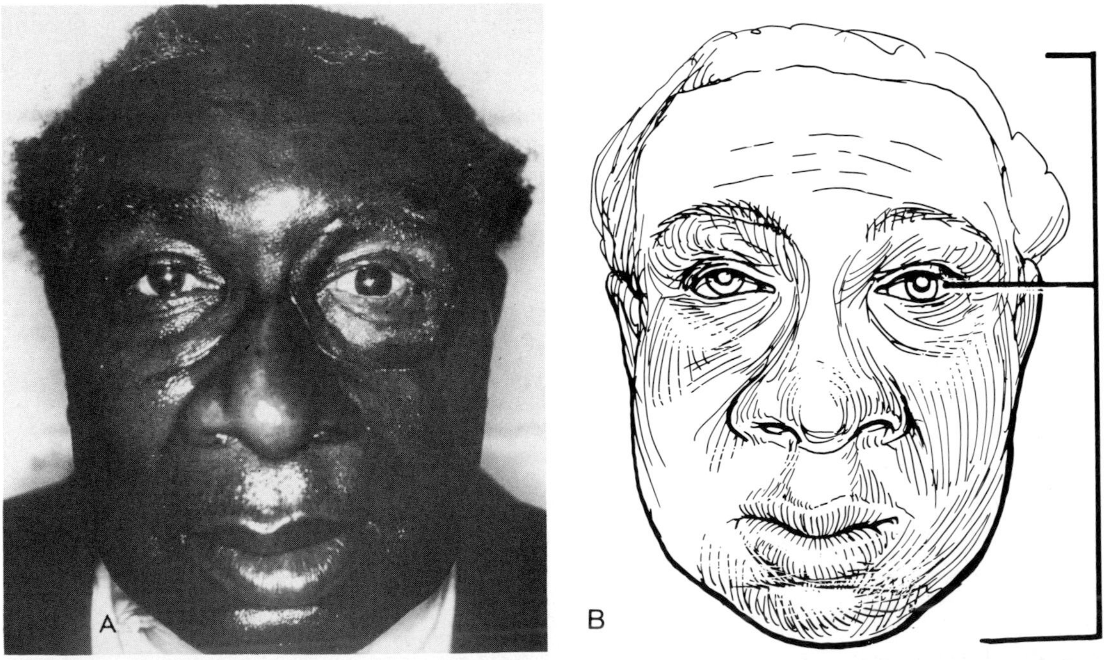

Figure 1–25. *A*, Patient with an unusually low cranial vault. Note also the position of the nostrils in relation to the medial canthi *B*, Drawing shows the high position of the eyes.

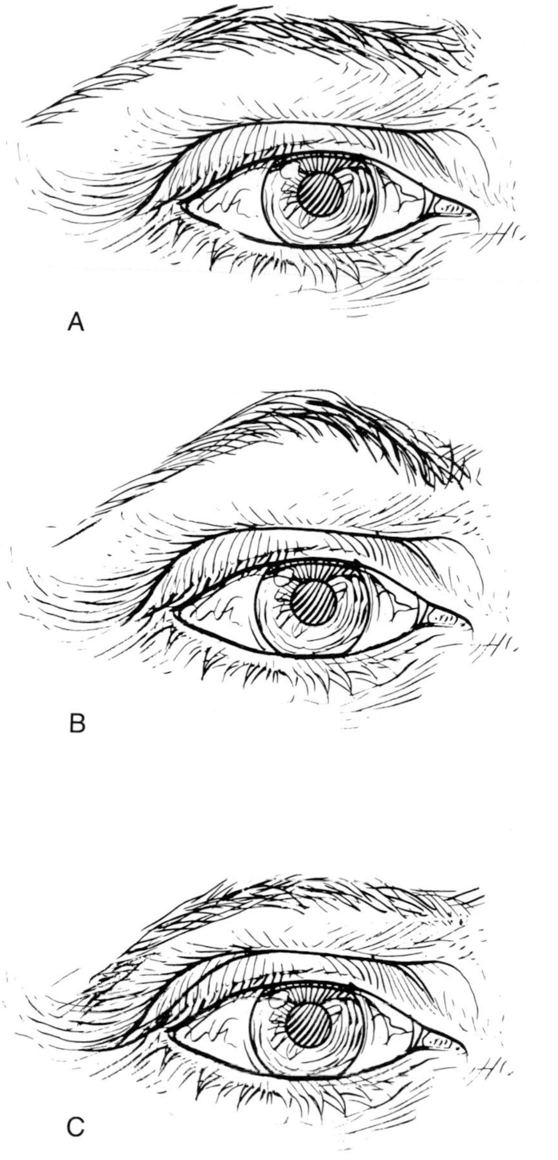

Figure 1–26. *A*, Preferred position of the eyebrow. *B*, *C*, Less attractive positions of the eyebrow.

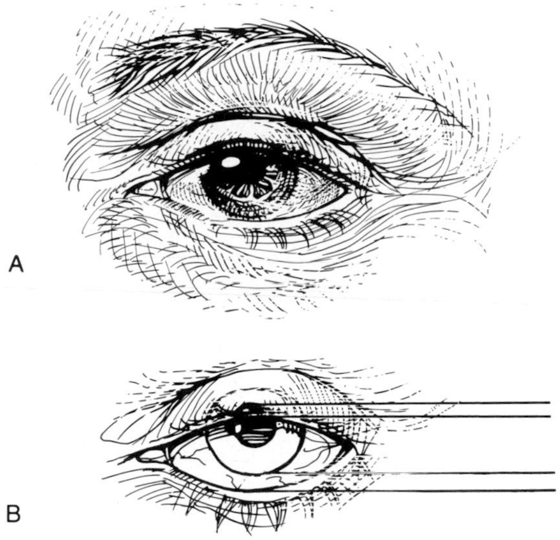

Figure 1–27. *A*, The upper lid should touch the pupil on forward gaze. The lower lid should touch the limbus. *B*, The sclera of the eye should not show between the limbus and the lower lid ("scleral show"). The lines designate deviation from the ideal.

rim of the orbital cavity. The repetition of three lines of the same curvature is not artistic and gives an uninteresting appearance (Fig. 1–26*B*). An older, more serious appearance is characteristic of individuals with brows slanting downward as they progress laterally (Fig. 1–26*C*).

On straightforward view, the rim of the upper eyelid should touch the edge of the pupil; the lower lid touches the limbus (Fig. 1–27*A*).

The appearance of the eye is, to a great extent, determined by the shape and size of the orbit and palpebral aperture. A superior tilt of the palpebral fissure from medial to lateral with some degree of bowing of the border of the lower eyelid gives the desirable "almond shape" of the eye. A large orbit gives the appearance of enophthalmos or "deep-set eyes" with a large supratarsal fold. Hypoplasia of the inferior orbital rim is associated with "scleral show" of the lower eyelid.

George Bridgman, long considered the finest instructor of life drawing in America, evolved a system of simplifying and blocking masses of human figures into geometric shapes and giving them increased definition. Constructive anatomy was an integral part of the course. Bridgman saw four distinct forms in the face: (1) the square or rectangular forehead; (2) the flat cheekbone area; (3) the triangular form of the lower jaw; and (4) an erect cylindrical form on which are placed the base of the nose and the mouth (Fig. 1–28*A–C*). Bridgman (1973) saw the nose as a wedge (Fig. 1–28*D*), with its root in the forehead and its base in the upper lip. He described two wedges meeting on the bridge of the nose (Fig. 1–28*E–G*) and tapering toward the forehead and the bulbous tip, and remarked that the bulb rises from the middle of the upper lip (septum), expands into a bulbous tip, flows over the sides, and flares out to form the wings of the nostrils.

Artists of the past taught that the upper

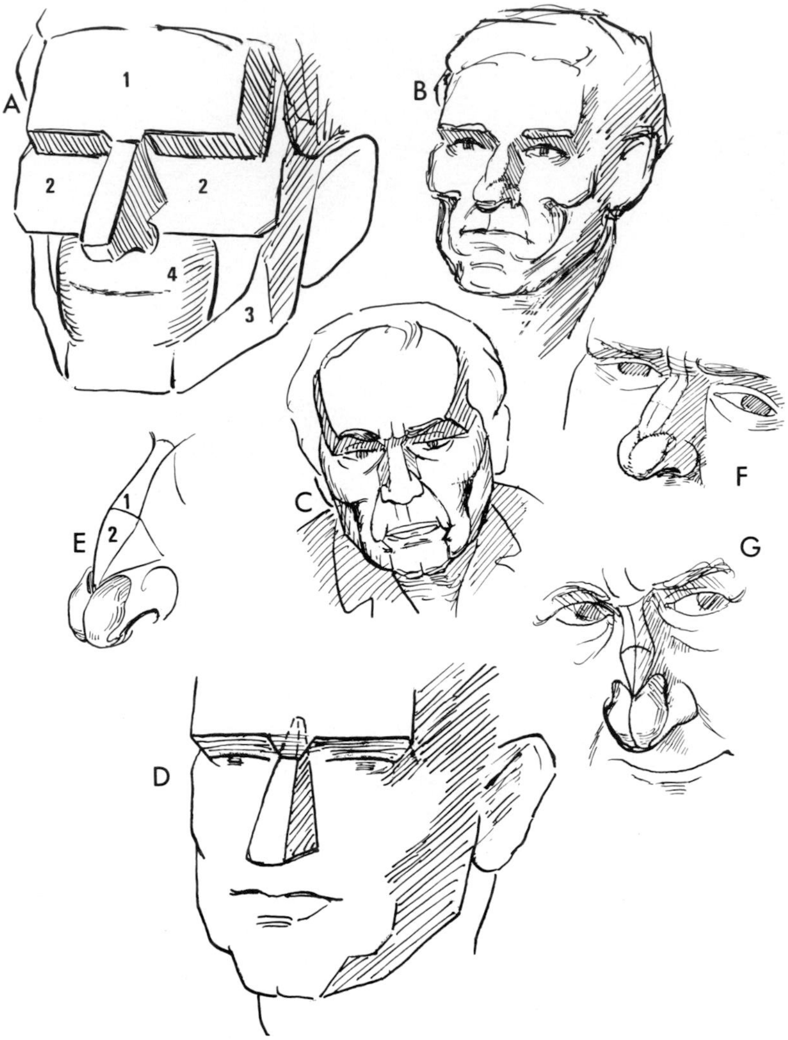

Figure 1–28. *A* to *C*, Geometric shapes in the face. *D*, The nose seen as a wedge inserting into the forehead. *E*, Two wedges shown meeting at the bridge of the nose. *F, G*, Variations in the nasal wedges (after Bridgman).

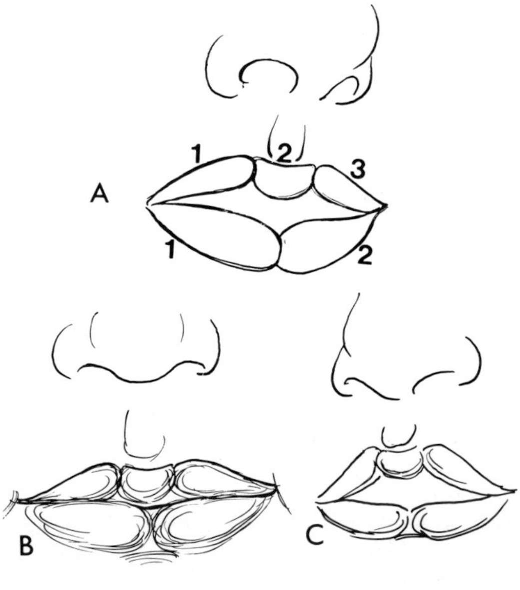

Figure 1–29. Diagram showing how to draw the lips: the prolabial and two lateral segments above; two segments below.

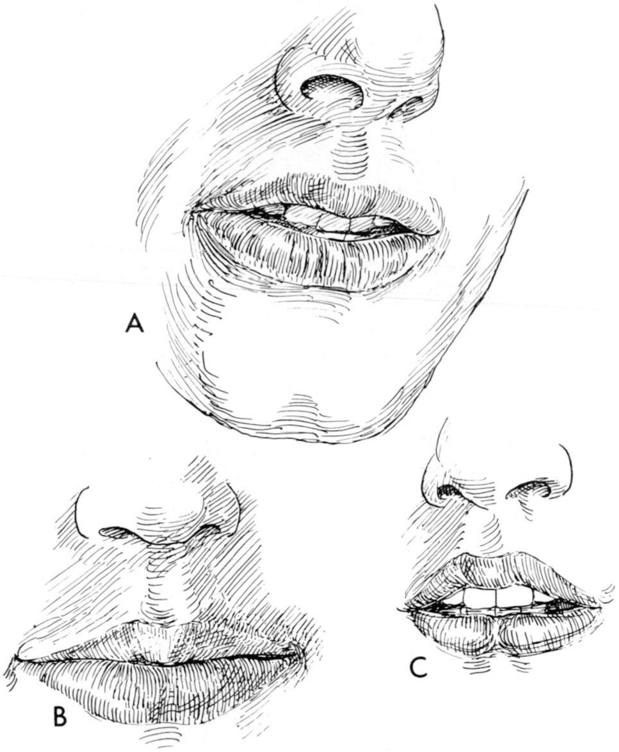

Figure 1–30. Drawings of the lips from the diagram in Figure 1–29.

lip is composed of three muscles and the lower lip of two muscles. They taught that the preliminary sketch should be diagrammed to show these divisions (Fig. 1–29) and thereby facilitate production of the finished product by giving the student a simple understanding of the subtle lip form. Figure 1–30 is a drawing of the lips diagrammed in Figure 1–29: *A*, lips of a young man; *B*, lips of a young woman; *C*, lips of a young girl.

Most artists have difficulty in drawing the ear because of a lack of understanding of its anatomy (Fig. 1–31*A*). It appears to be a complex structure because of the intricate convolutions. Simplification of the structure into an elongated "*C*" for the helix, a "*Y*" for the superior and inferior crura, the triangular fossa, and the concha, and a "*U*" for the lobule (Fig. 1–31*B*) renders it understandable (Fig. 1–31*C*). Any surgeon planning reconstruction of the ear should first practice drawing it or modeling it in clay.

The length of the body in relation to the head varies according to the artist. Leonardo claimed the head to be one-eighth the length of the body, the leg from the crest of the ilium to the base of the heel one-half the length of the body, and the distance from the fingertip to the center of the chin one-half the length of the body. At that time Leonardo was inter-

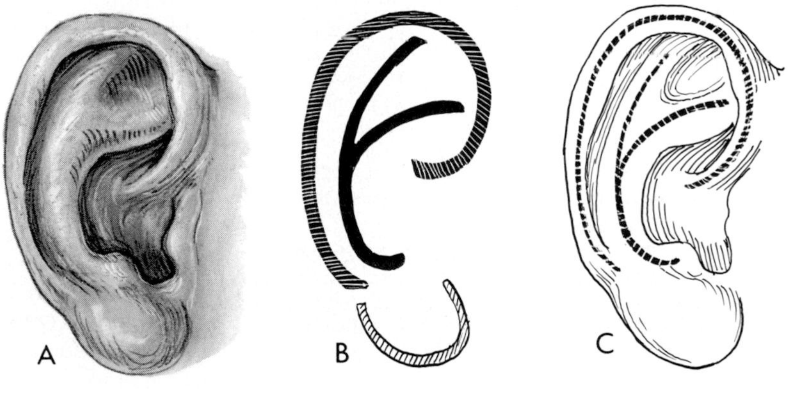

Figure 1–31. Simplifying the ear into an elongated "C" for the helix, a "Y" for the superior and inferior crura, the triangular fossa, and the concha, and a "U" for the lobule.

ested in the Platonian theory of the geometric representation of the universe as discussed in the book of Fra Luca Pacciola (circa 1445–1514), with whom Leonardo collaborated. According to the position in which one places the human body, the body may be enclosed within a square because of the equal dimensions of the arm-span and the body height when they are perpendicular to each other, in a circle when the limbs are more or less in abduction, and in a pentagon (the Pythagorean symbol of a microcosm). Leonardo's plates to this effect expressed an esthetic rule rather than an anthropologic fact, and he later abandoned that concept. Richer (1920) of the Ecole des Beaux Arts in Paris taught that the body length equaled 7½ heads (Fig. 1–32). Richer further divided the body into masses for study and analysis, as shown in Figure 1–33.

Figure 1–33*E* is a copy of a diagram by Lanteri of the Ecole des Beaux Arts, which shows his view of the circumscribed forms or masses of the face. It should be noted that

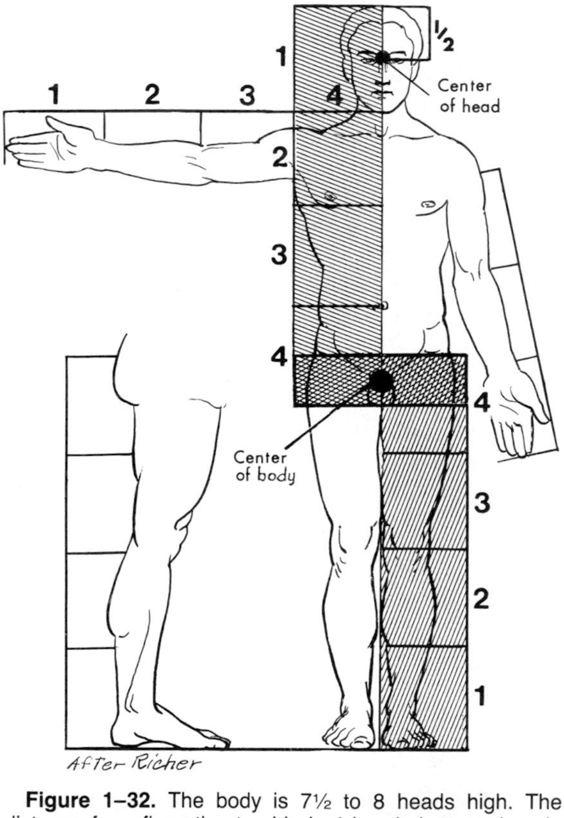

Figure 1–32. The body is 7½ to 8 heads high. The distance from fingertips to chin is 4 heads in men, less in women because of the narrower shoulders. (Adapted from Richer, P.: Morphologie de la Femme. Plon-Nourrit et Cie, 1920.)

both Lanteri and Bridgman regarded the infraorbital area as part of the flat zygomatic area, not as a separate mass, as the plastic surgeon would see it. Leonardo paid considerable attention to the infraorbital area in many drawings (see Fig. 1–19), emphasizing the area in older faces and in his own self-portrait.

PHOTOGRAPHY

Photography is essential as a diagnostic modality, as a means of evaluating the patient's self-image, as a record of the progress made in multiple-stage operations, and as a "before" and "after" record of the surgical result. Photographs are also increasingly important as medicolegal documents. They allow the patient to view himself in profile without mirror distortion, and also aid the surgeon when they are attached to the wall of the operating room for easy viewing.

Gillies, in his speech at the Congress banquet at the First International Society of Plastic Surgeons in Stockholm, said facetiously: "I have been asked to speak about the important advances in plastic surgery. I think the most important advance is photography!"

In facial surgery the photograph serves as a means of determining how the patient views himself and thus of learning to what extent the patient's perception of himself is realistic or unrealistic. In the severely disfigured patient, total rehabilitation often cannot be achieved; a comparison of preoperative and postoperative photographs will help the patient to perceive the improvement achieved. "Did I really look like that?" is his frequent comment.

Consistency in Medical Photography: Standards for Comparison. Any surgeon attending a scientific meeting or reading a professional journal will notice the frequent absence of any type of standard of comparison between preoperative and postoperative photographs of patients; the position, the lighting, and the exposure all vary. Often the preoperative photograph shows the patient in the position and under lighting and exposure that show the deformity at its worst; the postoperative view may be taken at an angle, with flat lighting, and with the most favorable photographic exposure. The surgeon or author does not mean to be dishonest, but he

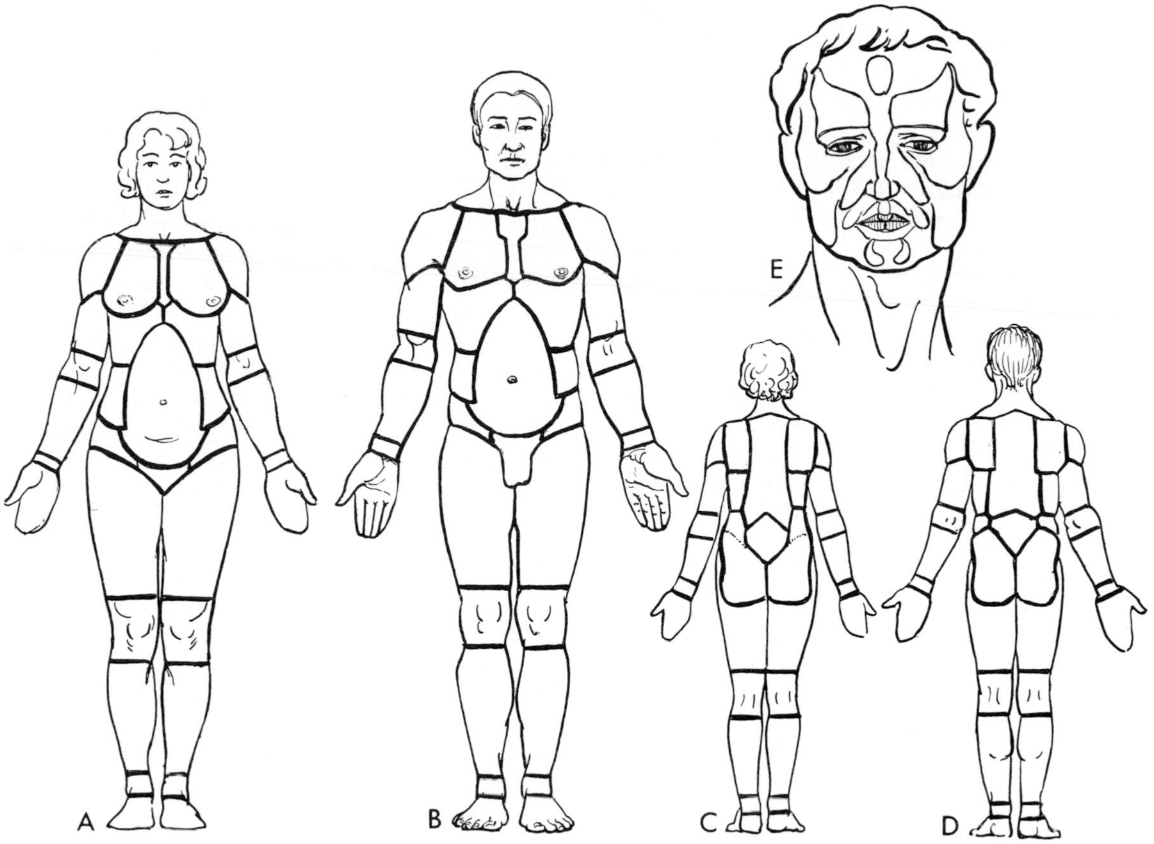

Figure 1–33. *A* to *D*, Divisions of the body surface for the purpose of artistic analysis (after Richer). *E*, Masses of the face (after Lanteri).

can convey that impression (Chapple and Stephenson, 1970). When the surgeon takes his own photographs with a direct flash attachment, he is bound to obtain differences in exposure, and he is also dependent upon the developer of the pictures.

It is always desirable to have a professional photographer but one is not always available. Some advice from Don Allen, the photographer of the Institute of Reconstructive Plastic Surgery since 1947, is pertinent (Morello, Converse, and Allen, 1977).

Role of the Medical Photographer. The medical photographer must ask himself the following questions: What is the purpose of the photographs? How do they differ from ordinary photography? The photographer must be closely associated with the field of medicine, usually through a hospital affiliation. Most of his work is governed by a strict set of rules. Photographers outside the medical field remark, with truth, that they are almost totally bound up by confining limitations. The main confining limitation is *consistency*, which is an absolute and a constant challenge.

A medical photograph must be an accurate, pictorial (visual) record relative to a certain condition. It may stand alone as a single photograph tied to a single date, or may be part of a continuing, comparable record of the progress achieved by staged surgical procedures over an indeterminate period. To ensure its reliability the photographer must be consistent in quality, position, and accuracy.

Color transparencies serve a dual purpose, since satisfactory black and white photographs can be made through internegatives. There are many good color processing laboratories available throughout the world to provide fast, quality service. Color transparencies are also useful in illustrating lectures.

Vast amounts of visual records would be lost if it were not for the color-loaded, single lens reflex camera in the hands of doctor, nurse, or technician. When the original color photograph or its black and white reproduction is not of top quality, the culprit more than likely is the lighting. Most of the camera units incorporate a single-source strobe light, which is almost always mounted close to the lens axis, a feature that tends to produce a photograph without the contour details obtained by adequate lighting. This is an unavoidable characteristic, but the fact that the unit will produce consistently good color and exposure makes the unit most valuable.

The four major factors relating to these goals are the studio, the camera, the patient, and the lighting.

The *studio* should be large enough (at least 8 × 12 ft) to make use of a focal length lens angle long enough to yield no distortion and to permit patients to be photographed full length. The walls and ceiling are painted off-white because color film tends to absorb any wall color. Windows are curtained to prevent outside light, and fluorescent lighting, which produces a green tint in color slides, is avoided. A light blue-green background is suitable for black and white and color photography. Appropriate eye level markers, or fixed points to help the patient in holding a given position, should be available. This requires a secure and comfortable chair of the correct height that can easily be moved.

The *camera* should be of the single-lens, reflex type with interchangeable lenses and good optics, capable of strobe-synchronization. The single-lens reflex helps to achieve a correct camera angle. There should be two camera bodies, one for color slides and the other for black and white film. The viewfinder of the camera should have a grid to aid alignment.

The *patient*, placed 3 ft in front of the background to eliminate shadows, should be photographed in a comfortable atmosphere, without make-up, distracting clothes, interfering hair, or jewelry. Long hair should be cleared from the face. The patient's face should be placed in a position in accord with the horizontal (Frankfort) and midsagittal planes of the face (see Fig. 1–17).

The *lighting* is usually achieved by employing a set of at least three studio-type strobe light heads equipped with modeling lights. Strict lighting rules produce constant results. One must remember that the camera does not lie, but the lighting can and will unless careful attention is given at all times to this aspect.

Illustrations. There are several basic views to demonstrate proper alignment, correct and consistent lighting, and relative magnification: full-face view (Fig. 1–34), submental views (two) (Fig. 1–35), matching three-quarter anterior views (two) (Fig. 1–36), and matching left and right profile views (Fig. 1–37).

Depending on the clinical problem, other photographic views can be obtained. In maxillofacial surgical reconstruction occlusal views (frontal and oblique) are essential (Fig. 1–38) and can be obtained in a longitudinal fashion. A facial palsy photographic series would include various functional views (Fig. 1–39). The cardinal fields of gaze should be obtained in patients with extraocular muscle dysfunction or in those undergoing orbital translocation surgery. Photographic close-up views of scars and skin lesions are critical for documentation purposes.

The production of each patient photograph must be guided by (1) proper positioning, (2) proper camera angle approach, (3) controlled lighting, (4) consistent photographic technique, and (5) proper laboratory finishing. The photographic laboratory offers the final control. Magnification and alignment must be maintained at this, the final stage.

The Black and White Print Versus the Color Transparency. If the photographs are taken under the conditions described above, a transparency is as accurate a document as a black and white print. However, the print has the advantage that (1) it can be more easily looked at with the patient; and (2) it can be placed on the wall of the operating room, where, because of its larger size, it can be readily and more accurately examined.

The increasing availability of video equipment renders it helpful to the surgeon in both operating room and office. It is the preferred method of documenting the efficacy of surgical procedures designed to restore function, as in the patient with facial palsy.

THE PLASTIC SURGEON AND THE INTEGUMENT

Although the plastic surgeon is concerned with repairing the skeletal framework, muscles, tendons, nerves, and vessels, he must, in order to ensure a successful result, obtain adequate cutaneous covering of his underlying surgical procedures. He must, therefore, be an expert in the management of soft tissue wounds, whether operative or traumatic in

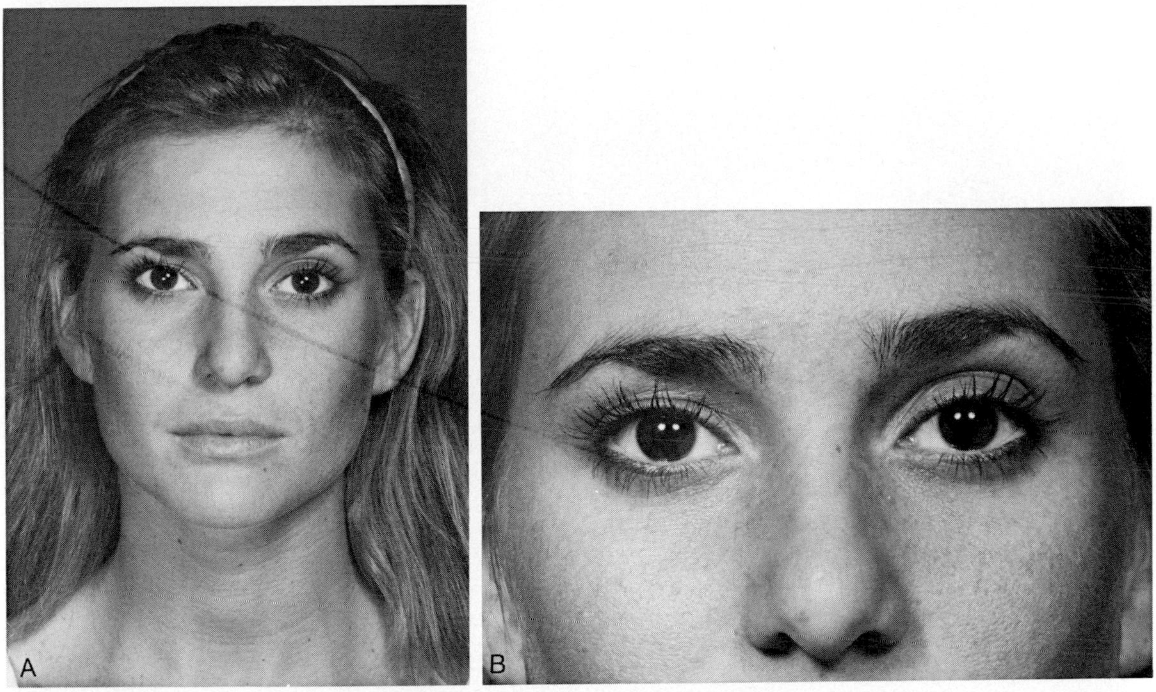

Figure 1–34. Various photographic views. *A*, Full-face (frontal). *B*, Forward eye gaze (close-up). The face is oriented according to the Frankfort horizontal and midsagittal planes. Note the brow asymmetry.

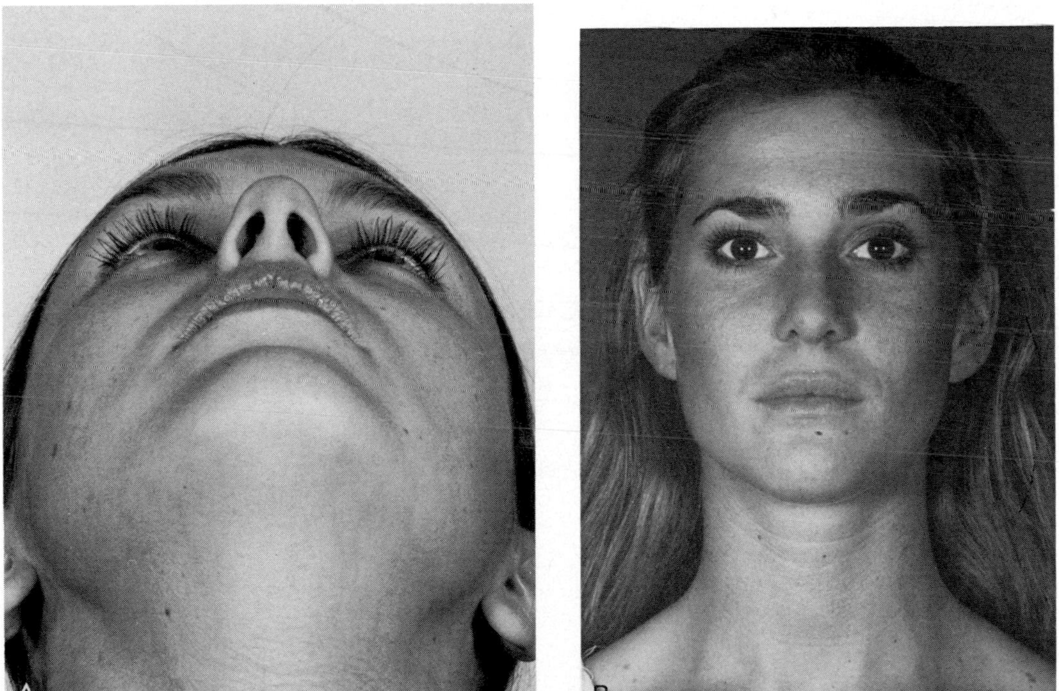

Figure 1–35. *A*, Base of the nasal pyramid. *B*, Face and neck view.

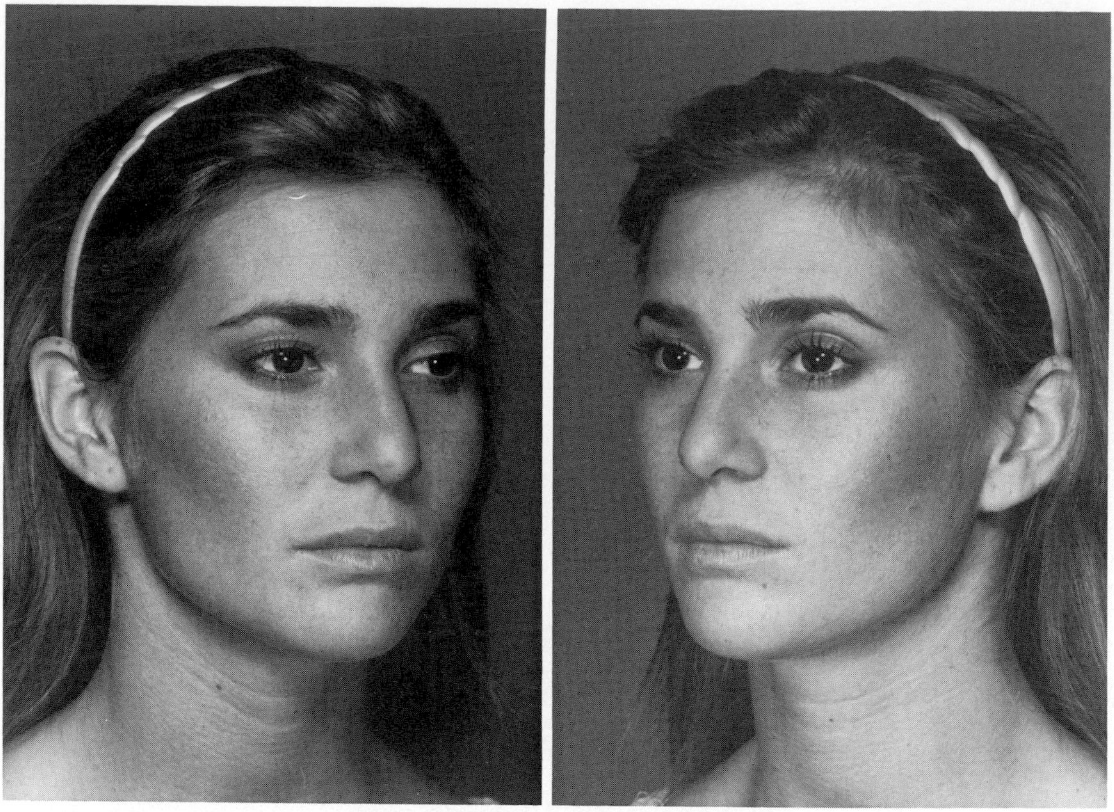

Figure 1–36. Three-quarters facial views.

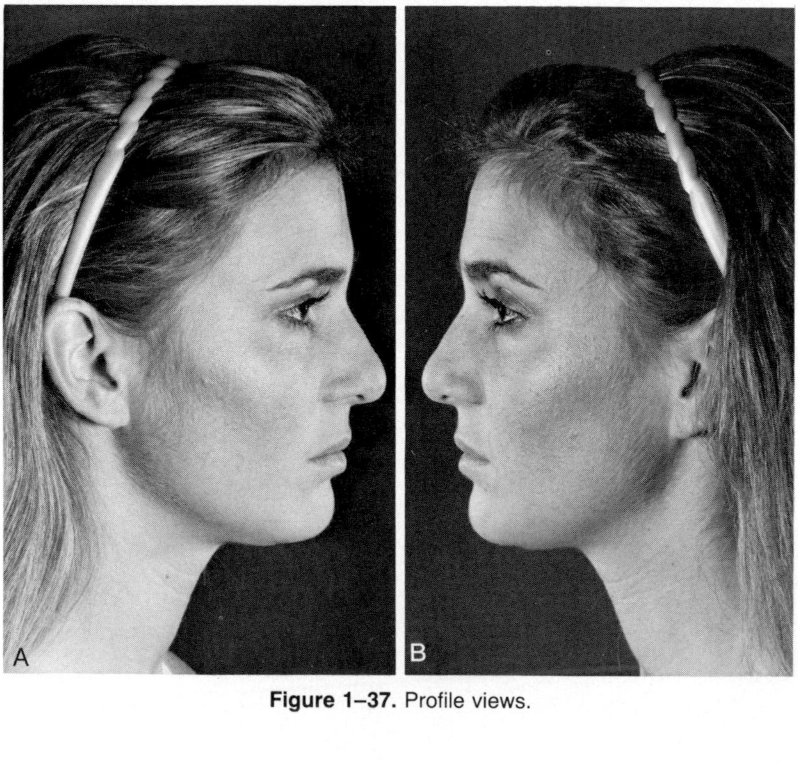

Figure 1–37. Profile views.

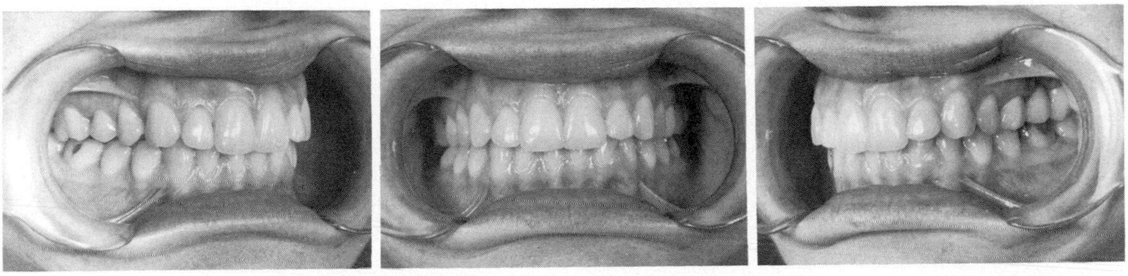

Figure 1–38. Occlusal (frontal and oblique) views.

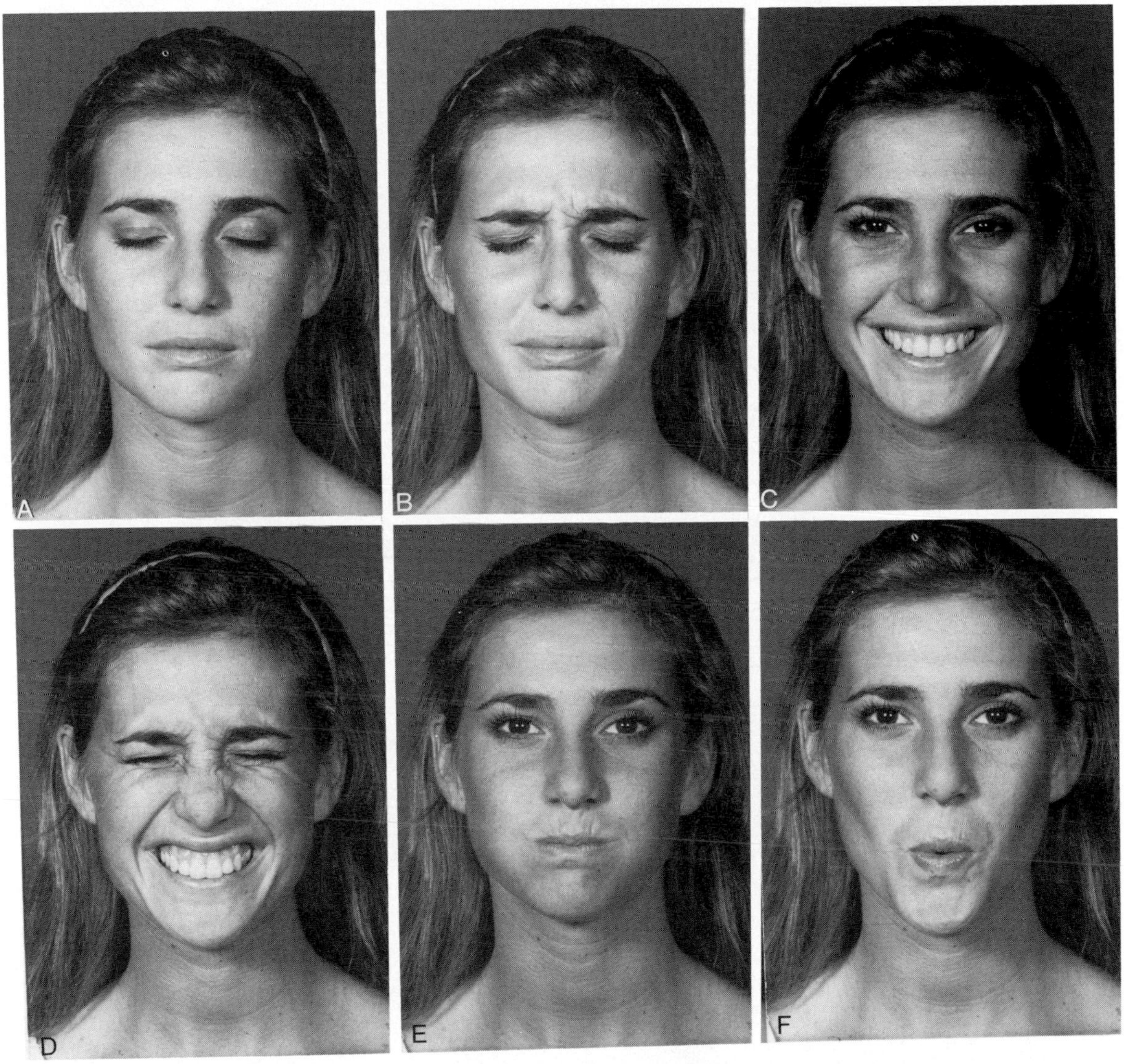

Figure 1–39. Facial palsy series. *A*, Eyelid closure. *B*, Forced eyelid closure. *C*, Mild smile. *D*, Forced smile. *E*, Test of lip competence. *F*, Pursing of lips.

origin. The skin is elastic, extensible, and resilient; these characteristics vary from birth to old age.

Lines of Skin Tension. Skin possesses a degree of elasticity owing to the presence of elastic fibers in the dermis. Elastic fibers are disposed in bundles with the collagen fibers, many of them looped spirally around collagen fibers, and are distributed through the dermis, becoming finer toward the surface of the dermis. The elasticity maintains the skin in a state of constant tension. This is demonstrated by the gaping of wounds following incision through the dermis, and also by the immediate contraction of skin grafts as they are removed from the donor site; the thicker the skin graft, the greater the amount of elastic tissue and associated contraction. The elasticity and extensibility of the skin also facilitates the shifting of skin flaps. Degeneration of the elastic tissue in the skin of the aged is a contributing factor in the relaxation of facial skin and the formation of excess skin folds.

The existence of lines of tension in the skin was first noted by Dupuytren (1832) in describing wounds of the skin made by penetrating instruments. He reported the case of a cobbler who committed suicide by stabbing himself with an awl; the awl was pointed at the tip and round in section, but the wounds in the cobbler's skin were linear in outline, as though made by the blade of a knife (see also Chap. 7).

Langer (1861) found that, following puncture of the skin in various parts of the body, the puncture holes, originally round, had a tendency to become an ellipse by the normal tension of the skin (Fig. 1–40). Langer considered that human skin was less extensible in the direction of the lines of tension than across them.

Langer's concept was not corroborated by practical experience, as some of Langer's (tension) lines were found to run across natural creases, wrinkles, and flexion lines. Other empirical findings about Langer's lines are that they exist in excised skin, that they do not correlate with the orientation of dermal collagen fiber orientation, and that they affect the mechanical and surgical properties of skin (Ksander, Vistnes, and Rose, 1977).

Practical experience has shown that wounds heal better and scars are less conspicuous when incisions are made within, or parallel to, natural flexion lines or lines of facial expression. Cox (1941) made sections of tissue removed from a wound incised parallel to a flexion line. Sections of skin made in two planes, one exactly at right angles and another exactly parallel to the long axis of a wound, indicated a striking difference in structure according to the plane of the section. Sections taken at right angles to the long axis of the wound showed a marked preponderance of connective tissue and elastic fibers cut transversely; sections parallel to the long axis of the wound showed that most fibers extended longitudinally.

Gibson (1967) has shown that, when skin is stretched, collagen and elastic fibers become aligned in the direction of the stretch

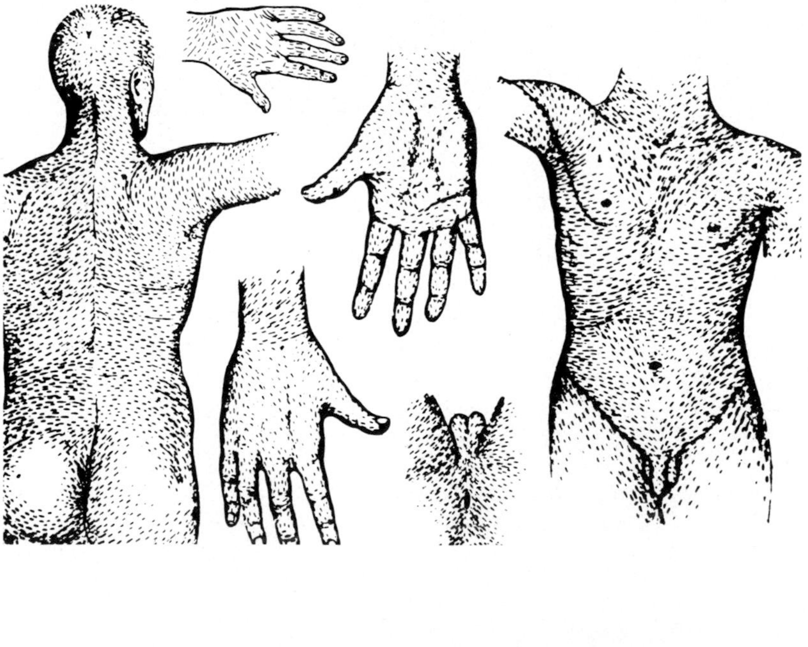

Figure 1–40. Langer's lines of the skin.

(see Chap. 7). This condition exists in the lines of expression or creases of flexion. Wounds within or parallel to these lines are less subject to tension from the activity of the underlying musculature that has produced the lines of tension.

Lines of Minimal Tension. In a cutaneous defect, maximal contraction results in a scar (contracture) whose long axis crosses the *lines of minimal tension* at right angles. The lines of minimal tension are the result of adaptation to function, the skin being constantly pulled and stretched by the underlying muscle and joint. The connective tissue, collagen, and elastic fibers are arranged in bundles that are perpendicular to the underlying muscles. A scar parallel to the lines is not subject to the intermittent pull of the subjacent muscles—hence the term "lines of minimal tension." A scar placed within a line of minimal tension or parallel to it is submitted to minimal tension during the period of healing. Borges (1973) preferred the term "relaxed skin tension lines" in describing these lines.

In the head and neck, the lines of minimal tension (Fig. 1–41) represent adaptation to two different types of functional mechanisms. The first type is represented by the *lines of habitual expression in the face*, such as the lines in the forehead, eyelids, and nasolabial folds and other lines of expression around the mouth. The second type, the *lines of skin relaxation* (such as the horizontal circular lines in the neck), results from movements of flexion and extension. Lines of relaxation, of flexion and extension, are formed in the various areas of the body—trunk, limbs, hands, and feet.

A scar that traverses the lines of minimal tension of the skin at right angles is subjected to constant changes in tension as a result of the activity of the underlying musculature; hypertrophy of the scar often develops. Only a slightly visible scar results when incisions in the neck are made within a skin fold or crease, or are parallel to the fold. Considerable width can be excised on either side of an incision parallel to or in the skin folds without materially increasing tension when the wound is closed, since the skin around the folds is loose and redundant.

Lines of Expression. Lines of expression are produced by repeated and habitual contraction of the underlying muscles of facial expression. In some regions a number of muscles act in unison. The nasolabial fold, for example, represents the area of junction between the skin of the lip, which is tightly bound to the underlying orbicularis oris muscle, and the more loosely bound skin of the cheek over the buccal fat pad. The nasolabial fold is also formed by muscular contraction of the zygomaticus, quadratus labii superioris, and caninus muscles, and in part by the risorius and buccinator muscles.

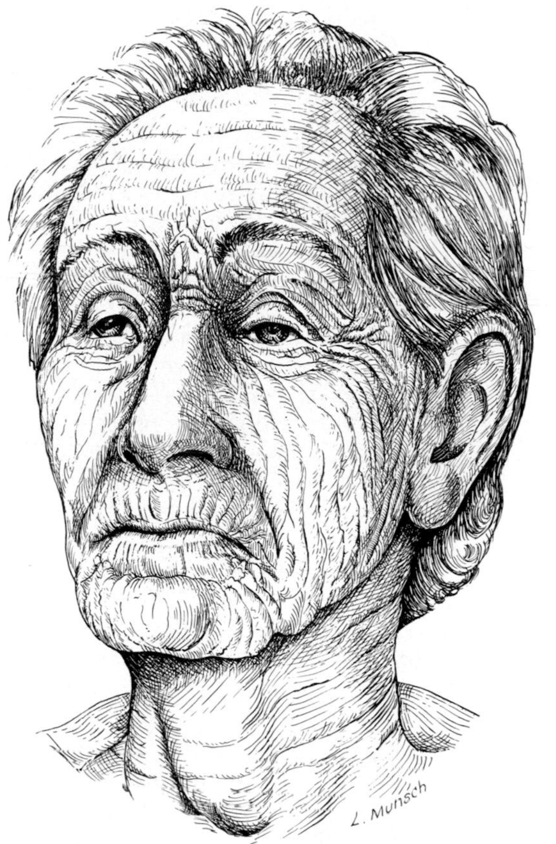

Figure 1–41. The lines of minimal tension of the face and neck.

The supraorbital wrinkle lines and the transverse lines of the forehead are caused by the contraction of the frontalis muscle, which is inserted into the skin of the lower forehead. In the upper eyelids, many fine perpendicular strands of fibers of the levator aponeurosis terminate in the dermis of the skin and along the tarsus to form the supratarsal fold. Similar insertions in the lower lid create the fine horizontal lines, which are accentuated by the contraction of the orbicularis oculi muscle. The sphincter action of the orbicularis oculi muscle is altered by its origin and insertion at two fixed points, the medial canthus and the lateral canthus. Contraction of the lateral portion of the muscle produces lines; wrinkles are at right angles to the action of the muscle. In the upper portion of the dorsum of the nose, the corrugator supercilii and orbicularis oculi muscles act somewhat antagonistically to the frontalis to form the almost vertical lines observed during the act of frowning.

The oblique lines on the side of the nose are a consequence of the action of the angular head of the quadratus labii superioris and the procerus muscles. The vertical lines in the lower part of the nose are caused by the contraction of the transverse portion of the nasalis muscle. Crease lines develop radially from the oral fissure. At the angles of the mouth, however, the combined action of the quadratus labii superioris and other muscles in this region causes the lines to blend with those of the nasolabial fold. The formation of the lines on the lateral aspect of the chin results from the action of the triangularis, quadratus labii inferioris, and mentalis muscles.

The transverse lines across the neck, located perpendicularly to the platysma muscle, separate folds of excess skin, permitting extension of the neck. Near the chest the horizontal neck lines assume a more oblique direction.

Every individual possesses lines of expression that become more apparent when the muscles contract. Wrinkles are less evident in young people; however, in old age skin creases and wrinkles are more numerous because the skin, through degenerative changes, has lost its elasticity and becomes redundant. Because the skin is less elastic and also redundant, it is incapable of assuming its smooth appearance at the termination of muscular contraction.

Choice of Site of Incision. The size and direction of an elective incision should always be chosen in relation to the lines of minimal tension. For example, when planning an incision in the thorax for the removal of costal cartilage, flexion of the thoracic skin shows the position of the skin folds, and the incision is placed in this position. When the incision thus placed does not provide the best exposure of the underlying structures, it is lengthened. Because of the better quality of scar obtained, the longer incision is still less visible than a shorter incision placed at right angles to the skin fold; in children, incisions in this area have a notable tendency to hypertrophy. No amount of care in suturing or in the approximation of wound edges will help if the scar is in a position unfavorable to minimal scarring, i.e., at right angles or oblique to the lines of minimal tension.

Although the lines of expression and flexion creases generally coincide with the lines of minimal tension and are the best guide to the placing of incisions, there are exceptions. On the hand, for example, wrinkles produced by hyperextending the thumb and flexing the metacarpal joint of the index finger do not represent the lines of minimal tension (Fig. 1–42). Another exception is the submental fold.

Anatomic Areas. Incisions in certain anatomic areas are particularly unfavorable and tend to heal in a hypertrophic manner. The most notable of these areas are the shoulder and the presternal area, which involves exceptional skin tension, expecially in women with pendulous breasts. Man, originally a quadriped, became a biped; in the erect position the upper extremities hang loosely, and the skin of the shoulder is thus placed under tension. Only in the elderly do anteroposterior folds appear in this area as the skin loses its elasticity and becomes lax.

The Influence of Age. During infancy and

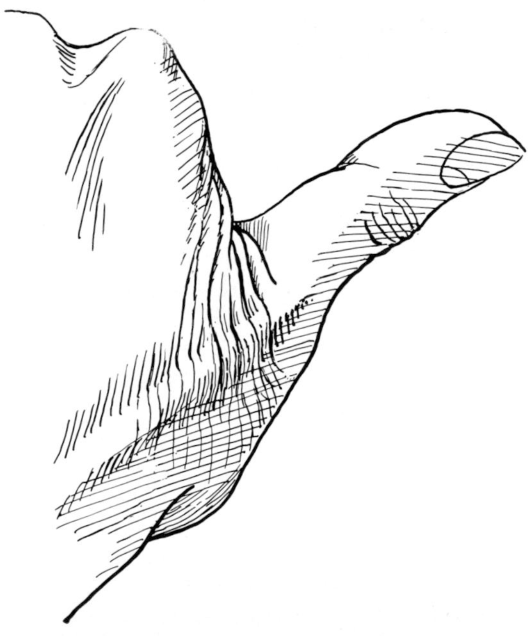

Figure 1–42. The lines produced by hyperextending the thumb and flexing the metacarpal joint of the index finger do not represent the lines of minimal tension.

the major part of childhood, the skin has its maximal elasticity; it is also padded by a type of adipose tissue, familiarly termed "baby fat," which maintains the skin at its maximal distention. As the aging process takes place, the skin loses much of its elasticity, and the subcutaneous fat changes in character and quantity; the skin folds and wrinkles increase with the progressive relaxation of the skin. In addition, cheek fat (Bichat) decreases markedly in volume.

The greater elasticity and extensibility of the skin in infants and young children make possible the use of large rotation and advancement flaps to cover defects. Conversely, scars in children tend to be thicker and wider. The aged patient with relaxed skin has a similar advantage, making possible types of reconstructive procedures that would not provide satisfactory results in young adults. One of the few compensations of old age is the inconspicuous scar, the result of the relaxation of the skin.

Types of Skin. Oily skin that contains hypertrophied and hyperactive sebaceous glands is unfavorable for satisfactory scar formation. The scars are usually wide, depressed, and irregular in outline. This type of skin is usually found over the distal nose, cheeks, and forehead.

Wide and unsightly scars also result in patients with fibroelastic diatheses such as the Ehlers-Danlos syndrome.

TIMING OF REPAIR

In the treatment of congenital deformities, a number of problems are posed. A major problem is the age at which surgical treatment should be administered. Some deformities must be remedied within a few days after birth, and a number of surgeons have made it their practice to repair a cleft lip in the newborn baby before the mother and child leave the hospital. Most prefer to wait until the child is 2 to 4 months old before performing the corrective surgery, feeling that the increase in the size of the structures will allow for more accurate repair and that the child then is also more physiologically equipped to withstand surgical trauma. In addition, the family has had time to comprehend the severity of the deformity. Other elective procedures are best postponed until the infant is at least 1 year old, as morbidity at this age is decreased; a postponement until the child is 4 years old may be advisable if the patient's cooperation is required. In microtia, it would be preferable to reconstruct a new auricle prior to school age in order to avoid psychologic trauma. However, construction of the auricle is easier when the child is 6 or 7 years of age because of the greater size of the donor costal cartilage.

In developmental malformations, it was the practice in the past to wait until completion of growth before undertaking reconstructive surgery. This philosophy had been the practice in craniofacial malformations, for example, although postponement of surgery often resulted in progressive accentuation of the malformation. Moreover, as in Crouzon's disease, the surgeon was waiting for craniofacial growth and development that would never be realized. In the interim there would be progressive deterioration in the child's psychologic status. Thus, there has been a tendency in craniofacial surgery centers in recent years to undertake surgical repair in younger patients.

Such a problem is also posed in treating the patient with a cleft palate; it has been felt by some that surgery interfered with growth and that postponement of operation was desirable in order to permit maxillary growth to progress unimpeded. Another variable to be considered was the fact that the child would not have satisfactory speech, with its associated sociologic problems, until the palate was repaired. A change of attitude in recent years has led to a more selective approach to the timing of reconstructive surgery during the growth and development of the patient.

The type of plastic surgery practiced in cancer patients differs from the definitive type of surgery done to repair congenital malformations or deformities following trauma. Preoccupation with the eradication of malignant disease predominates in the plan of treatment. However, attention should also be paid to reconstructing the resulting contour and functional defects as part of the "treatment of the whole patient."

In treating oromandibular cancer, if primary reconstruction is not performed after resection of the soft tissues of the lips, cheeks, floor of the mouth, and mandible, constant drooling is present and retention of food is difficult. Unable to feed himself, having to be fed through a tube, the patient has a repulsive appearance to onlookers and even to himself. Outwardly alive, he is inwardly dead.

In other types of cases—after resection of a malignant lesion of the nose, for example—primary reconstructive surgery may not be indicated. A secondary procedure to reconstruct the nose after an interval of a few months is preferable for several reasons. The excisional site can be examined for evidence of tumor recurrence and the patient also has time to adjust to the psychologic trauma of the surgical ablation.

CHOICE OF METHOD OF REPAIR

The quality of the repair often depends on the surgeon's operative skill and judgment in selecting the operative procedure. Sound clinical judgment in choosing the method of repair is one of the difficult aspects in teaching plastic surgery. The student of plastic surgery can peruse books and publications that contain descriptions, both textual and illustrative, of many operative procedures, but judgment comes only with years of clinical experience. In his remarkable *Principlization of Plastic Surgery,* Millard (1986) outlined 33 strategic principles based on his own professional experience and his training with Gillies.

Consideration of Age and Sex of Patient

Certain procedures are an excellent choice for the patient in the older age group, in whom the relaxed, aging tissues provide an ample supply of tissue to permit closure of the donor site with minimal tension and a relatively inconspicuous scar. Secondary deformities caused by the transfer of regional flaps to repair the defects are also of relatively lesser import in the aged patient, whose main problem may be solely functional. A similar technique may be totally inapplicable in the younger patient.

The method of repair is also influenced by the sex of the patient. For example, flaps may be transferred from the upper, anterior chest in male patients, a procedure that may not be cosmetically acceptable to the female. Cheek resurfacing in the adult male also demands the transfer of hair-bearing skin as from the adjacent neck area.

Camouflage versus Anatomic Restoration

Facial appearance may be improved by a type of camouflage exemplified by the procedure employed in malunited fracture of the zygoma. Contour is restored by an onlay bone graft or alloplastic implant in preference to attempting to reposition the zygoma, a more difficult surgical task in some cases.

On occasion, it is decided to redesign dentures in the edentulous patient rather than undertake a complicated jaw osteotomy with its attendant period of intermaxillary fixation.

Color and Texture Match

When transferring skin to the face, a satisfactory match in color, thickness, and texture is important, for the skin of the transplant must harmonize with the tissue surrounding the defect. The choice of tissue borrowed from another area of the body to repair a defect of the soft tissue of the face requires careful consideration. The texture and color of the skin of the face and neck differ from those of other areas. Unsuccessful matching of the skin results in a conspicuous "patch," which is even more accentuated during emotion or after sun exposure.

The Barter Principle

When the skin is borrowed from one area of the face to repair another, the secondary deformity may be discernible, but the procedure is often desirable because a closer match of tissue is obtained than when a flap is transferred from a distant area. The principle simplifies reconstruction and avoids conspicuous disparity in skin color and texture. In this process of "robbing Peter to pay Paul," the price paid is at the discretion of the surgeon. It seems obvious that good clinical judgment reduces the cost of the barter to a minimum. Remember, "Paul must also be able to pay Peter."

One example of the principle of barter is the use of a forehead flap for subtotal reconstruction of the nose. Forehead tissue is employed for this procedure because the best results in terms of color and texture match are obtained by the use of forehead skin. A major portion of the flap is replaced in its original site after dividing the pedicle, leaving a portion of the flap to form the reconstructed nose. A secondary defect remains on the forehead. This defect is repaired by the most suitable skin available in order to minimize the secondary deformity. Full-thickness skin removed from the supraclavicular area offers a suitable color match. The supraclavicular defect can usually be closed primarily. This is a good barter; by contrast, a split-thickness graft placed upon the forehead represents an unsatisfactory repair of the secondary defect.

Principle of Shifting the Defect

This principle is applied in the transfer of a defect to an area that is either less conspicuous or less important from a functional point of view. For example, a defect may require a flap of tissue from the adjacent skin in order to provide the optimal thickness of both skin and the underlying subcutaneous tissue. The procedure is accomplished by closing the primary defect with an adjacent rotation flap; the secondary defect is then repaired by a skin graft or another local flap. For example, when a flap is raised from the preauricular area and transferred to a zygomatic defect, skin of suitable color and texture is provided, in addition to the subcutaneous tissue removed with the flap from over the parotid-masseteric fascia. The secondary defect can be repaired by a full-thickness retroauricular graft; the vascularization of the graft is assured and the esthetic result is excellent. The deficiency in the subcutaneous tissue is less obvious in the preauricular area, a less conspicuous portion of the face than the zygomatic area.

Another example of the principle of shifting the defect is the reconstruction of a median defect of the lower lip by shifting the remaining lateral portions of the lower lip to the midline and repairing the laterally situated secondary defects by Estlander flaps from the upper lip.

Autogenous versus Alloplastic Material

In general, autogenous grafts are preferred to alloplastic material, especially in a heavily scarred or poorly vascularized recipient site. While the ease of procurement of alloplastic material cannot be denied, the technique suffers the disadvantages of infection and possible extrusion through the overlying soft tissue. However, the long-term success of Silastic rubber in chin augmentation and in increasing the profile of the Oriental nose has been high. The choice of alloplastic versus autogenous material must be critically made by the surgeon.

Reasons for Postponing the Operation

Temporary or even indefinite postponement for reconstructive or esthetic surgery may occasionally be necessary for various reasons. Time may be needed for infection or inflammation to resolve or for the primary wound to heal, and there may be psychologic factors. Varying periods of time, depending on the vascularity of the region, should be permitted to elapse after the healing of the original wound before reconstruction is initiated. Latent infection disappears during this period, and gradual softening of scar tissue occurs by reestablishment of the hemic and lymphatic circulation.

The passage of time softens and smooths scars, skin grafts, and flaps, permitting the repaired tissues to adapt themselves to the underlying structures. The surgeon must allow sufficient time to elapse to permit revascularization and softening of scar before proceeding to a later stage in reconstruction. There is the famous adage attributed to Gillies: "Never do today what can better be done tomorrow."

The initial tendency to hypertrophic scarring diminishes with the passage of time; this is particularly true in burn deformities. Reconstructive procedures are more successful after the tendency to hypertrophic scarring has lessened.

After other types of traumatic injuries, at least six months should elapse before the secondary repair of scars, skin grafts and flaps, and bone and cartilage grafts is undertaken. The exception to this rule is the functional defect such as the lip injury associated with drooling and problems in mastication. Secondary corrective operations on the nose should be postponed for at least six months.

PLASTIC SURGICAL TECHNIQUE

The modern plastic surgeon has at his disposal an armamentarium including special needleholders, delicate forceps, skin hooks, fine-caliber needles with swedged on synthetic or absorbable suture, magnification, and many other instruments that are used manually or driven mechanically. The basic principles of plastic surgery techniques have been admirably reviewed in the English language by McGregor (1975), Grabb and Smith (1979), and Millard (1986).

The making of incisions with the scalpel at right angles to the skin, careful hemostasis with fine-tipped hemostats, gentleness in handling the tissues to avoid devitalization: these are points of technique that are well known but cannot be overstressed. Hematoma is one of the most frequent causes of failure in plastic surgical operations. The use of precise electrocoagulation, with fine-tipped instruments grasping the bleeding vessel, is an efficient and rapid method of obtaining hemostasis. Small, flat, perforated catheters attached to a suction apparatus and placed under widely undermined skin flaps have reduced the incidence of hematoma and infection.

Figure 1–43. "The figure-of-eight sutures fit for cloven or harelips; as also the dilination of the Needle about whose ends the thred is wrapped over and under, to and again." (From Johnson, T.: The works of that famous chirurgion Ambrose Parey, London, 1649, Richard Cotes and Willi Dugard. Illustration is a copy of Paré's original woodcut.)

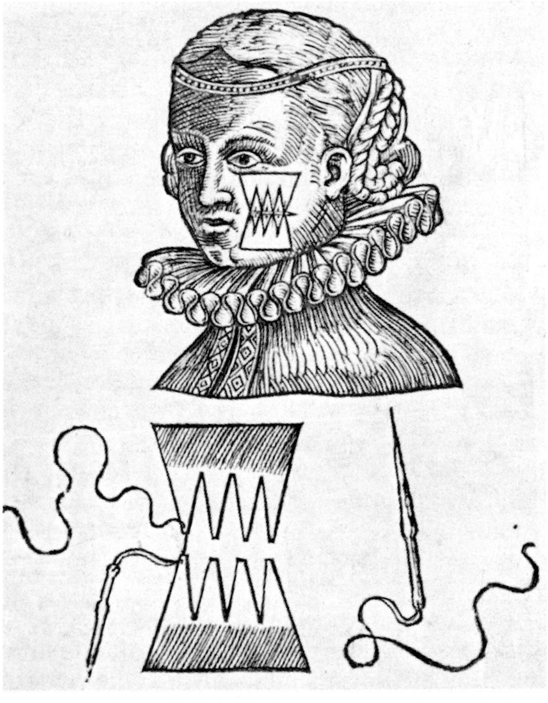

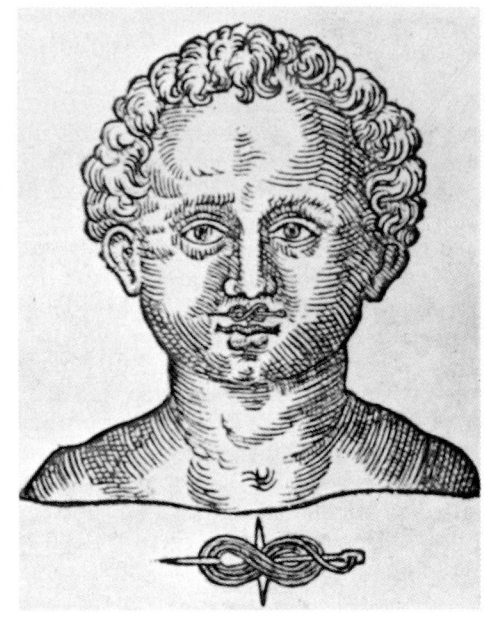

Figure 1–44. Method of using a dry suture to splint and draw together the edges of a cheek wound, as described by Ambroise Paré. (From Johnson, T.: The works of that famous chirurgion Ambrose Parey, London, 1649, Richard Cotes and Willi Du-gard. Illustration is a copy of Paré's original woodcut.)

Suturing

Various techniques were used in the period of Ambroise Paré (1575). Figures 1–43 and 1–44 are redrawn from Paré's works. Figure 1–43 represents the "twisted suture" (la suture entortillée); a straight needle penetrated both edges of the wound and suture material was twisted in a figure-of-eight fashion around the ends of the needle. This technique was employed until the discovery of anesthesia in the nineteenth century, and was used in early cleft lip repairs. Another technique shown by Paré approximates the wound edges by means of sutures passed through cloth glued to the skin surface (la suture agglutinée) (Fig. 1–44). These methods of suturing wounds were still used until the first part of the nineteenth century. Approximation of the wound edges, or reinforcement of the sutured wound, was revived by the introduction of porous papertape Steri-strips (Fig. 1–45).

Precise approximation of skin edges without undue tension ensures primary healing with minimal scarring. The *everting interrupted suture* is the most frequently employed type of suture in plastic surgery (Fig. 1–46). The needle penetrates the epidermis close to the incision line, diverging from the edge of the wound in order to encircle a larger amount of dermis and tissue in the depths of the wound than at the surface. The path of the needle is similar to the outline of a laboratory Erlenmeyer flask. In this manner the suture everts as well as approximates (Fig. 1–47).

The *inverting suture* is required in approximating the skin in the construction of a tube flap or in establishing a skin fold in the upper lid by inverting the skin edge toward the upper edge of the tarsus (Fig. 1–48). Inversion is obtained by changing the pathway of the needle to encircle a larger amount of tissue at the surface of the wound than in the depth of the wound; inversion is also obtained by placing the sutures superficially in the skin. The disadvantage of the inverting suture is

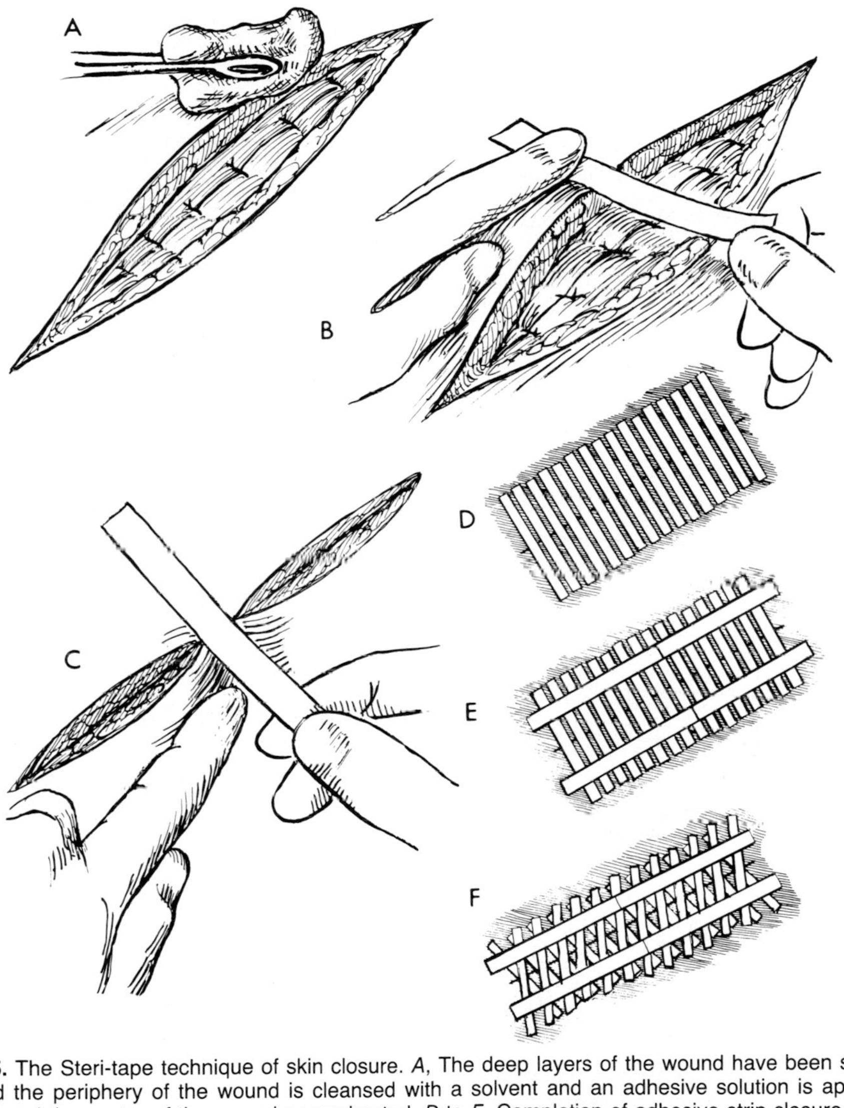

Figure 1–45. The Steri-tape technique of skin closure. *A*, The deep layers of the wound have been sutured. The skin surface around the periphery of the wound is cleansed with a solvent and an adhesive solution is applied. *B*, *C*, First strip is applied and the center of the wound approximated. *D* to *F*, Completion of adhesive strip closure.

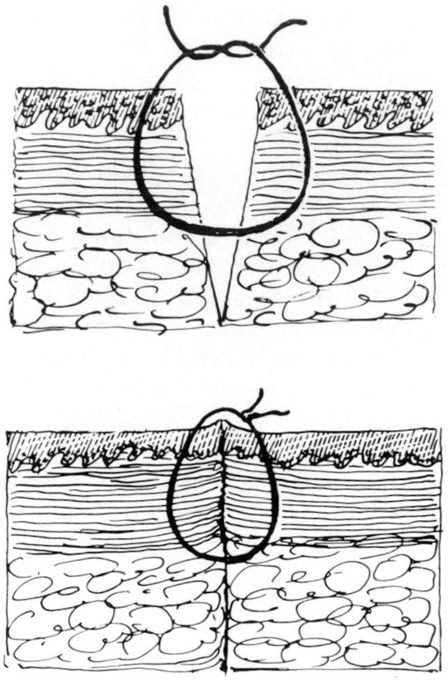

Figure 1–46. The everting interrupted suture: correct manner of placing a suture to produce eversion. The needle should be placed to form a wider loop deep in the tissue to obtain eversion. The outline of the suture path is similar to an Erlenmeyer flask.

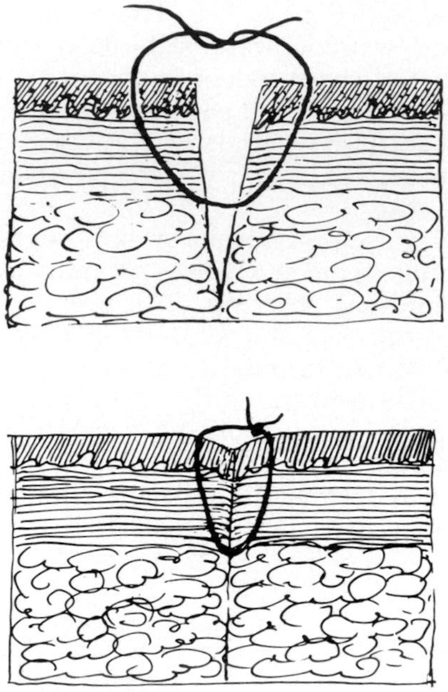

Figure 1–48. Inverting suture: placing the suture to produce inversion. Inversion of wound edges is produced when the suture loop is wider superficially than it is deep in the tissues.

the progressive widening of the resulting scar.

Subcuticular buried sutures are placed on the undersurface of the cutis (dermis) with the knot downward beneath the dermis; these are useful approximating sutures if tension is present and a widened scar is feared (Fig. 1–49).

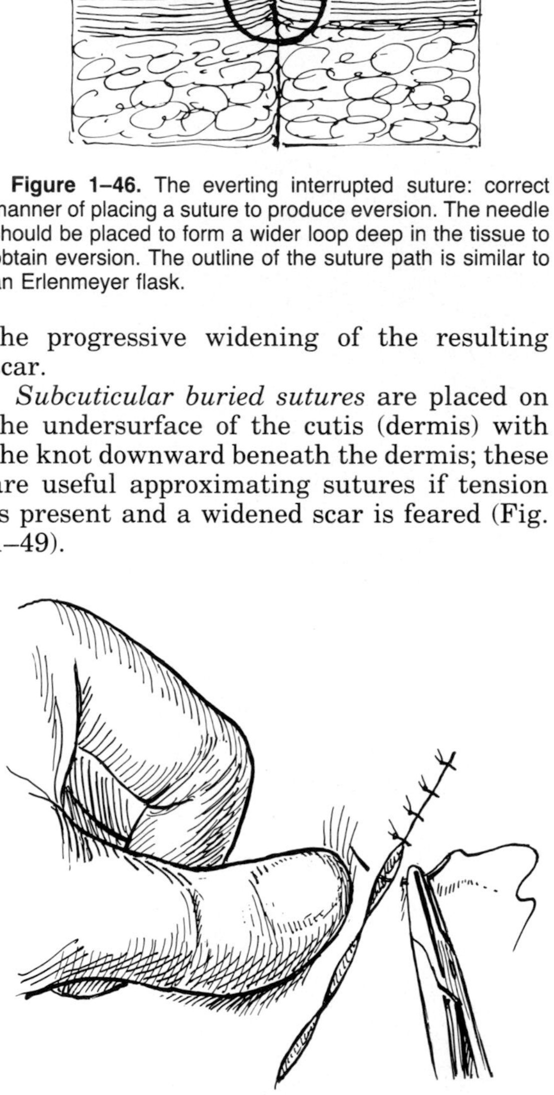

Figure 1–47. Placing interrupted sutures. Eversion can often be obtained by slight thumb pressure, by lightly applied fine tooth forceps, or by means of a skin hook.

Special sutures such as *vertical mattress sutures* (Fig. 1–50) are also useful to evert the wound edges or maintain the skin coapted to the underlying fascial layer. They are rarely indicated on the face.

The *horizontal mattress suture with a dermal component* (Fig. 1–51), the suture being placed through the undersurface of the dermis, is useful at the scalp-skin junction if there is tension. The dermal component avoids suture marks in the skin. The suture also gives excellent approximation of the edge of a skin flap to the edge of the recipient site; the dermal component is placed through the dermis of the flap. The suture assists in joining a thicker wound edge to a thinner wound edge and equalizing the level of the epithelial layers. It is especially indicated in the closure of the retroauricular scalp incision of the facialplasty.

In some areas, as satisfactory an approxi-

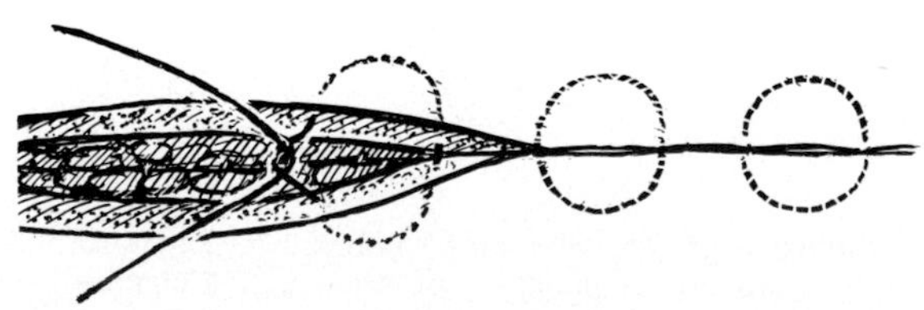

Figure 1–49. Interrupted subcuticular sutures.

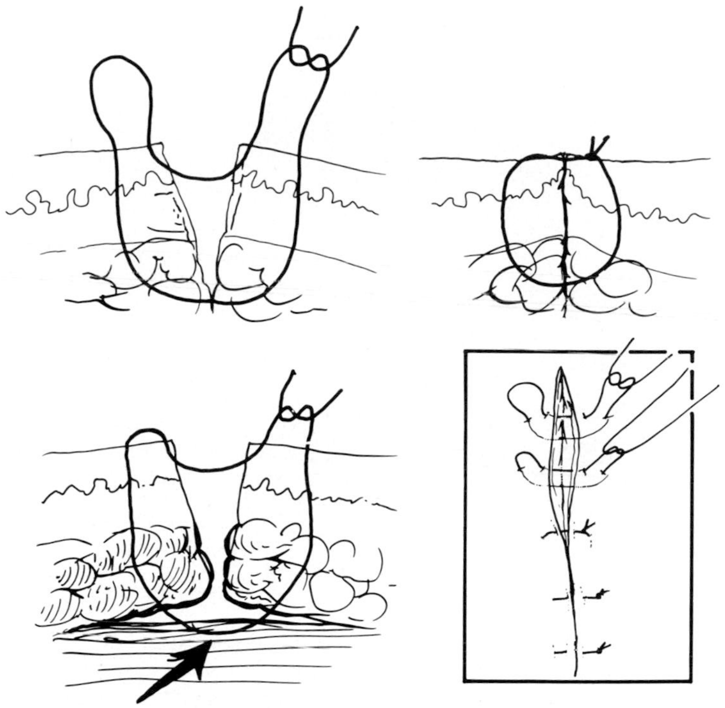

Figure 1–50. The vertical mattress suture.

mation can be obtained by a carefully inserted *continuous running suture* as by interrupted sutures (Fig. 1–52) provided that each suture penetration is carefully executed.

The *removable continuous intradermal suture* (Fig. 1–53) is of particular value in children, whose skin is normally under greater tension than that of the adult and in whom suture marks are apt to occur. Each suture should penetrate the undersurface of the dermis 1 or 2 mm from the wound edge in order to obtain slight eversion and satisfactory approximation. The continuous subcuticular suture may be left in place for a longer period, thus ensuring the maturation of collagen in the wound without danger of suture marks. A precaution must be taken in using a subcuticular suture: the suture must be looped through the skin at intervals, depending on the length of the wound and the area of the body in which it is located. If this precaution is not taken, the suture may resist removal. The protruding ends of the suture are buried by means of the procedure illustrated in Figure 1–54 if the suture cannot be withdrawn.

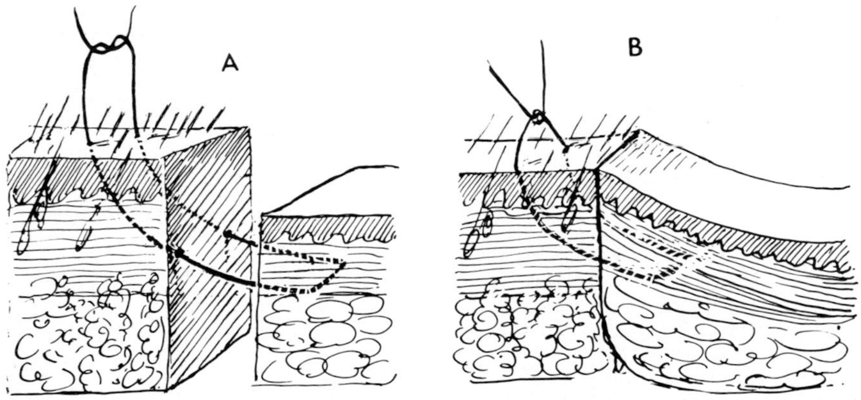

Figure 1–51. Horizontal mattress suture with an intradermal component. *A*, *B*, Eversion of thinner skin to obtain satisfactory approximation with thicker scalp tissue.

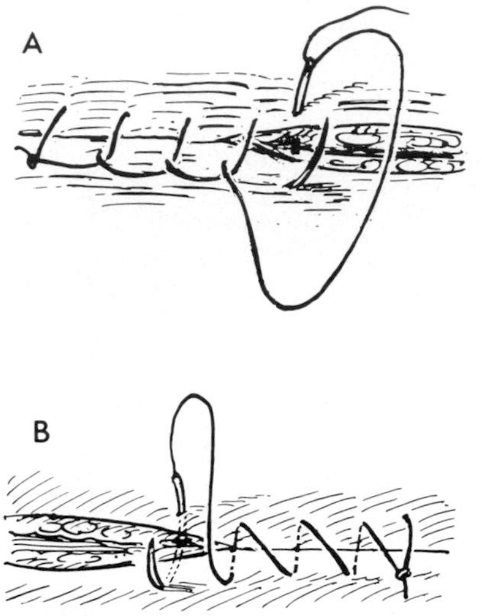

Figure 1–52. Continuous running suture. *A*, Continuous locking suture. *B*, Continuous nonlocking suture.

Subcutaneous sutures are also employed to obtain layer-by-layer closure in deep wounds to eliminate dead space and to help relieve tension in an advancement flap.

Variations in Technique of Wound Suturing. It may be advisable to leave a base of scar tissue and suture the wound edges over the base after excising the superficial portion of a depressed scar (Fig. 1–55). An ingenious technique to diminish tension on skin is that advocated by Millard (1970) (Fig. 1–56). A flap of subcutaneous fat may also be advanced from beneath one wound edge to augment a thinner opposing wound edge.

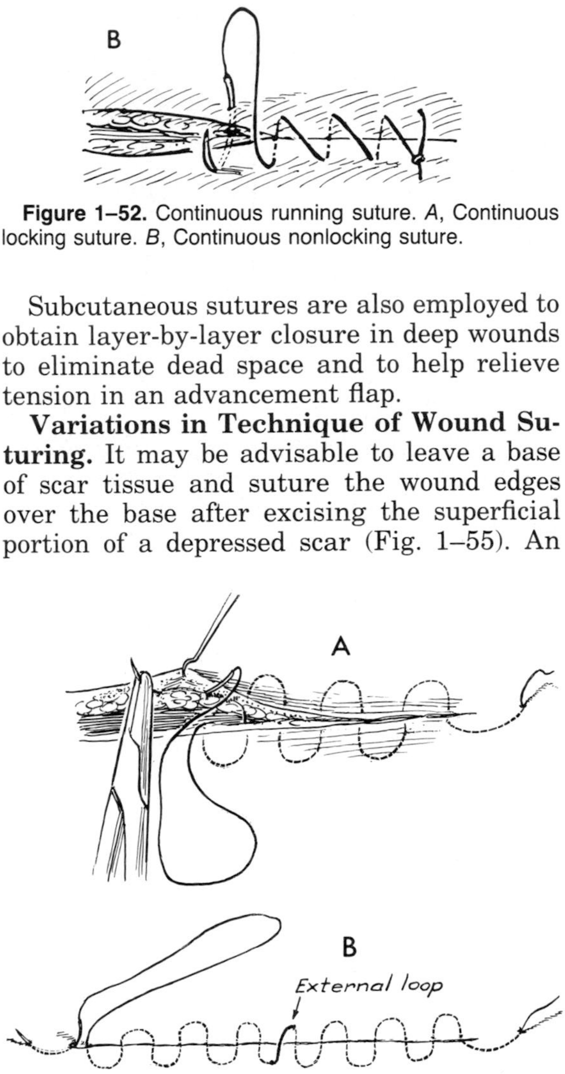

Figure 1–53. The removable continuous subcuticular suture. *A*, The suture has been placed through the epidermal surface and is introduced into the wound through the dermis. A hook everts the wound edge, permitting the needle to penetrate the undersurface of the dermis. *B*, The subcuticular sutures are being completed and the needle is being brought out through the epidermis. Note that the suture is brought out through the skin halfway across the wound (or more often in longer wounds) to facilitate its eventual removal.

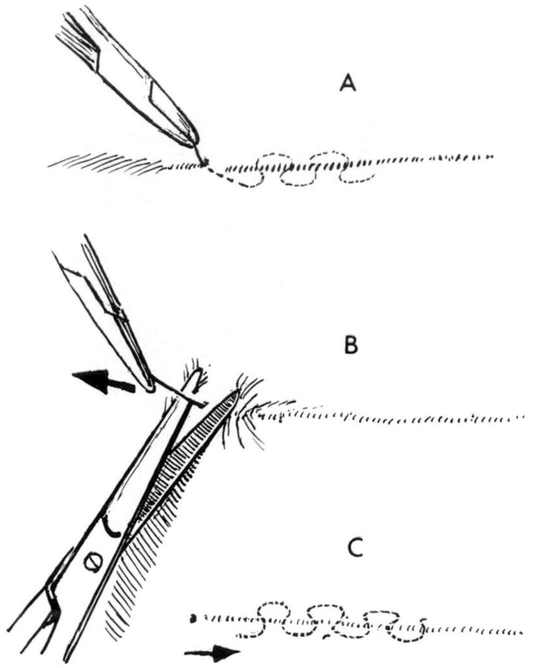

Figure 1–54. What to do if a subcuticular suture cannot be removed or a portion of it ruptures during removal. *A*, The protruding end is grasped with a hemostat. *B*, Traction is exerted by the hemostat, and pressure is applied on the skin by the blades of scissors. *C*, The end of the suture retracts under the skin.

"Depuckering" the Pucker. When the two sides of an elliptic wound are of equal length, the wound may be closed without a resulting pucker at one end. If the two sides are unequal or if the ellipse has a wide curvature, a pucker or "dog-ear" is inevitable. The problem is to "depucker" without unduly extending the length of the wound. The technique shown in Figure 1–57 has given satisfactory results.

Pressure Dressings

A pressure dressing reduces the size of a dead space, prevents hematoma formation, and immobilizes skin grafts, especially in a concave recipient site. The need for a compressive dressing varies according to the type of operation and the area in which it is performed. In most skin grafting procedures,

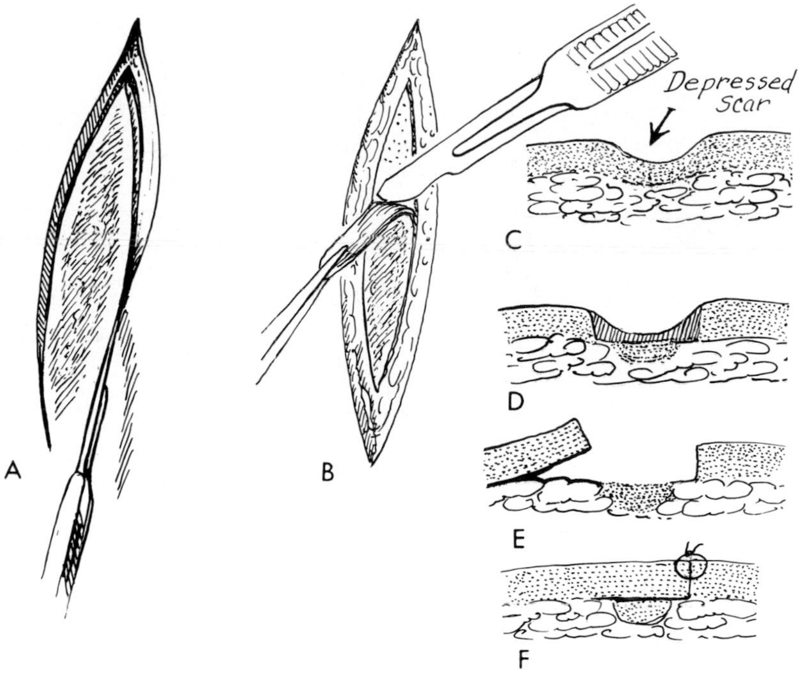

Figure 1–55. Partial excision of the scar. *A, B*, In a depressed scar it may be advisable to leave a base of scar tissue and suture the wound edges over the base, excising the superficial portion of the scar. *C*, Sectional view illustrating the depressed scar. *D*, Crosslined area illustrates the excised portion of the scar. *E*, The undermining of one side of the wound. *F*, The wound edge has been advanced over the scar and sutured to the contralateral side.

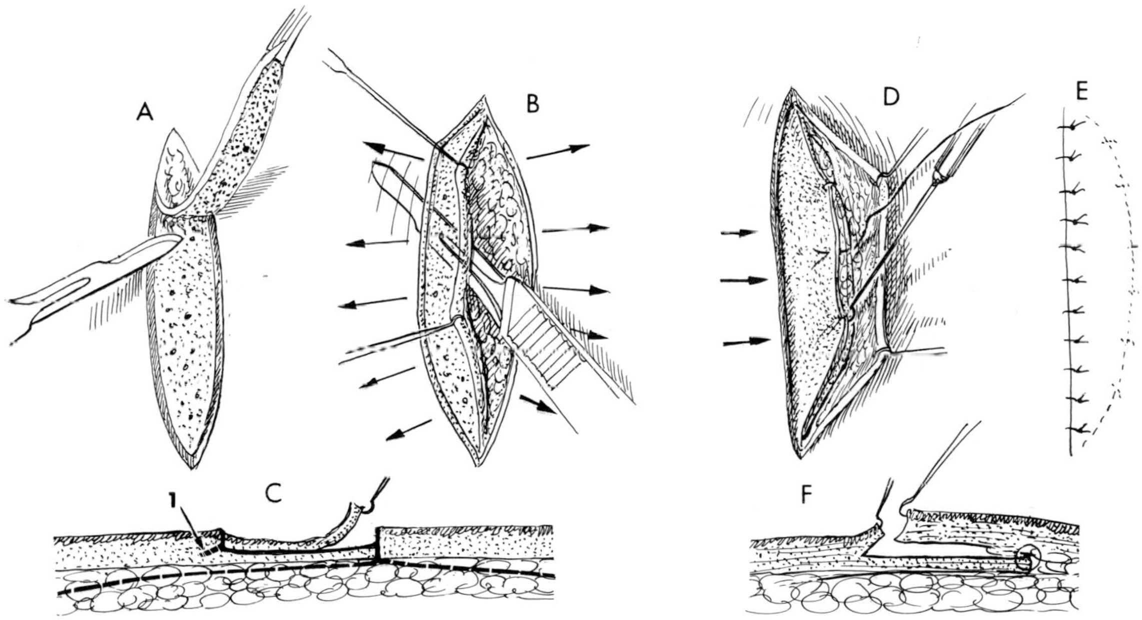

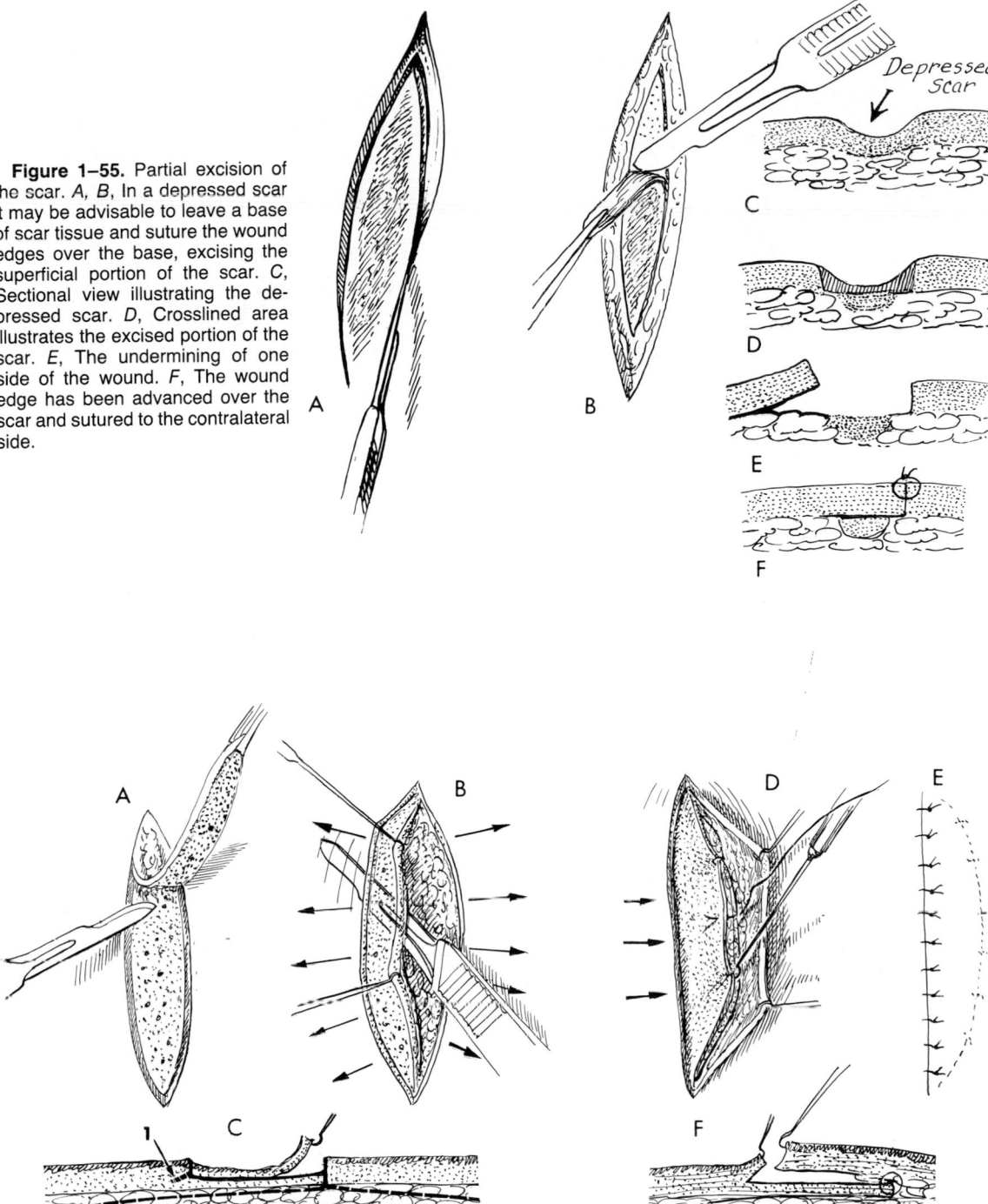

Figure 1–56. The use of scar tissue after split-thickness excision of the scar to diminish tension on the sutured wound. *A*, Partial excision of scar. *B*, Remaining scar tissue is undermined. *C*, Split-thickness excision of scar. Note the short incision (1) made to facilitate the advancement flap. *D to F*, Flap of dermal scar is advanced and sutured subcutaneously into the undermined area on the opposite side of the scar. The purpose of this technique is to release tension from the sutured wound. (After Millard, D. R.: Scar repair by double-vested principle. Plast. Reconstr. Surg., *45*:616, 1970.)

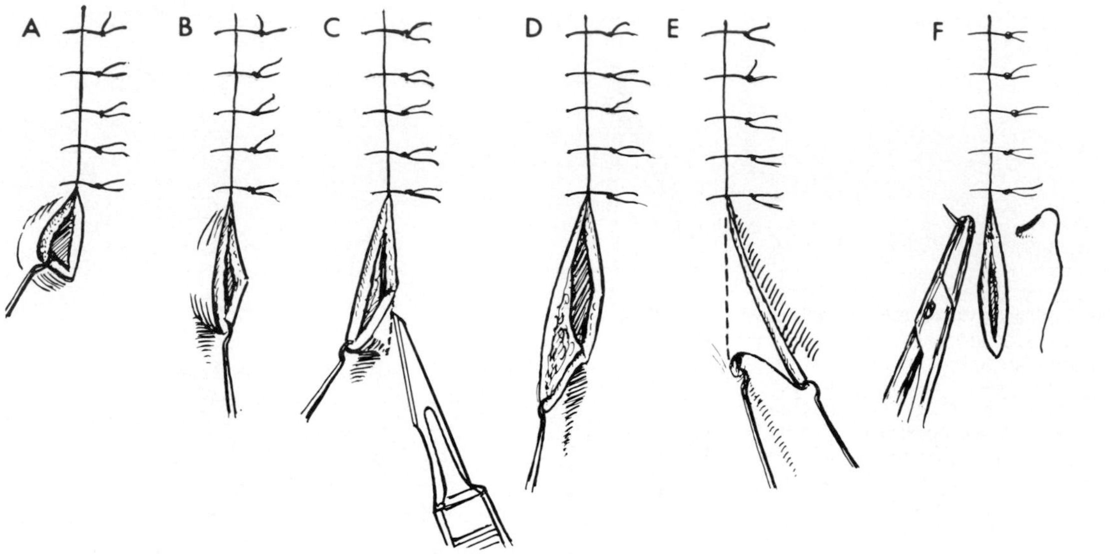

Figure 1–57. "Depuckering" the pucker (or removal of a dog-ear). *A*, The excess tissue is retracted by a hook. *B*, A hook is placed at the end of the incision. *C*, The hook retracts the tissue laterally, and a sharp, pointed blade (#11) makes an incision in direct prolongation of the sutured wound. *D*, The resultant flap is retracted. *E*, The flap of excess tissue is overlapped over the proposed line of suture. Note the hook exerting traction at the end of the incision line. The dotted lines indicate the line of incision for the removal of the excess tissue. *F*, The elongated wound is sutured.

the compressive or bolus dressing may be the most important part of the operation, ensuring as it does the close coaptation of the graft to the recipient site. Skin grafting may be done without a compressive dressing in certain selected cases in which careful observation ensures that the graft remains in contact with the recipient bed. Compressive dressings are not necessary in certain types of procedures in which only the integument is involved, and may be dispensed with if they are uncomfortable to the patient. The open method of treatment (Wallace, 1949) may be preferable to treat burns or abraded areas. A pressure dressing may also be unnecessary when the wound has been closed without undermining the edges of the wound.

Suction catheters have replaced pressure dressings in areas where they are difficult to apply, e.g., the scapular region or cervical area following the elevation of skin flaps for a neck dissection. It should be emphasized that, while hematoma is one of the most frequent complications in plastic surgery, suction devices will not *prevent* a large hematoma formation.

Transplantation

"To transplant" (from the latin verb *transplantare*) designates the removal of a colony of living cells from a donor area and its transfer to a recipient site where it is capable of propagating a lineage of living cells. The term is employed for the transfer of tissues or an organ from one part of the body to another, or from one individual to another. The term "graft" (from the French *greffe*) is essentially synonymous with the term "transplant."

Various terms have become accepted to define the modes of transplantation: *autograft* designates a graft transferred from one area to another in the same individual; *allograft* ("homograft") defines a graft transplanted between individuals of the same species; *xenograft* ("heterograft") indicates the transplantation of tissue between individuals of different species.

The term *isograft* is usually employed to designate an allograft between highly inbred (genetically pure) strains of animals. *Syngenesiotransplantation* is the grafting of tissue, not between two individuals of ordinary genetic diversity, as in the allograft, but between individuals of close genetic relationship. *Brephoplasty* (May, 1934) indicates the grafting of embryonic tissues.

Replantation designates the surgical procedure whereby tissue or a structure is replaced in its original site. The term *implantation* is employed in this text to designate the insertion into the tissues of a foreign, relatively inert material referred to as an "inorganic implant" (see Chap. 20).

Two methods of skin transplantation are available, mediate and immediate. In *mediate* transplantation of skin, the survival of the transplant is ensured by a pedicle to which it remains attached until vessels have grown into the flap from the recipient site–hence the term "skin flap" (see Chap. 9).

In *immediate* transplantation of skin, a portion of skin is completely detached from its vascular connections, and revascularization of the transplant is accomplished by vascular connections and ingrowth of vessels from the host site; this type of free transplant is known as a "skin graft" (see Chap. 8). The development of microvascular surgery has permitted the immediate transfer of a skin flap, the *microvascular free flap* (see Chap. 12).

Transplantation of other tissues, such as dermis (Chap. 14), fat (Chap. 14), fascia (Chap. 14), tendon (Chap. 15), muscle (Chap. 16), nerve (Chap. 19), cartilage (Chap. 17), and bone (Chap. 18) is discussed in individual chapters.

There are specific indications for the use of inorganic implants as useful adjuncts to other surgical procedures (Chap. 20).

The Full-Thickness Defect, the Straight Line, and Wound Tension: Three Enemies of the Plastic Surgeon

The first enemy is a wound devoid of integument. The wound contracts; the result is a contracture with deformity and functional impairment. If it cannot contract, the wound may progress toward an indolent ulcer. *Consequently the full-thickness defect is to be repaired.* Skin covering should always be provided by direct approximation, the application of a skin graft, or the transfer of a flap. In the reconstruction of a full-thickness defect of the cheek or the nose, for example, a lining as well as a surface covering should be provided.

The *straight line*, situated neither within nor parallel to a line of minimal tension, is the second enemy of the plastic surgeon, since contraction along the straight line causes distortion and contracture and results in hypertrophy of the resulting scar. The straight line must be interrupted by a Z-plasty or W-plasty in order to distribute the contractile forces in more than one direction. This principle is the basis of techniques developed to avoid contraction of straight scars that run at variance with the lines of minimal tension. The Z-plasty is the plastic surgeon's best friend, and the W-plasty can also be helpful. The straight line, when situated in a favorable site (along a line of minimal tension) and when the wound edges are sutured meticulously, is not an enemy: the resulting hairline scar is inconspicuous.

Wound tension should be avoided at all costs. Undermining the wound edges is helpful but usually gives only partial relief of tension. Disruption of wounds, cross-hatching stitch marks, widening and thickening of scars, and necrosis of flaps are the consequences of excessive wound tension. Skin grafts or skin flaps are required when direct approximation of the wound edges cannot be achieved without undue tension.

THE Z-PLASTY

One of the most widely employed techniques in plastic surgery is the Z-plasty, characterized by the transposition of two triangularly shaped flaps (Fig. 1–58). The Z-plasty serves three purposes: (1) lengthening of a linear scar contracture; (2) dispersal of the scar, thus breaking up the straight-line scar; and (3) realigning the scar within the lines of minimal tension. Elongation and interruption of the straight line and release of the linear scar contracture prevent its recurrence.

Development of Z-Plasty. Borges (1974) has researched the origin and development of the Z-plasty. The first procedures consisted of a single transposition flap, hardly what we could call a true Z-plasty. Such procedures were described by Fricke (1829), Horner (1837), Serre (1842), and Denonvilliers (1854). These procedures involved the transposition of a flap from the temporal area or from the cheek to correct ectropion of the lip or eyelid. McCurdy published a number of articles on what he called the "Z-plastic method" between 1898 and 1924. Although his first Z-plasty procedures were not true Z-plasties, he is credited with the current popularization of the Z-plasty technique. Berger in 1904 was the first to describe a true Z-plasty.

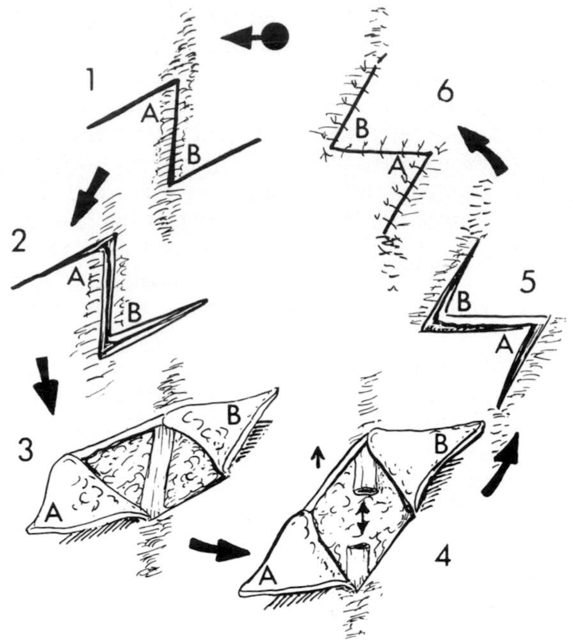

Figure 1–58. Z-plasty technique (after McGregor). *1*, Central limb designed along the scar. Both limbs are equal in length. Angles A and B are 60°. *2, 3*, Flaps are incised and elevated. *4*, Release of deeper portion of the scar. *5*, Transposition of triangular flaps. *6*, Wounds are approximated. Note lengthening and new direction of the scar.

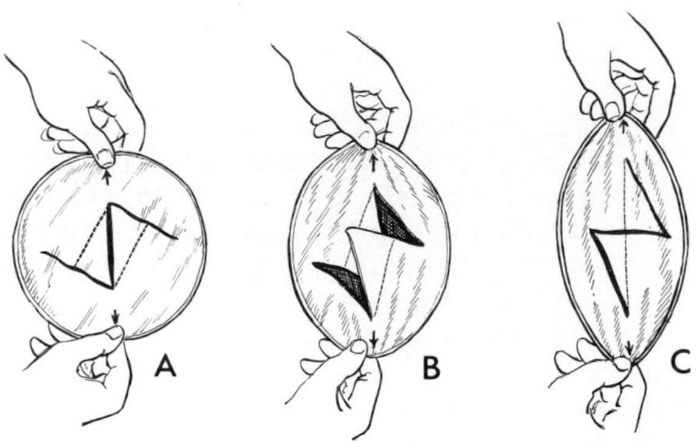

Figure 1–59. Elongation obtained by the Z-plasty (after Limberg).

The first description of multiple Z-plasties was by Morestin in 1914. The flaps were incised and allowed to shift in place without undermining. According to Woolf and Broadbent (1972), the geometric principles involved in the Z-plasty were first described by Limberg in 1929. Limberg's classic book (1946) contains a description of the many applications of the Z-plasty technique. Davis and Kitlowski (1939) reviewed their experience with use of the Z-plasty, and Davis reviewed the practical applications of the principle in 1946. McGregor (1957) also discussed the theoretical basis of the Z-plasty. The books of Kazanjian and Converse (1959, 1974) and of Grabb and Smith (1968, 1979) have also discussed this technique in considerable detail. Borges (1973) published a book, the subject matter of which is entirely devoted to the Z- and W-plasties.

Technique of Z-Plasty. In the classic Z-plasty the two triangular flaps of skin and subcutaneous tissue of equal size and depth are delimited by the three incisions of equal length cut at a 60-degree angle (see Fig. 1–58); the line of contracture is thus broken and also lengthened (Fig. 1–59). The length of the central limb and the angles of the Z determine the size of the flaps. The longer the central limb, the more lengthening is obtained, all the limbs being of the same length (Fig. 1–60). If the incisions outlining the Z-plasty are not of the same length, puckering of the flaps results (Fig. 1–61). (See exceptions under Variations in the Z-plasty Technique.)

In addition to its lengthening effect, the value of the Z-plasty lies in the redistribution of tension and dispersal of the scar (Fig. 1–62).

A Z-plasty in the middle of a long scar breaks the continuity and elongates the scar. Multiple Z-plasties (Fig. 1–63) have been employed successfully in linear, contracted scars and are preferred to a single, large Z-plasty, especially in the face.

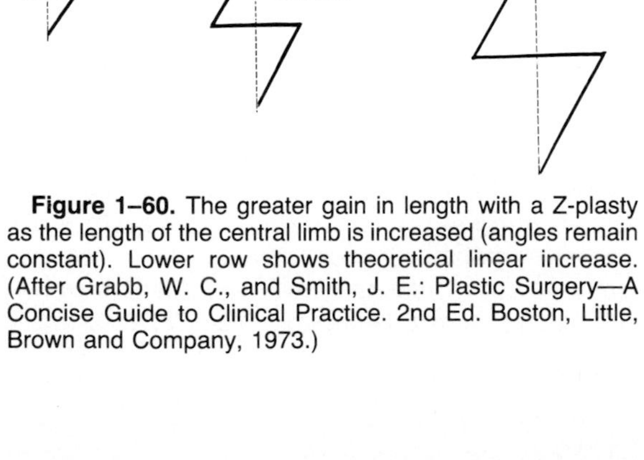

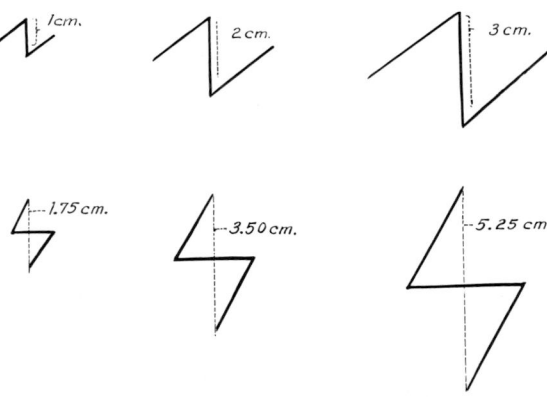

Figure 1–60. The greater gain in length with a Z-plasty as the length of the central limb is increased (angles remain constant). Lower row shows theoretical linear increase. (After Grabb, W. C., and Smith, J. E.: Plastic Surgery—A Concise Guide to Clinical Practice. 2nd Ed. Boston, Little, Brown and Company, 1973.)

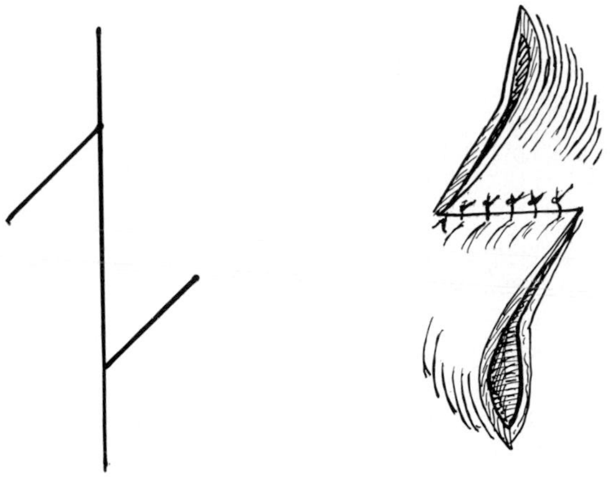

Figure 1–61. Puckering of the flaps results when the central member and limbs of the Z-plasty are of unequal length.

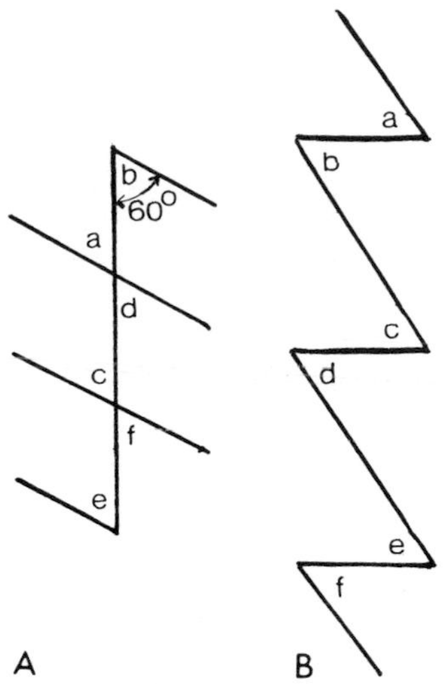

Figure 1–63. Multiple Z-plasty technique (after Davis and Kitlowski, 1939). *A*, Design. *B*, Final appearance following transposition of flaps. The technique is preferred to a single large Z-plasty in the revision of long, linear scars, especially on the face.

Staige Davis had noted (1931) that release of scar contracture by means of the Z-plasty technique resulted in an improvement in the quality of scar tissue, the tissue becoming softer and better appearing. He reaffirmed this observation in subsequent papers (Davis and Kitlowski, 1939; Davis, 1946). A modification of collagen structure has been demonstrated in the scarred area following a Z-plasty procedure (Longacre and associates, 1966). Both depressed scars and hypertrophic scars often become inconspicuous following excision and the interruption of the linear contracture by one or multiple Z-plasties.

Amount of Elongation According to the Z-Flap Design. Much has been written about the degree of elongation obtained by varying the angles of the segments of the Z-plasty. While the geometric calculations appear accurate on paper, there are too many unpredictable factors in the patient to make them reliable. Theoretical considerations, although demonstrable on a piece of rubber sheeting or chamois skin, where the tension is equally distributed, are useless from a clinical point of view. Skin tension varies because of the presence of scar tissue that is unequally distributed and is not of the same thickness on both sides of the contracture. In the usual clinical situation when one needs to elongate an area because of distortion of landmarks or web formation (often after burns), one employs the most useful Z-plasty angle, which is usually 60 degrees. Greater elongation can be obtained by the use of wide flaps (see The Four-Flap Z-plasty).

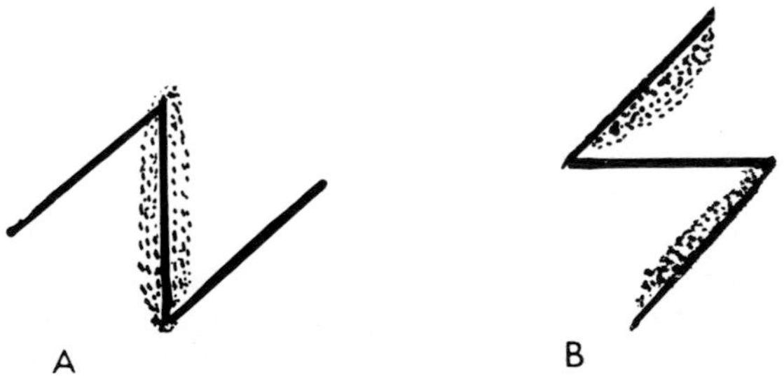

Figure 1–62. Dispersal of scar follows transposition of the flaps in a Z-plasty (stippled area represents scar tissue).

Use of Z-Plasty to Realign the Scar within Lines of Minimal Tension. The Z-plasty (or W-plasty) should not be used if the scar does not cross a line of minimal tension. Resection by elliptic incision (fusiform excision) is preferred in this situation.

It takes courage to increase deliberately the length of a clean linear scar, even though it is unsatisfactory because it crosses the lines of minimal tension. No amount of care in meticulously suturing the wound will help if the scar is in an unfavorable position.

The application of the Z-plasty principle for the realignment of a scar crossing a line of minimal tension is most useful but requires careful consideration. The angles of the Z-flaps vary according to the obliquity of the scar in relation to the lines of minimal tension, and may be considerably less than 60 degrees. The more oblique the scar, the more

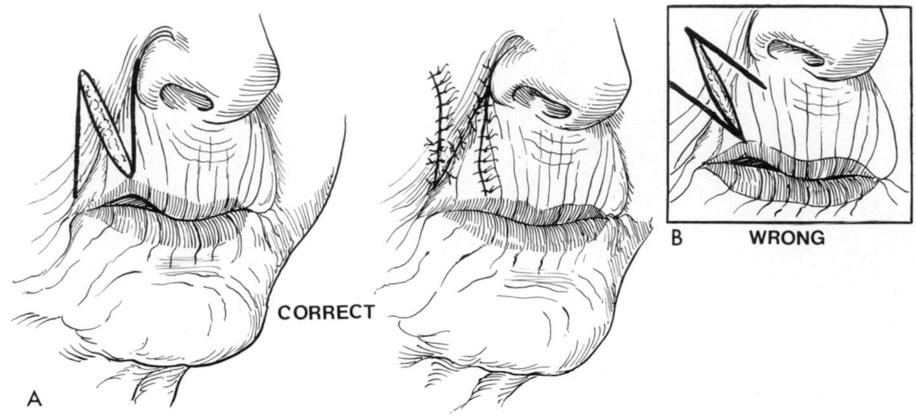

Figure 1–64. The angles of the Z-flaps vary according to the obliquity of the scar and its relation to the line of minimal tension; the more oblique the scar, the more acute the angle of the Z-flaps. *A*, Note that the scar is traversing the nasolabial fold obliquely. The flaps have been designed. The angles are less than 60 degrees. *B*, Flaps have been transposed. The Z was designed so that the ends of the limbs fall into the nasolabial fold. *Insert*, wrong design of the Z-plasty: the limbs of the Z cross the lines of minimal tension. (After Borges, A. F., and Alexander, J. E.: Relaxed skin tension lines, Z-plasties on scars and fusiform excision of lesions. Br. J. Plast. Surg., *15*:242, 1962.)

acute is the angle of the Z-flaps. This concept is illustrated in Figure 1–64. In the realignment of a scar crossing the nasolabial fold, the angles of the Z-flaps may be more acute. It is necessary to design the Z so that the ends of the limbs fall into the nasolabial fold.

The closer the scar is directed toward a right angle crossing of the lines of minimal tension, the more do the angles of the Z-plasty limbs approach 60 degrees.

In the design of any Z-plasty, the limbs should follow the lines of minimal tension (Fig. 1–65*A*). Thus, after transposition, the limbs follow the lines of minimal tension. If the design were made in the opposite direction, the Z would cross the lines of minimal tension (Fig. 1–65*B*).

Figure 1–66*B* illustrates the advantage of two small Z-plasties over one large Z-plasty (Fig. 1–66*A*) in breaking up the scar into smaller components separated by normal tissue. Figure 1–66*C* illustrates a Z-plasty whose central limb is placed in the middle of a long scar; as stated earlier, an improvement is achieved by the lengthening, relaxation, and interruption of the longitudinal tension.

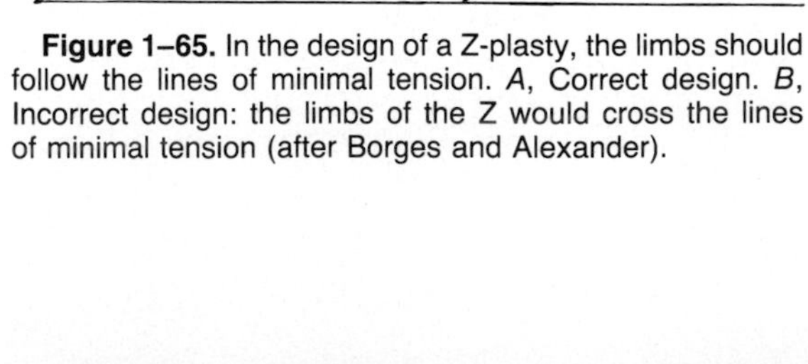

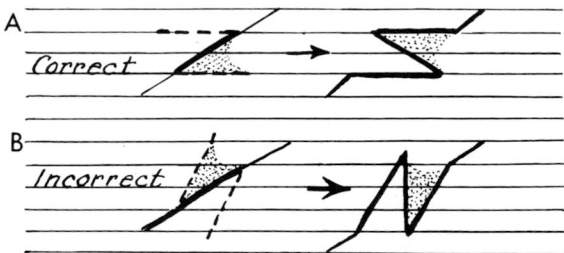

Figure 1–65. In the design of a Z-plasty, the limbs should follow the lines of minimal tension. *A*, Correct design. *B*, Incorrect design: the limbs of the Z would cross the lines of minimal tension (after Borges and Alexander).

Variations in Z-Plasty Technique

Unequal Triangles. Triangles of an unequal size are indicated in the Z-plasty when the skin on one side of the central segment is loose and the other side requires more elongation, particularly in burn patients when the resection of the scar tissue on that side is not indicated (Fig. 1–67). This is an application of the "half-Z" procedure, which consists of a flap fitted into an incision made in the opposing wound edge and is a technique for lengthening the short side (Fig. 1–68). One incision is made almost at right angles to the border of the defect on the short side, while the other forms a more acute triangular flap on the long side. The width of the base of the triangular flap determines the amount of lengthening of the short side, into which it is inserted. This technique can be employed only when the tissues are soft and pliable. The length of the limbs of the Z-plasty may also vary when the irregular scar requires lengthening and relaxation (Fig. 1–69). The S-plasty (Fig. 1–70), a variation of the Z-plasty, is employed in cervical con-

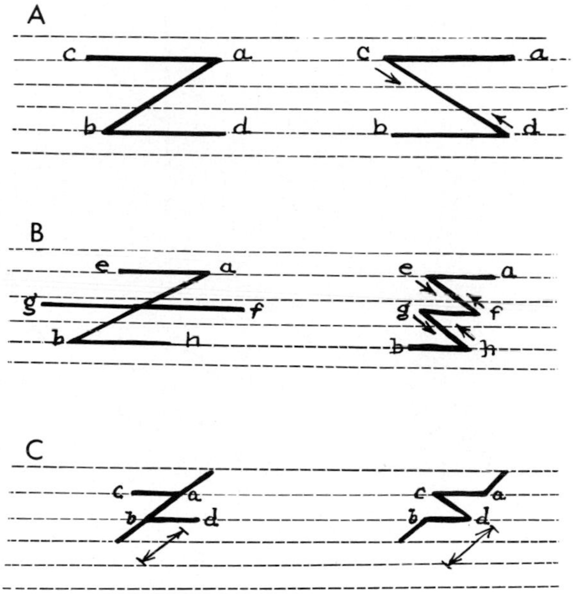

Figure 1–66. *A*, Inadequacy of a single large Z-plasty. The direction of the scar (central limb) is reversed, but its direction is not improved in relation to the lines of minimal tension and its length is not broken up into smaller scars. *B*, If one designs two or more Z-plasties, the long scar is divided into smaller, less contractile segments. *C*, A Z-plasty in the middle of a long scar interrupts the longitudinal contraction of the scar and elongates it (after Borges and Alexander).

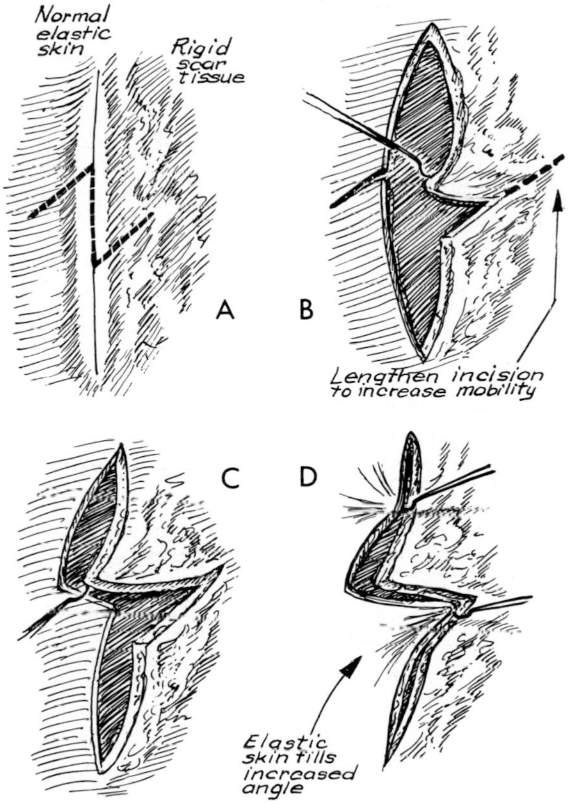

Figure 1–67. Z-plasty with flaps of unequal size. *A*, Scarred area in which one bank consists of thin, elastic skin, whereas the other bank contains thick, rigid, scarred skin. *B*, Central scar has been excised. The Z-flap on the scarred bank has been elongated to provide greater mobility. *C, D*, Transposition of flaps.

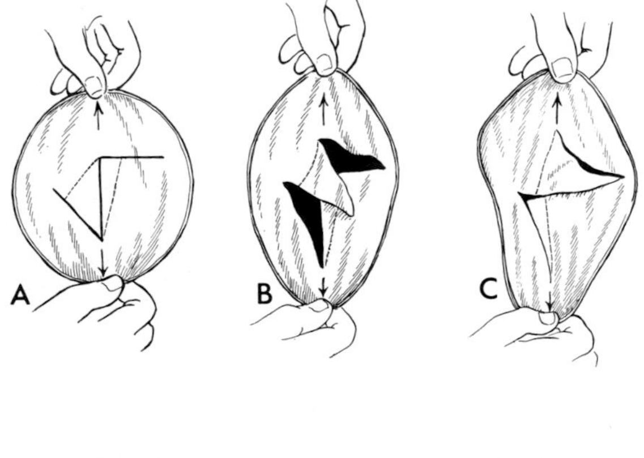

Figure 1–68. Half-Z technique. *A*, Arrows indicate direction of elongation; Z-incision is indicated. *B*, Preparation of Z-flaps. *C*, Elongation obtained by Z-plasty technique (after Limberg, 1946.) The insertion of the triangular flap into the horizontal incision elongates the right bank (in drawing) more than the left bank.

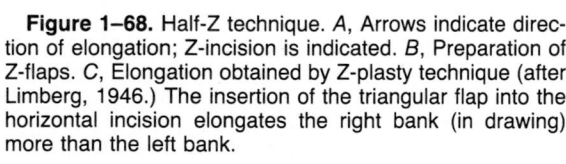

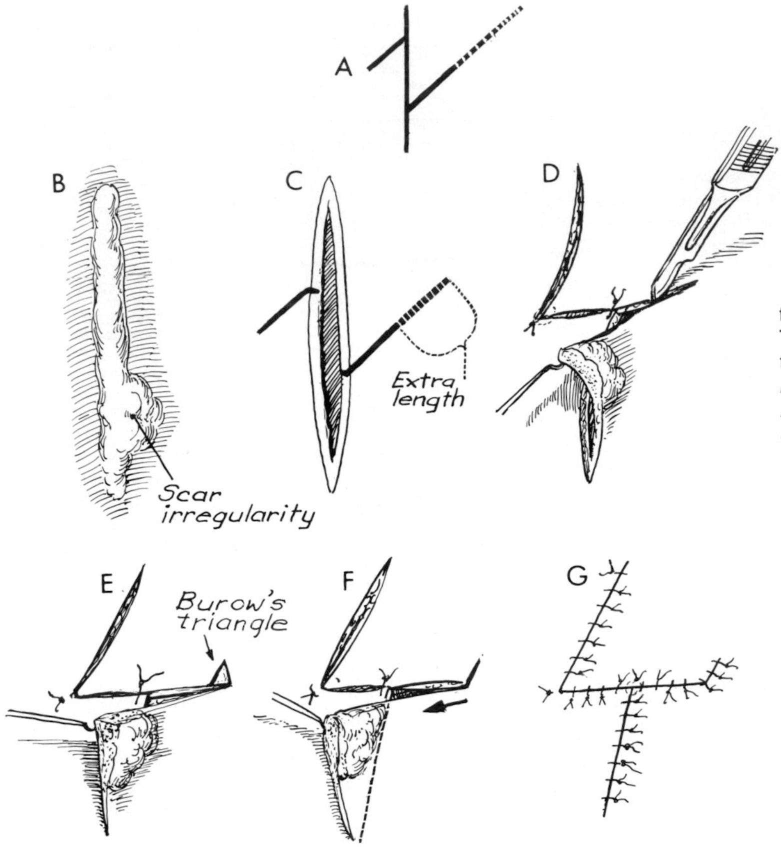

Figure 1–69. Z-plasty with unequal triangles. *A*, Z-plasty. *B*, Scar tissue. *C*, The main portion of the scar is excised through elliptical incisions. Z-flaps (*A* to *D*) are outlined. *D*, Flaps are transposed. Additional scar tissue excision is required as indicated. *E*, In order to avoid a pucker, a small Burow's triangle is excised as indicated in *E*. The flap containing scar tissue is advanced. *F*, Scar tissue is excised. *G*, Completion of Z-plasty with unequal triangles.

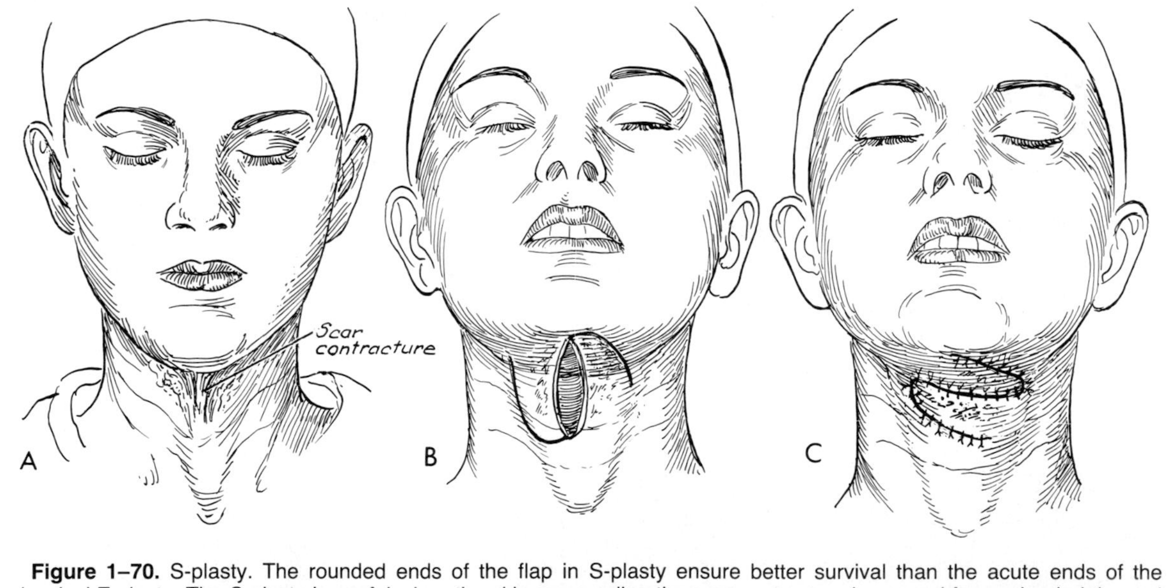

Figure 1–70. S-plasty. The rounded ends of the flap in S-plasty ensure better survival than the acute ends of the classical Z-plasty. The S-plasty is useful when the skin surrounding the scar contracture is scarred from a healed thermal burn. *A*, Scar contracture of neck. *B*, S-plasty. *C*, The S-plasty has been completed.

tractures, as the tips of the flaps are less susceptible to necrosis than those with the acute angle of the classic Z-plasty. It is especially indicated when the involved area includes healed, burned skin or skin graft (Converse, 1964).

Double Opposing Z-Plasties. Double opposing Z-plasties (Fig. 1–71) are particularly effective in interrupting a line of contracture when the anatomic position of the contracture does not permit the use of large flaps, such as in the medial canthal region for the correction of epicanthal folds (Converse and Smith, 1966). Double opposing Z-plasties are also useful in diminishing the size of the Z-plasty flaps when the vascularization of the flaps is precarious, such as is frequent in

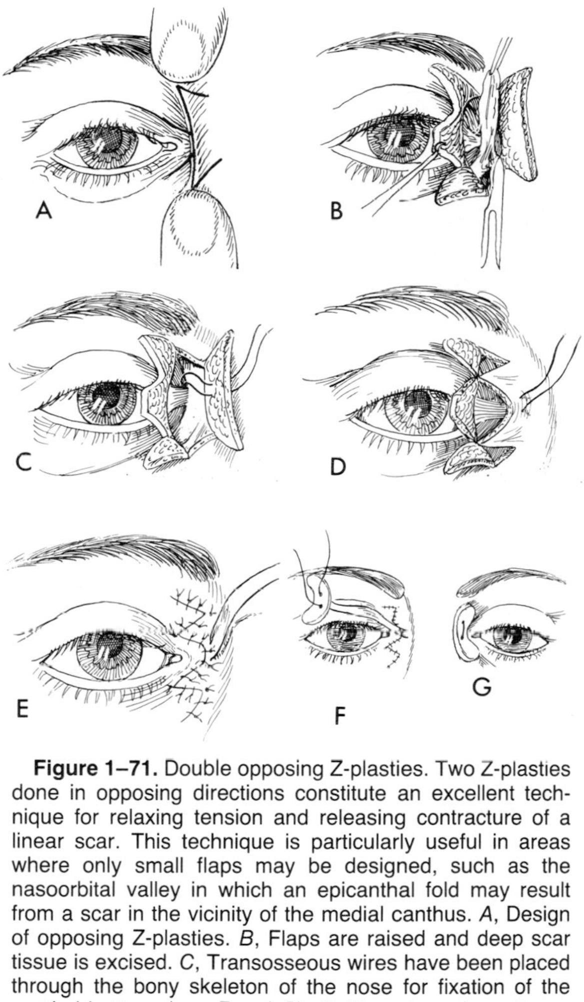

Figure 1–71. Double opposing Z-plasties. Two Z-plasties done in opposing directions constitute an excellent technique for relaxing tension and releasing contracture of a linear scar. This technique is particularly useful in areas where only small flaps may be designed, such as the nasoorbital valley in which an epicanthal fold may result from a scar in the vicinity of the medial canthus. *A*, Design of opposing Z-plasties. *B*, Flaps are raised and deep scar tissue is excised. *C*, Transosseous wires have been placed through the bony skeleton of the nose for fixation of the canthal buttons (see *F* and *G*). *D*, Flaps have been transposed. *E*, Double opposing Z-plasties completed. *F, G*, Canthal buttons maintained by through-and-through wiring.

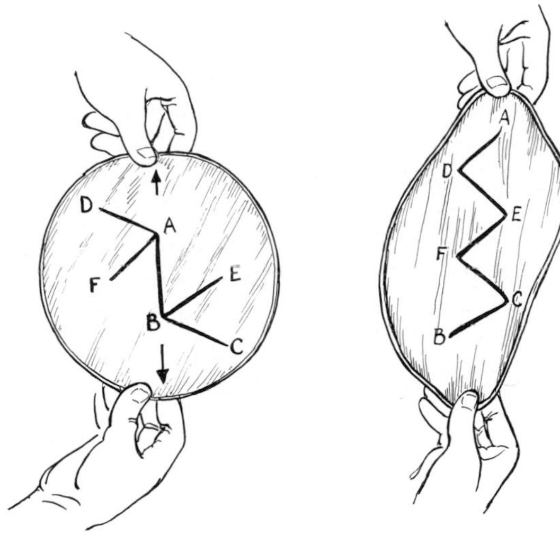

Figure 1–72. The Limberg *(left)* design of the four-flap Z-plasty. The technique consists of outlining wide angle flaps, which are then divided into separate flaps converting the usual two-flap Z-plasty into a four-flap design *(right)*. Elongation obtained after transfer of the four flaps.

burn contractures. Double opposing Z-plasties with small flaps are as effective in contracture release as the single Z-plasty with larger flaps.

The Four-Flap Z-Plasty. The four-flap Z-plasty was described in Limberg's book in 1946 (Fig. 1–72). It has been utilized to achieve a maximal gain in length with the ease of the classic 60-degree angle flaps and without the difficulty of transfer of flaps with a wider angle.

The technique consists of outlining wide angle flaps, each flap being divided into two separate flaps, thus converting the usual two flap Z-plasty into a four-flap Z-plasty.

A modification was introduced by Iselin (1962). His "plastie en Z rectifiés" was used to correct a contracture of the thumb web.

Iselin's technique has been employed by Woolf and Broadbent (1972) for a contracted web space in the hand (Fig. 1–73), for axillary contractures following burns (Fig. 1–74), and for minor cases of syndactyly. Furnas (1965) has studied the four-flap Z-plasty in considerable detail (Fig. 1–75) and has suggested a number of applications of the technique (stenosis of the external auditory canal or a tracheal stoma).

Other multiple flap variations of the Z-plasty have also been described: a five-flap (Hirshowitz, Karev, and Levy, 1977) and a six-flap (Tolhurst, 1985) Z-plasty.

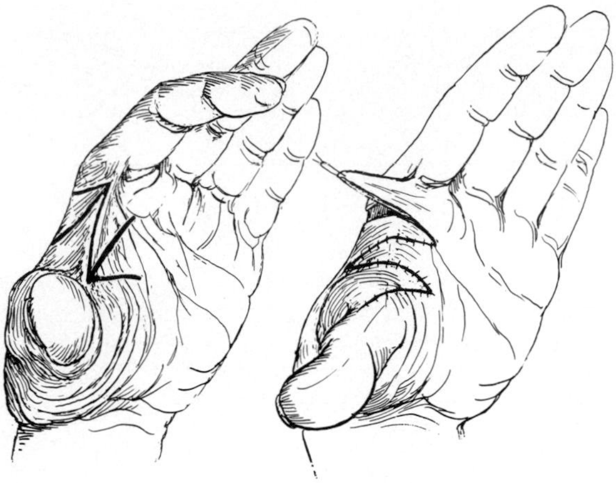

Figure 1–73. Application of the four-flap technique for a contracted web space in the hand. *Left*, Design of the four-flap Z-plasty. *Right*, After transfer of the flaps (after Woolf and Broadbent).

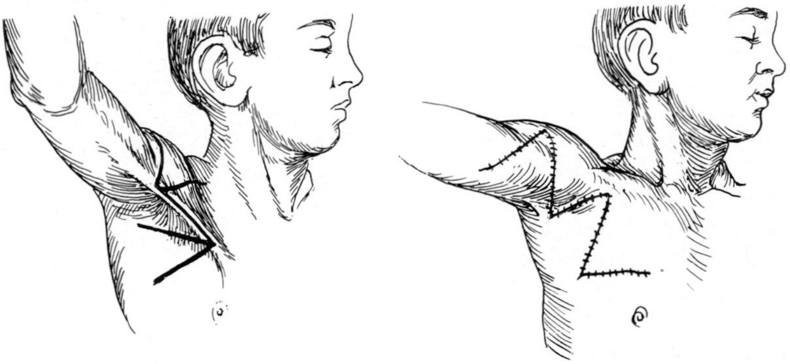

Figure 1–74. Application of the four-flap technique to correct an axillary contracture following a thermal burn. *Left*, Design of the four-flap Z-plasty. *Right*, Correction obtained after transfer of the flaps.

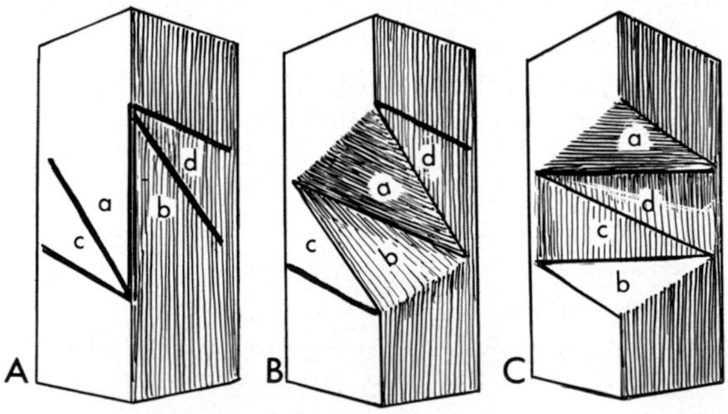

Figure 1–75. Four-flap Z-plasty, showing three interlocking tetrahedrons. *A*, Flaps in initial position ($a = b =$ 45° tip angle, $c = d =$ 30° tip angle. *B*, Transposition of *a* and *b* demonstrates first tetrahedron. *C*, Additional transposition demonstrates third tetrahedron (after Furnas).

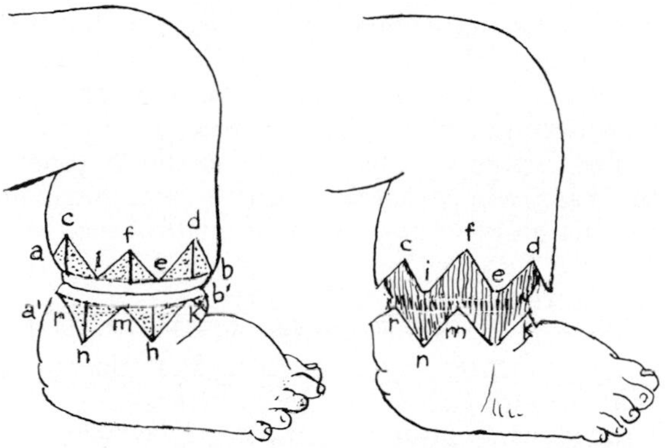

Figure 1–76. Ombrédanne's technique to relieve a congenital constricting band of the lower extremity. *Left*, Design of the flaps. *Right*, After excision of the constricting band, the flaps are ready to be sutured (after Borges).

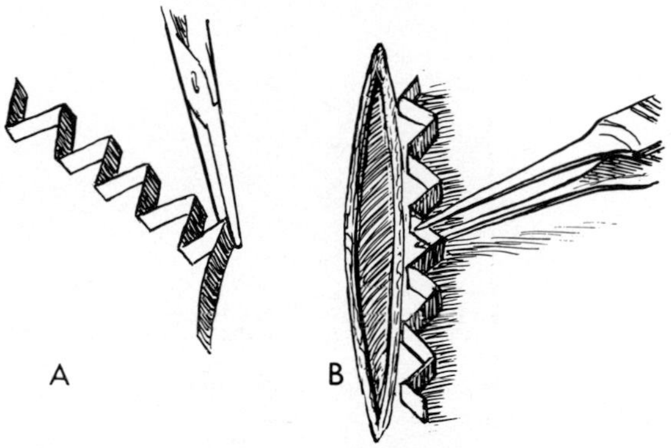

Figure 1–78. *A*, A metal pattern can be employed to assist in designing the W-plasty. A piece of metal is bent into a series of angles by means of a hemostat. *B*, One side of the metal pattern is painted with Bonney's blue solution by means of a cotton-tipped applicator. The pattern is then applied to the skin, leaving an imprint.

THE W-PLASTY

The W-plasty (Borges, 1959) consists of the imbrication of triangles of skin on each side of the excised scar.

A surgical technique resembling the W-plasty was described by Ombrédanne in 1937 and was employed by him to correct a congenital constricting band of the lower extremity (Fig. 1–76).

Hazrati (1952) described a compound right-angle Z-plasty. Borges (1973) has pointed out that this technique might well represent the missing link between the multiple Z-plasties and the W-plasty technique (Fig. 1–77).

In order to produce triangles of equal size, a metal pattern can be employed (Fig. 1–78). A large hemostat bends the soft metal band into a series of 60-degree angles. The size of the triangle is determined by the width of the limb of the particular hemostat.

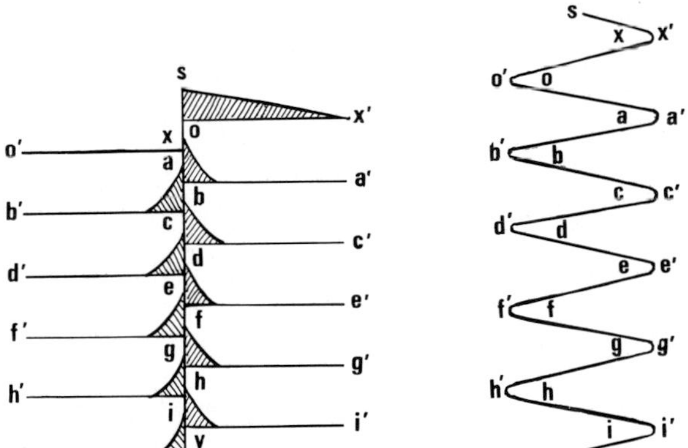

Figure 1–77. The compound right angle Z-plasty (after Hazrati). *Left*, Design of the compound right angle Z-plasty. *Right*, After transfer of the flaps (after Borges).

The pattern is painted with surgical ink and applied to one side of the scar; a similar procedure is repeated on the opposite side of the scar. The metal pattern is not essential, as the design can easily be made freehand by the operator.

At the end of the scar, the triangles are smaller and the length of the limbs of the W are tapered (Fig. 1–79*A*). With a sharp-pointed scalpel, the limbs of the W-plasty are incised on each side alternatively. In this fashion the tissues are firmer and easier to incise than if one entire edge is prepared before incising the opposing edge. After each triangle is outlined, the tip of the triangle on the contralateral side should be placed at the midpoint of the base of the opposing triangle (Fig. 1–79*B*).

Each triangular flap is approximately 5 mm in length and has an angle of approximately 55 degrees in vertical or almost vertical scars (scars that cross the lines of minimal tension at right angles). As the inclination of a scar in relation to the minimal tension lines becomes more acute, the angles of each triangular flap become more obtuse (Fig. 1–79*B*). Borges (1971) advocated gradually increasing the angles until they reach 90 degrees, when the scar traverses the lines of minimal tension at an angle of more than 60 degrees.

A continuous subcuticular suture of 4-0 monofilament nylon should be employed to approximate the angles. The subcuticular suture should be placed halfway between the apex and the base of each triangle in order to avoid buckling of the flaps. Additional

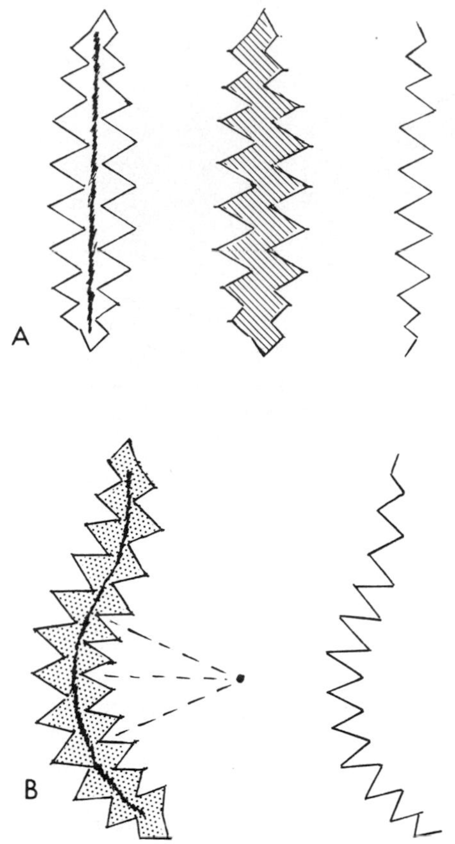

Figure 1–79. W-plasty. *A*, W-plasty for repair of a straight scar. Triangles become smaller at the end of the scar, and the length of the limbs of the flap is tapered to avoid puckering. *B*, On a curved scar, the angles of the inner aspect of the curve should be more acute than the angles of the outer aspect of the curve (after Borges).

approximation is obtained with interrupted 6-0 nylon sutures.

Indications and Contraindications for Z- and W-Plasties. The Z-plasty and W-plasty techniques have two common denominators: they break up the straight linear scar into smaller components, and they improve the direction of the scar in relation to the lines of minimal tension.

The Z-plasty has the advantage that it elongates a contractile scar, changes the direction of the scar (when correctly done), and places it more nearly parallel to the lines of minimal tension. It also has the advantage of utilizing all of the available skin, as it is possible in some cases to perform the Z-plasty without excising the scar, if tissue is scarce. The change that takes place in the character and quality of the scar when tension is relaxed was mentioned earlier in the chapter. Since the Z-plasty elongates the linear scar, it thereby relaxes tension; it also permits readjustment of displaced tissue.

The Z-plasty is preferable to the W-plasty in areas where there is either too much or too little skin tension. A horizontal scar extending across the cheek, lower lip, or chin can be repaired by a W-plasty.

The main disadvantage of the Z-plasty, when improperly designed and/or placed, is that it elongates the scar excessively and enlarges the area it occupies. However, the Z-plasty nearly always improves the condition for which it is applied. The longer segments of the Z-plasty, which are especially apparent on the face, are another disadvantage over the W-plasty. It is possible to counteract this danger by Z-plasties with smaller limbs, such as the double opposing Z-plasty, and by multiple Z-plasties. In oblique scars traversing the lines of minimal tension at an angle of less than 30 degrees, a Z-plasty procedure is preferable to a W-plasty. When the scar is almost parallel to the lines of minimal tension, the entire scar or the major portion of the scar should be excised by elliptic incisions parallel to the lines of minimal tension. The wound is closed by direct approximation.

The W-plasty also has the advantage of having smaller triangular limbs, which break up the scar into smaller components and relieve the bowstring effect.

When the W-plasty is employed, there is no displacement of anatomic landmarks, as there is no transposition of tissue. W-plasties are indicated on scars of the face that are perpendicular or nearly perpendicular to the lines of minimal tension. They also have the ability to restore the normal contour of the scarred cheek.

The W-plasty has the disadvantage of increasing rather than decreasing the tension in the area of the scar because of the necessary sacrifice of tissue. It should be reserved, therefore, for scars surrounded by plentiful tissue. When elongation of the linear scar is required, the Z-plasty is always preferable.

If irregularities (and not hypertrophic scars) in the surface area persist following either a Z- or W-plasty, a single (or a repeated) dermabrasion at a suitable interval after the operation improves the surface contour.

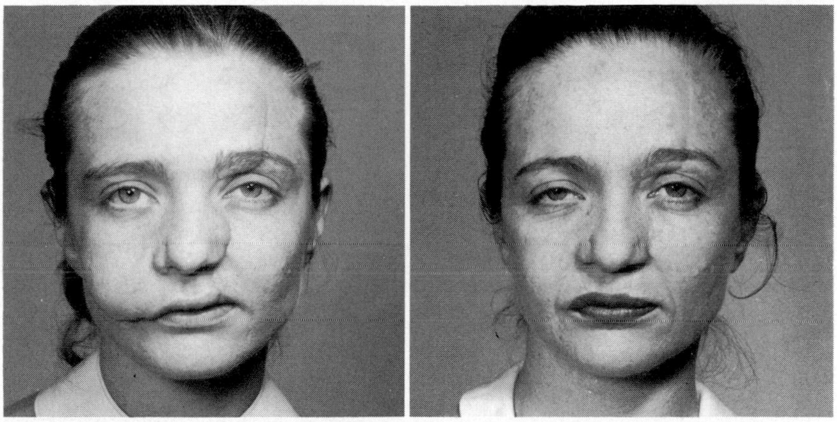

Figure 1–80. Z-plasty and W-plasty in scars resulting from avulsion of facial soft tissue. *A*, Massive partial avulsion of the soft tissues of the face. The flap sheared from the facial skeleton extended from the left side of the forehead through the left eyebrow and upper eyelid downward along the lateral wall of the nose, through the upper lip on the left side, through the right angle of the mouth backward to an area situated immediately in front of the right auricle. Massive lymphatic obstruction resulting from the scar caused long-term lymphedema. *B*, Final result obtained.

Z-Plasty and W-Plasty in Depressed Scars of Partially Avulsed Trapdoor Flaps. The patient seen in Figure 1–80*A* suffered a massive partial avulsion of the soft tissues of the face when she was projected through the windshield of the automobile in which she was a front seat passenger when it was involved in a head-on collision with another vehicle.

Lymphatic obstruction by the deeply penetrating scar resulted in long-term lymphedema of the soft tissues of the face, which accentuated the deep indentation produced by the scar. Interdigitation between edematous and normal tissue bordering the scar by a combination of Z-plasty and W-plasty, as well as excision of the scar, resulted in amelioration of the trapdoor scars (Fig. 1–80*B*).

THE V-Y ADVANCEMENT

The V-Y advancement is a helpful technique in lengthening certain anatomic structures such as the columella or in correcting notching of the lip (Fig. 1–81). It was probably first described by Blasius (1848) for the correction of a contracture of the anterior neck. A V-shaped incision is made through the skin; the skin on either side of the V is advanced in the direction of the apex of the V; and the incision is closed as a Y.

REPEATED (SERIAL) PARTIAL EXCISIONS (Morestin, 1915; Davis, 1929; Smith, 1950)

Partial excision may be preferable in the eradication of pigmented nevi or of wide scars in which total excision and suture cannot be accomplished without tension. Multiple repeated (serial) partial excisions are indicated in areas surrounded by loose tissue. Serial excisions are done at suitable intervals, provided that sufficient loose tissue is available and that distortion of the eyelids, nose, or lips does not result; distortion must be avoided. Wide undermining of the surrounding skin is essential.

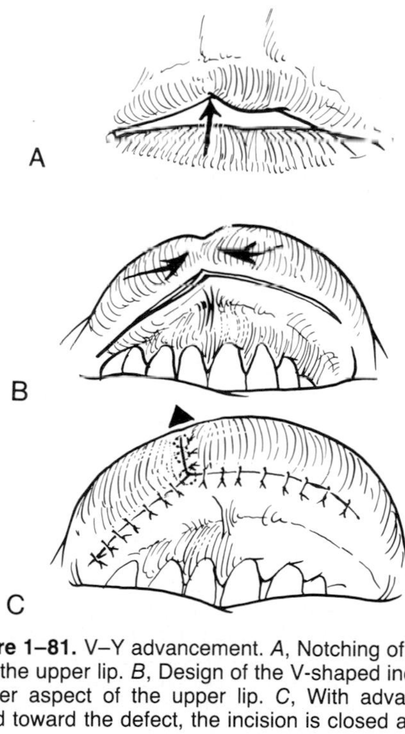

Figure 1–81. V–Y advancement. *A*, Notching of the right side of the upper lip. *B*, Design of the V-shaped incision on the inner aspect of the upper lip. *C*, With advancement directed toward the defect, the incision is closed as a Y.

The technique of multiple partial excision has its best application in infants, in whom the skin is more elastic than in adults; closure of the resulting defect is thus facilitated. In aged patients the looseness of skin and excess of skin also favor this technique.

With the development of skin expansion techniques, the indications for serial excisions have probably decreased.

REFERENCES

Ammon, F. A. von, and Baumgarten, M.: Die plastische Chirurgie nach ihren bisherigen Leistungen Kritisch dargestellt. Berlin, Reimer, 1842.

Bakamjian, V. Y.: A two-stage method for pharyngoesophageal reconstruction with a primary pectoral skin flap. Plast. Reconstr. Surg., *36*:173, 1965.

Balch, C. M., and Marzoni, F. A.: Skin transplantation during the pre-Reverdin era, 1804–1869. Surg. Gynecol. Obstet., *144*:766, 1977.

Baronio, G.: Degli Innesti Animali. Stamperia e Fonderia del Genio. Milan, 1804.

Berger, P.: Autoplastie par dédoublement de la palmure et échange des lambeaux. *In* Berger, P., and Banzet, S. (Eds.): Chirurgie Orthopédique. Paris, G. Steinheil, 1904, p. 180.

Bert, P.: De la Greffe Animale. Paris, J. B. Ballière et Fils, 1863.

Bhishagratna, K. K.: An English translation of the Sushruta samhita based on original Sanskrit text. 3 Vols. Calcutta, Bose, 1916, p. 107.

Blair, V. P.: Surgery and Diseases of the Mouth and Jaws. St. Louis, MO, C. V. Mosby Company, 1912.

Blair, V. P.: The delayed transfer of long pedicle flaps in plastic surgery. Surg. Gynecol. Obstet., *33*:261, 1921.

Blair, V. P.: Reconstructive surgery of the face. Surg. Gynecol. Obstet., *34*:701, 1922.

Blair, V. P., and Brown, J. B.: Use and uses of large split skin grafts of intermediate thickness. Surg. Gynecol. Obstet., *49*:82, 1929.

Blandin, P. F.: De l'autoplastie, ou restauration des parties du corps, qui ont été détruites, à la faveur, d'un emprunt fait à d'autres parties plus ou moins éloignées. Thesis, Urtubie, Paris, 1836.

Blasius, E.: Gaumennaht Staphylorraphie. *In* Handbuch der Chirurgie. Vol. 2. Halle, E. Anton, 1839–1843.

Blasius, E.: Beiträge zur praktischen Chirurgie. Berlin, A. Forstner, 1848.

Borges, A. F.: Improvement of antitension-line scars by the W-plastic operation. Br. J. Plast. Surg., *12*:29, 1959.

Borges, A. F.: Historical review of the Z- and W-plasty revisions of linear scars. Int. Surg., *56*:182, 1971.

Borges, A. F.: Elective Incisions and Scar Revision. Boston, Little, Brown & Company, 1973.

Borges, A. F.: The five single Z-plasties. Va. Med. Monthly. *101*:618, 1974.

Borges, A. F., and Gibson, T.: The original Z-plasty. Br. J. Surg., *22*:237, 1973.

Bridgman, G.: Complete Guide to Drawing from Life. New York, Sterling Publishing Company, 1973.

Brown, J. B., and McDowell, F.: Skin Grafting. Philadelphia, J. B. Lippincott Company, 1939.

Bünger, C.: Gelungener Versuch einer Nasenbildung aus einem völlig getrennten Hautstück aus dem Beine. J. Chir. Augenh. Berlin, 1823.

Burget, G. C., and Menick, F. J.: The subunit principle in nasal reconstruction. Plast. Reconstr. Surg., *76*:239, 1985.

Burkhardt, J.: The Civilization of the Renaissance in Italy. New York, Harper & Brothers, 1929.

Carpue, J. C.: An account of two successful operations for restoring a lost nose from the integuments of the forehead. London, Longman, 1816.

Chapple, J. G., and Stephenson, K. L.: Photographic misrepresentation. Plast. Reconstr. Surg., *45*:135, 1970.

Clarkson, P.: Sir Harold Gillies. Br. Med. J., *2*:641, 1966.

Converse, J. M.: New forehead flap for nasal reconstruction. Proc. R. Soc. Med., *35*:811, 1942.

Converse, J. M.: Victor Veau (1871–1949). The contributions of a pioneer. Plast. Reconstr. Surg., *30*:225, 1962.

Converse, J. M.: Introduction to plastic surgery. *In* Converse, J. M (Ed.): Reconstructive Plastic Surgery. 1st Ed. Ch. 1, p. 16, Fig. 1–17. Philadelphia, W. B. Saunders Company, 1964.

Converse, J. M.: The classic reprint: La réduction graduelle des difformités tégumentaires, by H. Morestin, M. D., Paris (Bull. et mém. Soc. chir. Paris, *41*:1233, 1915). Translated from the French. Plast. Reconstr. Surg., *42*:163, 1968.

Converse, J. M.: Kazanjian and Converse. Surgical Treatment of Facial Injuries. 3rd Ed. Baltimore, Williams & Wilkins Company, 1974.

Converse, J. M., and Smith, B.: Naso-orbital fractures and traumatic deformities of the medial canthus. Plast. Reconstr. Surg., *38*:147, 1966.

Cox, H. T.: The cleavage lines of skin. Br. J. Surg., *29*:234, 1941.

Daniel, R., and Taylor, G. I.: Distant transfer of an island flap by microvascular anastomosis. Plast. Reconstr. Surg., *52*:111, 1973.

Davis, J. S.: Plastic Surgery—Its Principles and Practice, Philadelphia, P. Blakiston's Son & Company, 1919.

Davis, J. S.: Removal of wide scars and large disfigurements of the skin by gradual partial excision with closure. Ann. Surg., *90*:645, 1929.

Davis, J. S.: Relaxation of scar contractures by means of the Z-, or reversed Z-type incision; stressing use of scar infiltrated tissues. Ann. Surg., *94*:871, 1931.

Davis, J. S.: The story of plastic surgery. Ann. Surg., *113*:641, 1941.

Davis, J. S.: Present evaluation of the merits of the Z-plasty operation. Plast. Reconstr. Surg., *1*:26, 1946.

Davis, J. S., and Kitlowski, E. A.: The theory and practical use of the Z-incision for the relief of scar constriction. Ann. Surg., *109*:1001, 1939.

Davis, J. S., and Traut, H. F.: Origin and development of blood supply of whole thickness skin grafts. Ann. Surg., *82*:871, 1925.

Delagenière, H.: Greffes Ostéo-périostiques. J. Chir., *17*:305, 1921.

Delpech, J. M.: Chirurgie Clinique de Montpellier, ou Observations et Réflexions Tirées des Travaux de Chirurgie de cette Ecole. Paris, Gabon et Cie, 1823–1828.

Denonvilliers, C. P.: Présentation de Malades. Bull. Soc. Chir. (Paris), *5*:35, 118, 1854.

Desault, P. J.: Oeuvres Chirurgicales ou Exposé de la Doctrine et de la Plastique. Vol. 2. Paris, Megegnon, 1798.

Diderot, D.: Encyclopédie, ou Dictionnaire Raisonné des Sciences, des Arts et des Métiers, par une Société des gens de lettres. Vol. 1. Paris, 1751.

Dieffenbach, J. F.: Die operative Chirurgie. Leipzig, F. A. Brockhaus, 1845–1848.

Dupuytren, G.: Leçons orales de clinique chirurgicale,

faites à l'Hôtel-Dieu de Paris. Paris, G. Baillière, 1832–1834.
Edgerton, M. T.: The role of plastic surgery in academic medicine. Presidential address. Plast. Reconstr. Surg., *54*:523, 1974.
Esser, J. F. S.: Esser Inlay (Epithelial Inlay). Leiden, Brill, 1940.
Farkas, L. G.: Anthropometry of the Head and Face in Medicine. New York, Elsevier, 1981.
Filatov, V. P.: Plastie à tige ronde. Vestnik oftal., No. 5, 1917.
Finochietto, E.: Presentaçion de instrumentos. Prensa Med. Argent., *6*:356, 1920.
Firenzuola: Opere di Firenzuola, Milan, 1802.
Fomon, S.: Surgery of Injury and Plastic Repair. Baltimore, Williams & Wilkins Company, 1939.
Fricke, J. C. G.: Bildung neuer Augenlider (Blepharoplastik) nach Zerstörung und dadurch hervorgebrachter Auswartwendung derselben. Hamburg, Perthes & Basser, 1829.
Furnas, D. W.: The tetrahedral Z-plasty. Plast. Reconstr. Surg., *35*:291, 1965.
Gentleman's Magazine: A communication to the editor, Mr. Urban, signed B. L. and dated Oct. 9, 1794. Vol. 64. Part Two, pp. 891–892; engraved illustration between pp. 882 and 883. London, Nichols, 1794.
German, W., Finesilver, E. M., and Davis, J. S.: Establishment of circulation in tubed skin. Arch Surg., *26*:27, 1933.
Gibson, T.: Biochemical properties of skin. Surg. Clin. North Am., *47*:279, 1967.
Gibson, T., and Medawar, P. B.: The fate of skin homografts in man. J. Anat., *77*:299, 1943.
Gillies, H. D.: Plastic Surgery of the Face. London, Oxford University Press, 1920.
Gillies, H. D., and Millard, D. R., Jr.: Principles and Art of Plastic Surgery. Boston, Little, Brown & Company, 1957.
Gnudi, M. T., and Webster, J. P.: The life and times of Gasparo Tagliacozzi. New York, Herbert Reichner, 1950.
Grabb, W. C., and Smith, J. E.: Plastic Surgery—A Concise Guide to Clinical Practice. Boston, Little, Brown & Company, 1968. 3rd Ed., 1979.
Graefe, C. F. von: Rhinoplastik; oder, Die Kunst den verlust der Nase organisch zu ersetzen in ihren früheren Verhältnissen erforscht und durch neue Verfahrungsweisen zur höheren Vollkommenheit gefördert. Berlin, In der Realschulbuchhandlung, 1818.
Harii, K., Ohmori, K., and Ohmori, S.: Hair transplantation with free scalp flaps. Plast. Reconstr. Surg., *53*:410, 1974.
Hazrati, E.: Compound right angle Z-plasty. Plast. Reconstr. Surg., *10*:133, 1952.
Hemingway, E.: A Moveable Feast. New York, Charles Scribner's & Sons, 1964, p. 82.
Hirshowitz, B., Karev, A., and Levy, Y: A 5-flap procedure for axillary webs leaving the apex intact. Br. J. Plast. Surg., *30*:48, 1977.
Horner, W. E.: Clinical Report on the Surgical Department of the Philadelphia Hospital, Blockley, for the Months of May, June, and July, 1837. Am. J. Med. Sci., *21*:99, 1837.
Iselin, M.: La plastie en Z rectifiés. Ann. Chir. Plast., *7*:295, 1962.
Ivy, R. H.: War injuries of the face and jaws (Internatl. Abstr. Surg.). Surg. Gynecol. Obstet., *27*:101, 1918.
Ivy, R. H.: Plastic and reconstructive surgery of the face. Internatl. Abstr. Surg., *36*:1, 1923.
Ivy, R. H.: War injuries of the face and jaws (Internatl. Abstr. Surg.). Surg. Gynceol. & Studies of the College of Physicians of Philadelphia, *16*:42, 1948.
Jobert (de Lamballe), A. J.: Traité de Chirurgie Plastique. Paris, J. B. Baillière et fils, 1849.
Joseph, J.: Nasenplastik und sonstige Gesichtsplastik nebst einem Anhang uber Mammaplastik: Ein Atlas und Lehrbuch. Leipzig, Berlin, 1928.
Kazanjian, V. H., and Converse, J. M.: The Surgical Treatment of Facial Injuries. Baltimore, Williams & Wilkins Company, 1949. 2nd Ed., 1959. 3rd Ed., 1974.
Klasen, H. J.: History of Free Skin Grafting. Berlin, Springer-Verlag, 1981.
Krause, F.: Ueber die Transplantation gosser, ungestielter Hautlappen. Dtsch. Gesell. Chir. Verhandl., *22*:46, 1893.
Ksander, G. A., Vistnes, L. M., and Rose, E. H.: Excisional wound biomechanics, skin tension lines and elastic contraction. Plast. Reconstr. Surg., *59*:398, 1977.
Labat, L.: De la rhinoplastie, art de restaurer ou de refaire complètemente le nez. Thesis, Paris, 1834.
Langer, C.: Zur Anatomie und Physiologie der Haut. Sitzungsb. Acad. Wissensch., *45*:223, 1861.
Lawson, G.: On the successful transplantation of portions of skin for the closure of large granulating surface. Lancet, *2*:708, 1870.
LeFort, L.: Blépharoplastie par un lambeau complétement détaché due bras et reporté à la face. Insuccès. Bull. Soc. Chir. (Paris), *1*:39, 1872.
Lexer, E.: Die freien Transplantationen. Stuttgart, F. Enke, 1919.
Lexer, E.: Die gesamte Wiederherstellungschirurgie. Leipzig, J. A. Barth, 1920.
Limberg, A. A.: Skin plastic with shifting triangular flaps. Translated from the Russian. Leningrad Trauma Institute, *8*:62, 1929.
Limberg, A. A.: Matematicheskie Osnovuy Mestnoy Plastiki Na Poverchnosti Chelovecheskogo Tela, Medgiz, 1946.
Liston, R.: Practical Surgery. London, J & A Churchill, 1831–1837.
Longacre, J. J., Seghers, M. J., Berry, H. K., Wood, R. W., Munick, L. H., et al.: L'ultrastructure de collagène et la relation avec la correction des cicatrices hypertrophiques. Ann. Chir. Plast., *9*:111, 1966.
Macgregor, F. C.: Transformation and Identity. The Face and Plastic Surgery. New York, Quadrangle, New York Times Book Company, 1974.
Majno, G.: The Healing Hand. Cambridge, Harvard, 1975.
Malgaigne, J. F.: Manuel de Médecin Opératoire. Paris, G. Baillière, 1849.
Malt, R. A., and McKhann, C. F.: Replantation of severed arms. J.A.M.A., *189*:716, 1964.
Mauclaire, P.: Les Greffes Chirurgicales. Vol. 1. Paris, G. Baillière, 1922.
May, H.: Erich Lexer. A biographical sketch. Plast. Reconstr. Surg., *29*:141, 1962.
May, R. M.: La greffe brephoplastique sous-cutanée de la thyroide chez le rat. Comptes rendus. Acad. Sci., *199*:807, 1934.
McCarthy, J. G.: The postresidency fellowship in plastic surgery: Its evolution and future. Plast. Reconstr. Surg., *76*:790, 1985.
McCurdy, S. L.: Manual of Orthopedic Surgery. Pittsburgh, Nicholson Press, 1898.
McCurdy, S. L.: Plastic operations to elongate cicatricial contractions across joints. Cleveland Med. J., *3*:123, 1904.
McCurdy, S. L.: Z-plastic surgery. Surg. Gynecol. Obstet., *16*:209, 1913.

McCurdy, S. L.: Z-plastic surgery. Int. J. Surg., *30*:389, 1917.
McCurdy, S. L.: Correction of burn scar deformity by the Z-plastic method. J. Bone Joint Surg., *6*:683, 1924.
McGregor, I. A.: The theoretical basis of the Z-plasty. Br. J. Plast. Surg., *9*:256, 1957.
McGregor, I. A.: Fundamental Techniques of Plastic Surgery and Their Surgical Applications. 6th Ed. Baltimore, Williams and Wilkins Company, 1975.
McLean, D., and Buncke, J.: Autotransplant of omentum to a large scalp defect, with microsurgical revascularization. Plast. Reconstr. Surg., *49*:268, 1972.
Medawar, P. B.: The behavior and fate of skin autografts and skin homografts in rabbits. J. Anat., *78*:176, 1944.
Millard, D. R.: Scar repair by double-vested principle. Plast. Reconstr. Surg., *45*:616, 1970.
Millard, D. R.: Principlization of Plastic Surgery. Boston, Little, Brown & Company, 1986.
Miller, C. C.: Cosmetic Surgery: The Correction of Featural Imperfections. Chicago, Oak Printing Company, 1907.
Morello, D. C., Converse, J. M., and Allen, D.: Making uniform photographic records in plastic surgery. Plast. Reconstr. Surg., *59*:366, 1977.
Morestin, H.: De la correction des flexions permanentes des doigts consectives aux panaris et aux phlegmons de la paume de la main. Rev. Chir., *50*:1, 1914.
Morestin H.: La reduction graduelle des difformités tégumentaires. Bull. Mém. Soc. Chir. Paris, *41*:1233, 1915.
Murray, J. E., Merrill, J. P., and Harrison, J. H.: Renal homotransplantation in identical twins. Surg. Forum, *6*:432, 1955.
Natvig, P.: Jacques Joseph, Surgical Sculptor. Philadelphia, W. B. Saunders Company, 1982.
Nélaton, C., and Ombrédanne, L.: Rhinoplastie. Paris, G. Steinheil, 1904.
Nélaton, C., and Ombrédanne, L.: Les Autoplasties. Paris, G. Steinheil, 1907.
O'Brien, B., MacLeod, A., Hayhurst, J., et al.: Successful transfer of a large island flap from the groin to the foot by microvascular anastomoses. Plast. Reconstr. Surg., *52*:271, 1973.
Ollier, L.: Greffes cutanée ou autoplastique. Bull. Acad. Méd., *1*:243, 1872.
Ombrédanne, L.: Maladie Amniotique. *In* Ombrédanne, L., and Mathieu, P. (Eds.): Traité de Chirurgie Orthopédique. Vol. 1. Masson et Cie, Paris, 1937, p. 44.
Padgett, E. C.: Calibrated intermediate skin grafts. Surg. Gynecol. Obstet., *69*:779, 1939.
Paré A.: Les oeuvres de M. Ambroise Paré conseiller et premier chirurgien du roy. Avec les figures et portraicts tant de l'anatomic que des instruments de chirugie, et de plusieurs monstres. Le tout divisé en vingt-six livres, comme il est contenu en la page suyvent. Paris, G. Boune, 1575.
Peer, L. A.: Transplantation of Tissue. Cartilage, Bone, Fascia, Tendon and Muscles. Vols. I & II. Baltimore, Williams & Wilkins Company, 1955, 1959.
Pollock, G. C.: The operation of skin transplantation; clinical remarks. Lancet, *2*:669, 1870.
Reverdin, J. L.: Greffes épidermiques; expérience faite dans le service de M. le docteur Guyon, à l'Hôpital Necker, pendant 1869. Bull Soc. Impériale Chir. Paris, Series 2, Vol. 10, published in 1870.
Richer, P.: Morphologie de la Femme. Plon-Nourrit et Cie, 1920.
Rogers, B. O.: Personal communication, 1974.
Rogers, B. O.: Nasal reconstruction 150 years ago: aesthetic and other problems. Aesth. Plast. Surg., *5*:283, 1981.
Roux, P. J.: Quarante années de practique chirurgicale. Vol. I, Chirurgie réparatrice. Paris, Masson et Cie, 1854.
Sabbatini, P.: Cenno storico dell'origine e progressi della rinoplastica e cheiloplastica, seguita dalla descrizione di queste operazioni sopra un solo individuo. Bologna, Belle Arti, 1838.
Sanvenero-Rosselli, G., and Boggio-Robutti, G. (Eds.): Transactions of the Fourth International Congress of Plastic and Reconstructive Surgery, Rome, October, 1967. Amsterdam, Excerpta Medica Foundation, 1969.
Serre, M.: Traité sur l'art de restaurer les déformités de la face, selon la méthode par deplacement, ou méthode française. Montpellier, L. Castel, 1842.
Sheehan, J. E.: Plastic Surgery of the Orbit. New York, Macmillan Publishing Company, 1927.
Smith, F.: Nelson's Looseleaf Reconstructive Surgery. Springfield, IL, Charles C Thomas, 1928.
Smith, F.: Plastic and Reconstructive Surgery. Philadelphia, W. B. Saunders Company, 1950.
Steinschneider, E.: Beitrage zur Kieferschusstherapie. Berlin, Urban, 1917.
Symonds, J. A.: The Renaissance in Italy. New York, Cerf (The Modern Library), 1935.
Szymanowski, J. von: Handbuch der operativen Chirurgie. Braunschweig, F. Viewig u. Sohn, 1870.
Tagliacozzi, G.: De Curtorum chirurgia per Insitionem. Venice, Gaspare Bindoni, 1597.
Tessier, P., Guiot, G., Rougerie, J., Delbet, J. P., and Pastoriza, J.: Osteotomies cranio-naso-orbital-faciales. Hypertelorisme. Ann. Chir. Plast., *12*:103, 1967.
Thiersch, C.: Ueber die feineren anatomischen Veränderungen bei Aufheilung von Haut auf Granulationen. Arch. Klin. Chir., *17*:318, 1874.
Tolhurst, D. E.: A variation of the six-flap Z-plasty theme. Plast. Reconstr. Surg., *75*:911, 1985.
Velpeau, A. A. L. M.: Nouveau Eléments de Médecin Opératoire. Paris, J. B. Baillière, 1839.
Velpeau, A. A. L. M.: New Elements of Operative Surgery. 3rd American Ed. from last Paris Ed. Translated by P. S. Tousend under supervision of Valentine Mott. New York, Wood, 1951.
Velter, E.: Plaies pénétrantes du crane par projectiles de guerre. Paris, A. Maloine et Fils, 1917.
Verneuil, A.: Mémoires de Chirurgie. Paris, B. Masson, 1877–1888.
Voltaire, François Marie Arouet de: Oeuvres complètes. Vol. 42, pp. 413–414. Paris, Imprimerie de la Société littéraire-bibliographique, 1785. (Dictionnaire philosophique. Vol. 6.)
Wallace, A. B.: Treatment of burns; return to basic principles. Br. J. Plast. Surg., *1*:233, 1949.
Warren, J. M.: Rhinoplastic Operations. With Some Remarks on the Autoplastic Methods Usually Adopted for the Restoration of Parts Lost by Accident or Disease. Boston, Clapp, 1840.
Warren, J. M.: Surgical Observations with Cases and Observations. Boston, Ticknor & Fields, 1867.
Webster, J. P.: In Memoriam, Vilray Papin Blair. Plast. Reconstr. Surg., *18*:83, 1956.
Wilflingseder, G.: Personal communication, 1975.
Wolfe, J. R.: A new method of performing plastic operations. Med. Times and Gazette, *1*:608, 1876.
Woolf, R. M., and Broadbent, T. R.: The four-flap Z-plasty. Plast. Reconstr. Surg., *49*:48, 1972.
Zeis, E.: Handbuch der plastischen Chirurgie (nebsteiner Vorrede von J. F. Dieffenbach). Berlin, Reimer, 1838.

2

M. Michael Cohen, Jr.

Dysmorphology, Syndromology, and Genetics

Most chapters dealing with medical genetics that appear in surgical textbooks impress readers as an afterthought included for the sake of completeness. A glance through the typical contents of such a chapter—an analysis of complex pedigrees and the study of chromosomal anomalies—usually leaves the relationship between genetic and surgical concerns unexplained. This chapter is designed to be read by surgeons. It bridges the gap between medical genetics and surgery by emphasizing the *anatomic* basis of dysmorphology and syndromology, and by relegating formal genetics to an appendix for consultation at the end of the chapter.

The same anomaly can be viewed from different perspectives: anatomic and genetic. For example, craniosynostosis can be viewed from these two perspectives (Table 2–1). When the main interest is the clinical description, growth and development, or surgical management of craniosynostosis, the perspective is anatomic. Within this context, the particular suture that is synostosed is of primary importance. From the perspective of genetics, classification of various syndromes on the basis of the particular suture synostosed can be misleading. Because patients with the same genetic condition may have fusion of different sutures, the specific suture synostosed is of secondary importance in this context. The clinical geneticist is mainly concerned with the overall pattern of anomalies, both major and minor, throughout the body (from which the diagnosis of specific syndromes follows) and with those family members affected (from which genetic counseling follows). Thus, seemingly small differences between syndromes with craniosynostosis may sometimes be very important. Furthermore, from the genetic point of view, cranio-

Table 2–1. Two Perspectives on Craniosynostosis

Anatomic Perspective	Genetic Perspective
Specific suture synostosed of primary importance	Specific suture synostosed of secondary importance
Clinical description	Overall pattern of anomalies
Growth and development	Which family members affected
Surgical management	

From Cohen, M. M., Jr.: Craniosynostosis: Diagnosis, Evaluation, and Management. New York, Raven Press, 1986.

synostosis and syndromes with craniosynostosis should not be classified on the basis of which sutures are synostosed (Fig. 2–1). It is important to emphasize that, although anatomic and genetic means of classifying craniosynostosis may overlap, both perspectives are equally valid and depend on context. Conditions that are anatomically similar can be grouped together for surgical purposes even though their etiologies may be different; their pathogenetic bases and phenotypes may, however, be similar or identical (Cohen, 1986).

The outline of this chapter is as follows. First, the principles of dysmorphology are presented. Single birth defects, the building blocks of many syndromes, can be categorized as malformations, deformations, and disruptions. It is practical to distinguish between these classes of anomalies because the clinical implications of each are different. The interrelationships between anomalies are also discussed. Finally, minor anomalies and their implications are considered.

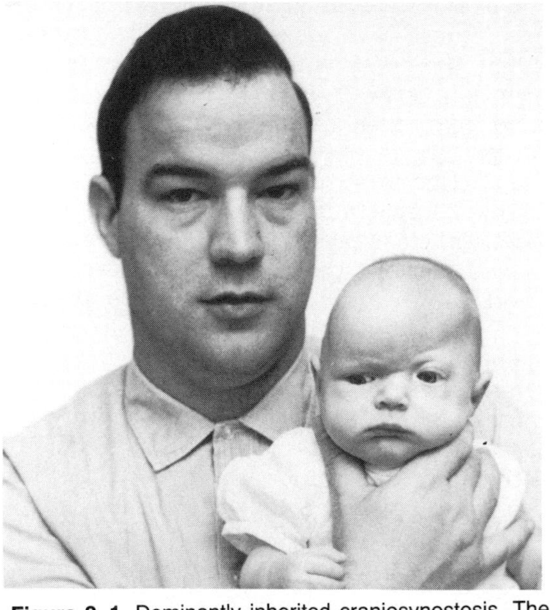

Figure 2–1. Dominantly inherited craniosynostosis. The father has sagittal synostosis. The infant has unilateral coronal involvement. (From Anderson, F. M., and Geiger, L.: Craniosynostosis; a survey of 204 cases. J. Neurosurg., *22*:229, 1965.)

The principles of syndromology are considered second. The process of syndrome delineation and its rationale are described. Syndromologists have a twofold interest:

1. *Patient care*, which includes clinical and laboratory evaluation, overall diagnosis, and patient counseling for the medical aspects of the disorder and its implications for the risk of recurrence.
2. *Etiology and pathogenesis*, which include:
   a. The frequent discovery of etiologic heterogeneity from family histories and genetic studies.
   b. The implication that etiologic heterogeneity may sometimes indicate pathogenetic heterogeneity.
   c. The process of syndrome delineation, which aids in the classification of disorders for the proper study of pathogenesis.

After an analysis of selected craniofacial anomalies, there follows a short appendix of formal genetics, which includes human cytogenetics and chromosomal anomalies, monogenic inheritance patterns, and multifactorial inheritance.

A number of other relevant subjects for surgeons cannot be addressed within the scope of this chapter: dysmorphic growth and development (Cohen, 1981, 1982, 1986); clinical approach to syndrome diagnosis (Cohen, 1982); syndrome prototypes (Cohen, 1986); and neoplastic aspects of syndromology (Cohen, 1982).

PRINCIPLES OF DYSMORPHOLOGY

Anomalies, the building blocks of various syndromes, are divided into three types: *malformations, deformations*, and *disruptions* (Fig. 2–2). Syndactyly is a malformation caused by intrinsically abnormal development during the embryonic period. Clubfoot is a deformation that can result from mechanical compression during the fetal period. Digital amputation with an aberrant tissue band is caused by disruption of otherwise intrinsically normal development. Most anomalies observed at birth can be sorted into one of the three basic categories. This is a practical approach, because the clinical implications of each category are different.

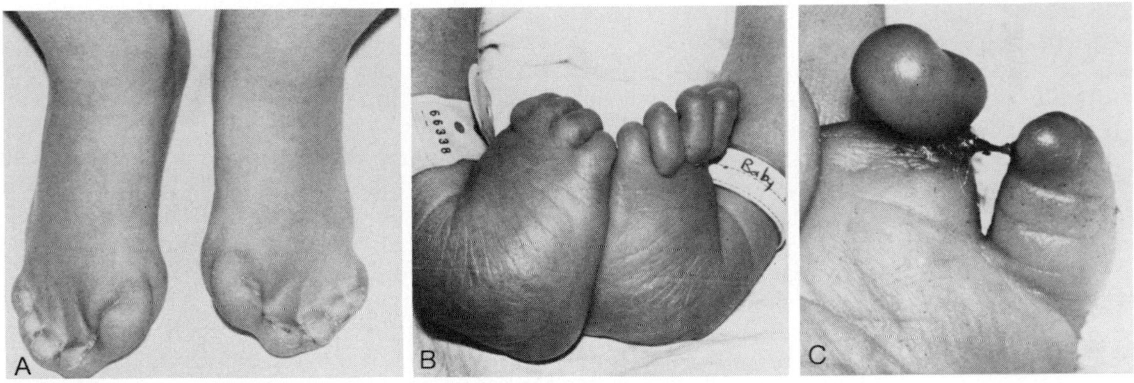

Figure 2–2. Three types of anomalies. *A,* Syndactyly, a malformation. *B,* Clubfoot, a deformation. *C,* Digital amputation in association with aberrant tissue band, a disruption. (From Cohen, M.M., Jr.: The Child with Multiple Birth Defects. New York, Raven Press, 1982.)

Malformations

A malformation may be defined as a morphologic defect of an organ, part of an organ, or a larger area of the body, resulting from intrinsically abnormal development (Spranger and associates, 1982). Approximately 3 per cent of newborns have significant malformations, and approximately 1 per cent have multiple malformations. There are three classes of malformations: incomplete morphogenesis, redundant morphogenesis, and aberrant morphogenesis.

The most common class is incomplete morphogenesis, in which a developmental arrest occurs, as in renal agenesis. If the ureteric bud fails to contact the metanephric blastema or if the blastema fails to respond to it, the kidney does not form. Other types of incomplete morphogenesis, with examples, are listed in Table 2–2.

Redundant morphogenesis is less common. In this class of malformations, the redundant structure passes through the same stage of morphogenesis at the same time as its normal counterpart. An example is an ear tag in the presence of an otherwise normal ear. Such a tag may be interpreted as a supernumerary auricular hillock.

Aberrant morphogenesis is rare and has no counterpart in normal morphogenesis. A mediastinal thyroid gland serves as an example, because it is never found in this location at any stage of normal morphogenesis. Because the classification of malformations in Table 2–2 is not all-inclusive and because nothing is implied about mechanisms, it is a classification of convenience rather than of scientific merit.

Malformations may be relatively simple or complex. The later the defect is induced, the simpler is the malformation. Malformations

Table 2–2. Abnormal Morphogenesis Resulting in Malformations

Types of Abnormal Morphogenesis	Examples of Malformations	Relative Frequency as a Class
Incomplete morphogenesis		
Lack of development	Absent nostril, renal agenesis	Common
Hypoplasia	Microcephaly, micrognathia	
Incomplete closure	Cleft palate, iris coloboma	
Incomplete separation	Syndactyly	
Incomplete septation	Ventricular septal defect	
Incomplete migration	Exstrophy of cloaca	
Incomplete rotation	Malrotated gut	
Incomplete resolution of early form	Choanal atresia, Meckel's diverticulum	
Persistence of early location	Low-set ears, undescended testes	
Redundant morphogenesis	Supernumerary ear tag, polydactyly	Uncommon
Aberrant morphogenesis	Mediastinal thyroid gland, paratesticular spleen	Rare

From Cohen, M. M., Jr.: The Child With Multiple Birth Defects. New York, Raven Press, 1982.

initiated earlier during organogenesis tend to have more far-reaching consequences. A malformation sequence may be defined as multiple defects derived from a known or presumed structural defect (Spranger and associates, 1982). The primary defect triggers a chain of secondary and tertiary events, resulting in what appear to be multiple anomalies.

Three malformation sequences are illustrated in Figure 2–3. In holoprosencephaly, the first malformation sequence, the embryonic forebrain fails to cleave sagittally into cerebral hemispheres, transversely into telencephalon and diencephalon, and horizontally into olfactory and optic bulbs. Holoprosencephaly varies in its degree of severity. Holoprosencephaly is associated with facial dysmorphism, which also varies from mild to severe expression (Fig. 2–4). One eye or closely set eyes, proboscis formation, single nostril nose, and median cleft lip may be observed in variation and combination. All malformations trace their origin developmentally to a primary defect in morphogenesis, probably an abnormality in the prechordal mesoderm (Cohen, 1982).

The second malformation sequence (see Fig. 2–3) is meningomyelocele in which spina bifida, a malformation, leads to congenital hip dislocation and clubfoot, two deformations.

Finally, the Robin sequence can be considered as a malformation sequence in some instances, such as in the partial trisomy 11q syndrome (Aurias and Laurent, 1975). With the dysmorphic development and growth deficiency that accompany most chromosomal syndromes, the initiating event in the Robin sequence in this syndrome may be intrinsic mandibular hypoplasia.

Malformations may be minimally or maximally expressed. For example, bifid uvula is a minimal expression of cleft palate. More complex malformations also may be minimally or maximally expressed, as seen in holoprosencephaly and its attendant facial dysmorphism (see Fig. 2–4) (Cohen, 1982).

NONSPECIFICITY OF MALFORMATIONS

Malformations are nonspecific. Each may occur as an isolated defect; each may also occur as a part of various syndromes. Cleft

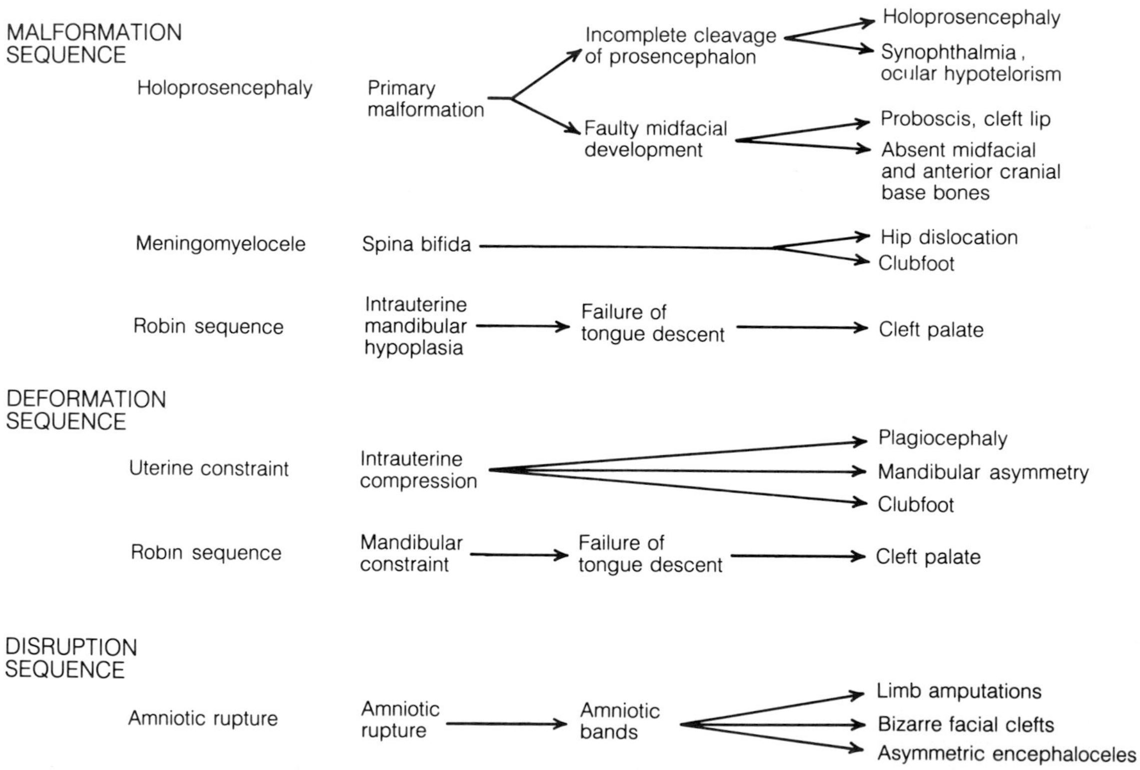

Figure 2–3. Malformation, deformation, and disruption sequences. (From Cohen, M.M., Jr.: The Child with Multiple Birth Defects. New York, Raven Press, 1982.)

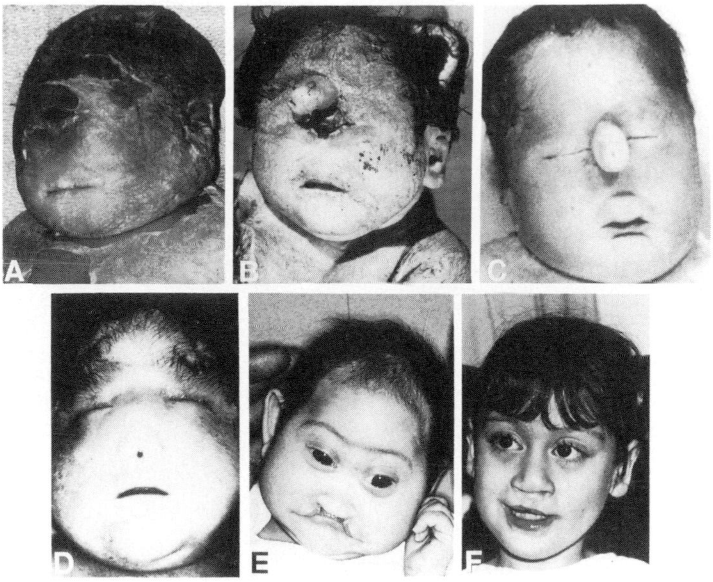

Figure 2–4. Spectrum of dysmorphic facies associated with variable degrees of holoprosencephaly. *A,* Cyclopia without proboscis formation (note the single, centrally located eye). *B,* Cyclopia with proboscis. *C,* Ethmocephaly (orbital hypotelorism with proboscis located between the eyes). *D,* Cebocephaly (orbital hypotelorism with single-nostril nose). *E,* Median cleft lip, flat nose, and orbital hypotelorism. *F,* Orbital hypotelorism and surgically repaired cleft lip. (*A* and *F* from Cohen, M.M., Jr., and Hohl, T.H.: Etiologic heterogeneity in holoprosencephaly and facial dysmorphia with comments on the facial bones and cranial base. *In* Bosma, J. F. (Ed.): Development of the Basicranium. U.S. Dept. of Health, Education, and Welfare, Bethesda, MD, 1976, pp. 384–388. *B, C,* and *D* from Cohen, M.M., Jr., Jirasek, J.E., Guzman, R.T., Gorlin, R.J., and Peterson, M.Q.: Holoprosencephaly and facial dysmorphia: nosology, etiology, and pathogenesis. *In* Bergsma, D. (Ed.): Orofacial Structures. Baltimore: Williams & Wilkins for the National Foundation—March of Dimes Birth Defects Foundation BD:OAS VII(7):125–135, 1971, with permission from the copyright holder. *E* from DeMyer, W., and Zeman, W.: Alobar holoprosencephaly with median cleft lip and palate: clinical, electroencephalographic, and nosologic considerations. Confin. Neurol., *23*:1, 1963. S. Karger AG, Basel, Switzerland.)

palate, for example, may occur alone or as part of the autosomal dominant Stickler syndrome, a condition characterized by high myopia, retinal detachment, and abnormalities of bones and joints. Because malformations occur with various frequencies in different syndromes, they are facultative rather than obligatory; they may or may not be present in a given example of a condition in which they are known to be features (Opitz, Herrmann, and Dieker, 1969; Cohen, 1976). Although patients with the Rubinstein-Taybi syndrome usually have broad thumbs, some of them have normal thumbs. Two common features of the Beckwith-Wiedemann syndrome are macroglossia and omphalocele, yet cases are known in which both malformations are absent. Pathognomonic anomalies for various syndromes are rare. Since anomalies are both nonspecific and facultative for various disorders, syndrome diagnosis is made not from any one anomaly but from the overall pattern of anomalies.

MALFORMATION SYNDROMES

A malformation syndrome may be defined as several malformations thought to be pathogenetically related in the same individual. A true malformation syndrome is characterized by embryonic pleiotropy in which a pattern of developmentally unrelated malformation sequences occurs; that is, the malformations that make up the syndrome occur in embryonically noncontiguous areas. They are not related to one another at the descriptive embryonic level, but at a more basic level the malformations have or are presumed to have a common cause and are thus pathogenetically related. The difference between a malformation sequence and a malformation syndrome is illustrated in Figure 2–5. When holoprosencephaly occurs alone, it is a malformation sequence, but when it occurs with multiple noncontiguous anomalies in trisomy 13 syndrome or with multiple noncontiguous anomalies in the autosomal, recessively inherited Meckel syndrome, it is a malformation syndrome composed of several malformation sequences.

Malformation syndromes lack biochemical definition. The highest state in malformation syndrome delineation is a known-genesis syndrome of the pedigree or chromosomal type. Pedigree syndromes may involve mutant embryonic proteins that are switched off before birth, thus masking the basic defect. Many other malformation syndromes remain unknown-genesis syndromes of the provisionally unique- or recurrent-pattern type.

Deformations

A deformation may be defined as an abnormal form or position of a part of the body

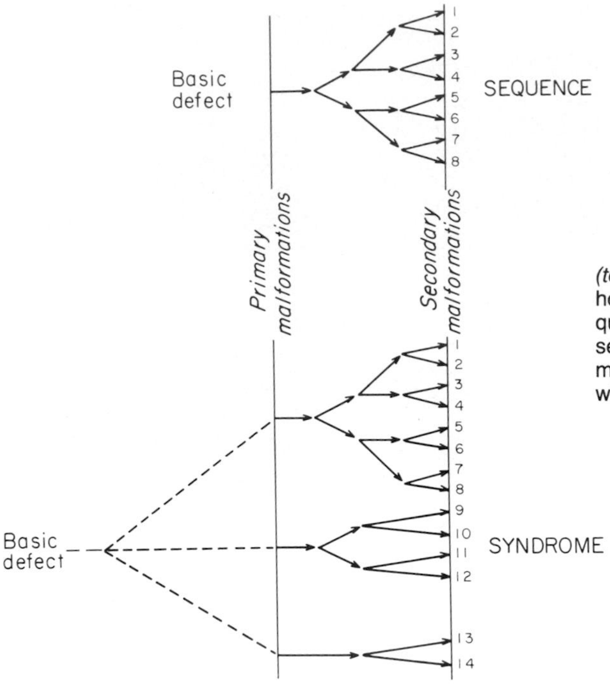

Figure 2–5. Comparison of a malformation sequence *(top)* with a true malformation syndrome *(bottom)*. Isolated holoprosencephaly is an example of a malformation sequence. The combination of holoprosencephaly, ventricular septal defect, and polydactyly, caused by trisomy 13, is a malformation syndrome. (From Cohen, M.M., Jr.: The Child with Multiple Birth Defects. New York, Raven Press, 1982.)

caused by nondisruptive mechanical forces (Fig. 2–6) (Spranger and associates, 1982). Approximately 2 per cent of newborns have deformations. Important examples include clubfoot (see Fig. 2–2), congenital hip dislocation, and congenital postural scoliosis. Deformations arise most often during late fetal life. Since the most common cause is intrauterine molding by mechanical forces, the musculoskeletal system is usually affected. The most important factor contributing to deformations is lack of fetal movement, whatever the cause. Deformations may result from mechanical, malformational, or functional causes (Table 2–3).

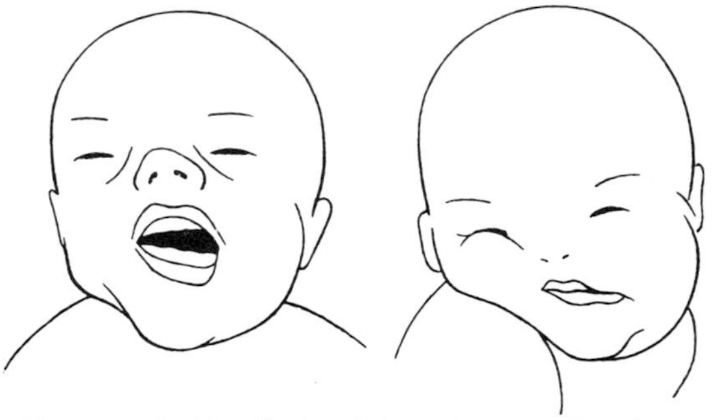

Figure 2–6. Mandibular deformation resulting from a lateroflexed position of the head in utero with the shoulder pressed against the mandible for a prolonged period. (Courtesy of Mead Johnson Nutritional Group, Evansville, IN 47721.)

Mechanical causes of deformations are most common. Correlating various pregnancy factors known to be statistically associated with the occurrence of congenital deformations, Dunn (1976) postulated how such factors might be interrelated (Fig. 2–7). First pregnancies tend to be associated with unstretched uterine and abdominal muscles, re-

Table 2–3. Causes of Deformations

Extrinsic
Mechanical
Unstretched uterine and abdominal muscles
Small maternal size
Amnionic tear
Unusual implantation site
Uterine leiomyomas
Unicornuate uterus
Bicornuate uterus
Twin fetuses
Intrinsic
Malformational
Spina bifida
Other central nervous system malformations
Bilateral renal agenesis
Severe hypoplastic kidneys
Severe polycystic kidneys
Urethral atresia
Functional
Neurologic disturbances
Muscular disturbances
Connective tissue defects

From Cohen, M. M., Jr.: The Child With Multiple Birth Defects. New York, Raven Press, 1982.

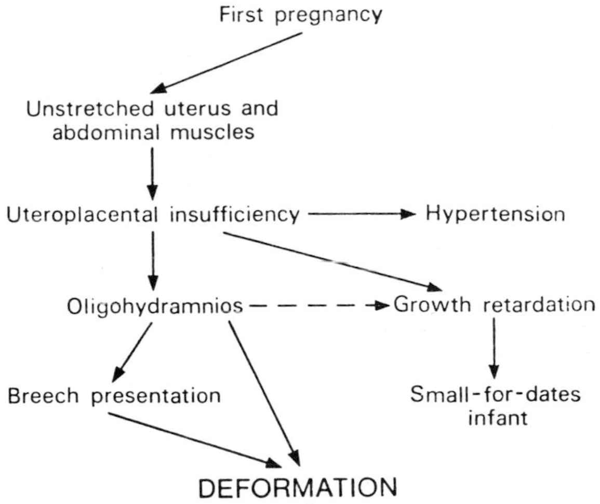

Figure 2–7. Sequence of events leading to intrauterine deformation. (From Dunn., P.M.: Congenital postural deformities. Br. Med. Bull., *32*:71, 1976.)

sulting in uteroplacental insufficiency, which in turn can lead to oligohydramnios. Breech presentation is common, since the uterus is too compressed to allow the fetus to rotate into the cephalic position. Uterine restraints on fetal movement allow mild but persistent extrinsic forces to deform the fetus. For the first few days after birth, infants with deformities usually can be folded into their atypical prenatal postures. The close correspondence on radiographic examination between the abnormal posture of the fetus before delivery and the posture of the infant after birth has been observed repeatedly. Such posture has been named the position of comfort by Chapple and Davidson (1941).

If postural deformities have a mechanical origin, more than one deformation might be expected to occur in some patients. In a study of approximately 4500 newborns, Dunn (1976) noted that one-third of newborns with deformations had two or more deformities. A deformation sequence can be specified as multiple deformations derived from a known or presumed mechanical factor or previous structural defect (Spranger and associates, 1982). Figure 2–3 illustrates two deformation sequences. In the first example, intrauterine compressive forces led to three deformations (plagiocephaly, mandibular asymmetry, and clubfoot) in the same patient. In the second example, micrognathia, caused by intrauterine constraint, led to failure of tongue descent, resulting in cleft palate. Thus, the Robin sequence may be considered on a malformational or a deformational basis, depending on whether the initiating event causing intrauterine micrognathia is mandibular hypoplasia or extrinsic mechanical forces acting on the mandible (Cohen, 1982).

In a study of newborns, Dunn (1976) found that 7.6 per cent of malformations were associated with deformations. When this relationship occurred, the malformations primarily involved the central nervous system and the urinary tract, and most often the deformations were secondary to the malformations. Both central nervous system and urinary tract malformations cause deformations by interfering with fetal movements. A malformation sequence can result in two deformations (see Fig. 2–3). Spina bifida, a malformation, leads to congenital hip dislocation and clubfoot since the malformations may produce partial paralysis of the legs. The resultant muscular imbalance is an intrinsic deforming force that limits the ability of the fetus to kick and hence to change position, thus altering the direction along which extrinsic deforming forces may be acting. Hip dysplasia, hip dislocation, and clubfoot may be explained on this basis, as may the hypoplastic lower limbs (a growth disturbance caused by deficient innervation).

To protect the fetus from extrinsic forces, there must be sufficient amnionic fluid. Some amnionic fluid crosses the amnion as a transudate, but most is produced by fetal urine. Any malformation of the urinary tract that significantly reduces the output of fetal urine results in a lack of amnionic fluid, thus producing the deformities of the Potter sequence (Fig. 2–8). Malformations such as bilateral renal agenesis, severe hypoplastic kidneys, severe polycystic kidneys, or urethral atresia can cause primary oligohydramnios and its results. A severe caudal axis malformation sequence such as sirenomelia, in which the kidneys and genitalia are both missing, also produces oligohydramnios and the deformed face and hands of the Potter sequence (Cohen, 1982).

Functional causes of deformations include forms of congenital hypotonia and neuromuscular types of arthrogryposis. Congenital hypotonia may be accompanied by micrognathia, microglossia, prominent lateral palatine ridges, abnormal flexion creases, pes planovalgus, and other deformities. The arthrogryposes are characterized by congenital immobility of the limbs and fixation of the joints in certain positions (Cohen, 1982).

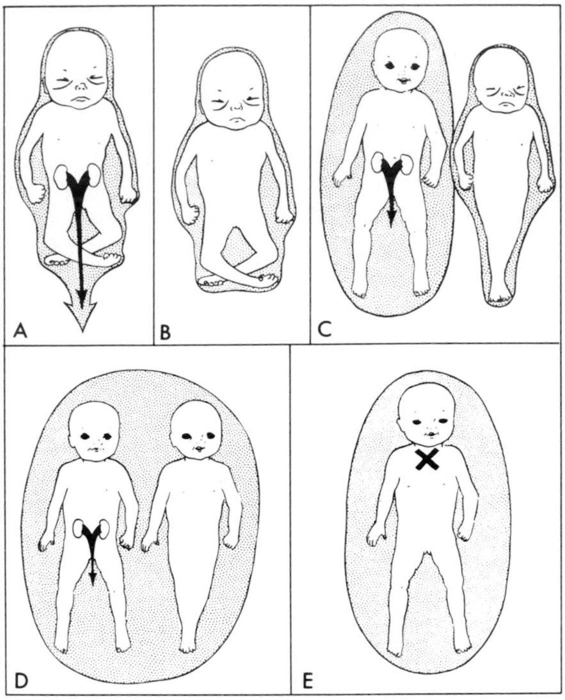

Figure 2–8. Oligohydramnios has different causes and leads to the facial and limb deformities of the Potter sequence. Normally, small amounts of amnionic fluid cross the amnion as a transudate, but most amnionic fluid results from fetal urination. *A,* Amnionic tear with chronic leakage of fluid leading to oligohydramnios, Potter facies, and limb positioning defects. Both kidneys are present and urination is normal. *B,* Bilateral renal agenesis resulting in the Potter sequence. *C,* Monozygotic twins with separate amnions. The fetus on the left has kidneys, and sufficient fetal urine is contributed to the amnionic fluid to protect the fetus from the deformities of the Potter sequence. The fetus on the right has sirenomelia in which both kidneys and genitalia are absent. Since there is no urinary contribution to the amnionic fluid, compression results in the facial and upper limb deformities of the Potter sequence. *D,* Monozygotic twins sharing a common amnionic sac. Although the fetus on the right has sirenomelia, the Potter deformities are absent because the fetus on the left provides sufficient urine in the amnionic fluid to protect the co-twin from the deformations of the Potter sequence. *E,* The fetus has bilateral renal agenesis and therefore does not contribute fetal urine to the amnionic fluid. Absence of the Potter sequence is based on a neurologic swallowing deficit because amnionic fluid crossing the amnion remains external to the fetus, protecting it from extrinsic deforming forces. (From Cohen, M.M., Jr.: The Child with Multiple Birth Defects. New York, Raven Press, 1982.)

COMPARISON OF MALFORMATIONS AND DEFORMATIONS

The characteristic features of malformations and deformations are contrasted in Table 2–4. Malformations tend to arise during the embryonic period at the time of organogenesis and are primary errors of morphogenesis. Deformations, on the other hand, tend to arise during the fetal period and are changes in the shape of previously normal parts. Thus, deformations tend to affect intact regions. A clubfoot is not an organ defect but a regional defect, since the limbs have already formed. With simple clubfoot, for example, five digits and the proper number of phalanges and metatarsals are present. This is not true of malformations such as ectrodactyly or polydactyly (Cohen, 1982).

A degree of perinatal mortality accompanies every statistical survey of malformations, because of the high frequency of central nervous system and cardiovascular anomalies. In contrast, the perinatal mortality rate tends to be low in surveys of deformations (Cohen, 1982).

Finally, spontaneous correction or correction by posturing is possible in many deformations. Dunn (1976) noted that 90 per cent of deformations correct spontaneously after birth. That self-correction occurs so commonly is not surprising, because after birth the infant is no longer subject to intrauterine constraining forces. Tibial torsion present in newborns, for example, undergoes spontaneous correction in most cases. With deformations, the degree to which self-correction is possible depends on how long during fetal life the constraining forces were acting, and on how severe the deformation was. Postural correction is feasible in many cases of scoliosis, congenital hip dislocation, and clubfoot. In contrast, spontaneous correction of malformations is rare, except for small septal defects, and correction by posturing is impossible.

TIME OF ONSET OF MALFORMATIONS AND DEFORMATIONS

Although the distinction between malformations and deformations based on embry-

Table 2–4. Comparison of Malformations and Deformations

	Malformation	Deformation
Time of occurrence	Embryonic period	Fetal period
Level of disturbance	Organ	Region
Perinatal mortality	+	−
Spontaneous correction	−	+
Correction by posture	−	+

From Cohen, M. M., Jr.: The Child With Multiple Birth Defects. New York, Raven Press, 1982.

onic and fetal periods is useful, rigid adherence to these time periods can be misleading. Malformations arise most commonly during the embryonic period, but some malformations such as cleft soft palate and hypospadias arise during the fetal period. Others may also be defined as a delay or error in perinatal transition, as with patent ductus arteriosus. Rarely, morphogenesis may fail to take place during the postnatal period, as in agenesis of the third molars.

The timing of malformations is summarized in Table 2–5. It is incorrect to speak of a malformation necessarily being caused *at* the specific time that it arose during development. Technically, the only statement that can be made about cause in relationship to embryonic timing is that something happened *before* the latest point in time at which a given malformation might arise (Warkany, 1971). The cause of the malformation might have occurred at that time, but it might have been earlier.

This principle is illustrated by any monogenic malformation syndrome. For example, suppose a patient with the Meckel syndrome has encephalocele, polycystic kidneys, polydactyly, ventricular septal defect, and cleft palate. As is true of many malformation syndromes, the embryonic timing of each of these malformations is different. The only statement that can be made about cause is that something must have happened before the earliest induced malformation. In the case of the Meckel syndrome, the earliest malformation occurred at four weeks of development, but because the syndrome has autosomal recessive inheritance, the abnormality was present earlier than four weeks of development, specifically at the zygotic stage of development. Two mutant genes in the homozygous state were present at the time.

It has already been stated that deformations arise most commonly during the fetal period. The fetus is especially prone to deformation because of its skeletal plasticity and rapid rate of growth in a potentially constraining intrauterine environment. That rapid growth can be a factor in prenatal deformations is easily realized because a fetus of 28 weeks doubles its body weight in six weeks. In contrast, during postnatal growth a 5 year old boy requires six years to double his body weight. Deformations, however, may arise during the postnatal period, as in cases of progressive scoliosis, for example, or in patients with severe cerebral palsy who develop craniofacial deformity, scoliosis, and contractures. Postnatal deformities also may be induced deliberately, as in the Chinese footbinding practice in young girls, and in the Chinook Indian practice of splinting the head between boards during infancy to form a pointed skull. The same principles are used by orthopedic surgeons and orthodontists who correct deformities by postural means.

Disruptions

A disruption is a morphologic defect of an organ, part of an organ, or a larger region of the body, resulting from a breakdown of, or an interference with, originally normal development (Spranger and associates, 1982). An amputation of a digit in utero caused by an aberrant tissue band serves as an example, as do other band-caused disruptions such as ring constriction and distal pseudosyndactyly (Torpin, 1968; Baker and Rudolph, 1971).

Another possible disruptive cause of limb reduction defects may be early severe compression in utero secondary to bicornuate uterus, leiomyomas, or early amnionic rupture (Graham and associates, 1980). Similar limb reduction anomalies have resulted from vascular compromise produced by compression in rat fetuses subjected to amnionic puncture (Kennedy and Persaud, 1977). In a disruption sequence, multiple defects are derived from one disruptive factor. Aberrant tissue bands can produce a dramatic disrup-

Table 2–5. Timing of Malformations

Period	Frequency of Malformations	Examples
Embryonic	Common	Anencephaly, cleft lip, syndactyly
Fetal	Less common	Hypospadias, posterior cleft palate
Perinatal	Uncommon	Patent ductus arteriosus, cryptorchidism
Postnatal	Rare	Agenesis of third molars

From Cohen, M. M., Jr.: The Child with Multiple Birth Defects. New York, Raven Press, 1982.

tion sequence (see Fig. 2–3) consisting of asymmetric encephaloceles, bizarre facial clefts, and limb amputations (Fig. 2–9) (Jones and associates, 1974).

Disruptions tend to be sporadic occurrences in contrast to malformations and deformations, both of which may recur in some instances. No two cases of a given disruption are alike. Examples of a given disruption tend to be more variable than those of a given malformation or deformation. Finally, disruptions can be interpreted mistakenly as embryonic malformations when, in fact, they arise later during intrauterine life. For example, an open calvarial defect caused by disruption from the results of amnionic rupture may be mistaken for anencephaly, a malformation with a risk of recurrence (Cohen, 1982).

INTERRELATIONSHIPS BETWEEN MALFORMATIONS, DEFORMATIONS, AND DISRUPTIONS

It should be recognized that although the distinctions between malformations, deformations, and disruptions are useful for clinical purposes, the three classes of anomalies are interrelated and may even overlap in some instances (Fig. 2–10). It is not always possible to assign an anomaly to one specific class. For example, some types of malocclusion are both malformational and deformational and cannot be clearly assigned to one class or the other. It has already been observed that malformations can result in deformations, as with the deformational components of the meningomyelocele sequence. It has also been stated that some anomalies, such as the Robin sequence, may be malformational or deformational, depending on the initiating factor. Sometimes the same mechanism can result in different classes of anomalies. For example, intrauterine compression during the fetal period may result in deformations, but when severe compression is present earlier during the embryonic period, disruptions may be produced. Cases of limb and body wall deficiency have both disruptive and deformational components (Miller and associates, 1981). In this condition, amniotic rupture sequence can lead to two types of disruptions: (1) compression-related defects such as limb deficiency, body wall deficiency, and neural tube defects; and (2) band- or adhesion-related defects such as craniofacial clefts. Deformations resulting from compression may include severe scoliosis, retroflexion of the neck, and ear deformities.

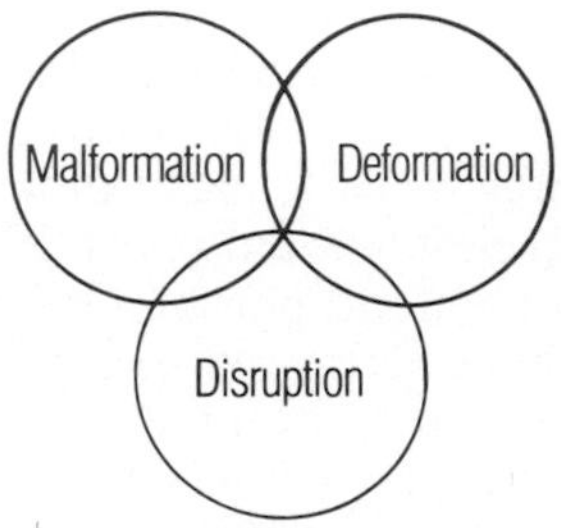

Figure 2–10. Interrelationships between malformations, deformations, and disruptions. (From Cohen, M.M., Jr.: The Child with Multiple Birth Defects. New York, Raven Press, 1982.)

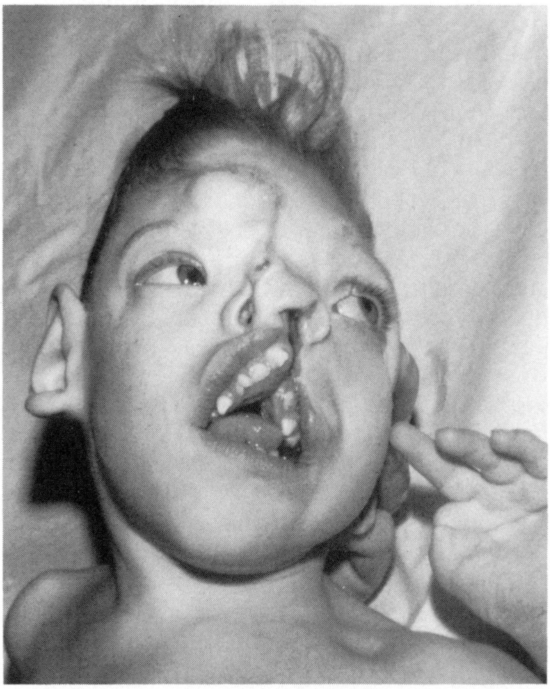

Figure 2–9. Disruptive process. Bizarre facial clefting and asymmetric encephaloceles, the result of aberrant tissue bands. (From Cohen, M.M., Jr.: The Child with Multiple Birth Defects. New York, Raven Press, 1982.)

Minor Anomalies and Their Significance

A distinction can be made between major and minor anomalies (Fig. 2–11). Major anomalies, such as omphalocele, tetralogy of Fallot, and cleft lip, are of obvious surgical, medical, or esthetic importance. Minor anomalies, such as upslanting palpebral fissures,

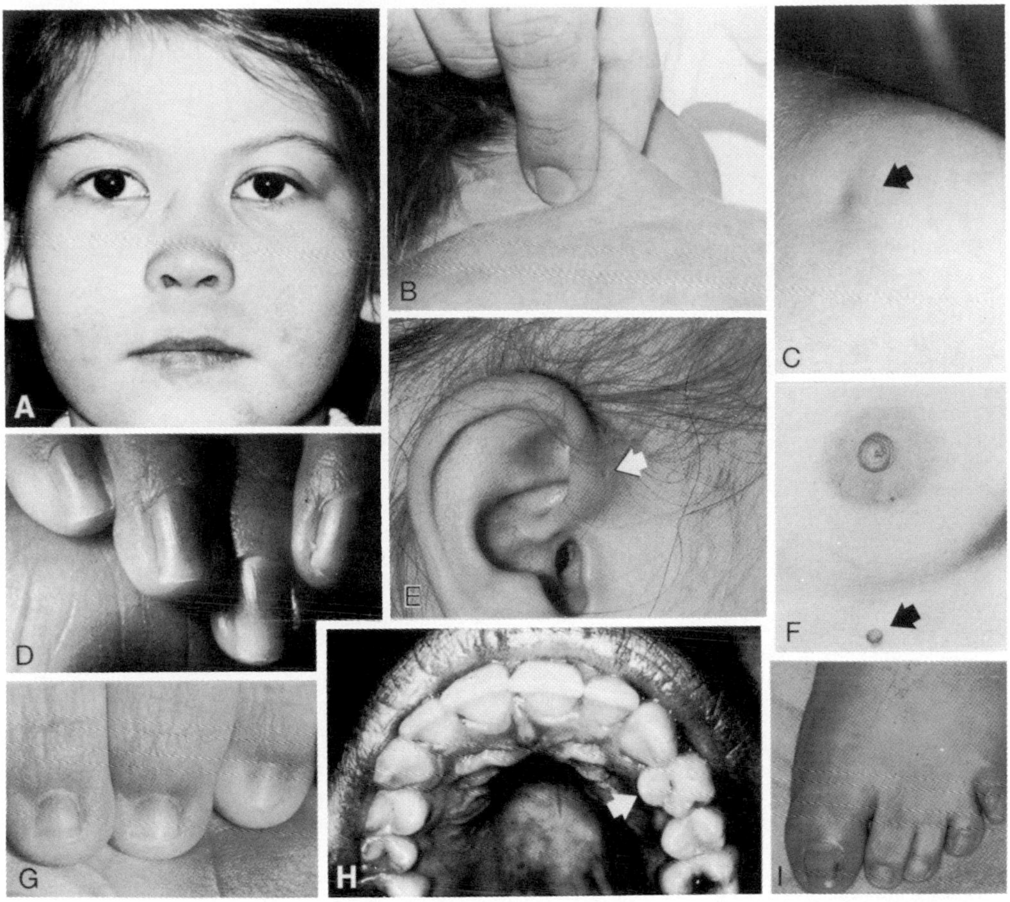

Figure 2–11. Selected minor anomalies. *A,* Epicanthic folds. *B,* Loose skin on the posterior neck. *C,* Acromial dimple. *D,* Hyperconvex fingernails. *E,* Ear pit. *F,* Supernumerary nipple. *G,* Small, deeply set nails. *H,* Accessory cusp on tooth. *I,* Partial soft tissue syndactyly. (From Cohen, M.M., Jr.: The Child with Multiple Birth Defects. New York, Raven Press, 1982.)

lack of helical fold, and clinodactyly, are not of serious surgical or medical significance, although in some instances they may be of esthetic concern, as in the case of prominent epicanthic folds. A representative but by no means exhaustive list of minor anomalies is presented in Table 2–6. Because minor anomalies may serve as indicators of altered morphogenesis and may sometimes imply more serious structural defects, they may provide valuable diagnostic clues for specific patterns of malformation (Fig. 2–12).

The occurrence of single minor anomalies is common in the general population, being found in approximately 15 per cent of all newborns. Of great interest is the occurrence of major malformation in association with 90 per cent of all newborns with three or more minor anomalies (Marden, Smith, and McDonald, 1964). The implication is clear. Any newborn with three or more minor anomalies should be carefully evaluated for possible hidden major malformations, such as cardiac, renal, or vertebral defects. Before significance is ascribed to any minor anomaly, it should be ascertained whether it is present in any other member of the family.

Minor anomalies occur with high frequency in many malformation syndromes. For example, in trisomy 21 syndrome, 79 per cent of all malformations detectable by clinical examination are minor anomalies; in trisomy 18 syndrome, 38 per cent; in trisomy 13, 50 per cent; and in the Turner syndrome, 73 per cent (Smith and Bostian, 1964). Thus, minor anomalies serve as diagnostic aids for many malformation syndromes.

Finally, 42 per cent of patients with idiopathic mental retardation have three or more malformations, of which 80 per cent are mi-

Table 2–6. Minor Anomalies

Head	**Neck**
Aberrant scalp hair patterning	Mild webbed neck
Flat occiput	Branchial cleft fistula
Bony occipital spur	**Hands**
Third fontanel	Rudimentary polydactyly
Eyes	Duplication of thumbnail
Epicanthic folds	Single palmar creases
Epicanthus inversus	Unusual dermatoglyphics
Upward-slanting palpebral fissures	Clinodactyly (5)
Downward-slanting palpebral fissures	Short fingers (4,5)
Short palpebral fissures	**Feet**
Dystopia canthorum	Syndactyly (2–3)
Minor hypertelorism	Gap between toes (1–2)
Minor hypotelorism	Short great toe
Minor ptosis	Recessed toes (4,5)
Coloboma	Thickened nails
Ears	Prominent calcaneus
Primitive shape	**Skin**
Lack of helical fold	Hemangioma (other than face or neck)
Asymmetric size	Pigmented nevi
Posterior rotation	Mongoloid spot (whites)
Small ears	Depigmented spot
Protuberant ears	Unusual placement of nipples
Absent tragus	Accessory nipples
Double lobule	Café-au-lait spot
Auricular tag	**Body**
Auricular pit	Diastasis recti
Narrow external auditory meatus	Umbilical hernia
Nose	Minor hypospadias
Small nares	Deep sacral dimple
Notched alas	**Skeletal**
Oral regions	Cubitus valgus
Borderline small mandible	Prominent sternum
Incomplete form of cleft lip	Depressed sternum
Bifid uvula	Shieldlike chest
Aberrant frenula	Genua valga
Enamel hypoplasia	Genua vara
Malformed teeth	Genu recurvatum

Adapted from Marden, P. M., Smith, D. W., and McDonald, M. J.: Congenital anomalies in the newborn infant, including minor variation. J. Pediatr., *64*:357, 1964.

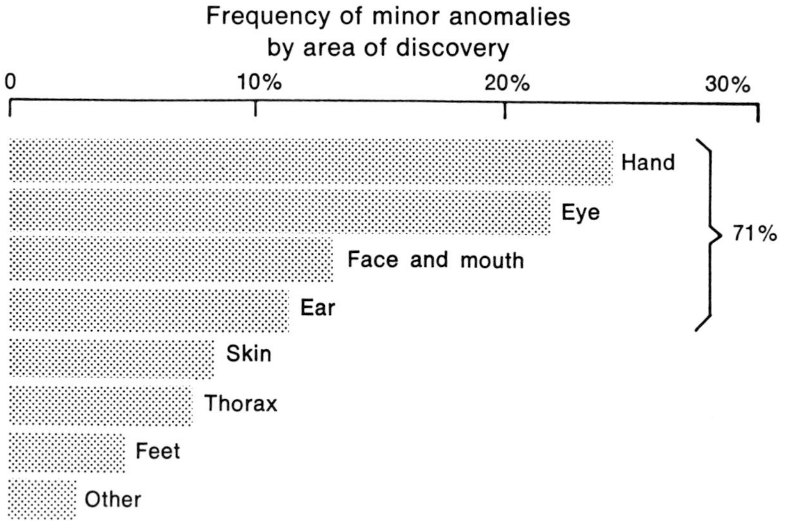

Figure 2–12. Frequency of minor anomalies by region. Of all minor anomalies, 71 per cent occur in the head and neck region and on the hand. (Redrawn from Smith D.W., and Bostian, K.E.: Congenital anomalies associated with idiopathic mental retardation. J. Pediatr., *65*:189, 1964.)

Table 2–7. Significance of Minor Anomalies

Fact	Implication
In newborns with three or more minor anomalies, 90% have major anomaly	Search for occult major anomaly
Minor anomalies present in many multiple congenital anomaly syndromes	Aid in diagnosis
42% of idiopathic mental retardation cases have three or more anomalies of which 80% are minor anomalies	Aid in prognosis

From Cohen, M. M., Jr.: The Child With Multiple Birth Defects. New York, Raven Press, 1982.

nor. Thus, the presence of minor anomalies may be considered an aid in determining the prognosis of mental deficiency. The significance of minor anomalies is summarized in Table 2–7.

PRINCIPLES OF SYNDROMOLOGY

Approximately 1 per cent of all newborns have multiple anomalies, or syndromes. Of these, only 40 per cent can be diagnosed as having specific, recognized syndromes (Marden, Smith, and McDonald, 1964); the other 60 per cent represent unknown entities that need to be further delineated. Although many syndromes are individually rare, in the aggregate they constitute a significant portion of medical practice. The process of syndrome delineation can be divided into the following stages:

1. *Unknown-genesis syndromes*
   a. Provisionally unique-pattern syndromes
   b. Recurrent-pattern syndromes
2. *Known-genesis syndromes*
   a. Pedigree syndromes
   b. Chromosomal syndromes
   c. Biochemical defect syndromes
   d. Environmentally induced syndromes

Unknown-Genesis Syndromes

In an unknown-genesis syndrome, the cause is simply not known.

PROVISIONALLY UNIQUE-PATTERN SYNDROMES

In a provisionally unique-pattern syndrome, several anomalies are observed in the same patient to the extent that the clinician does not recognize the overall pattern of defects from his own experience, nor from searching the literature, nor from consultation with the most learned colleagues in the field. The infant shown in Figure 2–13 has craniosynostosis with a cloverleaf skull and anomalies of the brain, limbs, and genitalia. The findings are summarized in Table 2–8. The patient's condition represents a provisionally unique-pattern syndrome. Most likely the anomalies have a common cause, although an unknown one, rather than different causes acting independently. The probability that such anomalies occur in the same patient by chance becomes less likely the more anomalies the patient has and the more infrequently the anomalies occur individually in the general population (Cohen, 1982).

If a second example comes to light, the condition is no longer unique. A provisionally unique-pattern syndrome is a one-of-a-kind syndrome to a particular observer at a par-

Table 2–8. Provisionally Unique-Pattern Syndrome

- Skull
  - Craniosynostosis with partially fused metopic, sagittal, left lambdoidal, and right coronal sutures
  - Asymmetric cloverleaf skull
- Brain
  - Polymicrogyria
  - Hypoplastic frontal lobes
  - Absent olfactory tracts and bulbs
  - Herniation of cerebellum into cervical spinal canal
  - Hydrocephaly
- Face
  - Orbital hypotelorism
  - Orbital proptosis
  - Epicanthal folds
  - Low nasal bridge
  - Short, upturned nose
  - Small, downturned mouth
  - Narrow palate
  - Low-set, posteriorly angulated ears
- Limbs
  - Duplication of thumb
  - Small fifth fingers
  - Limited knee extension
  - Metatarsus adductus
- Genitalia
  - Micropenis
  - Bifid scrotum
- Other
  - Agenesis of cervical thymic lobes
  - Bilateral bilobed lungs

From Cohen, M. M., Jr.: Craniosynostosis: Diagnosis, Evaluation, and Management. New York, Raven Press, 1986.

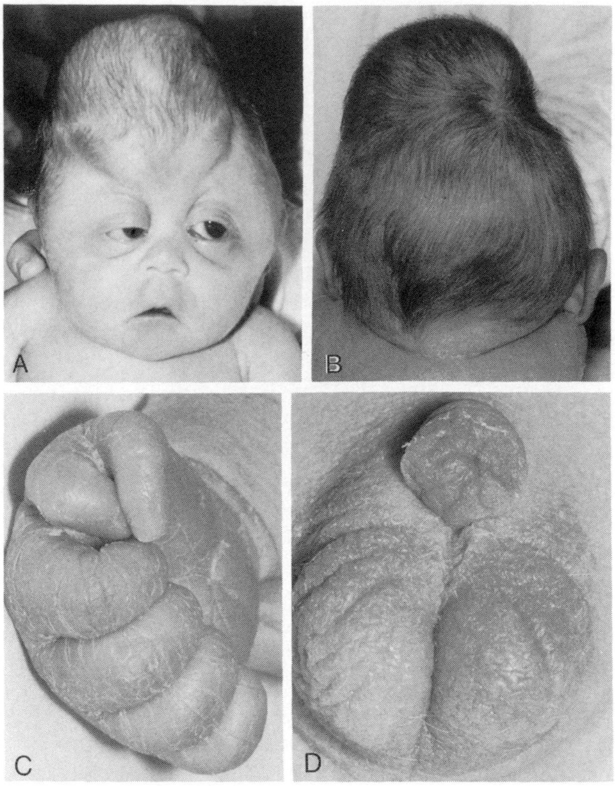

Figure 2–13. Example of a provisionally unique-pattern syndrome. *A, B,* Craniosynostosis, cloverleaf skull, and facial anomalies. *C,* Preaxial polydactyly. *D,* Micropenis and bifid scrotum. (From Cohen, M.M., Jr.: On the nature of syndrome delineation. Acta Genet. Med. Gemellol. (Roma), *26*:103, 1977.)

ticular point in time. There may be a nineteenth century description of a similar example that has escaped his attention. There may also exist instances of the syndrome in different parts of the world where they are as yet unrecognized. Thus, many syndromes that appear to be unique at the time at which the initial patient is discovered are no longer unique when two or more other examples become known. Conversely, some syndromes may indeed be truly unique (Cohen, 1982).

All provisionally unique-pattern syndromes should be published. In practice, they are usually filed away and hardly ever published because their significance is a mystery to clinicians and to journal editors alike. However, the publication of a provisionally unique-pattern syndrome is like an advertisement with a red flag—it reaches a large audience, and may prompt one or more clinicians to react by publishing similar cases. When this occurs, the process of syndrome delineation is under way.

RECURRENT-PATTERN SYNDROMES

A recurrent-pattern syndrome can be defined as a similar or identical set of anomalies in two or more unrelated patients. The Weaver syndrome is an example of an early recurrent-pattern syndrome (Fig. 2–14, Table 2–9). The same abnormalities in two or more patients suggest, but do not prove, that the pathogenesis may be the same. At the recurrent-pattern stage of syndrome delineation, the etiology is still not known. In general, the validity of a recurrent-pattern syndrome increases the more abnormalities there are in the syndrome and the more patients who are known to be affected.

At the recurrent-pattern stage of syndrome delineation, the number of findings is usually expanded as the number of patients increases. However, because the etiology remains unknown at this point in time, other examples of the syndrome tend to be selected because they most closely resemble the first case. This results in an artificial homogeneity of cases, which emphasizes the most severe aspects of the syndrome. Thus, readers should be wary of estimated frequencies given in review articles and textbooks for various anomalies that occur in a recurrent-pattern syndrome; they tend to be overestimates that can affect the prognostic risk counseling for possibly developing some feature of the syndrome, such as mental retardation.

Table 2–9. Comparison of Features of Two Patients with Recurrent-Pattern Syndrome

Feature	Patient 1	Patient 2
Growth		
Excessive growth of prenatal onset	+ + +	+ + +
Accelerated osseous maturation	+ + + +	+ + + +
Performance		
Hypertonia	+ +	+
Hoarse, low-pitched cry	+ +	+ +
Developmental delay	?	?
Excessive appetite	+ +	+ +
Craniofacial		
Wide bifrontal diameter	+ + +	+ + +
Flat occiput	+	+
Large ears	+ + +	+ + +
Orbital hypertelorism	+ +	+ +
Long philtrum	+ +	+
Relative micrognathia	+	+
Limbs		
Hands		
Prominent finger pads	+ +	+ +
Simian crease	−	+
Camptodactyly	+ +	+
Broad thumbs	+ +	+
Thin, deep-set nails	+ +	+ +
Feet		
Clinodactyly	+	+
Talipes equinovarus	+ +	−
Short fourth metatarsals	+	−
Limited early elbow and knee extension	+	+
Widened distal femurs and ulnas	+ +	+ +
Skin		
Excessive, loose skin	+ +	+ +
Inverted nipples	+	+
Thin hair	+	+
Other		
Umbilical hernia	+ +	+
Inguinal hernias	+ +	−

+ through + + + + = present, in varying degrees of severity; − = absent; ? = uncertain.

From Weaver, D. D., and associates: A new overgrowth syndrome with accelerated skeletal maturation, unusual facies, and camptodactyly. J. Pediatr., *84*:547, 1974.

Known-Genesis Syndromes

In known-genesis syndromes, several anomalies are causally related on the basis of (1) occurrence in the same family or, less conclusively, the same mode of inheritance in different families; (2) a chromosomal defect; (3) a specific defect in an enzyme or structural protein; or (4) an environmental factor.

PEDIGREE SYNDROMES

The term pedigree syndrome refers to known genesis on the basis of pedigree evidence alone; the basic defect itself remains undefined, although the condition is known to represent a monogenic disorder. An example is the autosomal dominantly inherited Crouzon syndrome, characterized by craniosynostosis, ocular proptosis, and midface hypoplasia (Fig. 2–15).

CHROMOSOMAL SYNDROMES

Chromosomal syndromes are cytogenetically defined. An example is trisomy 13 syndrome, which is characterized by alobar holoprosencephaly, microphthalmia, median cleft lip, polydactyly, congenital cardiac defects, and other anomalies (Fig. 2–16).

BIOCHEMICAL DEFECT SYNDROMES

In biochemical defect syndromes, the specific enzymatic defects of recessive disorders are known. The term is also meant to include specific defects in structural proteins as these become known in some of the dominant disorders. The Hurler syndrome, characterized by α-L-iduronidase deficiency, is an autosomal recessive, enzymatically defined syndrome. In this mucopolysaccharidosis, the facial appearance becomes coarse and the sagittal and lambdoid sutures may be prematurely synostosed (Fig. 2–17).

ENVIRONMENTALLY INDUCED SYNDROMES

These syndromes are defined in terms of environmental factors or causative teratogens. An example is the fetal alcohol syndrome. Infants born to mothers who are chronic alcoholics during their pregnancies have an increased risk of having prenatal onset growth deficiency persisting into postnatal life, microcephaly, mental deficiency, narrow palpebral fissures, mild maxillary hypoplasia, long philtrum, joint deformities, cardiac malformations, and other anomalies (Fig. 2–18).

Comments on Syndrome Delineation Process. The process of syndrome delineation is summarized in Figure 2–19. Generally, a syndrome can be placed in one of the categories discussed above. Occasionally, a syndrome may be delineated in a one-step delineation, thus bypassing several of the stages mentioned earlier. For example, if a new chromosomal abnormality is discovered during the laboratory investigation of a patient clinically defined as having a provision-

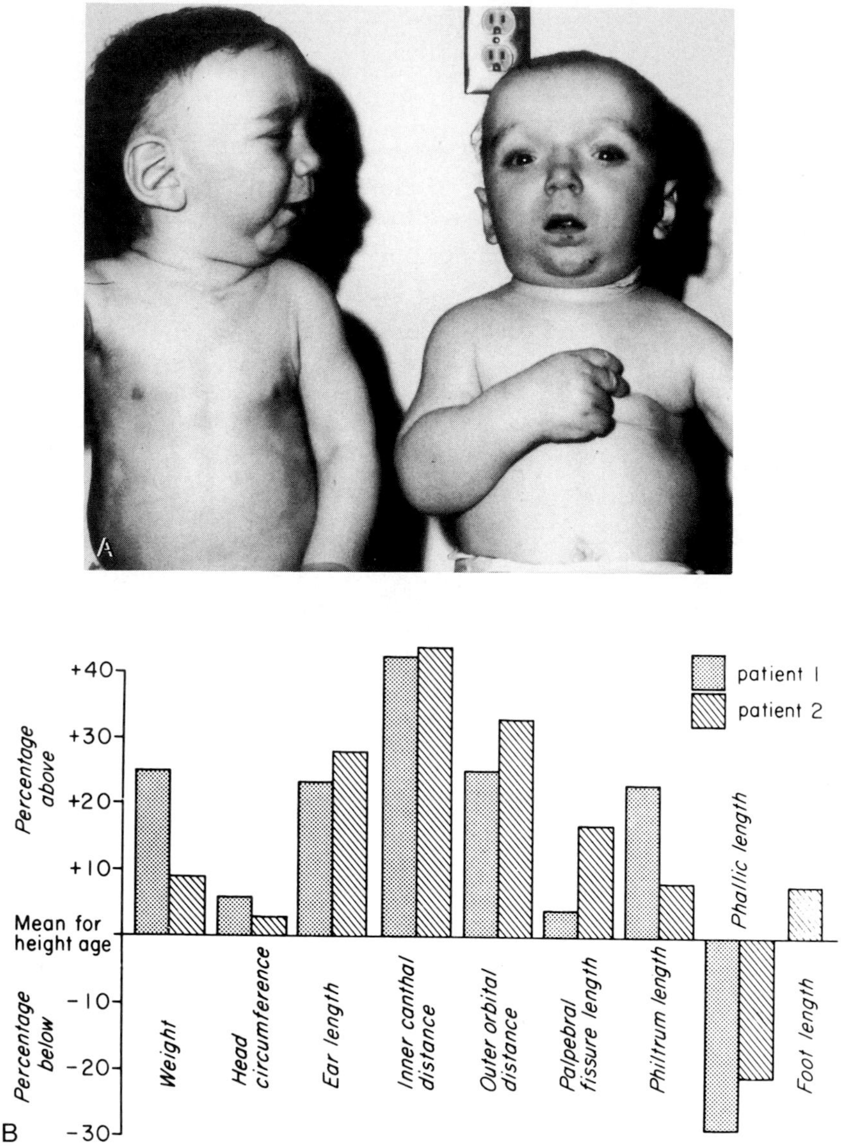

Figure 2–14. Examples of a recurrent-pattern syndrome in two patients. *A,* Note the similarity. *B,* Note the similarity of measurement patterns.

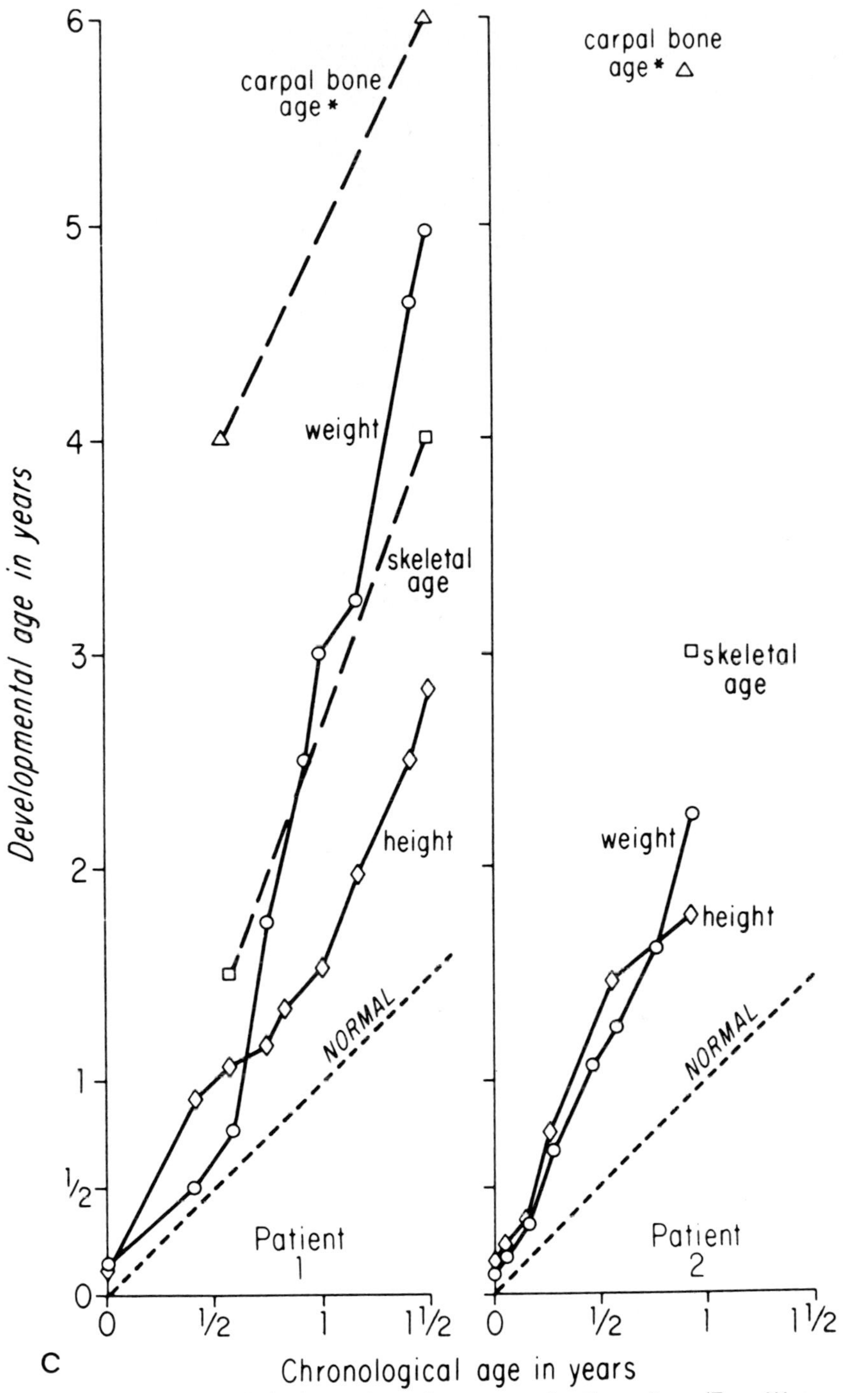

Figure 2–14 *Continued C,* Note the similarity in accelerated osseous maturation pattern. (From Weaver, D.D., Graham, C.B., Thomas, I.T., and Smith, D.W.: A new overgrowth syndrome with accelerated skeletal maturation, unusual facies and camptodactyly. J. Pediatr., *84*:547, 1974.)

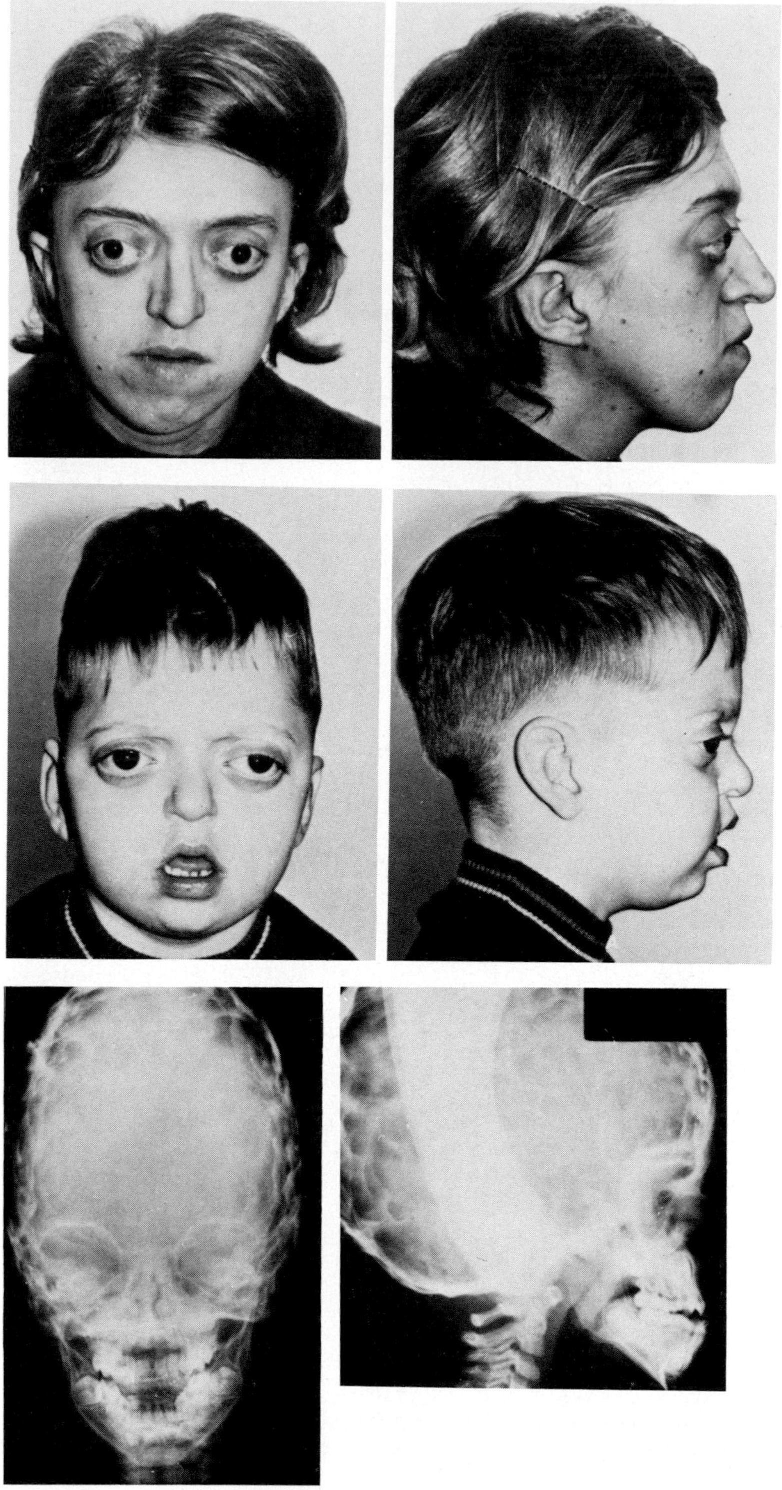

Figure 2–15. Pedigree syndrome example. Crouzon syndrome in a mother and son. Note brachycephaly, ocular proptosis, maxillary hypoplasia, and beaked nose. *Bottom*, Cephalometric roentgenograms of the son. Note brachycephaly, increased digital markings, and maxillary hypoplasia. (From Cohen, M.M., Jr.: Craniosynostosis: Diagnosis, Evaluation, and Management. New York, Raven Press, 1986.)

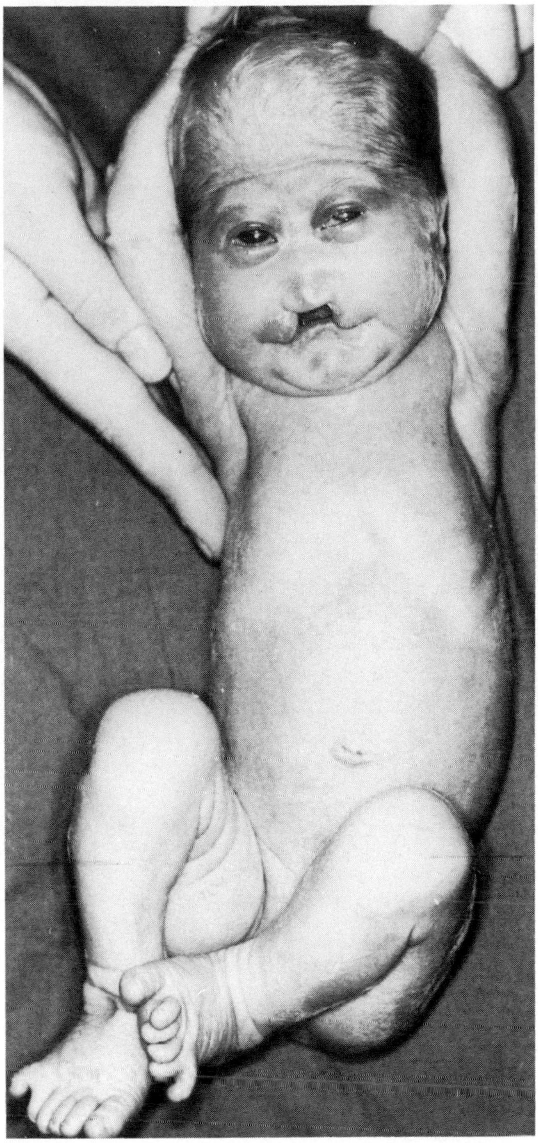

Figure 2–16. Example of a chromosomal syndrome: trisomy 13 syndrome. Orbital hypotelorism, flat nose, median cleft lip, and polydactyly. (From Conen, P.E., Erkman, B., and Metaxotou, C.: The "D" syndrome. Report of four trisomic and one D/D translocation case. Am. J. Dis. Child., *111*:236, 1966. Copyright 1966, American Medical Association.)

ally unique-pattern syndrome, the patient represents a known-genesis syndrome of the chromosomal type in a one-step delineation. However, the variability in clinical expression must await the discovery of more patients. In other instances, such as a large dominant pedigree with many affected individuals, variability can be determined in one step (Cohen, 1982).

Provisionally unique-pattern syndromes occur with some frequency. Further delineation often occurs, given sufficient time. A truly unique-pattern syndrome may occur with a chromosomal anomaly involving two or more breaks. The condition may be sporadic or may segregate within a family. Since the chance of an identical duplication-deficiency syndrome occurring in another family is slight, the syndrome may be considered unique to an affected individual or an affected family (Cohen, 1982).

Sporadic Occurrence and Syndrome Delineation. It should be emphasized that sporadicity per se does not necessarily mean that a condition is nongenetic. In the early stages of syndrome delineation, a number of sporadic instances of a new recurrent-pattern syndrome might represent a monogenic disorder. Because of the small size of the human family, more than one-half of all families in which both parents are heterozygous carriers for a given autosomal recessive disorder have

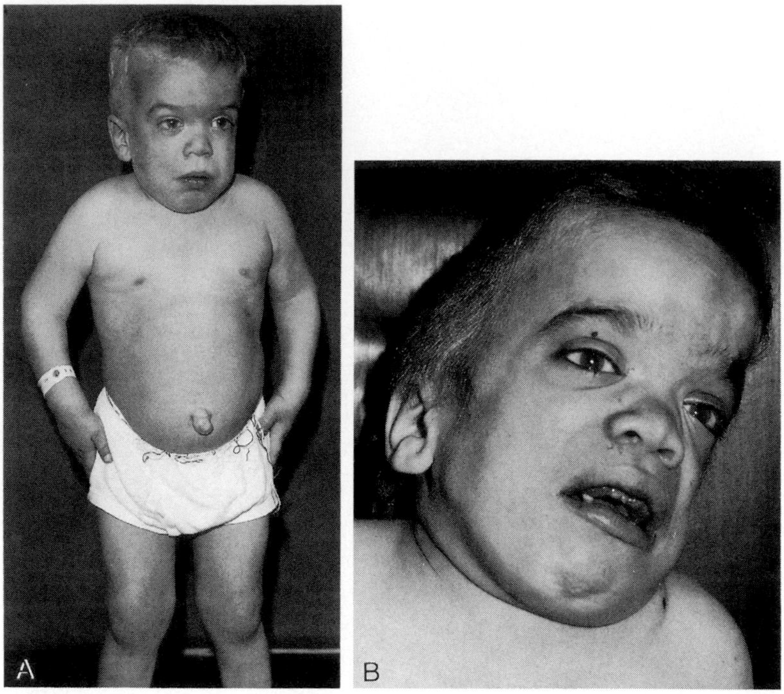

Figure 2–17. Example of a biochemical defect syndrome: Hurler syndrome. *A,* 10 year old patient with coarse facial features and umbilical hernia. *B,* The same patient at 18 years of age. Note the progressive coarsening of the facial features, corneal clouding, and open mouth. The skull shape resulted from premature closure of the sagittal and lambdoid sutures. (From Smith, D.W.: Recognizable Patterns of Human Malformation. 3rd Ed. Philadelphia, W. B. Saunders Company, 1982.)

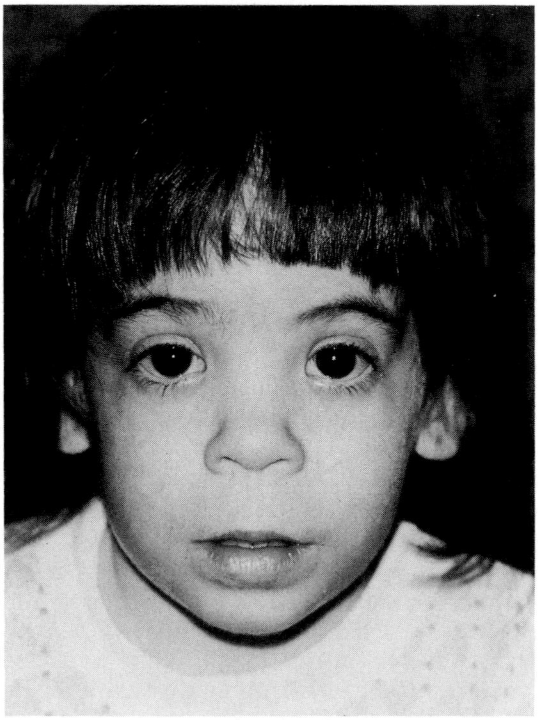

Figure 2–18. Example of an environmentally induced syndrome: the fetal alcohol syndrome. Microcephaly, narrow palpebral fissures, mild maxillary hypoplasia, and short nose. (From Clarren, S.K., and Smith, D.W.: The fetal alcohol syndrome. N. Engl. J. Med., *298*:1063, 1978. Reprinted by permission of The New England Journal of Medicine.)

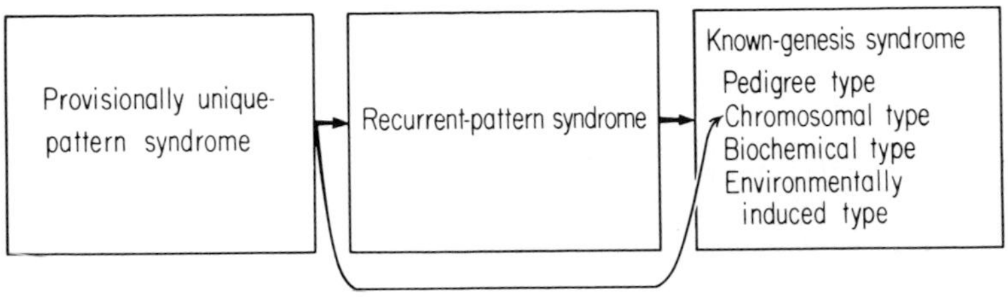

Figure 2–19. Summary of the process of syndrome delineation. (From Cohen, M.M., Jr.: The Child with Multiple Birth Defects. New York, Raven Press, 1982.)

only one occurrence of the disorder per family. Sporadic occurrences of a syndrome can also represent fresh mutations for an autosomal dominant disorder in which the genetic fitness is dramatically reduced. Most instances of the Apert syndrome (a known autosomal dominant disorder) are sporadic because the severe physical malformations and the mental deficiency (present in some cases) diminish the person's desirability as a mate (Fig. 2–20). In the few known instances in which mating has occurred, dominant transmission of the disorder has been observed (Fig. 2–21).

Differences Between Syndromology and Classical Medicine. The similarities and differences between syndromology and classical medicine are illustrated in Figure 2–22. In classical medicine, there are two general categories to consider. In the first category, clinical presentations become all-important, and the challenge lies in proper evaluations, from which diagnosis and treatment follow. In the second category, research is conducted on various disease entities to elucidate mechanisms of etiology and pathogenesis. Although some disorders are well understood and others are poorly understood, classical medicine assumes that almost all disease categories have at least been described. Only rarely does a new disease entity, such as legionnaires' disease, come to light.

Syndromology, like classical medicine, deals with the first two general categories. However, a third category becomes apparent, since the condition of many patients examined by the syndromologist represents a provisionally unique-pattern syndrome. Thus, the syndromologist is always asking, "Does the patient represent a known disease category or an unknown disease category?" Clinicians not trained in syndromology or medical genetics usually become uncomfortable with this concept, since they are not used to dealing with "new diseases" (Cohen, 1982).

Pace of Syndrome Delineation. The process of syndrome delineation has progressed at an extremely rapid pace during the past one and one-half decades. For example, in 1971, 72 syndromes with orofacial clefting were known. By 1978, 154 were known and today, over 300 such syndromes are recognized. Eighteen craniosynostosis syndromes were described in 1975, but today 64 syndromes are recognized. Even with the complex craniofacial anomalies such as holoprosencephaly, 41 syndromes are known today compared with 10 in 1971 (Cohen, 1982, 1986, in press) (Table 2–10).

Significance of Syndrome Delineation. The significance of syndrome delineation cannot be overestimated. As an unknown-genesis

Table 2–10. Syndrome Delineation for Two Craniofacial Anomalies Over Time

Syndrome Delineation Involving Craniosynostosis

Etiology	*1975*	*1979*	*1986*
Chromosomal	0	11	14
Monogenic	12	26	31
Autosomal dominant	(5)	(12)	(13)
Autosomal recessive	(7)	(12)	(13)
X-linked	(0)	(2)	(2)
Inheritance pattern unclear	(0)	(0)	(3)
Environmentally induced	1	2	3
Unknown genesis	5	18	10
Miscellaneous	—	—	6
Total Syndromes	18	57	64

Syndrome Delineation Involving Holoprosencephaly

Etiology	*1971*	*1982*	*1986*
Chromosomal	5	13	17
Monogenic	5	12	18
Holoprosencephaly	2	5	8
Autosomal dominant	(0)	(1)	(4)
Autosomal recessive	(2)	(4)	(4)
Arhinencephaly	3	7	10
Autosomal dominant	(1)	(2)	(3)
Autosomal recessive	(0)	(2)	(4)
X-linked recessive	(2)	(3)	(3)
Environmental	0	1	1 + (?7)*
Unknown genesis	0	5	5
Total syndromes	10	31	41

*Seven suspected or suggested teratogens not added in total syndrome estimate.

From Cohen, 1982, 1986, in press. Criteria for inclusion or exclusion of a syndrome differ slightly in different yearly estimates, but most of the increase is due to syndrome delineation per se.

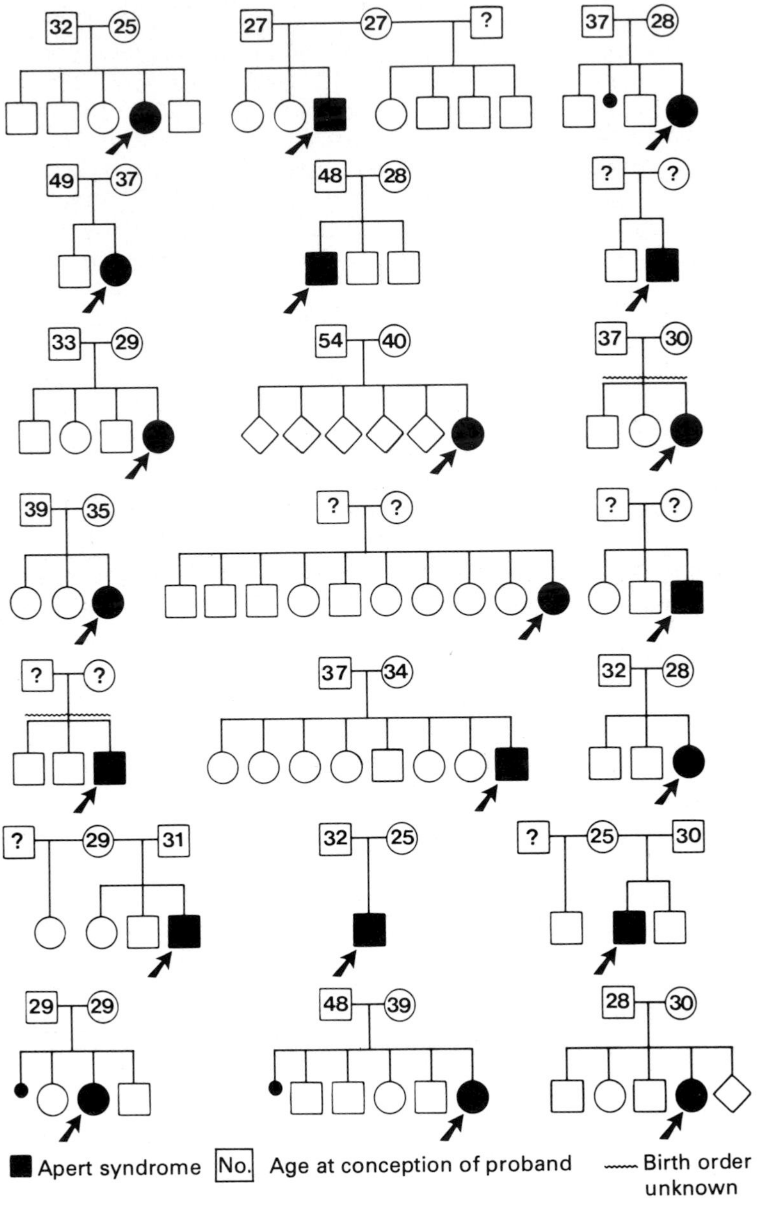

Figure 2–20. Sporadic occurrences of the Apert syndrome represent fresh mutations for an autosomal dominant disorder in which genetic fitness is dramatically reduced. (From Cohen, M.M., Jr.: An etiologic and nosologic overview of craniosynostosis syndromes. *In* Bergsma, D. (Ed.): Malformation Syndromes. New York: American Elsevier Publishing Co. for the National Foundation—March of Dimes Birth Defects Foundation BD:OAS XI(2):137–189, 1975, with permission from the copyright holder.)

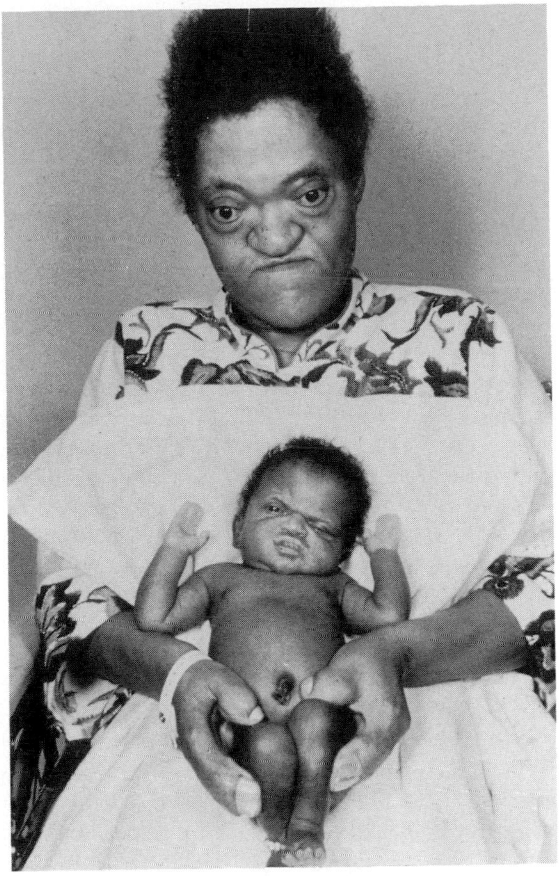

Figure 2–21. Dominant inheritance of the Apert syndrome. An affected mother and child. (From Roberts, K. B., and Hall, J. G.: Apert's acrocephalosyndactyly in mother and daughter: cleft palate in the mother. *In* Bergsma, D. (Ed.): Orofacial Structures. Baltimore: Williams & Wilkins for the National Foundation—March of Dimes Birth Defects Foundation BD:OAS VII(7):262–264, 1971, with permission from the copyright holder.)

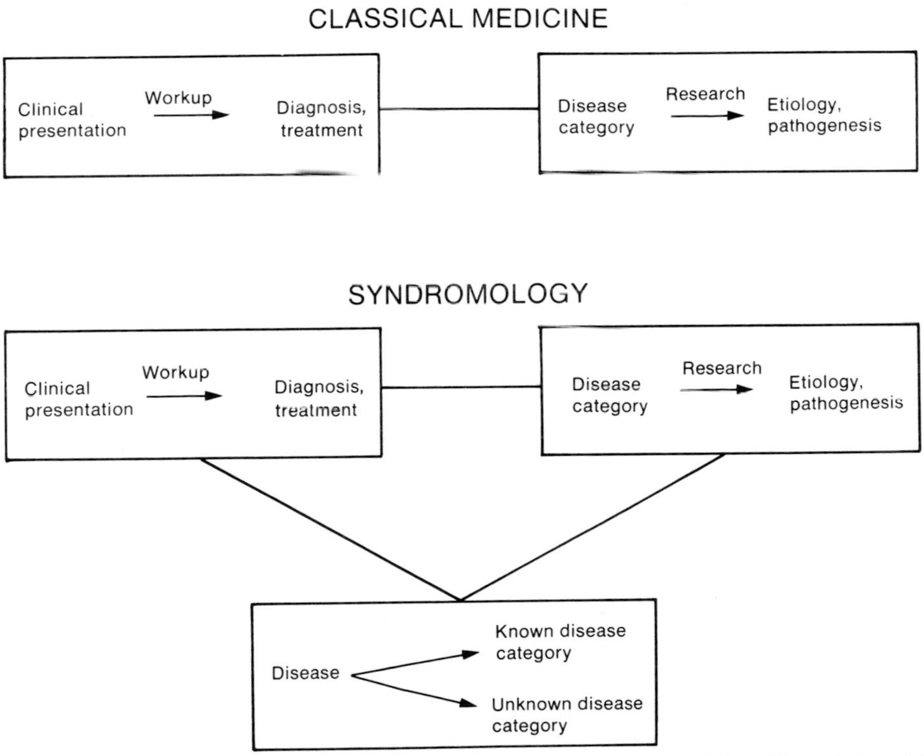

Figure 2–22. Similarities and differences between syndromology and classical medicine. (From Cohen, M.M., Jr.: The Child with Multiple Birth Defects. New York, Raven Press, 1982.)

syndrome becomes delineated, its phenotypic spectrum, its natural history, and its inheritance pattern or risk of recurrence become known, allowing for better patient care and family counseling. If the phenotypic spectrum is known, the clinician can search for suspected defects that may not be immediately apparent, but which may produce clinical problems at a later date, such as a congenital heart defect in the Carpenter syndrome. If a certain complication can occur in a given syndrome, such as a Wilms tumor in the Beckwith-Wiedemann syndrome, the clinician is forewarned to monitor the patient for possible development of neoplasia. Finally, if the recurrence risk is known, the parents can be counseled properly about future pregnancies, as in the autosomal recessively inherited Meckel syndrome, a condition in which encephalocele is combined with polydactyly, polycystic kidneys, and other anomalies. Recurrence risk counseling is especially important if the risk is high, and if the disorder is severely handicapping or disfiguring and carries a risk of mental retardation, as in a potential parent who has Apert syndrome. Such counseling is also of importance if the condition is not compatible with life, as in Elejalde syndrome, or would mean a dramatically shortened life span, as in the Ives-Houston syndrome. Thus, syndrome delineation fosters good patient care; the overall treatment program gains rationality. With a provisionally unique-pattern syndrome, in contrast, the treatment program and overall management frequently leave something to be desired (Cohen, 1982).

ANALYSIS OF SELECTED CRANIOFACIAL ANOMALIES

The etiology and pathogenesis of selected craniofacial anomalies will now be considered from the perspective of syndromology. Unfortunately, most discussions of craniofacial anomalies assume that there is only one mechanism for each anomaly that remains to be elucidated, and that once this is done, alternative hypotheses will be shown to be incorrect. This is Model I illustrated in Figure 2–23; the phenotype (*P*) is said to have one cause (*X*).

Syndrome delineation and clinical evidence to date strongly suggest that most craniofacial anomalies are pathogenetically heterogeneous—that several different mechanisms may be responsible for the same malformation. This reasoning follows from the process of syndrome delineation in which a given malformation—e.g., cleft palate—is shown to have multiple causes. The finding of etiologic heterogeneity strongly suggests pathogenetic heterogeneity (Cohen, 1982).

The more complicated version of mechanisms responsible for craniofacial anomalies is illustrated in Model III of Figure 2–23. Because the phenotype (*P*) is known to be etiologically heterogeneous (*A, B, C*), the pathogenesis may also be heterogeneous (*X, Y, Z*). Although any given craniofacial malformation can be shown to be etiologically heterogeneous, in some instances the pathogenesis may prove to be the same, as illustrated in Model I (*X*) or similar, as illustrated in Model II (X, X_1). However, the burden of proof should be that conditions known to be etiologically heterogeneous are not pathogenetically heterogeneous but homogeneous (Cohen, 1982).

The specific craniofacial anomalies to be analyzed from this perspective include the Robin sequence, unilateral craniofacial microsomia, and craniosynostosis.

Robin Sequence. The Robin sequence (see also Chap. 63) consists of micrognathia, cleft palate, and glossoptosis (Fig. 2–24*A, B*). The pathogenesis is usually thought to be based

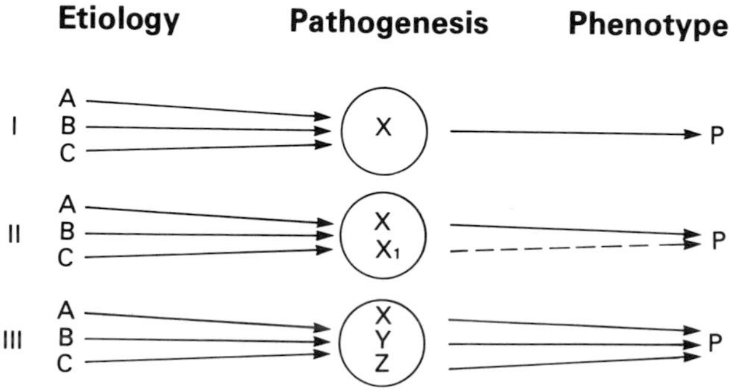

Figure 2–23. Possible relationships between etiology, pathogenesis, and phenotype (From Cohen, M.M., Jr.: The Child with Multiple Birth Defects. New York, Raven Press, 1982.)

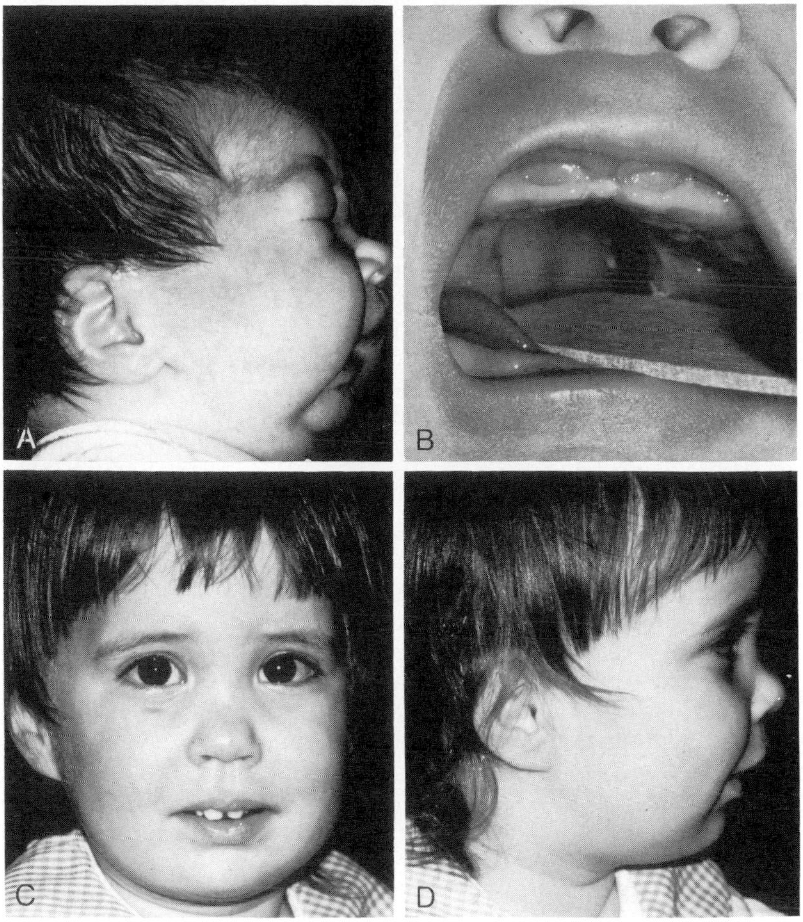

Figure 2–24. Robin sequence. *A, B,* Patient showing micrognathia and U-shaped cleft palate. *C, D,* The same patient showing mandibular catch-up growth. (From Cohen, M.M., Jr.: Syndromology's message for craniofacial biology. J. Maxillofac. Surg., *7*:89, 1979.)

on a small mandible that prevents the normal descent of the tongue. Thus, the tongue interferes with palatal fusion. The mandible often exhibits significant catch-up growth in time (Fig. 2–24*C, D*).

The syndromology perspective on the Robin sequence adds considerably to the understanding of the pathogenesis. Table 2–11 lists some syndromes in which the Robin sequence is one feature. The etiology of each condition is different. Thus, the Robin sequence is probably pathogenetically heterogeneous. The autosomal dominantly inherited Stickler syndrome (Herrmann and associates, 1975) is the most common syndrome associated with the Robin sequence. Since abnormalities of bones and joints occur in Stickler syndrome, the major pleiotropic effect appears to be on connective tissue. Thus, in this condition, the Robin sequence may result from intrinsic mandibular hypoplasia and failure of connective tissue penetration across the palate. Another condition that may include the Robin

Table 2–11. Conditions Associated with the Robin Sequence

Monogenic syndromes
Beckwith-Wiedemann syndrome
Camptomelic syndrome
Cerebrocostomandibular syndrome
Diastrophic dysplasia
Donlan syndrome
Myotonic dystrophy
Persistent left superior vena cava syndrome
Radiohumeral synostosis syndrome
Spondyloepiphyseal dysplasia congenita
Stickler syndrome
Chromosomal syndromes
Partial trisomy 11q syndrome
Teratogenically induced syndromes
Fetal alcohol syndrome
Fetal hydantoin syndrome
Fetal trimethadione syndrome
Unknown-genesis syndromes
Digitopalatal syndrome
Femoral dysgenesis–unusual facies syndrome
Martsolf syndrome
Robin–amelia syndrome

From Cohen, M. M., Jr.: The Child With Multiple Birth Defects. New York, Raven Press, 1982.

sequence is partial trisomy 11q syndrome (Aurias and Laurent, 1975). With the growth deficiency that accompanies most chromosomal syndromes, there may not be significant mandibular catch-up growth in patients with partial trisomy 11q syndrome who survive. Therefore, to include such patients in a mandibular growth study of the Robin sequence would yield erroneous data.

Some examples of the Robin sequence have been associated with oligohydramnios (Herrmann and Opitz, 1974). It is thought that reduced amniotic fluid results in compression of the chin against the sternum, restricting mandibular growth and impacting the tongue between the palatal shelves. Because micrognathia is based on intrauterine molding, mandibular catch-up growth is expected after birth when intrauterine deforming forces are no longer acting. Poswillo (1973) has produced a phenocopy of the Robin sequence in rats by puncturing the amniotic sac prior to palatal closure. Some experimental animals also had deformities of the limbs, ranging from clubfeet to ring constrictions and intrauterine amputations. Such limb abnormalities have also been associated with the Robin sequence in humans (Routledge, 1960; Smith and Stowe, 1961).

The Robin sequence has also been associated with congenital hypotonia (Herrmann and Opitz, 1974). If neurogenic hypotonia occurred before complete closure of the palate, it is conceivable that the Robin sequence might result from lack of mandibular exercise. Different etiologic and pathogenetic possibilities are summarized diagrammatically in Figure 2–25 (Cohen, 1982).

Unilateral Craniofacial Microsomia. Unilateral craniofacial microsomia is a well-known condition affecting aural, oral, and mandibular growth (Fig. 2–26*A*, *B*) (see also Chap. 62). The disorder may be mild or severe and involvement is limited to one side in most cases, but bilateral involvement also occurs, with more severe expression on one side (Gorlin, Pindborg, and Cohen, 1976). Poswillo (1973) reported a phenocopy in mice following maternal administration of triazene, and in monkeys following maternal ingestion of thalidomide. He proposed that pathogenesis was based on embryonic hematoma formation arising from the anastomosis that precedes formation of the stapedial artery stem. Variation in the severity of unilateral craniofacial microsomia was found to depend on the size and extent of hematoma formation, large hematomas interfering more severely with branchial arch growth by taking longer to resolve than small hematomas.

It seems most probable that unilateral craniofacial microsomia is both etiologically and pathogenetically heterogeneous. Hematoma formation has heterogeneous causes, including hypoxia, hypertension, pressor agents, salicylates, and anticoagulants (Poswillo, 1973). Although embryonic hematoma formation may explain some human cases of unilateral craniofacial microsomia, it probably does not explain all cases. For example, familial instances are known (Gorlin, Pindborg, and Cohen, 1976), and in some cases affected relatives may have only preauricular tags (Figs. 2–26*C*, *D*, 2–27). It is difficult to conceive of any basic mechanism causing hematoma formation to explain these cases. In minimally affected individuals, the ear and mandible are well formed; the preauricular tag seems to represent an accessory auricular hillock, an example of embryonic redundant

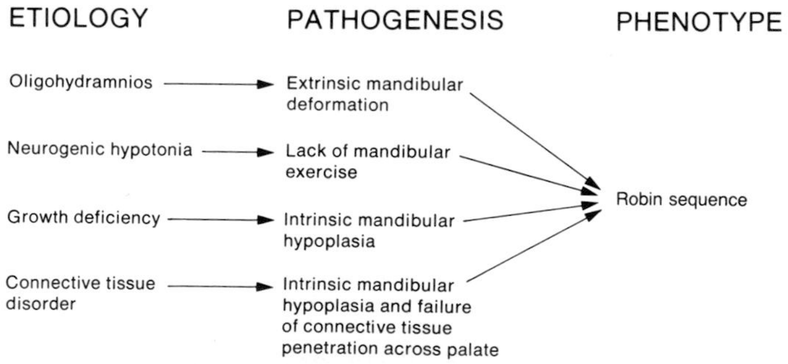

Figure 2–25. Etiologic heterogeneity suggests pathogenetic heterogeneity in the Robin sequence. The following pathogenetic possibilities should be considered. 1, Oligohydramnios results in decreased amniotic fluid, compressing the chin against the sternum and thus restricting mandibular growth. 2, If hypotonia restricts mouth opening during early fetal life before complete palatal closure, the Robin sequence might result from lack of mandibular exercise. 3, Growth deficiency, as observed in chromosomal syndromes such as the partial trisomy 11q syndrome, may produce the Robin sequence by intrinsic mandibular hypoplasia. 4, In a connective tissue disorder such as the Stickler syndrome, the Robin sequence may result from intrinsic hypoplasia and failure of connective tissue penetration across the palate. (From Cohen, M.M., Jr.: Syndromology's message for craniofacial biology. J. Maxillofac. Surg., 7:89, 1979.)

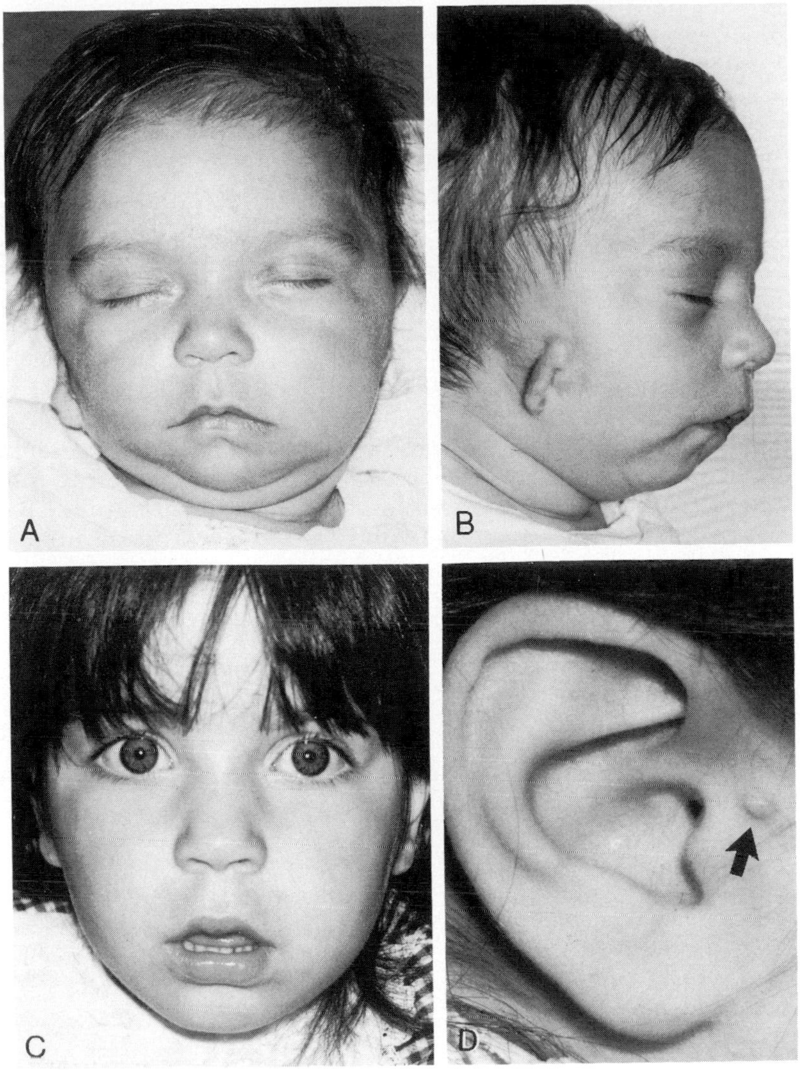

Figure 2–26. *A, B,* Unilateral craniofacial microsomia. *C, D,* The sister of the patient shown in *A* and *B.* Note the preauricular tag, representing an accessory auricular hillock. The ear is otherwise normal. (From Cohen, M.M., Jr.: Syndromology's message for craniofacial biology. J. Maxillofac. Surg., 7:89, 1979.)

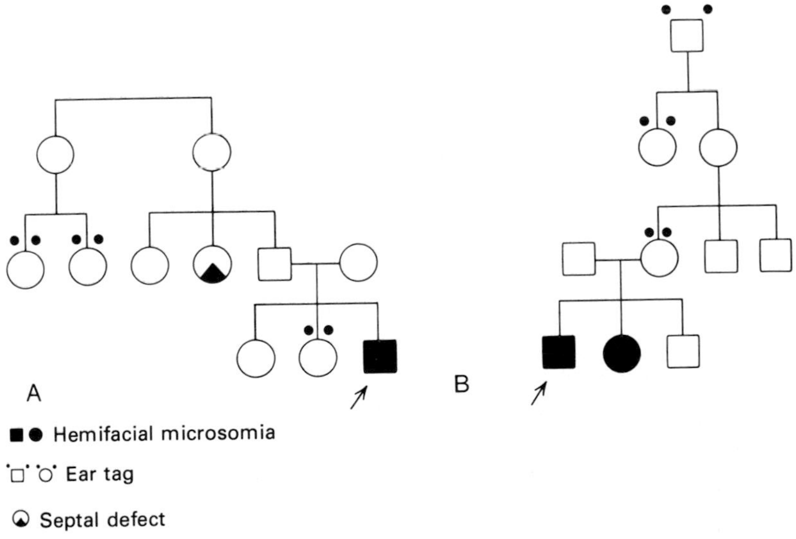

Figure 2–27. Pedigrees with unilateral craniofacial microsomia in which minimally affected relatives have only preauricular tags. *A,* The family of the proband and sister shown in Figure 2–26. *B,* Family from Pruzansky, S.: Clinical investigation of the experiments of nature. ASHA Report, *8*:62, 1973.

morphogenesis. To postulate separate pathogenetic mechanisms to explain instances of unilateral craniofacial microsomia and accessory ear tags in the same family (see Figs. 2–26, 2–27) seems unnecessarily complicated. The most frugal hypothesis should take into account that the two pedigrees in Figure 2–27 represent a single entity that is variably expressed and genetically transmitted.

Unilateral craniofacial microsomia is known to occur either as an isolated defect or together with a variety of other anomalies (Gorlin, Pindborg, and Cohen, 1976). A recurrent-pattern syndrome has been described consisting of unilateral craniofacial microsomia, occipital encephalocele, hypoplastic lung, vertebral anomalies, and renal agenesis (Fig. 2–28) (Cohen and associates, 1980). These malformations most likely have a common (but unknown) cause rather than being caused by different factors acting independently. Whatever mechanism is responsible for one malformation should be responsible for the other malformations. To date, there is no experimental evidence that hematoma formation can cause encephaloceles or renal agenesis. Therefore, it seems unlikely that hematoma formation has anything to do with the pathogenesis of this recurrent-pattern syndrome.

Some cases of the amniotic band spectrum of disruptions have been noted to simulate unilateral craniofacial microsomia (Hall, 1979). In such instances, unilateral craniofacial microsomia possibly may be caused by intrauterine compression secondary to oligohydramnios. Kennedy and Persaud (1977) extracted amniotic fluid from pregnant rats

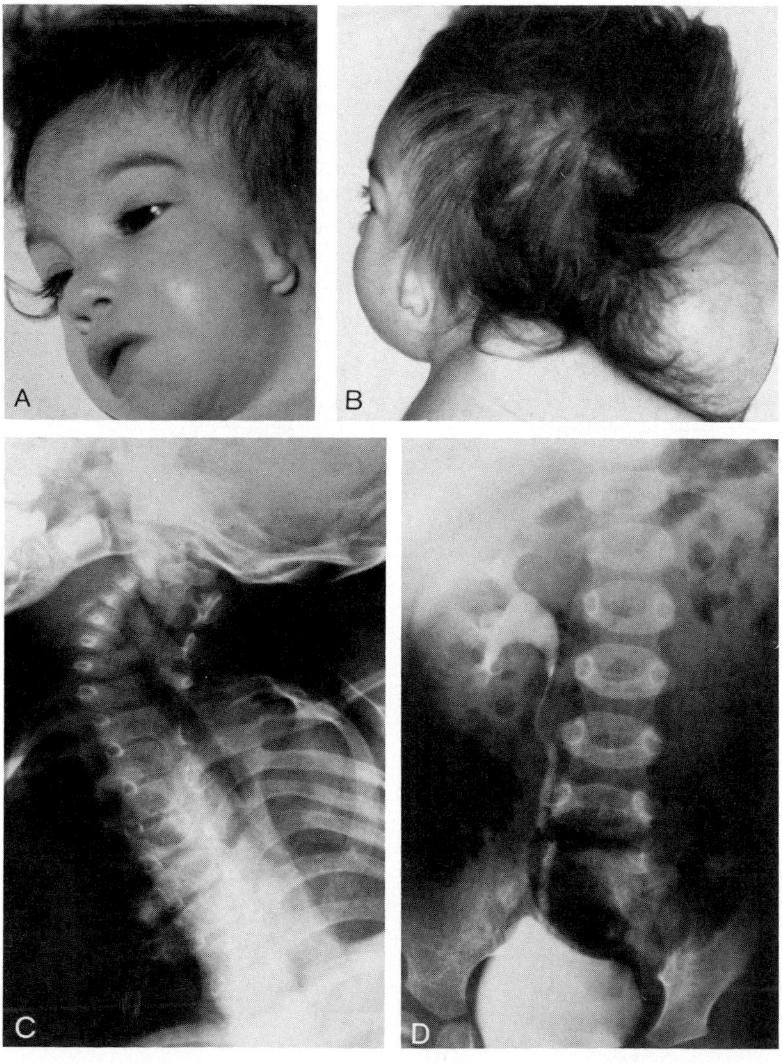

Figure 2–28. Patient with recurrent-pattern syndrome consisting of *(A)*, unilateral craniofacial microsomia, *(B)*, occipital encephalocele, *(C)*, hypoplastic left lung and vertebral anomalies, and *(D)*, unilateral renal agenesis. (From Cohen, M.M., Jr.: Syndromology's message for craniofacial biology. J. Maxillofac. Surg. 7:89, 1979.)

at 16 days of gestation and studied the embryos at various times thereafter. On histologic examination, they found hemorrhage and edema followed by tissue necrosis in the cartilage and mesenchymal preskeleton of the developing limbs. Thus, the observed reduction defects and amputations of the limbs resulted from venous stasis, hypervolemia, and embryonic oxygen deficiency caused by intrauterine compression. Kennedy and Persaud (1977) did not give a detailed histologic evaluation of the branchial arch region, but they did note that micrognathia was observed in addition to subcutaneous hemorrhages in the head region. Thus, intrauterine compression might be construed as a possible mechanism for producing hematoma formation in the branchial arch region, resulting in unilateral craniofacial microsomia. Since human unilateral craniofacial microsomia may be observed occasionally with limb reduction defects (Gorlin, Pindborg, and Cohen, 1976), the association appears to have a common pathogenesis compatible with the hypothesis of Poswillo (1973). If unilateral craniofacial microsomia is ever observed with frank amniotic band-related limb abnormalities, this too would be compatible with Poswillo's hypothesis.

Craniosynostosis. Three classic theories have been advanced to explain craniosynostosis. Virchow (1851) believed that it was a primary malformation and that the associated cranial base deformity was secondary to craniosynostosis. The converse was postulated by Moss (1959): the cranial base malformation was the primary anomaly, resulting in secondary premature fusion of the cranial sutures. In speculating on the pathogenesis of the Apert syndrome, Park and Powers (1920) postulated a primary defect in the mesenchymal blastema that led to both craniosynostosis and an abnormal cranial base.

Currently, the theory of Moss (1959) is the most popular of the three. Unfortunately, most discussions of craniosynostosis assume that there is a single pathogenetic mechanism that remains to be elucidated, and that after this is accomplished, alternative hypotheses will be shown to be incorrect. Syndrome delineation and clinical evidence to date strongly suggest that craniosynostosis is pathogenetically heterogeneous. At least 64 different syndromes have been recognized in which craniosynostosis is a feature, excluding secondary forms of synostosis (see Table 2–10). Some are known to be and others are presumed to be etiologically heterogeneous. Such etiologic heterogeneity, of course, suggests the possibility of pathogenetic heterogeneity. Thus, all three theories are probably correct; each may be implicated in some, but not all, cases of craniosynostosis.

According to Moss's theory (1959), spatially malformed lesser sphenoidal wings in coronal synostosis, and spatially malformed cribriform plate and crista galli in sagittal synostosis, are viewed as primary abnormalities that, at the points of dural attachment, transmit aberrant tensile forces upward through the dura, leading to premature fusion of the overlying sutural tissues.

Many familial instances of isolated (nonsyndromic) craniosynostosis have been observed (Cohen, 1977). Most examples are compatible with autosomal dominant transmission. In some families, involvement is variable, some family members having fusion of the sagittal suture, some having fusion of the coronal suture, and still others having synostosis of both coronal and sagittal sutures (see Fig. 2–1). It is difficult to conceive of dramatically different primary abnormalities of the cranial base occurring in the same family as a dominant trait. Thus, a different pathogenetic mechanism from the one proposed by Moss (1959) may be operative in such families.

A primary abnormality of the cranial base as the cause of craniosynostosis in the Apert syndrome has been proposed by Moss (1959) and supported by Stewart, Dixon, and Cohen (1977). However, clinical evidence to date indicates that the pathogenetic mechanism for craniosynostosis in this syndrome may possibly be unique. Features of the Apert syndrome include progressive calcification and fusion, with time, of the bones of the hands, feet, and cervical spine (Schauerte and St-Aubin, 1966). Progressive generalized bony dysplasia with ankylosis of joints, as well as progressive limitation of motion at these joints, have been documented (Harris, Beligere, and Pruzansky, 1977). Finally, progressive overcalcification of the cartilaginous portion of the nasal septum and stylohyoid ligaments has also been observed (Harris, Beligere, and Pruzansky, 1977). The most frugal hypothesis would be that whatever mechanism is responsible for progressive calcification throughout the body is also responsible for premature craniosynostosis in the Apert syndrome. Because neither the cranial base nor the points of dural attachment can be invoked to explain progressive calcification elsewhere, it is probable that they have nothing to do with craniosynostosis in the Apert syndrome either.

Graham, deSaxe, and Smith (1979) hypothesized that human prenatal head constraint may be responsible for some cases of craniosynostosis. They noted that some mothers of infants with isolated sagittal synostosis gave a history of early descent of their abdominal silhouette and severe pelvic pressure during the last one to three months of gestation. These symptoms were interpreted as a sign of early descent of the fetal head into the lower pelvis.

Graham, deSaxe, and Smith (1979) noted that fetal head constraint in lateral dimension could limit growth stretch at the sagittal suture, resulting in ridging of the suture. They pointed out that fetal head constraint as a possible cause of sagittal synostosis was compatible with two epidemiologic facts. First, synostosis of the sagittal suture is the most common type, and in most instances the patient is otherwise normal. Thus, a significant proportion of such cases might be explained on the basis of long-standing molding forces. Second, strikingly more males than females are affected by sagittal synostosis. This finding may be related to more rapid growth and larger head size of males during the last trimester of pregnancy. An experimental animal study lends support to the hypothesis of Graham, deSaxe, and Smith (1979). Koskinen-Moffett (1986) produced prenatal synostosis of the coronal and squamosal sutures in mouse pups by closing the uterine cervix with a surgical clip to delay birth for several days and thus crowd the fetuses.

Lack of growth stretch at the sutures may also be implicated in three malformations in which premature craniosynostosis may occur as a complicating feature. First, sutural fusion may accompany some cases of microcephaly (Duggan, Keener, and Gary, 1970). Lack of central nervous system growth may result in lack of growth stretch across the sutural areas, producing secondary craniosynostosis. Second, several reports have linked shunted hydrocephaly to craniosynostosis (Andersson, 1966; Kloss, 1968). Medium and low pressure systems may be implicated, in which growth stretch at the sutural areas suddenly becomes totally deficient. Finally, some cases of encephalocele have been associated with craniosynostosis (Lorber, 1967). Such "blow-out" lesions may sometimes result in lack of growth stretch across the sutures.

Premature craniosynostosis may result from several dysmetabolic states. It has been observed to accompany hyperthyroidism (Figs. 2–29, 2–30) during childhood (Menking and associates, 1972; Penfold and Simpson, 1975; Johnsonbaugh and associates, 1978). Sutural fusion may be caused by primary thyroid hyperplasia, but more commonly results from excessive thyroxine treatment for congenital hypothyroidism.

Premature sutural fusion may also occur in the Hurler syndrome (see Fig. 2–17), which is characterized by α-L-iduronidase deficiency. The craniosynostosis involves the sagittal and lambdoid sutures (Gorlin, Pindborg, and Cohen, 1976).

Craniosynostosis has been observed in various etiologically distinct forms of rickets, including vitamin D deficiency rickets, simple hypophosphatemic rickets, hypophosphatemic-hypocalcemic-aminoaciduric rickets, hypophosphatemic-aminoaciduric-cirrhotic rickets, azotemic osteodystrophy, and hypophosphatasia. The extent of synostosis is related to

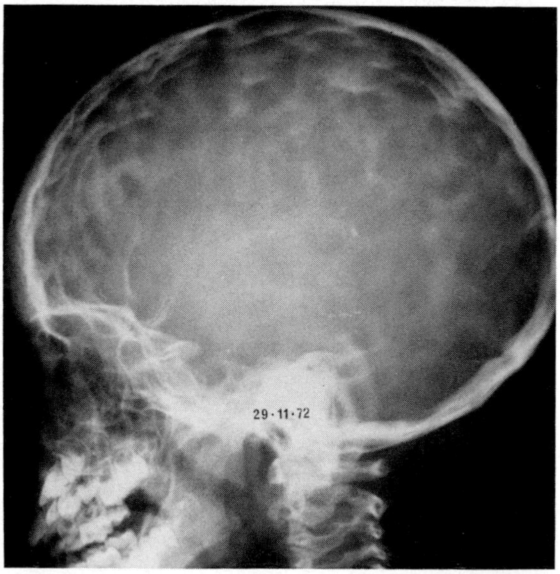

Figure 2–29. Craniosynostosis secondary to excessive thyroxine treatment. Skull radiograph showing changes consistent with complete symmetric synostosis in a 4 year old patient. (From Penfold, J.L., and Simpson, D.A.: Premature craniosynostosis—a complication of thyroid replacement therapy. J. Pediatr., *86*:360, 1975.)

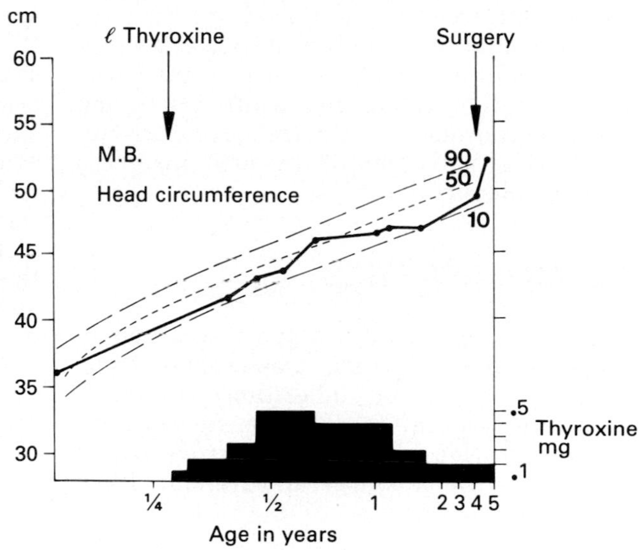

Figure 2–30. Craniosynostosis secondary to excessive thyroxine treatment. Note the acceleration of the head circumference during a period of intensive thyroxine replacement therapy, and resumption of growth following neurosurgical intervention to relieve the sutures. (From Penfold, J.L., and Simpson, D.A.: Premature craniosynostosis—a complication of thyroid replacement therapy. J. Pediatr., *86*:360, 1975.)

the severity of the rachitic process. Premature sutural fusion was observed in approximately one-third of 59 rachitic children under 9 years of age in the study of Reilly and associates (1964).

Craniosynostosis may occur in various hematologic disorders (Fig. 2–31). Hyperplasia of the marrow with compensatory bony overgrowth of the calvaria can "lock" the sutures. Conditions known to result in premature fusion of sutures include the thalassemias, sickle cell anemia, congenital hemolytic icterus, and polycythemia vera (Dykstra and Halbertsma, 1940; Duggan, Keener, and Gay, 1970).

Premature fusion of sutures may accom-

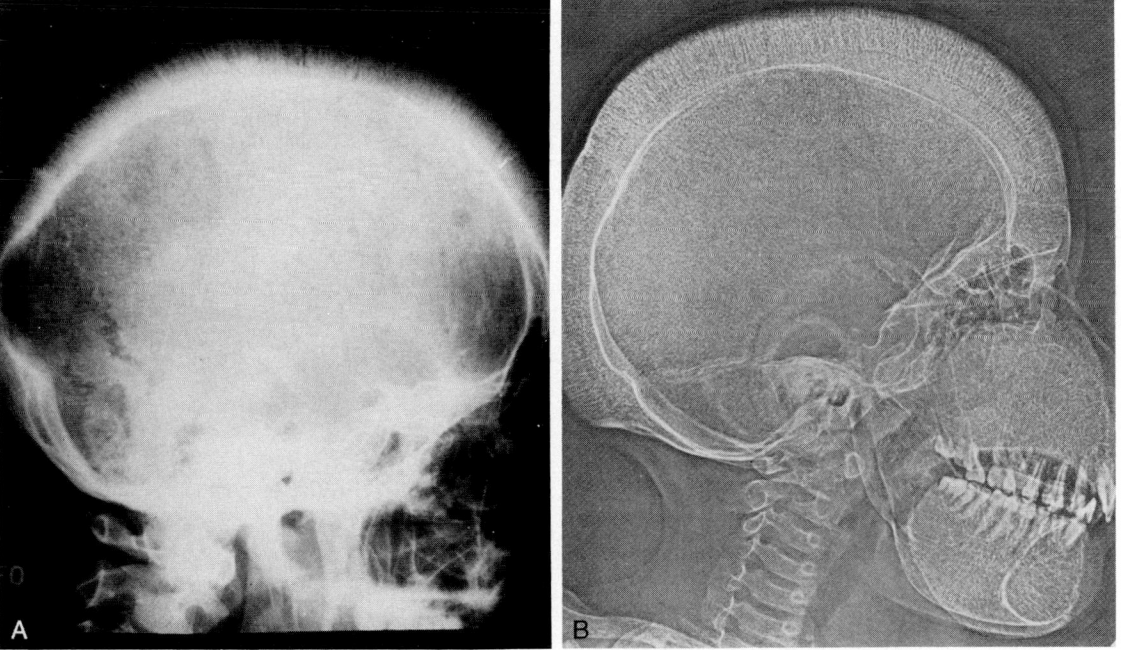

Figure 2–31. *A,* Skull roentgenogram of a patient with sickle cell anemia. Note the hair-on-end appearance of the ectocranial bone deposition. *B,* Xeroradiograph of thalassemia. Note the thickening of the skull. Hyperplasia of the marrow results in compensatory bony overgrowth. (From Cohen, M.M., Jr.: Craniosynostosis: Diagnosis, Evaluation, and Management. New York, Raven Press, 1986.)

pany a variety of miscellaneous disorders as an occasional abnormality: ataxia-telangiectasia (Robinson, 1962), the epidermal nevus syndrome (Moynahan and Wolff, 1967), and the Job syndrome (Smithwick and associates, 1978). The pathogenesis in such instances remains obscure.

FORMAL GENETICS

This section provides a short appendix to human cytogenetics and chromosomal abnormalities, monogenic inheritance patterns, and multifactorial inheritance. Several references provide more comprehensive coverage (Kelly, 1980; Emery and Rimoin, 1983; Thompson, 1986).

Cytogenetics and Chromosomal Anomalies

Chromosome studies can be carried out in a variety of clinical situations. Chromosomes are visible only when cells divide in mitosis or meiosis. Cell culture methods have greatly extended the range of possible tissues and types of cells from which dividing cells can be obtained: small lymphocytes, fibroblasts, amnionic fluid cells, and even viable cells from spontaneous abortions, embryos, and fetuses for a number of hours after death.

Many techniques have revealed the underlying structural features of chromosomes. Human chromosomes are grouped by size and centromere location; the latter may be metacentric, submetacentric, or acrocentric (Fig. 2–32). Characteristic banding patterns of the chromosomes permit identification of each individual chromosome (Fig. 2–33, Table 2–12). The karyotype or chromosomal constitution of any cell is abbreviated by three symbolic parts, each separated by a comma: the number of cells observed, the number of sex chromosomes and their type, and specific description of any unusual chromosome or chromosomes. Table 2–13 lists a few of the symbols commonly used. Numerical abnormalities reflect the total number of chromosomes (Fig. 2–34). Sex chromosome aneuploidy is described both numerically and in the sex chromosome constitution. Three examples are:

46,XX	Normal female with 46 chromosomes and two X chromosomes.
47,XXY	Klinefelter syndrome with 47 chromosomes, two X chromosomes, and one Y chromosome.
47,XY,+21	Trisomy 21 syndrome with 47 chromosomes, a normal male sex chromosome constitution, and one extra 21 chromosome.

Structural abnormalities of chromosomes include deletions (Fig. 2–35), duplications, inversions, and translocations. Referring to the symbols in Table 2–13 and the banding pattern numbers of chromosome 5 in Table 2–12, the following is an example of a structural abnormality:

46,XY,del(5)(p13) 46,XY,del(5) (qter → p13):	Normal number of chromosomes with normal male sex chromosome constitution and deletion of the short arm of chromosome 5.

The first set of symbols represents the short designation for the cri du chat syndrome. This form identifies the chromosome involved in the deletion and the breakpoint. The second set of symbols represents the detailed desig-

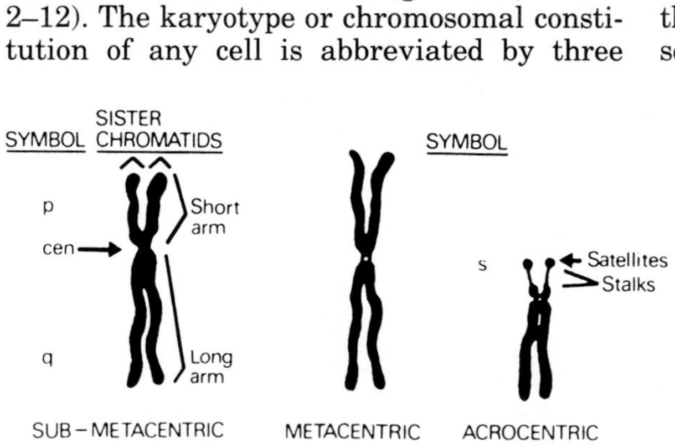

Figure 2–32. General morphology of human chromosomes. (From Lubs, H.A., and Ing, P.S.: Human cytogenetic nomenclature. *In* Emery, A.E.H., and Rimoin, D.L. (Eds.): Principles and Practice of Medical Genetics. Vol. I. Edinburgh, Churchill Livingstone, 1983, pp. 162–169.)

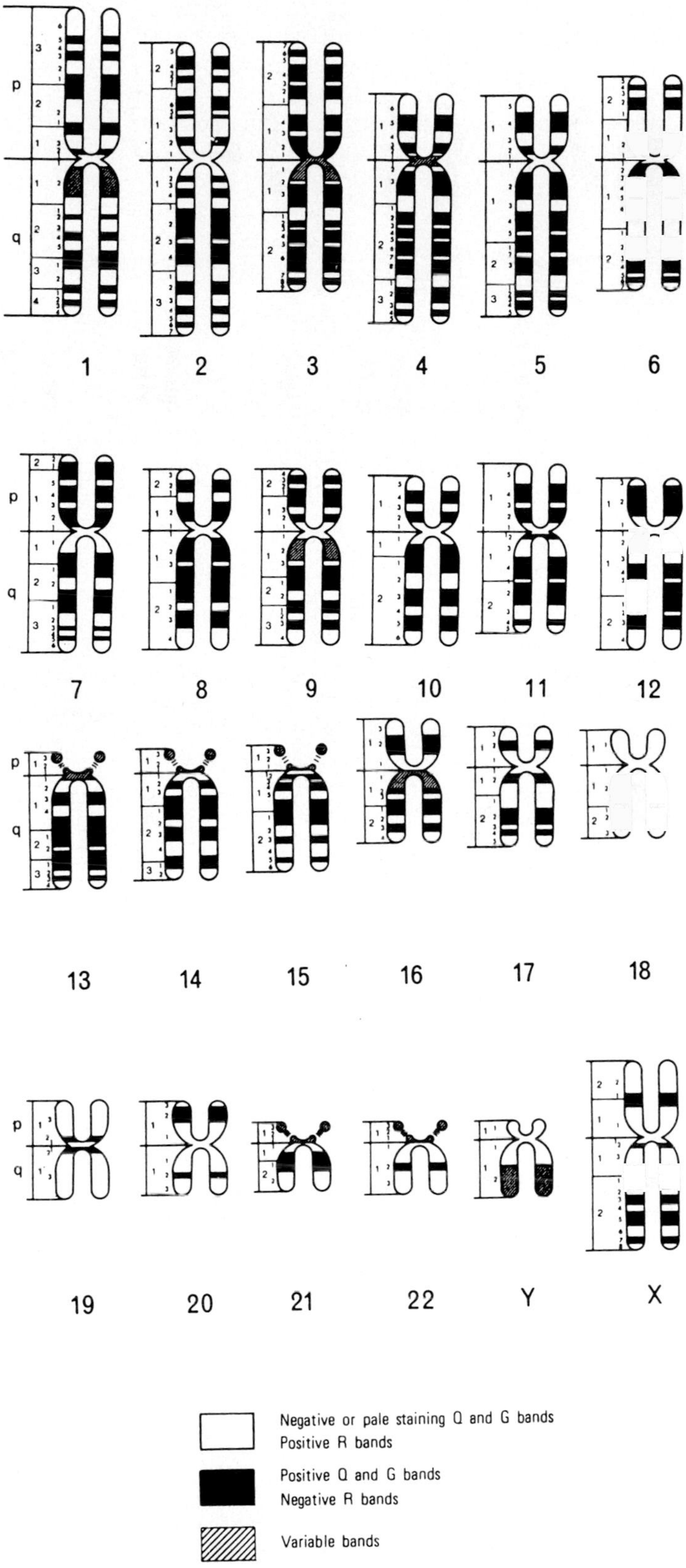

Figure 2–33. Diagrammatic representation of the human karyotype. Designations under the chromosomes indicate chromosome numbers and sex chromosomes. Numbers on the lefthand side of each chromosome refer to bands. Short arm of chromosome is indicated by *p*; long arm by *q*. For the meaning of banding patterns at the bottom of the diagram, consult Table 2–12. (From Paris Conference, 1971.)

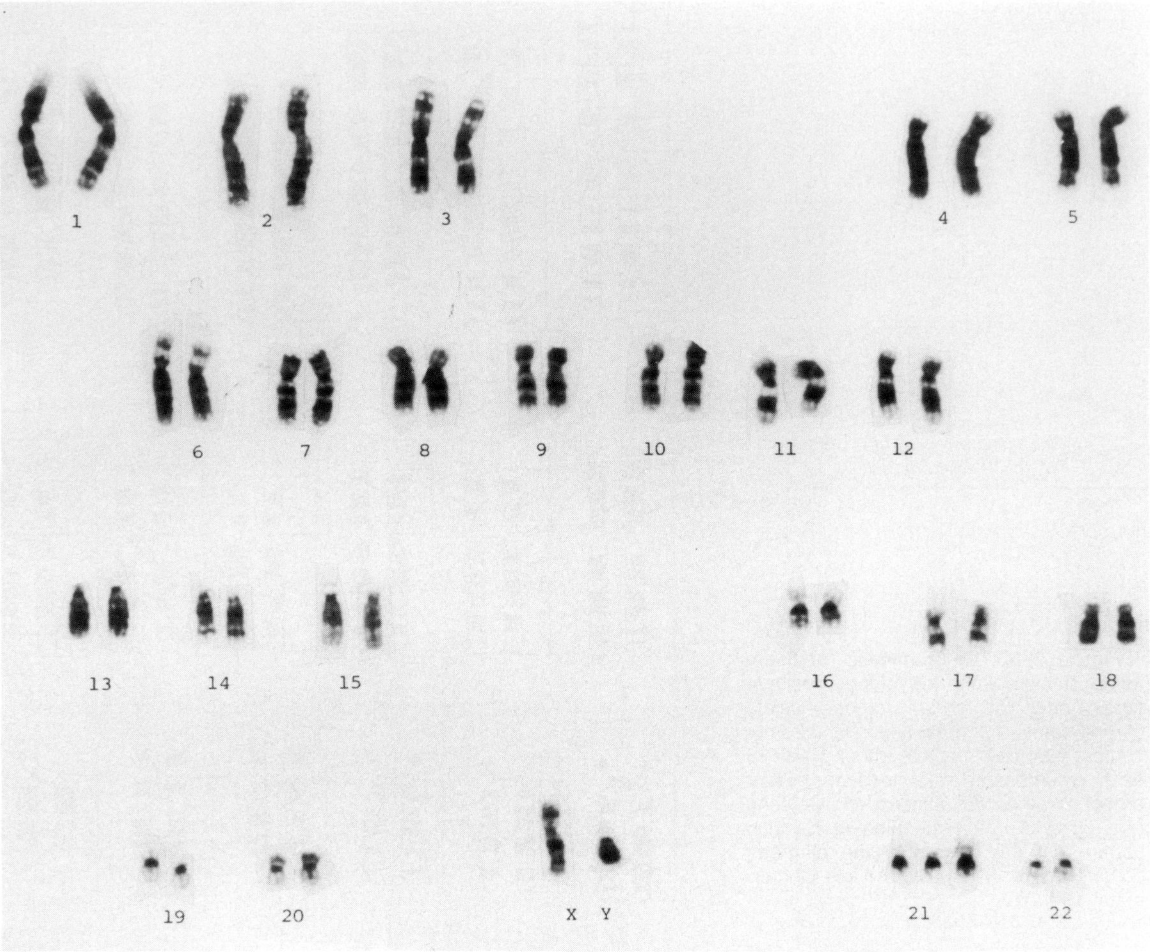

Figure 2–34. Human karyotype with banding showing Down syndrome (47,XY,+21).

Table 2–12. Chromosome Banding

Type	Stain	Area Stained	Effect
Q-banding	Quinacrine	Chromosome arms; mostly repetitive AT-rich DNA	Under UV light, distinct fluorescent banded pattern for each chromosome
G-banding	Giemsa	Chromosome arms; mostly repetitive AT-rich DNA	Distinct banded pattern for each chromosome; same as Q-banding pattern except single additional band near centromere of chromosomes 1 and 16
R-banding	Variety of techniques	Chromosome arms; mostly unique GC-rich DNA	Reverse banding pattern of that observed with Q- or G-banding
C-banding	Variety of techniques	Centromere region of each chromosome and distal portion of Y chromosome; highly repetitive, mostly AT-rich DNA	Largest bands usually on chromosomes 1, 9, 16, and Y; chromosomes 7, 10, and 15 have medium-sized bands; size of C-bands highly variable from person to person

Table 2–13. Some Karyotype Symbols and Their Meanings*

Symbol	Meaning
p	Short arm
q	Long arm
,	Separates chromosome number from sex constitution and sex constitution from description of unusual chromosome
cen	Centromere
s	Satellite
del	Deletion
dup	Duplication
t	Translocation
inv	Inversion
ter	Terminal end of a chromosome
:	Used to describe a break
: :	Describes breakage and reunion
→	Indicates from __ to __

*These are only a few of the common symbols used; there are many others. From Paris Conference, 1971.

nation and identifies the abnormal chromosome from end to end. The colon indicates that the segment closest to the 5p13 band is deleted. Both forms represent the same chromosomal anomaly. In publications, it has been recommended that the detailed form be given first, from then on using only the short form. In laboratory reports, the short form is used (Lubs and Ing, 1983).

Consider the symbols used for a Down syndrome translocation:

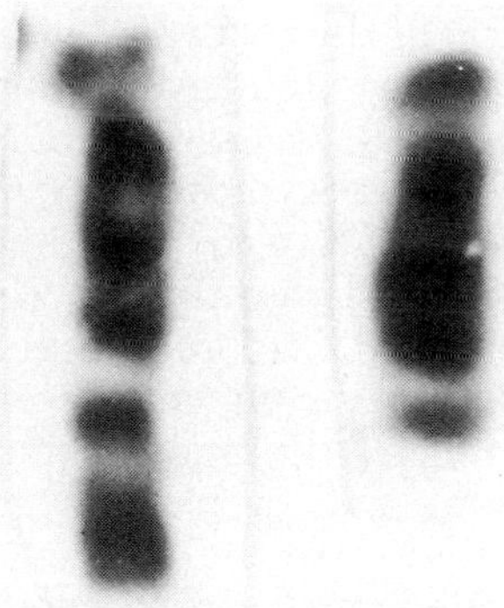

Figure 2–35. Deletion of long arm of chromosome 18 *(right)* del(18)(q22.1).

45,XX,t(4;21)(p11;q11) 45,XX,t(14:21) (14qter → 14p11: 21q11 → qter)	One chromosome appears to be missing; the sex constitution is female; and translocation between chromosomes 14 and 21 results in two chromosomes becoming one by centric fusion.

The first set of symbols represents the short designation for the balanced translocation; the second set represents the detailed designation.

Chromosome studies should be performed on all patients with a suspected chromosomal syndrome to confirm the diagnosis. Family studies may be indicated with structural rearrangements. For example, with translocation-type Down syndrome, it is important to know if the translocation arose de novo or if one parent is a translocation carrier. In the latter situation, the parent is at increased risk for having another child with translocation-type Down syndrome.

Chromosome studies should also be carried out on any patient with multiple malformations when the overall diagnosis is unknown. The criteria listed in Table 2–14 may be used to help decide whether a chromosome study should be performed. The following generalizations should be kept in mind when using the criteria. First, chromosomal aberrations usually have adverse effects on *many* parts of the body. Consequently, an individual with only two anomalies, such as an atrial septal defect and clinodactyly, is unlikely to have a chromosome problem. Second, most people with unbalanced autosomes have growth deficiency of prenatal or postnatal onset and mental retardation. Thus, any individual with normal growth parameters and normal psychomotor development is not, as a rule, a candidate for chromosome study. Exceptions to both generalizations include some sex chromosome disorders that may have few, if any, recognizable anomalies. Other exceptions include very small deletions or duplications (Jones and Jones, 1983).

Monogenic Inheritance Patterns

In medical genetics, autosomal dominant inheritance involves a rare gene, so that

Table 2–14. Indications for Chromosome Studies*

Features

Scalp
1. Scalp defect (usually occipital) (Tri-13, 4p-)
2. Posterior hair whorl over posterior fontanel (Tri-21)

Ears (small) (Tri-21, 18q)

Eyes
1. Upslanting palpebral fissures (Tri-21, 18q-)
2. Microphthalmos, anophthalmos (Tri-13) (13q-)
3. Cyclops or severe hypotelorism (Tri-13, 18p-)
4. Coloboma (iris) (4p-, cat eye syndrome)
5. Retinoblastoma (13q-)

Nose—neonatal high nasal bridge (Tri-13, 21q-, 13q-)

Philtrum—very short (4p-)

Tongue
1. Cat-cry (5p-)
2. Small mouth that is hard to open (Tri-18)
3. Fishmouth with downturned corners (4p-, 5p-, 13q-)

Mandible prominent (multiple X syndromes, 18q-)

Neck—webbed (XO Turner syndrome and multiple X syndromes, Tri-8)

Short *sternum* (Tri-18)

Abdomen
1. Duodenal atresia (Tri-21)
2. Pyloric stenosis (21q-)
3. Multicystic kidneys (XO Turner)
4. Polycystic kidneys (Tri-13)
5. Omphalocele (Tri-18, triploidy)

Anal atresia (cat eye syndrome, 13q-, Tri-18, Tri-8)

External genitalia—scrotalization of phallus (Tri-13)

Extremities
1. Edema (XO Turner)
2. Radial hypoplasia including thumb abnormalities (Tri-18, 13q-, 4p-)
3. Radioulnar synostosis (multiple-X syndromes, XXY)
4. Overlapping fingers with nail dysplasia (Tri-18)
5. Dermatoglyphics
   (a) all low arches (Tri-18)
   (b) all ulnar loops (Tri-21)
   (c) tibial arch (Tri-21)
6. Vertical sole creases (Tri-8)
7. Rocker-bottom feet with prominent heels (Tri-13, Tri-18)

Skin
1. Keloids in caucasians (XO, 21q-)
2. Hemangiomas in unusual places that persist (XO Turner)

Miscellaneous: (less specific but useful when combined with other features)
1. Gynecomastia (XXY)
2. Preauricular or helical pits (cat eye syndrome)
3. Single umbilical artery (Tri-18)
4. Polydactyly (Tri-13)
5. Ambiguous genitalia

*Brackets list examples of chromosomal disorders that (frequently) have that particular feature.

Courtesy of B. D. Hall, Lexington, KY.

affected individuals are heterozygotes. An affected individual produces two kinds of gametes, one with a normal gene, one with an abnormal gene (Fig. 2–36). Thus, offspring of an affected individual have a 50 per cent chance of being affected. An autosomal dominant pedigree is illustrated in Figure 2–37. Dominant disorders are transmitted from generation to generation without skips, and both sexes have an equal chance of being affected. Notice that there are two instances of male to male transmission, which rule out X-linked inheritance. The ability of an autosomal dominant gene to be transmitted from generation to generation depends on the genetic fitness of the affected individual. For example, a pedigree similar to the one in Figure 2–37 might characterize a family with mandibulofacial dysostosis. In achondroplasia, the genetic fitness is reduced so that although some dominant pedigrees may be observed, many instances occur sporadically, resulting from new mutations. As shown in Figure 2–20, most cases of Apert syndrome occur sporadically because the malformations and mental deficiency (present in some cases) diminish the patients' desirability as mates.

Other features frequently found with autosomal dominantly inherited genes are incomplete *penetrance* and *variable expressivity*. Penetrance refers to the gene's ability to be expressed at all. In Figure 2–38, an autosomal dominant pedigree is shown with two instances of incomplete penetrance. Although the incompletely penetrant individuals do not show the trait, they are carriers for the disorder, with a 50 per cent risk of transmitting the gene to their offspring. A genetic trait may be variably expressed, ranging from mild to severe. For example, a parent with mandibulofacial dysostosis might exhibit only mildly downslanting palpebral fissures and mild zygomatic hypoplasia. On the other hand, her affected child might have severe downslanting of the palpebral fissures, absent zygomatic arches, and severe micrognathia.

With autosomal recessive inheritance, both parents are phenotypically normal but are heterozygous carriers for the abnormal gene. Parents produce two different kinds of gametes—one normal, one abnormal (Fig. 2–39). There is a 25 per cent chance of having an affected child. Of the phenotypically normal children, some will be heterozygous carriers for the disorder, like their parents.

Because offspring have a 25 per cent chance of being affected, sibships of two or more children may be found (Fig. 2–40). Both sexes have an equal chance of being affected. More remote ancestors as well as the parents are normal, as a rule. An increased percentage of pedigrees may have consanguinity. The rarer

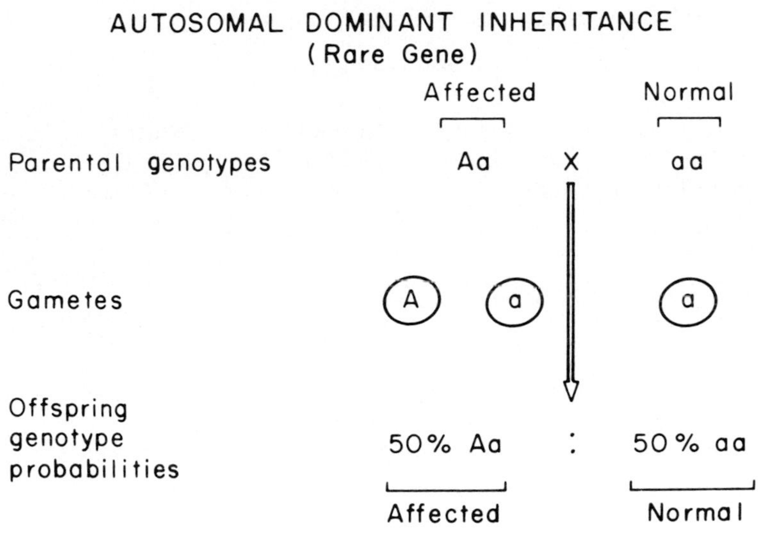

Figure 2–36. In autosomal dominant inheritance, an affected individual has a 50 per cent chance of having an affected offspring.

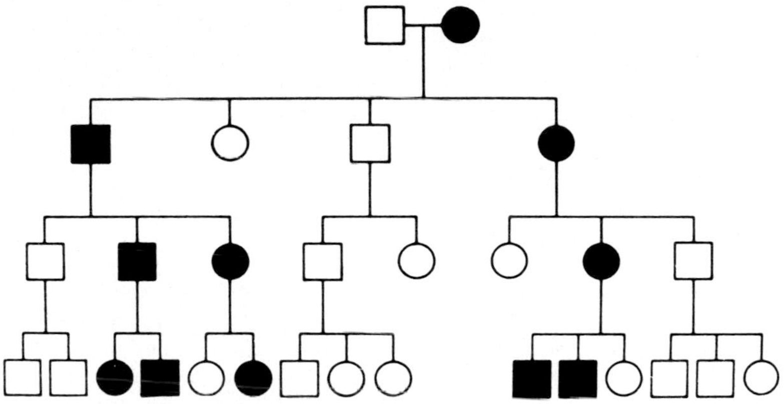

Figure 2–37. Autosomal dominant pedigree showing vertical transmission and male to male transmission.

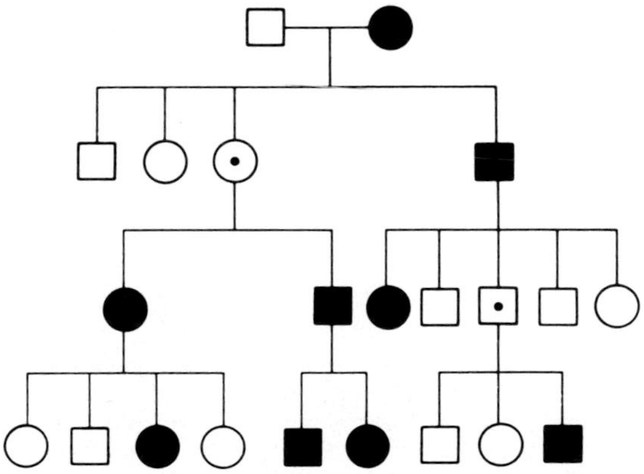

Figure 2–38. Autosomal dominant inheritance showing incomplete penetrance. Dots indicate genetic carriers for the abnormal gene who are phenotypically normal.

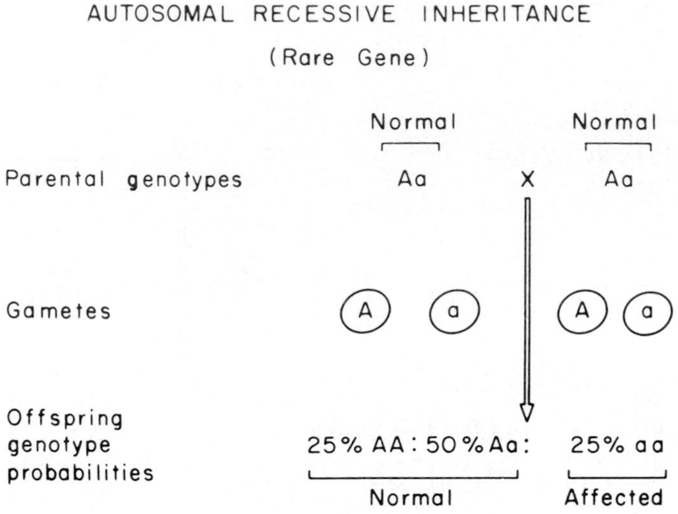

Figure 2–39. In autosomal recessive inheritance, both parents are phenotypically normal carriers who have a 25 per cent risk of having an affected offspring.

the gene is in the population, the more consanguineous pedigrees are likely to be found. Figure 2–41 shows how consanguinity increases the probability of homozygosity for the abnormal gene. Examples of autosomal recessive syndromes include the Morquio syndrome and the Ellis–van Creveld syndrome.

In X-linked recessive inheritance, both parents are phenotypically normal. The mother is a carrier for the abnormal gene and is able to produce two kinds of gametes, one with a normal gene, one with the abnormal gene. Offspring genotype probabilities are illustrated in Figure 2–42. Half of the males are affected and half of the females are phenotypically normal carriers for the gene. An X-linked recessive pedigree is shown in Figure 2–43*A*. The gene is transmitted from generation to generation in a diagonal pattern. Affected males do not produce affected offspring and are themselves the offspring of normal female carriers. In the population as a whole, more males tend to be affected. When females are affected, they are the offspring of an affected father and a normal carrier mother. In such instances, the parents are often related.

An example of an X-linked recessive disorder is the common type of hypohidrotic ectodermal dysplasia. A typical X-linked pedigree is found in Figure 2–43*A*, showing affected males and female carriers. The same pedigree is slightly altered in Figure 2–43*B* to look more like an X-linked dominant pedigree. This pattern fits if the disorder is defined as *any* degree of hypohidrosis. Since

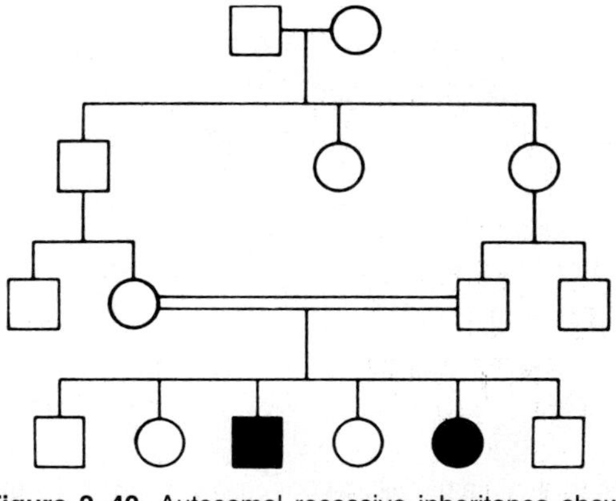

Figure 2–40. Autosomal recessive inheritance showing an affected brother and sister, normal parents, and normal grandparents. Note that the maternal grandfather and the paternal grandmother are siblings, resulting in parental consanguinity indicated by the double horizontal line.

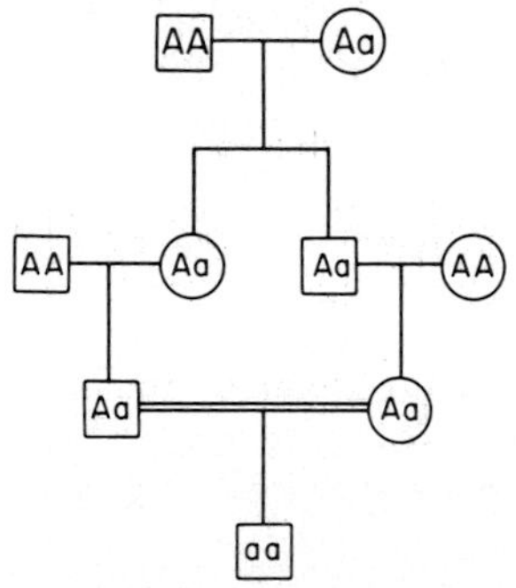

Figure 2–41. Affected homozygote *(aa)*, parental consanguinity indicated by the double horizontal line between two heterozygous parents, two heterozygous grandparents who are brother and sister, and the heterozygous great grandmother.

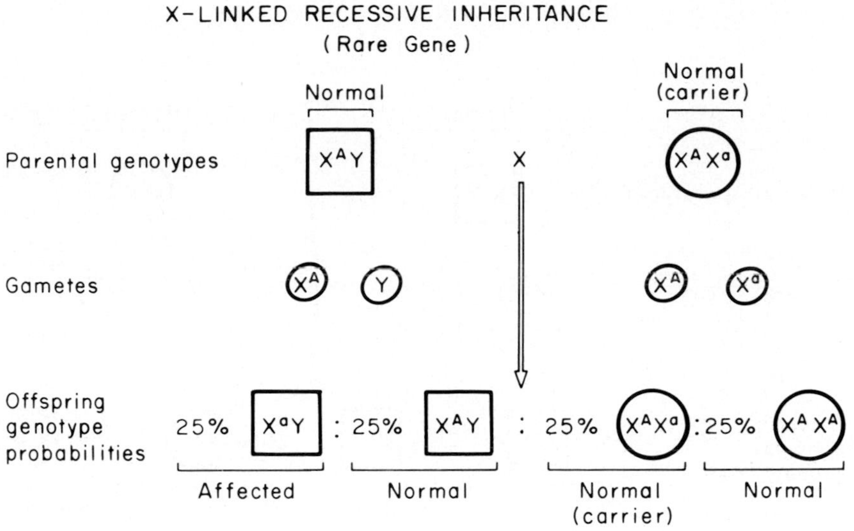

Figure 2–42. Parental genotypes, types of gametes, and offspring genotype probabilities in X-linked recessive inheritance.

carrier mothers do, in fact, have a patchy sweat gland distribution, they can be defined as being affected.

For X-linked dominant inheritance, parental genotypes, types of gametes, and offspring genotype probabilities are illustrated in Figures 2–44 and 2–45. A typical X-linked dominant pedigree is shown in Figure 2–46. Such a condition is transmitted from generation to generation without skips. All daughters of an affected male will be affected, but no sons of an affected male are affected. For affected females, offspring of either sex have a 50 per cent chance of being affected. X-linked dominant conditions are usually more severely expressed in males than in females, and in the population as a whole, more females tend to be affected. An example of an X-linked dominant condition is vitamin D resistant rickets.

Finally, the parental genotypes, types of gametes, and offspring genotype probabilities for X-linked dominant inheritance, lethal in the male, are illustrated in Figure 2–47. Only females are affected. The deficiency of males is expressed as an excess number of abortions in the offspring of affected females. The condition is transmitted from mother to daughter. An example of an X-linked dominant condition, lethal in the male, is the oral-facial-digital syndrome, Type I.

Multifactorial Inheritance

Multifactorial inheritance results from a combination of genetic and environmental factors. Such traits are primarily quantitative and continuous in nature. In the threshold model of multifactorial inheritance, the

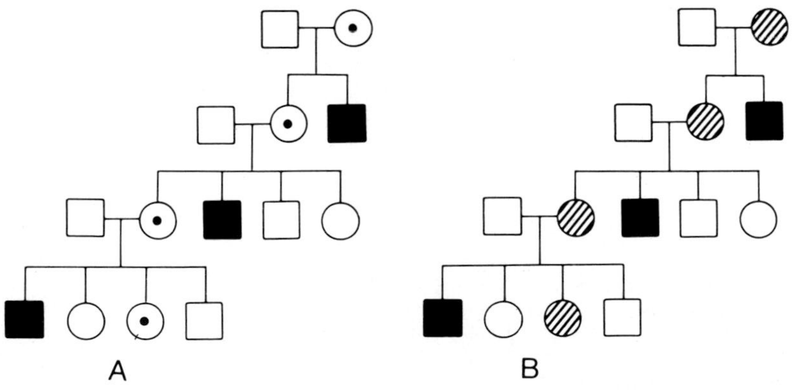

Figure 2–43. *A,* X-linked recessive pedigree (dots indicate female carriers). *B,* X-linked semidominant inheritance (disorder minimally defined so that female carriers are considered affected).

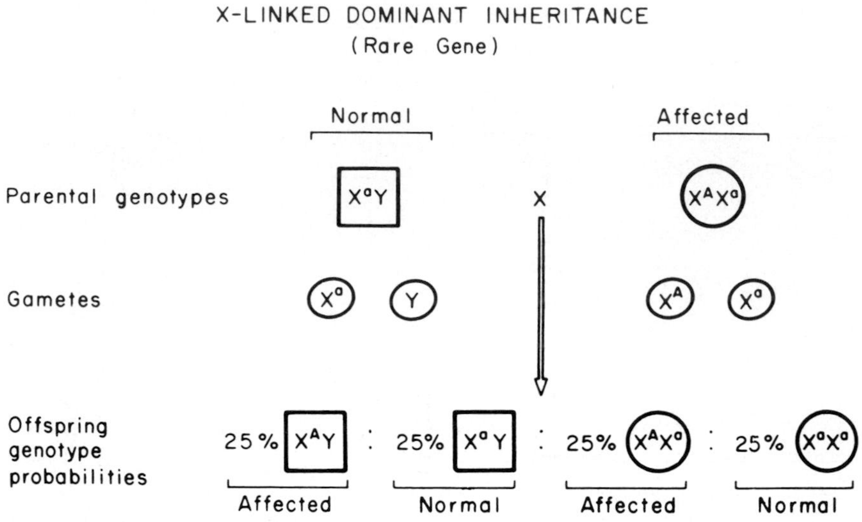

Figure 2–44. Parental genotypes, types of gametes, and offspring genotype probabilities in X-linked dominant inheritance (when the female is affected).

total liability of expression of the trait in question is reflected in the population as a normally distributed curve. Expression of the trait is restricted to those individuals who exceed a threshold of liability. Examples of multifactorial inheritance include cleft lip palate and anencephaly.

Multifactorial traits have a number of characteristics. First, the risk in relatives is greater than the frequency of the disorder in the general population. The magnitude of the difference in the risk is less as the frequency of the malformation increases in the population. Thus, first degree relatives such as siblings and offspring are most likely to be affected since on the average, they share 50 per cent of their genes in common. Second degree relatives such as aunts, uncles, nieces, and nephews are less likely to be affected since they share only 25 per cent of their genes in common. Third degree relatives such as first cousins are even less likely to be at risk since they share only 12.5 per cent of their genes in common.

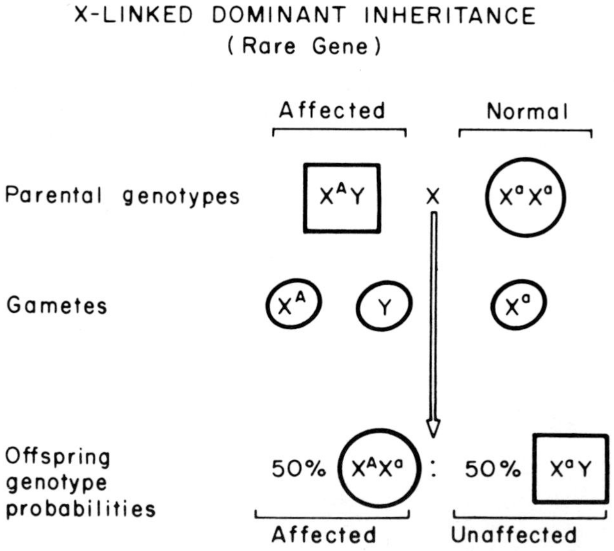

Figure 2–45. Parental genotypes, types of gametes, and offspring genotype probabilities in X-linked dominant inheritance (when the male is affected).

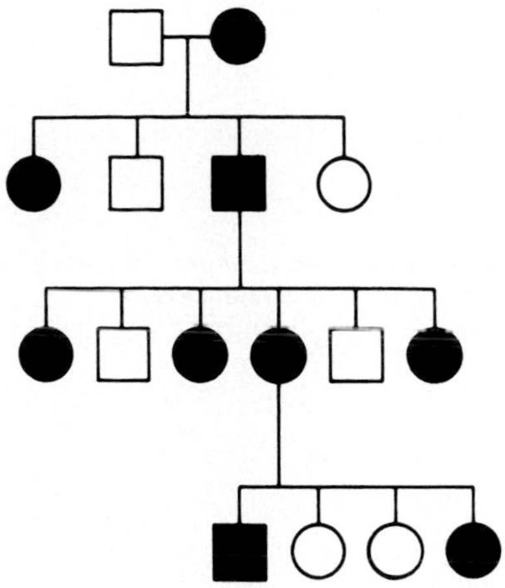

Figure 2–46. X-linked dominant pedigree. Note the vertical transmission and lack of male to male transmission. All daughters of an affected male are affected.

Second, the risk of the trait in question increases with each additional family member affected. The recurrence risk for a second affected child with a cleft lip palate is approximately 4 per cent if both parents are normal; the risk increases to approximately 16 per cent if one parent is also affected. Third, the more severe the malformation, the greater is the risk to the relatives. The risk for a second affected child is higher if the proband has bilateral cleft lip palate than if the proband has unilateral cleft lip. Fourth, if sex differences exist in the frequency of the trait in question, the risk to relatives is greater when the trait occurs in the less frequently affected sex. For example, cleft palate occurs less frequently in males than in females. The risk for cleft palate is greater in siblings of males with cleft palate than in siblings of females with cleft palate. Finally, an increase in parental consanguinity is to be expected with multifactorial causation.

Sporadicity

Earlier, it was emphasized that sporadic occurrence per se does not necessarily indicate that the condition in question is nongenetic. Figures 2–48 and 2–49 show some examples of sporadic occurrence with autosomal dominant and autosomal recessive disorders. Sporadic occurrence is found most frequently with multifactorial disorders. Sporadicity also occurs with *variant additive patterns*.

At times, it may be difficult to distinguish between a true multiple anomaly syndrome, which is a form of discontinuous variability with respect to normal first degree relatives, and a variant additive pattern, which is a

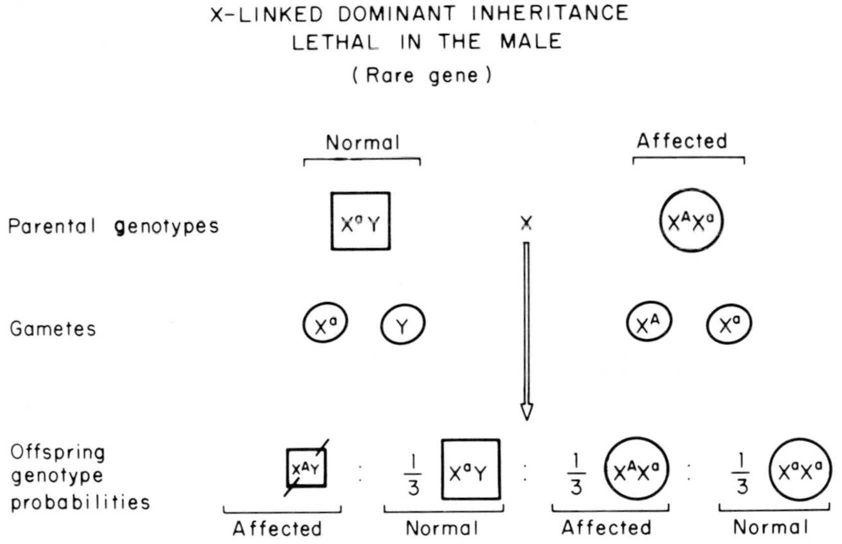

Figure 2–47. Parental genotypes, types of gametes, and offspring genotype probabilities in X-linked dominant inheritance (lethal in the male). Note that since the affected males are aborted, inheritance is from mother to daughter. An affected female has a one-third chance of having an affected daughter, a one-third chance of having a normal daughter, and a one-third chance of having a normal son.

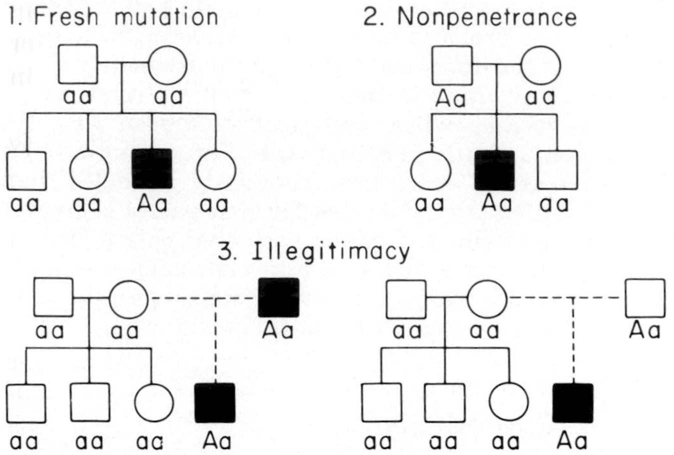

Figure 2–48. Examples of sporadicity in autosomal dominant inheritance.

form of continuous variability with respect to such relatives. A variant additive pattern usually consists of several minor anomalies and often a major anomaly in the same individual, so that the pattern of morphologic findings in that individual is statistically unusual for the general population but biologically normal for the individual's family, with the possible exception of the major anomaly. A variant additive pattern is an unusual chance pattern that can be identified in the population because the minor anomalies that make up the pattern in the proband may be observed separately in various relatives. Thus, the pattern is not caused by a monogenic or chromosomal abnormality, but by a variety of different genes acting independently. In this context, the minor anomalies in the proband and his or her family should be regarded as normal, morphologic variants.

The parents often explain that their child is not at all abnormal but simply resembles other members of the family. Facial comparison may be particularly telling. Many variant additive patterns do not have a major anomaly. When a major anomaly occurs in addition by chance, the likelihood of referral to a syndromologist increases. Care must be taken not to overdiagnose a variant additive pattern as a true multiple anomaly syndrome of presumed unitary etiology.

A typical example of a variant additive pattern is a proband with downslanting palpebral fissures, ear pits, mandibular prognathism, clinodactyly, cubitus valgus, and ventricular septal defect. In the examination of the proband's relatives (Fig. 2–50), the father is noted to have downslanting palpebral fissures and cubitus valgus, the mother is found to have ear pits and clinodactyly, and both the brother and the maternal grand-

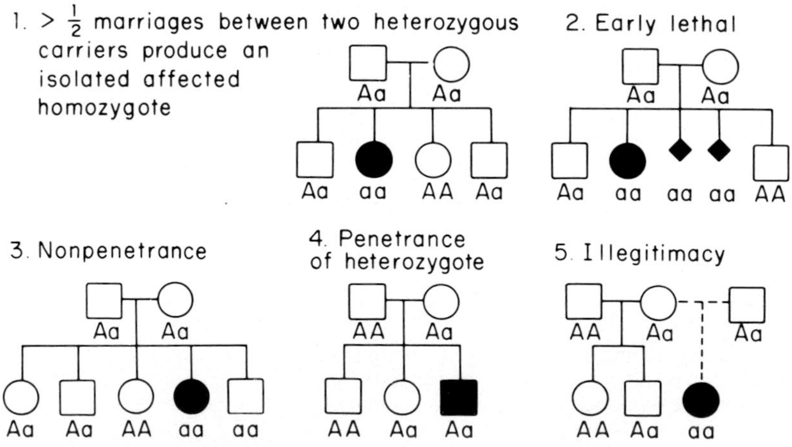

Figure 2–49. Examples of sporadicity in autosomal recessive inheritance.

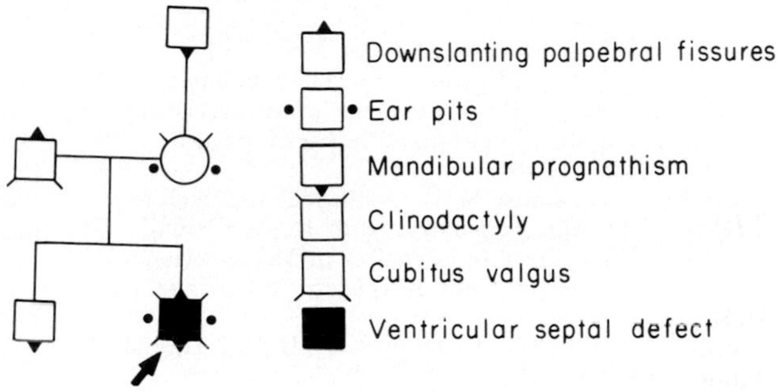

Figure 2–50. Variant additive pattern. Note that all features of the pattern observed in the proband except the ventricular septal defect are dispersed in various members of the family. (From Cohen, M.M., Jr.: On the nature of syndrome delineation. Acta Genet. Med. Gemellol. (Roma), *26*:103, 1977.)

father are observed to have mandibular prognathism. Thus, all the features except the ventricular septal defect are dispersed in various members of the family as minor anomalies. They happened to come together in the proband by chance in addition to one major anomaly—a ventricular septal defect. The probability of all these anomalies coming together in future offspring in this family is slight, although various individual anomalies or combinations of anomalies may recur. For example, of three future offspring, a first might have ear pits; a second, ventricular septal defect, clinodactyly, and downslanting palpebral fissures; a third, mandibular prognathism and cubitus valgus. Thus, a variant additive pattern may be considered unique to an affected individual or to an affected family. In this particular family, genetic counseling should take into account a multifactorial recurrence risk of a ventricular septal defect (Cohen, 1982).

REFERENCES

Anderson, F. M., and Geiger, L.: Craniosynostosis; a survey of 204 cases. J. Neurosurg., *22*:229, 1965.

Andersson, H: Craniosynostosis as a complication after operation for hydrocephalus. Acta Paediatr. Scand., *55*:192, 1966.

Aurias, A., and Laurent, C.: Trisomie 11q. Individualisation d'un nouveau syndrome. Ann. Genet., *18*:189, 1975.

Baker, C. J., and Rudolph, A. J.: Congenital ring constrictions and intrauterine amputations. Am. J. Dis. Child., *121*:393, 1971.

Chapple, C. C., and Davidson, D. T.: A study of the relationship between fetal position and certain congenital deformities. J. Pediatr., *18*:483, 1941.

Clarren, S. K., and Smith, D. W.: The fetal alcohol syndrome. N. Engl. J. Med., *298*:1063, 1978.

Cohen, M. M., Jr.: Dysmorphic syndromes with craniofacial manifestations. *In* Stewart, R. E., and Prescott, G. H. (Eds.): Oral Facial Genetics. St. Louis, C. V. Mosby Company, 1976, pp. 500–662.

Cohen, M. M., Jr.: Genetic perspectives on craniosynostosis and syndromes with craniosynostosis. J. Neurosurg., *47*:886, 1977.

Cohen, M. M., Jr.: A critical review of cephalometric studies of dysmorphic syndromes. Proc. Finn. Dent. Soc., *77*:17, 1981.

Cohen, M. M., Jr.: The Child with Multiple Birth Defects. New York, Raven Press, 1982.

Cohen, M. M., Jr.: Dysmorphic growth and development and the study of craniofacial syndromes. J. Craniofac. Genet. Dev. Biol. (Suppl.), *1*:43, 1985.

Cohen, M. M., Jr.: Craniosynostosis: Diagnosis, Evaluation, and Management. New York, Raven Press, 1986.

Cohen, M. M., Jr.: Epidemiology, genetics, and syndromology of holoprosencephaly. Teratology (in press).

Cohen, M. M., Jr., Zellweger, H., Waziri, M., Hanson, J. W., and Jones, K. L.: A recurrent-pattern syndrome of branchial arch anomalies, encephalocele and renal anomalies. Morphogenesis and Malformations Meeting, San Diego, CA, 1980.

Conen, P. E., Erkman, B., and Metaxotou, C.: The "D" syndrome. Report of four trisomic and one D/D translocation case. Am. J. Dis. Child., *111*:236, 1966.

DeMyer, W., and Zeman, W.: Alobar holoprosencephaly (arhinencephaly) with median cleft lip and palate: clinical, electroencephalographic, and nosologic considerations. Confin. Neurol., *23*:1, 1963.

Duggan, C. A., Keener, E. B., and Gay, B. B.: Secondary craniosynostosis. Am. J. Roentgenol., *109*:227, 1970.

Dunn, P. M.: Congenital postural deformities. Br. Med. Bull., *32*:71, 1976.

Dykstra, O. H., and Halbertsma, T.: Polycythemia vera in childhood. Am. J. Dis. Child., *60*:907, 1940.

Emery, A. E. H., and Rimoin, D. L.: Principles and Practice of Medical Genetics. Edinburgh, Churchill Livingstone, 1983.

Gorlin, R. J., Pindborg, J. J., and Cohen, M. M., Jr.: Syndromes of the Head and Neck. 2nd Ed. New York, McGraw-Hill Book Company, 1976.

Graham, J. M., Jr., deSaxe, M., and Smith, D. W.: Sagittal craniostenosis: fetal head constraint as one possible cause. J. Pediatr., *95*:747, 1979.

Graham, J. M., Miller, M. E., Stephan, M. J., and Smith, D. W.: Limb reduction anomalies and early in utero limb compression. J. Pediatr., *96*:1052, 1980.

Hall, B. D.: Syndromes and situations simulated by amniotic bands. Birth Defects Conference, Chicago, June 24–27, 1979.

Harris, V., Beligere, N., and Pruzansky, S.: Progressive generalized bony dysplasia in Apert syndrome. Birth Defects, *14*:1975, 1977.

Herrmann, J., France, T. D., Spranger, J. W., Opitz, J. M., and Wiffler, C.: The Stickler syndrome (hereditary arthroophthalmopathy). Birth Defects, *11*:76, 1975.

Herrmann, J., and Opitz, J. M.: Naming and nomenclature of syndromes. Birth Defects, *10*:69, 1974.

Johnsonbaugh, R. E., Bryan, R. N., Hierlwimmer, U. R., and Georges, L. P.: Premature craniosynostosis: a common complication of juvenile thyrotoxicosis. J. Pediatr., *93*:181, 1978.

Jones, K. L, and Jones, M. C.: A clinical approach to the dysmorphic child. *In* Emery, A. E. H., and Rimoin, D. L. (Eds.): Principles and Practice of Medical Genetics. Vol. I. Edinburgh, Churchill Livingstone, 1983, pp. 152–161.

Jones, K. L., Smith, D. W., Hall, B. D., Hall, J. G., Ebbin, A. J., et al.: A pattern of craniofacial and limb defects secondary to aberrant tissue bands. J. Pediatr., *83*:90, 1974.

Kelly, T. E.: Clinical Genetics and Genetic Counseling. Chicago, Year Book Medical Publishers, 1980.

Kennedy, L. A., and Persaud, T. V. N.: Pathogenesis of developmental defects induced in the rat by amniotic sac puncture. Acta Anat., *97*:23, 1977.

Kloss, J. L.: Craniosynostosis secondary to ventriculoatrial shunt. Am. J. Dis. Child., *116*:315, 1968.

Koskinen-Moffett, L.: In vivo experimental model for prenatal craniosynostosis. J. Dent. Res., *65*, Special Issue, Abstr. 980, 1986.

Lorber, J.: The prognosis of occipital encephalocele. Dev. Med. Child. Neurol. (Suppl.), *13*:75, 1967.

Lubs, H. A., and Ing, P. S.: Human cytogenetic nomenclature. *In* Emery, A. E. H., and Rimoin, D. L. (Eds.): Principles and Practice of Medical Genetics. Vol. I. Edinburgh, Churchill Livingstone, 1983, pp. 162–169.

Marden, P. M., Smith, D. W., and McDonald, M. J.: Congenital anomalies in the newborn infant, including minor variation. J. Pediatr., *64*:357, 1964.

Menking, M., Wiebel, J., Schmidt, W. U., Schmidt, W. T., Ebel, K. D., and Ritter, R.: Premature craniosynostosis associated with hyperthyroidism in 4 children with reference to 5 further cases in the literature. Monatsschr. Kinderheilkd., *121*:106, 1972.

Miller, M. E., Graham, J. M., Jr., Higginbottom, M. C., and Smith, D. W.: Compression-related defects from early amnion rupture: evidence for mechanical teratogenesis. J. Pediatr., *98*:292, 1981.

Moss, M. L.: The pathogenesis of premature cranial synostosis in man. Acta Anat., *37*:351, 1959.

Moynahan, E. J., and Wolff, O. H.: A new neurocutaneous syndrome (skin, eye, brain) consisting of linear nevus, bilateral lipodermoids of the conjunctiva, cranial thickening, cerebral cortical atrophy, and mental retardation. Br. J. Dermatol., *79*:651, 1967.

Opitz, J. M., Herrmann, J., and Dieker, H.: The study of malformation syndromes in man. Birth Defects, *5*:1, 1969.

Park, E. A., and Powers, G. F.: Acrocephaly and scaphocephaly with symmetrically distributed malformations of the extremities. Am. J. Dis. Child., *20*:235, 1920.

Penfold, J. L., and Simpson, D. A.: Premature craniosynostosis—a complication of thyroid replacement therapy. J. Pediatr., *86*:360, 1975.

Poswillo, D.: The pathogenesis of the first and second branchial arch syndrome. Oral Surg., *35*:302, 1973.

Pruzansky, S.: Clinical investigation of the experiments of nature. ASHA Report, *8*:62, 1973.

Reilly, B. J., Leeming, J. M., and Fraser, D.: Craniosynostosis in the rachitic spectrum. J. Pediatr., *64*:396, 1964.

Roberts, K. B., and Hall, J. G.: Apert's acrocephalosyndactyly in mother and daughter: cleft palate in the mother. Birth Defects, *7*:262, 1971.

Robinson, A.: Ataxia-telangiectasia presenting with craniostenosis. Arch. Dis. Child., *37*:652, 1962.

Routledge, R. T.: The Pierre Robin syndrome. A surgical emergency in the neonatal period. Br. J. Plast. Surg., *13*:204, 1960.

Schauerte, E. W., and St-Aubin, P. M.: Progressive synostosis in Apert's syndrome (acrocephalosyndactyly) with a description of roentgenographic changes in the feet. Am. J. Roentgenol., *97*:67, 1966.

Smith, D. W.: Recognizable Patterns of Human Malformation. 3rd Ed., Philadelphia, W. B. Saunders Company, 1982.

Smith, D. W., and Bostian, K. E.: Congenital anomalies associated with idiopathic mental retardation. J. Pediatr., *65*:189, 1964.

Smith, J. L., and Stowe, F. R.: The Pierre Robin syndrome. Pediatrics, *27*:128, 1961.

Smithwick, E. M., Finelt, M., Pahwa, S., Good, R. A., Nespitz, C. K., et al.: Cranial synostosis in Job's syndrome. Lancet, *1*:826, 1978.

Spranger, J. W., Benirschke, K., Hall, J. G., Lenz, W., Lowry, R. B., et al.: Errors of morphogenesis: concepts and terms. J. Pediatr., *100*:160, 1982.

Stewart, R. E., Dixon, G., and Cohen, A.: The pathogenesis of premature craniosynostosis in acrocephalosyndactyly (Apert's syndrome)—a reconsideration. Plast. Reconstr. Surg., *59*:669, 1977.

Thompson, M. W.: Thompson and Thompson Genetics in Medicine. 4th Ed. Philadelphia, W. B. Saunders Company, 1986.

Torpin, R.: Fetal Malformations Caused by Amnion Rupture During Gestation. Springfield, IL, Charles C Thomas, 1968.

Virchow, R.: Über den Cretinismus, namentlich in Franken, und über pathologische Schädelformen. Verhandl. Phys. Med. Gesellsch. Würzburg, *2*:231, 1851.

Warkany, J.: Congenital Malformations: Notes and Comments. Chicago, Year Book Medical Publishers, 1971.

Weaver, D. D., Graham, C. B., Thomas, I. T., and Smith, D. W.: A new overgrowth syndrome with accelerated skeletal maturation, unusual facies, and camptodactyly. J. Pediatr. *84*:547, 1974.

3

Suzanne B. Housman

Psychosocial Aspects of Plastic Surgery

In 1949 the total number of plastic surgery procedures performed in the United States was 15,000 (Macgregor, 1974). In 1986 590,550 esthetic procedures and 1,259,500 reconstructive plastic surgery procedures were carried out in the U.S. (see Tables 3–1, 3–2). Some people can cope with or compensate for disfigurement or unattractiveness, but others are resorting to plastic surgery in increasing numbers as techniques improve and availability and public awareness increase.

From the literature on the psychologic and sociologic aspects of plastic surgery, a curious fact emerges: most of it has been written by plastic surgeons. On the one hand, this finding may indicate an increased sensitivity by plastic surgeons, to psychic forces as they pertain to esthetic form as compared with other surgeons concerned mainly with survival and functional issues. References to the plastic surgeon as a "30 minute psychiatrist" (Anderson, 1974), "psychosurgeon," and even "psychiatrist with a knife" (Rozner, 1973) are not without foundation. On the other hand, they may indicate an increased need for involvement of psychiatrists and social scientists in the treatment of the patient undergoing plastic surgery. Goin and Goin (1981a) referred to the need to "tame" a psychiatrist, i.e., to train one to work in this highly specialized field, which not only includes Diagnostic and Statistical Manual (DSM III-R) (American Psychiatric Association, 1987) diagnoses but also requires a sensitivity to the issues of change in body image and physical attractiveness. It also requires a practical knowledge of the possibilities and, more important, the limitations of plastic surgery (Edgerton and Knorr, 1971; Olley, 1974).

Another obvious flaw in the literature is the paucity of well-designed research studies, especially those that include a control group.

PHYSICAL ATTRACTIVENESS

Of paramount concern to the plastic surgeon is patient selection. How can one predict who will benefit the most, and whether the risk is worth the gain, while at the same time weeding out the psychologically unstable? The interpretation of who represents the latter has been greatly modified (reduced) over

Table 3–1. Plastic Surgery Procedures Performed in 1984 and 1986 by ASPRS Members

		1986		1984	% Increase/ Decrease
Esthetic Surgical Procedures					
Abdominoplasty		32,300		20,900	55
Blepharoplasty		84,700		73,900	15
Breast augmentation		93,500		95,000	(2)
Chemical peel		15,600		16,200	(4)
Dermabrasion		26,300		23,500	12
Forehead lift		15,900		—	—
Hair transplant		2,800		4,500	(38)
Mastopexy		17,200		16,200	6
Mentoplasty (chin augmentation)		15,300		17,500	(13)
Otoplasty		14,900		13,200	13
Rhinoplasty		82,200		70,500	17
Rhytidectomy (face lift)		66,900		54,400	23
Suction assisted lipectomy (SAL)		99,350		55,900	78
Thigh	30,800		17,500		
Abdomen	23,850		13,600		
Buttocks	18,600		14,900		
Face	26,100		9,900		
Surgical body contouring		23,600		16,000	48
Total Esthetic		590,550		477,700	24
Reconstructive Surgical Procedures					
Breast reconstruction		57,200		98,800	
Breast reduction		48,600		37,700	
Cleft lip/palate		24,200		21,000	
Other congenital anomalies		17,250		18,200	
Dog bites		25,900		22,300	
Emergency Room care		187,800		160,500	
Hand		192,200		166,300	
Lacerations		168,700		144,300	
Primary burn care		20,400		23,200	
Reconstruction		136,450		130,500	
Head/neck	26,300		31,400		
Lower extremity	24,150		22,500		
Trunk	16,200		13,200		
Trauma	69,800		63,400		
Scar revision		82,000		79,600	
Tumor removal		208,500		201,800	
Head/neck	106,900		119,800		
Other	101,600		82,000		
Other		90,300		284,500	
Total Reconstruction		1,259,500		1,388,700	
Total (esthetic and reconstructive)		1,850,050		1,866,400	

From American Society of Plastic & Reconstructive Surgeons, Inc., May, 1987.

time as more and more patients have elected for cosmetic change. Why do people opt for change in physical form? Why has the exercise of this option become more socially and culturally acceptable? There is much comment in the plastic surgical literature on the presumed social and psychologic rewards of being physically attractive, but the documentation of why this is so is to be found in the social science literature, much of which represents well-designed, controlled studies. These studies show that physical attractiveness has a statistically significant effect on self-esteem and other measures of psychic well-being—beauty is *not* skin deep. For reviews of the literature, see *Clinics in Plastic Surgery*, July 1982, and *Psychological Aspects of Facial Form*, 1981).

Benefits start accruing to the physically attractive from birth. Nurses of premature infants award a higher intellectual prognosis to attractive babies (Corter and associates,

Table 3–2. Male Esthetic Surgery

Procedures	Number of Operations Performed In 1986	Percentage Performed on Men	Number Performed on Men
Abdominoplasty	32,300	7	2,264
Blepharoplasty	84,700	18	15,244
Chemical peel	15,600	4	624
Dermabrasion	26,300	27	7,096
Forehead lift	15,900	10	1,590
Hair transplant	2,800	95	2,650
Mentoplasty (chin augmentation)	15,300	18	2,759
Otoplasty	14,900	44	6,547
Rhinoplasty	82,200	25	20,558
Rhytidectomy (face lift)	66,900	10	6,693
Suction Assisted Lipectomy (SAL)	99,350	6	5,966
Thighs	30,800	3	924
Abdomen	23,850	9	2,146
Buttocks	18,600	3	557
Face	26,100	9	2,349
Surgical body contouring	23,260	6	1,415

From American Society of Plastic & Reconstructive Surgeons, Inc., May, 1987.

1980). Parents have higher expectations of success for their attractive children (Adams and LaVoie, 1975), and as a consequence provide more quality parenting (Boukydis, 1981; Hildebrandt, 1981).

These infants also receive more visual attention from adults (Hildebrandt and Fitzgerald, 1977) and are less likely to be judged antisocial (Dion, Berscheid, and Walster, 1972). Other authors have shown that preschool children aged 3 to 4 years are potentially influenced by the good looks of their playmates in that they ascribe to them greater social attributes (Dion, 1973; Dion and Berscheid, 1974; Adams and Crane, 1981).

By elementary school age, both parents believe their attractive sons will respond to inductive reasoning as a disciplinary style (Adams and LaVoie, 1975), and women caregivers are more likely to punish unattractive young boys (Dion, 1974). Teachers give more attention, information, and opportunities to physically attractive children (Adams and LaVoie, 1977). In addition, they are more likely to be referred for special educational assistance, when indicated (Barocas and Vance, 1974).

And what of the young adult? One of the first and best known studies is that of Walster and associates (quoted in Kalick, 1978) on dating. The researchers found that the *only* significant predictor of a partner's liking and desire to date again, whether the person was male or female, was the degree of physical attractiveness. This factor was more important than IQ, academic achievement, or other personality measures. Allen and Meredith (described in Allen and Wroble, 1978) reported that physically attractive women were more likely to receive dates, whether or not they were trustworthy or independent (two qualities for which the investigators tested). As dating progressed, physical attractiveness became *more*, rather than less, important (Mathes, 1975). Dion, Berscheid, and Walster (1972), when presenting young men and women with head and shoulder photos of other young men and women of varying degrees of attractiveness, asked for speculation regarding personalities and life events. In every case the more physically attractive were more highly rated (a finding that other investigators have since corroborated). The more physically attractive were perceived to be more kind, sociable, outgoing, sensitive, strong, modest, and poised and more sexually warm and exciting. It follows that they were more likely to get better jobs, have better marriages, and have happier and more fulfilling lives. This study was appropriately entitled "What is beautiful is good." Of special note is that these views prevailed whether the rater or ratee was male or female, findings indicating that physical attractiveness influences the lives of young men as well as young women.

What effect does all this have on the physically attractive person's self-image? The answer is increased self-esteem (Berscheid and associates, 1971; Mathes and Kahn, 1975; Allen and Wroble, 1978), which leads to increased socialization (Berscheid and associates, 1971; Krebs and Adinolfi, 1975; Allen and Wroble, 1978) with greater assertiveness and social skills (Jackson and Huston, 1975; Goldman and Lewis, 1977).

Additional studies have borne out these assumptions. The physically attractive are more likely than the unattractive to receive job offers, given equal qualifications (Dipboye, Fromkin, and Wiback, 1975; Cash and associates, 1977). Once hired they receive higher evaluations (Landy and Sigall, 1974) and receive greater credit for success (Seligman, Pascall, and Takata, 1981). For example, in a psychotherapeutic setting, patients who perceive their therapists as attractive tend to improve more rapidly (Shapiro and associates, 1976). Therapists tend to view their attractive patients as more responsive to therapy; the unattractive are more likely to be referred for psychiatric hospitalization (Barocas and Vance, 1974). However, Cash and associates (1977) showed that therapists underestimate the psychologic problems of their attractive clients and give them less attention.

What is the response of the unattractive? Dion and Stein (1978) found that unattractive fifth and sixth grade boys mostly used threat and command to influence their peers, whereas attractive boys were assertive but not aggressive. Attractive rape victims are perceived by unattractive women to be responsible for their own victimization (Baunach, 1981).

In summary, the physically attractive enter life with a halo effect and receive preferential treatment from cradle to adult life. The positive reinforcement for an attractive appearance tends to confirm the assumptions of the nurse in the nursery, the parents, and the teachers alike. It is *not* meant to imply that the physically attractive are better people than the unattractive, but that they are offered far greater opportunities for success and happiness.

The Spectrum of Beauty

The concept of beauty may translate across cultures but its interpretation may not. For example, tattooing may be considered an art form, as in the Far East, or a stigmatizing brand, as in Nazi concentration camps, street gangs, or contemporary prisons. Voluntary keloid scarification beautifies the Nigerian but deforms the American black. Distention of the neck, lips, and earlobes enhances the desirability of the African woman, and nose piercing that of the Muslim woman, whereas Western women merely pierce their ears. As with beauty, interpretations of deformity may vary. The Greeks left their deformed infants to die on a hillside, whereas pre-Columbans practiced head molding and induced spinal deformities in their infants, rewarding the dwarfed and hunch-backed with privilege (Rees and Daniller, 1969). One may also speculate that being born female may be considered a type of "deformity," in view of worldwide historical preference for the male. Greek mythology refers to the Amazons, a fierce group of women who preferred to cut off their right breasts rather than have them interfere with drawing a bow (Rees and Daniller, 1969). Feet binding was a vogue in China at the turn of the century, as was rib removal to enhance the waist contour of nineteenth century Europeans. Chests were bound in Western women in the 1920's. Circumcision and clitorectomy may be religious rites, symbols of group membership, or measures taken to bring health. Hair may be cut for fashion or shorn in bereavement; fingers may be amputated out of respect for a Sensai or in memory of the dead. Cleft (hare) lip may superstitiously be thought to result from a woman petting a rabbit during pregnancy; other birth deformities being the result of a full moon, an eclipse of the sun, or an earthquake. Thus, people seek to impose meaning on things they do not understand, with whatever information is available to them.

The inner esthetic norms are far more restrictive than the statistical norms of the individual species. Thus, a flattened nose becomes "pugnacious," a weak chin a sign of a weak character, and "bags under the eyes" a sign of debauchery. Even signs of childbirth and normal aging are becoming less and less tolerated as youthfulness becomes synonymous with capacity (Reich, 1969).

As one moves from one culture to another, a change may be elicited in the direction of conformity to the new culture. To be physically or behaviorally out of sympathy with one's culture can be disastrous. The Hopi Indians deliberately drove offenders in their community to insanity by the punishment of derisive laughter (Macgregor, 1970). The American Shakers practiced shunning, the ancient Greeks and modern East Europeans exile. In Western culture names and noses are changed in an effort to assimilate (Macgregor, 1967b). Before the "black is beautiful" rallying call of the 1960's, skin was chemically lightened and hair was straightened. The *ready-to-wear* concept encourages a standardized figure (Reich, 1975). The presence or absence of cosmetics, body paint, nail polish, hair dyes and bleach, hair straighteners and permanents, and finally jewelry and clothes are all variations on the same theme. One adorns and physically alters the body to obtain various rewards or punishments, to enhance beauty or ward off evil spirits or disease. It might be argued that these efforts represent voluntary or self-induced "mutilations" of the normal healthy body. The key to the discussion "deformity versus cosmetic" is the individual motivation, *beauty being in the eye of the beholder*. "Vanity as an impulse has without doubt been of far more benefit to civilization than modesty has ever been" (Courtiss, 1980). For a far more extensive review of crosscultural differences, including photographic illustrations, see Rees and Wood-Smith (1973).

RELIGION AND PLASTIC SURGERY

Taylor, Litin, and Litzow (1966) reviewed Western cultural values as regards plastic surgery from a religious viewpoint. Under Jewish law the Talmud permits physicians to heal, but whether that sanction includes cosmetic surgery is unclear. However, women are encouraged to enhance their physical attractiveness, although this is frowned on for men. Extreme objection exists to mutilation of the human body without strong medical reason. Protestants, on the other hand, feel that whatever contributes to man's total effectiveness and happiness in normal life relationships is acceptable. The Catholic point of view is perhaps best summarized by the address of Pope Pius XII in 1959 to the Italian Congress of Plastic Surgeons (Taylor, Litin, and Litzow, 1966): "Remember that your vision should go beyond tissues and outward forms and reach the soul, whose interior beauty you will teach others to appreciate." He saw plastic surgery as being ". . . at the top of the medical profession for its beneficial work in restoring harmony and propriety to body and occasionally the spirit" (Robertson, 1967). However, plastic surgery was viewed as unlawful when its purpose is to increase seductiveness, gratify vanity, or help a criminal escape justice.

PATIENT SELECTION

Plastic surgery has its roots in the reconstruction of traumatic, deforming injury and in the repair of birth defects. Only later was surgical revision of body parts for purely esthetic reasons included in the field. To quote Greer (1984), "understanding the motives, espectations, and desires of a patient seeking . . . surgery is at least as important as manual dexterity for achieving consistent, satisfying results." With this in mind, one can review the history of patient selection for plastic surgery.

The plastic surgery patients receiving the most study have been those with minor defects, those requesting multiple operations, and psychiatric patients. As mentioned, the definition of the last-named has been greatly altered over time as awareness of patient motivation has been enhanced. Many patients who carried a psychiatric label presented seeking correction of minor defects. Because of a conditioned fear of such patients, surgeons, who one would presume could recognize an alteration in "anatomic perfection," would turn them away. A series of studies was performed by Hay and associates in England (Hay, 1970; Hay and Heather, 1973) in which photographs of patients with minor defects were shown to an independent panel of raters, with random photos of nurses serving as controls. Although the raters were blind to the study, they were consistently able to pick out the patients seeking surgery (rhinoplasty), rating them as more disfigured than the controls. Although on psychologic testing the rhinoplasty patients were found to be more disturbed than the controls, there was no correlation between the degree of psychologic disturbance and the degree of deformity, thus supporting the argument that the degree of deformity is not a reason for rejecting the patient for surgery. In cases of doubt, Hay (1970) recommended referring the patient to a psychiatrist for general improvement in adjustment rather than appraisal of the physical lesion. He believed that, if accepted for treatment, these patients usually did well both in plastic surgery and psychotherapy. This finding supports that of Edgerton, Jacobson, and Meyer (1961) and others (Olley, 1974) in which 16 per cent of their "psychotic" patients improved with surgery, suggesting that even patients with *real* psychiatric diagnoses can possibly benefit from corrective surgery, as long as they are also followed by intensive psychiatric support. Suitable patients should have a *realistic* appraisal of the possibilities and limitations of surgery, regardless of the degree of psychologic disturbance (Clarkson and Stanford-Clark, quoted in Editorial, Med. J. Aust., 1974). The authors are not endorsing *all* psychiatric patients for plastic surgery. Surgery should *not* be performed on patients with untreated schizophrenia, psychotic affective disorders, or paranoia, or patients about whom the surgeon has a "gut feeling" (Mohl, 1984). When in doubt, the patient should be referred to a psychiatrist. An excellent account of what the surgeon should ask the psychiatrist was presented by Anderson (1974), and it is summarized as follows: Is the patient mentally ill? If so, can surgery proceed, and with what precautions? Can surgery accomplish what may be the patient's hidden fancies? The initial reason for which a patient seeks surgery may not be the real reason, i.e., the patient may be fearful of refusal of surgery (Reich, 1969). At the same time, it is also wise for the surgeon to attend to his own fantasies of omnipotence (Schulman, 1980). Belfer, Mulliken, and Cochran (1979) discovered unconscious motivation in four of their patients only postoperatively, when the patients shifted from a passive and withdrawn posture to an active one by seeking divorce. In general, patients who can clearly articulate their motives for cosmetic surgery are better surgical candidates than those who cannot (Mohl, 1984).

There are additional critical questions. Will the stress of surgery lead to breakdown or decompensation? If surgery may proceed, what should be the precautions? Postoperative psychiatric depression is usually a temporary phenomenon and is not uncommon after surgery. Dugas (1983) recommended including postoperative depression as a possibility in the preoperative informed consent. In addition, he recommended giving the guilt-ridden postoperative patient preoperative pictures for jealous or worried friends or family to see. Is the patient litigious, accusatory, or angry with hospital and staff? If the decision for surgery is reached, one might include in the consent clauses the fact that the patient has been truthful and agrees to follow postoperative orders. One should include permission to use photos in the consent, and counsel about residual and possibly new scars. One might also include the patient's recognition of normally occurring facial asymmetries that surgery may not correct, especially those of the ears, nostrils, eyes, and brows (Gorney and Harries, 1974). There are also naturally occurring asymmetries of the left versus the right side of the face, which are due to differing growth rates and varying hemispheric innervation of the muscles of expression (Borod and Koff, 1984).

Another important question is whether the patient is likely to change his mind or regret the decision because of shaky motivation or unrealistic expectations. Such a patient is "doctor shopping," with a bag full of magazine photographs of a presumed optimal result, or may be seeking consultation only because of pressure from others. This type of patient may be the perfectionist who wants immediate magical improvement (Olley, 1974). The patient may presume inordinate postoperative financial or social gain, or may expect to capture the attention of an unappreciative husband. A final question is whether the patient can accept less than perfection. Anderson (1974) counseled the surgeon that "the enemy of good is better," and admonished against the "rescue complex" of the physician who believes that he can accomplish anything. "Many plastic surgeons have the desire to create beautiful people, the 'Pygmalion complex,' thus obscuring the wish to cure and the need to cure. When such a patient and surgeon meet, the indication for treatment is solely their mutual satisfaction" (Macgregor, 1971).

One is encouraged to refer to another plastic surgeon if there is a poor "personality fit" with the patient (the strongest motivator for litigation) and one is advised not to make "deals" (Mohl, 1984). When rejecting a patient for surgery, it is recommended that the surgeon consult with the patient's family physician who referred him, as to who should inform the patient, and possibly refer the patient for psychiatric evaluation (Wray, 1986). The patient should be gently informed why he is rejected, without wasting his time by referring him to another plastic surgeon to avoid confrontation.

According to Swanson (cited in Lubkin,

1975), patients with psychiatric problems show an increased incidence of surgical complications such as wound infection, thrombophlebitis, ileus, and pulmonary infection. However, others (Greer, 1984) reported that patients do better postoperatively after a psychiatric consultation, i.e., they are more pleased with the surgical result. Greer (1984) promoted the value of the psychiatric consultation, even when it takes place up to six and 12 weeks postoperatively.

Age Considerations. What special consideration should be given the patient on the basis of age? When is the best time for surgery, given a choice? Ramsay (cited in Lubkin, 1975) studied patients before surgery and noted that, overall, 73 per cent experienced fear, whether scheduled for major or minor surgery. Fear of anesthesia was greater than fear of surgery by 4 to 1. Of children four to 12 years of age, 55 per cent were frightened, as were 82 per cent of the 22 to 62 year old patients, and 57 per cent of the 62 to 82 year olds. Lubkin (1975, citing a personal communication from Nictern) reviewed the two critical periods of childhood, being from 4 to 6 years of age and at puberty, the so-called ages of individualization and separation from parents. The younger child experiences panic regarding small cuts and bruises. Castration fears also appear. Sleep disturbances, such as nightmares threatening bodily destruction, are common, as is fear of going to sleep and death. The 4 to 6 year old child is most vulnerable to bodily assault, maximally via surgery, and yet the same children present for surgery "just before school." Lubkin (1975) recommended childhood surgery when the patient is under 4 years old, if possible. Knorr, Hoopes, and Edgerton (1968), on the other hand, believed that the adolescent is more concerned with body image change than any other group. They are satisfactory plastic surgery candidates as they can integrate the surgical change (into an already changing body image) better.

Spira and associates and Pick and associates (quoted in Meyer and associates, 1973) supported this conclusion in their studies of adolescent prisoners who demonstrated a lower recidivism rate after plastic surgery. In the study of adult prisoners provided with plastic surgery (Schuring and Dodge, 1967) a five year follow-up of surgical versus nonsurgical controls showed no significant difference in recidivism. Other investigators (Kurtzberg and associates, 1967) reported significant findings on neuropsychologic testing, namely, that inmates requiring plastic surgery were more disturbed than control prisoners, which suggests that real or imagined handicap aggravates psychopathic manifestations.

Another patient population that has been much commented on consists of males presenting for cosmetic surgery. Whereas women have been culturally encouraged to seek improvements in physical attractiveness, men have been expected to be rugged, "roughing it out" being equated with masculinity. Men aged "gracefully," women "fell apart." In view of the differing cultural stereotypes, men presenting for cosmetic surgery years ago might have been perceived as eccentrics or insecure. As cultural mores have changed, however, more men are presenting for plastic surgery. According to statistics published by the American Society of Plastic and Reconstructive Surgeons (1987), men now represent 25 per cent of rhinoplasties, 10 per cent of face lifts, 18 per cent of blepharoplasties, and 18 per cent of mentoplasties (see Table 3–2). The most common is the operation for hair transplant for correction of male pattern baldness, 95 per cent being for men, followed by otoplasty (44 per cent).

Dysmorphophobia. This term, although frequently used in the plastic surgery literature in England, has rarely appeared in the American literature and does not appear in the DSM III-R (Diagnostic and Statistical Manual of the American Psychiatric Association, 1987). It refers to a subjective feeling of ugliness in a person of normal appearance. Andreason and Bardash (1977) addressed this issue and raised the question of whether dysmorphophobia represents a symptom or a disease. They described the dysmorphophobic patients as follows: They are usually young (late teens or early 20s), are perfectionistic, and have both schizoid and narcissistic personality traits. They have mixed obsessive and schizoid traits, and are self-centered. They seek to enhance their beauty and intelligence rather than achieve success in their vocational careers, social lives, or relationships. Their IQ's are usually normal or above normal. They may have ideas of references regarding their "deformity" (e.g., a 20 year old patient requested a face lift, but there were no overt delusions or psychotic features). There is no information regarding etiology, clinical course, or prognosis, but one wonders whether these patients appear with differing labels such as the polysurgery or mania operativa patient, or even the transsexual or hidden self-mutilator. The surgeon should be ever alert for such personality traits, because these patients will require psychiatric assistance.

THE FACE

The face contains the majority of the sense organs and, along with the hand, has the greatest cortical representation; it is essential for communication and gesture. We "speak" with our lips, our eyes, our hands, as well as with all the other muscles of facial expression. A mute person can still produce the "spoken word" via the graceful interplay of the muscles of the face and upper extremities. A differing neuroanatomy exists for *posed* expressions such as surprise, horror, and frowning (Van Gelder, cited in Borod and Koff, 1984) as opposed to the expressions of sadness, contempt, disdain, smiling, doubt, irony, horror, and surprise. Whether neural fibers are crossed or uncrossed has been well defined (Miehlke and Van Gelder, cited in Borod and Koff, 1984). For *spontaneous involuntary* emotional expression, although there is some consensus pertaining to origins, the pathways are unclear. There is also the interplay of genetics and psychosocial environment as to when and what one voluntarily expresses, as well as which stimuli can elicit a spontaneous facial expression. We enhance nature's message by adorning or covering the face, such as in crowning or veiling. We "face the world . . . speak face to face," and "face ourselves" in the mirror each day. In order to communicate more easily we keep our faces as well as our hands uncovered. In women, and less so men, bareness may extend to the breasts and legs. Whether one chooses to address this concept from an anatomic, anthropologic, psychiatric, psychologic, or sociologic perspective, one is "talking" about the same thing, human expression. Body image is a derivative of these interplays. In medicine those with the greatest power to enhance or detract from this capacity are the plastic surgeon, neurosurgeon, and psychiatrist, while the social scientists also have a great deal to offer.

The patient with cleft lip and palate or the burn patient is not discussed in this chapter. For excellent reviews of these topics, see McWilliams (1982) for the former and Bernstein (1976) and Goodstein (1985) for the burn patient.

The development of craniofacial rehabilitation teams in the 1970's (Tessier, 1971; Converse and associates, 1974) prompted a close collaboration between the plastic surgeon and the psychologist, psychiatrist, or social scientist. Although the primary purpose of such multidisciplinary groups was to provide clinical service, to assess psychologic status and prognosis, and to counsel, interest also developed in research that could shed more light on such matters as the role of facial disfigurement on psychosocial development, cognitive changes, and body image as well as the effects of surgery on patients at different age levels (Lefebvre and Munro, 1978; Belfer, Mulliken, and Cochran, 1979; Kapp-Simon, 1981; Pillemer, 1981; and Pertschuk and Whitaker, 1985, 1988).

Pertschuk and Whitaker (1985), in a study of children with craniofacial deformities and a group of controls, found that children with craniofacial deformities had problems with self-concept, anxiety, introversion, and home and classroom behavior. These problems, although pervasive, were rarely profound, i.e., they rarely revealed severe limitations. Group analysis based on age (children 6 to 13 years old) also showed no statistical differences. The children were seen preoperatively and none had received any psychologic treatment. The authors speculated that the improvement in facial appearance might sensitize the patient to residual impairments. Macgregor had observed in 1953 that the mildly deformed tended to exaggerate the degree of deformity, while those classed as severely deformed were inclined to minimize the degree of deformity. The former also complained more, were less resigned, and more insistent that others should feel as they did regarding the defect. After surgery, the group with craniofacial deformity still had persistent deficits in self-concept and extroversion, but they showed improvement in previously inhibited and hyperactive behavior and a trend toward decreased aggression. They also exhibited consistent improvement in psychosocial adjustment and behavior in the home and school.

Most studies dealing with the psychosocial aspects of facial disfigurement can be criticized because the affected individuals have been studied at only one point in their psychosocial development, usually in a clinical setting. Such reports provide only limited information on the adjustment of patients with facial deformity to improvement in self-esteem, on vocational training, on changes in the attitudes of family members or spouses, and on the subsequent need for psychotherapeutic intervention.

One of the few longitudinal or long-term studies was that of Macgregor (1979), which focused on the quality of lives of individuals with facial deformity who underwent corrective surgery, yet retained some of the stigmata of the deformity. At the time of entry into the original project, the ages of the 16 participating individuals ranged from 18 months to 33 years. There were eight males and eight females, two of whom were married. As to the severity of their disfigurements, nine were classified as marked and seven as gross. Eleven had congenital deformities; five had acquired disfigurement as a result of trauma or disease. Because their surgical and cosmetic problems were complex (many patients had multiple deformities), all would require a series of plastic surgical procedures extending in some cases over a period of years.

At the time of the follow-up study the age range within the group was from 22 to 58 years. Fourteen were married and 12 had children. Four women whose faces were still noticeably marred had been married and divorced but were remarried.

Because of reconstructive surgery, the facial deviation of nine patients could now be evaluated as slight or moderate, and that of five, originally classified as gross, could be evaluated as marked. Although patient interviews and analysis of data were still to be completed, some measurable items had begun to emerge. For example, practically all were self-supporting or supported by a spouse. In terms of education, all but four had completed high school and seven had earned college or graduate degrees. Of the 14 patients who were married, the disfigurement in all but one had played a decisive role in the selection of partners. Because opportunities for dating and marriage were either nonexistent, limited, or perceived as limited, all but one had married someone from a lower social or educational level, someone from another religion, or an individual who was also handicapped. All seemed to feel that they must be content with any willing partner.

Although it would seem that on the whole the patients had made satisfactory adjustments, the conclusions are statistically correct but misleading. A series of in-depth interviews and sentence completion tests, however, made it possible to learn what kinds of adaptations had been made and at what cost, and what had been the quality of each individual's life.

Perhaps one of the most striking findings of the study was that all 16 patients had managed in one fashion or another to cope with their disfigurement. Everyone indicated that this had been a formidable task. Over the years all patients experienced episodes of turmoil and crisis related to their appearance. Periods of depression (two children and one adult actually attempted suicide), during which personality and emotional and social functioning were noticeably impaired, were not uncommon. Despite the precariousness of their everyday lives, all had managed to survive.

Various methods were employed by the patients to cope with their social barriers (real and perceived), including blatant defiance and complete withdrawal from any form of social interaction. The latter represented extreme methods of behavioral adaptation, but most exhibited a pattern of social withdrawal. Even married patients tended to confine themselves to their immediate family—"My home is my haven." None of the patients ever accepted their deformity or position in life; frustration, disappointment, and a sense of impotence persisted. They were also angry in a general sense at a society that made them expend so much valuable energy to overcome or counter the social deprivations of that environment.

Down Syndrome

A relatively new area of interest to plastic surgeons and social scientists alike is the rehabilitation of the child with Down syndrome. Techniques are now available to reduce the stigmata of the syndrome such as the epicanthal folds, the slanting of the palpebral fissures, the depressed nasal bridge, and the hypoplastic cheeks and chin (see Chap. 64). Both tongue and hearing problems may interfere with speech, language, and consequently cognition. It is important to recall that the degree of mental retardation among these patients varies from borderline low average to severely low IQ (Mearig, 1985). When considering the intellectual capacities of the children, one must bear in mind the functional as well as the psychosocial deprivations consequent upon their facial disfigurements.

In a study by Lemperle and Radu (cited in Rozner, 1983), 102 patients with Down syndrome were followed for at least one year postoperatively. The conclusions were that 75 per cent benefited from surgery in that they were able to keep their mouths closed, had improved speech and eating function, had less inflammation and friability of the lips, had fewer respiratory infections, and had improved mood and self-confidence. However, only 15 per cent of families with an affected child seek surgical rehabilitation (Rozner, 1983).

A study was conducted by Pueschel, Monteiro, and Erickson (1986). Questionnaires were sent to 146 parents of children with Down syndrome, 118 pediatricians, 256 family practitioners, and eight plastic surgeons. The questions concerned aspects of the child's life, health, and psychosocial environment and the attitude of the respondents toward surgical correction of the Down syndrome stigmata. Responses were received by 51 per cent of the parents via questionnaire, 63 family practitioners, and *all* the plastic surgeons. The results are summarized as follows: Significantly fewer parents than physicians noted eating, chewing, and drooling problems. Significantly fewer parents felt that the facial characteristics impaired mental and social development or acquisition of skills. While 62 per cent of the physicians thought the facial stigmata had a negative effect on the child, only 28 per cent of the parents agreed. Whereas physicians (54 per cent) thought teachers had decreased expectations because of the stigmata, only 24 per cent of the parents felt the same. Most strikingly, whereas only 4 per cent of the physicians considered that the children were accepted by society, 85 per cent of the parents felt they were. Ninety-two per cent of the parents and 76 per cent of the physicians expressed concern regarding the risk of surgery. Both groups thought that the parents' wishes and doctors' recommendations were equally important regarding the decision to undergo surgery, but 50 per cent of the parents (versus 33 per cent of the physicians) felt that the child should give consent. Sixty-one per cent of the parents refused surgery outright; 26 per cent were undecided; and 13 per cent believed that surgery was beneficial regardless of the child's age. The physicians were split equally for and against surgery, while seven of eight of the plastic surgeons were in favor. In defending their positions against surgery, parents used such phrases as, "Our child is beautiful . . . We love him just the way he is."

The contradictory nature of the results makes interpretation difficult, since what appears obvious to the physician is illusory to the parents, who presumably know the child and his or her environment better. The parents are more educated and accepting of the child owing to self-help groups and increasing social acceptance. On the other hand, parents may feel that the obvious stigmata of Down syndrome protect the child from undue pressure to perform. The fact that it is a relatively common anomaly worldwide, and possibly one that elicits sympathy, may in fact offer protection to the child. Another factor is that the parents are uneducated regarding surgical technique, risk, and result. As the variables of the family's religion and prenatal amniocentesis were not studied, one cannot determine what role, if any, they played.

THE NOSE

Prominently displayed on the face between the eyes, the "windows to the soul," is the nose. Its presence is appreciated both on confrontation and in profile. Stereotyped, the nose may be considered an index of character and has been the elicitor of countless jokes (Macgregor and Schaffner, 1950).

In a Johns Hopkins survey of young women seeking rhinoplasty, most of whom were Jewish, Meyer and associates (1960) concluded that the patients suffered from a conflict in sexual identification and ambivalence in identification with their parents. They had as objectives the need to modify the contour of a nose that was said to resemble that of their fathers. In another study (Edgerton, Jacobson, and Meyer, 1961), 71 per cent of 98 patients received an unhealthy psychiatric diagnosis. Nevertheless, in a follow-up study six months later 94 per cent expressed satisfaction with the surgical results. The study by Reich (1969) of 750 cosmetic surgery patients not only confirmed these findings but added credence to the view that looking "normal" releases one's energy for more constructive ends (Macgregor and associates, 1953).

Macgregor should be credited with shifting the emphasis away from psychologic explanation of the motivations of the plastic surgery patient and emphasizing the sociologic-cultural ramifications of deviations in facial appearance (Macgregor, 1947; Macgregor and Schaffner, 1950). In a classic study of the social and cultural components in the motivations of patients seeking rhinoplasty (Macgregor, 1967b), she noted that more than half (72 per cent) of the reported 89 patients were first or second generation Americans (Table 3–3). Most of the patients were young single adults of both sexes of upper-lower and lower-middle socioeconomic status. Most had not attained an educational level beyond high school. The series was divided into two groups. Group I patients (46) sought nasal surgery to modify or eradicate ethnic visibility because of perceived prejudice and discrimination. They desired to "look American." Group II patients (35) looked at nasal surgery as a means of avoiding undesirable personality characteristics stereotypically ascribed to certain types of noses. They wanted to be identified with "what I am—not what I look like" or they wished to look more attractive in a society that rewards youth and beauty.

Burk, Zelen, and Terino (1985) recalled *previous* psychodynamic interpretations of the female patients who sought a rhinoplasty as being unconsciously ambivalent regarding their mothers, while more strongly identifying with their fathers. Their requests were viewed as a desire to change the symbol of the paternal penis and thus strengthen their identification with their mother. Their diagnoses were *presumed* to be those of obsessive and schizoid personalities. Men, on the other hand (Hill and Silver, cited in Lubkin, 1975), were felt to be unconsciously homosexual, tailoring a nose too reminiscent of a painfully masculine father. As previously mentioned, in the studies by Hay (1970) and Hay and Heather (1973), 28 of their 45 patients identified with neither parent. Those that did were equally divided, and this might be explained by the genetics of family resemblance. On follow-up (Hay and Heather, 1973), patients with minor and major repairs did equally well.

In a study of prison inmates who requested plastic surgery (Kurtzberg and associates, 1967), the rhinoplasty patients had the highest level of depression and scored highest on the Minnesota Multi Personality Index (MMPI) scale of psychopathologic deviation. In addition, *all* the sex offenders requesting plastic surgery wanted rhinoplasties. Connolly and Gipson (1978) carried out a 15 year follow-up of 187 patients who had rhinoplasties between 1955 and 1960 (judged minor deformities). They studied only those patients who were considered by a family physician to be psychologically disturbed, and they were compared with controls. Of 101 patients compared, two of six patients who were diagnosed as schizophrenics had doubts regarding their gender.

In 1978 Kalick presented photographs drawn from plastic surgery journals of college-age women before and after rhinoplasty, with and without mentoplasty. The presumed psychosocial benefits and personality varia-

Table 3–3. Immigrant Status, Ethnocultural Background, Religion

	Number	Percentage
Immigrant status		
First generation American	8	9
Second generation American	56	63
Third generation American	13	15
Old white American	3	3
Negro American	1	1
Non–United States citizen	6	7
Not ascertained	2	2
Total	89	100
Ethnocultural background		
Jewish	33	37
Italian	23	25
Armenian, Greek, Iranian, Lebanese, Syrian	9	10
American (old white, 3; Negro, 1)	4	5
Austrian, German	4	5
Irish	4	5
Polish, Russian	3	3
Other	9	10
Total	89	100
Religion		
Catholic	40	45
Jewish	31	34
Protestant	10	11
Other	4	5
No affiliation	4*	5
Total	89	100

*The statements of two of these patients were interpreted as a repudiation of their parents' religion, which was Jewish. However, when Jews are discussed as an ethnocultural group in this study, these two patients are included.

Data from Macgregor, 1967b.

bles were speculated on by university men. After surgery, the women were presumed by the raters to be milder, more sensitive, and more sexually warm and responsive than before surgery. They were also believed to be more competent marriage partners and more likely to marry the person of their choice after surgery. They were perceived to be happier postoperatively, and the raters were more likely to want to meet or work with them. The raters were blind to the type of surgery. The results of the study suggest that cosmetic surgery patients, even those who are not judged unattractive preoperatively, should start to reap the benefits of their improved physical appearance soon after surgery, as all patients were judged more attractive postoperatively.

An excellent research design is that of Cash and Horton (1983), who repeated Kalick's 1978 study but eliminated some of the latter's confounding variables. All patients in the study had had a rhinoplasty, and pre- and postoperative photographs, including frontal and lateral views, were projected lifesize for equal-time viewing at equal intervals. Standardized grooming and cosmetics were employed for all subjects. The authors did not mention whether standardized lighting was used for each subject or whether facial expression was controlled. The raters, both male and female, were blind to the type of plastic surgery. The patients were of various ages, but the raters were all of university age. The results of various speculations regarding the patients' personalities again showed a "halo effect" of physical attractiveness and personality. The influence of the raters' sex was minor. The presumed age of the patient was also unrelated to the outcome. Sixty-four per cent of the patients were considered more attractive postoperatively. Among those judged more attractive, the patients' age and sex were not factors, and this designation was not related to the preoperative level of attractiveness.

The number of rhinoplasties performed in the United States increased by 17 per cent between 1984 and 1986 (see Table 3–1), but the degree of patient satisfaction remained unchanged, ranging between 76 and 92 per cent (Reich, 1975; McKinney and Cook, 1981), depending on such factors as positive or negative reinforcement from family and friends postoperatively, or the need for further surgical revision. McKinney and Cook (1981) found a higher rate of postoperative dissatisfaction among women in the fifth decade, who usually had not been referred by a physician, and a trend for widowed and divorced females to be more dissatisfied.

THE EAR

Although the nose is prominently placed on the face, the ear is more often adorned, and many cultures pierce the ears of female infants. Hall (cited in Macgregor, 1978), studying children's attraction to body parts, found an inordinate amount of attention paid to the ears, their own and others. When malformed, the ears elicit such ridiculing epithets as "Dumbo . . . jughead . . . rabbit ears." In Western culture the short and limited type of men's hairstyles make an ear deformity more apparent. However, women with deformed ears must also limit their range of hairstyles and forgo ear adornment. Macgregor (1978) poignantly documented the effects of ear deformity on children and the beneficial effects of surgical correction. Otoplasty increased by 13 per cent between 1984 and 1986; men made up 44 per cent and women 56 per cent of patients (see Tables 3–1, 3–2).

THE AGING FACE

As the impression of the patient seeking a rhinoplasty has been modified with changing cultural values, so has that of the patient desiring a face lift. Whereas men were considered shallow and insecure by some (Rozner, 1973), and face lift surgery was regarded as a reinforcement of the patient's masochistic strategy to avoid confronting depression and aging (Edgerton and Knorr, 1971; Meerlo, cited in Macgregor, 1976; Web and associates, quoted in Burk, Zelen, and Terino, 1985), other investigators began to recognize the psychic healing potential offered by such surgery. By the late 1960's it was recognized that up to 20 per cent of patients seeking a face lift were successful businessmen, motivated to improve their appearance in the competitive marketplace, or divorced or widowed men desiring to impress younger girlfriends (Baker and Gordon, 1969). An attitude was beginning to take hold that patients presenting for face lift were, in fact, individuals more alert to cultural values and conscious of the economic and psychosocial benefits of being more attractive (Robertson, 1967).

A word of caution, however, is necessary concerning surgery for the older population. There is a general impression that postoperative depression is more frequently observed in this group than in patients who have undergone other types of esthetic surgery (Goin and Goin, 1981b). Goin and associates (1980) studied 50 women who underwent face lift surgery and compared them with controls. In terms of the MMPI (Minnesota Multi Personality Index), 14 per cent showed preoperative evidence of low-score depression, and 54 per cent showed evidence of some type of psychologic disturbance apparent *only* to a psychiatrist. Women with lasting depressions beginning immediately in the postoperative period were independent and self-reliant and wanted to be in control of their lives. As their characters discouraged nurturing, they received little postoperative emotional support. They hated the aging process, over which they had no control, and expected surgery to stop it. Conversely, those women who developed a continuing depression by two weeks postoperatively were passive-dependent individuals who did not want to change their lives. They were the only ones whose depression was also related to disappointment with the surgical results.

Four patients who were in the midst of bereavement before surgery improved afterward. Although the point was not fully discussed by the authors, some of their predictors of satisfactory results contradicted the existing literature, on matters such as "good" patients scoring higher than average on the paranoid scale of the MMPI, and having a history of previous cosmetic surgery (type and amount unspecified). However, high paranoia scores may actually lend credence to a controversial study by Leeb, Bowers, and Lynch (1976) on the recall of the consent by 100 patients (elective reconstructive surgery, esthetic surgery, and emergency room patients) seven days later. These authors found that patients who rated themselves as "very nervous" as opposed to "calm" had a statistically improved retention of the consent, 48 per cent versus 30 per cent. The study indicated that nervousness, rather than causing decreased attention and therefore memory, might in fact represent hypervigilance, a characteristic of paranoia. In contrast to these findings, Burgoyne and associates (cited in Goin and Goin, 1981b) reported the intraoperative evolution of transient paranoid delusions toward the surgeon, secondary to local anesthesia and intravenous sedation, based on overheard conversations. Another study (Briggs and Ogg, 1973) reported preoperative anxiety, agitation, and confusion ending in refusal of surgery, owing to the effects of premedication, and there is even a report of the rare complication of postrhytidectomy psychosis (Schweitzer and Hirschfeld, 1984).

Nevertheless, the number of face lifts increased by 23 per cent from 1984 to 1986 (Table 3–1), supporting Goin's statement that "Grandma (or Grandpa for that matter) isn't sitting at home in a rocking chair anymore . . . She's out playing tennis, shopping . . . in the business world" (American Society of Plastic and Reconstructive Surgeons, 1987). And she is increasingly doing it with a more attractive face.

THE BREAST

The female breast is the universal symbol of nourishment, love, sexuality, comfort, and femininity, the primary focus of male admiration in a "mammarized" world (Grossman, 1976). Its importance has been emphasized in cave drawings as well as in fashion, and it is a stronger sexual stimulus to the male than the female genitalia (Kinsey, 1948, cited in Baker, Kolin, and Bartlett, 1974). The plastic surgeon has the ability to augment or reduce the effects or, in the case of reconstruction after mastectomy, "conjure up a trompe l'oeil: an anatomical illusion to delight the visual senses . . ." (Ward, 1981).

Augmentation

Augmentation may be desired for a variety of reasons, including a unilateral congenital abnormality, a unilateral acquired childhood abnormality, primary hypoplasia, or (most frequently) postlactational involution.

The average woman seeking augmentation is married, educated, and a middle class mother in her 30's who seeks "normal" breasts (Baker, Kolin, and Bartlett, 1974). She is frequently referred by a pleased friend or relative. In the United States, she is psychiatrically as stable as other women (Shipley, O'Donnell, and Bader, 1977; Sihm, Jagd, and Pers, 1978). *In the past,* it was felt that an augmentation request by the adolescent or adult woman represented unconscious guilt regarding affectionate and sexual feelings for her father, with the consequent punishment of small breasts (Edgerton and associates, quoted in Burk, Zelen, and Terino, 1985). She was considered to have hysterical character traits, with a tendency toward depression (Edgerton and associates, quoted in Burk, Zelen, and Terino, 1985). Another study found that these patients had a remarkably increased incidence of gynecologic surgery and described the patients as socially outgoing with considerable energy, impulsive, insecure, and inadequate, with few lasting relationships (Baker, Kolin, and Bartlett, 1974). Commonly these women are embarrassed regarding the small breast size, often refusing to appear naked before others and rejecting sexual breast play (Baker, Kolin, and Bartlett, 1974; Ohlsén, Pontén, and Hambert, 1979; Beale, Lisper, and Palm, 1980).

The husbands frequently discourage surgery with such comments as "I love you just the way you are . . . ," yet after surgery they are pleased with the results, as evidenced by an increase in sexual frequency (Baker, Kolin, and Bartlett, 1974; Grossman, 1976). Postoperative patients often report an increase in the number of orgasms and an increased desire for breast play, and a few report having orgasms for the first time (Baker, Kolin, and Bartlett, 1974; Ohlsén, Pontén, and Hambert, 1979). It is surprising how a relatively small change in breast size can cause such satisfaction, with the results surpassing expectations and the patient's satisfaction exceeding that of the surgeon (Baker, Kolin, and Bartlett, 1974; Sihm, Jagd, and Pers, 1978; Ohlsén, Pontén, and Hambert, 1979; Beale, Lisper, and Palm, 1980; Beale and associates, 1984). One study, in which five of 37 patients reported increased nipple sensation after surgery, also noted that 30 of the 37 patients had decreased nipple sensation postoperatively but were unaware of this until a physician recorded it on examination (Ohlsén, Pontén, and Hambert, 1979). Operations for breast augmentation decreased in number by 2 per cent between 1984 and 1986 (see Table 3–2).

Reduction

People seeking reduction resemble breast augmentation patients in many ways. In the preoperative period they have a distorted body image and low self-esteem; postoperatively they feel increasingly self-confident, more feminine, and more sexually attractive compared with controls (Hollyman and associates, 1986). The patient's satisfaction exceeds that of the surgeon. A German study even reported that visible esthetic faults, such as broad scars, hypertrophy, inverted nipples, and decreased nipple sensation, were overlooked by the patient (Muller, 1974). Most of the patients also had relief of back pain that had been secondary to weighty breasts.

Another fact that emerges from the histories of both sets of women (augmentation and reduction candidates) before surgery, *as well as from controls*, is a distortion of body image. In one study 10 per cent of patients seeking breast augmentation had developed a different sense of "normal," becoming aware after surgery that other women in general do not have very large breasts (Beale and associates, 1984). On the other hand, the breast reduction patient, in the preoperative period, overperceives the size of her breasts, her waist, and less so her hips, as compared with controls (Hollyman and associates, 1986). It should be noted that the controls also overestimated waist and hip size. The former studies were conducted in Sweden, whereas the latter were done in the United Kingdom. Crosscultural differences may make a difference but, unfortunately, similar studies have not been carried out in the United States for comparison. No studies questioned patients regarding the size of the breasts of their mothers or other significant females.

Reconstruction after Mastectomy

Breast cancer is the most common malignancy of women in the United States and represents 10 per cent of all cancers reported, 90,000 cases being reported each year in the United States (Goin and Goin, 1981b). Nine million women will develop breast cancer during their lifetime (Goldberg, Stolzman, and Goldberg, 1984). Many women resist breast examination because of the fear of mutilation (Snyderman and Starzynski,

1969). Women with intraductal cancer have a three to five times greater than average chance of cancer in the other breast, with a risk of 1 per cent per year. Women who have first-order relatives with breast cancer before menopause have a 50 per cent chance of developing breast cancer (Goin and Goin, 1981a). In 1973 Hackett (cited in Lubkin, 1975) analyzed 563 patients with regard to the length of delay before seeking medical treatment. The results were startlingly similar to those of a 1924 study by Simmons and Daland (cited in Lubkin, 1975), despite years of public education. The results are summarized as follows: most breast cancers were discovered on routine physical examination; 10 to 20 per cent of patients *never* sought a physician; 30 per cent of patients saw a physician four weeks after the lesion was detected; and anxious patients delayed longer, *especially* those exposed to public propaganda. The delay was conscious and deliberate in the case of many. Finally, women who had a family history of breast cancer were *less* likely to consult a physician, as they presumed it was "hopeless."

Whereas it was previously thought that a woman must mourn the loss of her breast by experiencing its absence before proceeding to the adaptive aspects of her life (Klein, cited in Wellisch and associates, 1985), up to 96 per cent of mastectomy patients prefer reconstruction to be carried out as quickly as possible, i.e., a one-stage procedure including mastectomy and reconstruction (Goin and Goin, 1981a; Teimourian and Adham, 1982; Levinson, 1984; Goldberg, Stolzman, and Goldberg, 1984; Stevens and associates, 1984; Wellisch and associates, 1985). In general, patients prefer reconstruction whether it be done immediately (Goin and Goin, 1981a) or up to 25 years after the mastectomy (Teimourian and Adham, 1982). However, the National Cancer Institute revealed that in 1980 only 25 per cent of women in the United States were aware of the possibility of reconstruction (cited in Schain, Jacobs, and Wellisch, 1984). Remarkably, the numbers of procedures increased by 39 per cent between 1981 and 1984 (American Society of Plastic and Reconstructive Surgeons, 1987).

There is a disparity between the patients' and the surgeons' satisfaction with the surgical results. A survey of 100 general surgeons in Melbourne, Australia indicated that 43 per cent of the surgeons considered that reconstruction was "not worth the time and effort involved . . ." (cited in Mendelson, 1980). Goin and Goin (1981b) described a "pseudoacceptance" by the unreconstructed mastectomy patient, wherein the patient admits to a hidden depression described as "disgusting self-pity," while appearing adjusted to friends. Older patients were more embarrassed to seek reconstruction as "it is not supposed to matter," but "no woman should be forced to retire her breasts due to some cultural or age stereotype" (Schain, Jacobs, and Wellisch, 1984). Some patients, aware of the possibility of reconstruction, may refuse it by playing the martyr while unconsciously feeling guilt for considering such self-centered surgery after being given the "gift of life." In this way, they superfunction in an attempt to overcome adversity (Schain, Jacobs, and Wellisch, 1984). The tendency of some surgeons to downplay reconstruction is unfortunate, since the studies supporting breast reconstruction indicate patient delight in having "reverse mastectomy," making additional comments such as "feeling whole again, balanced, complete, and feeling symmetrical."

There is now evidence that 30 to 50 per cent of mastectomy patients experience "phantom breast," a finding that may explain why those reconstructed immediately perceived the "new breast" as immediately theirs, whereas the delayed reconstruction patients take longer to incorporate the reconstructed breast (Goin and Goin, 1981a,b). Perhaps, the cortex of the brain is easily fooled because it is asleep while this "switch" takes place, with little sensory input. The patient undergoing delayed reconstruction may more resemble the stroke victim who experiences slow return of function; in this case, "recovering" the weight and volume of the reconstructed breasts results in a return of a sense of symmetry and balance. The importance of sensory input may supersede the importance of the visual, esthetic result, thus explaining the disparity between the patient's satisfaction and that of the surgeon.

It is appropriate to end this topic by relating the feelings of a patient who wrote a letter to one of the plastic surgery journals (Levinson, 1984) after undergoing breast reconstruction. Besides promoting reconstruction, she cautioned plastic surgeons not to consider nipple reconstruction as just an "extra" but rather as a needed step in the return to a "wholly attractive body" (Millard, Devine, and Warren, 1971, citing Boulton and Holukohly). She experienced increased optimism and felt more whole and symmetric, "not like a broken mannequin." Her "real" (reconstructed) breast also lessened the fears of an 18 year old daughter, and she noted that, if the possibility of reconstruction were more widely known, more women would carry out self-examinations and seek earlier treatment. She ends her appeal with: "Few events in my life have rivaled the intensity of this medical experience that compassionately combined the brilliant skills of both science and art."

THE GENITALIA

Male Impotence

In the past it was commonly believed that up to 90 per cent of male impotence was psychogenic. It is now known that more than 50 per cent is organic in nature, the leading endocrinic cause being diabetes mellitus (30 to 60 per cent), in which impotence can be the first symptom (Bodner, 1985). Bodner (1985) made a review of the anatomy, physiology, and causes and an evaluation of impotence. Although the diabetic recipient of a penile implant has been the most comprehensively studied (Beaser and associates, 1982), the results in nondiabetic recipients are comparable. Beaser and associates (1982) carried out a review of the history of implants and the various types available.

A summary of the results of penile implants (Martin and Montague, 1982; Beaser and associates, 1982; Bodner, 1985; Peterson and associates, 1985) reveals that 81 to 95 per cent of patients are satisfied postoperatively; the implant did not affect the patient's ability to ejaculate; and 91 per cent were able to experience penetrating orgasms postoperatively (versus 66 per cent preoperatively). There was increased sexual frequency following surgery, and a significant correlation between the patient's and the partner's satisfaction and response. These women are comparable with the husbands of mastectomy patients in that only 62 per cent of the women were enthusiastic before surgery, as opposed to 83 per cent or more after surgery. Beaser and associates (1982) described a widow who on follow-up said that the prosthesis had made the couple's last years together more enjoyable. Most satisfied patients are between the ages of 40 and 60 years (91 per cent), whereas older and younger men are less satisfied, 71 and 70 per cent, respectively (Beaser and associates, 1982).

Regarding patient selection, the favorable candidate is presumed to be one who recognizes ambivalence regarding the surgical procedure, has a mature relationship with his partner, has had a sexual relationship both before and after the onset of impotence, and enjoys satisfactory mental health (Berg and associates, 1984). It is advisable to include the partner in pre- and postoperative discussion and education (Beaser and associates, 1982; Berg and associates, 1984). The patient who is more likely to be dissatisfied, regardless of the surgical outcome, is one with a diagnosis of primary psychogenic impotence in whom the fears of sexual failure predominate over performance (Martin and Montague, 1982). These patients are more likely to exhibit hysterical expectations toward surgery, e.g., increased orgasms or a change in the overall size of the penis (Berg and associates, 1984).

Penile Reconstruction

The conditions leading to penile reconstruction are as follows: congenital malformations, infection, lymphatic obstruction, trauma, and cancer; the incidence of cancer is 0.3 per cent in the United States (Boxer, 1975). All involve loss of tissue and utilize reconstruction techniques developed for Sex Reassignment Surgery (SRS) (see Chap. 88).

Penile agenesis is rare, occurring in one in 50,000 births, 35 cases being reported in the literature by 1975 (Boxer, 1975). The consensus is that the genetic male should have orchiectomy and be reared as a female (Boxer, 1975, citing Brosman, Sterling, Young, and associates). It was emphasized that the decision regarding sex reassignment should be made *rapidly* (one day after birth at the latest), and preferably the staff should make the final decision regarding sex change *before* the parents become aware of the anomaly. These authors also recommended assigning one physician as the spokesperson to the family, as representing a united staff decision and thereby avoiding confusion. The physician should be available to the family for consultation in the future. If follow-up is unlikely, the authors recommended immediate orchiectomy to avoid virilization at puberty. The reasons for early sex reassignment are multiple and include the avoidance of parental confusion; parental attitudes in early life regarding the sexual identity of their child influence the way in which they handle their children's bodies, and will affect the child's evolution of body image (Meyer, 1982). It should be noted that male infants achieve erection in utero, as visualized on ultrasound, and they manipulate their penises by 1 year of age (Meyer, 1982, citing Galenson and associates). The infant's genitalia receive much stimulation in diapering, cleaning, and elimination, a further contribution to gender evolution and body image. An infant with agenesis of the phallus can be surgically converted to a female and later receive estrogen supplements at puberty, the patient's physique thereby developing normal-appearing female breasts and contour. Young and associates (1971) also recommended reassignment as female, since the patient's genitalia are less open to scrutiny by peers, both in childhood and later in public rest rooms and locker rooms.

Penile Replantation

Engelman and associates (1974) reviewed the literature on penile replantation, which included 11 cases plus one of their own. Follow-up data were available on only ten of the 12 cases, owing to the young ages of two of the patients. All the ten cases were deemed successful, with preservation of urination, erection, intromission, ejaculation, and partial sensation (with one exception to the last-named). (See also Male Genital Mutilation later in this chapter.)

Vaginal Reconstruction

Surgical reconstruction of the female genitalia can be the consequence of various anomalies (see Chap. 87). Although the etiologies may differ, there is a similar resultant anatomic anomaly, i.e., congenital adrenal hyperplasia, male and true, and thus the same surgery (Jones, 1974). Although the rationale for early surgery pertains to females as well as to males, reconstruction may have to be delayed until up to 18 months of age, at which time the surgeon can more easily identify the vagina and handle the tissues in surgery. Jones (1974) described ablation of the small penis and total clitorectomy for an enlarged clitoris, since otherwise a remaining stump can result in pain.

Money (1975) reviewed 45 cases of genetic males raised as females, 43 secondary to congenitally defective penises and two with infantile ablatio penis. Follow-up data are available on most of the patients. One of the patients with ablatio penis happened to be an identical twin. Money (1975) used nine year follow-up data on this twin, as well as additional information on matched pairs of female hermaphrodites followed by the Johns Hopkins Clinic, to substantiate his theory that gender identity is sufficiently incomplete at birth to permit successful reassignment of a genetic boy to a girl. In support of this, he also mentioned that vaginoplasty permits a normal sex life, including orgasmic response, whereas phalloplasty does not allow a normal sex life and also requires more extensive surgery.

Transsexuals

The term "transsexual" was first introduced by Cauldwell in 1949 (Meyer and Reter, 1979) and refers to a person who wishes to be the opposite sex. Surgery as an attempt to "reassign" a patient sexually was first performed by Abraham in 1931 (Meyer and Reter, 1979), but it was not until the celebrated Christine Jorgensen case in 1952 that transsexualism became a topic of debate for both the public and the press. There has been an extensive body of literature since then, emanating mostly from Sweden (Lundström, Pauly, and Walinder, 1984; Lindemalm, Korlin, and Uddenberg, 1986) and the Johns Hopkins group in the United States (Edgerton, 1984). Serious research began after Benjamin's classic postoperative study of transsexuals, 87 per cent of whom were satisfied with the results (cited in Lothstein, 1982). Pauly's (1968) study of 121 patients, concluding that postsurgery patients were ten times more socially and emotionally stable than those who received no surgery, provided the impetus for continued surgical correction (Lothstein, 1982).

It is impossible to review all the transsexual literature, not only because of the volume but also because of the confusion and frustration inherent in trying to interpret it. No one can agree on what the term "transsexualism" actually signifies, and the debate continues as to whether the treatment of choice for a patient who thus labels him- or herself is *sex reassignment surgery* (SRS) or psychotherapy. Arguments both for and against sex reassignment are based on rhetoric versus hard data, with a lack of scientific evidence to support views or even diagnosis (Lothstein, 1982, 1984). Nothing can account for the overall reported "subjective" success rate after surgery of 68 to 100 per cent.

The Diagnostic and Statistical Manual (DSM) III-R (American Psychiatric Association, 1987) defines transsexualism as a feeling of discomfort and inappropriateness regarding one's assigned sex, with a wish to be rid of one's genitals and to gain the primary and secondary sex characteristics of the opposite sex. The person must have reached puberty; the disturbance must be continuous (not limited to periods of stress) for at least two years; there must be an absence of intersex or genetic abnormality; and it must not be due to any other mental disorder such as schizophrenia.

Sex reassignment surgery (SRS) was most frequently practiced in the 1960's and 1970's. However, this came to an abrupt end with a controversial publication and press release by Meyer and Reter in 1979; the media "distortion" resulted in the closing of the Johns Hopkins Gender Dysphoria Clinic (Lothstein, 1982). In this study the authors compared postoperative sex reassigned (male to female) patients with preoperative males, labeling the latter a control group in terms of job, education, and marital and domestic stability. The two groups were compared and the conclusion given was that, although the postoperative patients were more subjectively satisfied, "surgery confers no objective advantage in terms of social rehabilitation." Criticisms of this publication have been multiple, especially of the design of the study and the use of the preoperative patients, most of whom went on to surgery, as a control group (Fleming, Steinman, and Bocknek, 1980; Lothstein, 1982).

However, the most serious criticisms concerned the finality of the assertions of Meyer and Reter (1979) and the value judgments underlying their results (Fleming, Steinman, and Bocknek, 1980). Critics agreed that there was abuse of surgery owing to its widespread availability without proper diagnosis or psychotherapy support, but they felt there was insufficient evidence to warrant the termination of surgery or the research program (Fleming, Steinman, and Bocknek, 1980; Lothstein, 1982). At the initiation of this debate there were presumed to be an estimated 30,000 transsexuals worldwide, with approximately 10,000 residing in the United States (Lothstein, 1982, citing Berger and associates, 1977).

Major current theories regarding the etiologies of transsexualism were reviewed by Meyer (1982), and they include the biological/imprint hypothesis, the nonconflictual identity hypothesis, and the conflict/defense hypothesis. In the first two theories, psychotherapy is presumed to be ineffectual and surgery palliative. The conflict/defense hypothesis views psychotherapy as possibly beneficial and regards surgery as palliative collusion with the patient's symptoms. However, contrary to this view, Fisk (1978) cited four of his patients, previously psychotic, who were "cured" by crossdressing and the promise of SRS. At the opposite end of the pole is Edgerton (1984), whose support of sex "confirmation" surgery is based on the fact that *none* of his patients, some of whom he followed for 20 years, regretted undergoing SRS.

In a study of the sexuality of the postoperative transsexual patient (male to female), it was noted that one-third of the patients were sexually active pre- and postoperatively, and more than one-half experienced an orgasm postoperatively, although only one-third were considered to have satisfactory sexual adjustment (Lindemalm, Korlin, and Uddenberg, 1986). The authors also cited a study of castrated sex offenders wherein 11 of 35 nonestrogenized men (31 per cent) were still able to engage in sexual intercourse (Heim, cited in Lindemalm, Korlin, and Uddenberg, 1986). Lothstein (1982, citing Hastings and Blum) reported 12 of 25 patients who postoperatively experienced multiple orgasms.

The ratio of males to females requesting SRS varies, one study of over 700 patients reporting a ratio approaching 1 to 1 (Dixen and associates, 1984). Earlier research documented a ratio of 4 to 1 (male to female) (Dixen and associates, 1984, citing Pauly, and Randal). It may be speculated that the recent increase in women presenting for surgery could be attributed to improved surgical techniques or the feminist movement. Although in general there is a paucity of information on the female-to-male patient, it appears that this patient is more stable both sexually and psychosocially than the male-to-female counterpart. This finding stands despite the female-to-male's greater difficulty in "passing" for the opposite gender, and despite previously inferior surgical techniques (Dixen and associates, 1984). Early predictions of psychosis in and litigation from these patients have also proved to be unfounded (Meyer and Hoopes, 1974).

SELF-MUTILATION

This topic includes breast and genital surgery, as well as that of the extremities. Some might argue that transsexualism should be included since the patient's wish for self-mutilation is carried out by the hands of the surgeon. *Mania operativa*, wherein the patient seeks repeated unnecessary and unsuccessful surgical procedures, may also fall within this category. There is universal agreement among all authors, regardless of the anatomic location chosen by the patient for self-mutilation, that most patients are *not* attempting suicide at the time of the incident. The majority feel no pain during the mutilatory act. Most are in a tense emotional state before the act, followed by a depersonalized state in which they feel numb (as during the time when the self-mutilating act is carried out). There is a release of tension and resolution of depersonalization immediately after the act. Most self-mutilators repeat the act, although they may vary their choice of anatomic site. There are some striking differences between male and female self-mutilators: genital mutilation is more common in the male and the wrist in the female; both sexes have in common the general theme of confusion regarding sexual identity.

Male Genital Mutilation

In 1963 Blacker and Wong reviewed the world literature on male auto-castration, noting 40 cases reported since 1901. Until 1951 most were brief reports on an unusually violent event with little information about the patient's development and personality. A later review by Greilsheimer and Groves (1979) added an additional 16 cases, including one of their own. Data on two patients who recently underwent successful penile replantation at Bellevue Hospital are included (Housman, 1988).

The review by Greilsheimer and Groves (1979) included four of the patients who underwent penile replantation and were previously reported by Engelman and associates (1974). All the operations were successful but one patient subsequently committed suicide. Also included is Engelman's case, a self-mutilator who underwent successful penile replantation and was doing well at follow-up 18 months later.

The results reported by Greilsheimer and Groves (1979) may be summarized as follows: The reasons for penile auto-amputation are reflected as a wish to be or have the delusion of being female (mostly schizophrenics and transsexuals), homosexual feelings, real or imagined somatic illness, and problems with heterosexual feelings. Other mentioned variables include religiosity, psychotic symptoms, and failure in the male role. Mutilation as part of a suicide attempt was surprisingly uncommon. Only five patients had a history of suicide attempts, and only one committed suicide.

The review also noted the "stunningly negative effects on health caregivers," i.e., ward staff, making the patients feel guilty or worthless. Nurses were loath to enter the patient's room, and were pessimistic regarding the clinical outcome, despite the confidence expressed in the literature. The authors recommended that the psychiatric consultant attend to the staff as well as the patient.

Self-Amputation of Upper Extremities

Stewart and Lowrey (1980) reviewed four cases of upper extremity auto-amputation and criticized the replantation literature, in which there is little mention of the psychiatric symptoms of the self-mutilator. Their first patient, a 37 year old mother of three, amputated her right hand, quoting scripture: "If thy right hand offend thee, cut if off." The second patient, a 53 year old man, amputated his right hand, expressing the motive that caring for his ailing mother was "just too much for two hands." He was the only patient in the series to deny suicidal ideation at the time. The third patient was a 57 year old man who amputated eight of his fingers, initially saying it was an accident; he later went on to commit suicide. The final patient was a 53 year old married executive with two children who took a butcher knife to his neck, abdomen, and chest and both wrists, with partial disarticulation of both wrist joints. He was subsequently relieved that he had not killed himself but admitted to being suicidal at the time. All four of the reported individuals were depressed, none being schizophrenic.

The authors (Stewart and Lowrey, 1980) criticized the fact that psychiatric consultations are usually requested for patients undergoing penile replantation but not for those receiving other types of replantation.

Greilsheimer and Groves (1979) stressed the importance of what the patient did with the amputated part in terms of prognosis, i.e., did he throw it away or arrive at the emergency room clutching it in his hand? Did he immediately inform someone or casually seek attention two days later, as in one case?

Mania Operativa

This topic closely follows self-mutilation. As previously mentioned, the patient's request for repeated amputations (or other surgical procedures, including cosmetic surgery) may represent a hidden wish to self-mutilate. Under the category of mania operativa can also be found the Münchausen patient, although no extremity amputees carry this diagnosis thus far (Hunter and Kennard, 1982), and the SHAFT syndrome patient (*s*ad, *h*ostile, *a*nxious, *f*rustrating, and *t*enacious), who clings to the health care system (Hunter and Kennard, 1982, citing Wallace and Fitzmorris).

Hunter (1985) considered patients requesting amputation and reamputation at higher levels to be self-mutilators who fall into three categories: (1) amputation after a minor tissue injury; (2) amputation after minor fracture, patients often complaining of severe chronic pain, stump pain, and also difficulties with prosthesis and rehabilitation; and (3) amputation after multiple knee operations. Citing Wood, Hunter (1985) noted that only 35 per cent of 95 patients had pain relief after amputation if the chief preoperative complaint was chronic pain. Others (Parsons, Brown, and Sirota, 1981, citing Devaul and Faillace) reported that family members of the surgery-prone patient also had a higher than expected incidence of repeated surgery. In addition, the type of surgery requested was sometimes similar to that experienced by the parents. Parsons, Brown, and Sirota (1981) noted that in the case of one of their patients, who viewed amputation as nonstressful, there was an increased incidence of amputation among family members.

Hunter and Kennard (1982) noted that the diagnosis of these patients may be difficult, being secondary to associated drug or alcohol abuse, self-mutilation, hypochondriasis, or a sociopathic personality. In addition, the patient may have a grudge against society, physicians, or the hospital, and may be seeking secondary financial gain. The surgeon should remember that, although it is natural for a physician to sympathize with a complaint of pain, he can end up a court of law if he deceives the patient or the public. However, it is not a criminal offense for a patient to deceive the physician (Hunter, 1985). The surgeon who suspects mania operativa should be encouraged to obtain the patient's old records and to call a psychiatrist for consultation. The patient should not be confronted. Unfortunately, the prognosis is not good, many patients being so driven to amputation that they increase its likelihood by active or passive means (Parsons, Brown, and Sirota, 1981).

AMPUTATION AND REPLANTATION

How does one deal with the loss of a limb or other body part? Parkes (1975) compared the responses of 37 male versus 9 female amputees (lower extremities) and then compared the nine female amputees to 21 women recently widowed, postulating that mourning a limb resembled mourning a spouse. Women amputees had a statistically significant longer persistence of visual memories of the lost limb than did the males (78 per cent versus 27 per cent) for up to 13 months after injury, when the study was terminated. The author speculated that this finding is the result of women being more aware of their appearance than men. It should also be mentioned that because a woman's leg is exposed, she receives more visual sensory stimulation and psychosocial input regarding its appearance. Female amputees suffered less change in their financial status than did males (11 per cent versus 59 per cent).

In the comparison of widows with female amputees, both were noted to experience grief as reflected in an initial numbing followed by a restless pining and preoccupation with the loss, with clear visual memories of the lost husband or object as well as a sense of his or its presence. Seventy-five per cent of widows experienced illusory and hypnagogic phenomena, i.e., auditory and visual sensations; the latter increased over time, perhaps because the lost husband could not be replaced, whereas 85 per cent of amputees described painful or unpleasant cutaneous and proprioceptive phenomena and all but one experienced *phantom limb*. Three months after the loss the amputees had a greater sense of presence than the widows, the author speculating that this might be the result of an absence of formalized mourning ritual for the lost limb. Although the widows expressed more initial distress, they were more improved at the one year follow-up, with two-thirds of the widows working (versus one-third of the amputees).

Other investigators (Frank and associates, 1984) found that the older amputees fare better than younger amputees, showing less depression and fewer psychiatric symptoms. The symptoms not only are more prevalent in the younger amputee but also increase with time after amputation. Phantom pain at the one year follow-up was found in 20 per cent in one sample, and was thought to be associated with depression and a rigid, compulsive, self-reliant personality, whereas the low rate of emotional disturbance in the remainder of the groups was attributed to stoic denial (Lindesay, 1986).

Child amputees, aged 4 to 15 years, were studied by Turgay and Sonuvar (1983) with two months to nine years follow-up. They found that the child, family, and staff go through similar stages after amputation: shock, denial, protest, anger, and finally acceptance. The findings are similar to those reported by Parkes (1975). They found that the younger the child, the more likely is there to be misunderstanding regarding limb loss, e.g., the idea of punishment. Given the opportunity to talk, the child can pass quickly through the denial stage, although all maintain some degree of resentment and protest. There is also some collusion from parents to child, the latter becoming fixated in loss and mourning in an attempt to comfort the parents. Parents may react in various ways: e.g., suppressing anger toward the child; feeling pseudo-relief after amputation despite a poor prognosis such as when cancer is present; showing anger toward the staff; or being overcritical, possibly as a secondary factor to their own heightened sense of self-condemnation. Younger staff are more likely to experience depression, with guilt, a sense of failure, and even nightmares. The staff may defend against this reaction by not talking openly with the child or by rushing from a discussion of impending amputation to talking about a prosthesis. A psychiatrist or social worker can help to address these issues with all concerned.

Schweitzer and associates (1986) reviewed 38 upper extremity replantations. The amputations were secondary to industrial (42 per cent), domestic (29 per cent), and motor vehicle (13 per cent) accidents. The mean age of the patients was 34 years. Replantation failed in 21 per cent of the cases. Predisposing factors were alcohol and drugs (16 per cent) and personality traits such as poor impulse control, masochistic or counterphobic tendencies, or extreme action orientation. Twenty-four per cent had sustained previous injuries requiring hospitalization, and 53 per cent demonstrated significant discrepancy between the physical outcome and functional results. Thirteen of the 20 recently stressed patients showed adverse reactions such as guilt, remorse, and nightmares. Eleven per cent of patients were diagnosed as having adjustment disorder with anxious mood and 24 per cent as having adjustment disorder with depressed mood, the depression generally lasting several weeks.

Fear for survival of the replant was common, patients expressing uncertainty and constant apprehension and hypervigilance over the replanted part. Like the stroke victim, the patients complained that it did not feel like theirs, some thinking it was the property of a nurse or doctor. Others mourned the part or nurtured it like a newborn. There was a transient sense of hopelessness, despair, sadness, and pessimism regarding the future as the replanted part was reincorporated into the body schema. Schweitzer and associates, citing Muslin (1971), compared the replantation patient to the organ transplant patient in that there was an initial foreign body stage, followed by a stage of partial reincorporation, and finally complete incorporation.

REFERENCES

Adams, G. R., and Crane, P.: Cited in Chapter 2. *In* Lucker, W., Ribbens, K. A., and McNamara, J. A., Jr. (Eds.): Psychological Aspects of Facial Form. Ann Arbor, MI, Center for Human Growth and Development, University of Michigan, 1981.

Adams, G. R., and LaVoie, J. C.: Parental expectations of educational and personal-social performance of childrearing patterns as a function of attractiveness, sex, and conduct of the child. Child Study J., *5*:125, 1975.

Adams, G. R., and LaVoie, J. C.: Teacher expectations: a review of student characteristics used in expectancy formation. J. Instruct. Psych. Mono., *4*:1, 1977.

Allen, B. P., and Wroble, S.: Social Behavior: Facts and Falsehoods about Common Sense. Chicago, Nelson Hall, 1978.

Allen, B. P., and Wroble, S.: Attractive people like themselves better than unattractive people–most of the time: self descriptions employing the AGT. Quoted by Berscheid, E. *In* Lucker, W., Ribbens, K. A., and McNamara, J. A., Jr. (Eds.): Psychological Aspects of Facial Form. Ann Arbor, MI, Center for Human Growth and Development, University of Michigan, 1981.

American Psychiatric Association: Diagnostic and Statistical Manual of Mental Disorders. 3rd Ed., Revised. Washington, DC, American Psychiatric Association, 1987.

American Society of Plastic and Reconstructive Surgeons: Plastic Surgery Procedures Performed in 1986 by ASPRS Members. Chicago, May, 1987.

Anderson, J. R.: Philosophical considerations in revising cosmetic surgical operations. Otolaryngol. Clin. North Am., *7*:57, 1974.

Andreason, N. C., and Bardash, J.: Dysmorphophobia: symptom or disease? Am. J. Psychiatry, *134*:763, 1977.

Arndt, E. M., Travis, F., Lefebvre, A., Niec, A., and Munro, I. R.: Beauty and the eye of the beholder: social consequences and personal adjustments for facial patients. Br. J. Plast. Surg., *39*:81, 1986.

Baker, J. L., Jr., Kolin, I. S., and Bartlett, E. S.: Psychosexual dynamics of patients undergoing mammary augmentation. Plast. Reconstr. Surg., *53*:652, 1974.

Baker, T. J., and Gordon, H. L.: Rhytidectomy in males. Plast. Reconstr. Surg., *44*:219, 1969.

Baker, W. Y., and Smith, L. H.: Facial disfigurement and personality. J.A.M.A., *112*:301, 1939.

Barker, R. G., Wright, B. A., and Meyerson, L.: Adjustment to Physical Handicap and Illness: A Survey of the Social Psychology of Physique and Disability. Bulletin 55. New York, Social Science Research Council, 1953.

Barocas, R., and Vance, F. L.: Referral rate and physical attractiveness in third grade children. Percept. Mot. Skills, *39*:731, 1974.

Baunach, P. J.: Quoted in Chapter 2, 1974 citation. *In* Lucker, W., Ribbens, K. A., and McNamara, J. A., Jr. (Eds.): Psychological Aspects of Facial Form. Ann Arbor, MI, Center for Human Growth and Development, University of Michigan, 1981.

Beale, S., Hambert, G., Lisper, H. O., Ohlsén, L., and Palm, B.: Augmentation mammaplasty: the surgical and psychological effects of the operation and prediction of the result. Ann. Plast. Surg., *13*:279, 1984.

Beale, S., Lisper, H. O., and Palm, B.: A psychological study of patients seeking augmentation mammaplasty. Br. J. Psychiatry, *136*:133, 1980.

Beaser, R. S., Van der Hoek, C., Jacobson, A. M., Flood, T. M., and Desautels, R. E.: Experience with penile prosthesis in the treatment of impotence in diabetic men. J.A.M.A., *248*:943, 1982.

Belfer, M. L., Harrison, A. M., Pillemer, F. C., and Murray, J. E.: Appearance and the influence of reconstructive surgery on body image. Clin. Plast. Surg., *9*:307, 1982.

Belfer, M. L., Mulliken, J. B., and Cochran, T. C., Jr.: Cosmetic surgery as an antecedent of life change. Am. J. Psychiatry, *136*:199, 1979.

Berg, R., Mindus, P., Berg, G., and Gustafson, H.: Penile implants in erectile impotence. Outcome and prognostic indicators. Scand. J. Urol. Nephrol., *18*:277, 1984.

Bernstein, N. R.: Emotional Problems of the Facially Burned and Disfigured. Boston, Little, Brown & Company, 1976.

Berscheid, E.: An overview of the psychological effects of physical attractiveness. *In* Lucker, W., Ribbens, K. A., and McNamara, J. A., Jr. (Eds.): Psychological Aspects of Facial Form. Ann Arbor, MI, Center for Human Growth and Development, University of Michigan, 1981.

Berscheid, E., Dion, K., Walster, E., and Walster, G. W.: Physical attractiveness and dating choice: a test of the matching hypotheses. J. Exp. Soc. Psychol., *7*:180, 1971.

Berscheid, E., and Gangestad, A. B.: The social psychological indications of facial physical attractiveness. Clin. Plast. Surg., *9*:290, 1982.

Blacker, K. H., and Wong, N.: Four cases of autocastration. Arch. Gen. Psychiatry, *8*:169, 1963.

Bodner, D. R.: Impotence: evaluation and treatment. Primary Care, *12*:719, 1985.

Borod, J., and Koff, E.: Asymmetries in affective facial expression: anatomy and behavior. *In* Fox, N., and Davidson, R. (Eds.): The Psychology of Effective Development. Hillsdale, NJ, Lawrence Erlbaum Associates, 1984.

Boukydis, C.: Quoted in Chapter 2, 1977 citation. *In* Lucker, W., Ribbens, K. A., and McNamara, J. A., Jr. (Eds.): Psychological Aspects of Facial Form. Ann Arbor, MI, Center for Human Growth and Development, University of Michigan, 1981.

Boxer, R. J.: Reconstruction of the male external genitalia. Surg. Gynecol. Obstet., *141*:939, 1975.

Briggs, R. M., and Ogg, M. J.: Patients' refusal of surgery after Innovar premedication. Plast. Reconstr. Surg., *51*:158, 1973.

Brunswick, R. M.: A supplement to Freud's "History of an Infantile Neurosis." Int. J. Psychoanal., *9*:439, 1928.

Burk, J., Zelen, S. L., and Terino, E. O.: More than skin deep: a self-consistency approach to the psychology of cosmetic surgery. Plast. Reconstr. Surg., *76*:270, 1985.

Cash, T. F., and Horton, C.: Aesthetic surgery: effects of

rhinoplasty on social perceptions of patients by others. Plast. Reconstr. Surg., *72*:543, 1983.

Cash, T. F., Kehr, J., Polyson, J., and Freeman, V.: Role of physical attractiveness in peer attribution of psychological disturbance. J. Consult. Clin. Psychol., *45*:987, 1977.

Clifford, E.: Psychosocial aspects of orofacial anomalies: speculations in search of data. *In* Wertz, R. T. (Ed.): Orofacial Anomalies: Clinical and Research Implications. ASHA Reports No. 8. Washington, D.C., American Speech and Hearing Association, 1973.

Connolly, R. H., and Gipson, M.: Dysmorphophobia: a long-term study. Br. J. Psychiatry, *132*:568, 1978.

Converse, J. M., Wood-Smith, D., McCarthy, J. G., and Coccaro, P. J.: Craniofacial surgery. Clin. Plast. Surg., *1*:499, 1974.

Corter, C., Trehub, S., Boukydis, C., Ford, L., Clehoffer, L., and Minde, K.: Nurses' judgements of the attractiveness of premature infants. Infant Behav. Devel., *1*:373, 1980.

Courtiss, E. H.: Doctor, am I being vain? (editorial). Plast. Reconstr. Surg., *65*:819, 1980.

Dion, K. K.: Young children's stereotyping of facial attractiveness. Dev. Psychol., *9*:183, 1973.

Dion, K. K.: Children's physical attractiveness and sex as determinants of adult punitiveness. Dev. Psychol., *10*:772, 1974.

Dion, K. K., and Berscheid, E.: Physical attractiveness and peer perception among children. Sociometry, *37*:1, 1974.

Dion, K. K., Berscheid, E., and Walster, E.: What is beautiful is good. J. Pers. Soc. Psychol., *24*:285, 1972.

Dion, K. K., and Stein, S.: Physical attractiveness and interpersonal influence. J. Exp. Soc. Psychol., *14*:97, 1978.

Dipboye, R. L., Fromkin, H. L., and Wiback, K.: Relative importance of applicant sex, attractiveness and scholastic standing in evaluation of job applicant resumes. J. Appl. Psychol., *60*:39, 1975.

Dixen, J. M., Maddever, H., Van Maasdam, J., and Edwards, P. W.: Psychosocial characteristics of applicants evaluated for surgical gender reassignment. Arch. Sex. Behav., *13*:269, 1984.

Dugas, B.: Dealing with the dissatisfied patient. Plast. Surg. Nurs., *3*:33, 1983.

Edgerton, M. T.: The role of surgery in the treatment of transsexualism. Ann. Plast. Surg., *13*:473, 1984.

Edgerton, M. T., Jacobson, W. E., and Meyer, E.: Surgical-psychiatric study of patients seeking plastic (cosmetic) surgery: 98 consecutive patients with minimal deformity. Br. J. Plast. Surg., *13*:136, 1961.

Edgerton, M. T., Jr., and Knorr, N. J.: Motivational patterns of patients seeking cosmetic (esthetic) surgery. Plast. Reconstr. Surg., *48*:551, 1971.

Editorial: Cosmetic surgery. Med. J. Aust., *23*:763, 1974.

Engelman, E. R., Polito, G., Perley, J., Bruffy, J., and Martin, D. C.: Traumatic amputation of the penis. J. Urol., *112*:774, 1974.

Fisk, N.: Five spectacular results. Arch. Sex. Behav., *7*:351, 1978.

Fleming, M., Steinman, C., and Bocknek, G.: Methodological problems in assessing sex-reassignment surgery: a reply to Meyer and Reter. Arch. Sex. Behav., *9*:451, 1980.

Frank, R. G., Kashani, J. H., Kashani, S. R., Wonderlich, S. A., Umlauf, R. L., and Ashkanazi, G. S.: Psychological response to amputation as a function of age and time since amputation. Br. J. Psychiatry, *144*:493, 1984.

Freud, S.: From the history of an infantile neurosis. *In* Strachey, J. (Ed.): The Standard Edition of the Complete Psychological Works of Sigmund Freud. Vol. 17. London, Hogarth Press, 1955 (orig. publ. 1918).

Goffman, E.: Stigma: Notes in the Management of Spoiled Identity. Englewood Cliffs, NJ, Prentice-Hall, 1953.

Goin, J., and Goin, M. K.: Changing the Body. Psychological Effects of Plastic Surgery. Baltimore, Williams & Wilkins Company, 1981a.

Goin, M. K., Burgoyne, R. W., Goin, J. M., and Staples, F. R.: A prospective psychological study of 50 female face-lift patients. Plast. Reconstr. Surg., *65*:436, 1980.

Goin, M. K., and Goin, J. M.: Midlife reactions to mastectomy and subsequent breast reconstruction. Arch. Gen. Psychiatry, *38*:225, 1981b.

Goldberg, P., Stolzman, M., and Goldberg, H. M.: Psychological considerations in breast reconstruction. Ann. Plast. Surg., *13*:38, 1984.

Goldman, W., and Lewis, P.: Beautiful is good. Evidence that the physically attractive are more socially skillful. J. Exp. Soc. Psychol., *13*:125, 1977.

Goodstein, R. K.: Burns: an overview of clinical consequences affecting patients, staff, and family. Compr. Psychiatry, *26*:43, 1985.

Gorney, M., and Harries, T.: The preoperative and postoperative consideration of natural facial asymmetry. Plast. Reconstr. Surg., *54*:187, 1974.

Greer, D. M.: Psychiatric consultation in plastic surgery: the surgeon's perspective. Psychosomatics, *25*:470, 472, 1984.

Greilsheimer, H., and Groves, J. E.: Male genital self mutilation. Arch. Gen. Psychiatry, *36*:441, 1979.

Grossman, A. R.: Psychological and psychosexual aspects of augmentation mammaplasty. Clin. Plast. Surg., *3*:167, 1976.

Hay, G. G.: Psychiatric aspects of cosmetic nasal operations. Br. J. Psychiatry, *116*:85, 1970.

Hay, G. G., and Heather, B. B.: Changes in psychometric test results following cosmetic nasal operations. Br. J. Psychiatry, *122*:89, 1973.

Hildebrandt, K. A.: Quoted in Chapter 2. *In* Lucker, W., Ribbens, K. A., and McNamara, J. A., Jr. (Eds.): Psychological Aspects of Facial Form. Ann Arbor, MI, Center for Human Growth and Development, University of Michigan, 1981.

Hildebrandt, K. A., and Fitzgerald, H. E.: Gender bias in observers' perception of infant's sex: it's a boy most of the time. Percept. Mot. Skills, *45*:472, 1977.

Hill, G., and Silver, A. G.: Psychodynamic and aesthetic motivations for plastic surgery. Psychosom. Med., *12*:345, 1950.

Hollyman, J. A., Lacey, J. H., Whitfield, P. J., and Wilson, J. S.: Surgery for the psyche: a longitudinal study of women undergoing reduction mammaplasty. Br. J. Plast. Surg., *39*:222, 1986.

Housman, S.: Unpublished data, 1988.

Hueston, J. T.: Augmentation mammaplasty. Med. J. Aust., *1*:728, 1970.

Hunter, G. A.: Limb amputation and re-amputation in association with chronic pain syndrome. Prosthet. Orthot. Int., *9*:92, 1985.

Hunter, G. A., and Kennard, A. B.: Mania operativa: an uncommon unrecognized cause of limb amputation. Can. J. Surg., *25*:92, 1982.

Jackson, D. J., and Huston, T. L.: Physical attractiveness and assertiveness. J. Soc. Psychol., *95*:79, 1975.

Jones, E. E., Farina, A., Hosford, A. H., Marcus, H., Miller, D. T., and Scott, R. A.: Social Stigma: The Psychology of Marked Relationships. New York, W. H. Freeman & Company, 1984.

Jones, H. W., Jr.: Surgical construction of female genitalia. Clin. Plast. Surg., *1*:255, 1974.

Kalick, S. M.: Toward an interdisciplinary psychology of appearances. Psychiatry, *41*:243, 1978.

Kapp-Simon, K.: Psychological adaptation of patients with craniofacial malformations. *In* Lucker, W., Ribbens, K. A., and McNamara, J. A., Jr. (Eds.): Psychological Aspects of Facial Form. Ann Arbor, MI, Center for Human Growth and Development, University of Michigan, 1981, pp. 143–160.

Knorr, N. J., Hoopes, J. E., and Edgerton, M. T.: Psychiatric-surgical approach to adolescent disturbance in self image. Plast. Reconstr. Surg., *41*:248, 1968.

Krebs, D., and Adinolfi, A. A.: Physical attractiveness, social relations and personality style. J. Pers. Soc. Psychol., *31*:245, 1975.

Kurtzberg, R. L., Lewin, M. L., Cavior, M., and Lipton, D. S.: Psychologic screening of inmates requesting cosmetic operations: a preliminary report. Plast. Reconstr. Surg., *39*:268, 1967.

Landy, D., and Sigall, H.: Beauty is talent: task evaluation as a function of the performer's physical attractiveness. J. Pers. Soc. Psychol., *29*:299, 1974.

Lauer, E.: The family. *In* Macgregor, F. C., Abel, T. M., Bryt, A., Lauer, E., and Weissman, S.: Facial Deformities and Plastic Surgery: A Psychosocial Study. Springfield, IL, Charles C Thomas, 1953, pp. 103–129.

Leavell, H. R.: Medical progress: contributions of the social sciences to the solution of health problems. Reprinted in N. Engl. J. Med., *247*:885, 1952.

Leeb, D., Bowers, D. G., Jr., and Lynch, J. B.: Observations on the myth of "informed consent." Plast. Reconstr. Surg., *58*:280, 1976.

Lefebvre, A., and Munro, I.: The role of psychiatry in a craniofacial team. Plast. Reconstr. Surg., *61*:564, 1978.

Levine, S. B., and Shumaker, R. E.: Increasingly Ruth: toward understanding sex reassignment. Arch. Sex. Behav., *12*:247, 1983.

Levinson, J.: Breast reconstruction: a patient's view (letter). Plast. Reconstr. Surg., *73*:703, 1984.

Lindemalm, G., Korlin, D., and Uddenberg, N.: Long term follow-up of "sex change" in 13 male to female transsexuals. Arch. Sex. Behav., *15*:187, 1986.

Lindesay, J.: Validity of the General Health Questionnaire (GHQ) in detecting psychiatric disturbance in amputees with phantom pain. J. Psychosom. Res., *30*:277, 1986.

Lothstein, L. M.: Sex reassignment surgery: historical, bioethical, and theoretical issues. Am. J. Psychiatry, *139*:417, 1982.

Lothstein, L. M.: Psychological testing with transsexuals: a 30 year review. J. Pers. Assess., *48*:500, 1984.

Lubkin, V.: The public face or psychological and legal complexities in ophthalmic surgery. Br. J. Ophthalmol., *59*:593, 1975.

Lundström, B., Pauly, I., and Walinder, J.: Outcome of sexual reassignment surgery. Acta Psychiatr. Scand., *70*:289, 1984.

Macgregor, F. C.: The sociological aspects of facial deformities. Master's Thesis, University of Missouri, 1947, pp. 18–28.

Macgregor, F. C.: Some psychological hazards of plastic surgery of the face. Plast. Reconstr. Surg., *12*:123, 1953.

Macgregor, F. C.: Social Science in Nursing: Applications for the Improvement of Patient Care. New York, Russell Sage Foundation, 1960.

Macgregor, F. C.: Uncooperative patients: some cultural interpretations. Am. J. Nurs., *67*:88, 1967a.

Macgregor, F. C.: Social and cultural components in the motivations of persons seeking plastic surgery of the nose. J. Health Soc. Behav., *8*:125, 1967b.

Macgregor, F. C.: Social and psychological implications of dentofacial disfigurement. Angle Orthod., *40*:231, 1970.

Macgregor, F. C.: Selection of cosmetic surgery patients–social and psychological considerations. Surg. Clin. North Am., *51*:289, 1971.

Macgregor, F. C.: Transformation and Identity: The Face and Plastic Surgery. New York, Quadrangle, New York Times Book, 1974.

Macgregor, F. C.: Aesthetic plastic surgery—some caveats. Aesthetic Plast. Surg., *1*:71, 1976.

Macgregor, F. C.: A social science approach to the study of facial deformities and plastic surgery. *In* Converse, J. M. (Ed.): Reconstructive Plastic Surgery, 2nd Ed. Philadelphia, W.B. Saunders Company, 1977, pp. 565–584.

Macgregor, F. C.: Ear deformities: social and psychological implications. Clin. Plast. Surg. *5*:347, 1978.

Macgregor, F. C.: After Plastic Surgery: Adaptation and Adjustment. New York, Praeger Publishers, 1979.

Macgregor, F. C.: Social and psychological studies of plastic surgery: past, present and future. Clin. Plast. Surg., *9*:283, 1982.

Macgregor, F. C., Abel, T. M., Bryt, A., Lauer, E., and Weissman, S.: Facial Deformities and Plastic Surgery: A Psychosocial Study. Springfield, IL, Charles C Thomas, 1953.

Macgregor, F. C., and Schaffner, B.: Screening patients for nasal plastic operations: some sociologic and psychiatric considerations. Psychosom. Med., *12*:277, 1950.

Martin, L. M., and Montague, D. K.: Ejaculatory incompetence following penile prosthesis implantation in men with primary psychogenic impotence. Cleve. Clin. Q., *49*:93, 1982.

Mathes, E. W.: The effects of physical attractiveness and anxiety on heterosexual attraction over a series of 5 encounters. J. Marriage Fam. *37*:769, 1975.

Mathes, E. W., and Kahn, A.: Physical attractiveness, happiness, neuroticism, and self esteem. J. Psychol., *90*:27, 1975.

McKinney, P., and Cook, J. Q.: A critical evaluation of 200 rhinoplasties. Ann. Plast. Surg., *7*:357, 1981.

McWilliams, B. J.: Social and psychological problems associated with cleft palate. Clin. Plast. Surg., *9*:317, 1982.

Mearig, J. S.: Facial surgery and an active modification approach for children with Down syndrome: some psychological and ethical issues. Rehabil. Lit., *46*:72, 1985.

Mendelson, B. C.: The psychological basis for breast reconstruction following mastectomy (editorial). Med. J. Aust., *1*:517, 1980.

Meyer, E., Jacobson, E. E., Edgerton, M. T., and Canter, A.: Motivational patterns in patients seeking elective plastic surgery. I. Women who seek rhinoplasty. Psychosom. Med., *22*:193, 1960.

Meyer, J. K.: The theory of gender identity disorders. J. Am. Psychoanal. Assoc., *30*:381, 1982.

Meyer, J. K., and Hoopes, J. E.: The gender dysphoria syndromes. A position statement on so-called "transsexualism." Plast. Reconstr. Surg., *54*:444, 1974.

Meyer, J. K., Hoopes, J. E., Jabaley, M. E., and Allen, R.: Is plastic surgery effective in the rehabilitation of deformed delinquent adolescents? Plast. Reconstr. Surg., *51*:53, 1973.

Meyer, J. K., and Reter, D. J.: Sex reassignment. Follow-up. Arch. Gen. Psychiatry, *36*:1010, 1979.

Millard, D. R., Jr., Devine, J., Jr., and Warren, W. D.: Breast reconstruction: a plea for saving the uninvolved nipple. Am. J. Surg., *122*:763, 1971.

Mohl, P. C.: Psychiatric consultation in plastic surgery: the psychiatrist's perspective. Psychosomatics, *25*:471, 474, 1984.

Money, J.: Ablatio penis: normal male infant sex-reassigned as a girl. Arch. Sex. Behav., *4*:67, 1975.

Muller, F. E.: Late results of Strombeck's mammaplasty. A follow-up study of 100 patients. Plast. Reconstr. Surg., *54*:664, 1974.

Murray, J. E., Mulliken, J. B., Kaban, L. B., and Belfer, M.: Twenty years experience in maxillocraniofacial surgery. An evaluation of early surgery on growth, body function, and body image. Ann. Surg., *190*:320, 1979.

National Foundation for Facial Reconstruction: Statistics. New York, N.Y., 1986.

Ohlsén, L., Pontén, B., and Hambert, G.: Augmentation mammaplasty: a surgical and psychiatric evaluation of the results. Ann. Plast. Surg., *2*:42, 1979.

Olley, P. C.: Aspects of plastic surgery. Social and psychological sequelae. Br. Med. J., *3*:322, 1974.

Parkes, C. M.: Psychosocial transitions: comparisons between reactions of limb vs. loss of spouse. Br. J. Psychiatry, *127*:204, 1975.

Parsons, J. A., Brown, W. A., and Sirota, A. D.: Inappropriate amputation requests. Psychosomatics, *22*:822, 1981.

Pauly, I. B.: The current status of the change of sex operation. J. Nerv. Ment. Dis., *147*:460, 1968.

Pertschuk, M. J., and Whitaker, L.: Psychosocial adjustment and craniofacial malformations in childhood. Plast. Reconstr. Surg., *75*:177, 1985.

Pertschuk, M. J., and Whitaker, L.: Psychosocial outcome of craniofacial surgery in children. Plast. Reconstr. Surg., *82*:741, 1988.

Peterson, H. R., Best, J. D., Berger, R., Reenan, A., Porte, D., Jr., et al.: Attitudes of diabetic men after implantation of a semi-rigid penile prosthesis. Diabetes Care, *8*:156, 1985.

Pillemer, F. G.: Psychosocial Adjustment of Pediatric Craniofacial Patients Following Reconstructive Surgery. Doctoral Dissertation, Harvard University, 1981.

Pueschel, S. M., Monteiro, L. A., and Erickson, M.: Parents' and physicians' perceptions of facial plastic surgery in children with Down's syndrome. J. Ment. Defic. Res., *30*:71, 1986.

Redfield, R.: Relation of anthropology to the social sciences and humanities. *In* Kroeber, R. L. (Ed.): Anthropology Today: An Encyclopedic Inventory. Chicago, University of Chicago Press, 1953, pp. 728–738.

Rees, T. D., and Daniller, A.: Self-mutilation: some problems in reconstruction. Plast. Reconstr. Surg., *43*:300, 1969.

Rees, T. D., and Wood-Smith, D.: Cosmetic Facial Surgery. Philadelphia, W.B. Saunders Company, 1973.

Reich, J.: The surgery of appearance: psychological and related aspects. Med. J. Aust., *2*:5, 1969.

Reich, J.: Factors influencing patient satisfaction with the results of esthetic plastic surgery. Plast. Reconstr. Surg., *55*:5, 1975.

Roback, H. B., Felleman, E. S., and Abramowitz, S. I.: The mid-life male sex change applicant: a multiclinic survey. Arch. Sex. Behav., *13*:141, 1984.

Robertson, J. G.: Rhytidectomy combined with chemical peeling of the superficial cutaneous tissues. Int. Surg., *47*:576, 1967.

Rozner, L.: Attitudes to cosmetic surgery. Med. J. Aust., *2*:513, 1973.

Rozner, L.: Facial plastic surgery for Down's syndrome. Lancet, *1*:1320, 1983.

Safilios-Rothschild, C.: The Sociology and Social Psychology of Disability and Rehabilitation. New York, Random House, 1970.

Schain, W. S., Jacobs, E., and Wellisch, D. K.: Psychological issues in breast reconstruction. Intrapsychic, interpersonal and practical concerns. Clin. Plast. Surg., *11*:237, 1984.

Schulman, B. H.: Psychiatric assessment of the candidate for cosmetic surgery. Otolaryngol. Clin. North Am., *13*:383, 1980.

Schuring, A. G., and Dodge, R. E., Jr.: The role of cosmetic surgery in criminal rehabilitation. Plast. Reconstr. Surg., *40*:268, 1967.

Schweitzer, I., and Hirschfeld, J. J.: Postrhytidectomy psychosis: a rare complication. Plast. Reconstr. Surg., *74*:419, 1984.

Schweitzer, I., Rosenbaum, M. B., Sharzer, L. A., and Strauch, B.: Liaison consultation psychiatry with patients who have replantation surgery to the upper limb. Aust. N.Z. J. Psychiatry, *20*:38, 1986.

Seligman, C. N., Pascall, N., and Takata, G.: Citation from 1973, quoted in Chapter 3. *In* Lucker, W., Ribbens, K. A., and McNamara, J. A., Jr. (Eds.): Psychological Aspects of Facial Form. Ann Arbor, MI, Center for Growth and Development, University of Michigan, 1981.

Shapiro, A. K., Streuning, E., Shapiro, E., and Barten, H.: Prognostic correlates of psychotherapy in psychiatric out-patients. Am. J. Psychiatry, *133*:802, 1976.

Shipley, R. H., O'Donnell, J. M., and Bader, K. F.: Personality characteristics of women seeking breast augmentation. Plast. Reconstr. Surg., *60*:369, 1977.

Sihm, F., Jagd, M., and Pers, M.: Psychological assessment before and after augmentation mammaplasty. Scand. J. Plast. Reconstr. Surg., *12*:295, 1978.

Snyderman, R. K., and Starzynski, T. E.: Breast augmentation. Surg. Clin. North Am., *49*:303, 1969.

Stevens, L. A., McGrath, M. H., Druss, R. G., Kister, S. J., Gump, F. E., and Forde, K. A.: The psychological impact of immediate breast reconstruction for women with early breast cancer. Plast. Reconstr. Surg., *73*:619, 1984.

Stewart, D. E., and Lowrey, M. R.: Replantation surgery following self-inflicted amputation. Can. J. Psychiatry, *25*:143, 1980.

Taylor, B. W., Litin, E. M., and Litzow, T. J.: Psychiatric considerations in cosmetic surgery. Mayo Clin. Proc., *41*:608, 1966.

Teimourian, B., and Adham, M. N.: Survey of patients' responses to breast reconstruction. Ann. Plast. Surg., *9*:321, 1982.

Tessier, P.: The definitive plastic surgical treatment of the severe facial deformities of craniofacial dysostosis:

Crouzon's and Apert's diseases. Plast. Reconstr. Surg., *48*:419, 1971.

Turgay, A., and Sonuvar, B.: Emotional aspects of arm or leg amputation in children. Can. J. Psychiatry, *28*:294, 1983.

Updegraff, H. L., and Menninger, K. A.: Some psychoanalytic aspects of plastic surgery. Am. J. Plast. Surg., *25*:554, 1934.

Van Duyn, J.: Psyche and plastic surgery. South. Med. J., *58*:1255, 1965.

Ward, C. M.: Breast reconstruction after cancer–aesthetic triumph or surgical disaster? Br. J. Plast. Surg., *34*:124, 1981.

Wellisch, D. K., Schain, W. S., Noone, R. B., and Little, J. W., III: Psychosocial correlates of immediate versus delayed reconstruction of the breast. Plast. Reconstr. Surg., *76*:713, 1985.

Wray, R. C., Jr.: "The buck stops here" (editorial). Plast. Reconstr. Surg., *78*:85, 1986.

Wright, B. A.: Physical Disability–A Psychological Approach. New York, Harper & Row, 1960.

Young, H. H., 2nd, Cockett, A. T., Stoller, R., Ashley, F. L., and Goodwin, W. E.: The management of agenesis of the phallus. Pediatrics, *47*:81, 1971.

4

Brent V. Stromberg

Anesthesia

Although precise information is not available, approximately 1½ million surgical procedures are performed by plastic surgeons in the United States each year. Essentially, all of these require anesthesia. In many cases, the anesthesia and accompanying systemic sedation are administered by the surgeon. Even when the expertise of a trained anesthesiologist is available, a significant responsibility remains with the surgeon for preoperative and postoperative care and evaluation, as well as intraoperative participation with the anesthesiologist in the anesthetic care of the patient.

As rapid advances occur within the specialty of anesthesiology, it becomes not only more difficult, but also more important, that the surgeon remain well informed in anesthesia principles. The maintenance of a standard of anesthetic care equal to the highest level remains a requirement in every surgical procedure.

LEGAL ASPECTS

Although infrequently discussed in surgical texts, the legal implications of the actions of the plastic surgeon/anesthetist should be understood. The accepted standard of care by which the administration of anesthesia is judged is currently undergoing an evolution in legal circles.

It had been previously maintained that a practitioner should be held to the same standard of care as that generally available in his own community by members of his own specialty. However, the courts are now declaring that a physician should be considered, by reason of his medical training, to have access to continuing education opportunities, rapid patient consultation and transportation if necessary, and a standard of care equal to that in similar communities nationwide.

Although acknowledging that doctors practicing in small communities cannot be expected to have the facilities of those in larger communities, the courts have repeatedly declared that a physician should have adequate training to allow him to refer patients to others if he is not personally able to administer competent care.

A plastic surgeon is unlikely to be practicing in a locality without an anesthesiologist.

Few would limit the activities of a surgeon trained in local and regional anesthesia, but the standard of care for which he is responsible can be legally compared with that of the anesthesiologist. Thus, the plastic surgeon should at all times observe a high standard of care and skill. He is expected to practice standards commensurate with those of available anesthesiologists.

ANALGESIA AND SEDATION

The judicious use of analgesics and sedatives is a valuable adjunct to surgery. The current and appropriate trend in anesthesia practice is to minimize preoperative sedation, especially in the very young and the elderly. Although the pharmacologic preparation of the patient is no substitute for a thorough and appropriate psychologic preparation, the use of medication can be a valuable aid in the anxious patient. Patients electing surgery under local anesthesia are ideally prepared in such a way as to relieve anxiety and yet offer some analgesia, amnesia, and a sense of well-being while avoiding detrimental side effects. The achievement of this state requires psychologic and often pharmacologic preparation preoperatively.

The initiation of the psychologic preparation begins with the first visit to the surgeon. A complete history and physical examination does much to instill the patient's confidence in the surgeon. A thorough medical and surgical history is taken and a complete explanation of the procedure is given. The beneficial effect of the psychologic preparation of the patient during the preoperative interview has been documented (Egbert and associates, 1963). During this visit an initial appraisal can be made of the requirements for premedication sedation and analgesia. Various factors, such as the general physical status and condition of the patient, psychologic considerations, age, weight, perceived anxiety, previous adverse drug reactions, and other medical diseases (e.g., pulmonary, cardiovascular, hepatic, renal, or intracranial) may be important for determining the need for and amount of medication. It is important to individualize drug selection, the type of medication, the quantity, and the route of administration. This may be particularly true in the pediatric patient in whom the administration of premedication by an intramuscular injection may instill a significant amount of fear and anxiety, which may outweigh the further advantages to be obtained.

The premedication may begin the evening before surgery with an agent to facilitate the initiation of sleep. Commonly used agents are flurazepam (Dalmane) in 15 to 30 mg oral dosage or triazolam (Halcion) in a dose of 0.25 to 0.5 mg. The use of these mild agents can often be valuable in the preparation of the patient by allowing a relatively restful night's sleep. These agents have few side effects and there are few contraindications to their use.

Medications administered before the induction of surgery and those given as an adjunct during surgery usually consist of a combination of narcotic and a second agent, which is usually in the sedative/tranquilizer class. Commonly used agents and the usual dosage are indicated in Table 4–1.

Narcotic usage is generally confined to morphine and meperidine. Narcotics are extremely useful as premedications because they provide analgesia as well as a mild degree of sedation to reduce the usual preoperative anxiety. There are some undesirable side effects that may limit the applicability and dosage of narcotics in certain situations. Fortunately, most of the adverse effects can be reversed by the administration of naloxone (Narcan).

Comparison of the effects of morphine and meperidine can be helpful. It is important to note, however, that if these are given in appropriate dosage after a complete preoperative evaluation, significant side effects are rare. Morphine can produce venous dilation and a decreased heart rate sufficient to cause hypotension, particularly in the hypovolemic patient. Reversal of this effect with intravenous fluid administration is usually satisfactory. Occasionally, a vasopressor and narcotic reversal is required (Drews, Dripps, and Comroe, 1946). Meperidine can also act as a ve-

Table 4–1. Dosages of Commonly Used Preoperative Medications

Drug	Adult Dosage (mg)
Anticholinergics	
Atropine	0.3–0.6
Scopolamine	0.3–0.5
Barbiturates	
Secobarbital	50–100
Pentobarbital	50–100
Narcotics	
Morphine	5–10
Meperidine	50–100
Hypnotics	
Diazepam	5–10
Droperidol	2.5–5.0
Hydroxyzine	50–100
Midazolam	0.035–0.08

nous dilator and a myocardial depressant. If this agent is given in large dosages, this side effect can be severe. However, induction with small and appropriate doses in a sedated patient allows titration and rarely produces significant hypotension. Hypertension occasionally occurs in the awake patient and usually reflects an inadequate level of local anesthesia. Bradycardia can be produced by all narcotics but is most often associated with the use of morphine. When it does occur, it is treated with intravenous atropine (0.01 mg/kg). Bradycardia is considered to be vagally mediated and is rarely seen with the smaller doses of narcotics used for premedication and intraoperative supplementation of local anesthesia (Stanley and Webster, 1978).

Respiratory depression can be seen with all narcotics and is usually dose dependent (Bellville and Seed, 1960; Eckenhoff and Oech, 1960). The mechanism of respiratory depression is undoubtedly triggered through multiple pathways. Narcotics have been shown to depress both the pontine and the medullary centers of respiratory regulation. In addition, narcotics can decrease the respiratory center of the brain stem in its response to increasing levels of carbon dioxide (Bellville and Seed, 1960). The characteristic of narcotic-induced respiratory depression is a decreased respiratory rate initially. The depth of respiratory effort is maintained during the early phases of depression. Increasing narcotic levels at this point decrease both the respiratory rate and the tidal volume. Narcotics have been shown to stimulate a profound bronchoconstriction on occasion. This can be caused by a direct irritating effect on the smooth muscle of the bronchus, as well as indirectly by a histamine release (Adriani and Rovenstine, 1943). The cardiac and respiratory effects of the narcotics are somewhat age dependent, being more profound in the elderly patient (Foldes, Swerdlow, and Siker, 1964). Reversal of the cardiovascular effects can be obtained by the administration of small doses of naloxone (Narcan). The usual incremental dosages are 0.05 to 0.10 mg intravenously.

Use of a sedative is common and beneficial in most significant procedures performed under local anesthesia. The sedatives most often used in clinical practice are diazepam (Valium), droperidol (Inapsine), and lorazepam (Ativan). Occasionally, short-acting barbiturates such as secobarbital and pentobarbital are utilized. All these agents can be useful in decreasing anxiety and providing a smoother operative experience. Diazepam and lorazepam are benzodiazepine compounds. Although officially classified as minor tranquilizers, in increasing dosages they can provide a state of calmness, sedation, and unconsciousness (Greenblatt and Shader, 1974; Dundee, 1980). These agents are relatively free of significant cardiovascular or respiratory side effects when administered in the usual premedication dosages. Care must be utilized in the elderly and in patients with significant liver dysfunction because the metabolism of these agents occurs through the hepatic system (Klotz and associates, 1975). Intravenous administration of diazepam is followed rapidly by sedation (Eckenhoff and Oech, 1960). An interesting and useful effect of the benzodiazepine group of compounds is its ability to produce amnesia in an antegrade fashion (Brown, Main, and Lawson, 1968; George and Dundee, 1977); this property is present regardless of the route of administration.

A relatively new benzodiazepine is midazolam, a short-acting agent that acts predominantly as a central nervous system depressant. The effects are dose dependent. It is usually administered either intravenously or intramuscularly. Dosage recommended for adults is approximately 2 to 5 mg and it should be titrated carefully until the desired effect is obtained. It has a significant amnestic effect. The physiologic and side effects are similar to those of the other benzodiazepines. Midazolam can be used either as a preoperative medication in preparation for general anesthesia or as a sedating agent for local anesthesia. When used carefully in a monitored, titrated dosage it has been shown to be safe and effective, and it is rapidly becoming one of the more common agents utilized in its class.

Mild respiratory depression from the use of benzodiazepines is common. This is especially true when they are injected intravenously and it is secondary to a decrease in tidal volume incompletely compensated for with a slight increase in respiratory rate (Stovner and Endresen, 1966; Rao and associates, 1973). True apnea is uncommon but has been reported with the intravenous injection of as little as 10 mg of diazepam (Sadove, Balagot, and McGrath, 1965).

Droperidol is another agent that can be useful to sedate the perioperative patient. Chemically a butyrophenone, it gives a significant amount of sedation and provides an antiemetic effect. However, it has been shown to produce dysphoria in a small percentage of patients (Lee and Yeakel, 1975). In addition, it is a blocking agent for both alpha-adrenergic and dopinergic receptors. Thus, the administration of droperidol can lead to a decrease in blood pressure, especially in the hypovolemic patient. It may also exacerbate extrapyramidal symptoms in the patient with Parkinson's disease (Patton, 1975). However, the state of apparent apathy and mental detachment that the butyrophenones produce can be significantly helpful in medicating the patient (DeCastro and Mundeleer, 1959). This neuroleptanalgesia produces a drowsy indifferent patient. Again, the precise mechanism of action of droperidol is unclear but it is undoubtedly multifactorial. It has been shown to interfere with the dopamine, noradrenalin, serotonin, and gamma-aminobutyric acid pathways (Jansen, 1967; Morrison, 1974). Side effects are mostly related to the previously mentioned dysphoria. There is, however, a notable slight decrease in systemic blood pressure, which is probably secondary to the documented preferential blocking of the alpha-adrenergic system as well as to a slight myocardial depression (Puddy, 1971; Muldoon and associates, 1977). The use of droperidol may offer some limited protection against cardiac arrhythmias that are induced by catecholamine release (Long, Dripps, and Price, 1967). There is no noted effect on the hepatic, renal, or respiratory systems.

Barbiturates are occasionally used for sedation. These agents are beneficial because a significant amount of sedation with minimal cardiopulmonary effects is achieved. However, there is little analgesia associated with the use of barbiturates. Barbiturates in extremely large doses can produce a profound level of sedation, amnesia, and unconsciousness. However, in the doses used in local anesthesia, barbiturates not only fail to provide analgesia, but may in fact result in an actual increased sensitivity to peripheral pain (Robson, Davenport, and Sugiyama, 1965). Thus, it is important that a satisfactory local anesthesia be effected when barbiturates are utilized as the sedative, since the patient may actually experience an increase in perceived pain upon surgical manipulation. The cardiovascular effects of the barbiturates are predictable and grow in severity with increasing dosages. A peripheral vasodilation occurs principally on the venous side and causes a generalized myocardial depression (Eckstein, Hamilton, and McCammond, 1961). The latter results in a decrease in arterial blood pressure and cardiac output. In the patient who is less able to compensate for these changes, such as one who is chronically hypertensive or hypovolemic, this can be significant. In addition, barbiturates can be significant respiratory depressants. The action is predominantly at the respiratory center in the medulla where the responsiveness to increasing levels of carbon dioxide is decreased (Lee and Yeakel, 1975). A decrease in tidal volume is the predominant action of the barbiturates upon respiration. The respiratory rate usually is not affected until late.

Allergic reactions to the barbiturates are extremely rare. A skin rash has been reported but is distinctly uncommon (Guerra, 1980). On rare occasions, a reaction characterized by acute respiratory difficulty with laryngospasm, bronchospasm, and laryngeal edema can occur.

Barbiturates are relatively contraindicated in the patient with acute intermittent porphyria because of the likelihood of precipitating an acute attack.

The patient undergoing elective surgery either under local regional block or general anesthesia requires a considerable amount of psychologic preparation. Preoperative evaluation and examination are important to decrease the patient's anxiety regarding the upcoming surgery. Adequate preoperative preparation has also been shown to decrease the need for preoperative medication. However, the use of premedication, commonly consisting of a combination of analgesics and sedation, is important in the armamentarium of the surgeon to ensure a comfortable patient and a smooth operative course. The surgeon has several choices of agent: each one has distinct advantages and disadvantages, but a careful consideration of the patient and his requirements may help the surgeon to arrive at an ideal combination. It is also important for the surgeon to be familiar with the various agents and their side effects. It may be more effective to restrict usage to a few agents in each category than to make widespread experiments with multiple agents with which the surgeon has limited familiarity The oximetry intraoperative monitoring device is an essential component of any intravenous analgesia/sedation program.

LOCAL ANESTHESIA

Although the date of the first use of local anesthesia is unknown, the first purified local anesthetic agent, cocaine, was isolated by Niemann in 1860. This ester compound from the *Erythroxylon* coca bush was the first in a series of anesthetic agents isolated, and later synthesized. Karl Koller (1884) demonstrated the usefulness of cocaine in ophthalmologic procedures. Halsted (1885) reported the successful use of cocaine in over 1000 patients undergoing local anesthesia or regional blocks.

The early recognition of the toxicity of cocaine stimulated the search for safer agents. In 1899 procaine, also an ester molecule, was introduced as a safer anesthetic (Einhorn). Advances came rapidly, and by the first decade of the twentieth century the use of local anesthetics was relatively commonplace. The most significant development in the past 50 years has been the introduction of the first amide local anesthetic agent lidocaine in 1948 (Lofgren). Early attempts to utilize hydroxy compounds were disappointing as they proved to be highly irritating to the local tissue.

Mechanism of Action

Local anesthetics exert their principal effect at the nerve cell membrane. The exact mechanism of action is incompletely understood. In the normal resting state the concentration of intracellular sodium is kept low by an energy-requiring "sodium pump." The difference between inside and outside neurilemma levels of sodium maintains a difference in electrical potential across the membrane of 80 to 90 millivolts. When the nerve is excited, the membrane permeability to sodium increases significantly to allow a rapid influx of sodium into the cell with a reversal of membrane polarity. Thus, the propagation of the impulse occurs.

Two principal theories have been postulated to account for the mechanism of the permeability alteration to sodium. One theory is that the sodium molecule is too large to penetrate the pores of the membrane in the resting state. On excitation the membrane pores enlarge to allow the influx of sodium. Local anesthetics interact within the lipid membrane to block the opening of the pores to sodium, thus blocking nerve transmission.

A second theory suggests that local anesthetics work by displacing calcium ions from the axonal membrane. As the calcium-protein complex in the membrane forms an important constituent and is necessary for transmission of the nerve impulse, replacement of the cation with a stabilizing local anesthetic molecule increases membrane stability and decreases permeability to sodium with blockage of nerve impulse conduction.

Neither of these theories has been conclusively proved. Indeed, each may play a component part in the mechanism of action of local anesthetic agents.

Chemistry

Clinically used local anesthetic agents are weak organic bases. To increase water solubility, they are converted to salts, usually the hydrochloride salt. Thus, in the mildly basic body pH environment, the free base is again formed, which is the more active form of the drug. This finding explains, however, why local anesthetics are much less effective in an acidic environment, such as infected or inflamed tissues (Brown, 1981).

The formula of a local anesthetic agent is:

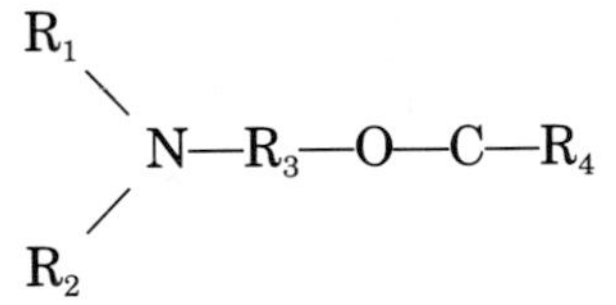

R_1 and R_2 represent hydrophilic amino groups; R_3 is a connecting group; R_4 is the lipophilic aromatic or hydrocarbon group.

The connecting group, R_3, may be either an ester or an amide. Procaine and lidocaine are representatives from each group.

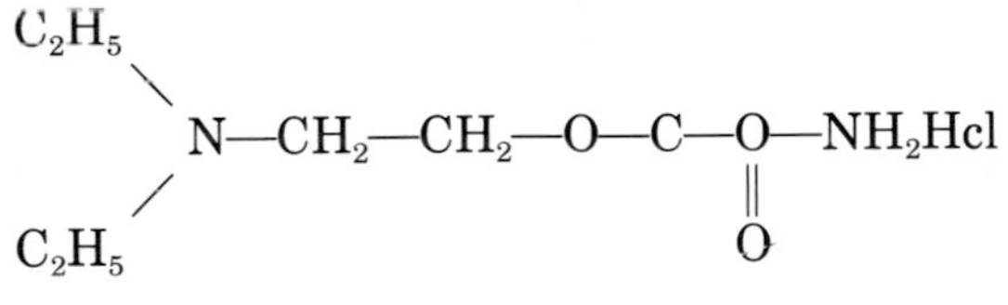

Procaine

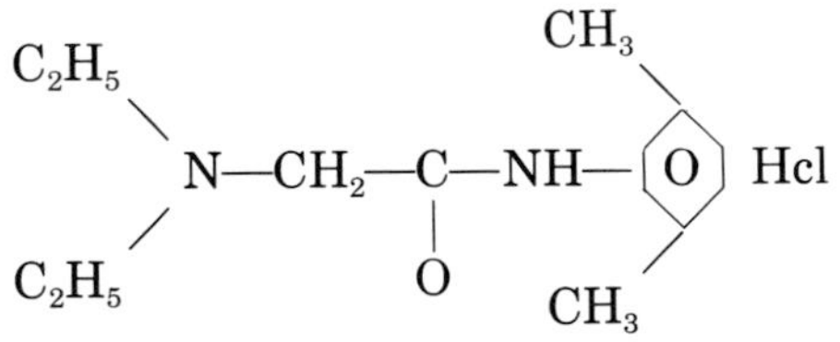

Lidocaine

Toxicity and Allergy

Although the thrust of anesthetic development and research has been to produce agents with increased potency and decreased toxicity, this generally has not been possible. As a rule, toxicity increases as potency increases.

Toxic reactions to local anesthetics are relatively common. True allergic reactions are extremely rare. The drug dosage required to produce central nervous system toxicity is shown in Table 4–2 (Covino and Vassallo, 1976).

Ester-type anesthetics (procaine, tetracaine) produce central nervous system stimulation (restlessness, agitation, and excitement) that may eventually lead to seizures.

Amide-type anesthetics (lidocaine, mepivacaine, bupivacaine) usually cause cortical depression (drowsiness, lethargy, sleep). If the amide dosage is significantly elevated, the cortical depression is followed by medullary stimulation (increased pulse rate, elevated blood pressure, elevated respiratory rate). The final stage of amide toxicity is generalized medullary depression with death secondary to respiratory depression (Steiner and Thompson, 1981).

True allergic reactions to local anesthetic agents are extremely rare and essentially confined to the ester group of agents. The amide group, although generally safe to give to a patient with a sensitivity to ester agents, should be given without preservatives, as methylparaben is often used and can cause an allergic reaction.

Although it is possible to carry out skin testing for sensitivity to the local anesthetic agents, the test is difficult to perform and interpret. For this reason its usefulness is somewhat controversial (Aldrete and Johnson, 1970; Incaudo and associates, 1978; de Shazo and Nelson, 1979; Fisher, 1979; Giovannitt and Bennett, 1979). However, at present an observed allergic reaction may represent a true anaphylactic reaction and should be treated as such. Allergic reactions are most likely the result of hapten formation (Giovannitt and Bennett, 1979).

Table 4–2. Central Nervous System Toxicity Dosage

Drug	Dose (mg/kg)
Ester Anesthetics	
Procaine	19
Tetracaine	2.5
Amide Anesthetics	
Lidocaine	6.5
Mepivacaine	10
Bupivacaine	1.6

In spite of the relative safety and frequency of usage, local anesthetic agents should be used with care. It is imperative that complete resuscitative equipment be immediately available when any local anesthetic is utilized.

REGIONAL ANESTHESIA IN HEAD AND NECK SURGERY

Efficiency in the administration of regional anesthesia in the head and neck area offers the plastic surgeon convenience and increased usefulness in a vast number of commonly performed procedures. Regional blocks provide one of the most widely used pain control methods in the head and neck area. With accurate patient assessment, as well as evaluation of the type of surgery to be performed, a minimum of risk and discomfort for the patient is ensured. Regional anesthesia by local infiltration of tissue and by nerve blocks has a success rate proportional to the accurate anatomic instillation of the anesthetic solution.

Although numerous variations of each type of nerve block exist and may be appropriate under different circumstances, the constant practice and application of a standard technique of each block yields the most consistent result. Properly administered, a regional block in the head and neck area should be successful in over 90 per cent of cases.

Patient Preparation

The choice of a type of anesthetic depends on many factors such as the patient's age, the medical and psychologic status, comprehension by the patient and the surgeon of the various procedures, the type of surgery to be performed, and the length of the proposed procedure. Two critical factors often inadequately evaluated are the patient's previous experience with regional blocks and the surgeon's efficiency in instilling the blocks. The patient's previous adverse experiences with regional block anesthesia may increase anxiety sufficiently to make a successful block extremely difficult. Conversely, a previous positive experience may greatly facilitate the administration of a successful block.

Patient preparation for regional anesthesia should follow routine protocols. A thorough medical history and physical examination should be standard. Preparation also includes a complete explanation of the procedure to be utilized to ensure a maximal degree of confidence on the part of the patient. An anxious patient is far more difficult to deal with than one who is optimistic and calm. Anxiety is often related to a fear of the unknown.

Preoperative restriction of oral intake is required; an interval of four to six hours is satisfactory in most cases to minimize nausea and vomiting, with the possible sequela of aspiration. In addition, there is always the possibility of an adverse reaction requiring intubation. Intubation with an empty stomach is less risky for the patient.

Preoperative sedation is often a useful adjunct and should always be considered. Many acceptable regimens exist that combine oral, intramuscular, and intravenous drugs, the use of which is often a matter of the surgeon's and the patient's preference. Anticholinergic agents are not required.

Attention to detail is extremely important in the preparation of the patient. Assurance of patient comfort and safety is paramount. With any procedure of significant length or complexity, an intravenous access route should be available. Moreover, supplementation of sedation as well as the administration of emergency drugs are facilitated if an intravenous line has previously been secured.

The instillation of a regional block in the head and neck area requires precise anatomic knowledge of the location of the nerve to be anesthetized and a safe approach. Any nerve that can be safely approached can be successfully blocked. Local infiltration of an anesthetic solution is also possible and follows the same general principles as local infiltration anesthesia in any anatomic area. Local infiltration anesthesia will not be further discussed here.

A significant number of acceptable anesthetic agents exist for regional nerve block anesthesia in the head and neck area. A complete list of all appropriate anesthetic agents that can be utilized in a regional nerve block is neither realistic nor appropriate. Numerous new agents become available on a yearly basis. The new agents usually offer a change only in the speed of metabolism, the relative strength, and occasionally the power of penetration. There is little intrinsic difference in either toxicity or effectiveness. Of all available agents, lidocaine remains the standard anesthetic agent for the head and neck area. It is much preferable for an individual surgeon to become comfortable with the use of one or two agents rather than to experiment with many types. The addition of vasoconstrictors, such as epinephrine or occasionally neosynephrine, prolongs the duration of action of the anesthetic and decreases toxicity by delaying its systemic uptake. This action allows for a more lengthy metabolism, and thus the total dosage may be augmented.

Regional Block of Scalp

The scalp is innervated by sensory branches from the trigeminal nerve as well as by cervical nerves. The forehead is principally supplied by the frontal nerve (supraorbital and supratrochlear) and by the zygomaticotemporal nerves. The temple receives its innervation from the temporal malar branch of the trigeminal nerve and from the auriculotemporal branch of the trigeminal nerve. The greater and lesser occipital nerves, which are distal branches of the cervical nerves, innervate the occipital and parietal regions. This series of nerves originates relatively deep in the soft tissue and rises to a subfascial plane in a line that encircles the head (Fig. 4–1). Although the precise location of each penetrating nerve is somewhat variable, the line of penetration into the subfascial area is relatively constant. Thus, blockage of the nerves of the scalp can be done effectively by instilling anesthetic solution in this line. Infiltration of an anesthetic solution easily anesthetizes the cranium, pericranium, fascia, subcutaneous tissue, and skin. The vascular supply to the scalp is in a similar distribution, and use of vasoconstrictors within the anesthetic solution significantly decreases bleeding during surgery in this area.

Instillation of an anesthetic solution follows a routine skin preparation. Depending on the surface to be anesthetized, an injection of 10 to 100 ml of 0.5 to 1.0 per cent lidocaine based on body weight with epinephrine, 1:100,000, is made. This is adequate anes-

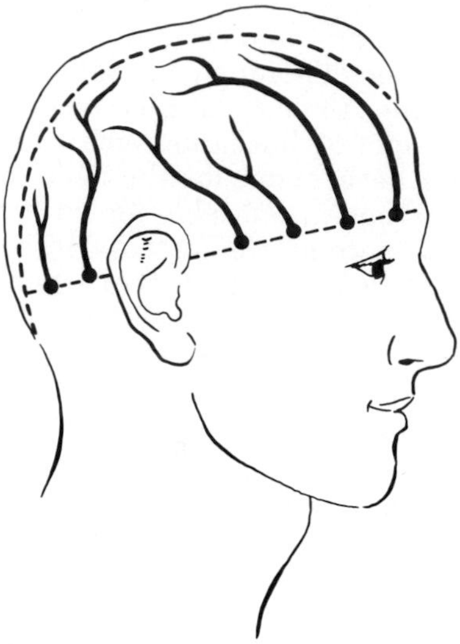

Figure 4–1. The sensory nerves to the scalp become subfascial in a relatively constant line encircling the head and passing through the occiput and glabella above the ears.

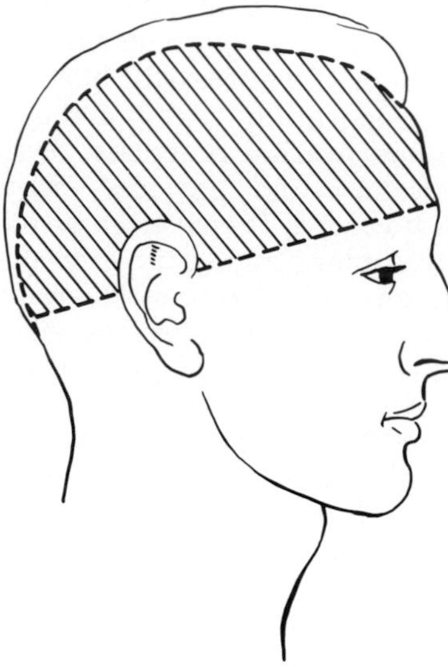

Figure 4–2. The regional anesthesia to the scalp is in a skullcap distribution.

thesia for one to two hours of surgery within five to 15 minutes after instillation. As previously mentioned, vasoconstrictive agents not only decrease bleeding but prolong the duration of anesthesia.

The anesthetic technique is carried out by defining a line that encircles the head and passes just above the ear and through the occiput and glabella. The injection should be into this area, to produce a wheal in the distribution to receive the surgery. Additional solution should be injected into the temporal fossa because of the increased muscle and soft tissue mass in this area. The area of anesthesia will be in a skullcap distribution after the block is complete (Fig. 4–2).

Regional Block of Forehead

The sensory innervation of the posterior scalp and facial areas is illustrated in Figure 4–3. The anterior portion of the scalp and face is innervated by branches of the trigeminal nerve. The posterior portions of the scalp as well as the neck and lower portion of the jaw are innervated by the cervical nerves.

Operations on the forehead and the scalp as far back as the lambdoid suture are made possible by regional block of the supratrochlear and supraorbital nerves. Regional blocks provide effective anesthesia in the forehead area. The location of these nerves can be aided by an understanding of the foramen through which they exit the bony structure of the skull (Fig. 4–4). Instillation of a few milliliters of 1 per cent lidocaine provides operative anesthesia within minutes. It is routinely safe to instill up to 10 ml of solution, although this quantity is usually not required. The addition of a vasoconstrictive agent is beneficial. The supraorbital notch

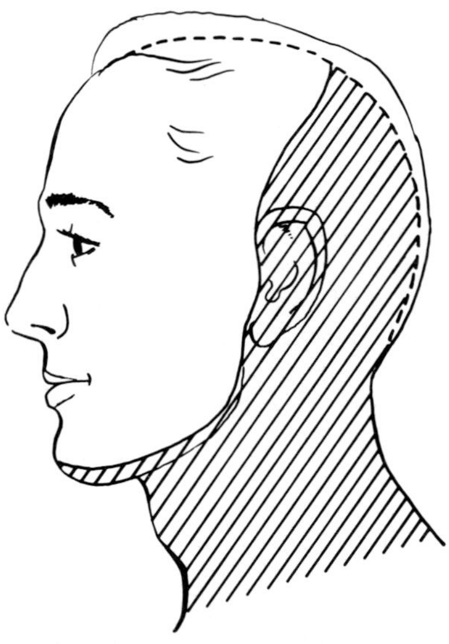

Figure 4–3. Sensory innervation of the head is divided into the face and anterior scalp, which is innervated by the trigeminal nerve, and the posterior scalp, neck, and portion of the lower jaw, which are innervated by the cervical nerves.

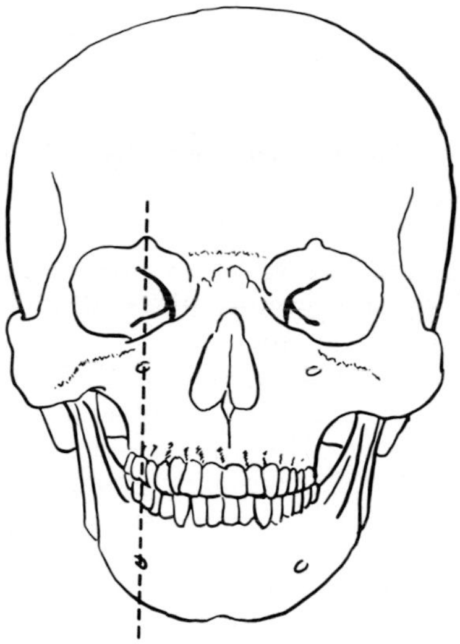

Figure 4–4. The supraorbital, infraorbital, and mental nerves exit the bony skull through foramina lying in a sagittal plane that also includes the pupil of the eye in a midgaze position.

can usually be palpated on the superior orbital rim. Injection of this area with 1 to 2 ml of anesthetic solution should produce paresthesias upon insertion of the needle. If paresthesias are not elicited, the solution can be injected when the needle strikes bone. Diffusion of the anesthetic agent provides relatively rapid anesthesia.

If anatomic palpation of the supraorbital foramen is difficult, it should be recalled that the supraorbital foramen, the infraorbital foramen, and the mental foramen lie on a straight line approximately 2.5 cm from the midline of the face. Therefore, location of one of these helps to determine the location of the others. The midline of the pupils routinely lies in this line (see Fig. 4–4).

Swelling and ecchymosis in the periorbital region are not unusual following this procedure, but are temporary and self-limited. Occasionally these signs last from several days to a week if the cause is hemorrhage.

Surgery near the midline of the forehead may require bilateral blocks.

Infraorbital and Alveolar Nerve Blocks

Blocks of the infraorbital and alveolar nerves can rapidly yield surgical anesthesia in the area of the lower eyelid, the lateral portion of the nose, the upper lip, the mucous membranes of the mouth, and the upper cuspid and incisor. Occasional temporary relief of dental pain is also possible.

The terminal portion of the maxillary nerve forms the infraorbital nerve. It emerges from the infraorbital foramen and divides into four branches: the inferior palpebral, the external nasal, the internal nasal, and the superior labial nerves (Fig. 4–5). The cutaneous sensory distribution is the lower eyelid, the lateral inferior portion of the nose, and the upper lip. The anterior superior alveolar nerve branches from this infraorbital nerve in the infraorbital canal to supply the upper incisor and cuspid teeth of the ipsilateral side.

Regional block of this nerve is possible with the instillation of 2 to 5 ml of 1 per cent lidocaine with epinephrine. This yields an adequate level of surgical anesthesia lasting approximately one hour. With the patient's head positioned perpendicular to the table, the infraorbital rim of the maxillary bone is located. The infraorbital foramen is then palpated. It is frequently difficult to palpate the foramen, and an approximation of 2.5 cm from the midline of the face is sufficiently accurate. This should lie just below the midline of the pupils, with the eyes in a straight forward gaze. The needle is inserted perpendicular to the skin, advanced, and stopped just inferior to the infraorbital rim (Fig. 4–6). Some texts describe advancing the needle into the foramen to elicit paresthesias. Although this may be done, it is unnecessary and risks injuring the nerve in the canal. Caution should be exercised to make the injection below the orbital rim and not within

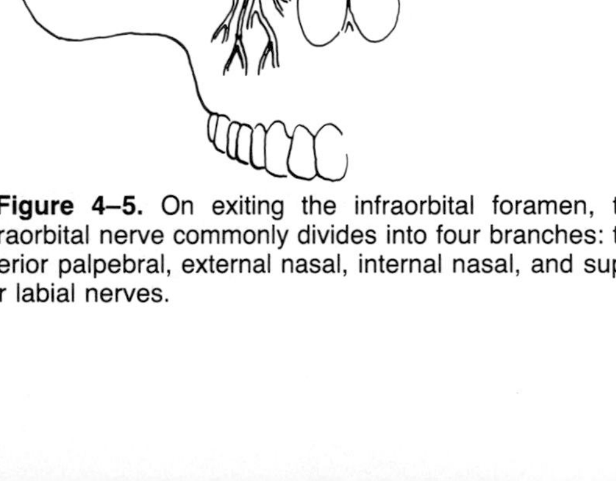

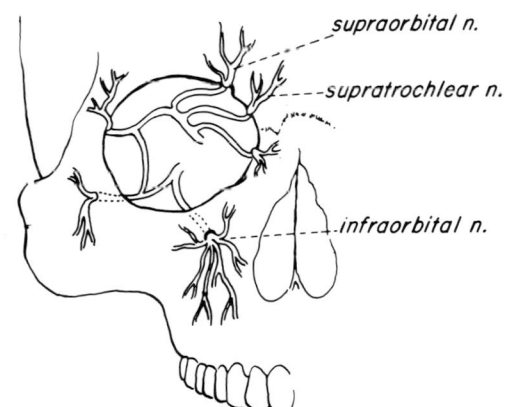

Figure 4–5. On exiting the infraorbital foramen, the infraorbital nerve commonly divides into four branches: the inferior palpebral, external nasal, internal nasal, and superior labial nerves.

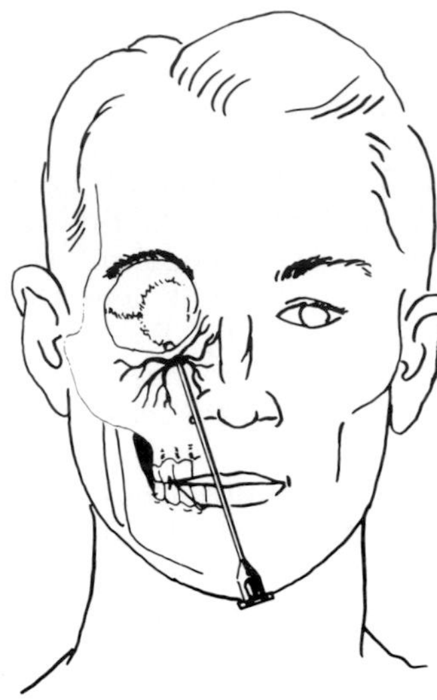

Figure 4–6. Infraorbital nerve block is obtained by inserting the needle as far as the infraorbital rim.

the orbital cavity. Paresthesias of the upper teeth as well as the upper lip may occur with advancement of the needle.

In addition to the routine complications of regional block, instillation of the anesthetic solution within the orbital cavity may produce a unique complication. If the needle is misplaced and the anesthetic solution is instilled within the orbit, the increase in intraorbital pressure may produce visual disturbances. Signs of increased pressure and hemorrhage into the orbital area include blurring of vision, diplopia, exophthalmos, loss of vision, and pain. These signs and symptoms routinely resolve as the anesthetic agent is absorbed, but may be of longer duration if the etiology is hemorrhage. If the local anesthetic solution alone is the cause, no specific treatment is indicated, since it is self-limiting. However, if the cause is felt to be secondary to hemorrhage (retrobulbar hematoma), a more complete ophthalmologic evaluation is indicated.

Anesthesia of the infraorbital nerve is extremely useful in many head and neck procedures. The distribution of complete surgical anesthesia is indicated in Fig. 4–7.

This nerve block is unusually easy to perform and complications are uncommon. Excellent anesthesia for surgery of the cheek and face results. For surgery near the midline of the face, bilateral blocks may be required. Although the quality of anesthesia is excellent, it disappears within 60 to 90 minutes. Reinstillation of this block can be performed in a cooperative patient.

Lower Incisor and Mental Nerve Blocks

The mandible and lower lips may be anesthetized by a regional block of the mental and lower incisor nerves.

The terminal branches of the inferior alveolar nerve forms the lower incisor and mental nerves. The mental nerve emerges from the mental foramen to provide sensation to the lower lips, the central mucous membranes, and the submental cutaneous area. The lower incisor nerve continues within the mandible to the symphysis to supply the incisor and bicuspid teeth (Fig. 4–8).

Instillation of this block is relatively safe and routinely successful. The mouth is closed to ensure laxity of the lips and cheeks. The cheek is retracted and the needle inserted into the mucous membrane between the bicuspids. The entry point is approximately 1 cm external to the buccal plate of the mandible. The needle is inserted at a 45 degree angle, aimed toward the apex of the root of the second bicuspid, and advanced until bone is contacted. Precise identification of the foramen is not routinely required. A successful block may be effected by the instillation of 0.5 to 1.0 ml of lidocaine. Usually, the needle is used to gently palpate the mandible until

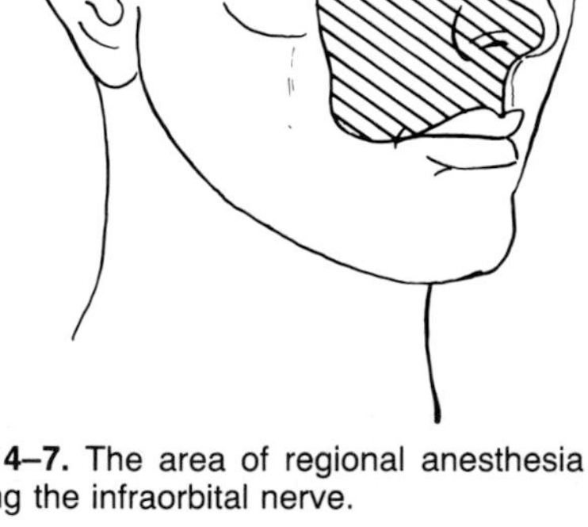

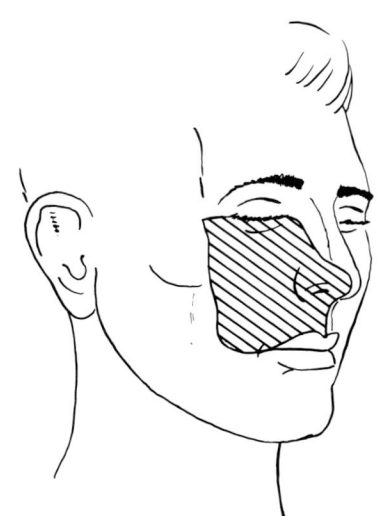

Figure 4–7. The area of regional anesthesia produced by blocking the infraorbital nerve.

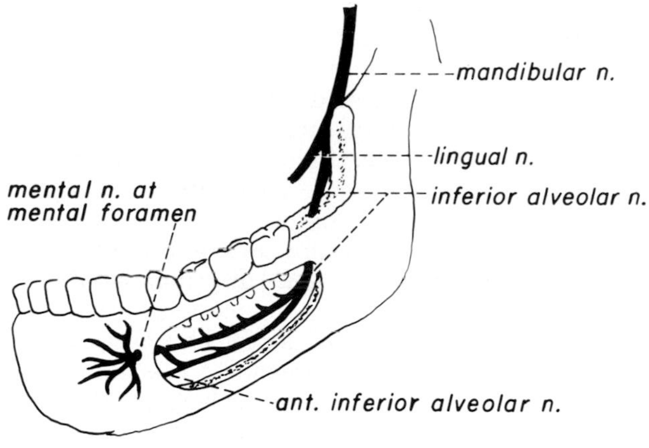

Figure 4–8. The anatomy of the inferior alveolar and the mental nerve.

the foramen is identified. An additional 0.5 to 1.0 ml of solution of lidocaine can be administered at that point. Surgical anesthesia is possible within five to ten minutes after injection.

Location of the mental foramen is important in this block. It is significant that the anatomic location varies according to the age of the patient. A young child has a foramen lying relatively close to the inferior border of the mandible below the first molar tooth. In an adult, the foramen lies in a plane midway between the upper and lower edge of the mandibular body below the second bicuspid. In an elderly patient with atrophy of the mandible, the mental foramen lies close to the upper margin of the mandible (Fig. 4–9).

Instillation of the anesthetic solution often elicits paresthesias in the distribution of the nerve, routinely described as electric-like shocks in the lower lip. As the needle and solution are further advanced, the paresthesias may be perceived in the anterior lower teeth.

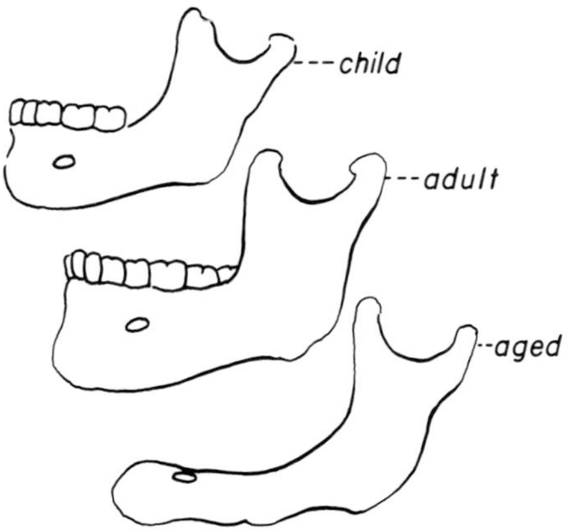

Figure 4–9. The location of the mental foramen varies with age and the status of the dentition.

If difficulty is encountered in locating the mental foramen, it should be recalled that it is in a vertical plane in line with the supraorbital notch, the infraorbital foramen, and the midpoint of the pupil (see Fig. 4–4).

It is important to aspirate before injecting the solution. When aspiration yielding blood occurs, as it does in 10 to 12 per cent of attempts, the needle should be repositioned. On occasions when the solution has been injected without repositioning the needle during a positive aspiration, intravenous and intra-arterial injections have occurred and produced acute overdose reactions. Intra-arterial injections have produced reversed flow in the artery, distributing anesthetic solution in the cerebral circulation.

Mandibular Nerve Blocks

Regional anesthesia of the mandible may be helpful during surgery and manipulation of the mandible. It is a useful technique to relax the masseter muscle in cases of trismus and neuralgia.

The mandibular branch is the third branch of the trigeminal nerve and is the largest of the three divisions. It exits from the skull through the foramen ovale and divides into a motor division and a larger sensory division. It courses opposite the mandibular notch between the coronoid and condyloid process of the mandible. Its sensory distribution is the pharynx, the lower teeth, the anterior two-thirds of the tongue, the mandible, and the postauricular regions. Numerous anatomic approaches have been described. However, it is perhaps most easily approached through the area of the infratemporal fossa just behind the pterygoid plate. At this point it courses in a downward direction. It can be one of the most helpful nerve blocks in the facial region. However, it also has the highest reported failure rate, being approximately 20 per cent in experienced hands.

Block of the mandibular nerve provides satisfactory anesthesia in the distribution of the inferior alveolar nerve, the mental nerve, and frequently the lingual nerve. This causes satisfactory surgical anesthesia of the mandibular teeth to the midline as well as the mucous membranes in this area and the anterior two-thirds of the tongue.

Successful utilization of this block depends on the correct identification of the anatomic site of injection. With the patient in the supine position, the mouth is opened widely. With palpation of the pterygomandibular raphe, the entry to the mucosa is located slightly lateral to this point. The retromolar fossa is palpated and the needle inserted into this area at a point parallel to the mandibular teeth at a 45 degree angle (Fig. 4–10). The advancing needle follows the posterior wall of the mandible. Paresthesias are often encountered but are not required. With the needle along the posterior wall, the injection is instilled. If the needle is situated either too low or too medial, paresthesias of the tongue secondary to stimulation of the lingual nerve may occur.

Sensory blocking with this injection provides complete anesthesia over the temporal region, the anterior two-thirds of the tongue, the mucous membranes, the lower lip, the temporomandibular joint, the salivary gland, and multiple local muscle groups. The area of cutaneous sensory anesthesia is illustrated in Figure 4–11.

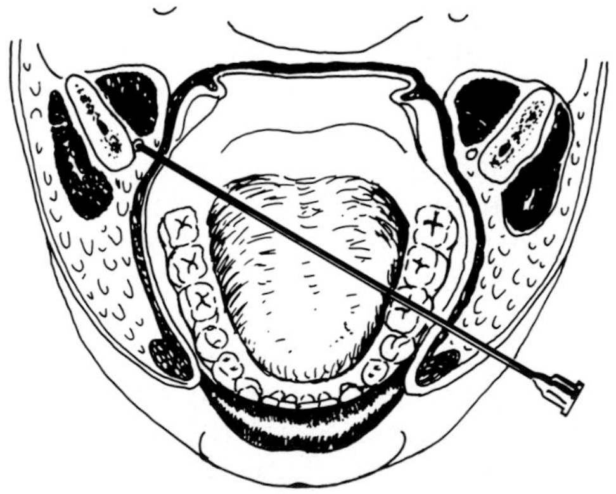

Figure 4–10. The mandibular nerve may be blocked by an intraoral approach along the posterior wall of the mandible (see text).

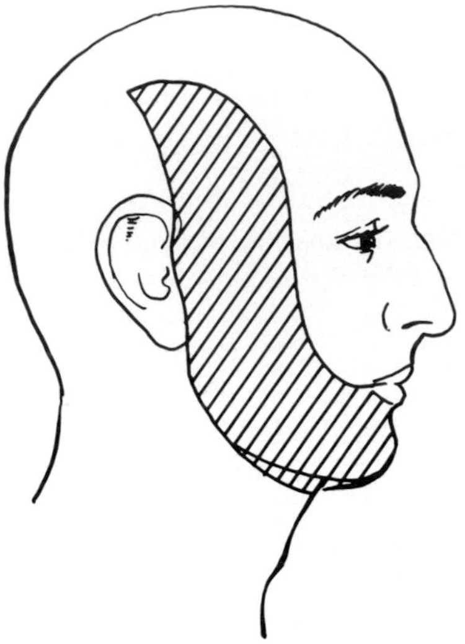

Figure 4–11. The cutaneous sensory block of the mandibular nerve produces surgical anesthesia over the inferior and lateral portion of the face.

It is important to aspirate before injection because of the multiple vessels in this area. If aspiration is negative, complications are rare. A hematoma in the region of injection is not uncommon; it is usually self-limiting and does not require therapy. Local pressure may be helpful in decreasing the size of the hematoma. Satisfactory surgical anesthesia for 60 to 90 minutes is possible. Although reinjection is feasible, more lengthy procedures are best performed with general anesthesia.

Regional Block of Maxilla

Surgical anesthesia and manipulation of the upper jaw and cheek are possible by means of regional block of the second division of the trigeminal nerve. The maxillary nerve exits the skull through the foramen rotundum. This foramen, situated in the greater wing of the sphenoid, is located slightly posterior and superior to the anterior ridge of the pterygoid plate. Subsequent to the emergence of the nerve from the fossa, it traverses the pterygoid palatine fossa to enter the orbit, and it is subsequently called the infraorbital nerve. Precise anesthetic blockage of this nerve provides anesthesia to the hemimaxilla.

Numerous anatomic approaches to this block have been described. Either an anterior or a lateral approach is effective. The anterior approach is made by palpating the anterior border of the coronoid process and the inferior margin of the malar bone. A long, fine needle is inserted perpendicular to the skin until contact is made with the maxillary bone. The needle is then withdrawn slightly and redirected superior and posterior to the fossa at a distance approximately 6 cm from the skin surface. Instillation of anesthetic solution is then performed after aspiration (Fig. 4–12). The anterior approach can also be made through an intraoral route. The approach is essentially the same except that the insertion of the needle is through the upper sulcus.

The lateral approach to the maxillary nerve block is by way of the sigmoid notch, and is begun by palpating the sigmoid notch with the patient's mouth slightly open and the jaw relaxed (Fig. 4–13). A small, external skin wheal is placed with the anesthetic solution. A long, thin needle is placed through the wheal and directed slightly anteriorly. At a depth of 4 to 5 cm the lateral pterygoid plate is encountered. The needle is then withdrawn slightly and reinserted in a more anterior and superior direction. This places the injecting needle anterior to the plate and into the sphenomaxillary fossa (Fig. 4–14). The needle is then advanced approximately 1 to 1.5 cm, the tip being placed in the vicinity of the maxillary nerve. After appropriate aspiration the solution is injected; paresthesias may be encountered. Figure 4–15 shows the areas of cutaneous anesthesia obtained by a maxillary block.

Complications with a maxillary nerve block are relatively predictable. Aspiration should

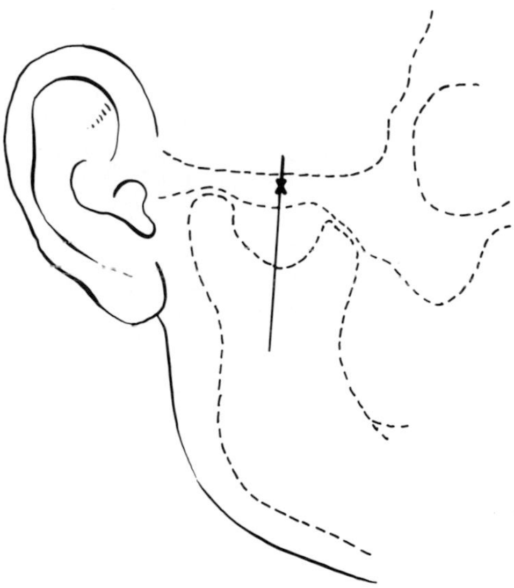

Figure 4–13. The lateral approach to the maxillary nerve block is initiated by palpating the sigmoid notch.

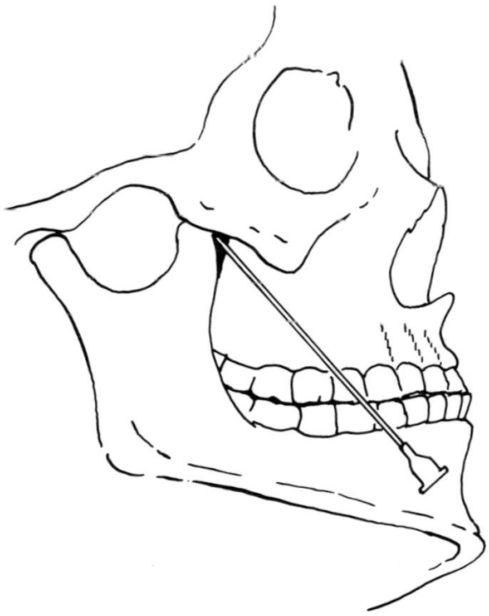

Figure 4–12. The anterior approach to the maxillary nerve block is superior and posterior to the coronoid process and the needle is directed into the sphenomaxillary fossa.

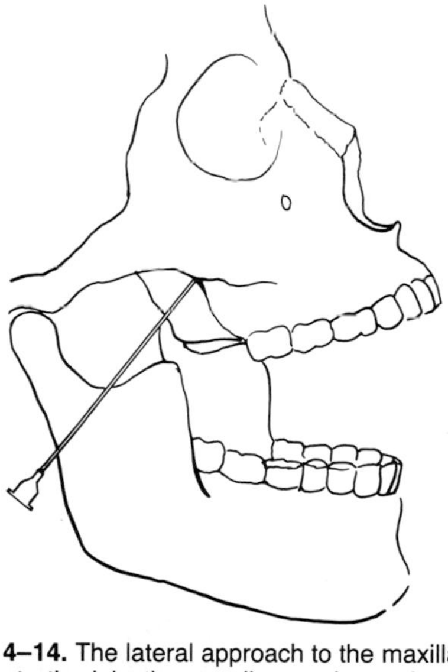

Figure 4–14. The lateral approach to the maxillary nerve block inserts the injecting needle anterior to the pterygoid plate and into the sphenomaxillary fossa.

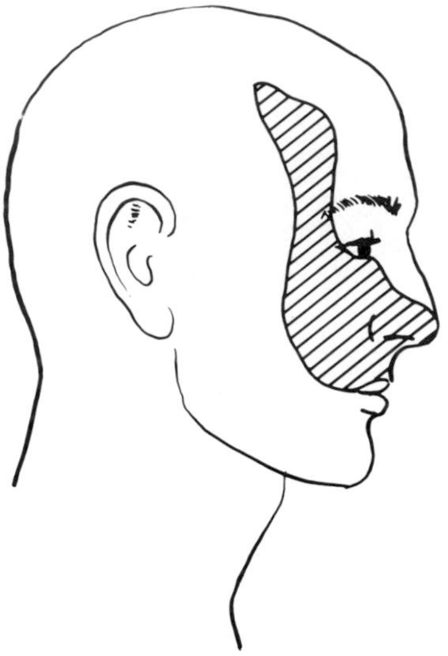

Figure 4–15. The cutaneous anesthesia produced by the maxillary nerve block.

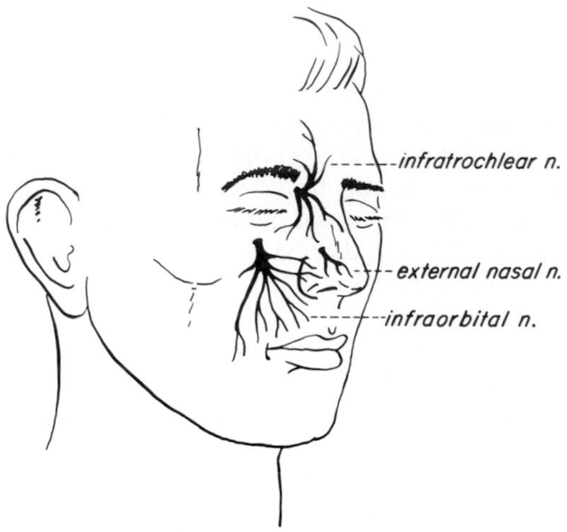

Figure 4–16. The cutaneous sensory nerve supply to the nose is predominantly from the infratrochlear, infraorbital, and external nasal nerves.

always be performed before injection of solution, and aspiration of blood precludes such injection. It is also possible to aspirate air through entry into the pharyngeal space. If either blood or air is encountered, the needle is redirected and the block may be safely continued.

Regional Block of Nose

Surgical anesthesia of the nose may be obtained by local infiltrating anesthesia, topical anesthesia through the mucous membranes, or regional blocks (see Chap. 35). A regional block of the nose is relatively easy but the technique suffers the disadvantage of lacking the wide infiltration of an epinephrine solution, which is helpful for vasoconstriction purposes.

Sensory innervation is predominantly derived from the infratrochlear nerve, the infraorbital nerve, and the nasal palatine and external nasal nerves (Fig. 4–16). Innervation of the anterior and internal portions of the nose is predominantly through branches of the sphenopalatine ganglion and the anterior ethmoidal nerves (Fig. 4–17).

Regional anesthesia of the external portion of the nose can be satisfactorily obtained by blockage of the previously described external innervation, as indicated in Figure 4–18. The use of 5 to 10 ml of 1 per cent lidocaine with epinephrine is adequate. Additional injections may be advisable to instill more epinephrine into the operative area.

A successful intranasal block is routinely obtained by the instillation of small cotton applicators dipped in a solution of 4 per cent cocaine. Placement of these on the inferior posterior nasal nerve, the nasopalatine nerve, and the superior posterior nasal nerve as well as branches of the ethmoidal nerve is successful. Precise localization of these nerves, as indicated in Figure 4–19, can minimize cocaine and anesthetic usage. On the other hand, the practice of packing the nose with plain gauze dipped in cocaine can also be utilized, although it is less precise anatomically.

Extreme caution should be used to avoid overdosage of the patient with cocaine. The practice of soaking nasal packing and cotton

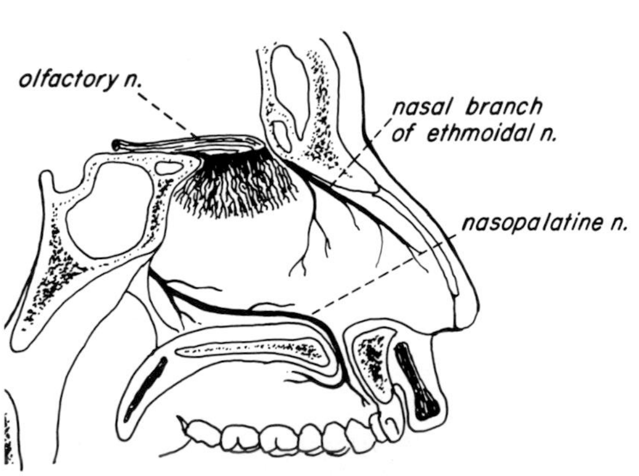

Figure 4–17. The innervation of the nasal cavity is through the ethmoidal and nasopalatine nerves.

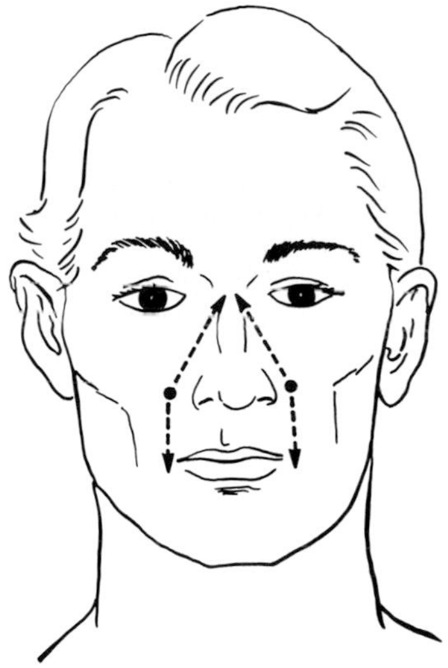

Figure 4–18. Technique for rapid nerve block of the external nose. The dotted lines indicate the path of the injecting needle.

with excessive amounts of cocaine to pack the nose should be avoided; it can lead to toxic systemic levels of cocaine through rapid absorption through the mucous membranes. Great care should be taken during the administration of cocaine, especially when other agents are also used. The simultaneous use of epinephrine, lidocaine, and cocaine in the nose must be approached with caution.

Regional Block of External Ear

Regional block of the external ear is relatively easily accomplished. Sensory innervation of the external ear is derived predominantly from the auriculotemporal nerve anteriorly and from the greater auricular nerve, the mastoid branch of the occipital nerve, and the occipital nerve itself posteriorly (Fig. 4–20). Although a satisfactory block can be obtained by infiltrating around the ear in a ringlike fashion, the use of an infiltration pattern, as indicated in Figures 4–21 and 4–22, gives a satisfactory level of anesthesia with a minimum of discomfort to the patient. The usual anesthetic solution is 1 per cent lidocaine with epinephrine 1:100,000.

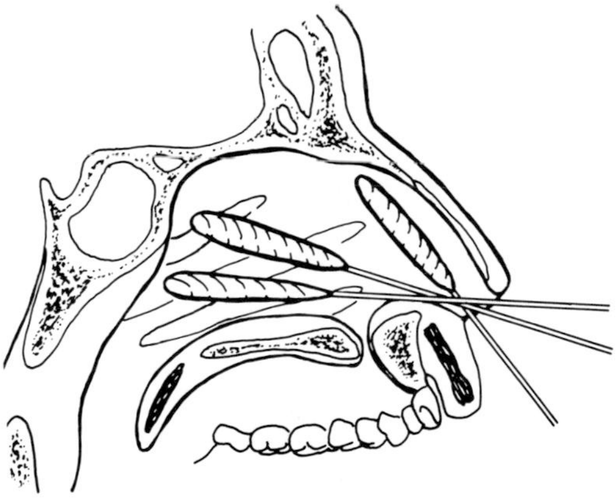

Figure 4–19. Nerve block of the internal portion of the nose can be achieved by the insertion of cotton applicators soaked in anesthetic solution.

Regional anesthesia of the upper extremity is discussed in Chapter 91.

GENERAL ANESTHESIA

The use of general anesthesia by the plastic surgeon is required not only in multiple operative sites but also in certain anatomic sites. The advantage of general anesthesia is that it makes possible the precise control of the patient's physiologic response as well as an increased control of pain and comfort for the patient. An overall understanding of the concepts of general anesthesia can only aid the surgeon in his preoperative assessment, intraoperative management, and postoperative care. Experienced anesthesiologists should be relied on to provide precise care and recommendations for the patient. Intraoperative therapeutic modification of the anesthetic state by means of relaxants, sedatives, diuretics, cardioactive drugs, reversal agents, and anesthetic drugs makes it possible to control the patient. In addition, the long-term medication taken by the patient for other reasons can also be administered during the anesthesia. Special techniques such as planned hypotension, hypothermia, or hyperventilation are also available.

The surgeon should work with the anesthesiologist to provide the utmost in patient safety and comfort. General anesthesia allows the patient the option of undergoing anesthesia in a much less stressful environment.

Multiple areas require special consideration on the part of the surgeon in relation to general anesthesia. The initial preoperative evaluation should be complete. It cannot be stressed too highly that the most critical aspect of the preoperative evaluation is a comprehensive history taking and physical examination. Numerous studies have been

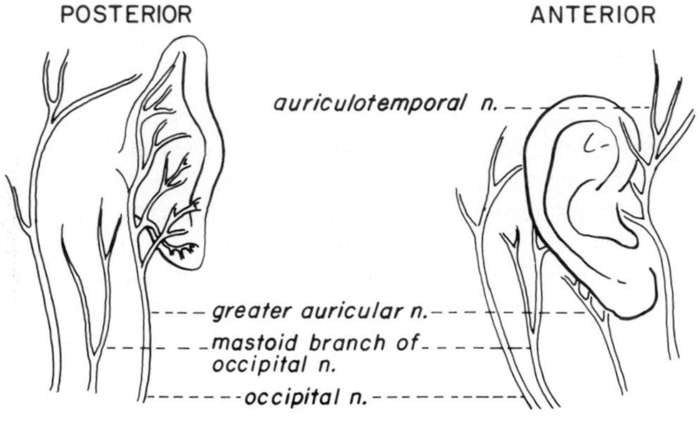

Figure 4–20. Sensory innervation of the external ear is predominantly derived from the auriculotemporal, greater auricular, mastoid branch of the occipital, and occipital nerves.

performed on the appropriateness of routine preoperative screening tests. These document that in the presence of a normal history and physical examination, no preoperative test has been shown to be universally beneficial.

Evaluation of the preoperative chest radiograph has been undertaken by multiple groups. Uniformly, the preoperative chest radiograph has been shown to be of no assistance in the decision to operate or in the choice of anesthesia (Royal College of Radiologists, 1979; Wood and Hoekelman, 1981; World Health Organization, 1983; Hubbell and associates, 1985; Tape and Mushlin, 1986). These studies demonstrated that in the patient with a normal history and physical examination, chest radiographs are not productive as a routine screening test. However, other studies have conclusively demonstrated that chest radiographs can be valuable in conjunction with either an abnormal medical history or physical examination referable to a pathologic chest condition. In addition, chest radiographs are recommended for patients undergoing an intrathoracic procedure.

Studies concerning the value of the electrocardiogram (ECG) yield similar results. Although abnormal ECG findings can be identified, usually in patients over 65 years of age, the impact of these findings either upon the scheduling of surgery or upon the intraoperative or postoperative management has not been found to be significant. An exception is the documentation of a cardiac or intrathoracic disorder, which makes ECG evaluation necessary. Current recommendations, based on prospective studies (Rabkin and Horne, 1983; Moorman and associates, 1985), are

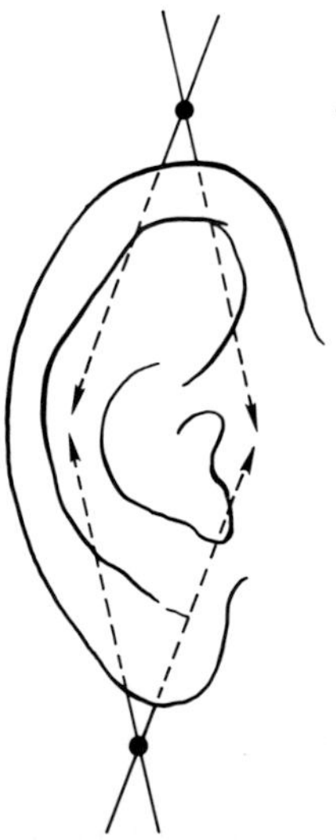

Figue 4–21. Method of regional anesthesia of the external ear. The arrows indicate the path of the injecting needle.

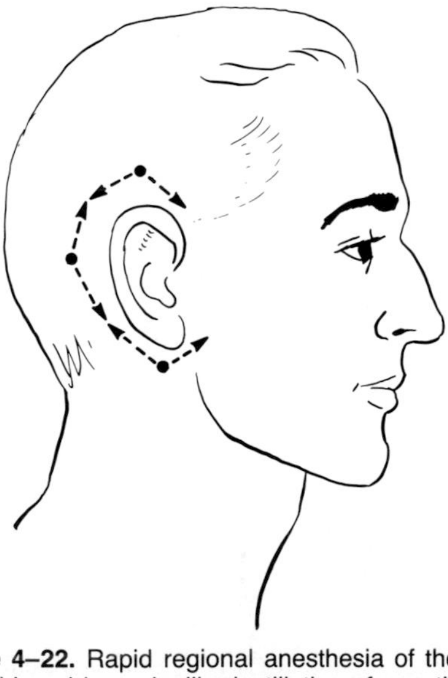

Figure 4–22. Rapid regional anesthesia of the external ear is achieved by a ringlike instillation of anesthetic solution. The arrows indicate the path of the injecting needle.

that ECGs should be obtained if there is evidence of a previous cardiac disorder. The usefulness of a baseline preoperative ECG has not been documented.

Evaluation of other routine laboratory tests yields similar results. The complete blood count, platelet count, leukocyte differential counts, serum chemistries, urinalysis, and activated partial thromboplastin and prothrombin time tests have all been shown to be not significantly beneficial in the patient with a totally negative medical history and physical examination (Korvin, Pearce, and Stanley, 1975; Shapiro, Hatch, and Greenfield, 1984; Kroenke and associates, 1986).

General Anesthesia Techniques

The primary consideration in any general anesthesia technique is the maintenance of an adequate airway. Endotracheal or nasotracheal intubation is generally used and is adequate. However, in difficult cases such as complex facial fractures, an elective tracheostomy may be necessary. The surgeon should also be prepared to carry out an emergency procedure if there is an unusual amount of swelling or trauma in the head and neck area. Occasionally, racemic epinephrine or steroids may be utilized to decrease tissue edema in these clinical situations. Intubation is usually performed when the patient arrives at the operating room, and this ordinarily requires visualization of the larynx. This type of direct laryngoscopy can also be utilized to assess trauma to the area in selected cases. Special fiberoptic instruments are available that may be used for nasotracheal intubation or bronchoscopy at the same time. They may also be utilized in situations of head and cervical spine trauma in which manipulation and hyperextension of the neck are ill advised. Other methods, such as preliminary digital intubation or a retrograde catheter technique, can be employed in circumstances of difficult intubation.

When a particular difficult intubation is anticipated or when the patient has eaten within the previous six to eight hours, the so-called awake intubation may be advised. During this procedure the patient may be mildly sedated, but he maintains his respiratory capacity and protective cough reflex. The procedure may be more frightening and uncomfortable for the patient but has the advantage of being safer.

Specific medications utilized during the course of general anesthesia are usually under the control of the anesthesiologist. Common intravenous medications include various narcotics, thiopental, etomidate, and ketamine, which offer various degrees of relaxation and analgesia. Under the careful monitoring of the anesthesiologist these agents are safe, but they all require continuous monitoring. Common inhalation anesthetics include nitrous oxide, halothane, enflurane, and isoflurane, which maintain the anesthetic level and decrease pain thresholds.

Multiple techniques and combinations of anesthetic agents are available. However, what is most important is that the anesthesiologist should have a plan available with which he feels comfortable. He should also be able to alter the plan intraoperatively if different conditions arise.

PEDIATRIC ANESTHESIA

Special anesthesia concerns are necessary for the pediatric patient, in whom preoperative preparation, intraoperative care, and postoperative considerations may be significantly different.

Preoperative preparation is similar in that an optimal physical and psychologic condition is essential. However, the possibilities of congenital anomalies, anemia (e.g., as in sickle cell disease), and recurrent pediatric illnesses should be considered (e.g., upper respiratory infection, otitis media). Attention should be given to the medical history with reference to premature birth, respiratory distress syndrome, and previous illnesses. Infants with a history of prematurity or respiratory distress syndrome should be strongly considered for inpatient monitoring, even for procedures that otherwise would be carried out on an outpatient basis. In these high risk infants, as many as one-third may experience postoperative respiratory problems (Steward, 1982).

Significant variation exists from institution to institution regarding preoperative oral intake and premedication orders. However, the guidelines listed in Table 4–3 are usually acceptable. It is important that the interval shown represents the time before surgery and not the time before the onset of the surgical day. Thus, a second or third patient on the operative schedule may be permitted to have oral fluids much later than the first patient.

Table 4–3. Preoperative Limitations of Oral Intake

Age	NPO
2–6 months	4 hours before surgery
6 months–2 years	6 hours before surgery
>2 years	8 hours before surgery

In general, younger children should be placed at the beginning of the operative schedule to minimize fluid problems and to optimize psychologic conditioning.

The preoperative psychologic response of a child is somewhat predictable and age dependent. Infants under 6 months of age generally have no psychologic difficulties at the time of surgery. Children aged between 6 months and 6 years may exhibit emotional stress from parental separation as well as from fear of pain or frightening experiences. Children aged between 6 and 12 years may fear the operation itself. Teenagers tend to minimize the fear of pain or surgery but become concerned about the anesthesia, the outcome, and the perioperative loss of control of the environment. Attention to psychologic preparation by the surgeon and anesthesiologist can do much to reduce the anxiety associated with the perioperative period.

Premedication should be used with care in the pediatric patient. There seems to be a general trend by anesthesiologists to minimize premedication in children and administer whatever is necessary in the operating room. The major concern is that of the small dosages required and often the small difference between the proper amount and overdosage. Physicians unaccustomed to pediatric drug dosages are advised to work closely with a pediatric anesthesiologist.

Useful premedications and appropriate dosages are set out in Table 4–4.

General anesthesia technique may take many acceptable forms and is appropriately customized to the patient and the procedure to be performed. There are two critical areas in which the surgeon must be involved. The first is monitoring and maintenance of an adequate airway. The requirement for frequently operating around the head and neck region, as well as the unusual head and neck positions (such as in cleft palate or intraoral surgery) and intraoperative changes in these positions, make vigilance mandatory. Maintenance or reestablishment of an adequate airway has priority over any other aspect of surgery.

The second area of concern to the surgeon is the maintenance of appropriate fluid and electrolyte metabolism. Prohibition of fluids for 24 hours may result in as much as a 10 per cent loss of body fluids in an infant. Thus, the time of fluid deprivation before surgery should be minimized. Clear liquids should specifically be offered to the child just before fluid restriction is begun. In addition, preexisting fluid and electrolyte abnormalities should be corrected before surgery. Fluid requirements are based on maintenance fluids plus replacement of losses. The most widely accepted method of estimating fluid requirements in children is based on caloric expenditure per body weight (Graves, 1982). This takes into account the observation that for children weighing less than 10 kg, 100 calories per kg are expended every 24 hours; the next 10 kg of weight require 50 calories per kg; weight over 20 kg demands 10 to 20 calories per kg; 1 ml of fluid is required per calorie. The maintenance volume is shown in Table 4–5.

Five per cent dextrose in 0.2 per cent sodium chloride closely approximates electrolyte requirements (3 mEq sodium, 2 mEq chloride per 100 ml fluid).

Table 4–4. Pediatric Preoperative Drugs and Dosages

Classification	Drug	Dose	Usual Route of Administration
Barbiturates	Secobarbital	2–6 mg/kg	PO, IM
	Pentobarbital	1–2 mg/kg	PO, IM
Narcotics	Morphine	0.1 mg/kg	IM
	Meperidine	1.0 mg/kg	IM
Sedatives	Diazepam	0.2–0.5 mg/kg	IV, IM
	Chlorpromazine	0.5 mg	PO, IM
	Hydroxyzine	1.0 mg–1 gm	IM
Anticholinergics	Atropine	0.02 mg/kg	IM
	Glycopyrrolate	0.01 mg/kg	IM

Table 4–5. Maintenance Fluid in Pediatric Patients

Body Weight	Daily Requirement	Hourly Requirement
0–10 kg	100 ml/kg	4 ml/kg
11–20 kg	1000 ml + 50 ml/kg over 10 kg	40 ml + 2 ml/kg over 10 kg
>20 kg	1500 ml + 20 ml/kg over 20 kg	60 ml + 1 ml/kg over 20 kg

Attention to blood loss is critical. A volume loss that would be insignificant in an adult may be critical in an infant. Rapid blood loss should be replaced with blood. Slower blood loss may be replaced with starch, Plasmanate, or lactated Ringer's solution, and the hematocrit and hemodynamic parameters should be monitored closely. It is generally recommended that the hematocrit be maintained above 30 per cent. Large blood losses and replacements require the monitoring of clotting parameters. Perioperative assurance of adequate fluids is still best obtained by monitoring blood pressure, pulse, and urinary output.

Intraoperative administration of epinephrine is helpful and relatively safe in infants. The arrhythmogenic potential of epinephrine is well documented, particularly with the concomitant usage of halothane. Although the maximal allowable dosage has not been determined, it has been shown that doses of up to 10 mg per kg of epinephrine can be safely used in pediatric patients who are not hypercapnic (Karl and associates, 1983).

KETAMINE

Although several intravenous anesthetic agents exist, ketamine has evolved as the most useful at the present time. Ketamine was first synthesized by Stevens in 1963 (Zsigmond and Domino, 1980) as 2-(2-chlorophenyl)-2-(methylamino) cyclohexanone HCl. It exists as two isomers, the dextrorotatory isomer being the more potent (Dundee and Wyant, 1974; Mariett and associates, 1977; Ryder, Way, and Trevor, 1978). Ketamine was approved for general clinical use in 1970.

Ketamine produces a "dissociative" anesthetic state. Electroencephalographic studies indicate a functional dissociation between the thalamoneocortical and limbic systems (Corssen, Miyasaka, and Domino, 1968). Thus, a state of unconsciousness occurs in which the patients exhibit analgesia and amnesia but have the clinical appearance of only mild sedation. The onset of anesthesia is rapid (20 to 60 seconds) and recovery from a single dose (2 mg/kg) requires 10 to 15 minutes.

Ketamine anesthesia maintains protective airway reflexes and is the only intravenous anesthetic that routinely produces cardiovascular stimulation. (Corssen and Domino, 1966). Blood pressure, heart rate, and cardiac output may be significantly increased (Dundee and Wyant, 1974; Zsigmond and Domino, 1980). The mechanism of stimulation is probably secondary to central nervous system sympathetic stimulation. Previous sedation of the central sympathetic system (such as earlier administration of halothane) blocks the ketamine stimulation (Stanley, 1973). Ketamine administration produces some antiarrhythmic effects (Dowdy and Kaya, 1968; Goldberg, Keane, and Phear, 1970) and has been recommended for patients undergoing cardiac procedures (Corssen and associates, 1970; Yoon, Zsigmond, and Kothary, 1975; Zsigmond and Domino, 1980). However, its tendency to produce tachycardia may stimulate tachyarrythmias (Cabbabe and Behbahani, 1985). A peripheral effect of ketamine has been postulated to explain the associated cardiovascular stimulation. The drug has been shown to desensitize peripheral arterial baroreceptors (Dowdy and Kaya, 1968). This effect would decrease the negative feedback impulses and result in increased pulse and blood pressure. Although the theory is sound, the relative contribution of desensitization versus sympathetic stimulation is unknown.

Ketamine anesthesia is relatively protective of the respiratory system. Upper airway protective reflexes are usually maintained (Taylor and Towey, 1971). The respiratory rate may be slightly depressed for the first few minutes (Podlesch and Zindler, 1967; Dundee and Wyant, 1974). Because of this effect, ketamine has enjoyed increasing popularity. However, with rapid administration or with narcotic premedication, apnea may be produced (Podlesch and Zindler, 1967). In addition, care must be exercised in patients with a full stomach. Studies have shown that despite a relatively active upper airway protective reflex, aspiration can occur (Taylor and Towey, 1971; Carson and associates, 1973).

The major limitation to a more widespread usage of ketamine has been the presence of the so-called emergence reactions, the occurrence of hallucination, delirium, and other psychic reactions, occasionally up to several weeks after administration (Fine and Finestone, 1973; Johnstone, 1973; Gallozzi, 1980). The reported incidence of adverse psychic emergence reactions varies up to 30 per cent (White, Way, and Trevor, 1982). Attempts to decrease this incidence have met with mixed results. The use of diazepam (Valium) preoperatively or concomitantly has been reported to decrease adverse reactions (McLean, 1971; Beekhuis, Klegon, and Kahn, 1978; Pandit, Kothary, and Kumar, 1980; Vinnik, 1980, 1981). A subsequent study reported a decreased incidence of unpleasant dreams or adverse reactions with ketamine (Cunningham and McKinney, 1983).

REFERENCES

Adriani, J., and Rovenstine, E. A.: The effect of anesthetic drugs upon bronchi and bronchioles of excised lung tissue. Anesthesiology, *4*:253, 1943.

Aldrete, J. A., and Johnson, D. A.: Evaluation of intracutaneous testing for investigation of allergy to local anesthetic agents. Anesth. Analg., *49*:173, 1970.

Beekhuis, G. J., Klegon, R. B., and Kahn, D. L.: Anesthesia for facial cosmetic surgery: low dosage ketamine-diazepam anesthesia. Laryngoscope, *88*:1709, 1978.

Bellville, J. W., and Seed, J. C.: The effect of drugs on the respiratory response to carbon dioxide. Anesthesiology, *21*:727, 1960.

Brown, P. R., Main, D. M., and Lawson, J. I.: Diazepam in dentistry: report on 108 patients. Br. Dent. J., *125*:498, 1968.

Brown, R. D.: The failure of local anaesthesia in acute inflammation. Some recent concepts. Br. Dent. J., *151*:47, 1981.

Cabbabe, E. B., and Behbahani, P. M.: Cardiovascular reactions associated with the use of ketamine and epinephrine in plastic surgery. Ann. Plast. Surg., *15*:50, 1985.

Carson, I. W., Moore, J., Balmer, J. P., and associates: Laryngeal competence with ketamine and other drugs. Anesthesiology, *38*:128, 1973.

Corssen, G., Allarde, R., Brosch, F., and associates: Ketamine as the sole anesthetic in open-heart surgery: a preliminary report. Anesth. Analg., *49*:1025, 1970.

Corssen, G., and Domino, F. F.: Dissociative anesthesia: further pharmacologic studies and first clinical experience with the phencyclidine derivative CI-581. Anesth. Analg., *45*:29, 1966.

Corssen, G., Miyasaka, M., and Domino, E. F.: Changing concepts in pain control during surgery: dissociative anesthesia with CI-581. A progress report. Anesth. Analg., *47*:746, 1968.

Covino, B. G., and Vassallo, H. G.: Local Anesthetics: Mechanisms of Action and Clinical Use. New York, Grune & Stratton, 1976.

Cunningham, B. L., and McKinney, P.: Patient acceptance of dissociative anesthetics. Plast. Reconstr. Surg., *72*:22, 1983.

DeCastro, G., and Mundeleer, P.: Anaesthesie sans sommeil, "la neuroleptanalgesia." Acta Chir. Belg., *58*:689, 1959.

de Shazo, R. D., and Nelson, H. S.: An approach to the patient with a history of local anesthetic hypersensitivity: experiences with 90 patients. J. Allergy Clin. Immunol., *63*:387, 1979.

Dowdy, E. G., and Kaya, K.: Studies of the mechanism of cardiovascular responses to CI-581. Anesthesiology, *29*:931, 1968.

Drews, J. H., Dripps, R. D., and Comroe, J. H.: Clinical studies on morphine. II. Effect of morphine upon the circulation of man and upon the circulatory and respiratory responses to tilting. Anesthesiology, *7*:44, 1946.

Dundee, J. W.: Benzodiazepines in anesthesia. *In* Aldrete, J. A., and Stanley, T. H. (Eds.): Trends in Intravenous Anesthesia. Chicago, Year Book Medical Publishers, 1980.

Dundee, J. W., and Wyant, G. M.: Intravenous Anaesthesia. Edinburgh, Churchill Livingstone, 1974, pp. 219–247.

Eckenhoff, J. E., and Oech, S. R.: The effects of narcotics and antagonists upon respiration and circulation in man. Clin. Pharmacol. Ther., *1*:483, 1960.

Eckstein, J. W., Hamilton, W. K., and McCammond, J. M.: The effect of thiopental on peripheral venous tone. Anesthesiology, *22*:525, 1961.

Egbert, L. D., Battit, G. E., Turndorf, H., and associates: The value of the preoperative visit by an anesthetist. J.A.M.A., *185*:553, 1963.

Einhorn, A.: Ueber die Chemie der localen Anaesthetica. München. Med. Wochenschr., *46*:1218, 1899.

Fine, J., and Finestone, S. C.: Sensory disturbances following ketamine anesthesia: recurrent hallucinations. Anesth. Analg., *52*:428, 1973.

Fisher, M. McD.: Intradermal testing in the diagnosis of acute anaphylaxis during anaesthesia—results of five years' experience. Anaesth. Intensive Care, *7*:58, 1979.

Foldes, F. F., Swerdlow, M., and Siker, S. S.: Narcotics and Narcotic Antagonists. Springfield, IL, Charles C Thomas, 1964, pp. 55–56.

Gallozzi, E.: Is there a place for the use of ketamine in plastic and reconstructive surgery? Ann. Plast. Surg., *4*:85, 1980.

George, K. A., and Dundee, J. W.: Relative amnesic actions of diazepam, flunitrazepam and lorazepam in man. Br. J. Clin. Pharmacol., *4*:45, 1977.

Giovannitt, J. A., and Bennett, C. R.: Assessment of allergy to local anesthetics. J. Am. Dent. Assoc., *98*:701, 1979.

Goldberg, A. H., Keane, P. W., and Phear, W. P.: Effects of ketamine on contractile performance and excitability of isolated heart muscle. J. Pharmacol. Exp. Ther., *175*:388, 1970.

Graves, S. A.: Pediatric blood and fluid therapy. *In* Thirty-third Annual Refresher Course Lectures of the American Society of Anesthesiologists, 1982, p. 224.

Greenblatt, D. J., and Shader, R. I.: Drug therapy. Benzodiazepines. N. Engl. J. Med., *291*:1011, 1239, 1974.

Guerra, F.: Thiopental forever after. *In* Aldrete, J. A., and Stanley, T. H. (Eds.): Trends in Intravenous Anesthesia. Chicago, Year Book Medical Publishers, 1980.

Halsted, W. S.: Practical comments on the use and abuse of cocaine; suggested by its invariably successful employment in more than a thousand minor surgical operations. N. Y. Med. J., *42*:294, 1885.

Hubbell, F. A., Greenfield, S., Tyler, J. L., Chetty, K., and Wyle, F. A.: The impact of routine admission chest x-ray films on patient care. N. Engl. J. Med., *312*:209, 1985.

Incaudo, G., Schatz, M., Patterson, R., Rosenberg, M., Yainamoto, F., and Hamburger, R. N.: Administration of local anesthetics to patients with a history of prior adverse reaction. J. Allergy Clin. Immunol., *61*:339, 1978.

Jansen, P. A. J.: The pharmacology of haloperidol. Int. J. Neuropsych., *3* (Suppl. 1):10, 1967.

Johnstone, R. E.: Letter: a ketamine trip. Anesthesiology, *39*:460, 1973.

Karl, H. W., Swedlow, D. B., Lee, K. W., and Downes, J. J.: Epinephrine-halothane interactions in children. Anesthesiology, *58*:142, 1983.

Klotz, U., Avant, G. R., Hoyumpa, A., and associates: The effects of age and liver disease on the disposition and elimination of diazepam in adult man. J. Clin. Invest., *55*:347, 1975.

Koller, C.: Vorläufige Mittheilung über locale Anästhesirung am Auge. Ber. Versomml. Ophth. Gesellsch., Stuttgart, *16*:60, 1884.

Korvin, C. C., Pearce, R. H., and Stanley, J.: Admissions screening: clinical benefits. Ann. Intern. Med., *83*:197, 1975.

Kroenke, K., Hanley, J. F., Copley, J. B., Matthews, J. I., Davis, C. E., et al.: The admission urinalysis: impact on patient care. J. Gen. Int. Med., 1:238, 1986.

Lee, C. M., and Yeakel, A. E.: Patient refusal of surgery following Innovar premedication. Anesth. Analg., *54*:224, 1975.

Lofgren, N.: Studies on Local Anesthetics: Xylocaine, A New Synthetic Drug. Stockholm, Ivar Haeggstroms, 1948.

Long, G., Dripps, R. D., and Price, H. L.: Measurement of antiarrhythmic potency of drugs in man: effects of dehydrobenzoperidol. Anesthesiology, *28*:318, 1967.

Marietta, M. P., Way, W. L., Castagnoli, N., Jr., and associates: On the pharmacology of the ketamine enantiomorphs in the rat. J. Pharmacol. Exp. Ther., *202*:157, 1977.

McLean, A. G.: Ketamine and diazepam in the adult patient. Med. J. Aust., *2*:338, 1971.

Moorman, J. R., Hlatky, M. A., Eddy, D. M., and Wagner, G. S.: The yield of the routine admission electrocardiogram. Ann. Intern. Med., *103*:590, 1985.

Morrison, J. D.: Neurolept techniques. *In* Dundee, J. W., and Wyant, G. M. (Eds.): Intravenous Anaesthesia. Edinburgh, Churchill Livingstone, 1974.

Muldoon, S. M., Janssens, W. J., Verbeuren, T. J., and Vanhoutte, P. M.: Alpha-adrenergic blocking properties of droperidol on isolated blood vessels of the dog. Br. J. Anaesth., *49*:211, 1977.

Niemann, A.: Quarterly J. Pract. Pharmacol., *9*:489, 1860. *From* Über eine neue organische Base in den Cocablättern. Göttingen, E. A. Hute, 1860, 52 pp.

Pandit, S. K., Kothary, S P., and Kumar, S. M.: Low-dose intravenous infusion technique with ketamine. Amnesic, analgesic and sedative effects in human volunteers. Anaesthesia, *35*:669, 1980.

Patton, C. M., Jr.: Rapid induction of acute dyskinesia by droperidol. Anesthesiology, *43*:126, 1975.

Podlesch, I., and Zindler, M.: Erste Erfahrungen mit dem Phencyclidinderivat Ketamine (CI-581), einen neuen intravenosen und intramuskularen Narkosemittel. Anaesthesist, *16*:299, 1967.

Puddy, B. R.: Effects of droperidol on the vasoconstriction produced by noradrenaline, histamine, sympathetic nerve stimulation and potassium ions in the isolated rabbit auricular artery. Br. J. Anaesth., *43*:441, 1971.

Rabkin, S. W., and Horne, J. M.: Preoperative electrocardiography: effect of new abnormalities on clinical decisions. Can. Med. Assoc. J., *128*:146, 1983.

Rao, S., Sherbaniuk, R. W., Prasad, K., and associates: Cardiopulmonary effects of diazepam. Clin. Pharmacol. Ther., *14*:182, 1973.

Robson, J. G., Davenport, H. T., and Sugiyama, R.: Differentiation of two types of pain by anesthetics. Anesthesiology, *26*:31, 1965.

Royal College of Radiologists: Preoperative chest radiography. National Study. Lancet, *2*:83, 1979.

Ryder, S., Way, W. L., and Trevor, A. J.: Comparative pharmacology of the optical isomers of ketamine in mice. Eur. J. Pharmacol., *49*:15, 1978.

Sadove, M. S., Balagot, R. C., and McGrath, J. M.: Effects of chlordiazepoxide and diazepam on the influence of meperidine on the respiratory response to carbon dioxide. J. New Drugs, *5*:121, 1965.

Shapiro, M. F., Hatch, R. L., and Greenfield, S.: Cost containment and labor-intensive tests: the case of the leukocyte differential count. J.A.M.A., *252*:231, 1984.

Stanley, T. H.: Blood pressure and pulse-rate responses to ketamine during general anesthesia. Anesthesiology, *39*:648, 1973.

Stanley, T. H., and Webster, L. R.: Anesthetic requirements and cardiovascular effects of fentanyl-oxygen and fentanyl-diazepam-oxygen anesthesia in man. Anesth. Analg., *57*:411, 1978.

Steiner, R. B., and Thompson, R. D. Local anesthesia. *In* Miller, R. D. (Ed.): Anesthesia. Edinburgh, Churchill Livingstone, 1981, pp. 195–497.

Steward, D. J.: Preterm infants are more prone to complications following minor surgery than are term infants. Anesthesiology, *56*:304, 1982.

Stovner, J., and Endresen, R.: Intravenous anaesthesia with diazepam. Proceedings of the 2nd European Congress on Anaesthesiology. Acta Anaesthesiol. Scand. (Suppl.), *24*:223, 1966.

Suchman, A. L., and Griner, P. F.: Diagnostic uses of the activated partial thromboplastin time and prothrombin time. Ann. Intern. Med., *104*:810, 1986.

Tape, T. G., and Mushlin, A. I.: The utility of routine chest radiographs. Ann. Intern. Med., *104*:663, 1986.

Taylor, P. A., and Towey, R. M.: Depression of laryngeal reflexes during ketamine anaesthesia. Br. Med. J., *2*:688, 1971.

Vinnik, C. A.: Is there a place for the use of ketamine in plastic and reconstructive surgery? Ann. Plast. Surg., *4*:86, 1980.

Vinnik, C. A.: An intravenous dissociation technique for outpatient plastic surgery: tranquility in the office surgical facility. Plast. Reconstr. Surg., *67*:799, 1981.

White, P. F., Way, W. L., and Trevor, A. J.: Ketamine—

its pharmacology and therapeutic uses. Anesthesiology, *56*:119, 1982.

WHO Scientific Group on the indications for and limitations of major x-ray diagnostic investigations: a rational approach to radiodiagnostic investigations. Geneva, Switzerland. World Health Organization, *689*:7, 1983.

Wood, R. A., and Hoekelman, R. A.: Value of the chest x-ray as a screening test for elective surgery in children. Pediatrics, *67*:447, 1981.

Yoon, M., Zsigmond, E. K., and Kothary, S. P.: A new anesthetic technique: analgesia with diazepam-ketamine-pancuronium in cardiac surgical patients. Comm. Anesth., *5*:10, 1975.

Zsigmond, E. K., and Domino, E. F.: Clinical pharmacology and current uses of ketamine. *In* Aldrete, J. A., and Stanley, T. H. (Eds.): Trends in Intravenous Anesthesia. Chicago, Year Book Medical Publishers, 1980, pp. 283–328.

5

Erle E. Peacock, Jr.
I. Kelman Cohen

Wound Healing

An understanding of the mechanisms of wound healing has increased dramatically during the past decade. Younger readers of this chapter will practice surgery in a generation in which the control of various healing processes should be more common than the treatment of beta-hemolytic streptococcal infection with penicillin. However, 50 years ago this infection was a virulent killer until Fleming made a rather simple laboratory observation and saved mankind from the horrors of major infections (Maurois, 1959). Today, wound healing abnormalities, rather than infection, are among the greatest causes of human disability, deformity, and even death. Although far more people suffer and even die each year from wound healing abnormalities than are saved by organ transplantation or cancer chemotherapy, research support has been meager in comparison with these more dramatic disease states (Trunkey, 1983). Perhaps this is because "wound healing" is a broad, multifaceted subject. The villain cannot be identified with a single word such as *cancer* or *hypertension*. In spite of these obstacles, considerable progress has been made.

What excites the student of wound healing today are the many findings over the past decade that *abnormal wound healing* may occur in previously unrecognized, as well as in recognized, conditions. Moreover, some of these conditions can now be corrected or at least improved by appropriate therapeutic intervention, and many other conditions are being biochemically defined in order to bring treatment within the clinician's immediate grasp. Most important, clinical surgeons and investigators are now beginning to realize that what was once considered normal and acceptable healing is neither normal nor acceptable. To say that a skin wound that remains closed represents normal healing is naive.

Most of the progress in the understanding of wound healing has been, and will continue to be, made in understanding and treating conditions such as keloid, cirrhosis, and tendon adhesion where tissue injury results in excessive scar formation. Equally important are problem wounds that fail to gain normal tensile strength, such as seen with nutritional deprivation, after trauma, or with some types of immunosuppression. These are associated with some form of decreased deposition of a normal collagen matrix. It is the opinion of the authors that attempts to accelerate normal healing are usually a waste of time and money. One cannot help but be cynical of the many studies in which wound manipulation has demonstrated a statistically significant increase in the rate of gain in strength, but on a range that has no clinical significance. Indeed, there is no known single biologic alteration that will accelerate the rate of tensile strength gain in a normally healing wound.

In contrast, the search for a spot weld of human tissue is not science fiction. Collagen, the major protein involved in providing tensile strength of the order required for normal use of a body part, can be made to polymerize or depolymerize predictably under a wide range of physiologic conditions. The authors predict that coaptation of wound edges with a spot weld of intrinsic collagen or a synthetic material that polymerizes rapidly will replace suture techniques, as practiced today.

Wound healing causes the plastic surgeon even more concerns than the usual problems of healing faced by all surgeons. *Appearance* and *function* are as important as *strength* to the plastic surgeon. Some areas, such as the surface of a tendon or a wound in a patient who forms keloids, present special problems. The statement, "I dressed the wound, God heals it" (Ambroise Paré) does not produce predictably successful repairs of tendons, nerves, or scars. Even the acceleration of retarded healing is not as important in most reconstructive and esthetic problems. It is the amount and quality of scar tissue, and ultimately its remodeling, that seem of greater importance. The biologic processes of greatest interest to the plastic surgeon are the *creation of the normal scar* (collagen synthesis, deposition, and remodeling) and *contraction* of the open wound.

The phenomenon of *epithelization* is important also in the normal resurfacing of a donor site or a partial-thickness burn wound. It must be remembered that *epithelization* is not the same as regeneration of skin. Skin is a complex organ and, like all others with the exception of liver, it does not regenerate to any extent. The mechanism by which more skin appears to be produced in such natural phenomena as pregnancy, breast development, obesity, or artificially induced models such as over a tissue expander, appears to be one of stretching, remodeling, or even alteration in the collagenous dermal architecture. Intussusceptive growth in adults does not play a role. The increased epithelial mitotic activity observed in expanded skin represents a normal response to expansion and *not* regeneration (Francis and Marks, 1977; Squier, 1980). Skin is known to grow only during development or until epiphyseal growth ceases.

Why, then, is the surgeon faced with the problem of human scar? In the course of higher development, man lost the ability to *regenerate* compound organs and has only the relatively simple, and often unsatisfactory, substitute of fibrous tissue repair to restore physical continuity. Unfortunately, repair in a general sense is regarded as beneficial, yet the method of restoring integrity with fibrous (collagenous) protein deposition may produce cosmetic and functional complications worse than the original wound (see Chap. 21). Similarly, the effect of overhealing on the function of internal organs may be disastrous. It is not the lye burn of the esophagus or the toxic injury of the liver that is fatal to patients, it is the scar (collagen deposition) that forms during tissue repair and results in dysphagia or fatal hepatic cirrhosis. Postoperative intestinal obstruction, stenosis of the bile ducts and ureter, adhesions around tendons, or the hard breast following silicone prosthesis implantation are all consequences of the reparative process in which contraction and fibrous protein synthesis are not controlled. If only the surgeon could prevent the primitive mammalian healing process of collagen deposition and regain the sophisticated regenerative capacities of "lower" forms of life on the phylogenic scale! Clearly, phylogenic regression would represent monumental progression.

The major biologic phenomena of wound healing will be discussed as separate entities. It should be remembered that "wound healing" per se is a broad term; each component to be described represents a discrete area worthy of a specific wound healing diagnosis. One should never describe a patient as having a wound healing problem. Every plastic surgeon must be specific. Problems should be described as those of epithelization, collagen metabolism, contraction, and so forth, *not* of wound healing.

EPITHELIZATION

The major function of epithelium is to act as a selective barrier between the body and the external environment. The epithelial barrier in humans prevents bacteria, toxic materials and some radiation from gaining access to the body—the *internal milieu* of

Claude Bernard. It also prevents or reduces the loss of fluids, electrolytes, and other substances from the internal milieu to the outer environment—the *external milieu.* Of course, the barrier function is not absolute. Toxic material, when applied in appropriate solvents, can penetrate, and ionizing radiation can penetrate epithelium if the wavelength and energy are sufficient to do so. Even without the addition of solvents, some pharmacologic agents such as nitroglycerin and beta-aminopropionitrile (BAPN) pass rapidly through skin and may have important clinical uses. In general, epithelium acts as a primary defense against a hostile environment and is a major factor in maintaining internal homeostasis.

Epithelization alone is sufficient only to provide total healing in partial-thickness wounds such as split-thickness skin graft donor sites and first and second degree burns. Healing of deep dermal injuries may even occur when there has been destruction of the epidermal basal layer, provided that hair follicles and sebaceous glands remain viable. These structures turn into virtual epithelial production factories, manufacturing the cells that will migrate to cover the deep partial-thickness injury. Unfortunately, the resulting "skin" is often devoid of sufficient hair follicles and sebaceous glands and, therefore, the "healed" skin is prone to infection. If any type of full-thickness wound, devoid of dermis, is allowed to "heal" by epithelization, it is doomed to failure. Epithelium is mainly composed of water, and a body area covered only by epithelium has little if any resistance to mechanical disruption (Fig. 5–1).

The process of epithelization can be divided into several separate events, including *cell dedifferentiation, mitosis,* and *migration,* which are responsible for resurfacing any denuded area with epithelial cells. *Contact inhibition* is the phenomenon that usually stops these processes.

Gillman and Penn (1956) reported that *cell dedifferentiation* was of prime importance in the resurfacing of a denuded area. Normally, at some point during cell differentiation the cell has no option but to continue performing a specialized function, and such an epithelial cell ultimately dies completely clogged with keratin. However, before reaching this stage the epithelial cell may dedifferentiate in the presence of tissue injury and undergo *mitosis.* The maximal increase in mitosis is usually noted 48 to 72 hours after injury (Bullough and Laurence, 1960; Sullivan and Epstein, 1963). *Migration* occurs as the motile epithelial cells move in a direction where contact will not occur (Fig. 5–2). This type of movement occurs until the cell dies or until it meets a cell of similar type. The migrating epithelial cells with ruffled membranes are coated with an adhesive surface and, when cells of similar type meet, adhesion occurs and the entire process reverts to a resting stage. This phenomenon is called *contact inhibition.*

The factor(s) that initiate epithelial cell migration, mitosis, epithelial cell-to-cell contact inhibition and cell maturation as well as dedifferentiation remain unclear. Human epithelial cell migration appears to be more than simple cell movement, since these cells climb over one another playing biologic leapfrog as they migrate (*epiboly*) (Stenn, 1981).

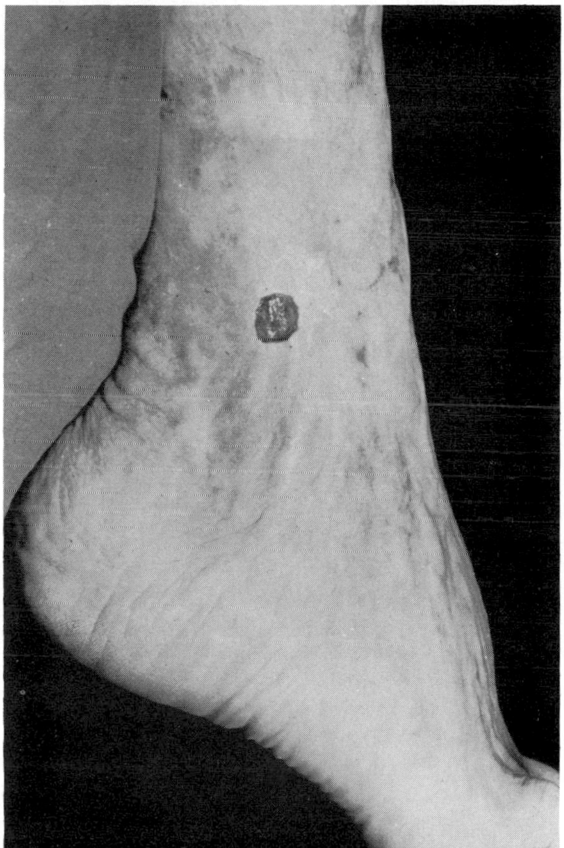

Figure 5–1. Typical recurrent ankle ulcer, which healed only by epithelization and by some degree of fibrous protein synthesis.

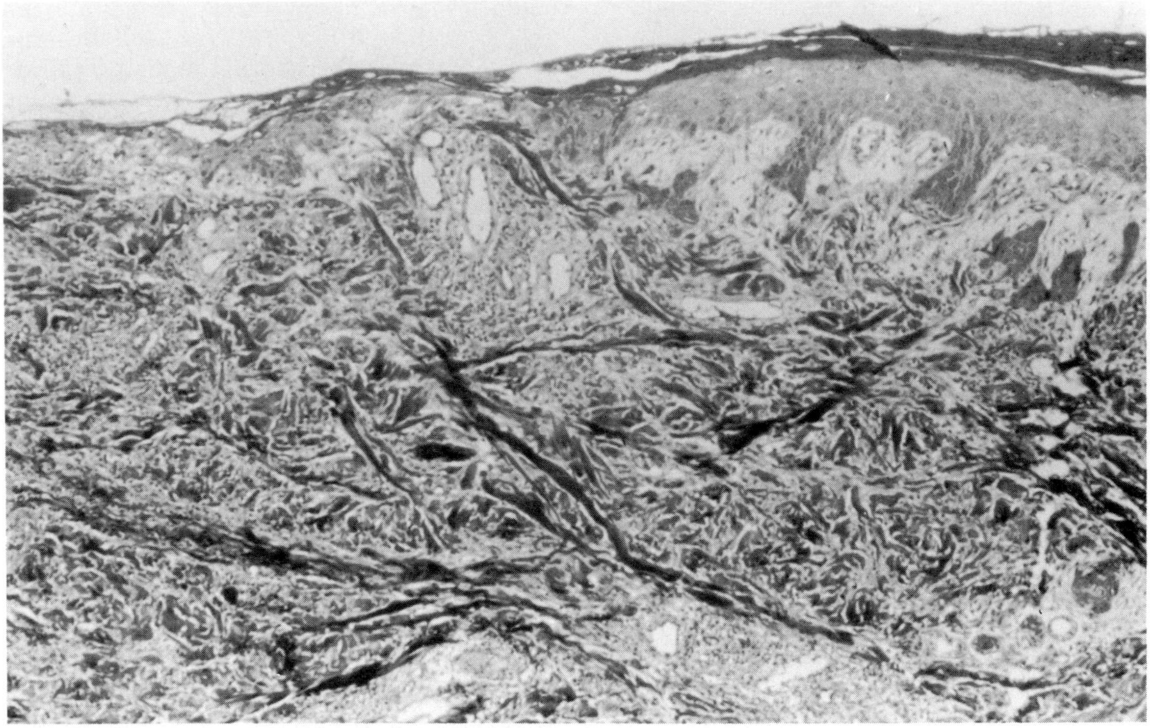

Figure 5–2. Microscopic appearance of advancing epithelial margin. The thickness of the epithelial margin is approximately 20 cells at the base *(right side of figure)* but diminishes to one cell thickness at the leading edge *(left side of figure).* This suggests that cell movement rather than mitosis is the predominant biologic mechanism involved.

Serum contains a factor, possibly derived from the platelet, that stimulates epithelial migration in tissue culture (Stenn, 1978). In addition, collagen appears essential for epithelial migration in tissue culture, as epithelial cells produce Type V collagen, and migration is prevented in the presence of proline analogues that inhibit epithelial collagen production (Stenn, Madri, and Roll, 1979). Therefore, collagen appears to be an essential lattice for epithelial cell migration. There is a controversy as to whether epithelial growth (mitosis and migration) is regulated by chalones, hormones, or both. A chalone is a substance or signal that *retards* activity, and when it is present, a steady state prevails (Marks, 1975). In its absence, events happen. Bullough and Laurence (1960) first described normal epithelial suppressor substances or chalones. Hormonal regulation has been ascribed to *epibolin,* which is required for epithelial migration, and epidermal growth factor (EGF), which is required for mitosis (Bertsch and Marks, 1974).

At the moment, there is no known catalyst to accelerate the process of epithelization. The maximal increase in mitosis is noted 48 to 72 hours after injury (Bullough and Laurence, 1960; Sullivan and Epstein, 1963). However, it is important for the surgeon to know that cell movement occurs more rapidly against two surfaces than against a single one. Thus, a cover provided by an artificial material or a natural dressing, such as a scab, provides more than protection for these delicate ameboid cells. The scab itself may be a very acceptable protection if it is not subjected to mechanical and chemical external trauma. The advancing edge of epithelial cells produces a collagenolytic enzyme that literally cuts through the interface between the scab and dermis to prepare a "carpet" of fibrous tissue ahead of the advancing epithelial cells (Grillo and Gross, 1964). Most important in choice of dressings is the observation of Rovee and associates (1972) that epithelium migrates best on a moist surface. Therefore, any donor site dressing that will prevent desiccation is preferable. Each year millions of dollars are spent on donor site dressing materials for which all sorts of claims are made that they promote more rapid healing (in this case epithelization). However, there are no *data* to validate that any one dressing material causes reepithelization of any split-thickness wound more rapidly than any other so long as the dressing material prevents wound desiccation. The most important influence the surgeon can exert is to take reasonable measures to ensure that epithelization is not inhibited. Such measures should include prevention of infection, protection from external trauma, and avoidance of chemical destruction of the epithelium by various drugs. The old maxim that one should never put on a wound that which one would not put in one's own eye holds true for the wound healing by epithelization.

Many substances have been studied for their epithelial stimulating powers. Although materials such as Scarlet Red may increase the peak at which epithelial mitotic activity occurs (Salomon, Diegelmann, and Cohen, 1974), there is no evidence that this or other materials increase epithelial migration or reduce the time when the wound is finally healed.

In a wound in which it is not possible for contact inhibition to occur because the area is too large for resurfacing by epithelization or because the area being covered is repeatedly traumatized, there is a continuous stimulation for epithelial cell dedifferentiation. During these long periods of stimulation to divide and become motile, some cells close to the wound margin may develop abnormal characteristics, including acceleration of the rate of mitosis. The almost inevitable end result of continued attempts to resurface a wound by epithelization alone is epidermal carcinoma (Fig. 5–3). For all practical purposes, any wound in which reepithelization is retarded long enough is in danger of malignant transformation, although the mechanisms by which this occurs are unclear. The length of time for such a complication to occur is extremely variable. For example, when the original wound is the result of radiant energy, the length of time required for carcinoma to develop is directly proportional to the wavelength of radiant energy. Thirty years may elapse before carcinoma develops in a burn scar (Marjolin's ulcer) when the radiation is of such a long wavelength as to almost be in the visible spectrum. In contrast, injury caused by x-ray or gamma wave radiation may produce a carcinoma in 12 to 24 months. Epithelial carcinoma caused by mechanical injury or occurring in chronic sinus tracts requires an even longer time interval to develop and is not as predictable as radiant energy–induced lesions.

Perhaps the best current study of epidermal hyperplasia is by Argyris (1981) who, using a mouse skin abrasion model, has demonstrated that increased cell proliferation is due to a shortening of the cell cycle, particularly the G_1 phase. In addition, hyperplasia is associated with increased cell loss as there is an increased rate of cell terminal differentiation and keratinization. Conversely, during regression of epidermal hyperplasia, the cell cycle and the length of the epidermal cell life return to normal. The mechanisms controlling these observations should lead to control of epidermal carcinoma.

A discussion of epidermal repair would not be complete without mention of the potential of using cultured epithelial cells to make "artificial skin." Yannas and associates (1982) and Burke and colleagues (1981) are among the pioneers in this field. Their product of silicone and collagen/ground substance, which is supplemented with the patient's epithelial cells, is now commercially being produced and should be available for general use in the near future. Gallico and colleagues (1984) have demonstrated that autogenous cultured epithelium replaced on the full-thickness wound of an infant not only grows, but also apparently forms a dermis-like layer beneath it, suggesting induction of dermal growth. This observation may open new vistas to management of full-thickness skin loss.

CONTRACTION

It is important to distinguish between contraction and contracture. *Contraction* is the active biologic process that decreases the dimension of the involved connective tissue. *Contracture* is the end result of the process of contraction. In large, open, full-thickness wounds left to heal without skin replacement, this phenomenon may be the salvation of patient and surgeon alike. For example, extremity amputations in the American Civil War were all left open to close by contraction because primary closure would have led to a high rate of morbidity and mortality from sepsis. The resulting contractures from these massive open wounds were usually strong and stable and could tolerate prosthetic

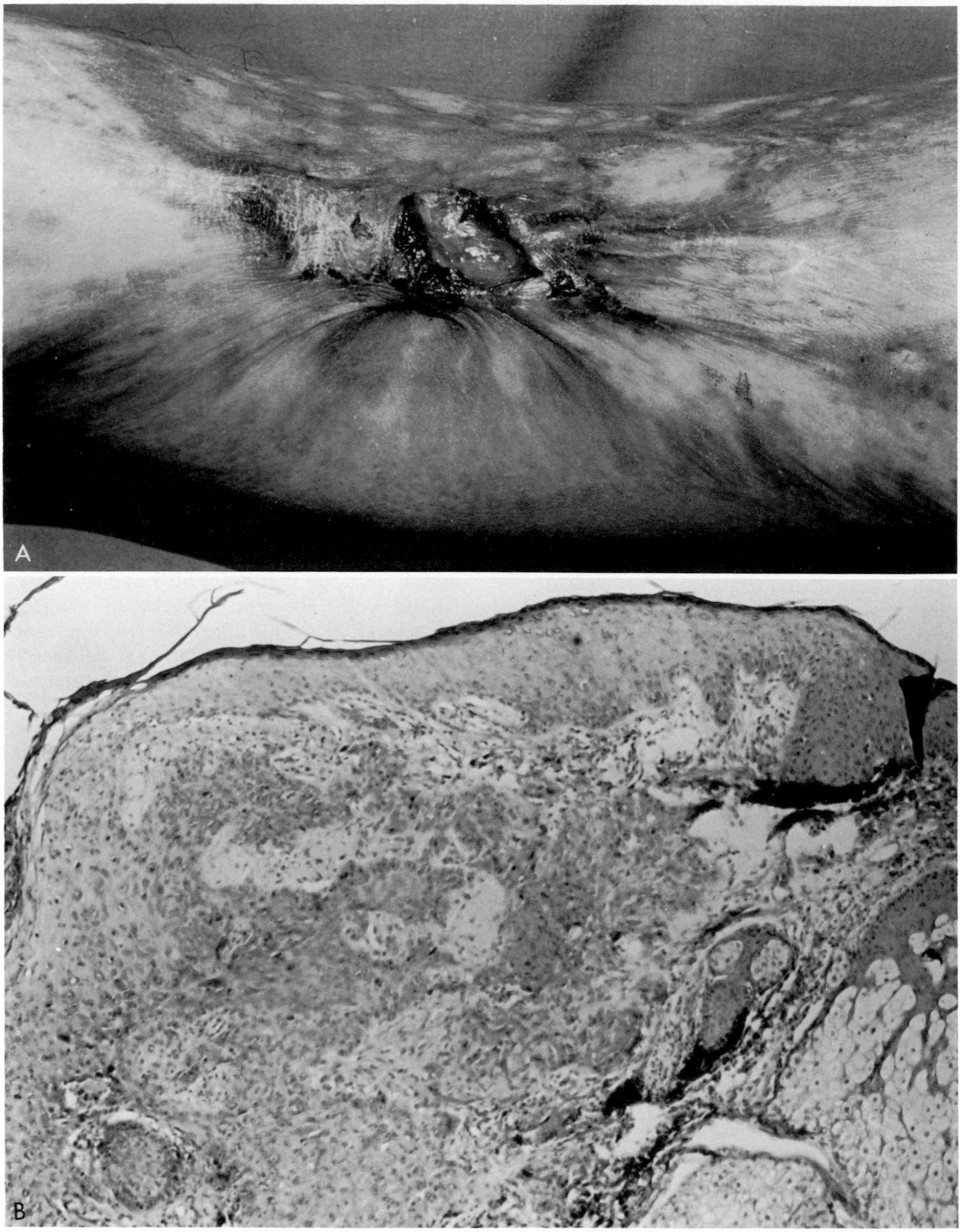

Figure 5–3. Epidermoid carcinoma developing in a 23 year old burn scar. *A,* Gross appearance. *B,* Microscopic appearance demonstrating piling up of excess epithelial cells rather than an edge of progressively diminishing thickness, as observed in the migrating cells in Figure 5–2.

weight bearing. In contrast, the process of contraction may lead to severe functional and esthetically deforming contractures such as burn scar contractures (Fig. 5–4). The contracture must be released surgically and the deformity recreated to cure the deformity. Contraction of the esophagus and biliary tract results in contractures that are disabling and lethal. Contraction around a breast prosthesis produces a contracture that has been one of the most aggravating complications faced by plastic surgeons and their patients for the past 30 years.

Although many investigators have made sound biologic observations on the etiology of contraction over the past 30 years, the cause and control have eluded clinical and investigative surgeons. Earlier observations (Watts, Grillo, and Gross, 1958; Grillo and Gross, 1959) suggested the "picture-frame theory" that the contractile process occurs beneath the advancing skin margin. Other studies indicated that contractile forces originated in the central granulation tissue (Van Winkle, 1967). Clearly, viable cells mediate the wound contraction process because radiation, cell toxins, and animal death all stop the contraction process (Rudolph, 1980).

A major advance in understanding wound contraction occurred with the discovery of a specialized form of mesenchymal cell called the myofibroblast (Gabbiani, Ryan, and Majno, 1971). This cell is a typical fibroblast with a well-developed endocytoplasmic reticulum that also possesses many of the features of a smooth muscle cell (Fig. 5–5). Such features include massive bundles of intracytoplasmic microfilaments, positive immunofluorescent labeling with human anti–smooth muscle serum, nuclear indentation indicative of contraction, and cell-to-stroma connections that would be necessary for cellular contraction to be imparted to whole tissue. Myofibroblasts are almost ubiquitous; they have been identified in virtually every type of tissue undergoing active contraction, including granulation tissue, tendon sheath, and palmar fascia in patients with Dupuytren's disease (Gabbiani and Majno, 1972), and in capsules around breast implants (Rudolph and associates, 1978). Therefore, many believe that wound contraction is almost entirely a cellular process that is not dependent on collagen synthesis or deposition. This hypothesis is confirmed by the finding that scorbutic and lathyritic animals undergo normal contraction (Grillo and Gross, 1959). However, the contracture produced in a scorbutic animal is much less stable than in a nonscorbutic one. Only a small force is required to release the contracture. One can conclude that, although the active process of contraction is not altered by inhibiting collagen synthesis or deposition, collagen provides the strength and integrity to maintain the contracture once it has occurred.

There is reason to question the hypothesis that this specialized fibroblast, the myofibroblast, is the engine of contraction. For example, some observers have noted that the quantity of myofibroblast-like cells is greater in the tissue after contracture has been completed (Rudolph and associates, 1978), suggesting that the myofibroblasts may not be the initiator of the process. In addition, Ehrlich (1984) has demonstrated that, although the fibroblast provides the force for contraction, the connective tissue matrix present within the area of tissue repair also plays an important role in the contractile process.

A major clinical goal of wound healing research is the ability to control wound contraction while simultaneously permitting

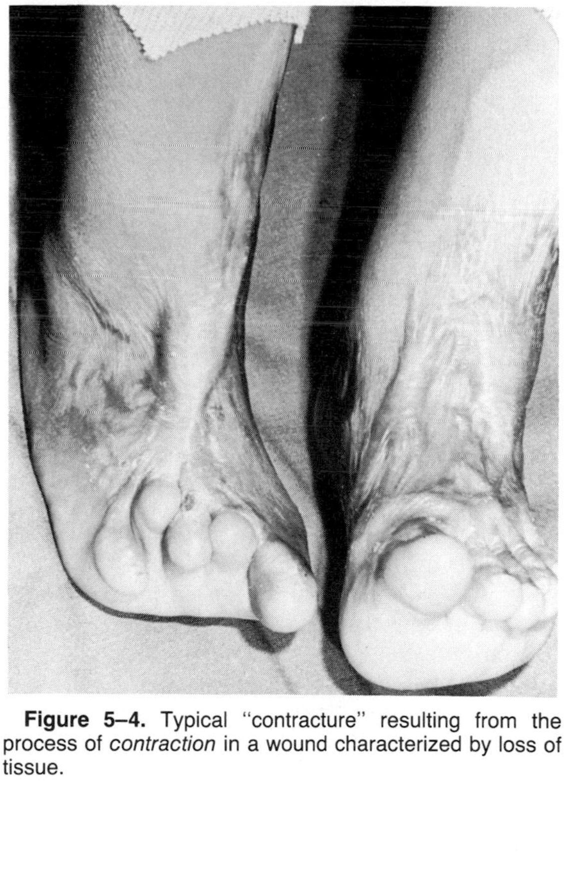

Figure 5–4. Typical "contracture" resulting from the process of *contraction* in a wound characterized by loss of tissue.

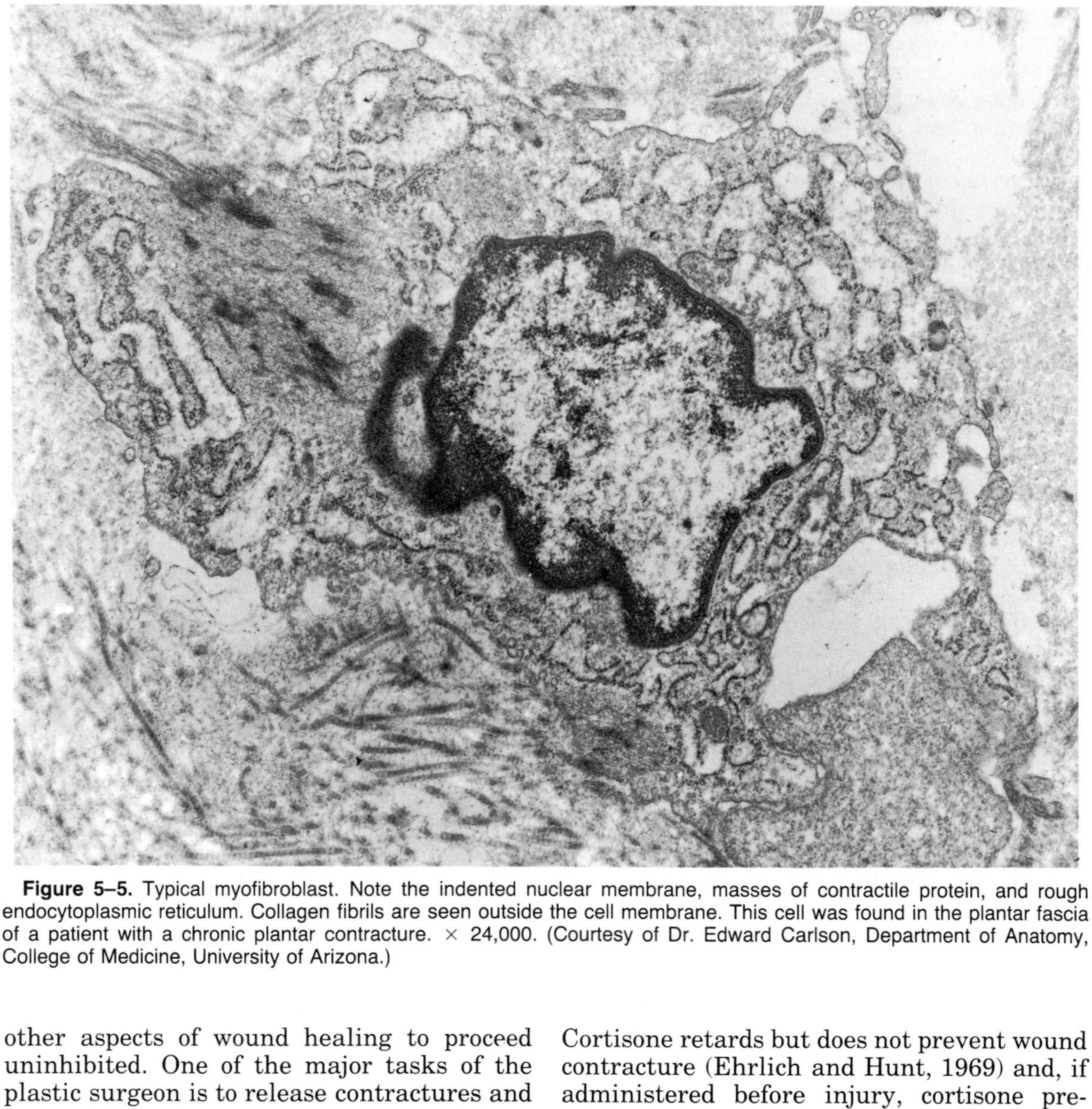

Figure 5–5. Typical myofibroblast. Note the indented nuclear membrane, masses of contractile protein, and rough endocytoplasmic reticulum. Collagen fibrils are seen outside the cell membrane. This cell was found in the plantar fascia of a patient with a chronic plantar contracture. × 24,000. (Courtesy of Dr. Edward Carlson, Department of Anatomy, College of Medicine, University of Arizona.)

other aspects of wound healing to proceed uninhibited. One of the major tasks of the plastic surgeon is to release contractures and prevent them from recurring by the addition of new tissue (graft or flap). Hopefully, this need will be obviated as the basic processes of contraction are elucidated. For example, granulation tissue contracts when stimulated by histamine, certain prostaglandins, or serotonin and wound contraction can be inhibited by the topical application of a smooth muscle inhibitor (Madden, Morton, and Peacock, 1974). Unfortunately, pharmacologic control by topical or systemic agents that are clinically efficacious has not been attained. For example, when Trocinate (thiphenamil hydrochloride) (a smooth muscle inhibitor) is removed from the wound site, contraction renews (Madden, Morton, and Peacock, 1974). Cortisone retards but does not prevent wound contracture (Ehrlich and Hunt, 1969) and, if administered before injury, cortisone prevents fibroblast and inflammatory cell migration into the wound. As vitamin A counteracts most of the deleterious effects of corticosteroids (Ehrlich and Hunt, 1969; Ehrlich, Tarver, and Hunt, 1973) but does not prevent epithelization, the short-term use of systemic steroids in the presence of vitamin A could inhibit contraction while allowing normal graft or flap healing to occur.

However, there is other information useful to plastic surgeons in the treatment of contraction. Application of a skin graft (split- or full-thickness) or skin flap on a contracting wound does not stop the contracting process but *may* reduce the amount of contracture (Rudolph, 1979). However, the application of a graft or flap in a contracting wound may be inadvisable without excision of the contracting wound. Placement of the graft or flap at the time at which the initial wound is created may help to retard contraction (Rudolph, 1980). When one observes clinically that the graft or flap has become ruffled or wrinkled, it is not the graft or flap that has contracted; rather, it is contracture of the underlying bed (Peacock and Van Winkle, 1970). Although the forces of contraction are strong and difficult to prevent by mechanical means, splinting and pressure have been reported to retard or prevent clinical contraction (Frank, Brahme, and Van de Berg, 1984). When fresh wounds are covered with a split- or full-thickness skin graft covered with a bolus dressing, contraction is lessened. Similarly, it is clinically difficult to predict if a long-standing contracture, which is released and covered with a skin graft, will contract again and produce a secondary contracture. Splinting of such wounds appears efficacious until remodeling of the wound bed and graft has occurred, the contractile cells in the connective tissue matrix of the wound have disappeared, and/or the matrix itself has returned to normal.

The age-old question is always raised. What contracts more—a full-thickness or a split-thickness graft? As already mentioned, it is the bed and not the graft that contracts. However, grafts do remodel, rapidly turning over the collagen present at the time of graft placement (Rudolph and Klein, 1973).

Finally, the results from wound contraction are one of the few fundamental processes in wound healing that can be predicted. All the surgeon has to do is grasp the wound edges with forceps and draw them together. Whatever deformity is produced by such a maneuver (such as displacement of an eyebrow) is identical to what results from the biologic process of wound contraction. The knowledge that skin does not regenerate but moves in a centripetal manner, as far as the redundant skin surrounding the wound permits, makes it possible to predict the exact deformity that will be produced if contraction occurs. In areas where skin is redundant, an amazingly large defect can be closed by movement of the skin edges. In areas where there is little or no redundant skin (such as over the anterior tibia, hand, face, or scalp of a young person), closure of the wound either does not occur completely or, even worse, does not occur without producing a deformity because the skin is stretched in an area where function requires relative laxity.

STRUCTURE AND SYNTHESIS OF FIBROUS PROTEIN AND MATRIX

Scar tissue collagen may produce success or failure for the surgeon. If insufficient scar tissue is deposited, morbidity and even mortality can result from the failure of structural integrity to be reestablished. In contrast, excessive scar formation is more often the bane of the plastic surgeon and other practitioners alike. The major component of scar tissue is the fibrous protein collagen. Considerable progress has been made during the past decade in our knowledge of collagen synthesis and degradation (collagenase), information that should lead to the control of scar formation in man.

Collagen is a large macromolecule, 300 nm in length, 15 nm in width, and with a molecular weight of approximately 300,000 (Fig. 5–6). It is composed of three coiled polypeptide chains (Miller, 1985) resulting from over 18 gene products arranged into at least 10 distinct types of collagen. Type I collagen, making up about 80 per cent of the collagen present in skin, has two similar chains called α_1 (I), and a third chain that is slightly dissimilar and is called an α_2 (I) chain. The primary structure carries an abundant sequence of amino acids in the form of a tripeptide: glycine-proline-hydroxyproline. Glycine is evenly distributed throughout the molecule, occurring as every third residue, but other amino acids are not evenly distributed. Hydroxyproline and hydroxylysine are found almost exclusively in collagen. However, small amounts are found in the C_1q component of complement and the enzyme acetylcholine esterase. If these proteins are absent, hydroxyproline serves as an indicator for the amount of collagen present and is usually an accurate method of quantitating collagen production and deposition.

An understanding of collagen metabolism from its inception is important to surgeons because there are several events in the basic synthetic pathway of the macromolecule that may affect clinical decisions. Collagen can be synthesized by a variety of cell types but, clearly, the most important is the fibroblast.

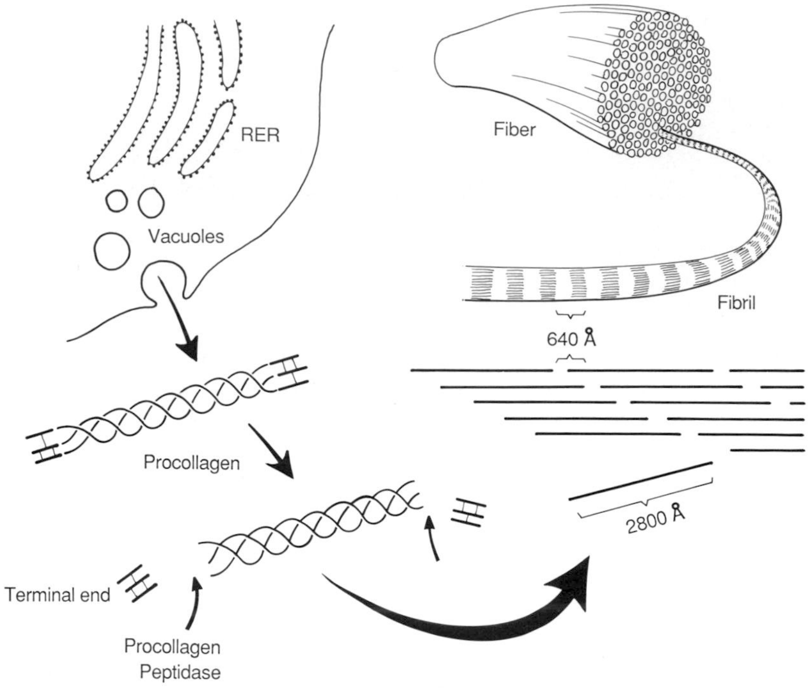

Figure 5–6. Diagram of the assembly of the components of a collagen fiber. (From Bryant, W.M., Greenwell, J.E., and Weeks, P.M.: Alterations in collagen organization during dilatation of the cervix uteri. Surg. Gynecol. Obstet., *126*:27, 1968. Reproduced by permission of Surgery, Gynecology and Obstetrics.)

Fibroblasts are derived from specialized stem cells normally found in the adventitia of small blood vessels (Grillo, 1963). They are not marrow-derived cells nor are they monocyte derived (Ross, Everett, and Tyler, 1970), as previously speculated by others (Moen, 1935; Allgower and Hulliger, 1960). Although normally a stellate or spindle-shaped cell, the fibroblast can assume almost any shape. When actively producing collagen, the fibroblast is characterized by the presence of an endoplasmic reticulum that takes the form of long intercommunicating cisternae with double rows of polysomes attached to membranes (Ross, 1968). The rough endoplasmic reticulum (RER) is the site of collagen synthesis. Before collagen synthesis can be initiated in the cytoplasm, the nuclear DNA must transfer the genetic message for collagen synthesis to occur in a proper fashion. This is accomplished by the transcription, processing, and transfer of mature mRNA to the ribosome. Messenger RNA then provides the proper pattern for collagen synthesis to occur. Although all cell types have the genetic information to produce collagen, this generally does not occur. What stimulates a particular cell to "express" its collagen genes remains speculative, although such questions are now being resolved. Genetic flaws, of course, can result in the production of abnormal collagens in such diseases as the various forms of Ehlers-Danlos syndrome (McKusick, 1972).

The hydroxylation of proline is a critical reaction in collagen formation and has always been of great interest to surgeons. Hydroxylation of proline does not occur until a large polypeptide has been produced (Uitto and Prockop, 1974). For proline hydroxylation to occur, precise cofactors, cosubstrates, and environmental conditions must exist. Cofactors of iron, copper, alpha-ketoglutarate, and ascorbic acid are required for molecular oxygen to hydroxylate proline in the presence of the enzyme prolyl hydroxylase (Hutton, Tappel, and Udenfriend, 1967; Uitto and Prockop, 1974). The role of the cofactors in vivo in the clinical control of collagen deposition is still under debate. To date, no safe clinical method has been found to selectively decrease or increase collagen production during the stage of synthesis. However, it is known that ascorbic acid deficiency or hypoxia can inhibit prolyl hydroxylation and hence production of normal collagen molecules. Similarly, either starvation or the administration of corticosteroids significantly decreases prolyl hydroxylase activity (Stein and Keiser, 1971).

The hydroxylation of lysine is equally important in collagen synthesis and occurs under similar conditions. The lack of appropriate hydroxylation of either of these amino acids results in the production of an abnormal collagen that does not produce normal wound strength and integrity. It will be degraded and it does not help in the formation of normal crosslinks. The lack of hydroxylysine is one of the forms of Ehlers-Danlos syndrome (McKusick, 1972).

Following hydroxylation, various sugar moieties are added to the molecule and these are important as intermolecular crosslinking occurs. The collagen molecule that is secreted from the cell is referred to as *procollagen* (Schofield, Uitto, and Prockop, 1974), which has large polypeptide chains attached to both its amino and carboxy terminal ends that must be cleaved by specific peptidases before intermolecular bonding can occur (Fig. 5–6). The old term *tropocollagen* refers to the triple helical molecule containing the short nonhelical segments that are an integral part of the molecule. These added peptides are thought to be present to ensure proper formation of the triple helical collagen structure. Hence, the C-terminal domain has been termed the "registration peptide" (Speakman, 1971). Absence of the procollagen peptidases in cattle produces a disease called dermatosporaxis, in which newborn calves have fragile skin that is easily wiped off (Lenaers and associates, 1971). A similar genetic enzymatic deficiency has been identified in patients with Ehlers-Danlos Type VII (McKusick, 1972).

After the amino and carboxy terminal peptides have been removed, the molecule is termed *collagen*. Each alpha chain containing approximately 1000 amino acids forms a left-handed helix owing to the orientation of proline residues in the intermolecular repeating triplets. The tertiary structure is produced by twisting of three alpha chains into a right-handed "super" helix. The tertiary structure is stabilized by the formation of various intramolecular crosslinks (hydrogen bonds, covalent bonds, and oppositely charged electrostatic groups) resulting in a rigid, rodlike molecule.

The primary collagen molecules crosslink with each other to form the fibrils and fibers that provide the tensile strength so important to the practice of clinical surgery. The molecules are aligned in a characteristic quarter-stagger overlay between molecules producing the 64 nm repeating periodicity seen in the ultrastructure bond pattern. The typical fibril that results (Fig. 5–6) may vary in size by the tension on the helical molecular structure.

Unidentified factors control the physical weave of the collagen fibrils and fibers to produce connective tissue scar of varying proportions and physical characteristics. A diagram of the various sequential stages of collagen arrangements is shown in Figure 5–6. Although many factors contribute to the final strength, elasticity, size, and shape of the scar, the physical weave is probably extremely important. For example, a nylon thread is relatively inelastic, yet a woven nylon stocking is very elastic. One can argue that the weave of collagen in tendon that is resistant to deforming forces must be quite different from that of an aortic wall, in which the same fibrils must accommodate pulsatile flow.

It has become clear that collagen is not just one molecule. Indeed, there are multiple genetic types of collagen and each type appears to be associated with a specific function or type of tissue (Amenta and associates, 1986). More than physical weave, collagen types may relate to mechanical tissue function. For example, rigid tendon, fascia, and bone are composed mainly of Type I collagen. Skin, which is more elastic, is 80 per cent Type I and 20 per cent Type III, suggesting that the more elastic the tissue, the greater is the quantity of Type III collagen. This teleologic argument is further strengthened by the finding that pulsatile blood vessels are mainly composed of 80 per cent Type III collagen with only 20 per cent Type I. The opposite relationship is present in skin, which is more rigid.

Significant collagen synthesis occurs much earlier (Diegelmann, Rothkopf, and Cohen, 1975; Cohen, Moore, and Diegelmann, 1979) than noted by Madden and Peacock (1968). This early collagen has now been identified as Types III (Clore, Cohen, and Diegelmann, 1979) and IV, and more recent evidence suggests that some of the Type IV collagen is made by inflammatory cells rather than by fibroblasts (Graham and associates, 1984a, b; Lindblad and associates, 1988).

Fibronectin is another high molecular weight extracellular glycoprotein (Ruoslahti, Engvall, and Hayman, 1981) that is important in tissue repair. Fibronectin appears early at the wound site (Kurkinen and associates, 1980) in association with fibrin, and its function is to facilitate adhesion, migration, and phagocytic processes of the leukocytes (Grinnell, 1984). This unusual glycoprotein also provides a primary substrate for the organization and deposition of collagen and matrix by the fibroblasts (Kurkinen and associates, 1980).

Finally, the role of ground substance in fibril formation is not clearly understood but is probably related to the control of the size and possibly the orientation of the fibrils and fibers (White, Shetlar, and Schilling, 1961). The actual sites at which glycoproteins combine with collagen (if indeed they do) or the interaction of these molecules remains unknown.

REMODELING OF COLLAGEN

Degradation of collagen is of equal importance as collagen production. As previously noted in normal tissue repair, collagen synthesis and collagen degradation are in a finely controlled state of equilibrium. Loss of this equilibrium results in abnormal tissue repair. The loss of equilibrium may be due to alterations in collagen degradation as well as collagen synthesis. Lack of collagen degradation could result in excessive deposition (i.e., keloid [Fig. 5–7], hypertrophic scar [Fig. 5–8], hepatic fibrosis). Excessive degradation could result in failure to heal or disruption of repaired wounds. What then is the degradative system of collagen remodeling (Figs. 5–9 and 5–10)? In 1964, Grillo and Gross first identified and measured the activity of an enzyme capable of depolymerizing collagen. Early work by Riley and Peacock (1967) noted the presence of the enzyme activity in a wide

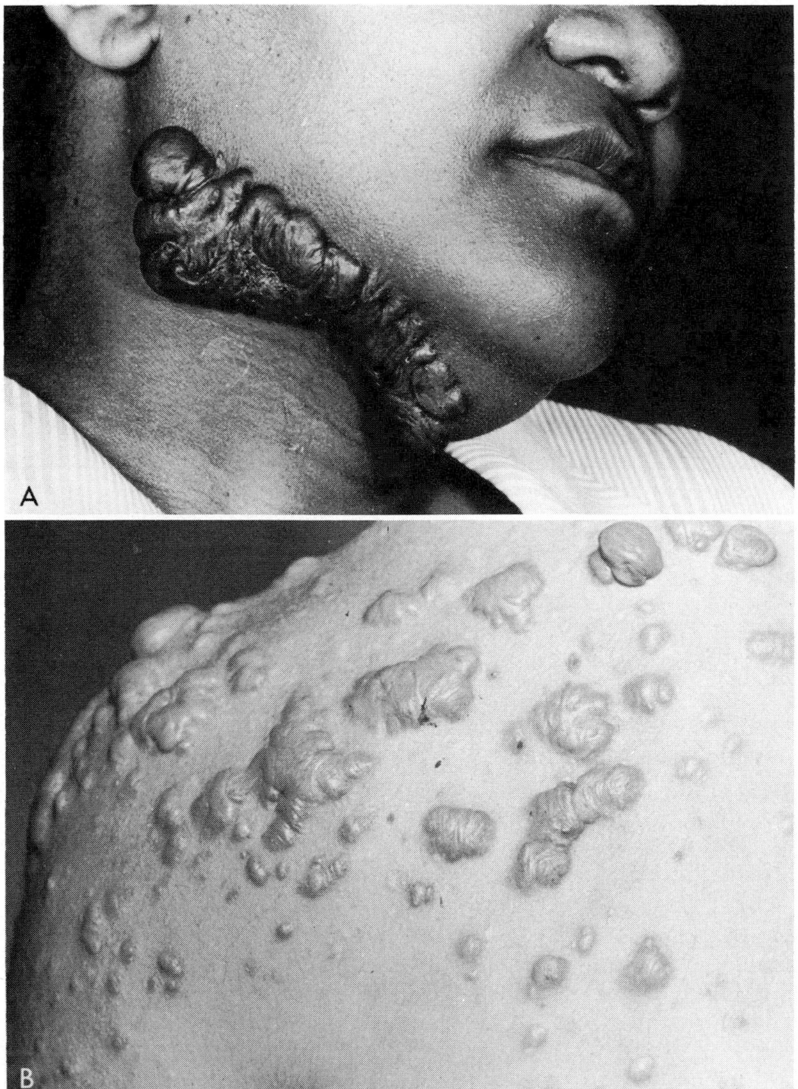

Figure 5–7. Overheating of a type classified as keloid. Keloids following healing of a transverse cervical laceration *(A)* and acute acne on the shoulder *(B)*. Note that the scars do not follow the outline of the original wound.

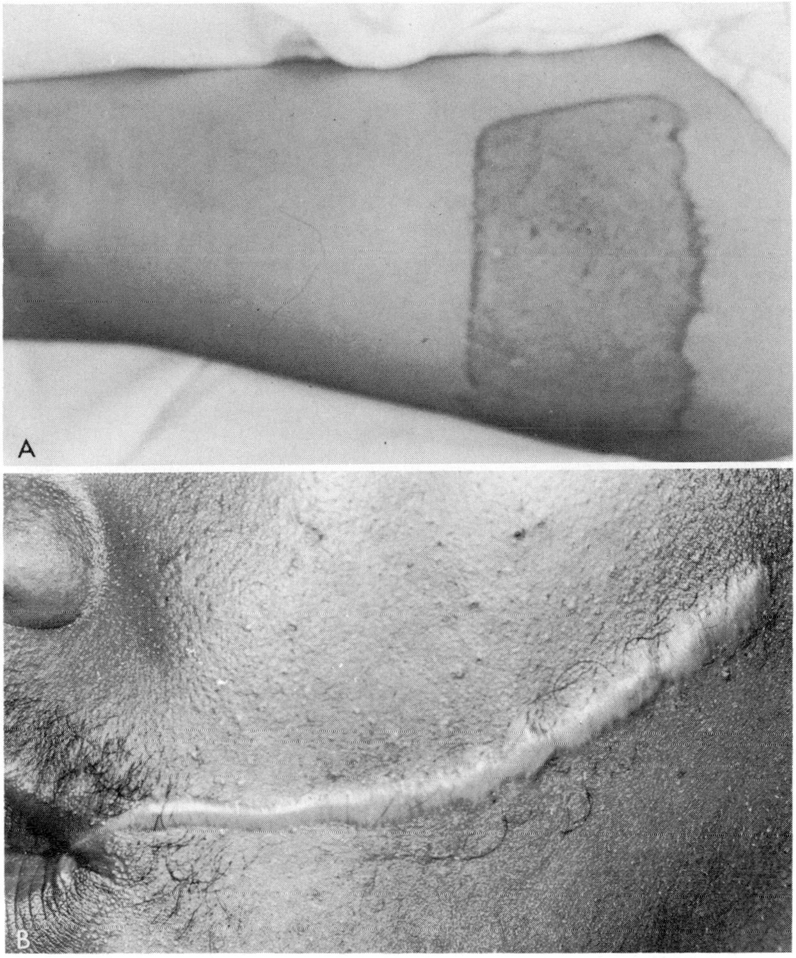

Figure 5–8. Overhealing of a type classified as hypertrophic scar. Note that the scar in the healed split-thickness skin donor site *(A)* and laceration of the cheek *(B)* follow the same general outline of the original wound.

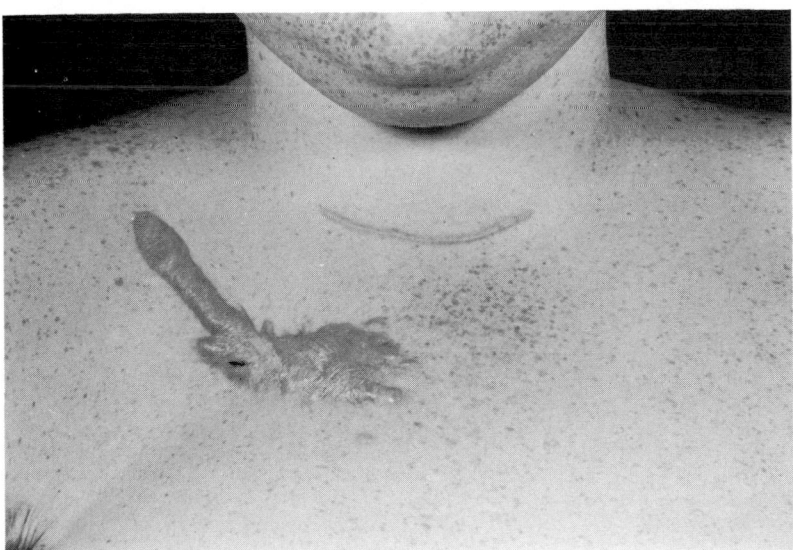

Figure 5–9. Remodeling of scars. Both wounds are one year old. The difference in appearance is primarily due to the remodeling process. No evidence of hypertrophic scar was present three weeks after injury. The hypertrophic scar in the pectoral wound developed over a nine month period, while normal scar development occurred in the tracheostomy incision.

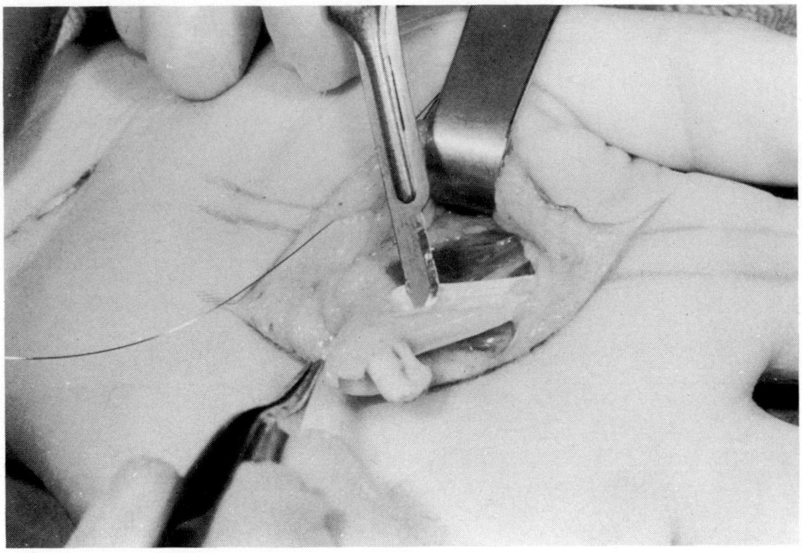

Figure 5–10. Scar tissue in the palm proximal to a finger injury. The newly synthesized collagen has remodeled around the distal end of a cut tendon to resemble normal tendon. This observation led pioneer hand surgeons to write and talk about "unsatisfied ends" and a tendon "sprouting filaments" that would attach to unmovable structures.

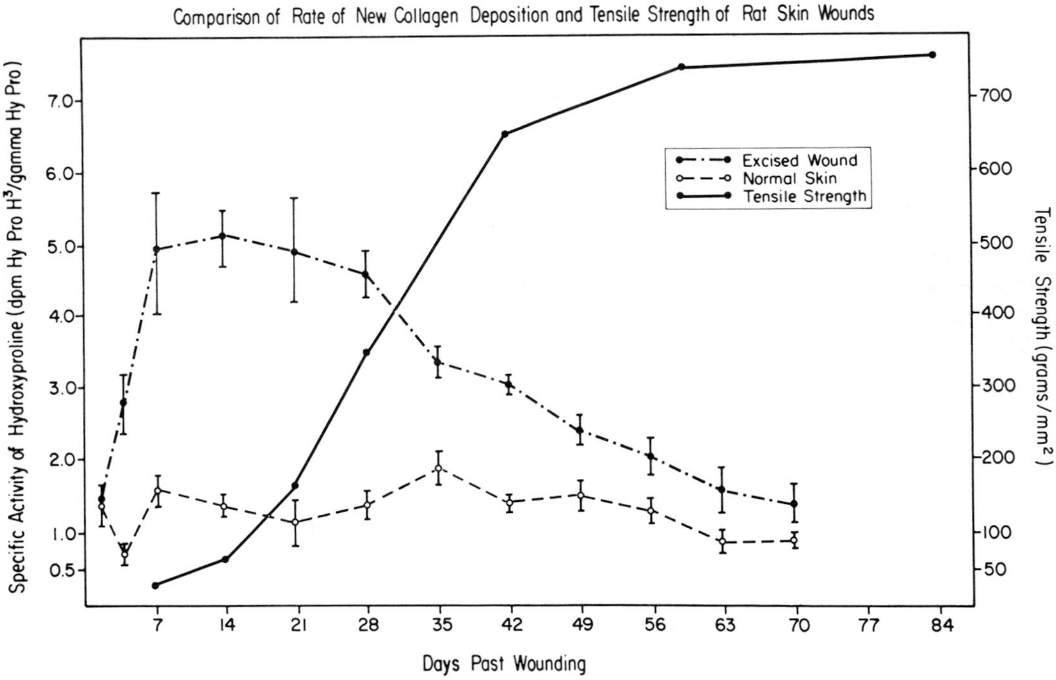

Figure 5–11. The relation of the rate of collagen synthesis to the gain of tensile strength of rat skin wounds. (From Madden, J. W., and Peacock, E. E., Jr.: Studies on the biology of collagen during wound healing. I. Rate of collagen synthesis and deposition in cutaneous wounds of the rat. Surgery, *64*:288, 1968. Tensile strength curve taken from Levenson, S. M., et al.: The healing of rat skin wounds. Ann. Surg., *161*:293, 1965.)

variety of human tissues. Since then, collagenase activity has been found in almost every tissue (Harris and Krane, 1974).

Rather than a single enzyme, it is now clear that there are a variety of collagenases. They are made by many cell types and they appear to have specific functions under set conditions (Werb, 1982). Unlike bacterial collagenase, which literally digests the entire collagen molecule, mammalian tissue collagenases are specific and cleave the collagen molecule at a point approximately three-quarters along the polypeptide chain. The two fragments of this cleavage (TC_a and TC_b) are thermally denatured at 37°C and can then be broken down further by a variety of peptidases and proteases until they are soluble in the plasmatic circulation. The degraded collagen can then be measured as hydroxyproline in blood or urine.

The measurement of collagenolytic activity in tissue remains a difficult challenge for the laboratory investigator. One cannot be sure that in vitro collagenase assays are always a true reflection of in vivo collagenase activity.

The relative timing of collagen synthesis and the changes in the physical properties of a healing cutaneous wound are illustrated in Figure 5–11. It is important to note that collagen synthesis has nothing to do with the gain in wound tensile strength. Tensile strength results from collagen crosslinking rather than collagen synthesis per se. Moreover, although there is a dramatic increase in wound tensile strength between the third and eighth week, wound strength *never* reaches that of normal skin. Histologic correlates are illustrated in Figures 5–12 and 5–13. Consideration of the scar in a clinically healed wound as a deposit of connective tissue, in or out of balance in terms of the ratio of collagen synthesis and deposition to collagenolytic activity, provides a theoretical explanation for many clinical phenomena previously unexplainable in cutaneous scars. The hypothesis also provides several avenues of approach to the control of scar formation (Peacock and Van Winkle, 1970).

As an example, one might consider three scars as variations in the equilibrium between collagen synthesis and degradation. These scars are a keloid, a relatively obscure cutaneous scar in a 42 day old wound, and a deteriorating scar in an ascorbic acid–deficient patient. While the scar in a normal 42 day old human cutaneous wound does not show any further increase or decrease in total collagen content, it should be noted that collagen synthesis, collagen deposition, and collagenolytic activity are greater than measured in unwounded skin. One must assume, therefore, that the rate of collagen synthesis and deposition and the rate of collagenolytic activity are in perfect equilibrium. If, through some genetic or other presently undefined factor, collagenolytic activity became less than the rate of collagen synthesis and deposition, or the rate of collagen synthesis and deposition became more, the scar would accrue more and more collagen until it developed the typical appearance of a keloid.

In keeping with the usual appearance of a keloid, the clinical manifestations would not appear for several weeks and would continue until mechanical or biologic factors, such as oxygen supply, brought the synthetic and lytic factors into equilibrium. If collagen synthesis were partially or completely depressed by removing a cofactor, such as ascorbic acid, collagenolytic activity would exceed collagen synthesis, and a previously healed wound would grow weaker until the normal stress caused by skin elasticity and muscular activity produced dehiscence (Cohen and Keiser, 1976).

This is precisely what happens in scorbutic animals and people whose wounds had healed before the onset of scurvy. It is known that ascorbic acid is not required to maintain the physical integrity of collagen under all circumstances. However, collagenous tissue in a state of dynamic equilibrium would obviously be altered dramatically by removing a cofactor needed for collagen synthesis. Between the extremes of dehiscence and keloid formation, other abnormalities could exist that would be explicable on the basis of unequal rates of collagen synthesis and destruction. Additional study of the factors that influence the rate of collagen synthesis and deposition and the rate of collagen destruction could be rewarding in understanding and controlling the deposition of scar after repair of a surface or deep injury.

FACTORS AFFECTING COLLAGEN METABOLISM

Five systems are activated by tissue injury, and influence collagen metabolism and ultimately the events of wound healing. These

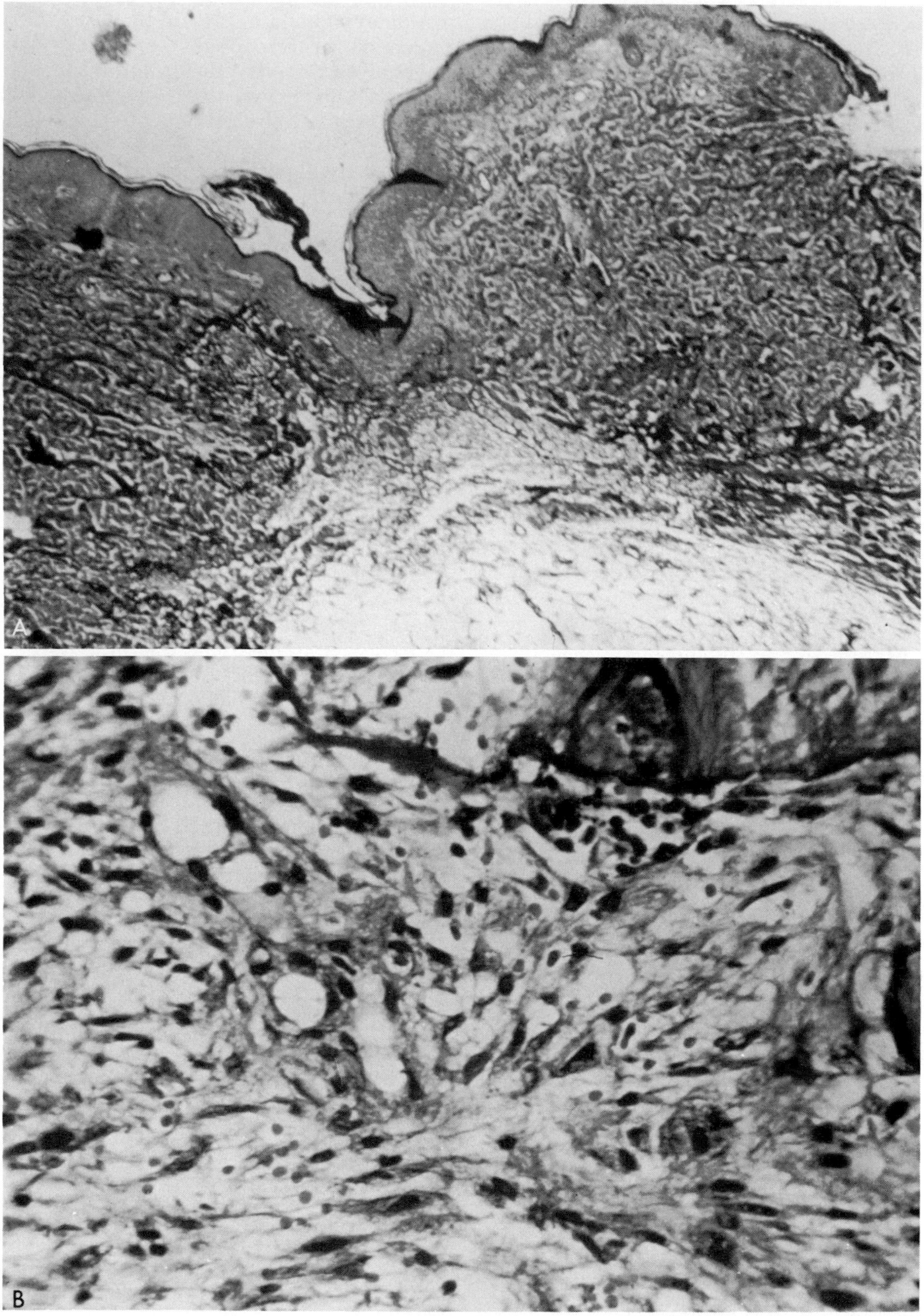

Figure 5–12. Low power *(A)* and high power *(B)* magnifications of seven day old healing cutaneous wound in a human patient. Note that purposefully oriented large collagen fibers span the gap, and only a fine reticulum of newly synthesized collagen can be identified.

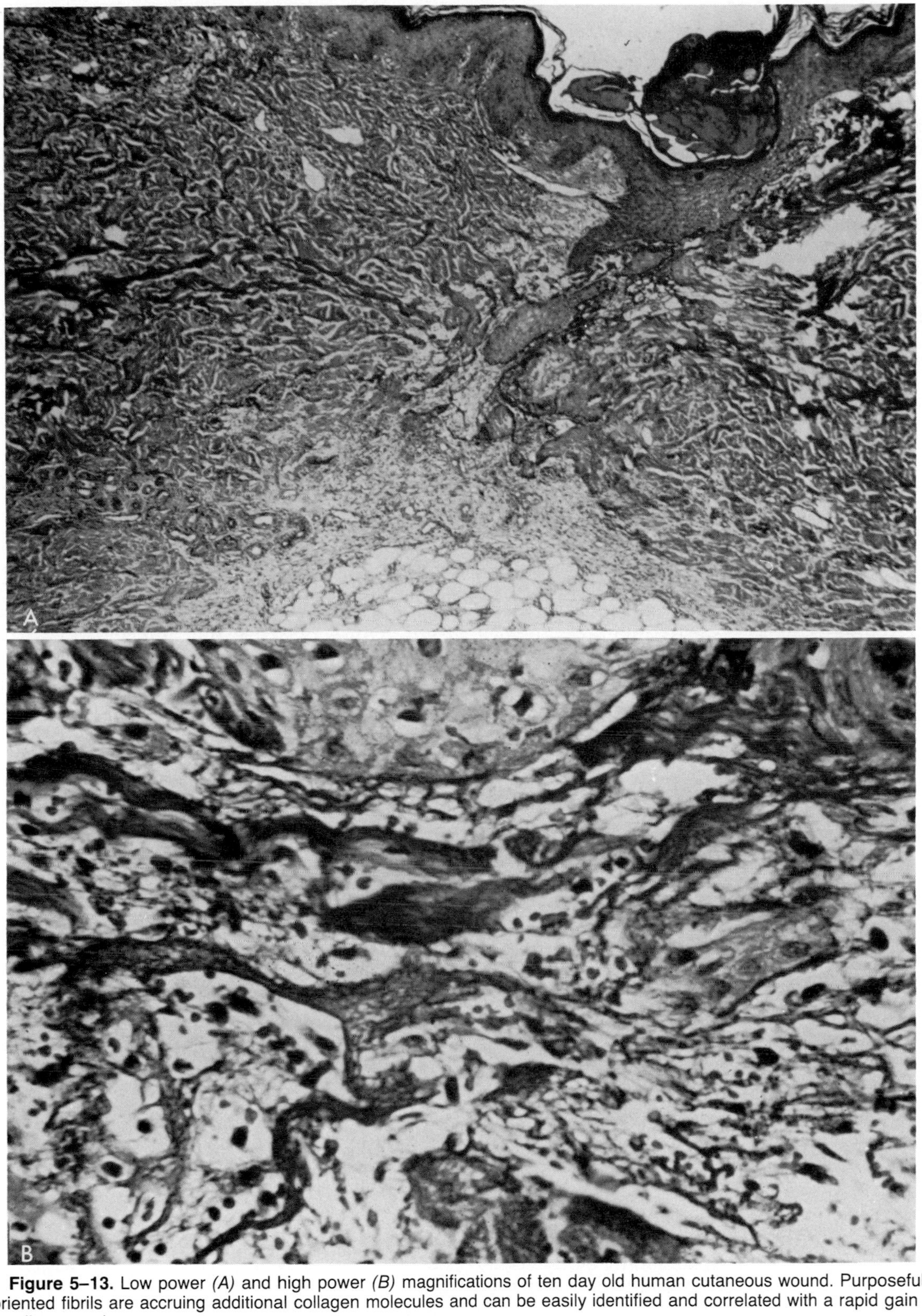

Figure 5–13. Low power *(A)* and high power *(B)* magnifications of ten day old human cutaneous wound. Purposefully oriented fibrils are accruing additional collagen molecules and can be easily identified and correlated with a rapid gain in tensile strength.

include *vascular changes, hemocoagulation,* and *inflammation.* The fourth system, *growth factors,* overlaps but is becoming of such major importance that it deserves a summary section alone. The final system is the *wound environment.*

Vascular changes are the first events following tissue injury and consist of a brief period of vasoconstriction followed by vasodilatation and leakage of plasma components around the endothelial cells. These events are modulated by the local release and interplay of histamine, bradykinin, prostaglandins (PGE_1, PGE_2, and PGA_2) as well as leukotrienes (Sedwick and Willoughby, 1985). These mediators not only affect endothelial cell capillary leak but also influence mesenchymal cells. For example, histamine appears to stimulate fibroblast proliferation (Russell, Russell, and Trupin, 1977; Topol, Lewis, and Benveniste, 1981).

Hemocoagulation occurs almost synchronously with the vascular changes. Fibrin formed during coagulation controls bleeding, and serves as a surface for the adherence and degranulation of platelets as well as a lattice for fibroblast migration (Graham and associates, 1984a, b). As platelets degranulate, they release the important wound healing modulator PDGF (platelet-derived growth factor), which is of vital importance in modulating mesenchymal cell proliferation (Ross and Vogel, 1978; Scher and associates, 1979). In addition, PDGF directs fibroblast chemotaxis (Seppä and associates, 1982) and enhances fibroblast collagenase activity (Bauer and associates, 1985). The coagulation cascade is most important in modulating the cellular events of inflammation and wound healing.

Initially, the *inflammatory* cells at the wound site are the same as those found in peripheral blood. True migration of inflammatory cells begins within a few hours when polymorphonuclear (PMN) cells make up the majority of inflammatory cells at the site of tissue injury (Simpson and Ross, 1972). It is now clear that migration of PMNs into the area of tissue injury is not a random event but that several locally released compounds are responsible for PMN migration. These include leukotriene B_4 (Bray, Ford-Hutchinson, and Smith, 1981), a product of the lipoxygenase pathway of arachidonic acid as well as the C_{5a} portion of complement (Wiggins, Giclas, and Henson, 1981). Such attractants produce a chemical gradient through which the PMNs migrate to localize at a site where damaged tissue digestion and bacterial digestion can be accomplished by the PMNs. While PMNs are not required for subsequent events in collagen metabolism (Simpson and Ross, 1972), they are important in the defense against infection and, hence, wound healing in general.

The macrophage arrives at the site of tissue injury 24 to 36 hours after injury and is the key inflammatory cell in modulating wound healing (Leibovich and Ross, 1975). Macrophages are derived from circulating monocytes attracted to the wound site by specific chemotactic agents such as lymphocyte-derived chemotactic factor (Altman and associates, 1973), *N*-formylmethionyleucylphenylalanine (FMLP) (Schiffmann, Corcoran, and Wahl, 1975), and collagen fragments. Attracted monocytes that have ingested debris are transformed into macrophages, and local macrophages are also recruited.

The monocyte-macrophage system of cells is somewhat complex. Macrophages secrete a host of biologically active products affecting many other cell types. However, the clinical significance of these multiple biologic products is difficult to judge at this time. They produce a PDGF-like factor (Martinet and associates, 1986), release a material that inhibits collagen synthesis at a transcriptional level (Narayanan, Voss, and Page, 1985), and are also capable of synthesizing collagen (Lindblad and associates, 1988) and fibronectin. Several authors have reported that the concentration of macrophage products can modulate fibroblast proliferation (Leibovich and Ross, 1975; Diegelmann, Cohen, and Kaplan, 1982). For example, it has been demonstrated that low concentrations of certain factors can stimulate fibroblast proliferation, whereas high concentrations inhibit this process.

Lymphocytes (T and B) are the final inflammatory cell type to populate the wound. The lymphokines T-cell release may inhibit or stimulate collagen synthesis, and stimulate MDGF secretion and macrophage collagenase production (Rosenbloom and associates, 1983; Duncan, Perlish, and Fleischmajer, 1984; Postlethwaite and associates, 1984). It is not surprising that, with fibroblasts residing in such a complicated environment in which so many mediators are present, the total clinical effect must be the sum total of these multifactorial influences.

Growth factors have been discussed throughout this section but are so important that they require emphasis. They will become potent clinical tools within the next decade. There are two categories of growth factors—chemotactic and hormonal. For example, PDGF, already discussed at length, is a chemotactic factor for fibroblasts and smooth muscle cells, attracting these cells to the site of platelet aggregation. As described above, activated macrophages produce a material identical to PDGF (Martinet and associates, 1986). Other investigators (DiCorleto and Bowen-Pope, 1983) have shown that endothelial cells can produce a PDGF-like factor. These observations are probably of clinical importance because they suggest that PDGF-like activity is needed for a prolonged period in the healing process, and the initial stimulus from PDGF is not sufficient. In fact, Grotendorst and associates (1982) have likened the platelet contribution to a kamikazi attack because these cells do not synthesize materials; they simply carry a load and, after they have released their "payload," their "mission" is complete. In contrast, macrophages and endothelial cells can synthesize a variety of materials over a prolonged period.

Several other growth factors have been termed "wound hormones." TGF-beta (transforming growth factor) is one of the more exciting of these materials (Sporn and Roberts, 1980; Sporn and associates, 1986). When injected locally, TGF-beta stimulates angiogenesis, fibroblast attraction, and collagen formation (Sporn and associates, 1983; Roberts and associates, 1986).

The *wound environment* includes factors already discussed in this section as well as several additional factors. For example, Hunt has stressed the importance of oxygen tension within the wound (Hunt and Pai, 1972; Hunt and associates, 1978; Knighton, Silver, and Hunt, 1981), since transient low wound tissue oxygen seems to stimulate cell migration, balance synthesis of angiogenic factor, and stimulate macrophage growth factor and thus collagenase production. Similarly, high lactate levels, the result of hypoxia, stimulate the macrophage to produce angiogenesis factor (Banda and associates, 1982). In addition, a moderate hyperoxic environment can actually increase the rate of open wound closure, probably as the result of increased epidermal activity rather than stimulation of wound contraction (Niinikoski, 1977). These data are not meant to suggest that wound hypoxia improves collagen deposition or ultimately healing. They merely note that these are normal wound events in the well-oxygenated host. What Hunt's work does stress is the need to maintain *normal* pO_2 in the wound environment if healing is to proceed normally (Hunt and Pai, 1972; Hunt and associates, 1978; Knighton, Silver, and Hunt, 1981). Moreover, Hunt stresses that arterial pO_2 may not be a reflection of wound tissue pO_2 and that, for example, decreased blood volume alone may result in a low wound tissue pO_2 in spite of a normal arterial pO_2. Therefore, he stresses maintenance of volume and monitoring of tissue pO_2 (a difficult feat with available devices).

Pharmacologic Agents: Corticosteroids

In spite of a vast literature, it is not totally clear how corticosteroids inhibit wound healing. However, some mechanisms are known. For instance, these agents inhibit fibroblast migration into the wound if an animal has been pretreated (Hunt and associates, 1969) and can inhibit prolyl hydroxylase activity (Cutroneo, Rokowski, and Counts, 1981; Cutroneo, Sterling, and Shull, 1986). Although corticosteroids inhibit this enzyme, they do not necessarily prevent collagen deposition. In addition, there is some speculation that corticosteroids increase collagenolytic activity (Houck and associates, 1968). Finally, these agents alter various aspects of the inflammatory response, which (as discussed) is the major modulator of the healing process.

Vitamin A appears to reverse the retardation of healing associated with corticosteroids (Hunt and associates, 1969; Stein and Keiser, 1971; Ehrlich, Tarver, and Hunt, 1973). Although the reason for this is unclear, vitamin A reverses the prolyl hydroxylation suppression of corticosteroids and is a cell membrane labilizer, while corticosteroids are a membrane stabilizer.

CHANGES IN PHYSICAL PROPERTIES OF COLLAGEN

Genetic Conditions

During the past decade a whole host of human diseases have been defined as having specific defects in collagen metabolism. In many respects, these are the only true collagen diseases. Most diseases classified as collagen diseases are poorly understood disease processes that may have only a secondary effect on collagen. The best example is the Ehlers-Danlos syndrome, which has now been clinically separated into at least ten separate clinical entities with the biochemical abnormality being described in at least three types (McKusick, 1972). For example, Type IV Ehlers-Danlos syndrome has a deficiency in Type III collagen, while Type VI Ehlers-Danlos is associated with lysyl hydroxylase deficiency. Another rare condition found primarily in cattle is dermatosparaxis, caused by a deficiency in the enzyme *procollagen peptidase* (Lenaers and associates, 1971). The list of the true collagen diseases should increase exponentially over the next decade because of an ever-growing sophistication in the detection of biochemical and immunologic collagen abnormalities.

Lathyrism

This is an example in which understanding a disease of healing may lead to improvement in the clinician's ability to control healing. Lathyrism was first described by Hippocrates as a disease in man associated with famine and, more commonly, in animals who have eaten the common ground pea or the flowering sweet pea of the plant genus *Lathyrus*. The disease processes that arose from ingestion of the sweet pea center on alteration in collagen metabolism and can be attributed to beta-aminopropionitrile (BAPN), which is the active collagen crosslink inhibitor contained in *Lathyrus*. The physiologic effects have been variable among species. For example, poultry with lathyrism usually succumb to rupture of a dissecting aortic aneurysm; young rats develop scoliosis, and older rats develop massive abdominal hernias.

Although many other lathyrogenic agents have been identified, BAPN is the most effective and widely studied in animal and man (Chvapil, 1982). Biochemically, it is a monoamine oxidase inhibitor and acts primarily to prevent oxidative deamination of the ϵ-amino group of lysine. This action, in turn, prevents formation of aldehydes and subsequent covalent crosslinking. The major biochemical difference between lathyrogenic and normal collagen is that the former has a considerable increase in alpha chains and a decrease in covalently bonded chains. The physical differences in tensile strength are enormous.

Similar physical effects are produced by penicillamine (β,β-dimethylcysteine), which is a known copper chelator used to treat Wilson's disease and cystinuria (Nimni and associates, 1969). However, the mechanism for its blockage of collagen crosslinking involves reaction with formed aldehyde groups (Levene, 1961). The end result is the same as that following BAPN in that tensile strength is decreased, and collagen crosslinks and deposition are inhibited.

The exciting question to ask is whether controlled lathyrism can be used to control scar in a clinical situation. Animal data have demonstrated that controlled lathyrism alters the physical properties of peritendinous adhesions and periarticular cartilage in immobilized joints. These findings suggest that inhibition of collagen crosslinking may be a useful method of controlling the physical properties of human scar tissues.

Peacock (1973) was the first to conceive of the use of crosslink inhibitors in human surgical conditions. The first attempts to produce controlled lathyrism in humans with systemic BAPN were halted because of liver enzyme changes and erythema multiforme, which apparently were the result of contaminants (Peacock and Madden, 1969). These complications have been eliminated by purified BAPN in FDA-supervised and controlled clinical trials as therapy for urethral stenosis and joint surgery of the hand. Because BAPN therapy of esophageal stenosis in dogs and joint stiffness in rats and dogs was successful, clinical trials of induced, controlled lathyrism in humans should be conducted (Madden and associates, 1973). At present, systemic BAPN is available only for FDA-controlled studies. However, D-penicillamine is more readily available and should be considered for clinical use.

Topical BAPN therapy has been used recently and shows great promise in ameliorating collagen-related functional disorders in close proximity to skin (Chvapil, 1986). Topically applied BAPN fumarate rapidly passes through skin, inhibiting collagen crosslinking in skin and subjacent structures (Fleisher and associates, 1981). Therefore, long-term application of low dose topical BAPN is possible without the systemic alteration in collagen crosslinking. Tendon adhesions, joint contractures, and temporomandibular joint ankylosis as well as keloid and hypertrophic scar may be treated effectively by this new modality. Clinical studies are under way in all these areas and early clinical results are promising. BAPN may also be used in combination with other collagen-controlling agents such as D-penicillamine and/or corticosteroids (Chvapil, 1982).

CLINICAL APPLICATION OF BIOLOGIC PRINCIPLES

The selection and placement of sutures in skin or any other tissue can be based, to some extent, on sound biologic principles. When two skin edges are coapted, there is a relatively prolonged period of increased collagen synthesis, degradation, and deposition in this wound as compared with normal skin. Because of this rapid remodeling, there is no suture material, either absorbable or nonabsorbable, to provide strength to allow the tension-closed wound to heal without widening. Every experienced plastic surgeon has encountered the wide scar, which is revised by using permanent dermal sutures, only to discover that a wide scar returns, yet the permanent suture is intact and in place. Clearly, the biologic phenomenon of wound remodeling has occurred, allowing the remodeling scar to widen around the intact permanent suture.

Contraction of skin grafts is not a clearly understood biologic process. However, two distinct phenomena must be considered. *Primary contraction* of the graft itself may occur as it remodels. Rudolph and Klein (1973) have demonstrated that there is a rapid turnover of collagen in both full- and split-thickness skin grafts. *Secondary contraction* is the biologic process by which the graft contracts because it is placed on an actively contracting bed. The latter is probably the most common factor in skin graft contracture. Clearly, the clinical observation of a wrinkled graft on a bed indicates that contraction has occurred beneath the graft, and the bed itself is the main cause of this problem. Obviously, both phenomena are usually important in the contraction process.

Selection of a skin graft thickness can be made with some biologic rationale, because full-thickness skin grafts apparently contract less than split-thickness grafts. In addition, immediate and long-term placement of stent dressings over skin grafts prevents the degree of contraction that occurs if the wounds are not treated with this compressive type dressing.

The treatment of split-thickness skin graft donor sites has also been the topic of subjective but heated debate. However, there is no evidence to suggest that any particular dressing is superior to another in terms of the length of healing time.

Although the basic biologic premise that skin is a complex organ that does not regenerate remains valid, the process of *tissue expansion* allows the harvesting of a greater area of skin as graft or flap from the same donor area. The expansion phenomenon does not imply "regeneration" but rather the physical stretching of skin with disruption of the macromolecular collagen fibers and remodeling of the collagen. On histologic study, there is dermal thinning, and electron microscopic study suggests an increased quantity of fibroblasts and myofibroblasts in the dermis. The epidermis does not appear to thin. This finding may be accounted for by increased mitotic activity in the expanded epithelium (Francis and Marks, 1977; Squier, 1980). The fact that epidermis remains of equal thickness after expansion should not be interpreted as "skin regeneration": it is not. Although excellent clinical results have been reported with tissue expansion (see Chap. 13), there are more questions than answers at the present time: hair growth, susceptibility to infection, contraction after transfer as a graft or flap, and sensibility changes are but a few.

How, then, does one select the proper graft and treat a particular wound? The choice may not always be easy. For example, the 2 cm cheek defect in a child that has healed by contraction and epithelization would classically be treated by release and application of a full-thickness skin graft from an area with satisfactory texture and color match. However, a properly placed and stented split-thickness graft might give an excellent result; tissue expansion might also be considered.

In contrast, in a 40 per cent body surface burn, the object is to resurface the wound as quickly as possible before fatal complications occur. Therefore, a thin graft would be used for a satisfactory "take" as well as for rapid donor site healing and the ability to reharvest additional thin grafts rapidly. One does not worry about skin color match and texture, factors of concern in the previous example of a facial deformity. Clearly, biologic considerations should always be exercised as the surgeon makes these clinical decisions.

TENDON HEALING

Although tendon healing is discussed in Chapter 15, a few comments are warranted in a wound healing chapter. The "one wound" concept is the key to an understanding of tendon healing. Tendons do not heal by a collagenous, spot-welding, end-to-end coaptation but the entire wound bed is involved in the healing process. The wound does not recognize that collagen should be deposited only at the tendon ends to increase tensile strength. The entire wound must heal with inflammation, collagen deposition, and remodeling. An understanding of these basic principles should assist the planning of both present and future mechanical and pharmacologic therapy.

Mechanical factors include selection of sutures, methods to approximate the tendon ends, and surgical manipulation of the sheath or sheath substitute as well as postoperative mechanical therapy (PT/OT). The biologic factors are the same as discussed throughout this chapter but, in the case of tendon repair, mechanical postoperative forces (exercise, early mobilization, etc.) are used to remodel the newly deposited collagen as well as pharmacologic agents that may accomplish the same goals. Arem and Madden (1976), in a classical experiment using subcutaneous sponges and magnets in rats placed in electromagnetic fields, clearly demonstrated that early mechanical force elongates newly synthesized collagen. This study provides the biologic basis to indicate why early postoperative hand therapy is beneficial. Although mechanical postoperative manipulation of the hand does not disrupt scar, it elongates scar throughout the wound, thereby allowing full range of motion through an attenuated scar. In the final analysis, it is tendon gliding and not the amount of collagen deposited that really matters in a functional sense. Pharmacologic intervention may also prove to be a promising way to improve tendon gliding. For example, topical BAPN on the skin of the repaired digit, combined with appropriate physical therapy, may lengthen the scar and improve function. The concept of early tendon motion and primary repair is based on biologic principles, as "no man's land" has become "every man's land."

Some of the major arguments over the past two decades on tendon repair now seem relatively unimportant. The arguments of extrinsic (Potenza, 1962; Peacock, 1965) versus intrinsic (Becker and associates, 1981; Graham and associates, 1984) healing are irrelevant. Both phenomena occur and are of equal concern. What may be of greatest biologic importance is the definition of the role of various cell types and wound agents on the healing of tendons. A clearer definition may result in better methods of pharmacologic control.

REFERENCES

Allgower, M., and Hulliger, L.: Origin of fibroblasts from mononuclear blood cells: a study on *in vitro* formation of the collagen precursor, hydroxyproline, in buffy coat cultures. Surgery, *47*:603, 1960.

Altman, L. C., Synderman, R., Oppenheim, J. J., and Mergenhagen, S. E.: A human mononuclear leukocyte chemotactic factor: characterization, specificity, and kinetics of production by homologous leukocytes. J. Immunol., *110*:801, 1973.

Amenta, P. S., Gay, S., Vaheri, A., and Martinez-Hernandez, A.: The extracellular matrix in an integrated unit: ultrastructural localization of collagen Types I, III, IV, V and VI, fibronectin, and laminin in human tissue placenta. Coll. Relat. Res., *6*:125, 1986.

Arem, A. J., and Madden, J. W.: Effects of stress on healing wounds: I. Intermittent noncyclical tension. J. Surg. Res., *20*:93, 1976.

Argyris, T. S.: The regulation of epidermal hyperplastic growth. CRC Crit. Rev. Toxicol., *9*:151, 1981.

Argyris, T. S., and Slaga, T. J.: Promotion of carcinomas by repeated abrasion in initiated skin of mice. Cancer Res., *41*:5193, 1981.

Banda, M. J., Knighton, D. R., Hunt, T. K., and Werb, Z.: Isolation of a nonmitogenic angiogenesis factor from wound fluid. Proc. Natl. Acad. Sci. USA, *79*:7773, 1982.

Bauer, E. A., Cooper, T. W., Huang, J. S., Altman, J., and Deuel, T. F.: Stimulation of *in vitro* human skin collagenase expression by platelet-derived growth factor. Proc. Natl. Acad. Sci. USA, *82*:4132, 1985.

Becker, H., Graham, M. F., Cohen, I. K., and Diegelmann, R. F.: Intrinsic tendon cell proliferation in tissue culture. J. Hand Surg., *6*:616, 1981.

Bertsch, S., and Marks, F.: Effect of foetal calf serum and epidermal growth factor on DNA synthesis in explants of chick embryo epidermis. Nature, *251*:517, 1974.

Bray, M. A., Ford-Hutchinson, A. W., and Smith, M. J. H.: Leukotriene B_4: an inflammatory mediator *in vivo*. Prostaglandins, *22*:213, 1981.

Bullough, W. S., and Laurence, E. B.: The control of epidermal mitotic activity in the mouse. Proc. Roy. Soc. Lond., *B151*:517, 1960.

Burke, J. F., Yannas, I. V., Quinby, W. C., Jr., Bondoc, C. C., and Jung, W. K.: Successful use of a physiologically acceptable artificial skin in the treatment of extensive burn injury. Ann. Surg., *194*:413, 1981.

Chvapil, M.: Experimental modifications of collagen synthesis and degradation and their therapeutic applications. *In* Weiss, J. B., and Jayson, M. I. V. (Eds.): Collagen in Health and Disease. Edinburgh, Churchill Livingstone, 1982.

Chvapil, M.: Personal communication, 1986.

Clore, J. N., Cohen, I. K., and Diegelmann, R. F.: Quantitation of collagen types I and III during wound healing in rat skin. Proc. Soc. Exp. Biol. Med., *161*:337, 1979.

Cohen, I. K., and Keiser, H. R.: Disruption of healed scars in scurvy—the result of a disequilibrium in collagen metabolism. Plast. Reconstr. Surg., *57*:213, 1976.

Cohen, I. K., Moore, C. D., and Diegelmann, R. F.: Onset and localization of collagen synthesis during wound healing in open rat skin wounds. Proc. Soc. Exp. Biol. Med., *160*:458, 1979.

Cutroneo, K. R., Rokowski, R., and Counts, D. F.: Glucocorticoids and collagen synthesis. Comparison of *in vivo* and cell culture studies. Coll. Relat. Res., *1*:557, 1981.

Cutroneo, K. R., Sterling, K. M., Jr., and Shull, S.: Steroid hormone regulation of extracellular matrix proteins. *In* Mecham, R. P. (Ed.): The Biology of the Extracellular Matrix. New York, Academic Press, 1986, pp. 119–176.

DiCorleto, P. E., and Bowen-Pope, D. F.: Cultured endothelial cells produce a platelet-derived growth factor–like protein. Proc. Natl. Acad. Sci. USA, *80*:1919, 1983.

Diegelmann, R. F., Cohen, I. K., and Kaplan, A. M.: Effect of macrophages on fibroblast DNA synthesis and proliferation. Proc. Soc. Exp. Biol. Med., *169*:445, 1982.

Diegelmann, R. F., Rothkopf, L. C., and Cohen, I. K.: Measurement of collagen biosynthesis during wound healing. J. Surg. Res., *19*:239, 1975.

Duncan, M. R., Perlish, J. S., and Fleischmajer, R.: Lymphokine/monokine inhibition of fibroblast proliferation and collagen production: role in progressive systemic sclerosis (PSS). J. Invest. Dermatol., *83*:377, 1984.

Ehrlich, H. P.: The role of connective tissue matrix in hypertrophic scar contracture. *In* Hunt, T. K., Heppenstall, R. B., Pines, E., and Rovee, D. (Eds.): Soft and Hard Tissue Repair: Biological and Clinical Aspects. New York, Praeger Press, 1984, Chap. 28.

Ehrlich, H. P., and Hunt, T. K.: The effects of cortisone and anabolic steroids on the tensile strength of healing wounds. Ann. Surg., *170*:203, 1969.

Ehrlich, H. P., Tarver, H., and Hunt, T. K.: Effects of vitamin A and glucocorticoids upon inflammation and collagen synthesis. Ann. Surg., *177*:222, 1973.

Fleisher, J. H., Misiorowski, R., Owen, J. A., and Chvapil, M.: Topical application of beta-aminopropionitrile. Life Sci., *29*:2553, 1981.

Francis, A. J., and Marks, R.: Skin stretching and epidermopoiesis. Br. J. Exp. Pathol., *58*:35, 1977.

Frank, D. H., Brahme, J., and Van de Berg, J. S.: Decrease in rate of wound contraction with the temporary skin substitute biobrane. Ann. Plast. Surg., *12*:519, 1984.

Gabbiani, G., and Majno, G.: Dupuytren's contracture: fibroblast contraction? An ultrastructural study. Am. J. Pathol., *66*:131, 1972.

Gabbiani, G., Ryan, G. B., and Majno, G.: Presence of modified fibroblasts in granulation tissue and their possible role in wound contraction. Experientia, *27*:549, 1971.

Gallico, G. G., 3rd, O'Connor, N. E., Compton, C. C., Kehinde, O., and Green, H.: Permanent coverage of large burn wounds with autologous cultured human epithelium. N. Engl. J. Med., *311*:448, 1984.

Gillman, T., and Penn, J.: Studies on the repair of cutaneous wounds. Med. Proc., *2*(Suppl. 3):121, 1956.

Graham, M. F., Becker, H., Cohen, I. K., Merritt, W., and Diegelmann, R. F.: Intrinsic tendon fibroplasia: documentation by *in vitro* studies. J. Orthop. Res., *1*:251, 1984a.

Graham, M. F., Diegelmann, R. F., Lindblad, W. J., Gay, R., Gay, S., and Cohen, I. K.: Effects of inflammation on wound healing: *in vitro* and *in vivo* studies. *In* Hunt, T. K., Heppenstall, R. B., Pines, E., and Rovee, D. (Eds.): Soft and Hard Tissue Repair: Biological and Clinical Aspects. New York, Praeger Press, 1984b, pp. 361–379.

Grillo, H. C.: Origin of fibroblasts in wound healing. An autoradiographic study of inhibition of cellular proliferation by local x-irradiation. Ann. Surg., *157*:453, 1963.

Grillo, H. C., and Gross, J.: Studies in wound healing. III. Contraction in vitamin C deficiency. Proc. Soc. Exp. Biol. Med., *101*:268, 1959.

Grillo, H. C., and Gross, J.: Collagenolytic activity and epithelial-mesenchymal interaction in healing mammalian wounds. J. Cell Biol., *23*:39A, 1964.

Grinnell, F.: Fibronectin and wound healing. J. Cell Biochem., *26*:107, 1984.

Grotendorst, G. R., Chang, T., Seppa, H. E., Kleinman, H. K., and Martin, G. R.: Platelet-derived growth factor is a chemoattractant for vascular smooth muscle cells. J. Cell Physiol., *113*:261, 1982.

Harris, E. D., Jr., and Krane, S. M.: Collagenases. N. Engl. J. Med., *291*:557, 1974.

Houck, J. C., Sharma, V. K., Patel, Y. M., and Gladner, J. A.: Induction of collagenolytic and proteolytic activities by anti-inflammatory drugs in the skin and fibroblast. Biochem. Pharmacol., *17*:2081, 1968.

Hunt, T. K., Conolly, W. B., Aronson, S. B., and Goldstein, P.: Anaerobic metabolism and wound healing: an hypothesis for the initiation and cessation of collagen synthesis in wounds. Am. J. Surg., *135*:328, 1978.

Hunt, T. K., Ehrlich, H. P., Garcia, J. A., and Dunphy, J. E.: Effect of vitamin A on reversing the inhibitory effect of cortisone on healing of open wounds in animals and man. Ann. Surg., *170*:633, 1969.

Hunt, T. K., and Pai, M. P.: The effect of varying ambient oxygen tension on wound metabolism and collagen synthesis. Surg. Gynecol. Obstet., *135*:561, 1972.

Hutton, J. J., Tappel, A. L., and Udenfriend, S.: Cofactor and substrate requirements of collagen proline hydroxylase. Arch. Biochem. Biophys., *118*:231, 1967.

Knighton, D. R., Silver, I. A., and Hunt, T. K.: Regulation of wound-healing angiogenesis—effect of oxygen gradients and inspired oxygen concentration. Surgery, *90*:262, 1981.

Kurkinen, M., Vaheri, A., Roberts, P. J., and Stenman, S.: Sequential appearance of fibronectin and collagen in experimental granulation tissue. Lab. Invest., *43*:47, 1980.

Leibovich, S. J., and Ross, R.: The role of the macrophage

in wound repair. A study with hydrocortisone and antimacrophage serum. Am. J. Pathol., *78*:71, 1975.

Lenaers, A., Ansay, M., Nusgens, B. V., and Lapière, C. M.: Collagen made of extended alpha chains, procollagen, in genetically defective dermatosporaxic calves. Eur. J. Biochem., *23*:533, 1971.

Levene, C. I.: Structural requirements for lathyrogenic agents. J. Exp. Med., *114*:295, 1961.

Lindblad, W. J., Gay, R. E., Gay, S., Diegelmann, R. F., and Cohen, I. K.: Immunohistochemical localization of Type IV collagen within healing dermal wounds. J. Histochem. Cytochem., submitted, 1988.

Madden, J. W., Davis, W. M., Butler, C., 2nd, and Peacock, E. E., Jr.: Experimental esophageal lye burns. II. Correcting established strictures with beta-aminopropionitrile and bougienage. Ann. Surg., *178*:277, 1973.

Madden, J. W., Morton, D., Jr., and Peacock, E. E., Jr.: Contraction of experimental wounds. I. Inhibiting wound contraction by using a topical smooth muscle antagonist. Surgery, *76*:8, 1974.

Madden, J. W., and Peacock, E. E., Jr.: Studies on the biology of collagen during wound healing. I. Rate of collagen synthesis and deposition in cutaneous wounds of the rat. Surgery, *64*:288, 1968.

Marks, F.: Isolation of an endogenous inhibitor of epidermal DNA synthesis (G_1 chalone) from pig skin. Hoppe-Seyler's Z. Physiol. Chem., *356*:1989, 1975.

Martinet, Y., Bitterman, P. B., Mornex, J.-F., Grotendorst, G. R., Martin, G. R., and Crystal, R. G.: Activated human monocytes express the c-sis proto-oncogene and release a mediator showing PDGF-like activity. Nature, *319*:158, 1986.

Maurois, A.: The Life of Sir Alexander Fleming (translated from the French by Gerard Hopkins). New York, Dutton, 1959, p. 293.

McKusick, V. A.: The Ehlers-Danlos syndrome. *In* McKusick, V. A. (Ed.): Heritable Disorders of Connective Tissue. St. Louis, C. V. Mosby Company, 1972.

Miller, E. J.: The structure of fibril-forming collagens. Ann. N.Y. Acad. Sci., *460*:1, 1985.

Moen, J. K.: The development of pure cultures of fibroblasts from single mononuclear cells. J. Exp. Med., *61*:247, 1935.

Narayanan, A. S., Voss, T., and Page, R. C.: Transcriptional regulation of fibroblast collagen synthesis by activated mononuclear cell supernatants. Biochem. Biophys. Res. Commun., *131*:1028, 1985.

Niinikoski, J.: Oxygen and wound healing. Clin. Plast. Surg., *4*:361, 1977.

Nimni, M. E., Deshmukh, K., Gerth, N., and Bavetta, L. A.: Changes in collagen metabolism associated with the administration of penicillamine and various amino and thiol compounds. Biochem. Pharmacol., *18*:707, 1969.

Peacock, E. E., Jr.: Biological principles in the healing of long tendons. Surg. Clin. North Am., *45*:461, 1965.

Peacock, E. E., Jr.: Thomas Orr Memorial Lecture: Biologic frontiers in the control of healing. Am. J. Surg., *126*:708, 1973.

Peacock, E. E., Jr., and Madden, J. W.: Some studies on the effects of beta-aminopropionitrile in patients with injured flexor tendons. Surgery, *66*:215, 1969.

Peacock, E. E., Jr., and Van Winkle, W.: Surgery and Biology of Repair. Philadelphia, W. B. Saunders Company, 1970.

Postlethwaite, A. E., Smith, G. N., Mainardi, C. L., Seyer, J. M., and Kang, A. H.: Lymphocyte modulation of fibroblast function *in vitro*: stimulation and inhibition of collagen production by different effector molecules. J. Immunol., *132*:2470, 1984.

Potenza, A. D.: Tendon healing within the flexor digital sheath in the dog. J. Bone Joint Surg., *44A*:49, 1962.

Riley, W. B., Jr., and Peacock, E. E., Jr.: The identification, distribution, and significance of a collagenolytic enzyme in human tissues. Proc. Soc. Exp. Biol. Med., *124*:207, 1967.

Roberts, A. B., Sporn, M. B., Assoian, R. K., Smith, J. M., Roche, N. S., et al.: Transforming growth factor type beta: rapid induction of fibrosis and angiogenesis *in vivo* and stimulation of collagen formation *in vitro*. Proc. Natl. Acad. Sci. USA, *83*:4167, 1986.

Rosenbloom, J., McArthur, W., Malamud, D., and Jimenez, S.: Characterization of a lymphokine produced by human T-cells which inhibits collagen synthesis. Cell. Immunol., *81*:192, 1983.

Ross, R.: The fibroblast and wound repair. Biol. Rev., *43*:51, 1968.

Ross, R., Everett, N. B., and Tyler, R.: Wound healing and collagen formation. VI. The origin of the wound fibroblast studied in parabiosis. J. Cell. Biol., *44*:645, 1970.

Ross, R., and Vogel, A.: The platelet-derived growth factor. Cell, *14*:203, 1978.

Rovee, D. T., Kurowsky, C. A., Labun, J., and Downes, A. M.: Effect of local wound environment on epidermal healing. *In* Maibach, H. I., and Rovee, D. T. (Eds.): Epidermal Wound Healing. Chicago, Year Book Medical Publishers, 1972.

Rudolph, R.: Inhibition of myofibroblasts by skin grafts. Plast. Reconstr. Surg., *63*:473, 1979.

Rudolph, R.: Contraction and the control of contraction. World J. Surg., *4*:279, 1980.

Rudolph, R., Abraham, J., Vecchione, T., Guber, S., and Woodward, M.: Myofibroblasts and free silicone around breast implants. Plast. Reconstr. Surg., *62*:185, 1978.

Rudolph, R., Guber, S., Suzuki, M., and Woodward, M.: The life cycle of the myofibroblast. Surg. Gynecol. Obstet., *145*:389, 1977.

Rudolph, R., and Klein, L.: Inhibition of mature ^{3}H-collagen destruction by triamcinolone. J. Surg. Res., *14*:435, 1973.

Ruoslahti, E., Engvall, E., and Hayman, E. G.: Fibronectin: current concepts of its structure and functions. Coll. Relat. Res., *1*:95, 1981.

Russell, J. D., Russell, S. B., and Trupin, K. M.: The effect of histamine on the growth of cultured fibroblasts isolated from normal and keloid tissue. J. Cell Physiol., *93*:389, 1977.

Salomon, J. C., Diegelmann, R. F., and Cohen, I. K.: Effect of dressings on donor site epithelialization. Surg. Forum, *25*:516, 1974.

Scher, C. D., Shepard, R. C., Antoniades, H. N., and Stiles, C. D.: Platelet-derived growth factor and the regulation of the mammalian fibroblast cell cycle. Biochim. Biophys. Acta, *560*:217, 1979.

Schiffmann, E., Corcoran, B. A., and Wahl, S. M.: *N*-Formylmethionyl peptides as chemoattractants for leucocytes. Proc. Natl. Acad. Sci. USA, *75*:1059, 1975.

Schofield, J. D., Uitto, J., and Prockop, D. J.: Formation of interchain disulfide bonds and helical structure during biosynthesis of procollagen by embryonic tendon cells. Biochemistry, *13*:1801, 1974.

Sedwick, A. O., and Willoughby, D. A.: Initiation of the inflammatory response and its prevention. *In* Bonta, I. L., Bray, M. A., and Parnham, M. J. (Eds.): Handbook of Inflammation. Amsterdam, Elsevier Science Publishers, 1985, p. 27.

Seppä, H., Grotendorst, G., Seppä, S., Schiffmann, E., and Martin, G. R.: Platelet-derived growth factor is chemotactic for fibroblasts. J. Cell Biol., *92*:584, 1982.

Simpson, D. M., and Ross, R.: The neutrophilic leukocyte in wound repair. A study with anti-neutrophil serum. J. Clin. Invest., *51*:2009, 1972.

Speakman, P. T.: Proposed mechanism for the biological assembly of collagen triple helix. Nature, *229*:241, 1971.

Sporn, M. B., and Roberts, A. B.: Peptide growth factors and inflammation, tissue repair, and cancer. J. Clin. Invest., *78*:329, 1980.

Sporn, M. B., Roberts, A. B., Shull, J. H., Smith, J. M., Ward, J. M., and Sodek, J.: Polypeptide transforming growth factors isolated from bovine sources and used for wound healing *in vivo*. Science, *219*:1329, 1983.

Sporn, M. B., Roberts, A. B., Wakefield, L. M., and Assoian, R. K.: Transforming growth factor-beta: biological function and chemical structure. Science, *233*:532, 1986.

Squier, C. A.: The stretching of mouse skin *in vivo*. Effect on epidermal proliferation and thickness. J. Invest. Dermatol., *74*:68, 1980.

Stein, H. D., and Keiser, H. R.: Collagen metabolism in granulating wounds. J. Surg. Res., *11*:277, 1971.

Stenn, K. S.: The role of serum in the epithelial outgrowth of mouse skin explants. Br. J. Dermatol., *98*:411, 1978.

Stenn, K. S.: Epibolin, a protein in human plasma that supports epithelial cell movement. Proc. Natl. Acad. Sci. USA, *78*:6907, 1981.

Stenn, K. S., Madri, J. A., and Roll, F. J.: Migrating epidermis produces AB_2 collagen and requires continual collagen synthesis for movement. Nature (London), *277*:229, 1979.

Sullivan, G. J., and Epstein, W. S.: Mitotic activity of wounded human epidermis. J. Invest. Dermatol., *41*:39, 1963.

Topol, B. M., Lewis, V. L., and Benveniste, K.: The use of antihistamine to retard the growth of fibroblasts derived from human skin, scar, and keloid. Plast. Reconstr. Surg., *68*:227, 1981.

Trunkey, D. D.: Trauma. Sci. Am., *249*:23, 1983.

Uitto, J., and Prockop, D. J.: Hydroxylation of peptide-bound proline and lysine before and after chain completion of the polypeptide chains of procollagen. Arch. Biochem. Biophys., *164*:210, 1974.

Van Winkle, W., Jr.: Wound contraction. Surg. Gynecol. Obstet., *125*:131, 1967.

Watts, G. T., Grillo, H. C., and Gross, J.: Studies in wound healing. II. The role of granulation tissue in contraction. Ann. Surg., *148*:153, 1958.

Werb, Z.: Degradation of collagen. *In* Weiss, J. B., and Jayson, M. I. V. (Eds.): Collagen in Health and Disease. Edinburgh, Churchill Livingstone, 1982, p. 121.

White, B. N., Shetlar, M. R., and Schilling, J. A.: The glycoproteins and their relationship to the healing of wounds. Ann. N.Y. Acad. Sci., *94*:297, 1961.

Wiggins, R. C., Giclas, P. C., and Henson, P. M.: Chemotactic activity generated from the fifth component of complement by plasma kallikrein of rabbit. J. Exp. Med., *153*:1391, 1981.

Yannas, I. V., Burke, J. R., Orgill, D. P., and Skrabut, E. M.: Wound tissue can utilize a polymeric template to synthesize a functional extension of skin. Science, *215*:174, 1982.

6

Alan R. Shons

Transplantation Biology

HISTORICAL BACKGROUND

The replacement of diseased, injured, or worn parts has been a dream of man for centuries. There are accounts of transplants from animals to man in Greek mythology. The legend of Cosmas and Damien recounts the transplantation of a leg from a Moor to a servant of the church whose own leg was amputated for cancer (Danilevicius, 1967).

The scientific foundation for clinical transplantation has been largely developed in the last 40 years, although brilliantly perceptive observations were made long before the modern era. Bert (1863) noted differing success rates in skin grafts within the same animal (autografts), between animals of the same species (allografts), and between animals of different species (xenografts). While Reverdin believed that skin grafts could be taken with equal success from the same individual or individuals of the same or different species, Lexer reported in 1911 that skin allografts were rejected in man, affirming the difference between autografts and allografts (Gibson, 1955). Schone (1912) suggested that "Transplantationsimmunität," i.e., transplantation immunity, was responsible for the failure of allografts. Shawan (1919) recognized the importance of blood groups in the rejection process. Holman (1924) made several important observations. He recognized that first set skin grafts between human beings sensitized the recipient and that second set grafts from the same donor precipitated a more extreme and rapid form of rejection. He also observed the specificity of sensitization produced by grafts from a single donor.

The immunologic basis of transplantation rejection had been defined by these early observations; however, doubts persisted. Loeb (1945) thought that individuality differences between donor and recipient, and not an immune process, were responsible for graft rejection. The conclusions of Loeb concerning individuality differentials were supported by the demonstrations of Padgett (1932), Brown (1937), and Converse and Duchet (1947) that skin grafts transplanted between monozygotic twins survived permanently.

The stage was set for clinical transplantation by the work of Gibson and Medawar (1943), which began with a description of events leading to the rejection of allografts in man and the more rapid rejection of second set grafts. Medawar's subsequent experimental work (1946a,b, 1948) proved: (a) that resistance to skin allografts is not innate—first set allografts have a brief period of acceptance; (b) that allograft sensitivity, once developed, is systemic; (c) that second set allografts are rejected in an accelerated fashion; and (d) that allograft rejection is donor specific.

THE ALLOGRAFT REACTION

Autografts survive indefinitely. Allograft survival is inversely proportional to the genetic disparity between donor and recipient. Grafts between individuals of different species (xenografts) are rejected most rapidly. Allografts are morphologically identical to autografts in the early post-transplant period if the recipient has not previously been sensitized to donor antigens.

Skin graft rejection has been used as a standard transplant model (Converse and Rapaport, 1956). Skin allografts and autografts appear similar for the first two days after grafting (see Chap. 8). Multiple dilated capillaries are noted without blood flow. By the third or fourth day, the dilated capillaries are replaced by small caliber vessels with rapid blood flow. The vessels persist in autografts. In allografts there is an infiltration of leukocytes into the perivascular spaces beginning at two to five days. Dilated vessels, thrombi, and punctate hemorrhages develop over the next two days. Blood flow ceases by the eighth or ninth day. Slough of the graft follows.

Second grafts from the same donor are rejected more rapidly. A "white graft reaction" occurs in which the graft is not vascularized if the second set grafts are applied within one week of the first set. A second set graft applied eight to 80 days after the first set will result in a four to five day rejection process. Second set grafts applied more than 80 days after the first set may undergo a rejection process similar to a first set rejection (Rapaport and Converse, 1957, 1958).

HISTOCOMPATIBILITY ANTIGENS

Graft rejection occurs because the recipient recognizes the donor tissue as foreign. Foreignness implies the existence of antigens on the graft that are different from the recipient. Antigens that can stimulate graft rejection are histocompatibility antigens. Many antigens can serve as histocompatibility antigens, blood group antigens being strong ones. Histocompatibility antigens are found primarily on cell surfaces, and their concentration varies among the several tissues of the body. There is great variability in the strength of histocompatibility antigens. Allograft survival may vary from one to 15 weeks in untreated recipients, depending on donor-recipient disparity. Studies by Rapaport and associates (1971) of similar antigens on human leukocytes and bacterial membranes suggest that histocompatibility antigens are composed of a wide range of determinants that may be individually specific or ubiquitous throughout nature.

HISTOCOMPATIBILITY GENETICS

The strongest transplantation antigens are the expression of a single chromosomal region called the major histocompatibility complex (MHC). The delineation of this complex began in the 1950's with the work of Dausset (1958). Leukoagglutinating antibodies were found in the sera of multiparous women and multiply transfused patients. Analysis of the reactivity patterns of the antisera against the cells of other individuals suggested the identification of antigens within the population that were the products of a polymorphic genetic locus. The antigens defined were termed human leukocyte antigens (HLA). In man the MHC is located on chromosome 6. All animals have a similar locus. In mice the strongest antigens are called H-2 antigens.

HLA antigens on cell surfaces can be detected in two ways. They may be defined by serologic reactions using typing sera obtained chiefly from multiparous women. Purified lymphocytes are obtained from heparinized blood by Ficoll-Hypaque gradient centrifugation. Specific antisera and complement are added in microtiter plates. Lymphocytes with specific alloantigens on the cell surface will be lysed or agglutinated. A second detection method measures the reactivity of host lymphocytes to donor lymphocytes. Lymphocytes from HLA-D different individuals mixed in culture respond by blast transformation, DNA synthesis, and proliferation. Purified lymphocytes obtained from heparinized blood are incubated with donor lymphocytes inactivated by radiation or mitomycin C. Tritiated thymidine is added to the culture and blast transformation of the responding lymphocytes is quantitated by the uptake of thymidine (Shons and associates, 1973). Antigens that can trigger the transformation of lymphocytes are called class II antigens. Antigens that cannot cause lymphocyte transformation are called class I antigens. Both class I and class II antigens can be detected by antisera.

Class I antigens are expressions of HLA-A and HLA-B loci. Class II antigens are the expression of the HLA-D locus. At each locus there are many alternative forms (alleles) of the gene. There are at least 18 alleles at the HLA-A locus, 32 at the HLA-B locus, and 10 at the HLA-D locus. Each person inherits one chromosome 6 from each parent, and thus everyone has two HLA antigen complexes. All HLA antigens are expressed codominantly on the cell surface. The known loci of the HLA complex are shown in Figure 6–1.

The relative positions of the loci have been determined; however, they are separated by considerable genetic material, the significance of which is not yet known. Some of the material controls the immune responsiveness of the individual. The susceptibility to a wide variety of diseases has been associated with certain HLA specificities (Goldman and Goldman, 1981). The correlation of several autoimmune diseases with HLA-DR3 (myasthenia gravis, Graves' disease, systemic lupus erythematosus) suggests that DR antigens are markers for adjacent immune response genes (Stastny and associates, 1983).

The HLA subloci on chromosome 6 are closely linked. Antigens from one chromosome constitute a haplotype. An individual normally inherits one haplotype from each parent. Genetic crossover can occur during meiosis to yield a recombinant haplotype between HLA-A and HLA-B antigens or between HLA-B and HLA-D antigens. Although the frequency of finding one allele at one HLA locus with another allele at a second HLA locus should be the product of the frequencies of the alleles in the population, this is not seen. Certain allele combinations are found in much higher than expected frequencies. This phenomenon is termed linkage disequilibrium and may be due to a selective advantage of certain haplotypes. Weak histocompatibility antigens are controlled by loci on chromosomes other than chromosome 6. Thus, allografts between unrelated HLA identical individuals will be rejected. The non–HLA determined histocompatibility antigens constitute a significant but undefined factor in clinical transplantation.

There is variability in HLA antigen expression among different cell types and even among different phases of the cell cycle. HLA-A and HLA-B antigens are expressed on most parenchymal cells, while HLA-D antigens are found primarily on macrophages, B lymphocytes, and dividing T lymphocytes.

The molecular structure of the class I and class II antigens has been well defined. Class I antigens consist of a two-chain molecule composed of a 44,000 MW glycoprotein determined by HLA genes in association with a 12,000 MW microglobulin determined by a gene on chromosome 15. The molecule is fixed to the cell membrane by the 44,000 MW chain containing 337 amino acid residues. Class II antigens consist of a two-glycoprotein chain molecule. The alpha chain is 34,000 MW and appears similar in structure among the different HLA-DR antigens. The beta chain is MW 29,000 and is noted to vary in structure among different HLA-DR antigens. It is likely that HLA-DR antigenic specificity resides in the beta chain (Schwartz, 1984).

HISTOCOMPATIBILITY TESTING

Transplant success correlates with the similarity of the antigenic mosaic of donor and recipient. Transplants between relatives are more successful than transplants between unrelated individuals, owing to the inevitable antigen sharing among relatives.

Two methods are used to assess antigenic differences between donor and recipient in human transplantation. *Leukocyte typing* is used to determine the HLA type of donor and

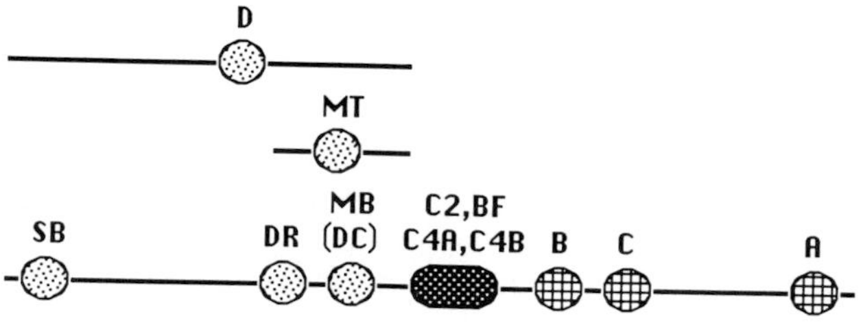

Figure 6–1. The HLA complex on chromosome 6. Class I loci are A, B, and C. Class II loci are SB, DR, MB(DC), MT, and D. The complement loci are C2, BF, C4A, and C4B. MT antigens may be molecules determined by DR and MB or they may have separate determinant loci. D lymphocyte activating determinants are controlled by several class II loci.

recipient. Standardized antisera obtained from multiparous women or multiply transfused patients can be used to characterize HLA-A, HLA-B, and HLA-D antigens on lymphocyte membranes. Lymphocytes, antisera, and complement are incubated. Lymphocytes that react with the antisera are killed and retain vital dyes indicating a positive test. Leukocyte typing is particularly useful in determining the best donor choice among family members. Because only major histocompatibility antigens are identified by this assay, it has limited usefulness for unrelated donor and recipient, owing to the many histocompatibility antigens not yet defined.

The *mixed lymphocyte culture (MLC) test* is used to detect the degree of histocompatibility between donor and recipient at the HLA-D/DR locus. The amount of stimulation of recipient lymphocytes by donor lymphocytes correlates with HLA-D/DR disparity, a critical factor in predicting allograft success. The assay requires several days, making it useful only for the study of living, related donor recipient pairs.

THE LYMPHOID SYSTEM

Allografts or xenografts are rejected by a complex immune mechanism based on the lymphoid system. A hematopoietic stem cell that arises in the yolk sac differentiates along a number of cell lines to yield all hematopoietic cells. The yolk sac stem cell differentiates into oligopotential progenitor cells of the myeloid series (basophils, neutrophils, eosinophils) and the lymphoid series. Lymphoid progenitor cells are influenced by the microchemical milieu of two central lymphoid organs, the thymus and the bursal equivalent tissues.

The thymus governs the development of cellular immunity responsible for delayed hypersensitivity and allograft rejection (Good and associates, 1966). As stem cells enter the thymic cortex and move to the thymic medulla, a series of differentiation steps occur in which there is an evolution of surface (T) molecules correlating with functional differentiation (Reinherz and Schlossman, 1980). The surface molecules can be detected by monoclonal antisera, and by this technique the functional subpopulations of lymphocytes can be identified. The development of capacity to respond to histocompatibility antigens is an important component of the intrathymic differentiation dependent on thymic stromal cells. Neonatal thymectomy seriously impairs the development of cellular immunity.

After leaving, the thymus T cells move to the peripheral lymphoid tissues, including spleen, lymph nodes, and Peyer's patches. T cell movement to the periphery is guided by interaction between surface molecules on the T cell and surface molecules on the venules (Gallatin, Weissman, and Butcher, 1983). T cells move preferentially to the paracortical regions of the lymph nodes.

Peripheral T cells can be divided into two subpopulations phenotypically based on T surface molecules. The two phenotypes are associated with distinct functional characteristics. Both populations carry the T1, T3, and T11 molecules. Cells that carry the T4 molecule are effector cells for hypersensitivity. T4 cells are helper cells for immunoglobulin synthesis as well as for the development of cytotoxic effector cells. T4 cells also aid in the induction of suppressor cells. Cells carrying the T8 molecule are cytotoxic effector cells and can act as suppressor cells, inhibiting immunoglobulin synthesis and delayed hypersensitivity reactions (Stobo, 1984).

Lymphoid cells that are not influenced by the thymus differentiate along another pathway controlled by the bursal system and are called B cells. In birds the bursa of Fabricius is a well-defined anatomic organ in the hindgut (Cooper, Peterson, and Good, 1965). An analogous organ in mammalians has not been found. In man, B cells are generated in the fetal liver. Stem cells then populate the bone marrow, where B cells are produced throughout life. B cells are located in the lymph node germinal centers and medullary cord lymphoid tissue.

B lymphocytes are responsible for humoral immunity. B lymphocyte differentiation begins with an antigen independent phase, followed by an antigen dependent phase. Immunoglobulins carried on the surface of B lymphocytes change in character with cell differentiation. The various immunoglobulin types can be identified by monoclonal antibodies (Kuritani and Cooper, 1982). Immature B cells display a high concentration of membrane-bound IgM. As differentiation proceeds, increasing amounts of IgG, which eventually becomes the predominant immunoglobulin, is noted (Abney and associates, 1978). Crosslinkage of membrane IgM on immature lymphocytes blocks subsequent differentiation and renders that particular clone inactive.

B cell differentiation may proceed to two end points. A plasma cell may form that has a short, four day life span and produces large amounts of an antigen specific immunoglobulin. Alternatively, B cells may progress to a resting state memory cell that can differentiate rapidly into a plasma cell upon further exposure to antigen (Levitt and Cooper, 1984).

THE MACROPHAGE SYSTEM

Mononuclear phagocytes arise from a multipotential stem cell in the bone marrow. Within the bone marrow, maturation from monoblast to monocyte occurs. Maturation involves progressive loss of proliferative capability and increasing functional capacity as measured by lymphocyte interaction and lysosome concentration. Monocytes migrate from the bone marrow to the circulation, then to an extravascular pool. Tissue macrophages arise from maturation of extravascular macrophages to serve multiple antigen recognition and processing functions. A complex of membrane receptors for both immune and nonimmune materials control macrophage response. Receptors for C3 complement, Fc immunoglobulin fragments, lymphokines, and complex carbohydrates have been identified (Cohn, 1978).

THE REJECTION MECHANISM—THE AFFERENT LIMB

The development of immunity and transplant rejection begins by exposure of the host to histocompatibility antigens of the graft. Histocompatibility antigens, being membrane components, are easily shed to the bloodstream or lymphatics (Najarian and associates, 1966). Most of the sensitization occurs in the peripheral lymphoid tissue of the host. A small component of the sensitization process takes place among the circulating lymphocytes. The specific site of cellular recognition is the small lymphocyte. In the last decade multiple complex cell interactions in lymphocyte activation have been defined.

The macrophage is necessary for lymphocyte activation. The macrophage traps antigens and presents them to T lymphocytes. The T lymphocyte and the cooperating macrophage must display the same major histocompatibility antigens (Ia antigens) on their cell surface. Only a subset population of macrophages carries the appropriate Ia antigen. Stimulated macrophages modulate the lymphocyte response by the production of interleukin 1 (IL 1), an immunologically nonspecific peptide of approximately 15,000 MW. IL 1 stimulates proliferation of T cells already activated by surface antigen contact. The substance is apparently a required cofactor for antigen induced lymphocyte proliferation (Oppenheim and Cohen, 1983). IL 1 has similar effects on B cells, enhancing replication and antibody production by both direct effects on the B cell and indirect effects through the stimulation of helper T cells.

T lymphocytes respond to antigen stimulation by proliferation and differentiation. Stimulation is a membrane mediated phenomenon. The membrane antigen receptor is known to be a disulfide linked heterodimer with chains of MW 49,000 and MW 43,000. Antigen specific heterodimers have been isolated and genes coding for the heterodimers have been identified (Meuer and associates, 1983). There are different functional subpopulations of the T cell that respond to different antigens. Class 1 antigens, i.e., the HLA-A and HLA-B antigens, are recognized by the cytotoxic T cells, which respond primarily by differentiation to a cell of killer capacity. Class II antigens, i.e., HLA-D antigens, cause the proliferation of helper T cells necessary for development of cytotoxic cells. Helper T cells produce interleukin 2 (IL 2), a 15,000 MW non–species specific protein known to promote and regulate cytotoxic T cell activity. The mechanism of helper T cell interaction with cytotoxic T cells is not clearly defined, but mediators such as IL 2 play an important role.

Antibody production is the end result of B lymphocyte activation. There are known to be multiple requirements for B cell stimulation. B cells are directed to leave the resting stage by antigen crosslinkage of immunoglobulin molecules. Helper T cells are required for antibody production. Helper T cells recognize HLA-D determinants on the resting B cell, then facilitate B cell differentiation. This implies the requirement of populations of similar HLA-D T and B lymphocytes. Helper T cells further facilitate B cell activity by the production of individual nonspecific soluble factors (Lawton, 1982).

The plasma cell is the fully differentiated antibody producing B cell. Each plasma cell produces an antibody of one immunoglobulin class and one specificity. In man, five immunoglobulin classes exist: IgG, IgM, IgA, IgD, and IgE. IgG is present in the highest serum concentration. Each IgG molecule is composed of four polypeptide chains: two light chains (MW 23,000) and two heavy chains (MW 50,000) linked by disulfide bonds. Amino acid analysis reveals that both heavy and light chains have a constant amino acid sequence at the C-terminal end and a variable amino acid sequence at the N-terminal end (Fig. 6–2). Antigen binding is associated with the two N-terminal ends on each IgG molecule. Secondary biologic properties (e.g., complement fixation) are associated with the C-terminal end. IgM immunoglobulins are large molecules (MW 850,000) that have five antigen combining sites. Each of the five subunits of IgM molecules resembles the IgG molecule, possessing two heavy and two light chains. IgG and IgM are the two immunoglobulin classes primarily involved in transplant rejection.

THE REJECTION MECHANISM—THE EFFERENT LIMB

Cell Mediated Responses

The presence of inflammatory cells at the site of graft rejection suggested to early investigators that the sensitized lymphocytes recognized and killed the graft. The rejection process is now known to be far more complex. The recognition of foreign tissue by lymphocytes and antibodies begins the activation of several enzyme systems that are in themselves destructive as well as effective in the recruitment of destructive cellular mediators (macrophages and polymorphonuclear leukocytes).

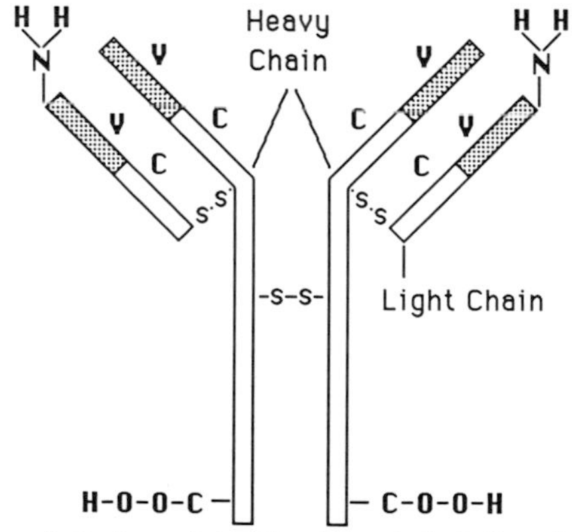

Figure 6–2. A model of the four-chain IgG molecule. V is the variable region. C is the constant region.

The lymphocyte response to histocompatibility antigens involves two cellular components. Precursor cytotoxic T lymphocytes recognize class I antigens, and class II antigens are recognized by precursor helper T lymphocytes. T helper lymphocytes produce a lymphokine (IL 2) that stimulates the production and function of cytotoxic T lymphocytes (Bach, Bach, and Sondel, 1976). IL 2 is one example of a variety of lymphokines that activate cellular immune mediators.

Migration inhibitory factor and chemotactic factor attract and immobilize macrophages, while macrophage activation factor stimulates macrophage graft destructive ability through stimulation of phagocytosis, pinocytosis, and cytotoxicity. Other lymphokines, including leukocyte inhibitory factor, have similar effects on leukocytes. Lymphokines that affect other cell lines include lymphotoxin, skin reactive factor, and interferon. The number of specifically sensitized cells may be increased through the production of transfer factor by sensitized lymphocytes. Transfer factor is a dialyzable DNase resistant molecule that can transfer specific antigen responsiveness to unsensitized lymphocytes.

Circulating antibody can mediate allograft rejection, but antibody is not required for allograft rejection. The antigen-antibody complex triggers several nonspecific effector mechanisms that cause graft destruction. The effector mechanisms are enzyme systems that attract active cells, degrade cell surfaces, increase vascular permeability, and cause clot formation.

The Complement System

The complement system is the primary mediator of antigen-antibody reactions. The system consists of at least 20 different plasma proteins within nine major subgroups existing in the circulation normally as inactive molecules. Activation of the system may occur by two different pathways. The classic pathway is activated by a complex of antigen and an antibody of subclass IgG1, IgG2, IgG3, and IgM. Activation occurs by the binding of complement component C1 to the Fc region of the immunoglobulin molecule. Nonimmunologic activation of the classic pathway can be effected by the direct binding of C1 to other substances such as DNA and C-reactive protein (Cooper, 1983).

The alternate or properdin complement activation pathway is triggered immunologically by antigen plus IgA or IgG molecules. The system is activated nonimmunologically by certain polysaccharides and lipopolysaccharides. The alternate pathway activates the complement sequence at the C3 level.

The several components of the complement system with component fragments serve a wide variety of functions. Fragments C3a, C4a, and C5a are anaphylatoxins. These peptides increase vascular permeability, cause histamine and lysosomal enzyme release, and are chemotactic (C5a). The terminal portion of the complement sequence, C5b-C9, must be bound to cell membranes to effect damage. The alteration may range from a change in charge to functional loss or membrane disruption (Fig. 6–3).

The Clotting System

Clot formation within an allograft can be initiated by two mechanisms. The intrinsic system is activated by antigen-antibody complex activation of Hageman factor (factor XII). The activation sequence continues through factors XI, IX, VII, and V to activation of prothrombin factor to form thrombin leading to fibrin polymerization. The extrinsic system is initiated by tissue thromboplastin release from cells damaged by antibody and complement or cytotoxic lymphocytes. Platelet phospholipids also promote clotting (Fig. 6–4).

The Kinin System

The kinin system is a third molecular cascade participating in the rejection process. Activated Hageman factor can lead to the formation of kallikrein, which acts on kininogen to produce bradykinin. The kinins, a group of active peptides, cause chemotaxis, dilate arterioles, increase capillary permeability, and cause smooth muscle contraction. Kinins are rapidly inactivated by plasma kinases.

The relative participation of cellular and humoral factors in allograft rejection is dependent on the preexisting state of sensitization of the host to antigens present within the graft. The time course and histologic features of first set allograft rejection are consistent with a primary cellular mechanism. A second set allograft is rejected faster, with histologic features indicating a greater participation of complement, clotting, and kinin factors. The rejection of grafts between species can be a very rapid process, one that has been shown to be primarily mediated by humoral factors (Shons, Moberg, and Najarian, 1972).

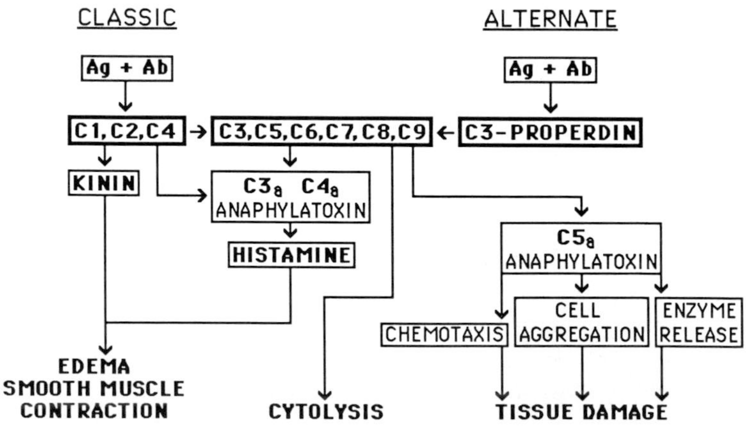

Figure 6–3. A diagram of the effect of complement system activation.

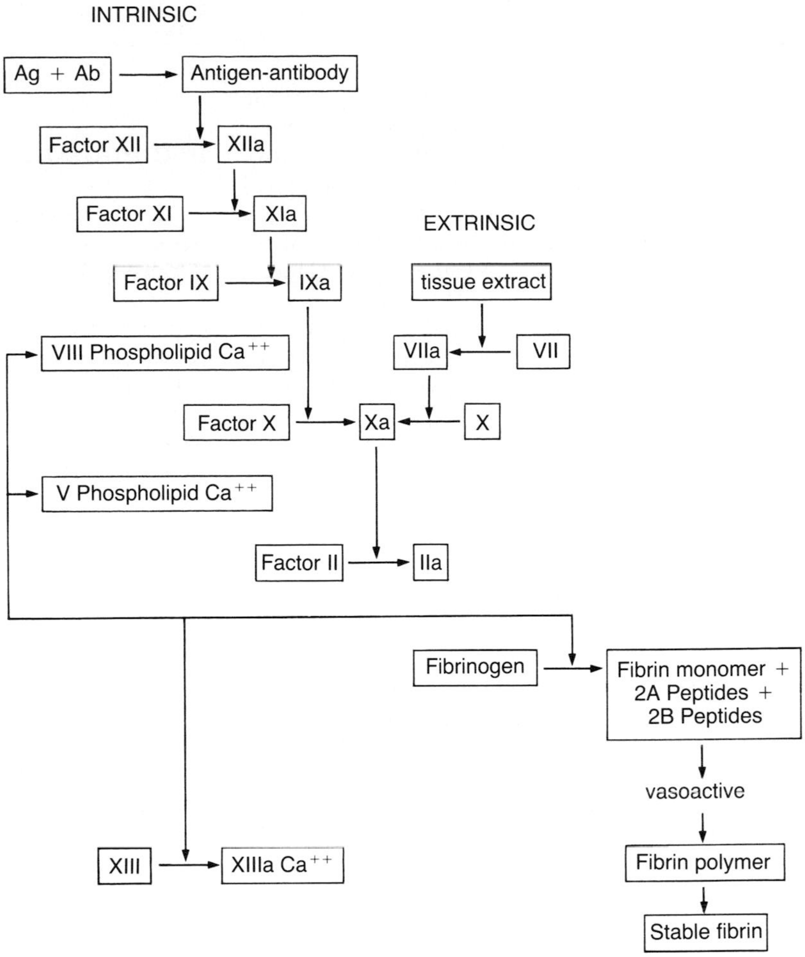

Figure 6–4. The clotting system. Antigen-antibody complexes initiate the intrinsic system. Tissue thromboplastin released from damaged cells initiates the extrinsic system.

MODIFICATION OF ALLOGRAFT REJECTION

Privileged Site

The rejection process can be modified by an immunologically privileged site, the induction of immunologic enhancement, immunologic tolerance, and immunosuppression.

Foreign tissue may provoke a lesser immunologic response in certain anatomic areas. The anterior chamber of the eye and the brain, both areas that lack lymphatic drainage, are immunologically privileged sites in which foreign tissue is well tolerated (Murphy and Sturm, 1923; Greene, 1941). The lack of lymphatic drainage was thought to block the afferent limb of the immune response by preventing sensitization. The reduced immune response is now known to be more complex. Subba Rao and Grogan (1985) have demonstrated reduced reactivity of spleen thymocytes in rats carrying allogeneic skin grafts in the anterior chamber. This finding suggests an active central immune regulation mechanism rather than a passive block of the sensitization process.

Immunologic Enhancement

Immunologic enhancement is the prolongation of graft survival in recipients previously immunized to antigens present in the graft. Enhancement has been attributed to the presence of antibodies that by some mechanism block graft destruction. The antibodies may mask foreign antigens, preventing the induction of cytotoxic T cells, and may inhibit the proliferation of sensitized cells. Alternatively, the antibodies may coat the graft cells, preventing destruction by the immune effectors.

Enhancement may be active or passive. Active enhancement follows host exposure to graft antigens. The timing of previous antigen exposure and subsequent graft as well as the form of antigen presentation are critically important. Accelerated rejection normally follows sensitization. The improved survival of kidney allografts in patients receiving pretransplant blood transfusions may be a clinical example of active enhancement (Opelz, Mickey, and Terasaki, 1981; Opelz, 1985). Passive enhancement is achieved by the transfer of immune serum or sensitized lymphocytes. The enhancing activity of serum lies in the IgG fraction.

Immunologic Tolerance

An ideal modification of the rejection process would be the induction within the host of a specific nonreactivity to antigens of the allograft. Immunologic tolerance is an immunologically unresponsive state induced by controlled exposure to antigen. Our understanding of this phenomenon began with the demonstration of Owen (1945) that, as a result of a prenatal exchange of red cell precursors, twin cattle retain throughout life a mixture of each other's erythrocytes, a condition called chimerism. Billingham and associates (1952) showed that chimeric cattle would accept skin grafts from each other but not from parents or siblings. Burnet and Fenner (1948) suggested that specific unresponsiveness would be achieved by antigen exposure in early life. Finally, Billingham, Brent, and Medawar (1956) demonstrated induction of immunologic unresponsiveness to histocompatibility antigens in mice by the neonatal injection of allogeneic cells.

Considerable experimental work has proved that immunologic tolerance can be obtained in specific animal models. The form of the antigen, dose, and route of administration are important variables. Large protein antigens are most effective. Particulate antigens such as bacteria cannot be used. Immunologic tolerance is more easily developed in the young or immunologically incompetent animal. Immunologic tolerance to the antigen mosaic of a tissue is harder to accomplish than is tolerance to a single antigenic determinant. The mechanism of tolerance may involve a complex interaction of T cell subpopulations. It has been suggested that suppressor cells are activated by exposure to alloreactive cells specific for tolerated antigens (Stephenson and Roser, 1985).

Immunosuppression

The success of clinical transplantation depends on nonspecific methods of immunosuppression that deplete or block proliferation of immunocompetent cells. Antigen specific methods of immunosuppression remain an intriguing laboratory pursuit.

Corticosteroids. Steroids are widely used in clinical transplantation. Their mechanisms of action are not well understood but their effectiveness is unquestioned. Steroids alone cannot prevent rejection, but in combination with other drugs they are effective in both preventing and reversing rejection. Steroids cross the cell membrane to bind with receptors in the cell cytoplasm. The steroid receptor complex then enters the nucleus to react with DNA. The lymphocyte is the cell most affected. DNA, RNA, and protein synthesis is reduced. Lymphocytolysis occurs in many of the affected cells. Maximal lymphopenia occurs four to six hours after a single dose of steroids. The reduction is greater in T cells than in B cells. Helper T cells are reduced more than suppressor T cells. The lymphopenia results from a combination of cytolysis and sequestration.

Steroids affect other cells important in allograft rejection. Chemotaxis and phagocytosis are reduced among neutrophils and macrophages. Steroid produced cell redistribution causes a temporary increase in circulating neutrophils by reducing endothelial margination. Steroid action on cells other than lymphocytes reduces primarily the nonspecific inflammatory component of allograft rejection (Fauci, 1979).

Antilymphocyte Globulin. Lymphocytes derived from thoracic duct drainage, peripheral blood, thymus, spleen, or lymph nodes can be used to produce in animals an antilymphocyte serum. The use of such a serum in clinical transplantation is controversial. However, its efficacy in preventing or ameliorating rejection has been proved, beginning with the work of Monaco, Wood, and Russell (1967). The rabbit and horse are most commonly used to produce human antilymphocyte serum. The active fraction of the serum is IgG, which can be purified as antilymphocyte globulin (ALG) and can be given intravenously, intramuscularly, or subcutaneously. The course of therapy is usually limited to the immediate pretransplant period plus a week or two after transplantation. The drug may also be used for short periods during rejection episodes.

The mechanism of action of ALG is poorly understood. The maximal effect is on the T lymphocyte and cell mediated immunity. There is little effect on antibody response. The long-lived T lymphocytes are coated with ALG and cleared from the circulation by the liver and spleen. Prolonged ALG administration depletes the paracortical T cell region of lymph nodes. ALG potentiates other immunosuppressive drugs.

The toxicity of ALG is related to its crossreactivity with other recipient antigens and the fact that the substance is a xenogeneic protein that can cause serum sickness. The crossreactivity can be reduced by absorption of the material with human platelets and red cell stroma. The immunosuppressive potency and the crossreactivity of each batch of ALG vary, and better assay methods are needed to assess these factors (Najarian and Simmons, 1971).

Radiation. Radiation can produce lymphopenia and suppress immunocompetent cell functions. High dose radiation produces changes in nucleic acids. DNA and cellular replication are particularly vulnerable. Cells possess repair mechanisms for radiation induced damage. However, the repairs may be inadequate in rapidly proliferating cells and cell death may result.

The immunosuppressive effects of radiation depend on the timing of radiation and antigen exposure. The maximal effect of radiation is achieved if it is given immediately preceding, during, or soon after antigen exposure. Late administration of radiation has little effect, since a stable population of sensitized cells has developed. In the clinical setting, radiation may be used to treat locally an organ undergoing a rejection episode (Johnson and associates, 1985).

Antiproliferative Drugs. Clinically useful immunosuppressant drugs inhibit lymphocyte proliferation by substituting for needed metabolites (antimetabolites) or by combining with cell components (alkylating agents).

The antimetabolite purine analogue, azathioprine (Imuran), is the most widely used drug in clinical transplantation. Azathioprine acts by competitive enzyme inhibition to block synthesis of inosinic acid, a precursor of adenylic and guanylic acid. DNA and RNA synthesis is reduced. The drug is primarily effective at blocking replicative functions, although other mechanisms of action have been suggested. The drug may also bind antigen receptor sites on T lymphocytes, rendering them nonfunctional. Liver and bone marrow toxicity is a side effect of the drug (Skinner and Schwartz, 1972).

Two other antimetabolites are effective immunosuppressants: the folic acid antagonists aminopterin and methotrexate, which prevent the conversion of folic acid to tetrahydrofolic acid. Their toxicity has prevented use in clinical kidney transplantation, although methotrexate is used in bone marrow transplantation.

Cyclophosphamide, an alkylating agent, is used in clinical bone marrow transplantation and it finds limited use in kidney transplant patients in whom the liver toxicity of azathioprine is a problem. Alkylating agents have an unstable ring as part of the molecular structure that combines with DNA, RNA, and structural proteins, rendering them faulty. Cell death may occur immediately or at the next mitosis. B lymphocytes and antibody production are affected more than T lymphocyte cell mediated immunity functions (Turk and Parker, 1979). Toxicity of cyclophosphamide is high, with manifestations among all systems that have rapidly dividing cell populations. Diarrhea, stomatitis, skin rash, anemia, and alopecia are seen.

Cyclosporine, a cyclic polypeptide, represents a new class of clinically useful immunosuppressants. Borel discovered the immunosuppressive properties of this fungal metabolite isolated from fungi Trichoderma polysporum and Cylindrocarpon lucidium (Borel and associates, 1977). The drug differs from conventional immunosuppressants in that it is not cytotoxic for lymphocytes and it has no antimitotic activity.

The mechanism of action of cyclosporine is unknown. The principal activity is directed at the T helper subpopulation of lymphocytes and cytolytic effector cells (Wiesinger and Borel, 1980). The action may be mediated by inhibiting the production or release of IL I from the macrophage antigen processing cells. This blocks IL 1 stimulation of T helper cells. Cyclosporine may also block IL 2 receptors on precursor T cells, preventing proliferation of cytotoxic T cells (Fig. 6–5). T suppressor cells are not affected. Cyclosporine does not affect neutrophils or macrophages and thus allows the maintenance of normal generalized immune defenses. B cell function also is not altered by cyclosporine.

Significant toxic side effects of cyclosporine are related to nephrotoxicity and hepatotoxicity. The toxicity is dose related and reversible. Bone marrow toxicity has not been a problem, in contrast to the experience with other immunosuppressants. An increased incidence of lymphomas has been reported in patients receiving cyclosporine. Owing to the higher incidence of many malignant conditions in immunosuppressed patients, the significance of the lymphoma incidence is not clear.

Clinical trials comparing cyclosporine and prednisone immunosuppression with azathioprine, prednisone, and ALG in kidney allograft recipients have shown a variable advantage of cyclosporine in first graft and patient survival (Najarian and associates, 1985). More dramatic advantages of cyclosporine are demonstrated in fewer rejection episodes, reduced infection rates, shorter hospitalization, and improved survival rates in second and third grafts (Morris, 1985).

COMPOSITE TISSUE TRANSPLANTATION

Clinical transplantation of organs essential for life has now reached a mature phase. Beginning with the first successful kidney transplant by Murray, Merrill, and Harrison (1956), steady progress in patient and graft survival has been achieved as a result of improvements in surgical technique and patient management. A breakthrough in preventing rejection has not occurred. The introduction of cyclosporine suggested a new era of immunosuppressants, yet serious and life-threatening side effects of immunosuppression persist.

The success of organ transplantation is somewhat surprising in view of the complexity of the problem. An 88 per cent two year patient survival rate and an 82 per cent two year graft survival rate in kidney allografts can be expected (Najarian and associates, 1985). A one year patient survival rate of 70 per cent is seen in liver transplants (Starzl and associates, 1985). The technically challenging heart-lung transplant yields a two year survival rate of 59 per cent in experienced hands (Jamieson and associates, 1985). Pancreas transplants are somewhat less successful, with a two year patient survival rate of 72 per cent and graft survival rate of 20 per cent (Sutherland and Kendall, 1985).

Dramatic success has been achieved in the techniques of microvascular tissue transfer and replantation, paralleling the developments in clinical organ transplantation. Plastic surgeons, once pioneers in the early days of organ transplants, are again looking to the world of allografts for possible solutions to reconstructive problems. With so many of the tools in hand, the legend of Cosmas and Damien is being examined in a new light. Buncke and associates (1982) successfully transplanted a full-thickness scalp flap between syngeneic twins (Fig. 6–6).

There is a resurgence of experimental work building a scientific foundation for eventual allotransplantation of nonvital body parts. The various components of composite tissue grafts have been studied and the most interesting data come from work involving limb allografts. The following discussion focuses on studies of cyclosporine immunosuppression.

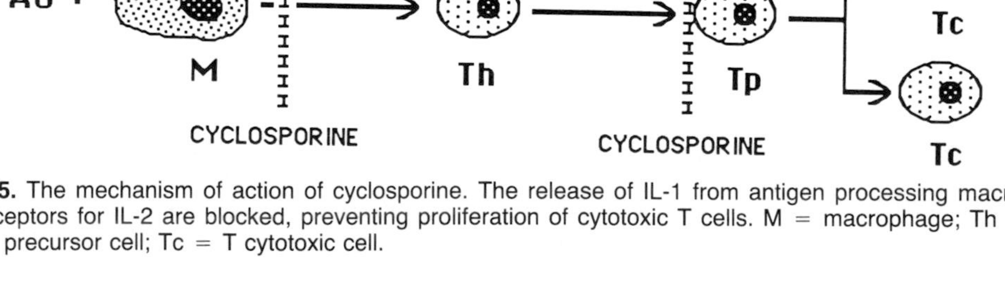

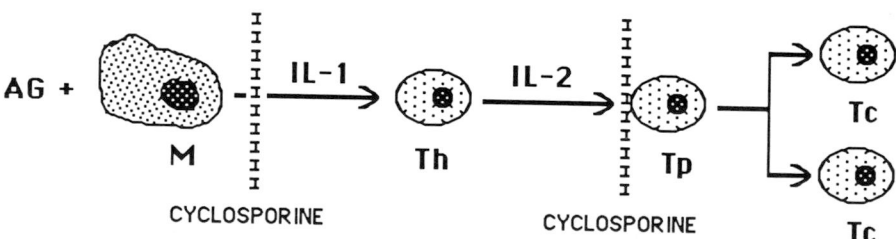

Figure 6–5. The mechanism of action of cyclosporine. The release of IL-1 from antigen processing macrophages is blocked. Receptors for IL-2 are blocked, preventing proliferation of cytotoxic T cells. M = macrophage; Th = T helper cell; Tp = T precursor cell; Tc = T cytotoxic cell.

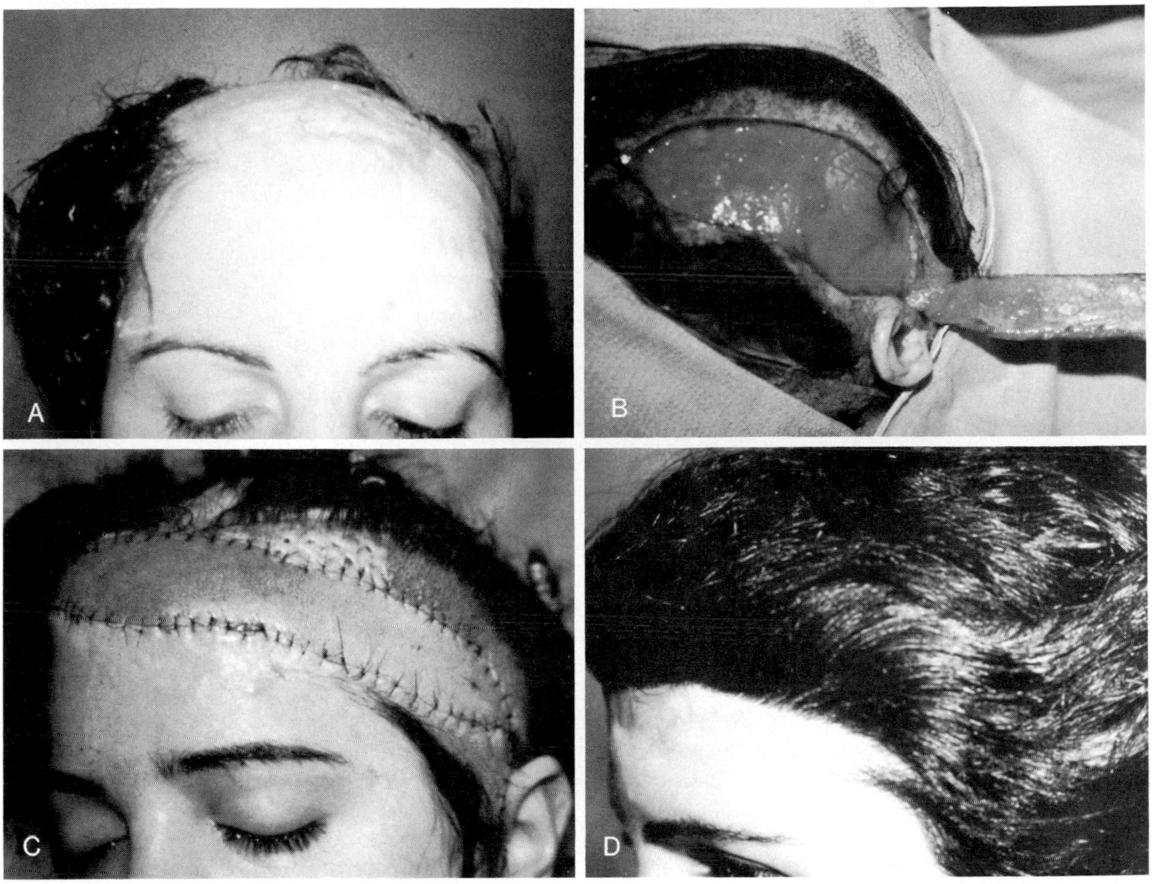

Figure 6–6. First transplantation of composite somatic tissue in humans (syngeneic) (Buncke and associates, 1982). *A*, Young woman missing over half of her scalp from an avulsion injury in a car collision. The defect was covered with a split-thickness skin graft. *B*, Microvascular free scalp flap from an identical twin before transfer with microvascular anastomosis of the superficial temporal vessels. *C*, Syngeneic free scalp flap in place on the recipient twin. *D*, Outgrowth of hair from the syngeneic scalp flap concealed the area of alopecia. Punch grafts and a second free flap from the twin provided additional coverage.

Bone Allografts

The first human bone graft (autograft) was performed by Von Walther in 1820 (Burchardt and Enneking, 1978). Bone autografts are now widely used in reconstructive surgery both as nonvascularized and vascularized transfers. Allogeneic and xenogeneic bone have been considered where donor sites are limited. The immunologic consequences of bone allotransplantation are not well defined. The cellular components of bone are strongly immunogenic, while the glycoprotein, collagen, and mucopolysaccharide bone matrix may elicit a minimal response. Marrow free bone matrix allografts do not provoke a regional lymph node response but they can sensitize the host, causing second set skin rejection (Burwell, 1963).

The mechanism of bone healing involving host cell repopulation of the inert transplant matrix has led to speculation that only short-term immunosuppression may be required for bone allografts. Burchardt, Glowczewskie, and Enneking (1981) compared six week with six month azathioprine immunosuppression in a dog allograft model. Bone healing was equivalent at one year. Most studies suggest that continuous immunosuppression is required to maintain integrity of the allograft except when only minor histocompatibility differences exist between donor and recipient. Cyclosporine was used in a rat model in a study of vascularized bone grafts. Bone healing occurred and graft viability was preserved during immunosuppression in transplants across major and minor histocompatibility barriers. Graft viability decreased when cyclosporine was discontinued in the major histocompatibility difference group, while graft viability was maintained across minor histocompatibility barriers (Halloran, Bushuk, and Stewart, 1983).

Nerve Allografts

A nerve graft that provides a Schwann cell conduit for recipient axon regeneration is similar to a bone graft in which a lattice is supplied by the graft for host cell ingrowth. The immunogenicity of the Schwann cell is greater than that of bone matrix, yet the temporary requirement for the graft material suggested the possibility of only short-term immunosuppression. Mackinnon and associates (1985) studied sciatic nerve allografts in a Lewis/ACI rat model without immunosuppression. An immunologic response was noted at eight days. By histological and electrophysiologic study, nerve regeneration was poor at five months post transplant. A cyclosporine study was performed by Zalewski and Gulati (1984). Two weeks after transplantation in nonimmunosuppressed rats the perineural sheaths and Schwann cells were destroyed. Axon regeneration was limited to the proximal graft area. After cyclosporine immunosuppression was used, nerve sheath integrity and axon regeneration continued for 12 weeks. When immunosuppression was stopped, the grafts rejected, indicating the immunologic vulnerability of donor Schwann cells even in the presence of host axons.

Skin Allografts

The skin allograft that was used to define transplantation genetics may also hold the key to success in composite allografts. Rejection seems to be different and more severe in skin than in any of the other tissues in a composite graft. Skin specific antigens not linked to the genes of the major histocompatibility complex may be a factor in the unique rejection process. Langerhans' cells present in the epidermis can stimulate a T cell response and may be an important component of graft sensitization of the host (Braathen and Thorsby, 1980). A complex reaction of T cell subsets has been shown at the rejecting skin allograft. Skin is infiltrated by cytotoxic lymphocytes while the graft bed is populated by T helper cells (Bhan, Mihm, and Dvorak, 1982). T helper cells can initiate graft rejection; cytotoxic T cells lack this ability (Loveland and McKenzie, 1982). Since only a few of the many cells infiltrating a graft at rejection are specifically sensitized, rejection may be primarily the result of a nonspecific inflammatory reaction mediated by sensitized T cell subsets (Ascher and associates, 1986).

Limb Allografts

The immunobiology of solid organ transplants is relatively simple since there is little variability in the rejection process among the closely related cell types within a single organ. The rejection process has been well defined histologically in kidney, heart, liver, and pancreas. The rejection process is uniform throughout, and modifications of rejection have a uniform effect throughout the graft. The wide variability of the composite tissues in a limb allograft leads to a wide variation in the rejection process and confuses the clinician's efforts at control.

The only reported human limb transplant was performed in 1964 in Ecuador. A cadaver forearm and hand were transplanted using prednisone, azathioprine, and local radiation immunosuppression. Initial success was followed by rejection at 14 days (Gilbert, 1964). Most laboratory work on limb transplantation has followed the first clinical trial.

Lapchinsky, Medevedeva, and Gadalina (1966) achieved prolonged survival of a canine limb allograft following crosstransfusion of the young recipient with donor animal blood. Goldwyn and associates (1966) reported a series of canine limb transplants using 6-mercaptopurine and azathioprine immunosuppression. Short-term success was obtained with the skin and muscle, which were noted to be the site of major rejection activity. Lance and associates (1971), using beagle dogs and continuous ALG, azathioprine, and hydrocortisone immunosuppression, obtained prolonged survival of limb transplants. The active rejection process in skin was noted and documented histologically in this series. The early canine series were all marred by problems with technique and infection.

The development by Shapiro and Cerra (1978) of a rat hind limb transplant model has led to major advances in the understanding of composite tissue transplantation. Rat limb allograft work began with a study by Doi (1979) who used Wistar to Fischer 344 limb allografts. Various combinations of prednisone, azathioprine, and 6-MP immunosuppression were used. Only the combination of azathioprine and prednisone prolonged limb survival over that of the controls. Twenty-four day graft survival was the maximum obtained in this series of transplants across a major histocompatibility barrier. Refinements of the rat limb transplant model have involved technical improvements, the use of cyclosporine, and more effective selection of the various well-defined genetic strains of laboratory animals. Donor and recipient strains that were matched at the major histocompatibility locus had been chosen to provide a moderate rejection process.

Preliminary work by Press, Sibley, and Shons (1983) was directed at the determination of appropriate cyclosporine dosage, one that would prolong graft survival yet avoid infectious complications. Prolongation of graft survival was not demonstrated in preliminary work using ACI to Lewis transplants with multiple combinations of prednisone and cyclosporine, a regimen proven effective in rat kidney and pancreas transplantation. Subsequently, a Fischer/Lewis donor recipient pair was used. The Fischer/Lewis combination constitutes a minor MLC incompatibility that differs at the RT-1C region. Without immunosuppression, rejection of ACI/Lewis grafts occurred at four days and rejection of Fischer/Lewis grafts at 11 days. A dosage of cyclosporine (2.5 or 1.25 mg/kg/day intraperitoneally combined with prednisone 4 or 6 mg/kg/day IP) provided prolonged graft survival (210 days). There was control but not complete obliteration of the rejection process. Higher cyclosporine doses would eliminate all cellular evidence of rejection in the first 14 to 21 days but animal deaths due to infection were common.

Gross and microscopic examination of the long-surviving limb allografts revealed marked differences between skin and other tissues. Beginning at 13 to 17 days, skin surface changes were noted. In some animals only mild erythema and scaling were observed. In others skin changes progressed to severe scaling and desquamation with healing of the surface by thin, hairless scar. The gross skin changes were noted in all animals and resolved by 30 days. Other tissues appeared grossly normal in the 13 to 30 day period.

On microscopic examination, changes were noted in all tissues at 13 to 30 days. Widespread lymphocyte infiltration was observed in skin, muscle, nerve, and blood vessels of the graft. Mononuclear inflammatory cells accompanied the lymphocytes. Macrophages and mast cells were prominent, especially in the dermis. Inflammatory cells were concentrated around the skin appendages and at the dermal-epidermal junction. Nonskin tissues reverted to normal appearance without cellular infiltrate after 40 days. The dermal mononuclear infiltrate persisted in skin throughout the period of longest survival. The skin of long-term survivors appeared variably scarred with loss of hair follicles and sweat glands.

Long-term survivors exhibited clinical evidence of sensory and motor nerve function. Animals with grafts surviving 54 to 215 days were able to extend the leg and plantar flex the foot. Protective sensibility was present. Electromyography confirmed nerve regrowth and end organ reinnervation (Press, Sibley, and Shons, 1986). Prolonged rat limb allograft survival (540 days) and functional recovery were also documented by Achauer and associates (1985) using Lewis X Brown Norway F-1 progeny to Lewis recipients. Cyclosporine, 8 to 25 mg/kg/day, was used for 20 days, then stopped or used intermittently.

Fritz and associates (1984) transplanted hind limbs heterotopically from ACI donors to Lewis recipients, a major histocompatibility barrier. Cyclosporine was given for one week, three weeks, or continuously. Only with continuous treatment did limbs survive for the long term. Kim and associates (1984) transplanted BUF hind limbs orthotopically to Lewis recipients, a major histocompatibility barrier, and showed marked prolongation of survival with cyclosporine maintenance. With a two month cyclosporine course, the limb survived 67 days. Rats treated with daily prednisone or azathioprine rejected the limb within eight days. Guzman-Stein and Shons (1987), in detailed studies of function, showed that orthotopic hind limb transplants sustained with cyclosporine developed sensory return, muscle tonus, active extension, flexion, and toe spread, functions that were almost equivalent to those of the autograft controls. Dorrler and associates (1986) applied a wide array of sophisticated methods of monitoring in evaluating a series of limb transplants in rabbits; the cyclosporine "wasting syndrome" was observed in some of the animals.

Egerszegi, Samulack, and Daniel (1984) have taken limb transplantation genetically closer to man by studying the transplantation of neurovascular free digital island flaps and hand transplants in the baboon. Long-term graft survival and functional recovery were achieved. Cyclosporine at doses higher than required for kidney transplants was necessary to prevent rejection, which was most evident in the skin. The cyclosporine dose was monitored to maintain serum trough levels of 800 ng/ml. During rejection episodes cyclosporine was increased to achieve serum trough levels of 1000 ng/ml and prednisone was added to the treatment protocol.

Vascularized Allografts of Bone and Muscle

Vascularized bone allografts have also been extensively investigated (Moore and associates 1984; Yaremchuk and associates, 1985). Because these allografts include vessels, tendons, connective tissue, and occasionally muscle, in addition to bone, they represent composite somatic tissue transplants of a non–skin-bearing type. In rat knee transplants, Paskert and associates (1987) showed prolonged survival after pretreatment with cyclosporine for seven days. Kesmarky and associates (1987), in transplanted hindlimbs in rats with major and minor histocompatibility barriers, showed that cyclosporine was needed for successful healing and incorporation of the allograft. Innis and associates (1987) compared vascularized and nonvascularized heterotopic bone allografts with strong histocompatibility barriers (Lewis to Brown Norway). They observed that vascularized bone allografts generated significant cell mediated and humoral responses as early as postoperative day five, while nonvascularized grafts showed a minimal humoral response. The implication was that the extensive clinical data available for nonvascularized bone allografts may not always be applicable to vascularized bone allografts.

Black and associates (1987) transplanted vascularized and reinnervated muscle units (gastrocnemius) from ACI rat donors to Lewis rat recipients. Partial return of function was seen. No difference was observed between the allotransplants and the syngeneic transplants.

Jones and colleagues (1987) performed vascularized gracilis allotransplants in dogs receiving a simultaneous heart transplant; cyclosporine with prednisone furnished immunosuppression. The skeletal muscle transplant and the cardiac muscle transplant showed a synchronous course of rejection, and the histologic patterns of biopsies of the transplanted gracilis muscle were predictive of events in the heart transplant.

Growth of Allografted Limbs

Halloran, Bushuk, and Stewart (1983) carried out orthotopic hindlimb transplants across major histocompatibility barriers and also across minor histocompatibility barriers. The transplanted limb was devoid of its foot and was divested of all skin (skin cover was provided by the recipient). Immunosupression was provided by an eight week course of cyclosporine without subsequent maintenance. Measurable growth of the bone was observed; more growth occurred in the presence of the minor histocompatibility barrier than with the major barrier. Kniha and associates (1988) studied the growth of forelimb allografts in young rabbits receiving a maintenance regimen of cyclosporine. The longitudinal growth of the humerus, ulna, and radius was substantial, averaging 75 to 80 per cent of the unoperated control bones. Hair growth and nail growth, response to pain stimuli, and function of the limb transplant on weight bearing were observed. Long-term studies were often abbreviated by a fatal "wasting syndrome," which appeared to be a toxic effect of cyclosporine, idiosyncratic to rabbits (Gratwohl and associates 1986). Siliski, Simpkin, and Green (1984) carried out vascularized orthotopic knee transplants fixed with miniplates in immature rabbits immunosuppressed with cyclosporine. Limited (±15 per cent of the control knee) bone growth was observed at the femoral and tibial epiphyseal plates in some rabbits, while somewhat increased growth (± 50 per cent of the control knee) was seen in others.

Gold and associates (1988a) transplanted non–skin-bearing vascularized forelimb allografts from Dutch rabbits to a subcutaneous position on the backs of New Zealand rabbits 2 to 2½ months old, and these were treated with an eight week course of cyclosporine. Growth was studied with serial radiographs and bone scans. Growth in the heterotopic forelimb continued in a pattern similar to that of the control limb, and continued after cessation of the cyclosporine until the bones were mature. The transplanted bone appeared viable on technetium scans at ten months. The results of this experiment suggest the possibility that non–skin-bearing somatic allografts may require only a limited period of treatment with cyclosporine to retain viability.

Primate Limb Allografts

Egerszegi, Samulack, and Daniel (1984) and Daniel and associates (1986) carried out upper limb allografts in outbred baboons, which included the hand and the distal forearm (Fig. 6–7). Difficulty was encountered in preventing rejection, and only one of the four hand transplants survived for a prolonged period (304 days). The surviving hand showed sensory return and motor function. Orthotopic neurovascular allografts of the skin of the index finger were also studied; the longest survival was 161 days.

Narayanan and associates (1988) carried out seven hand transplants in outbred baboons that were treated with a combination of cyclosporine and methylprednisolone. Five of the hand transplants were lost to acute rejection; one was lost to nonimmunologic complications. One hand survived for 296 days; satisfactory motor function and sensory return were observed.

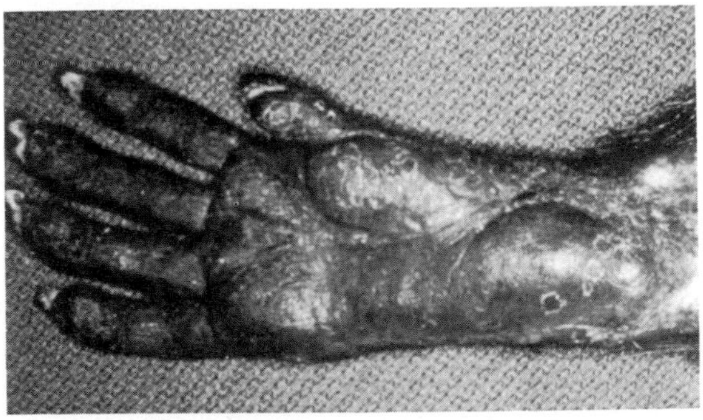

Figure 6–7. Hand allograft in an outbred baboon (Daniel and associates, 1986). The transplanted hand of a baboon 296 days postoperatively.

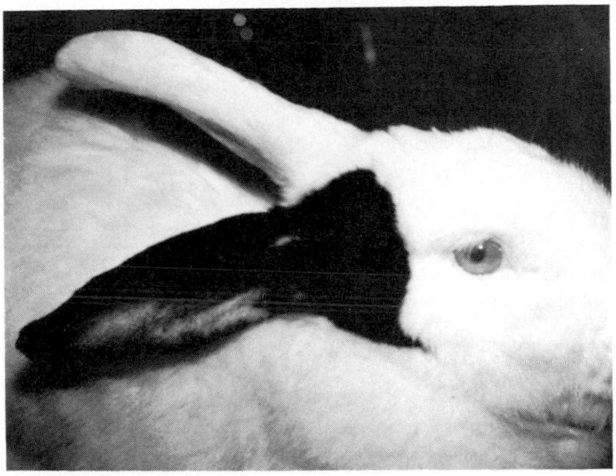

Figure 6–8. Ear-calvarium allograft in rabbit (Fudem and associates, 1985). Ear-calvarium-scalp modular transplant 36 days postoperatively (Dutch donor, New Zealand recipient).

Transplantation and Growth of Craniofacial Modules

Fudem and associates (1985) and Furnas and associates (1988) performed transplants of a module that incorporated the ear, scalp, and parietal bone in young rabbits receiving cyclosporine (Fig. 6–8). The vascular trunk of the module was provided by the common carotid artery and the internal jugular vein. Donors were Dutch rabbits and recipients were New Zealand rabbits. Growth in the length of the transplanted ear approximated that of the control ear, and growth of the calvarial segment approximated that of the control calvarium.

Hemimandibles with attached skin, cheek, and lip were transplanted from Dutch donor rabbits to New Zealand recipients (Furnas and associates, 1988; Randzio and associates, 1988) receiving cyclosporine. The vascular trunk of this hemimandibular module was the same as that of the ear-calvarium module. The longest survival was 100 days. Hair growth typically returned in one week. Mastication began soon postoperatively. The allografted mandibular body grew an average of 3.3 mm during the average 37 day study period, while the controls grew an average of 3.9 mm. The incisors and the first molars showed growth in length that was almost equal to that of the control.

A hemimaxilla-nose module (Furnas and associates, 1988) carried a high perioperative mortality rate because of a vulnerability to airway obstruction and blood loss. Young

Dutch rabbits were donors, and young New Zealand rabbits receiving cyclosporine were recipients. The module included half of the nose, the maxilla, the palate, and the maxillary incisors with attached mucosa and skin. The vascular trunk was the same as that of the preceding craniofacial modules. Survivors ate a soft diet by the fifth day. Hair growth was noted on the tenth day. The longest period of survival was 48 days, during which time the allografted maxilla increased 2.2 mm in length and 1.8 mm in height, and the anterior incisors grew 0.6 mm.

Hemimandibular transplants consisting of one-half of the mandible with the attached muscle, skin, and mucosa were transplanted in young outbred cynomolgus monkeys receiving cyclosporine (Gold and associates, 1988b) (Fig. 6–9). The common carotid artery and the internal jugular vein furnished the vascular trunk for the donor module. The donor carotid artery and jugular vein were anastomosed to the corresponding vessels in the recipient rabbit. Nerve repairs of the lower branches of the facial nerve and of the inferior alveolar nerve were performed. The four monkeys were observed for 13, 27, 63, and 65 days respectively. Hair growth began at day eight but was sparse. Two allografts showed severe, persistent rejection signs at two to three weeks despite the administration of methylprednisolone, and these monkeys were euthanized. The two longer-term survivors lived 63 and 65 days after the transplant. They chewed and ate a normal diet, and gained weight. Each had a rejection episode reversed with methylprednisolone. Mild rejection signs were seen in skin and muscle on histologic examination.

At the time of this writing, vascularized composite somatic tissue allografts are only experimental laboratory procedures. The side effects of current immunosuppression preclude the acceptance of a lifetime of treatment in exchange for replacement of a non–life-saving structure. However, a patient who needs replacement of both a vital organ and a somatic structure might be considered a

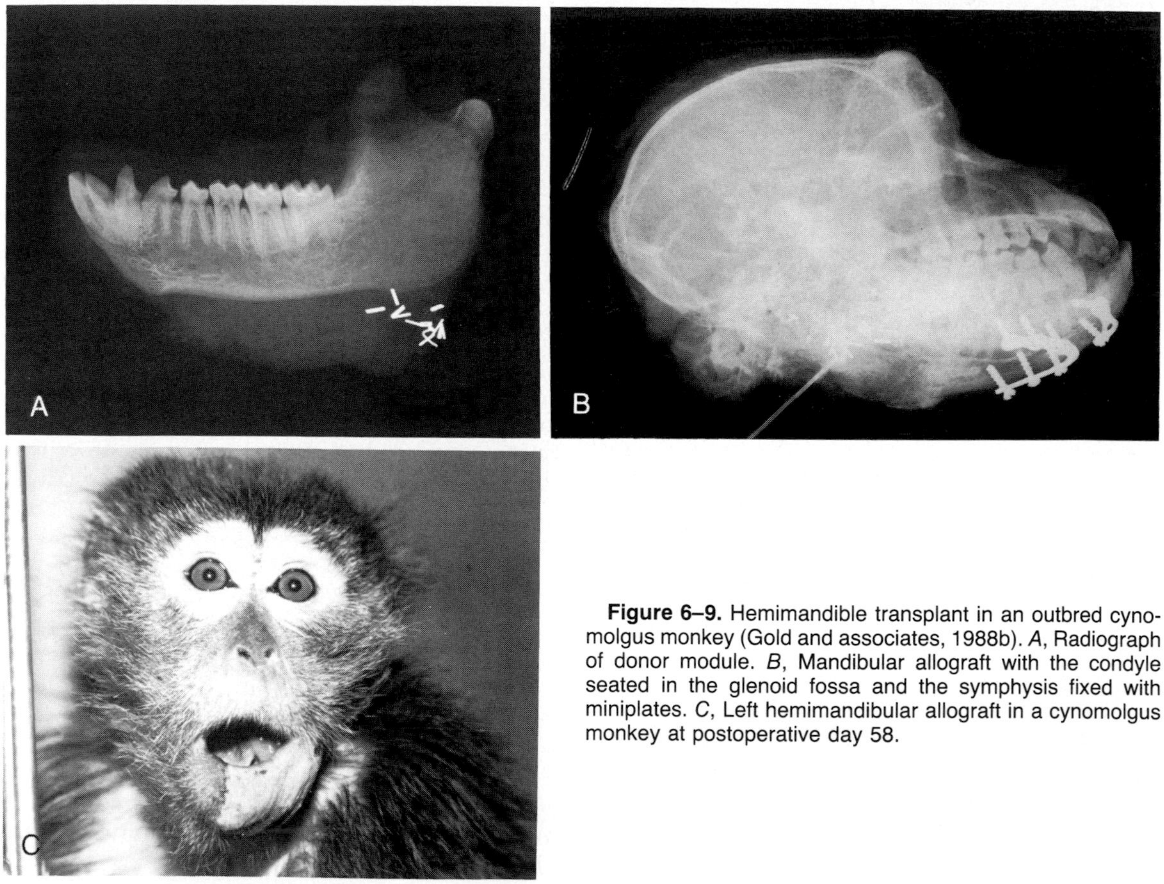

Figure 6–9. Hemimandible transplant in an outbred cynomolgus monkey (Gold and associates, 1988b). *A*, Radiograph of donor module. *B*, Mandibular allograft with the condyle seated in the glenoid fossa and the symphysis fixed with miniplates. *C*, Left hemimandibular allograft in a cynomolgus monkey at postoperative day 58.

Table 6–1. Orthotopic Composite Tissue Allografts Using Immunosuppression

Animal	Composite Tissue	Immuno-suppression	Maximal Graft Survival (days)	Function, Growth	References
Man	Forearm-hand	Steroid, AZA, Radiation	14	–	Gilbert, 1964
Mongrel dog	Limb	AZA, 6-MP	28	–	Goldwyn et al., 1966
Beagle dog	Limb	Steroid, AZA, ALG	300	+	Lance et al., 1971
Rat	Limb	Steroid, AZA, 6-MP	24	–	Doi, 1979
Baboon	Hand	Steroid, CYA	150+	+	Egerszegi et al., 1984
Rat	Limb	CYA	540+	+	Achauer et al., 1985
Rabbit	Mandible, ear, limb	Steroid, CYA	167	+	Fudem et al., 1985
Rat	Limb	Steroid, CYA	215	+	Press et al., 1986

AZA = azathioprine; ALG = antilymphocyte globulin; CYA = cyclosporine; 6-MP = 6-mercaptopurine.

potential candidate, since such a patient would already be committed to life-long immunosuppression.

The non–skin-bearing variety of somatic tissue transplant might prove to be a design that circumvents the need for permanent immunosupression. The behavior of the non–skin-bearing heterotopic forelimb transplants in rabbits suggests this possibility. Long-term primate studies are under way to illuminate this strategy further.

Representative series of orthotopic composite tissue allografts are summarized in Table 6–1.

REFERENCES

Abney, E. R., Cooper, M. D., Kearney, J. F., Lawton, A. R., and Parkhouse, R. M. E.: Sequential expression of immunoglobulin on developing mouse B lymphocytes: a systematic survey that suggests a model for the generation of immunoglobulin isotype diversity. J. Immunol., *120*:2041, 1978.

Achauer, B. M., Black, K. S., Hewitt, M. S., and Furnas, D. W.: Immunosurgery. Clin. Plast. Surg., *12*:293, 1985.

Ascher, N. L., Cahill, D. R., Hoffman, R. A., and Simmons, R. L.: Lymphocytes capable of mediating delayed-type hypersensitivity reactions accumulate within sponge matrix allografts. Surgery, *100*:321, 1986.

Bach, F. H., Bach, M. L., and Sondel, P. M.: Differential function of major histocompatibility complex antigens in T lymphocyte activation. Nature, *259*:273, 1976.

Bert, P.: Thèse pour le doctorat en médecine de la greffe animale. Paris, E. Martinet, 1863.

Bhan, A. K., Mihm, M. C., Jr., and Dvorak, H. F.: T-cell subsets in allograft rejection. In situ characterization of T-cell subsets in human skin allografts by the use of monoclonal antibodies. J. Immunol., *129*:1578, 1982.

Billingham, R. E., Brent, L., and Medawar, P. B.: Quantitative studies on tissue transplantation immunity. III. Actively acquired tolerance. Philos. Trans. R. Soc. Lond. (Biol. Sci.), *239*:375, 1956.

Billingham, R. E., Lampkin, G. H., Medawar, P. B., and Williams, H. L.: Tolerance to homografts, twin diagnosis and the freemartin condition in cattle. Heredity, *6*:201, 1952.

Black, K. S., Hewitt, C. W., Grisham, G. R., Caiozzo, V. J., Howard, E. B., and Achauer, B. M.: Two new composite tissue allograft models in rats to study neuromuscular functional return. Transplant. Proc., *19*:1118, 1987.

Borel, J. F., Feurer, C., Magnee, C., and Stahelin, H.: Effects of the new antilymphocytic polypeptide cyclosporin A in animals. Immunology, *32*:1017, 1977.

Braathen, L. R., and Thorsby, E.: Studies on human epidermal Langerhans cells: 1. Allo-activating and antigen-presenting capacity. Scand. J. Immunol., *11*:401, 1980.

Brown, J. B.: Homografting, with report of success in identical twins. Surgery, *1*:558, 1937.

Buncke, H. J., Hoffman, W. Y., Alpert, B. S., Gordon, L., and Stefani, A. E.: Microvascular transplant of two free scalp flaps between identical twins. Plast. Reconstr. Surg., *70*:605, 1982.

Burchardt, H., and Enneking, W. F.: Transplantation of bone. Surg. Clin. North Am., *58*:403, 1978.

Burchardt, H., Glowczewskie, F. P., and Enneking, W. F.: Short-term immunosuppression with free segmental fibular allografts in dogs. J. Bone Joint Surg., *63A*:411, 1981.

Burnet, F. M., and Fenner, F.: Genetics and immunology. Heredity, *2*:289, 1948.

Burwell, R. G.: Studies in the transplantation of bone. V. The capacity of fresh and treated homografts of bone to evoke transplantation immunity. J. Bone Joint Surg., *45B*:386, 1963.

Cohn, Z. A.: The activation of mononuclear phagocytes: fact, fancy and future. J. Immunol., *121*:813, 1978.

Converse, J. M., and Duchet, G.: Successful homologous skin grafting in a war burn using an identical twin as donor. Plast. Reconstr. Surg., *2*:342, 1947.

Converse, J. M., and Rapaport, F. T.: The vascularization of skin autografts and homografts. An experimental study in man. Ann. Surg., *143*:306, 1956.

Cooper, M. D., Peterson, R. D. A., and Good, R. A.: Delineation of the thymic and bursal lymphoid system in the chicken. Nature (Lond.), *205*:143, 1965.

Cooper, N. R.: Activation and regulation of the first complement component. Fed. Proc., *42*:134, 1983.

Daniel, R. K., Egerszegi, E. P., Samulack, D. D., Skanes, S. E., Dykes, R. W., and Rennie, W. R. J.: Tissue transplants in primates for upper extremity reconstruction: a preliminary report. J. Hand Surg., *11*:1, 1986.

Danilevicius, Z.: S.S. Cosmas and Damian. The patron saints of medicine in art. J.A.M.A., *201*:1021, 1967.

Dausset, J.: Iso-leuco-anticorps. Acta Haematol. (Basel), *20*:156, 1958.

Doi, K.: Homotransplantation of limbs in rats: a preliminary report on an experimental study with nonspecific immunosuppressive drugs. Plast. Reconstr. Surg., *64*:613, 1979.

Dorrler, J., Goring H., Gossman, R., Holzmann, T., Russe, I. et al.: Limb allograft survival under cyclosporine treatment. Transplant. Proc., *18*:1431, 1986.

Egerszegi, E. P., Samulack, D. D., and Daniel, R. K.: Experimental models in primates for reconstructive surgery utilizing tissue transplants. Ann. Plast. Surg., *13*:423, 1984.

Fauci, A. S.: Mechanisms of the immunosuppressive and anti-inflammatory effects of glucocorticosteroids. J. Immunopharmacol. *1*:1, 1979.

Fritz, W. D., Swartz, W. M., Rose, S., Futrell, J. W., and Klein, E.: Limb allografts in rats immunosuppressed with cyclosporin A. Ann. Surg., *199*:211, 1984.

Fudem, G. M., Davies, C. T., Powell, A., Wong, D., and Furnas, D. W.: Growth of vascularized somatic tissue allografts in young rabbits given cyclosporine. Surg. Forum, *36*:604, 1985.

Furnas, D. W., Randzio, J., Kniha, H., Fudem, G., Cruz, H. G., and Gold, M. E.: Growth of craniofacial and forelimb allotransplants in young rabbits. Transplant. Proc., *20*:332, 1988.

Gallatin, W. M., Weissman, I. L., and Butcher, E. C.: A cell-surface molecule involved in organ-specific homing of lymphocytes. Nature, *304*:30, 1983.

Gibson, T.: Zoografting: a curious chapter in the history of plastic surgery. Br. J. Plast. Surg., *8*:234, 1955.

Gibson, T., and Medawar, P. B.: The fate of skin homografts in man. J. Anat., *77*:299, 1943.

Gilbert, R.: Transplant is successful with a cadaver forearm. Med. Trib. Med. News, *5*:20, 1964.

Gold, M. E., Booth, K., Gruer, S., Kim, B., Chamberlin, D., and Furnas, D. W.: Growth of vascularized non–skin-bearing heterotopic forelimb allografts in young rabbits treated with cyclosporine: a preliminary report. Submitted for publication, 1988a.

Gold, M. E., Randzio, J., Kniha, H., Kim, B., Park, H., et al.: Transplantation of vascularized composite mandibular allografts in young cynomolgus monkeys. Submitted for publication, 1988b.

Goldman, J. N., and Goldman, M. B.: What the clinician should know about the major histocompatibility complex. J.A.M.A., *246*:873, 1981.

Goldwyn, R. M., Beach, P. M., Feldman, D., and Wilson, R. E.: Canine limb homotransplantation. Plast. Reconstr. Surg., *37*:184, 1966.

Good, R. A., Gabrielson, A. E., Peterson, R. D. A., Finstad, J., and Cooper, M. D.: The development of the central and peripheral lymphoid tissues—autogenetic and phylogenetic consideration. *In* Wolstenholme, G. E., and Porter, R. (Eds.): Ciba Foundation Symposium on Thymus and Autoimmune Disease. London, Churchill, 1966, p. 81.

Gratwohl, A., Riederer, I., Graf, E., and Speck, B.: Cyclosporine toxicity in rabbits. Lab. Anim., *20*:213, 1986.

Greene, H. S. N.: Heterologous transplantation of mammalian tumors. 1. The transfer of rabbit tumors to alien species. J. Exp. Med., *73*:461, 1941.

Guzman-Stein, G., and Shons, A. R.: Functional recovery in the rat limb transplant model: a preliminary study. Transplant. Proc., *19*:1115, 1987.

Halloran, P. F., Bushuk, M., and Stewart, J. A.: Effects of cyclosporine on the healing of vascularized and nonvascularized bone allografts in rodents. Transplant. Proc., *15*:3053, 1983.

Holman, E.: Protein sensitization in isoskingrafting. Is the latter of practical value? Surg. Gynecol. Obstet., *38*:100, 1924.

Innis, P. C., Randolph, M. A., Paskert, J. P., Burdick, J. F., Clow, L. C., et al.: Vascularized bone allografts: in vitro assessment of the cell mediated and humoral responses. Presentation, American Society for Reconstructive Microsurgery, San Antonio, TX, September 13, 1987.

Jamieson, S. W., Dawkins, K. D., Burke, C., Baldwin, J. W., Youseur, S., et al.: Late results in heart-lung transplantation. Transplant. Proc., *17*:212, 1985.

Johnson, H. K., Malcolm, H., Al-Abdulla, S., Fertman, S., Richie, R. E., et al.: The effect of local graft irradiation upon the reversal of cadaveric renal allograft rejection. Transplant. Proc., *17*:29, 1985.

Jones, N. F., Sank, A. C., Cherup, L. L., and Lorenc, Z. P.: Allotransplantation of vascularized skeletal muscle with cyclosporine immunosuppression. Presentation, American Society for Reconstructive Microsurgery, San Antonio, TX, September 13, 1987.

Kesmarky, S., Pan, Y. C., Randolph, M. A., Yaremchuk, M. J., and Weiland, A. J.: Vascularized bone allografting: the effect of cyclosporine in an orthotopic rat model. Presentation, American Society for Reconstructive Microsurgery, San Antonio, TX, September 13, 1987.

Kim, S. K., Aziz, S., Oyer, P., and Hentz, V. R.: Use of cyclosporin A in allotransplantation of rat limbs. Ann. Plast. Surg., *12*:249, 1984.

Kniha, H., Randzio, J., Gold, M. E., Fudem, G. M., Cruz, H. G., et al.: Growth of forelimb allografts in young rabbits immunosuppressed with cyclosporine. Ann. Plast. Surg., *22*:135, 1989.

Kuritani, T., and Cooper, M. D.: Human B cell differentiation. 1. Analysis of immunoglobulin heavy chain switching using monoclonal anti-immunoglobulin M, G and A antibodies and pokeweed mitogen-induced plasma cell differentiation. J. Exp. Med., *155*:839, 1982.

Lance, E. M., Inglis, A. E., Figarola, F., and Veith, F. J.: Transplantation of the canine hind limb. Surgical technique and methods of immunosuppression for allotransplantation. J. Bone Joint Surg. (Am.), *53*:1137, 1971.

Lapchinsky, A. G., Medevedeva, G. V., and Gadalina, I. D.: Homotransplantation of extremity to tolerant dogs. *In* Kovanov, B. B. (Ed.): Transplantation. Moscow, Moscow Press, 1966, p.6.

Lawton, A. R.: B lymphocyte development, heterogeneity and activation. Fed. Proc., *41*:2493, 1982.

Levitt, D., and Cooper, M. D.: Lymphocytes 11. B cells. *In* Stites, D. P., Stobo, J. D., Fudenberg, H. H., and Wells, J. V. (Eds.): Basic and Clinical Immunology. 5th Ed. Los Altos, Lange Medical Publications, 1984, p.76.

Loeb, L.: The Biological Basis of Individuality. Springfield, Charles C Thomas, 1945.

Loveland, B. E., and McKenzie, I. F. C.: Which T cells cause graft rejection? Transplantation, *33*:217, 1982.

Mackinnon, S. E., Hudson, A. R., Falk, R. E., and Hunter, D. A.: The nerve allograft response—an experimental model in the rat. Ann. Plast. Surg., *14*:334, 1985.

Medawar, P. B.: Immunity to homologous grafted skin. I. The suppression of cell division in grafts transplanted to immunized animals. Br. J. Exp. Pathol., *27*:9, 1946a.

Medawar, P. B.: Immunity to homologous grafted skin. II. The relationship between the antigens of blood and skin. Br. J. Exp. Pathol., *27*:15, 1946b.

Medawar, P. B.: Immunity to homologous grafted skin. III. The fate of skin homografts transplanted to the brain, to subcutaneous tissue and to the anterior chamber of the eye. Br. J. Exp. Pathol., *29*:58, 1948.

Meuer, S. C., Acuto, O., Hussey, R. E., Hodgdon, J. C., Fitzgerald, K. A., et al.: Evidence for the T3-associated 90K heterodimer as the T-cell antigen receptor. Nature, *303*:808, 1983.

Monaco, A. P., Wood, M. L., and Russell, P. S.: Some effects of purified heterologous anti-human lymphocyte serum in man. Transplantation, *5*:1106, 1967.

Moore, J. R., Phillips, T. W., Weiland, A. J., and Randolph, M. A.: Allogenic transplants of bone revascularized by microvascular anastomoses: a preliminary study. J. Orthop. Res., 1:352, 1984.

Morris, P. J.: Immunosuppression in renal transplantation. Transplant. Proc., *17*:1153, 1985.

Murphy, J. B., and Sturm, E.: Conditions determining the transplantability of tissues in the brain. J. Exp. Med., *38*:183, 1923.

Murray, J. E., Merrill, J. P., and Harrison, J. H.: Renal homotransplantation in identical twins. Surg. Forum, *6*:432, 1956.

Najarian, J. S., Fryd, D. S., Strand, M., Canafax, D. M., Ascher, N. L., et al.: A single institution, randomized, prospective trial of cyclosporin versus azathioprine-antilymphocyte globulin for immunosuppression in renal allograft recipients. Ann. Surg., *201*:142, 1985.

Najarian, J. S., May, J., Cochrum, K. C., Baronberg, N., and Way, L. W.: Mechanism of antigen release from canine kidney homotransplants. Ann. N.Y. Acad. Sci., *129*:76, 1966.

Najarian, J. S., and Simmons, R. L.: The clinical use of antilymphocyte globulin. N. Engl. J. Med., *285*:158, 1971.

Narayanan, K., Swartz, W. M., Stark, B., and Moller, A.: Allogeneic hand transplantations in primates. Presented at the International Organ Transplant Forum, Pittsburgh, September 1987.

Opelz, G.: Current relevance of the transfusion effect in renal transplantation. Transplant. Proc., *17*:1015, 1985.

Opelz, G., Mickey, M. R., and Terasaki, P. I.: Blood transfusions and kidney transplants: remaining controversies. Transplant. Proc., *13*:136, 1981.

Oppenheim, J. J., and Cohen, S.: Interleukins, Lymphokines and Cytokines. New York, Academic Press, 1983.

Owen, R. D.: Immunogenetic consequences of vascular anastomoses between bovine twins. Science, *102*:400, 1945.

Padgett, E. C.: Is iso-skin grafting practicable? South. Med. J., *25*:895, 1932.

Paskert, J. P., Yaremchuk, M. J., Randolph, M. A., and Weiland, A. J.: Prolonging survival in vascularized bone allograft transplantation: developing specific immune unresponsiveness. J. Reconstr. Microsurg., *3*:253, 1987.

Press, B. H. J., Sibley, R. K., and Shons, A. R.: Modification of experimental limb allograft rejection with cyclosporine and prednisone: a preliminary report. Transplant. Proc., *15*:3057, 1983.

Press, B. H. J., Sibley, R. K., and Shons, A. R.: Limb allotransplantation in the rat: extended survival and return of nerve function with continuous cyclosporin/prednisone immunosuppression. Ann. Plast. Surg., *16*:313, 1986.

Randzio, J., Kniha, H., Gold, M. E., Chang, T., Su, L., et al.: Growth of vascularized composite mandibular allografts in young rabbits. Submitted for publication, 1988.

Rapaport, F. T., Chase, R. M., Markowitz, A. S., McCluskey, R. T., Shimada, T., and Watanabe, K.: Cross-reactions in mammalian transplantation—with particular reference to streptococcal antigens and antibodies. Transplant. Proc., *3*:89, 1971.

Rapaport, F. T., and Converse, J. M.: Observations on the immunological manifestations of the homograft rejection phenomenon in man: the recall flare. Ann. N.Y. Acad. Sci., *64*:836, 1957.

Rapaport, F. T., and Converse, J. M.: The immune response to multiple-set skin homografts. An experimental study in man. Ann. Surg., *147*:273, 1958.

Reinherz, E. L., and Schlossman, S. F.: The differentiation and function of human T lymphocytes. Cell, *19*:821, 1980.

Schone, G.: Ueber Transplantationsimmunitat. Munch. Med. Wochenschr., *59*:457, 1912.

Schwartz, B. D.: The human major histocompatibility HLA complex. *In* Stites, D. P., Stobo, J. D., Fudenberg, H. H., and Wells, J. V. (Eds.): Basic and Clinical Immunology. Los Altos, Lange Medical Publications, 1984, p.55.

Shapiro, R. J., and Cerra, F. B.: A model for reimplantation and transplantation of a complex organ: the rat hind limb. J. Surg. Res., *24*:501, 1978.

Shawan, H. K.: The principle of blood grouping applied to skin grafting. Am. J. Med. Sci., *157*:503, 1919.

Shons, A. R., Etheredge, E. E., Schmidtke, J. R., and Najarian, J. S.: Mixed leukocyte response in human renal transplantation. Transplant. Proc., *5*:337, 1973.

Shons, A. R., Moberg, A. W., and Najarian, J. S.: Xenotransplantation. *In* Najarian, J. S., and Simmons, R. L. (Eds.): Transplantation. Philadelphia, Lea & Febiger, 1972, p. 729.

Siliski, J. M., Simpkin, S., and Green, C. J.: Vascularized whole knee joint allografts in rabbits immunosuppressed with cyclosporine A. Arch. Orthop. Trauma Surg., *103*:26, 1984.

Skinner, M. D., and Schwartz, R. S.: Immunosuppressive therapy. 1. N. Engl. J. Med., *287*:221, 1972.

Starzl, T. E., Iwatsuki, S., Shaw, B. W., Jr., and Gordon, R. D.: Orthotopic liver transplantation in 1984. Transplant. Proc., *17*:250, 1985.

Stastny, P., Ball, E. J., Dry, P. J., and Nunez, G.: The human immune response region (HLA-D) and disease susceptibility. Immunol. Rev., *70*:113, 1983.

Stephenson, S. P., and Roser, B.: The molecular basis of transplantation tolerance. Transplant. Proc., *17*:1145, 1985.

Stobo, J. D.: Lymphocytes. *In* Stites, D. P., Stobo, J. D., Fudenberg, H. H., and Wells, J. V. (Eds.): Basic and Clinical Immunology. 5th Ed. Los Altos, Lange Medical Publications, 1984, p. 69.

Subba Rao, D. S. V., and Grogan, J. B.: Cell-mediated immunity in rats bearing allogeneic skin in the anterior chamber of the eye. 1. Response to mitogens. J. Surg. Res., *38*:116, 1985.

Sutherland, D. E. R., and Kendall, D.: Clinical pancreas and islet transplant registry report. Transplant. Proc., *17*:307, 1985.

Turk, J. L., and Parker, D.: The effect of cyclophosphamide on the immune response. J. Immunopharmacol., *1*:127, 1979.

Wiesinger, D., and Borel, J. F.: Studies on the mechanism of action of cyclosporin A. Immunobiology, *156*:454, 1980.

Yaremchuk, M. J., Nettelblad, H., Randolph, M. A., and Weiland, A. J.: Vascularized bone allograft transplantation in a genetically defined rat model. Plast. Reconstr. Surg., *75*:355, 1985.

Zalewski, A. A., and Gulati, A. K.: Failure of cyclosporin A to induce immunological unresponsiveness to nerve allografts. Exp. Neurol., *83*:659, 1984.

7

Thomas Gibson

Physical Properties of Skin

It covers every inch of us from crown of head to toe
And through each tiny fragment the busy red cells flow
It's living, pulsing, breathing, percipiently sensing
One moment lying slack relaxed, another tautly tensing
It holds at bay bacterial germs, it keeps our innards in
That wondrous complex structure that is stratified squamous skin.

It's convex here and concave there and hardly ever flat
It moulds itself round muscles, it's padded out with fat
It hugs protruding members, lines every crease and crack
Tho' often tight there's aye excess when movement needs it slack
The curve of breast, of buttock, thigh, the cute up-tilted chin
There's nothing quite so cuddlesome as stratified squamous skin.

There's not another structure quite so well supplied with nerves
Whose every little ending some quick sensation serves
Of heat and cold, of wet and dry, the smarting sting of a lash
The pricklings of fear or the scratching urge of an itching nettle rash
The smooth caress of a lover's touch, the painful prick of a pin
There's nothing quite so sensitive as stratified squamous skin.

It's full of little sweating glands that help to keep us cool
It's not so good for keeping warm since losing all its wool
Oh! Here and there there's tufts of hair (Why did God put them there?)
But over all the rest of us we're starkly baldly bare
And isn't it a pity that to keep our warmth within
We have to cover up with clothes our stratified squamous skin.

It isn't only sweat of course exudes from out each pore
That's just the eccrine glands at work, there's apocrines galore
Who help to grease the flexures and in many ways complex
Produce those subtle odours that attract the opposite sex
Tho' many swamp their body smells with deodorants from tins
The connoisseur selects by scent his stratified squamous skins.

The biochemist looks at skin as just so many amines
Polymerising molecules and polypeptide proteins
The general surgeon looks at skin as something to be cut
And held in wide retraction while he searches for the gut
The plastic surgeon thinks of all the dollars he can win
By grafting and manipulating stratified squamous skin.

In childhood, adolescence, youth, it's smooth as baby's bot
Then wrinkles, creases, crow's feet form and age begins its rot

At first it's lovely, smooth and taut and then begins to flag
In middle age it starts to bulge and here and there to sag
The swelling paunch, the drooping breasts, the double triple chin
The ageing process best observed in stratified squamous skin.

But now's the time the plastic surgeon earns an honest buck
He cuts out all the excess skin, takes in a little tuck
Peels away the wrinkles with carbolic acid paste
Performs an apronectomy to narrow down the waist
Undermines his face lifts to abolish double chins
Thank God! he cries, for sagging wrinkled stratified squamous skins.

Skin has many biologic functions. We are concerned with its behavior as the material every surgeon handles and manipulates daily, usually quite intuitively and without any real appreciation of its underlying structure. This is partly due to the extreme variability of the physical properties of skin. They differ at the same site on different individuals; they differ at different sites on the same individual; they differ in different directions at the same site; and at any site they change remarkably with age. It is probably a truism that each piece of skin is uniquely constructed, and the uniqueness of its physical properties depends mainly on the twin fibrous networks of collagen and elastin, which constitute the bulk of the dermis, and the pattern of their interwoven architecture.

The structures of the collagen fibers in the dermis (Figs. 7–1 and 7–2) are extremely long compared with their diameter. In the relaxed state in young people they are markedly convoluted, but they become less so with age. They appear to be randomly oriented and intertwined one with another, yet when skin is stretched in any direction, the convolutions straighten out. Furthermore, as the load increases, an increasing number of fibers become aligned in the direction of the stretching force, until finally there is a structure of parallel fibers that is highly resistant to fur-

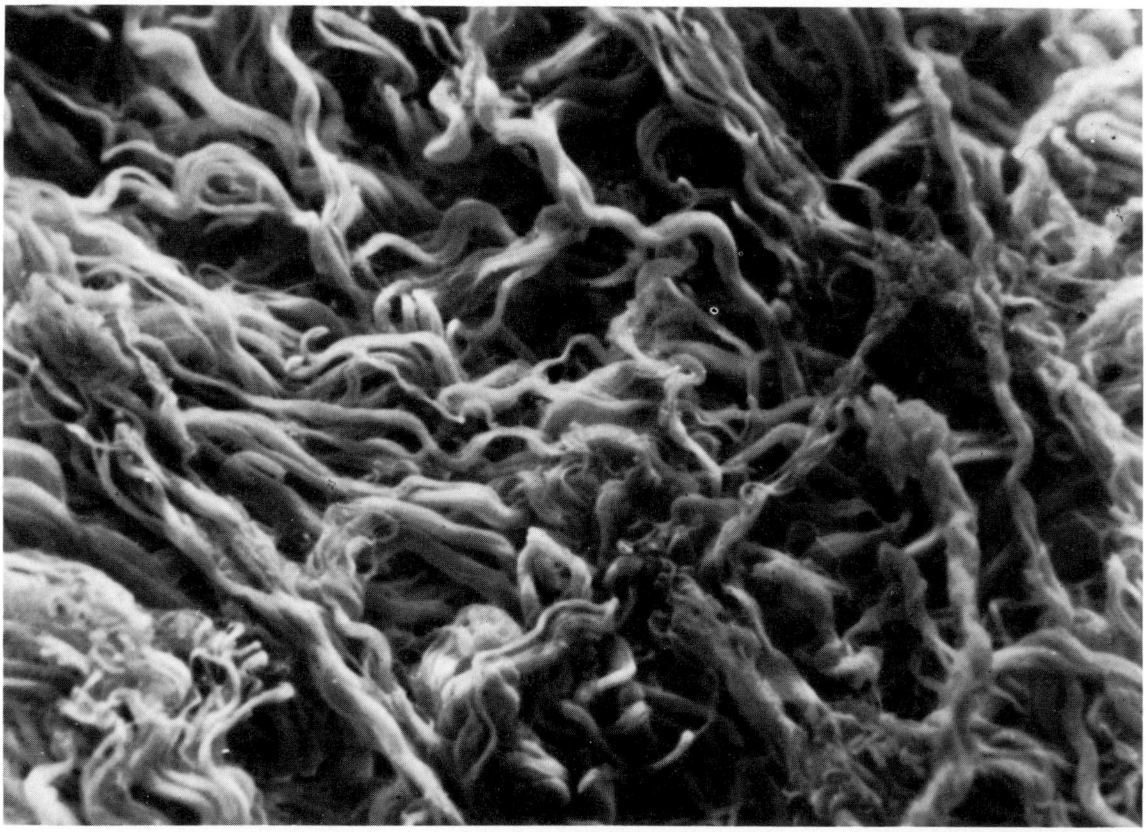

Figure 7–1. Scanning electron microscope (SEM) photograph of the collagen fibers of human dermis. (From Gibson, T., and Kenedi, R. M.: The structural components of the dermis. *In* Montagna, W., Bentley, J. P., and Dobson, R. L. (Eds.): The Dermis, 1970. Courtesy of Appleton-Century-Crofts, Publishing Division of Prentice-Hall, Inc., Englewood Cliffs, NJ.)

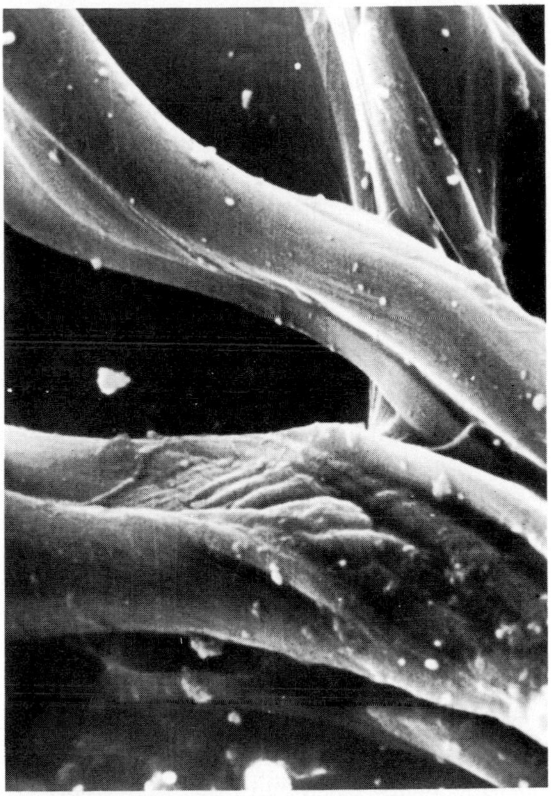

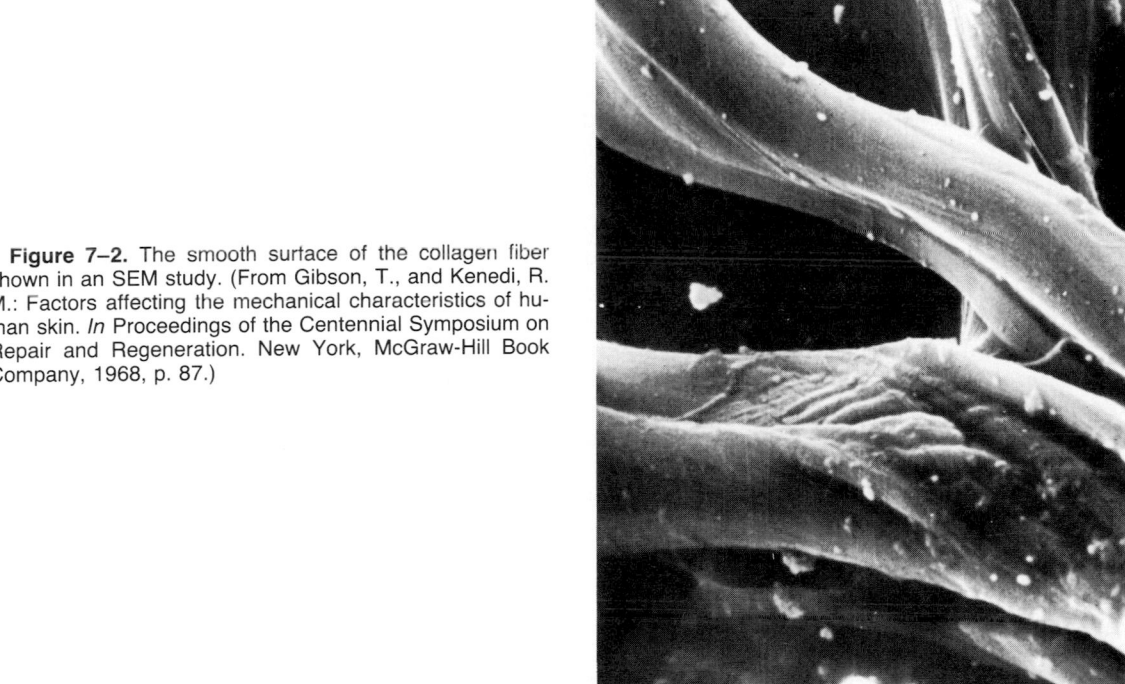

Figure 7–2. The smooth surface of the collagen fiber shown in an SEM study. (From Gibson, T., and Kenedi, R. M.: Factors affecting the mechanical characteristics of human skin. *In* Proceedings of the Centennial Symposium on Repair and Regeneration. New York, McGraw-Hill Book Company, 1968, p. 87.)

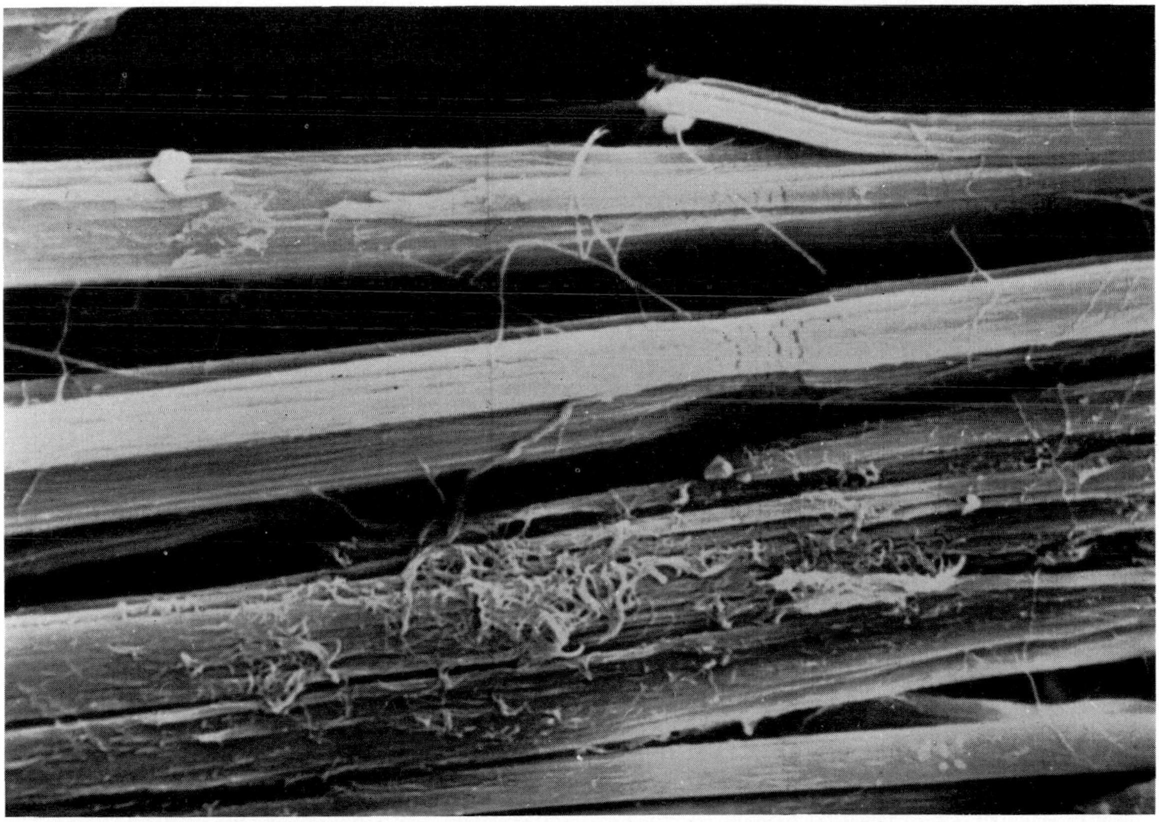

Figure 7–3. When skin is stretched, many of the fibers become aligned in a straight manner in the direction of stretch, thus imposing a limit on extensibility in that direction. (From Brown, I. A.: Structural and Mechanical Studies on Human Skin. Ph.D. Thesis, University of Strathclyde, Glasgow, 1971.)

ther extension (Fig. 7–3). This behavior underlies the typical stress-strain curve for skin (Fig. 7–4) and explains what every surgeon has observed: a certain amount of skin may be excised at any site and the wound closed easily, but there is a point beyond which no amount of additional tension on sutures effects closure.

Each collagen fiber is made up of hundreds of finer fibrils, and each fibril is in turn made up of several triple helical spiraled collagen molecules, twisted into "super coils" (see Chap. 5). Collagen shows structure within structure. The multiple, spring-like molecules resist extension, and the aggregated fibrils form a cable of great strength and limited extension, which is readily capable of bending in any direction as the fiber network moves. Finally the network provides free mobility to follow a wide range of body movements, but with a built-in limit to the amount of extension possible.

The collagen fibers illustrated are those that make up most of the thickness of the dermis. Near the epidermis, the fibers are much finer. The fine subepidermal fibers probably act as a damping link to protect the epithelial cells from the more acute and coarse movements of the collagen fiber network.

The elastic fibers of the dermis are much finer than the collagen fibers and, unlike the latter, have end-to-side junctions. Their function is to return the deformed collagen network to its relaxed condition. The elastic fibers are in part responsible for the tension naturally occurring in skin.

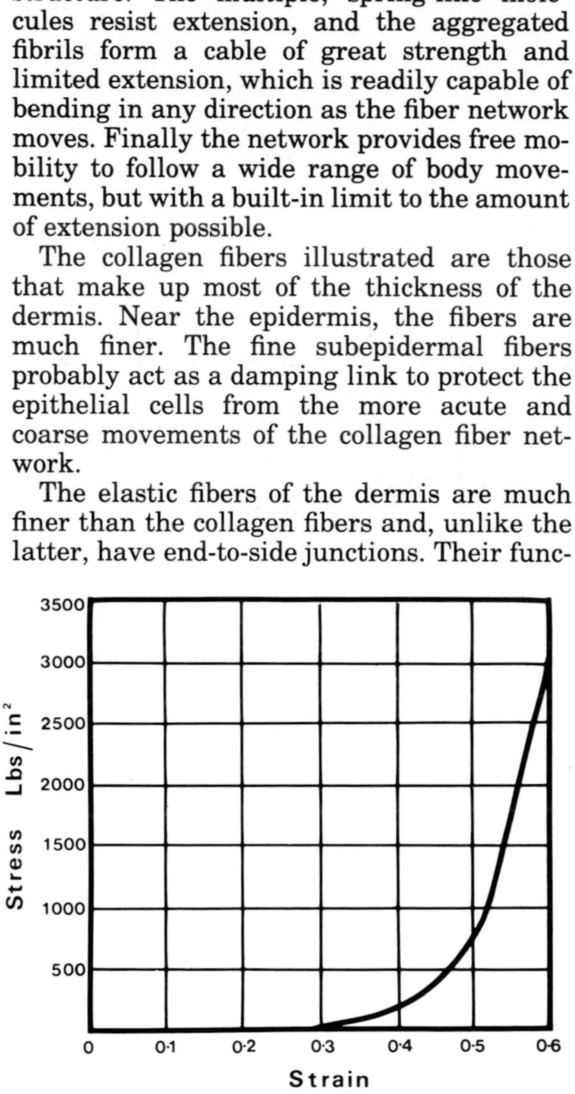

Figure 7–4. Typical stress-strain curve of human skin in tension. (From Gibson, T., and Kenedi. R. M.: The structural components of the dermis. *In* Montagna, W., Bentley, J. P., and Dobson, R. L. (Eds.): The Dermis, 1970. Courtesy of Appleton-Century-Crofts, Publishing Division of Prentice-Hall, Inc., Englewood Cliffs, NJ.)

Such a mobile microarchitecture requires a lubricant, and this is probably provided by the mucopolysaccharide ground substance and the tissue fluid lying around and between the fibers. It is noteworthy that each fibril in the fiber aggregate has a sheath of mucopolysaccharide that separates it from its fellows. Collagen does not exist in the body in a naked state; it is always associated with and covered by mucopolysaccharides.

Intertwined with the networks of collagen and elastin are three other networks: small blood vessels, nerve fibers, and lymphatics, respectively (Fig. 7–5). None of these structures contributes to the physical properties of skin, but their individual functions may be interfered with when the fibrous networks through which they pass are deformed. Thus, constriction of the blood vessels interferes with the blood supply and, if long continued, produces necrosis. Constriction of nerves causes pain, and interruption of the lymphatics results in edema.

The fibrous networks are transfixed in most parts of the body by a varying number of hairs (Fig. 7–6), which probably restrict the mobility of the dermis.

The physical properties of skin depend mainly on the patterns of the fibrous weave of the dermis. For descriptive purposes these can be divided into four groups: (1) viscoelastic properties, (2) skin tension properties, (3) skin extensibility, and (4) directional variations.

VISCOELASTIC PROPERTIES OF SKIN

There are basically two viscoelastic properties: "creep" and "stress relaxation." Creep occurs when a piece of skin is stretched and the stretching force is kept constant; the skin continues to extend, depending of course on the forces involved. Stress relaxation, the corollary of creep, occurs when a piece of skin is stretched for a given distance and that distance is held constant; the force required to keep it stretched gradually decreases (Fig. 7–7).

Time is required for creep and stress relaxation to occur. It is thus of paramount impor-

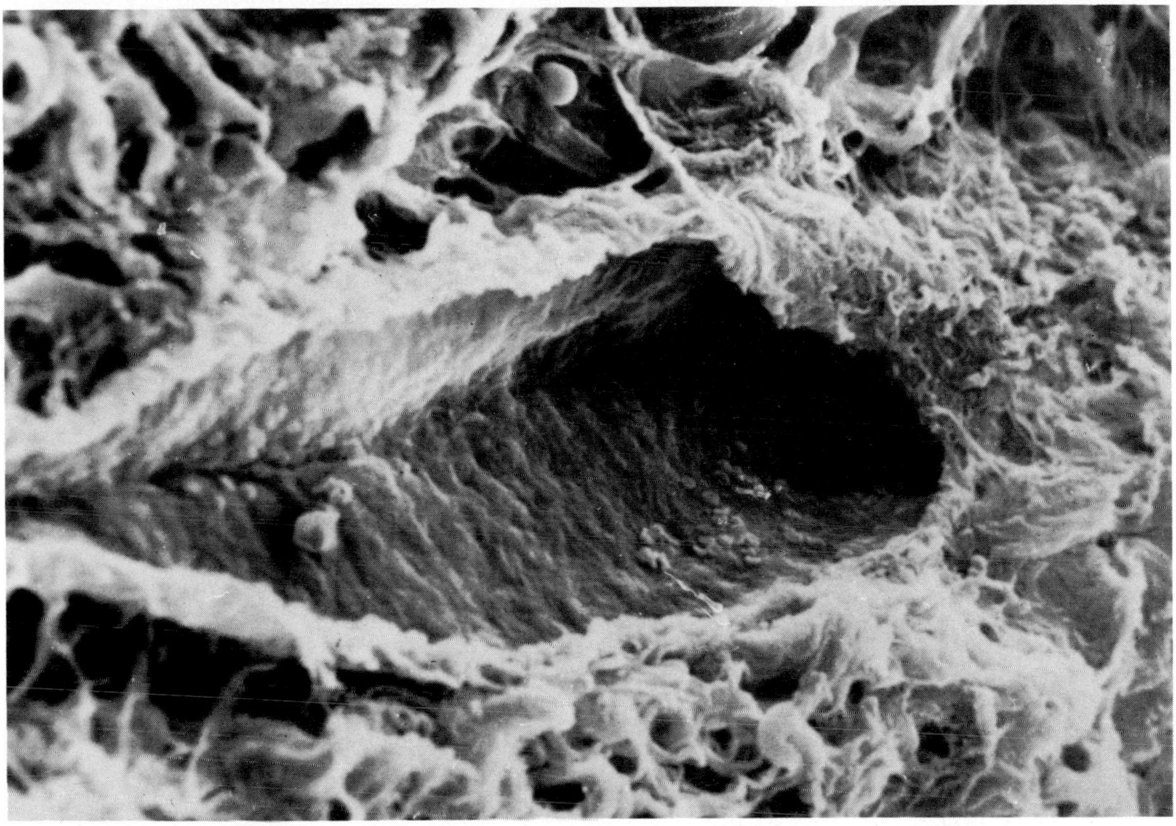

Figure 7–5. A small arteriole traversing the dermis. When the fiber network is deformed, the lumen may be obliterated, producing blanching and ultimately necrosis. (From Brown, I. A.: Structural and Mechanical Studies on Human Skin. Ph.D. Thesis, University of Strathclyde, Glasgow, 1971.)

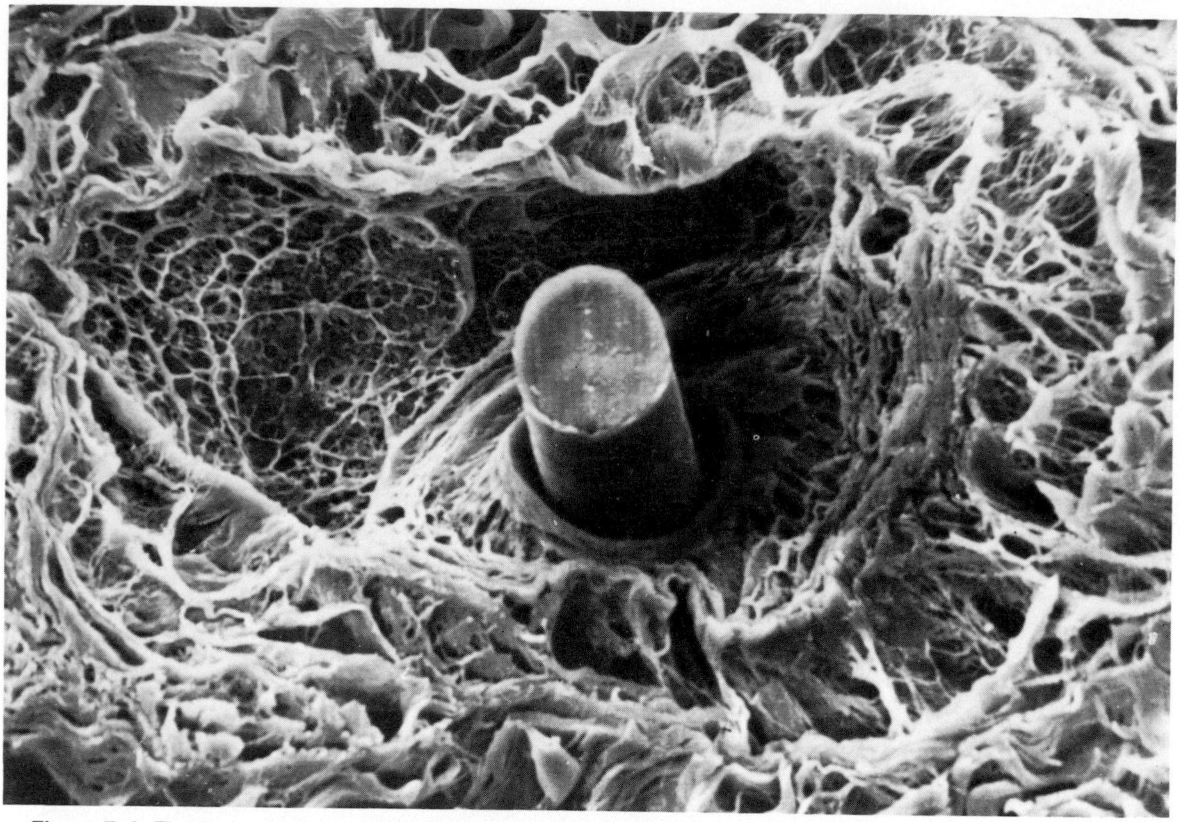

Figure 7–6. The fibrous networks are transfixed by hairs. A hair shaft surrounded by its follicle and by a sebaceous gland is shown attached to the main collagen network by fine fibrils. (From Brown, I. A.: A scanning electron microscope study of the effects of uniaxial tension on human skin. Br. J. Dermatol., 89:383, 1973.)

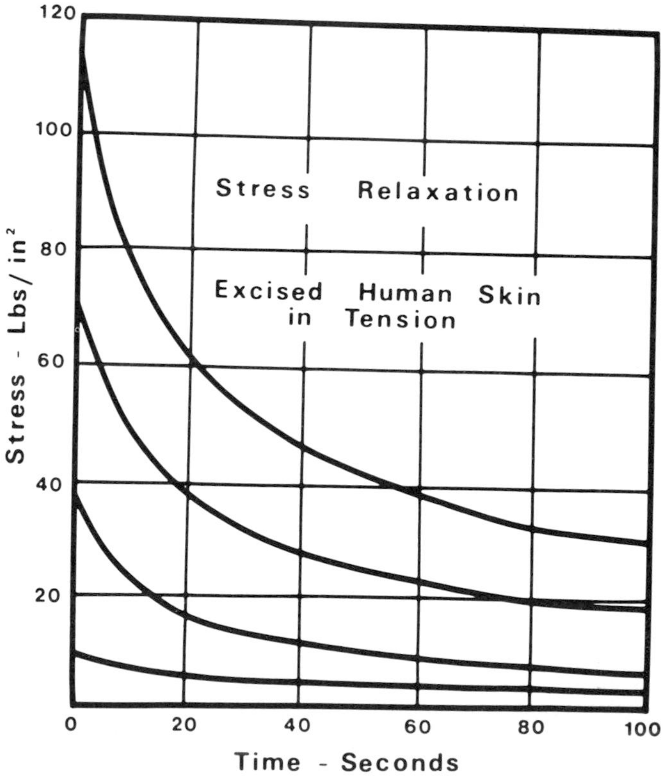

Figure 7–7. The stress relaxation that occurs in skin increases with the applied load. (From Gibson, T., and Kenedi, R. M.: The structural components of the dermis. *In* Montagna, W., Bentley, J. P., and Dobson, R. L. (Eds.): The Dermis, 1970. Courtesy of Appleton-Century-Crofts, Publishing Division of Prentice-Hall, Inc., Englewood Cliffs, NJ.)

tance that any measurements made of the physical properties of skin and its behavior under stress be made during a standard time. Failure to appreciate this variable in previous studies has caused confusion.

Creep is clinically important. It means that skin can be stretched by a significant, if small, amount. This can be of vital importance in such cases as the "just-too-small flap" or the "wound that just won't close." The usual technique is to place sharp, hooked retractors into the undersurface of the dermis on each side of the flap or wound, and to pull them in opposite directions with as much force as the surgeon and his assistant can extend, short of tearing the tissues, for at least a minute. It has been found that, if skin is "load cycled" (Fig. 7–8), the maximal extension is not usually obtained on the first loading. It is therefore advisable when trying to stretch skin to repeat the extension three or four times. One of the reasons for the viscoelasticity of skin is that, as the fibers in the dermis become aligned, tissue fluid and ground substance are progressively displaced from the network. The more fluid in the dermis, the greater is the amount of creep obtainable, and the phenomenon is particularly evident and useful when handling flaps that have recently been delayed or transferred.

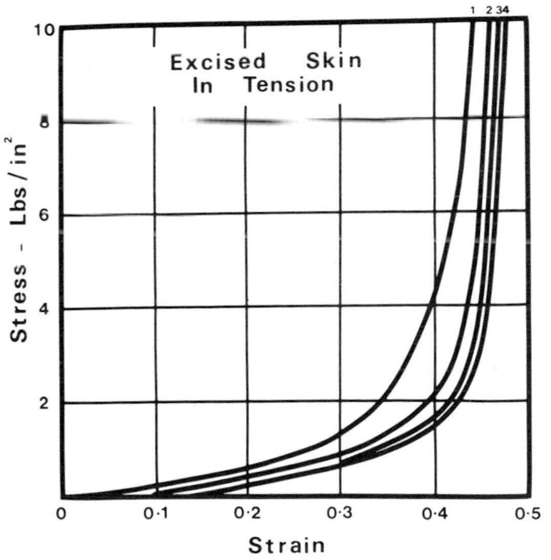

Figure 7–8. Repeated loading of skin shows varying curves until a stable state is attained in the region of curve 4. (From Gibson, T., and Kenedi, R. M.: The structural components of the dermis. *In* Montagna, W., Bentley, J. P., and Dobson, R. L. (Eds.): The Dermis, 1970. Courtesy of Appleton-Century-Crofts, Publishing Division of Prentice-Hall, Inc., Englewood Cliffs, NJ.)

Stress relaxation does not seem to have clinical relevance. It can, however, explain why the flap that appears to be sutured too tightly in the immediate postoperative period is often perfectly viable a few hours later.

SKIN TENSION PROPERTIES

The naturally occurring extensibility and tension in skin are often confused and referred to inaccurately as "elasticity." They are certainly interrelated; skin extends if increased tension is applied to it and, conversely, stretched skin is under increased tension. But they are distinct concepts and will be discussed separately.

Skin tension is of particular importance in wound healing. Clinical observation shows that it varies at different anatomic sites and in different directions at the same site. A sutured wound so oriented that the tension across it is maximal at that site is likely to produce a stretched hypertrophic scar. Plastic surgeons have learned to choose the direction of their incision wherever possible so that the tension across it is minimal and a fine linear scar is more probable.

Crease lines, whether caused by joint movement or by the play of underlying muscles, are tension lines in the sense that the tension across them must be virtually nil; otherwise, they would not have formed. The tension along a crease line is therefore higher than that across it. Sutured wounds that parallel creases are under the least possible tension at that site.

It would appear that there is a critical tension below which scars do not stretch but above which they do. Z-plasties around the head and neck often show a central limb that has stretched while the others have not, or vice versa.

Skin tension decreases with age, and the fine, almost undetectable scars that result in the lax skin of the elderly are well known; the same is true of the skin of the scrotum and the shaft of the penis. Conversely, there are areas, such as the shoulder and presternum, where the tension existing in all directions seems to be greater than the critical value, and stretched, if not hypertrophic, scars are almost inevitable.

The tension naturally present in skin is presumably a function of the elastic fiber network existing in a state of tension; collagen fibers have no power of retraction. In certain areas, gravity must contribute significantly to skin tension. The shoulder girdle is rather like a coat hanger supporting the skin of the chest and trunk, particularly in the female with the additional weight of the breasts. Such a condition may account for the high skin tension and stretched scars in the shoulder region. (See also the section on Langer's lines below.)

Unfortunately it has not so far been possible to devise a technique to measure tension in intact living skin, and absolute values to correlate with different kinds of scar remain unavailable.

Effect of Increased Tension on Normal Skin

A certain degree of increased tension can persist in skin for long periods without stretching the skin or producing any obvious effects. The normal skin immediately adjacent to a flexion contracture due to burn scarring does not stretch and correct the defect in spite of recurrent tension. Furthermore, in serial excisions of nevi, it can be shown (Gibson and Kenedi, 1967) that the increased tension imposed on the skin by the elliptic excision relaxes by only about 70 per cent after one year, and it is well known that over-enthusiastic serial excisions can produce permanent deformity.

With higher tensions one of three phenomena may occur, depending on the force applied: stretching, rupture (striae formation), or blanching of the skin.

The skin stretches in such conditions as lymphedema and adiposity, and in the most severe cases a linear stretch of nine to ten times may occur. "Stretch" is probably not the correct term, since the skin maintains its thickness and indeed may be thicker than normal. This type of stretching depends on biologic activity and growth and differs from the creep described above, which is purely physical in nature.

"Skin expansion" is becoming increasingly popular to obtain adequate local skin cover for breast prostheses (Radovan, 1982) and for a variety of other reconstructive purposes (Argenta, 1984). It involves the subcutaneous insertion of a silicone bag into which quantities of saline can be injected at intervals over a period of weeks. The overlying skin gradually "expands" until it is adequate for the purpose envisaged (see Chap. 13).

In this technique there is a combination of creep and biologic stretch. Argenta (1984) reported that within a period of 24 to 48 hours after injection, the overlying skin usually softens and can be moved over the prosthesis. This is the effect of creep, and thereafter creep and biologic stretch act together to provide sufficient *stretched* but otherwise normal local skin.

The dermis ruptures and striae form when an increasing load is applied at a faster rate than in skin stretch. Striae are found in the skin of the pregnant abdomen, in the skin covering the rapidly increasing fat deposits in Cushing's disease, and even in skin over the expanding muscles of enthusiasts taking body-building exercises (Glashan, 1963; Strivens, 1963). They lie as a rule at right angles to Langer's lines, which represent the direction of minimal extensibility. Whether they rupture or simply unravel from the weave has yet to be established. As Langer discovered, pregnancy imposes a different set of "lines" on a woman's abdominal skin from those of a nullipara.

Blanching of the skin occurs when the fibrous network is deformed to such an extent that the lumina of the dermal blood vessels are obliterated and blood flow is obstructed. If unrelieved, necrosis follows. Blanching may result from compression forces and can cause such lesions as pressure sores. It is probably more familiar to the plastic surgeon as the result of a tension force when skin flaps are sutured into defects slightly too large or skin is advanced too far after wide undermining. It should be remembered that in the examples mentioned—flaps and undermined skin—the force required to produce blanching is usually much less than that required in uncut skin.

A zone of blanching across a flap can usually be relieved if the force is not excessive, either by applying a stretching force and obtaining a modicum of *creep,* as described above, or by making a small incision just through the dermis in the center of, and at right angles to, the line of blanching. The latter maneuver divides the stretched, oriented fibers in the line of blanching and relaxes the collagen network. It has been found experimentally that 60 per cent more force can be applied before blanching recurs in a band that divides to enclose the small incision (Kenedi, Gibson, and Daly, 1965).

SKIN EXTENSIBILITY

Skin is extensible to allow for every possible body movement. Since none of our joints is universal, it follows that, on most parts of the body, skin extends more in some directions than in others. Skin extensibility is greatest in infancy. As skin is repeatedly stretched and relaxed throughout life, the ability of the elastic tissue matrix to return skin from its extended state to its fully relaxed state is gradually lost, and skin extensibility is replaced by skin laxity, which fulfills the same role of permitting free body movement. It is skin extensibility and skin laxity that permit many plastic surgical procedures, particularly the complete closure of skin defects without the need for importing tissue from a distance.

Skin extensibility, unlike skin tension, can be readily measured in vivo, and techniques vary from the approximation by the surgeon of picking up a fold between finger and thumb to the use of highly sophisticated and precise instruments.

Stark (1977) has mapped out the extensibility of skin and its orientation in young adults. For example, if measured when the subject is lying prone, the skin over the buttocks is about three times more extensible in a vertical direction (i.e., parallel to the spine) than it is across the buttocks. It thus provides adequate extensibility for full flexion of the hips. By contrast, over the tibia, skin has practically no extensibility; no neighboring joints require extensibility.

The results of accurate measurement may differ in vitro and in vivo: when skin is extended, it contracts by a similar amount at right angles to the direction of extension. Should the ability to contract be limited in vivo, as circumferentially around a limb, extension along the limb is similarly influenced. Furthermore, in vivo, skin is fixed to the underlying tissues to a varying degree, so that undermining usually permits additional extension, although at the expense of the blood supply.

DIRECTIONAL VARIATIONS IN SKIN PROPERTIES

Mention has already been made of certain directional variations in the physical properties of human skin, e.g., in skin tension and skin extensibility. Karl Langer (1819–1884) is widely known for his "lines," which in the past were misdrawn from textbook to textbook in a variety of ways, because few if any had seen or read his original work.

Langer's four articles on skin are entitled: I Cleavability (Die Spaltbarkeit); II Tension (Die Spannung); III Elasticity (Die Elasticität); IV Swelling capability (Das Quellungsvermögen). The last paper describes the effect of putting pieces of skin into acetic acid; in most instances the skin swelled more in one direction than in others. These four papers have been translated into English (Gibson, 1978). The following summarizes Langer's writings. The original papers deserve much further study.

Langer took up the observation of Dupuytren that a youth who attempted suicide by stabbing himself with a round-bodied awl produced linear clefts in the skin rather than round wounds. For most of his work, Langer used a 2 mm diameter awl, 20 to 25 mm long and ground to a sharp symmetric point. He was an anatomist in Vienna and his work was carried out in relatively fresh cadavers (Figs. 7–9 and 7–10).

Although Langer confirmed that clefts were formed in most areas of skin when stabbed, the idea of "lines" came later. When he had

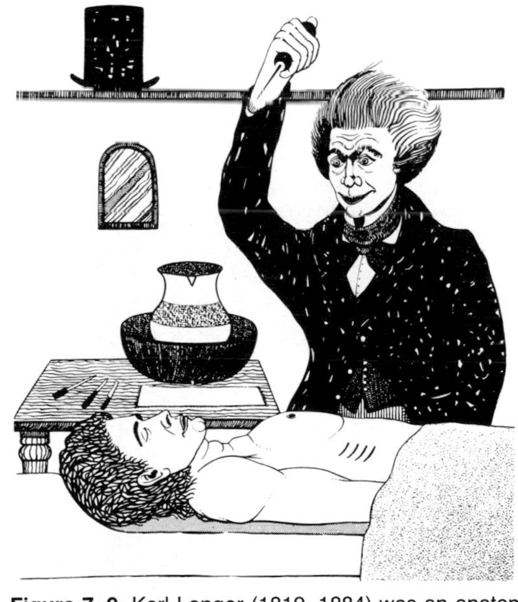

Figure 7–9. Karl Langer (1819–1884) was an anatomist in Vienna. His studies were carried out on fresh cadavers, which, surprisingly, produced results similar to those observable in the living.

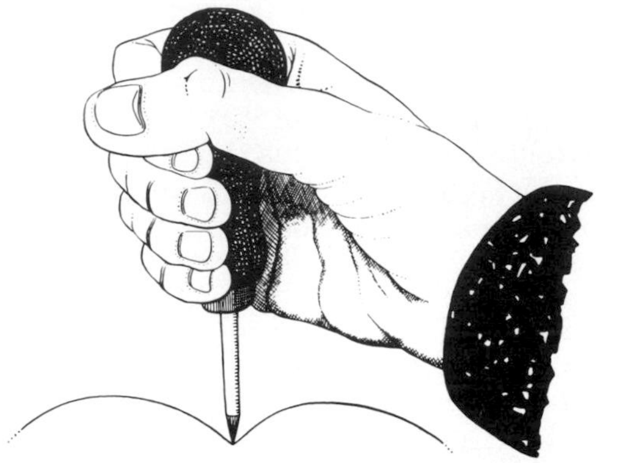

Figure 7–10. The instrument used to stab the skin was a 2 mm diameter awl sharpened to a point. Before piercing the skin, the point of the awl increases the skin tension in all directions. The collagen fibers that become aligned first are those which lie in the direction of minimum extensibility and which are then cleft by the point.

established the general direction of the clefts and the possibility that these were arranged in a linear fashion, he sited his stab wounds so that the clefts they produced followed the hypothetical pattern he had visualized: hence, the "lines" (Fig. 7–11) rather than an irregular collection of randomly sited clefts. Not all stab wounds produced clefts. When a pattern of lines met with another running in a different direction, stabbing along the junction produced irregular wounds usually triangular in shape. However, over most of the body's surface, clefts were produced.

Underlying this behavior is the arrangement of the fibers in the dermis. When Langer incised the skin at right angles to the lines on the front of the thigh, he could see with a lens that most of the fibers had been cut transversely or obliquely. Incised along the lines, the fibers ran mostly parallel to the cut (Fig. 7–12). From thin sections of the dermis cut parallel to the surface on the anterior thigh, Langer described a rhomboidal arrangement of the fibers. The longer and narrower the rhomboids, the more marked is the cleavage pattern; if the rhomboids are "squarer," less distinctive clefts are produced. Similar slices from the scalp showed a transversely cut hair follicle in each rhomboidal space (Fig. 7–13).

At the same time, Langer noted that completely excised strips of skin often retracted to a size less than that which they occupied in vivo. The fibers had then become curly or wavy in appearance and he concluded that, since wavy fibers could not be responsible for the retraction, some other substance must be involved. He had no technique for staining elastic fibers, but noted with his microscope an amorphous hyaline substance that he decided was the substance involved. He concluded: "Tension and retraction, fiber patterns and cleavage lines are thus interrelated and mutually dependent."

The fiber pattern in the dermis is not genetically determined. In the full-term fetus or neonate (Fig. 7–14) the cleavage lines encircle the limbs and trunk, apparently related to the expanding bulk of the fetus. By the age of 2½ years, the adult pattern of lines has been established (see Fig. 7–11), presumably by the increasing movement of the joints

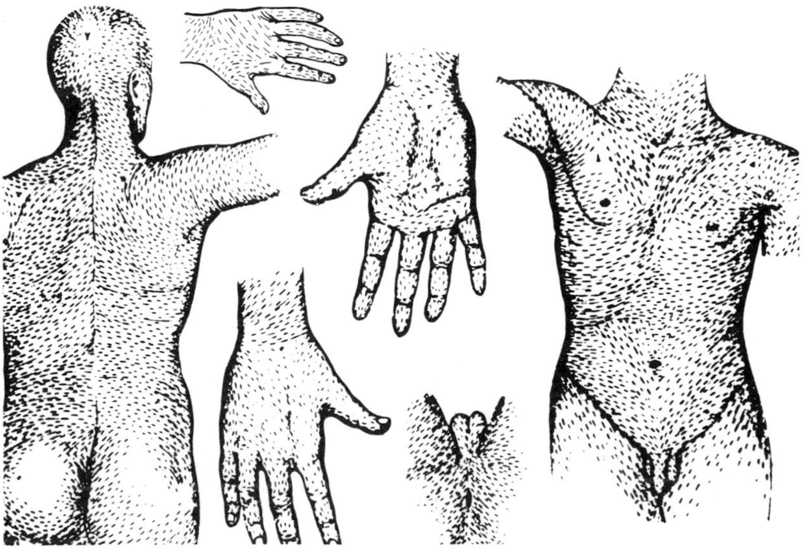

Figure 7–11. One of Langer's three illustrations of the cleavage lines. On the left side of each, the lines are from an adult cadaver; those on the right are from a 2½ year old boy. It is apparent that by this age a child already displays an adult pattern of lines. The other two plates are reproduced in Gibson, T.: Karl Langer (1819–1887) and his lines (editorial). Br. J. Plast. Surg., *31*:1, 1978.

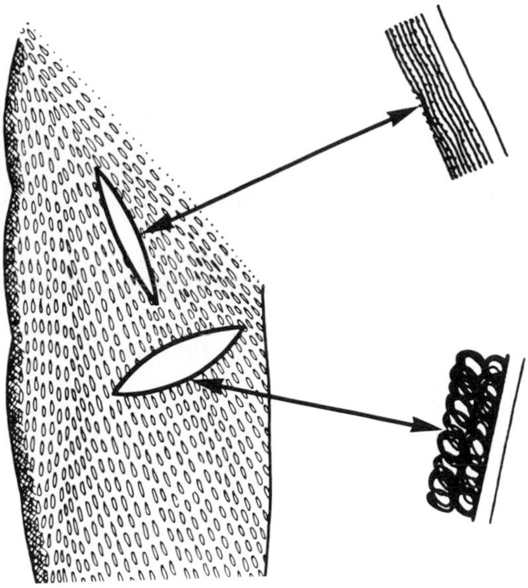

Figure 7–12. When the skin on the front of the thigh was cut along the cleavage lines, most of the fibers on the cut edge could be seen running parallel to the lines. When it was incised at right angles to the lines, most of the fibers had been cut transversely or obliquely.

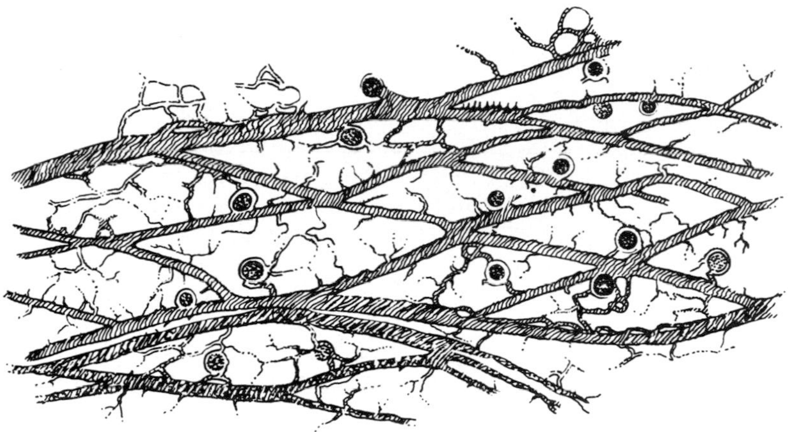

Figure 7–13. In situ, under normal tension Langer visualized the fiber pattern as rhomboidal. The long axes of the rhomboids lay along the cleavage lines. On the scalp, as illustrated, a transversely cut hair follicle lay in each rhomboidal space.

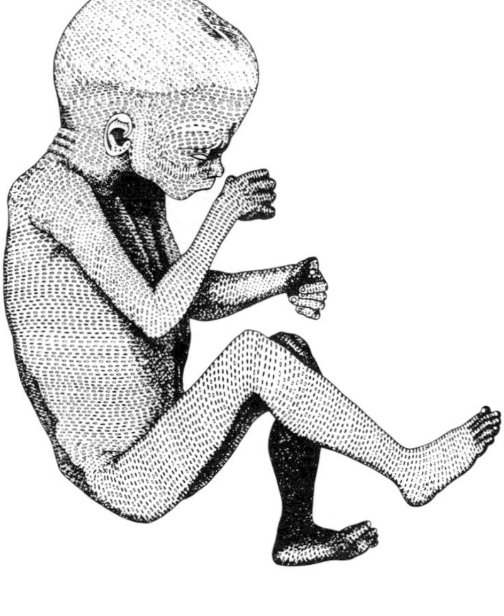

Figure 7–14. In the neonate the cleavage lines encircle the trunk and limbs and are probably related to the increasing bulk of the fetus. It is the activity of the joints in infancy that imposes the adult pattern. This is established by the age of 2½ years (see Fig. 7–11).

through their full range. The adult pattern can still be changed by anything that imposes new loads on the skin, such as pregnancy, obesity, or rapidly expanding tumors. In other words, the varying tensions in skin produce the fiber pattern, and not vice versa.

Cleavage Lines and Tension Lines. In his first paper Langer did not claim that his cleavage lines were tension lines, but in the second paper he showed that they were identical. He used a number of techniques, one of which is particularly ingenious. With a template he marked a circle on the skin and incised around the outline. The wound retracted to a varying degree. Langer made the fair assumption that the direction and degree of retraction were a function of skin tension. Thus, if the amount of retraction was the same in all directions around the incision, the skin tension was the same in all directions. If the tension was greater in one direction than another, the outer margin of the wound was drawn into an ellipse, the long axis of which lay in the tension line, while the central skin island also retracted into an ellipse but its long axis lay at right angles to the lines of tension (Fig. 7–15). An exaggerated sketch of this behavior is shown in Figure 7–16. Two instances in which the amount of retraction was the same all around the circle are interesting; on the central scalp there was very little retraction and thus little skin tension (Fig. 7–17), while over the sternum retraction was marked in all directions (Fig. 7–18). This may be related to the hypertrophic/keloid scars so commonly observed after even minor trauma.

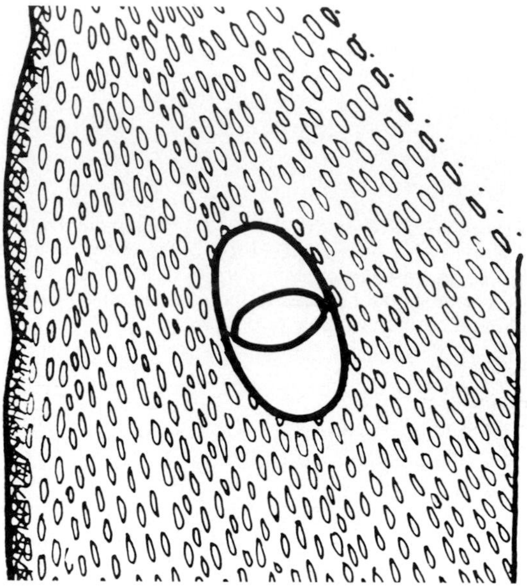

Figure 7–16. Retraction occurring on the front of the thigh when a circular outline has been incised. It is somewhat exaggerated, but illustrates that cleavage lines are tension lines and retraction lines.

Cleavage Lines and Skin Extensibility. Skin extensibility has already been described. It is easily measured in vivo (Stark, 1977) or

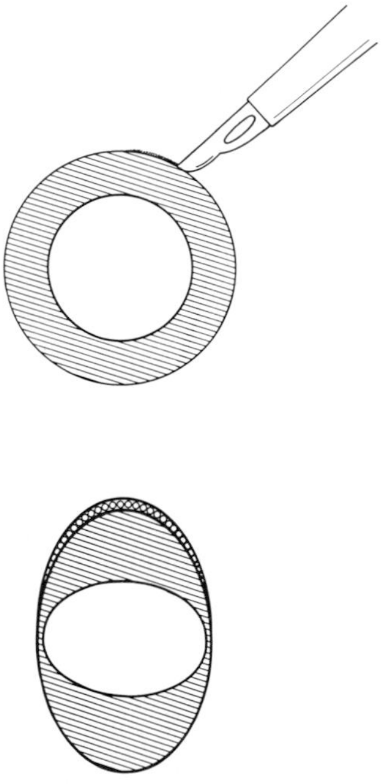

Figure 7–15. Langer incised around a circle marked on the skin. If skin tension was equal in all directions, the amount of retraction at all points around the wound was the same *(above)*. If skin tension was more marked in one direction, the outer skin margin was drawn out into an ellipse whose long axis lay along the tension lines. The central island retracted into an ellipse whose long axis was at right angles to the tension lines *(below)*.

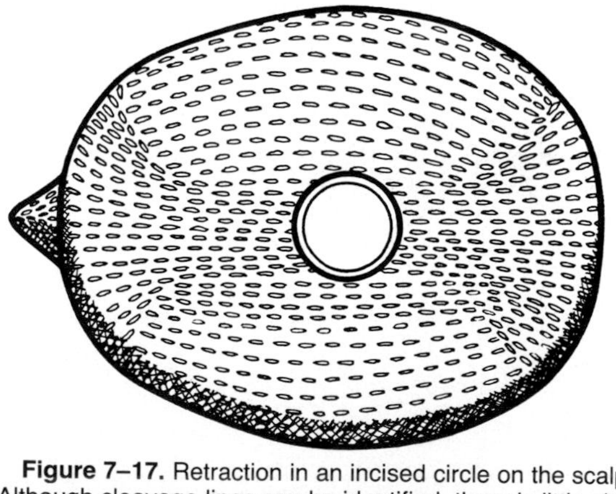

Figure 7–17. Retraction in an incised circle on the scalp. Although cleavage lines can be identified, there is little skin tension and only slight retraction of the wound in all directions.

in vitro. Highly sophisticated apparatuses can be applied to the skin via adhesive tapes for in vivo measurements, while excised specimens of skin can be stretched with great accuracy in such instruments as the Instron. Langer's experiments were carried out with the simplest techniques and are worth alluding to, since they underline what the author and his colleagues discovered, apparently de novo, a century later.

Langer tested skin from different parts of the body. He first stabbed the area a few times to ascertain the direction of the cleavage lines. Two 10 × 25 mm strips of skin were then excised, one of which ran parallel to the cleavage lines, the other at right angles to them. Of course, none of the initial stab wounds was included. The strips were held at each end by clamps and suspended within a glass tube containing a piece of wet paper to prevent drying. Two or three small pins thrust through the skin served as markers. The increase in distance between them, as weights were added to the open pan attached to the lower clamp, was a measure of the extension that resulted. Langer thus avoided the pitfalls of slip and shear, which can vitiate the results when the distance between the clamps is taken as measurement. An attached scale and a small telescope allowed an accuracy of 0.2 mm during measurements (Fig. 7–19).

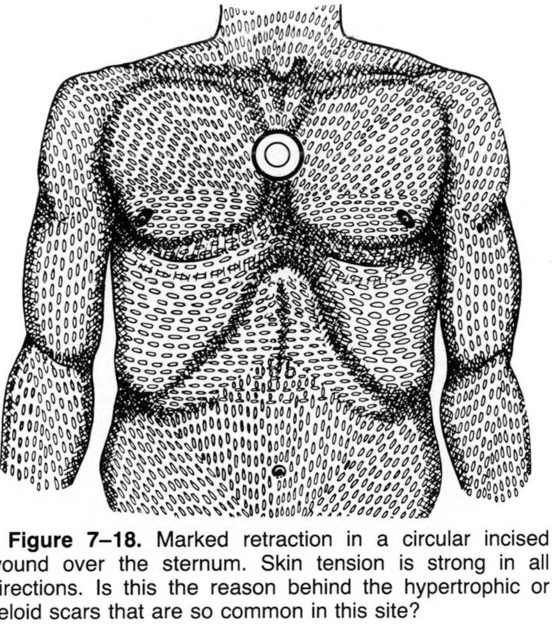

Figure 7–18. Marked retraction in a circular incised wound over the sternum. Skin tension is strong in all directions. Is this the reason behind the hypertrophic or keloid scars that are so common in this site?

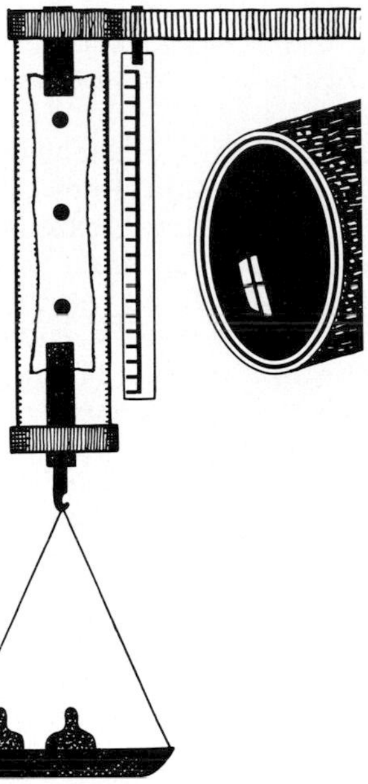

Figure 7–19. Measuring skin tension. A strip of skin is suspended between clamps in a glass tube. From the lower clamp is suspended a pan in which increasing weights may be placed. The markers are small pins driven through the skin, and the varying distance between them is measured by the attached scale and a small telescope. The results show that the extension across the cleavage lines is always greater than that along them.

Langer was aware of the viscoelastic properties of "creep" and "stress relaxation" (although he never knew the terms).

In order to allow for the extension which continued after the weight was applied and to obtain extension values which were as uniform as possible for the individual periods of loading, the loads were allowed to operate for initial time intervals: in some experiments for 2 minutes, in others 5. Further, I allowed 2 minutes to elapse after each loading before a new weight was applied.

He published many of his measurements in extenso and there are also a few graphs. The latter illustrate clearly the greater extension per unit load in transverse strips compared with those parallel to the cleavage lines. In addition they show that, as the load is increased, less and less extension occurs. His curves in fact have the same basic shape that the author and his colleagues observed with an Instron (see Fig. 7–4).

He wrote:

Two phases in the extension of a skin strip must be differentiated; the initial phase in which the fibers uncurl and the tissue is largely rearranged, and the terminal phase in which the extension affects mainly the fibers themselves.

In conclusion: Langer's lines are (1) cleavage lines, (2) tension lines, (3) retraction lines, and (4) minimal extensibility lines. Remember, however, that his results and those of the author and his colleagues were obtained in young adults. Increasing laxity replaces the skin tension of youth, and in the elderly such considerations rarely apply.

REFERENCES

Argenta, L. C.: Controlled tissue expansion in reconstructive surgery. Br. J. Plast. Surg., *37*:520, 1984.

Brown, I. A.: Structural and mechanical studies on human skin. Ph.D. Thesis, University of Strathclyde, Glasgow, 1971.

Brown, I. A.: A scanning electron microscope study of the effects of uniaxial tension on human skin. Br. J. Dermatol., *89*:383, 1973.

Gibson, T.: On the anatomy and physiology of the skin. An English translation of Langer's 4 papers cited below: I. The cleavability of the cutis. II. Skin tension. III. Skin elasticity. IV. Swelling capabilities of skin. Br. J. Plast. Surg., *31*:3, 9, 24, 39, 1978.

Gibson, T., and Kenedi, R. M.: Biomechanical properties of skin. Surg. Clin. North Am., *47*:279, 1967.

Gibson, T., and Kenedi, R. M.: Factors affecting the mechanical characteristics of human skin. *In* Dunphy, J. E., and Van Winkle, W., Jr. (Eds.): Repair and Regeneration: The Scientific Basis for Surgical Practice. New York, McGraw-Hill Book Company, 1969, p. 87.

Gibson, T., and Kenedi, R. M.: The structural components of the dermis. *In* Montagna, W., Bentley, J. P., and Dobson, R. L. (Eds.): The Dermis. New York, Appleton-Century-Crofts, 1970, p. 19.

Glashan, R. W.: Cutaneous striae. Br. Med. J., *1*:614, 1963.

Kenedi, R. M., Gibson, T., and Daly, C. H.: Bioengineering studies of the human skin I. *In* Jackson, S. F., Harkness, R., Partridge, S., and Tristram, G. (Eds.): Structure and Function of Connective and Skeletal Tissues. London, Butterworths, 1965, p. 388.

Langer, K.: Zur Anatomie und Physiologie der Haut I. Über die Spaltbarkeit der Cutis. S.-B. Akad. Wiss. Wien, *44*:19, 1861.

Langer, K.: Zur Anatomie und Physiologie der Haut II. Die Spannung der Cutis. S.-B. Akad. Wiss. Wien, *45*:133, 1862a.

Langer, K.: Zur Anatomie und Physiologie der Haut III. Über die Elasticität der Cutis. S.-B. Akad. Wiss. Wien, *45*:156, 1862b.

Langer, K.: Zur Anatomie und Physiologie der Haut IV. Das Quellungs vermögen der Cutis. S.-B. Akad. Wiss. Wien, *45*:156, 1862c.

Millington, P. F., Gibson, T., Evans, J. H., and Barbenel, J. C.: Structural and mechanical aspects of connective tissue. *In* Kenedi, R. M. (Ed.): Advances in Bio-medical Engineering. London, Academic Press, 1971, p. 189.

Radovan, C.: Breast reconstruction after mastectomy using the temporary expander. Plast. Reconstr. Surg., *69*:195, 1982.

Stark, H. L.: Directional variations in the extensibility of human skin. Br. J. Plast. Surg., *30*:105, 1977.

Strivens, T.: Cutaneous striae. Br. Med. J., *1*:263, 1963.

8

Ross Rudolph
Donald L. Ballantyne, Jr.

Skin Grafts

CLINICAL ASPECTS

Skin Anatomy

Skin, or integument, envelops the entire surface of the body, and its epithelium is continuous with that of the digestive, respiratory, and urogenital systems. It is an indispensable organ inasmuch as its total destruction is incompatible with survival. Skin serves as a barrier against the environment and is also the principal site of communication with the environment.

Skin plays an important role in regulating body temperature. Vasoconstriction of the skin capillaries reduces heat loss; vasodilation facilitates it. Heat loss occurs by evaporation of sweat. The entire cutaneous system can be considered a large glandular system (Montagna, 1962) because of the presence of holocrine (sebaceous) glands. Cells die as the epidermis is replaced, and keratin and sebum represent accumulations of the necrotic cells. The skin also contains many sensory nerve endings.

Skin is a compound organ. The two layers of the skin are derived from different embryonic layers and differ in character (Fig. 8–1). The outermost thinner layer is the epidermis; the innermost thicker layer is the dermis, which consists of connective tissue. The two layers are intimately connected by means of fine protoplasmic processes and elastic fibers that can be dissolved by a trypsin preparation (Rudolph and Milson, 1976). The epidermis contains no blood vessels; the dermis, acting as the nutrient base of the epidermis, is thus indispensable.

EPIDERMIS

The epidermis is a stratified squamous epithelium that covers the entire surface of the body. It differentiates early, having been recognized by Medawar (1953) in a 12 week old human embryo. The epidermis is composed of living malpighian stratum that rests upon the dermis and a desquamating dead superficial layer known as the stratum corneum. The cells of the malpighian stratum are arranged in layers that are not clearly defined and can probably be considered as separate steps in a continuous evolution from the basal to the outer cornified squamous layer. The basal layer, also called the stratum germinativum, is located adjacent to the dermis and its blood supply. In the stratum spinosum or prickle cell layer, which is superficial to the basal layer, the cells are larger and are joined by tiny fibrils known as tonofibrils. More superficially, the cytoplasm of the cells

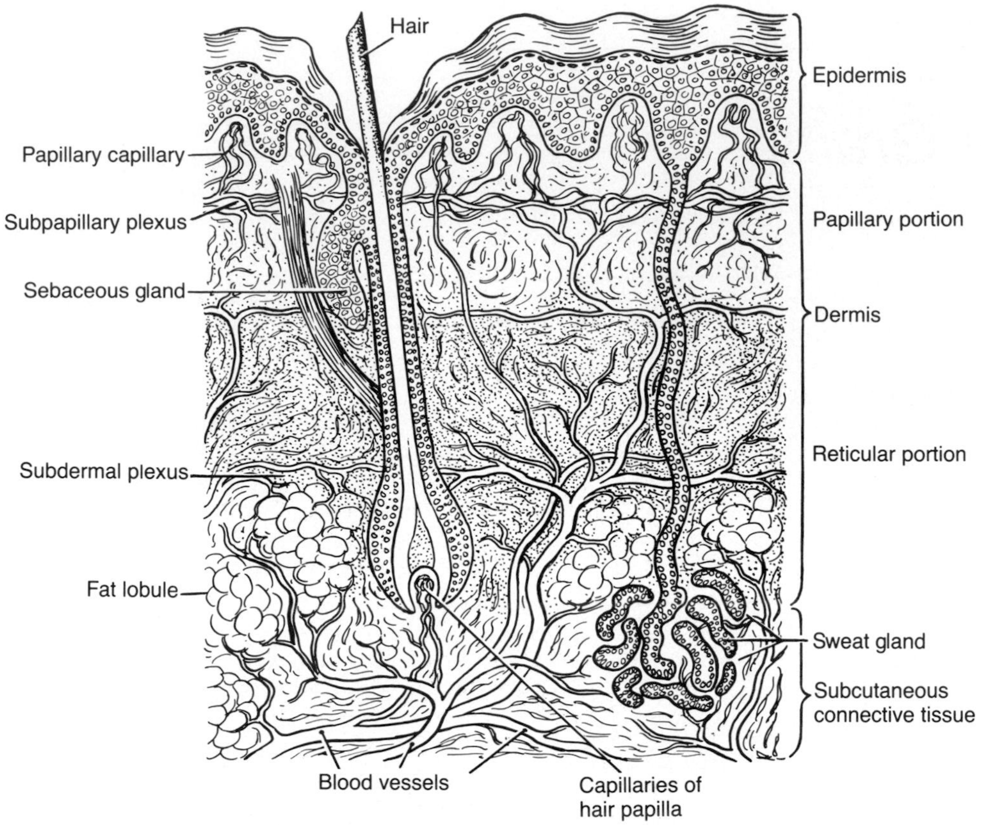

Figure 8–1. Section of human skin. (From Kazanjian and Converse.)

contains granules; the area is known as the stratum granulosum. The stratum lucidum, a clear band, separates this layer from the outer layer of the epidermis, which is the cornified stratum corneum. All these layers can be demonstrated in the thick skin of the palms and soles; the epidermis is considerably thinner elsewhere. The stratum corneum and stratum germinativum are the only layers consistently present in all parts of the body.

Epidermis undergoes growth and replacement throughout life (Storey and Leblond, 1951). New cells produced by mitosis in the basal layer exert a pressure that results in movement of the cells to the surface (Flemming, 1884); extruded cells are transformed into a horny material that forms the keratinized layers. The keratinization may be soft, as in the skin, or hard, as in the nails or hair cortex. It has been calculated that the renewal time of the malpighian layers is about 19 days. Thus, each epidermal cell spends an average of 10 days in its migration to the surface. The epidermis shows topographic differences that are remarkably persistent after transplantation. As the characteristics of transplanted skin do not change, the matching of skin from other areas of the body with the skin of the face is always difficult.

Epidermal tissue is subjected to trauma more often than other tissues of the body. The epidermis usually withstands environmental trauma, such as periodic exposure to solar radiation, wide variations in temperature, cuts, scratches, burns, bacteria, and viruses. The insoluble and tough keratinized superficial layers of the epidermis protect the body from the environment. Keratin does not cover the soft, stratified squamous epithelium of the oral and nasal cavities.

DERMIS

The dermis consists of two layers: a superficial or papillary layer and a deep or reticular layer (see Fig. 8–1).

The papillary layer, characteristic of man and less distinct in many mammals, contains widely separated, delicate, collagenous elastic and reticular fibers, enmeshed with capillaries and surrounded by ground substance.

The reticular layer is formed by dense, coarser, branching, collagenous fibers arranged in layers mostly parallel to the surface. Many fine furrows form a close network on the surface of facial skin. The small rhomboid ridges in which the orifices of the sweat glands are grouped, separated by fine grooves, depend on the arrangement of the dermal papillae in the dermis (Unna, 1883). The surface elevations are associated with the higher papillae and the furrows with the lower papillae.

Elastic tissue is distributed throughout the dermis and is closely interlaced in the reticular layer. The ground substance and interstitial fluid consist of extracellular fluid, derived largely from the blood plasma, and mucopolysaccharides, chiefly hyaluronic acid, chondroitin sulfates, and glycoproteins, in a varying degree of polymerization. The ground substance ordinarily has a gel-like consistency; the proportion of ground substance decreases with age, being replaced by fibrous intercellular tissue.

Connective tissue cells are sparsely distributed among the fibers. Fibroblasts are often associated with mast cells. Pigment-bearing cells, melanophages, are sparingly distributed in the dermis of normal skin.

DERMOEPIDERMAL JUNCTION

The dermoepidermal junction of human skin appears as an irregularly wavy line; the ridges or rete pegs project into the dermis, enclosing between them the vascularized dermal papillae. The keratinocytes, keratin-producing cells of the epidermis, which make up most of the epidermal cells, are attached to each other by desmosomes. Desmosomes are plaquettes of thickened cell membrane, each joined to the plaquette on the neighboring cell by three intermediary plaquettes seen by electron microscopy (Eriksson, 1972). The cells of the basal layer of the epidermis are attached to the basement membrane, a connective tissue layer, by half-desmosomes, so called because they have half the number of plaquettes. The basement membrane, on its dermal side, leads into a disorganized arrangement of "anchoring" fibrils (Braun-Falco, 1969).

HAIR FOLLICLES

Cells of the developing epidermis invade the dermis during embryonic development to form intradermal epithelial structures: the hair follicles, sebaceous glands, and sweat glands. These structures, principally the omnipresent sebaceous glands, are the source of an additional epidermal layer when the covering epidermis has been removed or destroyed, as in burns, abrasions, and donor areas of split-thickness skin grafts.

The downgrowth of epidermis into the underlying dermis begins early in the third month of fetal life. The fetus at about the sixth month has become covered with delicate hair (lanugo). This hair is shed before birth except in the eyebrows, eyelashes, and scalp, where it persists and becomes thicker. These hairs are replaced by coarser ones a few months after birth. A new hairy growth occurs over the rest of the body, covering it with a downy coat, the vellus. Coarse hair develops at puberty in the axilla, in the pubic region, on the face in males, and to a lesser extent on other parts of the body. A small bundle of smooth muscle fibers, the arrector pili, is attached to the connective tissue sheath of the hair follicle. Muscle contraction pulls on the hair follicle and acts on the sebaceous glands, expressing an oily secretion (Hamilton, 1951).

In transplanted skin the growth of hair in an area that should be hairless creates problems. Hair grows according to hair growth characteristics in the donor site, and is also known to grow later in skin grafts transplanted from a hairless donor site in children.

The skin of the eyelids contains no hair follicles. Hairs do not grow vertically from the skin but assume a slanting direction. This fact merits consideration when hair is being transplanted for the reconstruction of an eyebrow or for baldness; the incisions should be oblique in order to parallel the direction of the hair follicles.

SEBACEOUS (HOLOCRINE) GLANDS

Most sebaceous glands are appendages of hair follicles and open inside the pilosebaceous canal (see Fig. 8–1). These racemose or saccular glands are generally found on the underside of the hair follicles, but away from the hairs on the lips, buccal mucosa, and lacrimal caruncles. Sebaceous glands are at their largest size and greatest density in the skin of the forehead, nose, and cheeks, where their density attains 400 to 900 per sq cm of skin surface; in other areas of the body there may be fewer than 100 per sq cm. The lobules of sebaceous glands are solid masses of cells that gradually become filled with fat granules and finally disintegrate, giving forth an oily secretion known as sebum. This provides a lubricant for the hair, keeps the skin supple, protects it against friction, and makes it more impervious to moisture.

Doupe and Sharp (1943) have shown that the secretion of the sebaceous glands is the end product of cellular disruption and, in contrast to the secretion of sweat glands, is not under the control of the nervous system.

SWEAT (ECCRINE AND APOCRINE) GLANDS

Eccrine sweat glands are found over the general body surface of man except in the lips and some parts of the external genitalia; apocrine sweat glands tend to be concentrated in a number of areas, including the eyelids and axillae.

These are simple, tubular glands, usually coiled at the base of the dermis (see Fig. 8–1). The ducts of the sweat glands pass through the epidermis and open either at the sweat pores on the skin surface, or above the opening of the sebaceous glands in the hair follicle walls.

The density and distribution of sweat glands vary in different parts of the body. There are two distinct types of eccrine glands: those located in the palms of the hands and soles of the feet, and those of the whole body surface. The former are phylogenetically older and respond to emotional and mental stress, while the latter, which are found in significant numbers only in man and higher primates, are concerned with temperature regulation. The apocrine glands, which become active at puberty, secrete continuously. This activity is varied by emotion and hormonal changes as in menstruation and pregnancy. The secretions of eccrine glands are odorless, whereas those of the apocrine glands undergo bacterial decomposition and produce a characteristic odor.

Transplanted skin, temporarily severed from the nerve connections, lacks the lubrication normally supplied by the eccrine and apocrine glands and is therefore dry and more susceptible to injury. Bland creams, such as lanolin or cocoa butter, should be applied to grafted skin until reinnervation and function of the secreting glands are restored.

HYPODERMIS

Beneath the dermis is a fatty layer, or panniculus adiposus. Deep to the fatty layer is a discontinuous flat sheet of muscle, the panniculus carnosus, the main vestige of which in man is the platysma of the cervical region. In many animals the panniculus carnosus is well developed; its use, for example, allows horses to twitch off flies. The junction of dermis and subcutaneous adipose tissue is irregular. Domes of fat, the columnae adiposae, project into the lower layers of the dermis. Collagenous fiber bundles extend perpendicularly into the hypodermis and branch loosely to form the retinaculum cutis, which separates the lobules of fat. When skin sections are cut in a plane parallel to the skin surface at the junction between dermis and fat, the pattern is that of a collagen network with the fat protruding through the interspaces.

Many hair follicles, with their arrector pili muscles, are implanted into the summits of the fat domes, two or three to each dome. Most of the sweat glands are situated between the fat domes and the dermal collagen bundles. They are usually placed at a deeper level than the hair follicles; in the bearded area of the male face, however, hair follicles lie in the subcutaneous fat below the level of junction with the dermis. The irregular line of junction between dermis and fat and the presence of deeply situated epidermal structures account for the epithelization that follows burns of the face in which the cutaneous layer is apparently destroyed.

SKIN THICKNESS

Skin varies widely in thickness from region to region, and with age (Southwood, 1955). Skin is thickest in the trunk, palms, and soles and is thinnest in the eyelids and in the postauricular area. Men have thicker skin than females regardless of the anatomic area. Age is another important consideration, as the skin of children is quite thin. The dermis thickens gradually until the fourth or fifth decade, and after this the skin again thins. Thus, a given thickness of split-thickness graft harvesting may represent only a small portion of the total skin thickness from the back of an adult male, whereas on the thigh of an elderly emaciated female it may represent almost the entire skin thickness. Anyone contemplating cutting skin grafts must be aware of the differences in skin thicknesses and must take them into account in planning appropriate graft harvesting (Rudolph, 1976).

Skin Grafts

Skin is transplanted by completely detaching a portion of integument from its donor site and transferring it to a host bed, where it acquires a new blood supply to ensure the viability of the transplanted cells.

A skin graft consists of epidermis and dermis, the dermal component constituting either the entire thickness or only a portion of the dermis (Fig. 8–2); thus, skin grafts can be either full thickness or split thickness. A skin *autograft* (autogenous graft) is a graft transferred from a donor to a recipient site in the same individual. An *allograft* (homograft) is a transplant between genetically disparate individuals of the same species. A *xenograft* (heterograft) is a graft transplanted between individuals of different species. The term "isograft" is one employed in experimental transplantation to designate an allograft between highly inbred (genetically pure) strains of animals; such grafts may also be called "syngeneic."

Although Bünger in 1822 applied a skin graft from the thigh to the nose and Baronio (1804) had previously performed experimental skin grafts in sheep, the clinical importance of skin grafting was not appreciated until the latter part of the nineteenth century (see Chap. 1). Since that time, skin grafting has become a vital part of plastic and reconstructive surgery.

SELECTION

An important decision in skin grafting is selecting the ideal graft from the optimal donor site. The surgeon must first decide between full-thickness and split-thickness skin grafting, and this requires an understanding of the biology of grafts.

The earliest skin grafts were exceptionally thin split-thickness, composed of almost pure epithelium. Such grafts have little clinical applicability because the underlying wound contracts greatly and is unstable. Only if skin is in very short supply is epidermal grafting useful. The very thin skin grafts used by early surgeons (Ollier, 1872; Thiersch, 1874) have been replaced by thicker split-thickness grafts (Blair and Brown, 1929), which include all of the epidermis and a variable fraction of the dermis (see Fig. 8–2).

Split-thickness skin grafts may be applied to granulating wounds, since they require

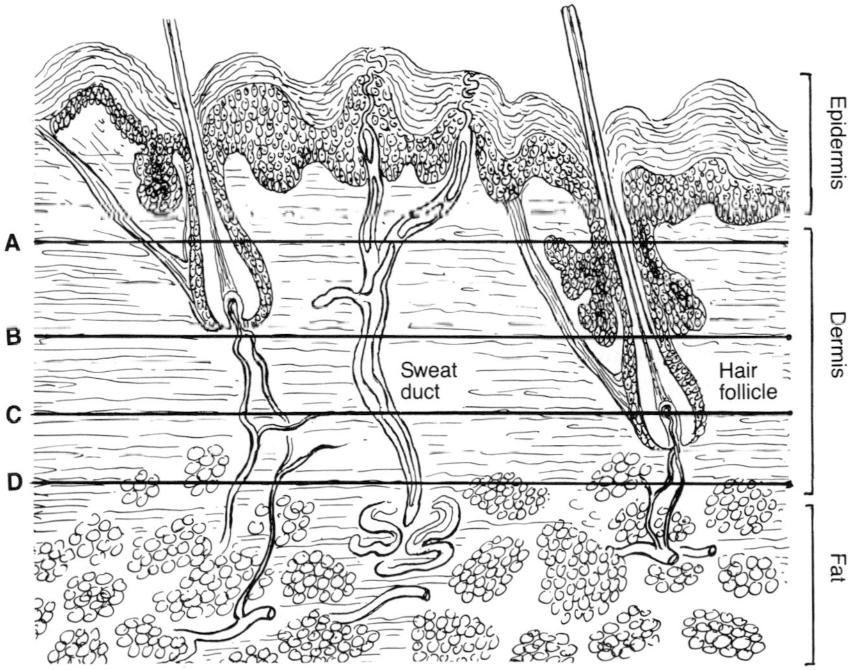

Figure 8–2. A section of skin to illustrate the comparative thickness of skin grafts. *A,* Line of section of the thin split-thickness (Thiersch) graft. *B,* Line of section of the split-thickness graft. *C,* Line of section of the thick split-thickness or three-quarter thickness graft. *D,* Line of section of the full-thickness graft. Note that the junction between the dermis and the subcutaneous tissue is irregular. The protrusions of the subcutaneous fat into the dermis are known as the columnae adiposae.

less ideal conditions for survival and can tolerate less vascularity than do full-thickness grafts. The average split-thickness skin graft used today is between 0.012 and 0.018 inch (0.30 to 0.45 mm).* Because blood vessels arborize as they ascend in the dermis, split-thickness skin grafts have a larger number of cut blood vessels on the undersurface and therefore a greater capacity to absorb nourishment from the wound bed.

The donor site for a split-thickness graft is able to heal spontaneously, since such grafts include only a portion of the dermis with a sufficient number of epidermal accessory structures left behind (see Fig. 8–2). If necessary, more split-thickness grafts can be harvested from the same site, an important consideration in patients with extensive skin loss. Wounds with questionable circulation or of large size are always covered with split-thickness skin grafts, despite the disadvantages of contraction, lack of growth in children, abnormal pigmentation, and occasional lack of durability (Rudolph, 1984).

Full-thickness grafts include the entire thickness of the skin, both epidermis and dermis. Such grafts resist contraction, grow in children, and have a texture and pigment appearance more similar to that of normal skin than do split-thickness grafts. Full-thickness grafts need excellent wound vascularity for survival, and in general are used on acute uncontaminated wounds of small size. A contaminated or large wound may be initially closed with a split-thickness graft, which is later replaced by a full-thickness graft to improve skin quality. Because they simulate normal uninjured skin, full-thickness grafts ideally would be used on all wounds that required skin grafting. However, this is obviously not possible, as wounds may be too large to be covered with full-thickness skin, too contaminated, or of poor vascularity, in which case split-thickness skin grafting is selected.

Choice of Donor Site. *Split-thickness skin grafts* can be taken from any area of the body, including the scalp and extremities (Fig. 8–3). Since the harvesting of split-thickness grafts does leave a scar, selection of the donor site should consider scar visibility as well as color match. When possible, split-thickness skin grafts should be taken from hidden areas such as the lateral buttock (Fig. 8–4) so that recreational clothing camouflages the scar, an equal consideration in both sexes. Lower extremity or trunk split-thickness grafts ideally should not be used in the face, as such grafts tend to have a yellowish-brownish color.

If split-thickness skin grafts are required for the face, skin harvested from "blush zones" such as the supraclavicular area and scalp is preferable. If the split-thickness grafts are cut superficially enough in a hairy area such as the scalp, hair should not grow in the recipient area nor should baldness develop in the donor area. Other areas such as the lateral neck and supraclavicular regions can serve as donor sites for facial split-thickness grafting, particularly in the elderly, ruddy-complexioned patient, and are best harvested with drum dermatomes.

A commonly used site for extremity or trunk skin grafts is the abdomen, as are the thighs and buttocks. If split-thickness grafts are required in hand reconstruction, i.e., for fingertips, they should be harvested from the upper inner arm, a cosmetically better location than the more accessible forearm.

Mucosal split-thickness grafts as in conjunctival replacement can be harvested from within the oral cavity using a specialized dermatome, the Castroviejo dermatome. Mucosal split-thickness grafts are selected when low friction and self-lubricating qualities are desired (Fig. 8–5). Since grafted skin always maintains the epidermal specificity of its donor site in humans (Briggaman and Wheeler, 1968), the demands of the recipient site influence the type of split-thickness graft chosen.

An important source of split-thickness grafts, occasionally overlooked in trauma situations, is avulsed or surgically removed skin. The patient with large areas of avulsed skin can have split-thickness grafts harvested from the otherwise discarded skin. Numerous techniques have been suggested, but the author has found most useful the sectioning of this skin into squares, which are then glued to a drum dermatome. The harvested split-thickness grafts from the otherwise useless avulsed skin can be placed on the denuded limbs or stored as necessary (Rudolph, Fisher, and Ninnemann, 1979; Rudolph, Earle, and Fratianné, 1975).

*Although medicine as a science has largely changed to the metric system, skin graft dermatomes in the United States and Great Britain continue to be marked in inches. Therefore, discussion of dimensions in this chapter will include inches as well as metric measurements.

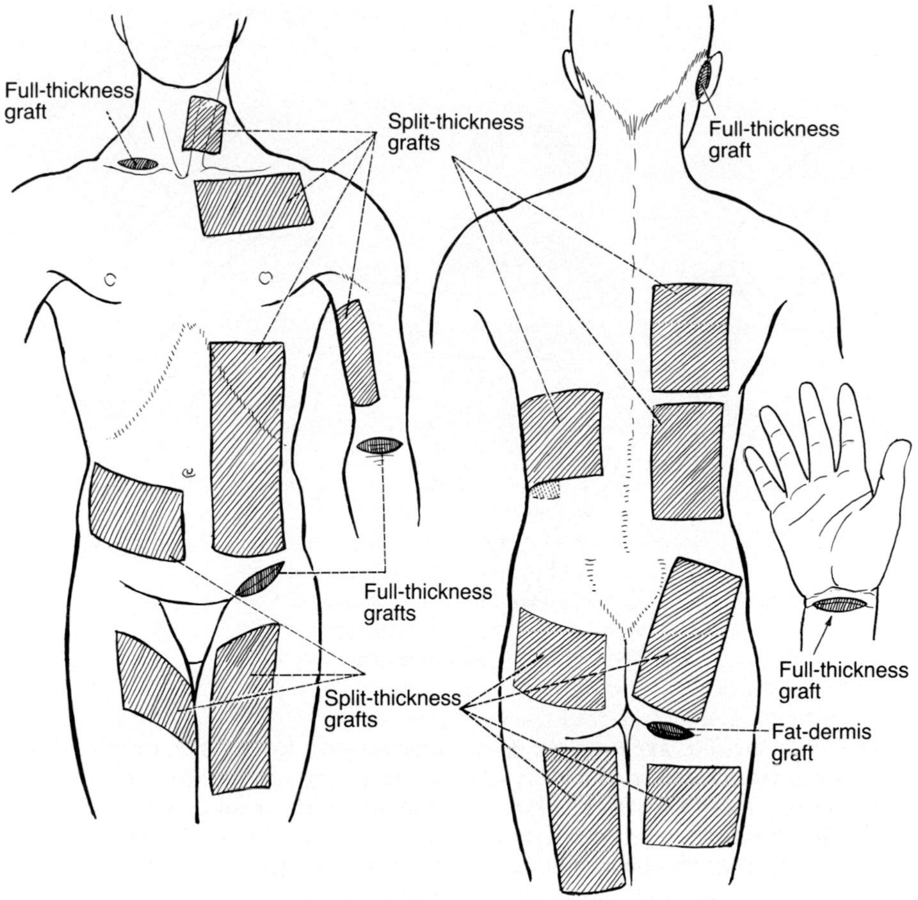

Figure 8–3. Available donor sites for skin grafts.

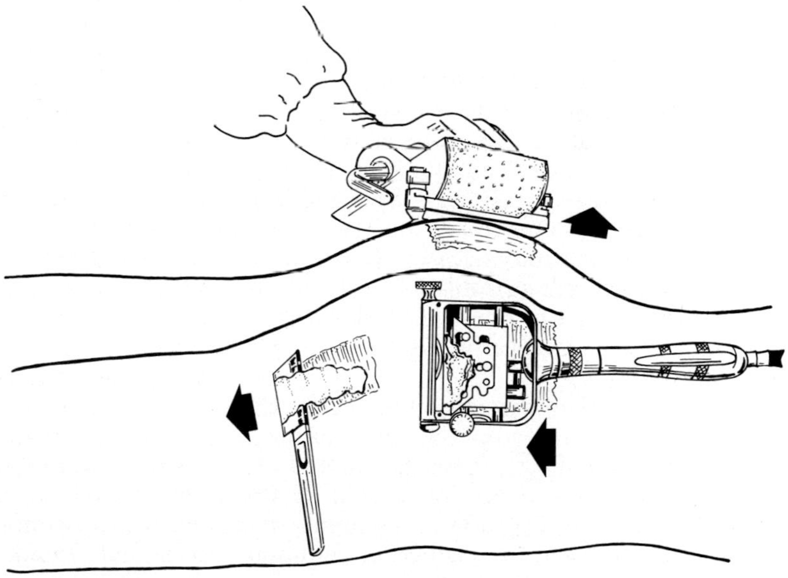

Figure 8–4. Split-thickness skin grafts should be harvested from relatively hidden areas such as the upper thighs and buttocks whenever possible. Drum dermatomes are generally used across a convex surface, while power dermatomes and hand-held knives are best used longitudinally on an extremity.

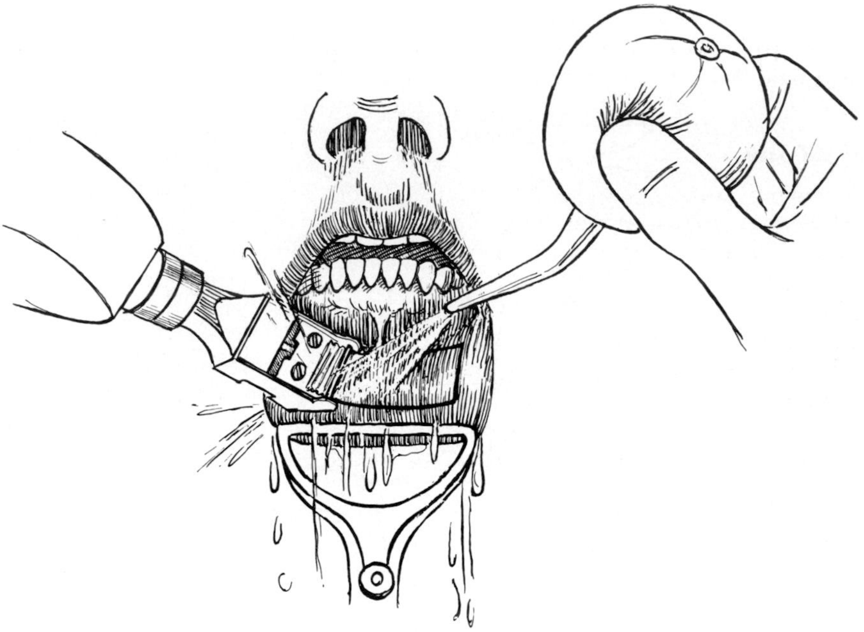

Figure 8–5. The Castroviejo dermatome.

Full-thickness skin grafts are almost always harvested from areas where the skin is thin (Rudolph, 1976) (see Fig. 8–3). Full-thickness grafts to the face are often taken from the upper eyelid, from the postauricular area, or from the supraclavicular region. Relatively large grafts (3 x 3 cm) can be harvested from behind the ear and the donor site closed primarily. Even larger grafts of postauricular skin may be harvested if the donor site is resurfaced with a split-thickness skin graft. Postauricular full-thickness skin grafts may remain slightly red, as do those from the supraclavicular area. The scarring of the supraclavicular area may be less desirable because of the relative exposure of this area. Full-thickness grafts from the central abdomen and trunk are rarely used as the skin is thick and prone to necrosis; hairless groin skin is thinner and may be used. Large areas of full-thickness skin suitable for grafting can be obtained from the dorsum of the foot, if the donor site is carefully closed with split grafting.

Other full-thickness donor sites include the prepuce and scrotum and the labia minora. These areas have dark pigmentation and are useful for reconstructing the areola of the breast. Full-thickness grafts of the nipple and areola may be used in reduction mammoplasty, or in reconstructing a breast after mastectomy for cancer, provided that the nipple is found to be free of tumor. However, because of the risk of seeding tumor, even if frozen sections are negative, the use of full-thickness nipple grafts from the breast with tumor has become less common. Full-thickness grafts of the areola and nipple may be obtained from the other breast in reconstruction after mastectomy.

Full-thickness grafts for resurfacing of fingertip defects can be taken from the flexor crease of the wrist, or even better, the elbow crease (see Fig. 8–3). Traumatically amputated digits may produce tissue appropriate for skin grafting when digital replantation is neither available nor appropriate. The amputated skin can be debrided of fat and applied as a full-thickness graft. The overlying thick keratin layer, which often causes curling, is also trimmed. Such full-thickness grafts of amputated digital skin may not always survive but may act as biologic dressings; patients are often very insistent that the amputated skin be replaced.

A final consideration in selecting a donor site for full-thickness skin is avoiding later hair growth (Vecchione, 1974). Since in most body locations the hair follicles lie within the dermis, unwanted hair can be transplanted if it is not avoided. Particularly in children, care must be taken to select an area that will in adult life be free of hair. This is especially important in the groin, to avoid pubic hair growing in an unwanted visible location.

CUTTING: SPLIT-THICKNESS GRAFTS

A variety of dermatomes are available for cutting *split-thickness grafts*. In general, air or electric powered dermatomes and the freehand knife are used to cut lengthwise on the extremity; drum dermatomes are used sidewise across the extremity, since the rolling maneuver required for graft cutting is best accomplished across a convex surface (see Fig. 8–4).

The harvesting of split-thickness skin grafts requires anesthesia, since such cutting is painful. With general anesthesia, the anesthesiologist should be alerted at the start of graft cutting as a lightly anesthetized patient may move. Local anesthetic solution can also be used. The donor site is marked and then thoroughly infiltrated with anesthetic solution, taking care not to skip areas in the donor site. An epinephrine-containing solution can be used to reduce blood loss. In addition, the blanching caused by epinephrine helps to identify the anesthetized areas. Regional blocks may be used as on the lateral thigh. Other techniques such as frost and surface anesthesia are less commonly used.

Power Dermatomes

Most split-thickness skin grafts in the United States are harvested with air or electric powered dermatomes, which can cut large amounts of skin rapidly. A power-driven dermatome uses a rapidly vibrating blade driven by an electric motor or gas turbine. The adjustable components work like a wood-cutting planer: a flat surface lies at the level of the knife blade and a smaller platform can be raised or lowered, depending on desired graft thickness. The width of the graft is determined by the width setting on the dermatome (Fig. 8–6).

The operating surgeon should check the dermatome to be sure that the sterile disposable cutting blade is inserted into the dermatome and secured with the fixation screws (Fig. 8–7). The thickness is determined by first closing the dermatome opening completely, then opening it by turning the setting knob to the appropriate thickness. The average split-thickness skin graft is cut at 0.015 inch; this can be checked by inserting a No. 15 Bard-Parker blade, which approximates that thickness. The width of the graft is set and the dermatome attached to the power source. The donor site is prepared with a surgical solution, ideally pHisoHex. If Betadine or some other sticky solution is used, it must be washed off, or the dermatome will stick to the skin and cut an irregularly shaped graft. The skin is thoroughly lubricated with sterile mineral oil to facilitate graft cutting. Experimental studies have shown that the mineral oil disappears from beneath the grafts within two to three weeks and causes no apparent interference with healing (Rudolph, 1976).

Cutting of the graft is accomplished by setting the dermatome flat on the skin, turning on the power, and advancing it flat across the skin surface with gentle downward pressure. An assistant can press on the skin in advance of the dermatome, although experienced operators may dispense with this step. An assistant can elevate the skin as it is cut from the dermatome, to allow graft thickness to be judged. The thicker the graft, the more opaque it is; an ideal skin graft is slightly translucent.

Graft thickness can also be judged by the type of bleeding observed at the graft donor site. Superficial grafts leave behind many small bleeding points; deeper cutting leaves fewer bleeding points, which bleed more, and grafts cut too deeply expose fat. Consideration of the underlying thickness of the skin *must* be taken into account when cutting a skin

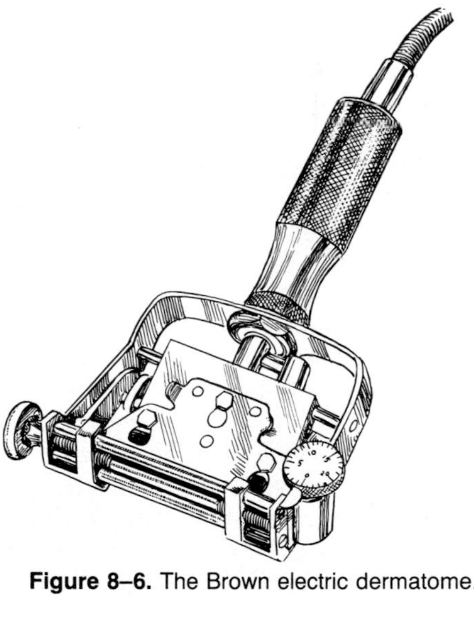

Figure 8–6. The Brown electric dermatome.

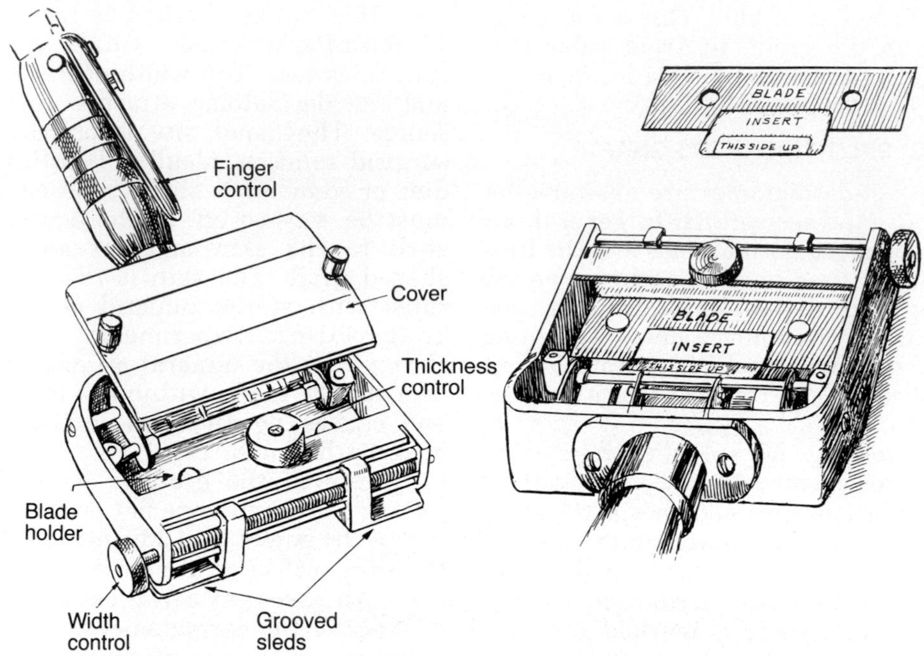

Figure 8–7. Air-driven dermatome. There are separate knobs to control the width and depth of the skin graft. A disposable blade is also provided.

graft with a dermatome, as cutting at a "standard" thickness may cut too deeply into a patient with thin skin. Placing the dermatome flat on the skin and maintaining that flatness makes rapid uniform harvesting of skin possible. Tilting the dermatome down may produce gouging and trenching of the skin.

The electric or gas powered dermatome can also be used in shaving scars where there is hypertrophy without contracture. With the instrument set at 0.025 to 0.031 inch, scar can be shaved off by repeated strokes until there is a thin sheet of scar overlying fat; this can be skin grafted. Power dermatomes can also be used in tangential excision of burns, with gradual removal of the burn eschar until bleeding points appear. Tangential excision is superior to a massive removal of eschar and underlying normal tissue with a dermatome set at a wide thickness, a procedure that can lead to excessive blood loss.

Castroviejo Dermatome. This small electric dermatome can be used for harvesting mucous membrane grafts for reconstruction of eyelid and socket deformities (see Fig. 8–5). The motor moves a small cutting head with the blade that controls the thickness of the cut. Another small electric dermatome is produced by the Davol Company, incorporating a disposable head (Fig. 8–8). The rechargeable handle drops into a sterile plastic bag, which is sealed. The disposable cutting heads are preset at 0.015 inch and are clipped into place. They are used with mineral oil lubrication and can produce satisfactory small grafts. The cutting blades on the small power dermatomes tend to lose their sharpness rapidly.

Drum Dermatomes

Reese Dermatome. The Reese dermatome (Fig. 8–9), a carefully machined instrument, is a modification of the Padgett-Hood dermatome. An accompanying set of shims permits careful calibration of the thickness of the graft. There is a disadvantage in that, if the graft is too thick or thin, it is difficult to change the calibration in the middle of a skin graft removal.

The skin is prepared by applying a topical antiseptic to the donor site, followed by a defatting agent, such as ether or acetone. The donor site is painted with the dermatome cement, care being exercised that the glue on the brush is not allowed to dry in order to avoid lumping of the prepared skin surface. If less than a full drum or a pattern graft is required, the desired shape can be outlined

Text continued on page 235

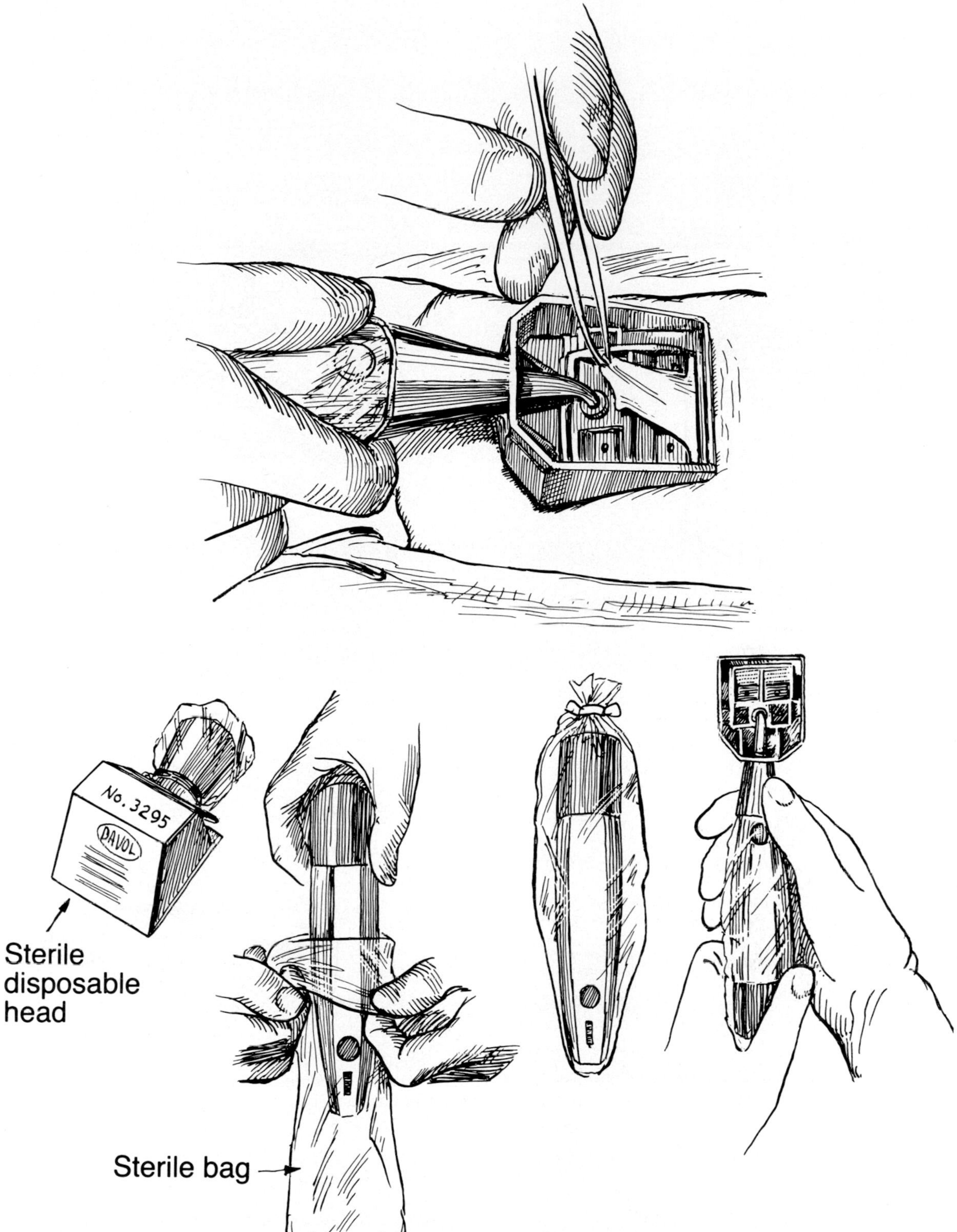

Figure 8–8. Disposable head dermatome (Davol). The instrument is powered by a rechargeable motor, which is placed in a sterile bag.

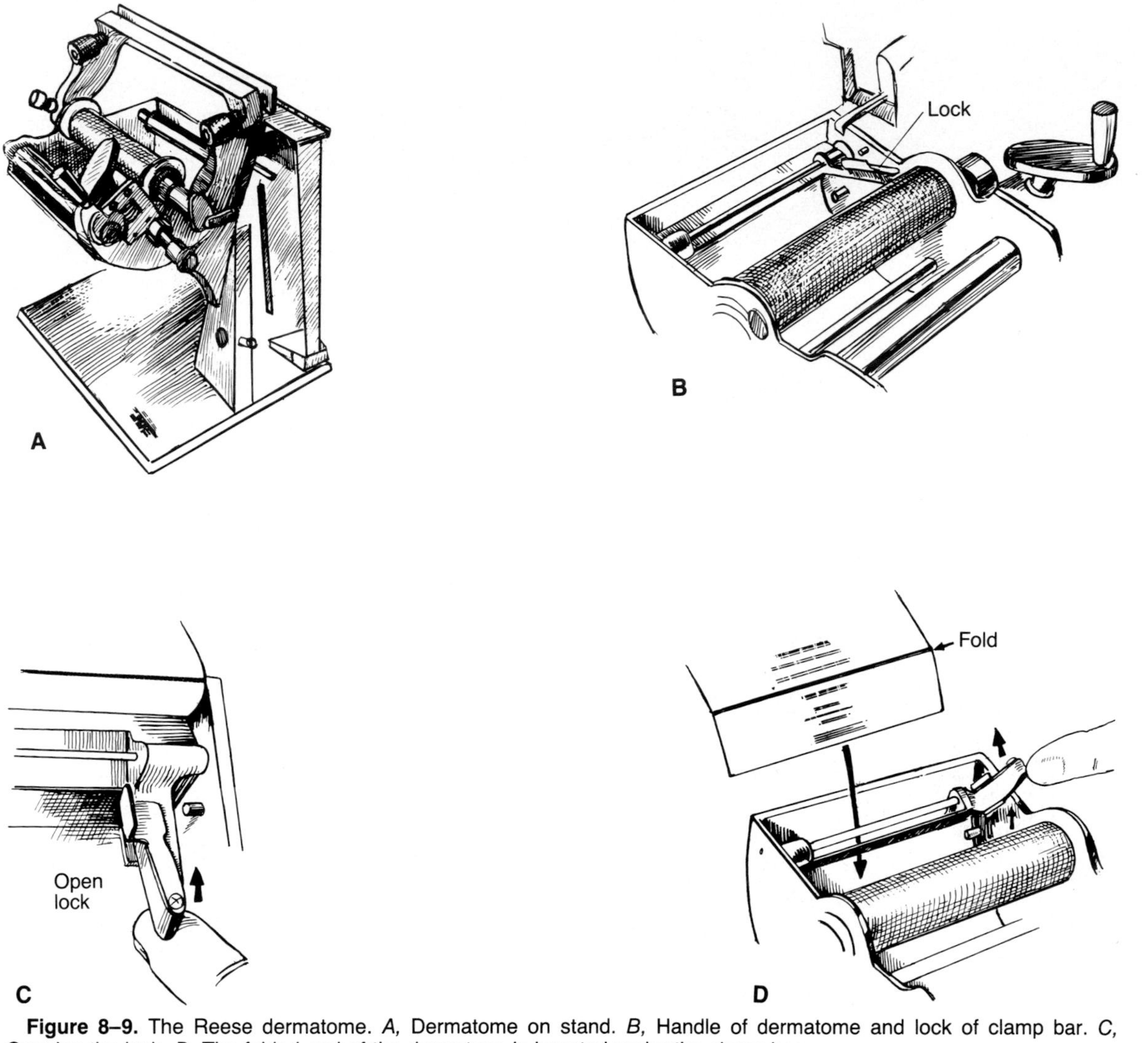

Figure 8–9. The Reese dermatome. *A,* Dermatome on stand. *B,* Handle of dermatome and lock of clamp bar. *C,* Opening the lock. *D,* The folded end of the dermatape is inserted under the clamp bar.

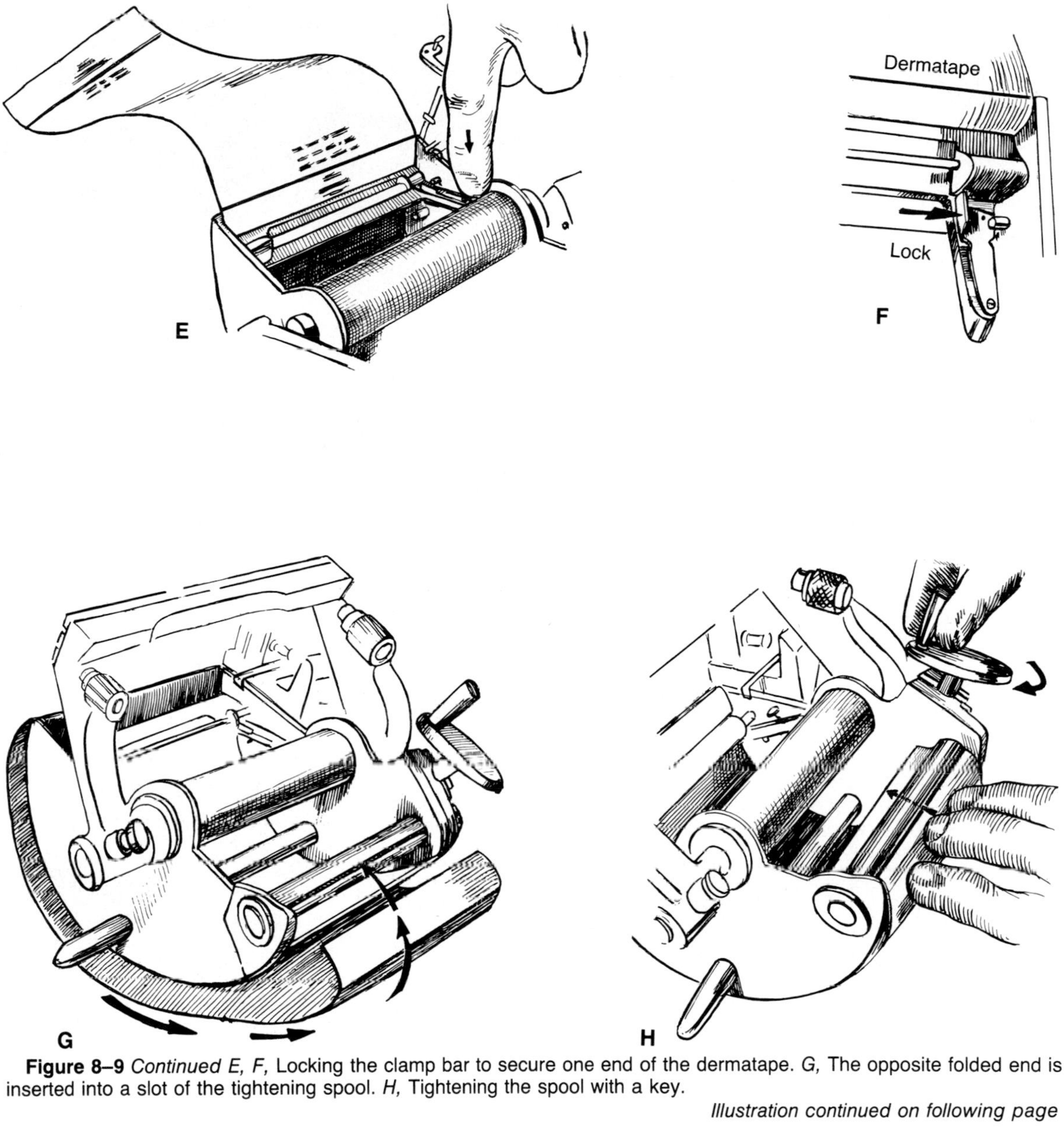

Figure 8–9 *Continued E, F,* Locking the clamp bar to secure one end of the dermatape. *G,* The opposite folded end is inserted into a slot of the tightening spool. *H,* Tightening the spool with a key.

Illustration continued on following page

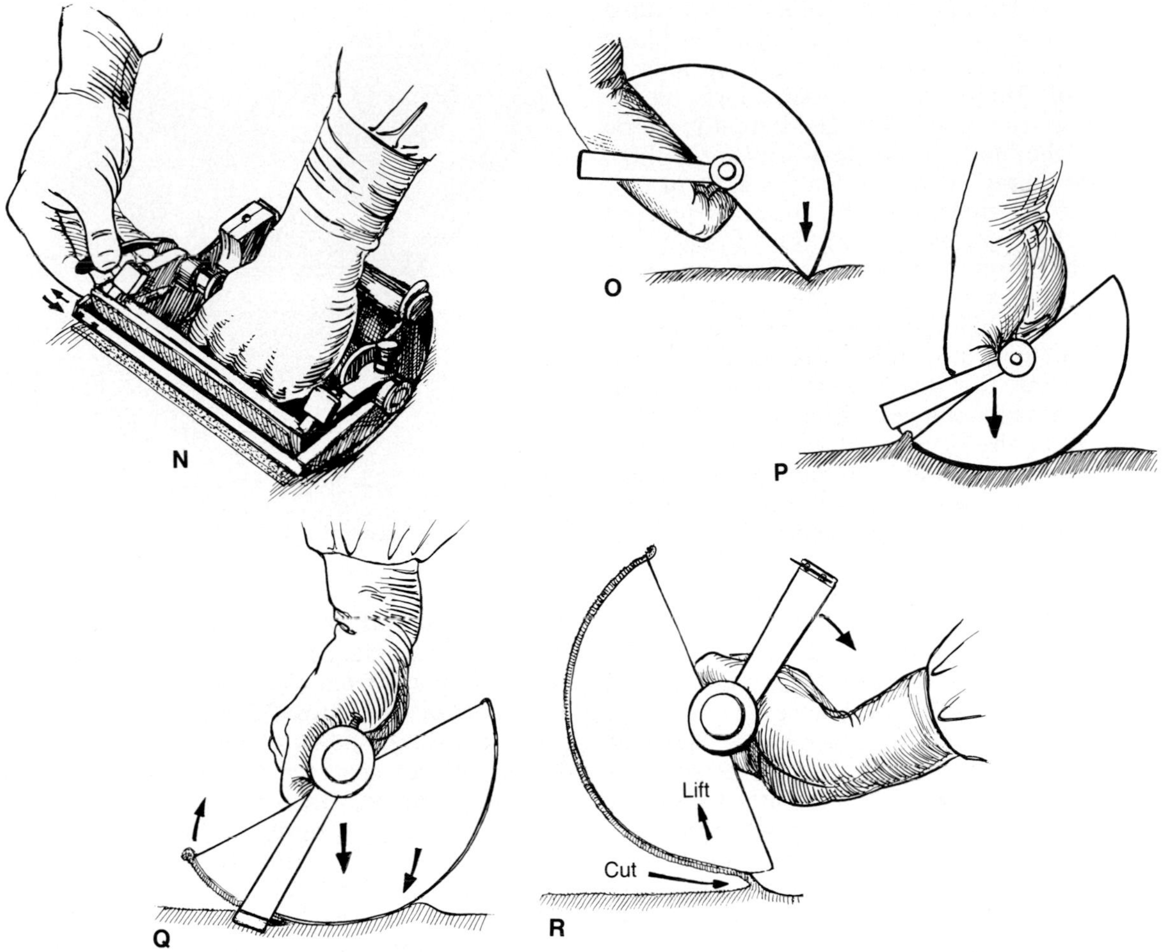

Figure 8–9 *Continued N,* Removal of the graft. *O,* Cross section view of initiating graft removal at the edge of the drum. *P,* Incorrect way of starting graft removal. *Q,* Proper way of advancing drum. Note direction of forces (*arrows*). *R,* The drum is lifted prior to cutting the graft through. (From Chase, R. A.: Atlas of Hand Surgery. Vol. I. Philadelphia, W. B. Saunders Company, 1973.)

with ink and the pattern painted with dermatome glue. Vaseline ointment can be applied around the pattern to avoid cutting into the surrounding tissue with the dermatome.

While the prepared donor site is drying (three minutes should elapse), the dermatome can be assembled. The dermatome sits in a stand that holds the full set of shims (Fig. 8–9*A*). The clamp bar that secures the laminated dermatape is opened. The dermatape is carefully folded at both ends along the black lines (Fig. 8–9*B, C, D*). One end of the dermatome is inserted beneath the clamp bar (Fig. 8–9*D*) so that the folded edge fits over the face margin of the drum. The clamp bar is returned to secure the dermatape and is locked in position (Fig. 8–9*E, F*). The opposite end of the dermatape is inserted into a slot in the tightening spool (Fig. 8–9*G*). The crank is then rotated to turn the spool and tighten the dermatape against the drum surface (Fig. 8–9*H*). The tape is incised along both free surfaces of the drum, and the outer cover is peeled back to expose the adhesive surface of the dermatape (Fig. 8–9*I*). A disposable blade and a shim of desired thickness are inserted into the blade clamp. Round nuts are tightened at either end to secure the blade clamp (Fig. 8–9*J, K*). While the instrument is being assembled, the skin is painted with glue in single strokes. Three minutes should elapse for drying of the adhesive (Fig. 8–9*L, M*).

To remove the skin, the instrument is first pressed against the donor site along its free edge (Fig. 8–9*N*) and then rotated slowly until the skin begins to fall away at the margins of the drum but still does not become detached (Fig. 8–9*O, P*). The cutting is started with almost no more forward force than is present in the weight of the blade assembly. The blade is moved from side to side while the drum is rotated slowly (dorsiflexion of the wrist) but held steady; at no time is the blade forced forward (Fig. 8–9*Q*). If there is any tendency for the skin to pull away at the margins, the drum is pressed more firmly against the skin and, in addition, is rotated slightly toward the cutting blade to roll the skin up in front of the cutting edge. If the blade tends to cut beyond the width of the drum, this is remedied by vertically lifting the drum away from the skin and/or having the assistant hold the skin away from the drum at each margin with a pair of hemostats. This complication can also be avoided by spreading mineral oil over the edges of the drum. The completion of the cutting can be effected by lifting the drum and graft away from the donor site and, with a few deft strokes of the blade, cutting the graft through (Fig. 8–9*R*); alternatively, the dermatome may be turned back and the graft severed from the bed with a knife.

The instrument is returned to the rack and the blade turned back to the protected position. The disposable blade should be immediately removed to avoid injury to the operating personnel. The graft is removed by gentle rubbing with a sponge gauze soaked in normal saline solution, leaving the glue on the dermatome.

When it becomes necessary to use a donor site such as the neck, chest, flank, or other areas of the body where there may be a depression or bony prominence, it is helpful to fill out such a depression or pad the prominence by injecting normal saline until it becomes level with the surrounding area. This technique permits the removal of grafts from any area of the body.

Padgett Dermatome. The Padgett dermatome, although lacking the precision of the Reese dermatome, is lighter and can be used more rapidly (Fig. 8–10). The distance between the blade and drum is calibrated in thousandths of an inch and is adjusted by turning a ratchet on one side of the blade arm. There is now available a plastic tape with glue on both surfaces. The outer protective cover is removed from the tape, and the latter is applied to the drum of the dermatome. The thickness of the cut must be increased approximately 0.004 inch to compensate for the thickness of the tape. The graft can be removed as outlined above for the Reese dermatome, and the skin graft can be easily removed from the tape.

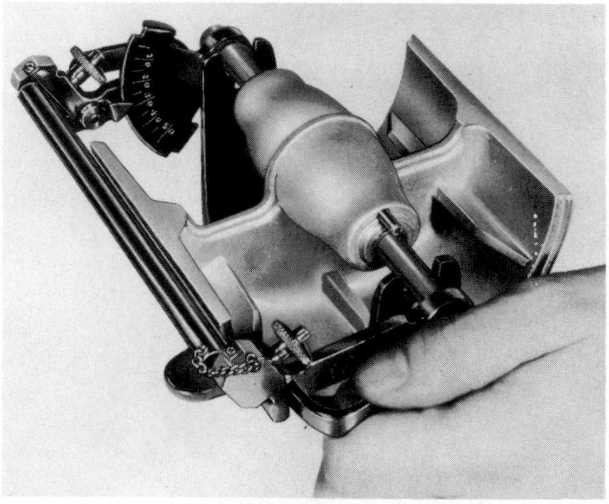

Figure 8–10. The Padgett-Hood dermatome. (Courtesy of Padgett Dermatome. Kansas City Assemblage Company, Kansas City, MO 64111.)

Selection of Drum Dermatomes. Practically speaking, the selection of which drum dermatome to use in a plastic surgical unit often depends on which one is available and sterile. However, a number of considerations aid in deciding which is preferable. The Reese dermatome provides only a 7 × 4 inch graft cutting size, whereas the Padgett dermatome is 8 inches long and comes in three widths: small—3 inches wide, medium—4 inches wide, and giant—5 inches wide. Both drum dermatomes allow harvesting of different thicknesses of split-thickness graft, but only the Padgett allows calibration while cutting is being accomplished. However, vigorous cutting with the Padgett dermatome can change the thickness of the graft unintentionally, a mishap that cannot occur with the Reese dermatome.

In terms of handling, the Padgett dermatome is lighter and is easy to handle, while the Reese is a heavier instrument. Each plastic surgeon must judge for himself which is more appropriate. While both types of drum dermatome require skin fixation, the Reese dermatome uses an adhesive tape that is applied to a drum and a glue that is applied to the skin surface. Most Padgett dermatomes depend on glue applied to both the drum and the skin surface, although adhesive tapes that fit the Padgett dermatome are also available. In either case, neutralization of glue by powder or petrolatum allows cutting of irregularly shaped grafts.

Freehand Cutting of Split-thickness Skin Grafts

Before the introduction of power-driven and drum dermatomes, all skin grafts were harvested with hand-held knives. These were long, sharp blades with an adapter over the blade that facilitated the cutting of the graft and controlled the graft thickness (Fig. 8–11). Such knives allowed cutting of very large pieces of skin. However, even in the best of hands the edges of the graft donor site were always irregular, a problem avoided with the power and drum dermatomes. With all such knife blades, the basic maneuver is a gradual back-and-forth movement, similar to that of cutting bread. Slicing is much more successful than pushing in cutting skin grafts. The large Humby-type knives are less used today, but smaller knives are often helpful in cutting small grafts (Goulian, 1968), particularly in an outpatient setting where a dermatome might not be easily available. The easy availability of the Goulian-type knife or razor blade should eliminate the use of pinch grafts. Such grafts were cut by piercing the skin with a needle, lifting it, and slicing it off. These grafts were thick in the center and thin on the edge, and left both unsightly donor and recipient areas. There is no modern use for pinch grafting.

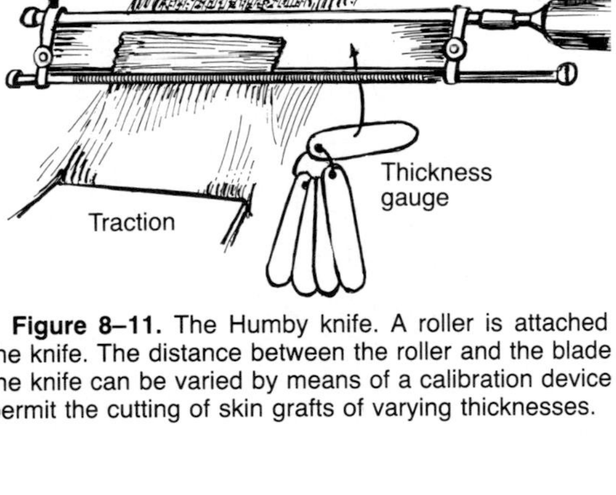

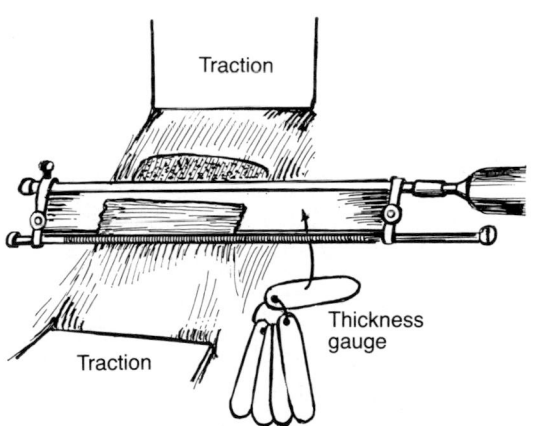

Figure 8–11. The Humby knife. A roller is attached to the knife. The distance between the roller and the blade of the knife can be varied by means of a calibration device to permit the cutting of skin grafts of varying thicknesses.

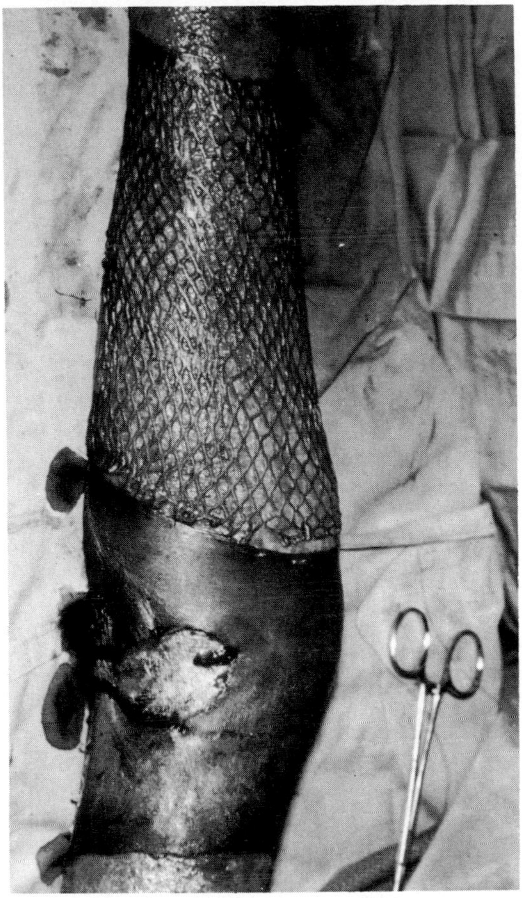

Figure 8–12. Mesh graft used to cover an extensive defect of the lower extremity.

Mesh Grafts

Mesh grafts are primarily useful in two situations: (1) when there is insufficient skin, as in a massive burn in which the skin graft must be expanded (Fig. 8–12); or (2) when a very convoluted surface must be covered with a graft where a sheet might not adhere well. Mesh grafts, particularly expanded ones, have significant disadvantages in healing. The expanded graft must heal in between the expansion by epithelization, and therefore the underlying wound may significantly contract. Mesh grafts are thus to be condemned in covering a joint or an area like the back of the hand, unless skin is in short supply in a life-threatening situation. Some surgeons advocate the use of mesh grafts to allow drainage, but generally a wound that is producing so much fluid that meshing is necessary is probably not yet ready for grafting, and meas-

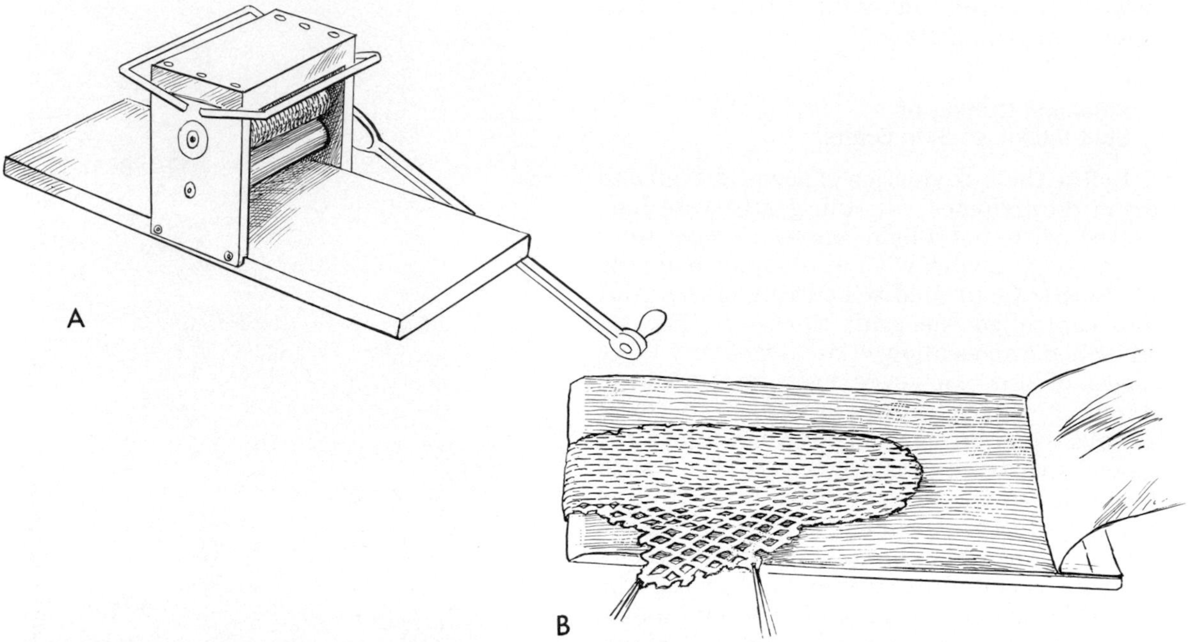

Figure 8–13. A, Zimmer skin graft mesher. B, At the completion of meshing. The graft sits on a disposable plastic sheet that had been advanced through the instrument. (From Chase, R. A.: Atlas of Hand Surgery, Philadelphia, W. B. Saunders Company, 1973.)

ures should be taken to control such drainage. Meshing does not prevent loss of a graft from hematoma, if bleeding is profuse at the time of skin grafting; delay of the grafting is more appropriate. If mesh grafting is used, a semiocclusive dressing is applied as there is less tendency for the graft edges to curl as they dry, and less desiccation of the underlying wound.

Meshing of split skin grafts is accomplished by placing the cut graft on a plastic carrier and carefully advancing it through a mechanical mesher by means of a crank (Fig. 8–13).

CUTTING: FULL-THICKNESS GRAFTS

Full-thickness grafts are cut free-hand with a scalpel; no dermatome is used. Such grafts must be relatively small and the donor site must be carefully selected. Usually a pattern of the defect to be grafted is made and transferred to the donor site where it is outlined (Figs. 8–14 and 8–15). If feasible, the pattern should be made after the excision, as the final defect is often larger than the pre-excision defect. It is important, particularly with an irregularly shaped pattern, to be sure that it is transferred with the desired side up and not in a reversed mirror image, as this can lead to a distorted graft.

The graft is harvested by cutting completely around the pattern and dissecting the skin at the level of the subcutaneous fat. This dissection can be facilitated by draping the graft over the surgeon's finger with a skin

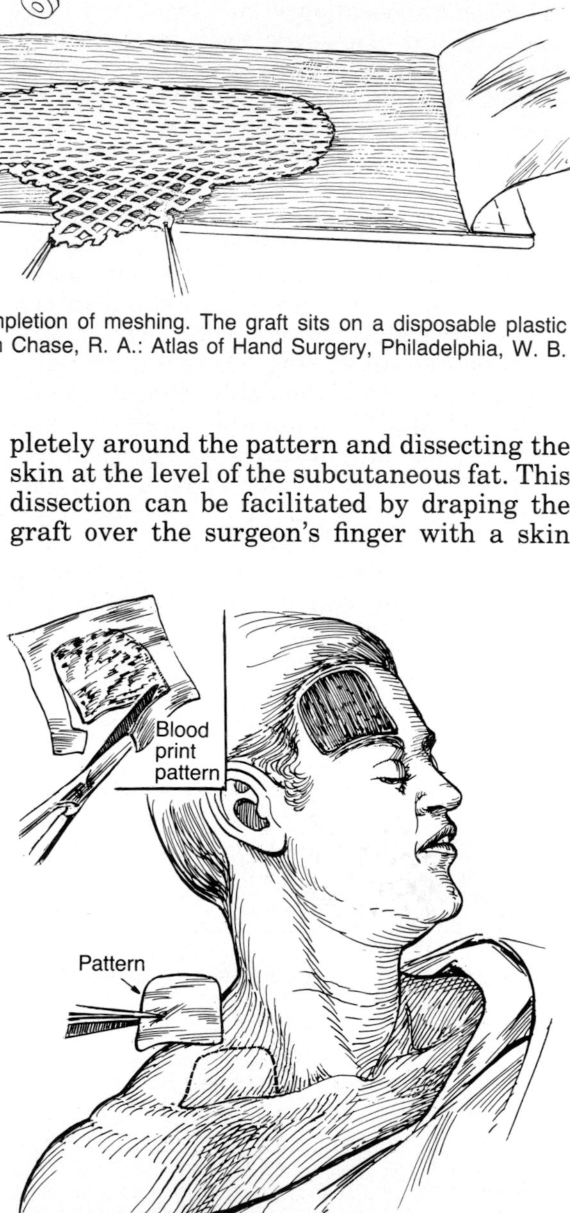

Figure 8–14. Removal of a full-thickness skin graft from the supraclavicular area. The graft was cut according to a pattern of the forehead defect.

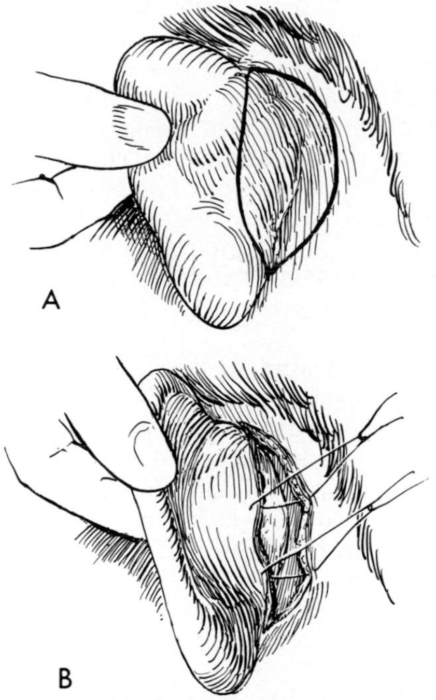

Figure 8–15. Retroauricular area as a donor site for a full-thickness skin graft. *A*, Proposed graft, including a portion of the retroauricular sulcus. *B*, The defect can usually be closed primarily.

hook, a maneuver that allows sensing of the thickness of the skin as the other hand cuts with the scalpel. Even after such harvesting, some fat usually remains on the undersurface of the graft. The fat can be removed by careful trimming with a sharp, curved scissors (Fig. 8–16). Constant wetting of the finger and graft with saline prevents the graft from curling on itself. The donor site is closed by undermining the skin edges and closing the wound primarily (see Fig. 8–15). On rare occasions a large full-thickness donor site may be closed by local flap rotation or resurfacing with a split-thickness skin graft.

Full-thickness mucosal grafts to reconstruct nasal and conjunctival defects can be harvested from the inner aspect of the cheek (Fig. 8–17). Care must be taken to avoid injury to the parotid duct. Nasal mucous membrane can be harvested from one side of the septum following submucosal injection of a vasoconstricting anesthetic solution; the exposed surface closes by epithelial migration. To support a lower eyelid, a composite graft of nasal mucous membrane with accompanying septal cartilage may be removed (see Chap. 34). This leaves the remaining perichondrial surface of the nasal septum intact to avoid perforation. A final type of mucous

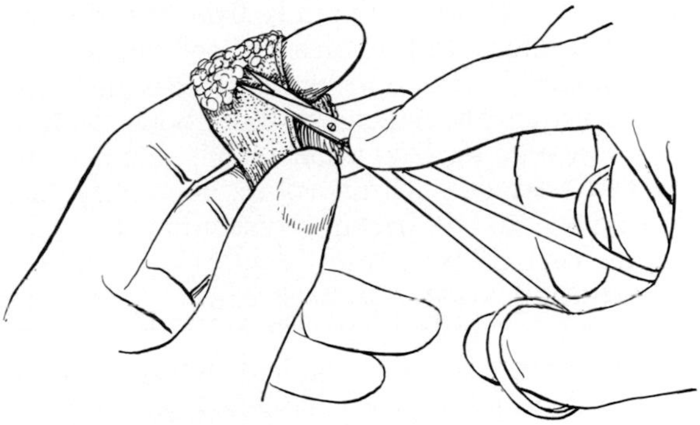

Figure 8–16. Defatting the undersurface of a full-thickness skin graft with a pair of scissors.

membrane grafting is that of conjunctival tissues to replace other conjunctiva. This graft can be taken more easily if the donor tissue is distended by submucosal injection of an anesthetic solution. Only the fornix should be used as a donor site, and only narrow ellipses of conjunctiva can be obtained because of the risk of eyelid contraction.

PREPARATION OF WOUND

Although considerable technical expertise is required to harvest the skin graft, no graft will succeed if the wound bed in which it is placed is inadequate. *Most skin graft failures can be ascribed to flaws in the recipient site, rather than to technical defects in the skin graft cutting.*

All skin grafts are parasites in that they

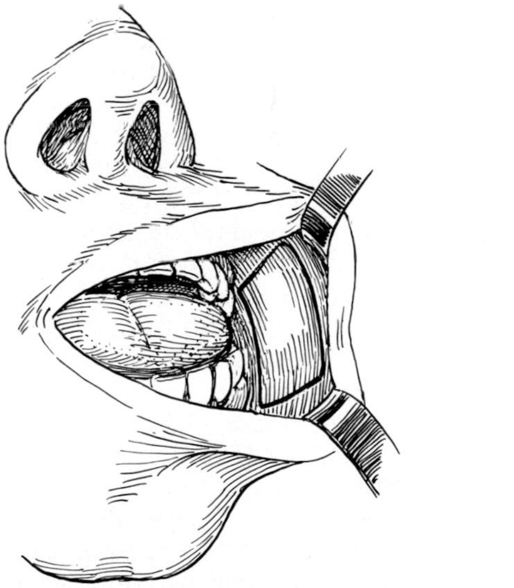

Figure 8–17. Full-thickness mucosal grafts can be procured from the inner aspect of the cheek.

must depend on blood supply from the wound bed. Therefore, tissue with limited blood supply—bone, cartilage or tendon—does not accept a skin graft. A surgeon faced with closing an avascular surface must either use a nonparasitic tissue such as a flap, or modify the wound so that it becomes vascular. For example, cortical bone may be debrided to allow granulation tissue to proliferate. Membranous bone that is relatively vascular, as in the denuded orbit of a radical maxillectomy, may accept a skin graft. Exposed cartilage is usually removed to allow skin grafting, although occasionally multiple perforations allow granulation tissue to form. Even chronic granulation tissue may not be sufficiently vascular to support skin grafts and should be resected down to better vascularized tissue.

The nature of the injury influences the ability of the wound to support a graft. A clean tissue avulsion may accept immediate skin grafting, whereas crushed or infected tissue is less likely to do so. Chronic wounds must be free of pus and should have a healthy, pink to beefy red appearance with an ideal wound pH of 7.4 or higher (Ye, 1957). Epithelial migration at the edges of the granulating surface may be a sign that the wound is ready for application of a skin graft. Hypertrophic "proud flesh" accepts a skin graft poorly and needs to be either trimmed or flattened with hypertonic (3 per cent) saline pressure dressings.

All granulation tissues contain bacteria, but not all are infected. The presence of more than 10^5 organisms per gram of tissue, as shown by quantitative bacteriology, almost always leads to loss of the graft (Robson and Krizek, 1973). Such quantitative bacteriology may help surgeons to decide whether or not a wound will accept a skin graft. A high bacterial count should be reduced judiciously with antibiotic and local wound therapy. Particular attention should be paid to eliminating *Streptococcus*. However, even a clean, healthy, granulating wound contains some bacteria, a situation that usually leads to use of a split-thickness rather than a full-thickness skin graft.

Wherever possible, underlying systemic conditions causing the wound should be corrected before skin grafting is attempted. For example, a venous stasis ulcer should be treated with appropriate attention to the venous pathology, such as vein stripping if indicated. A patient with a leg ulcer secondary to arterial occlusion should have arterial reconstruction done prior to skin grafting. Wounds that are exceptionally difficult to cover with a skin graft are those secondary to cancerocidal radiotherapy, and those resulting from vasculitis associated with autoimmune diseases such as rheumatoid arthritis. Radiation ulcers are best treated by excision and flap coverage, while the best therapy for ulcers from autoimmune diseases is to have the rheumatologist treat the basic disease more aggressively (Rudolph and Noe, 1983).

A chronic wound to be skin grafted must be free of necrotic tissue. This can be achieved by the use of sharp debridement followed by local treatment with wet soaks of half-strength Dakin's solution (0.25 per cent sodium hypochlorite). Other techniques, such as enzyme ointment or wet-to-dry dressings, are less effective.

Operating room treatment of the graft bed at the time of skin grafting is important in both acute and chronic wounds. Scrubbing the graft bed with detergents can increase the rate of infection (Edlich and associates, 1973). The wound should be cleaned with a more benign substance such as saline or Betadine solution. Surgical debridement may cause profuse bleeding, and hemostasis is essential for a graft to survive. Hemostasis can be achieved by electrocautery, ligation of vessels, or application of pressure. The use of hemostatic substances such as Oxycel or Gelfoam is hazardous when skin grafting is to be done, as they provide a nonvascular block between the recipient bed and graft. If electrocautery, ligation, and pressure have been tried for more than a reasonable time and bleeding is still profuse, it may be best to defer skin grafting until another day and apply dressings to the wound (Lehman and Saddawi, 1975). Placing a graft on a rapidly bleeding surface results in hematoma formation and graft loss.

GRAFT IMMOBOLIZATION AND POSTOPERATIVE CARE

For a skin graft to survive on its wound bed, it must adhere well enough to allow blood vessels to grow across the gap. In most cases of skin grafting, the optimal dressing is a *bolus* or *tie-over* dressing (Fig. 8–18). This is fashioned by placing sutures around the periphery to hold the graft onto the wound bed.

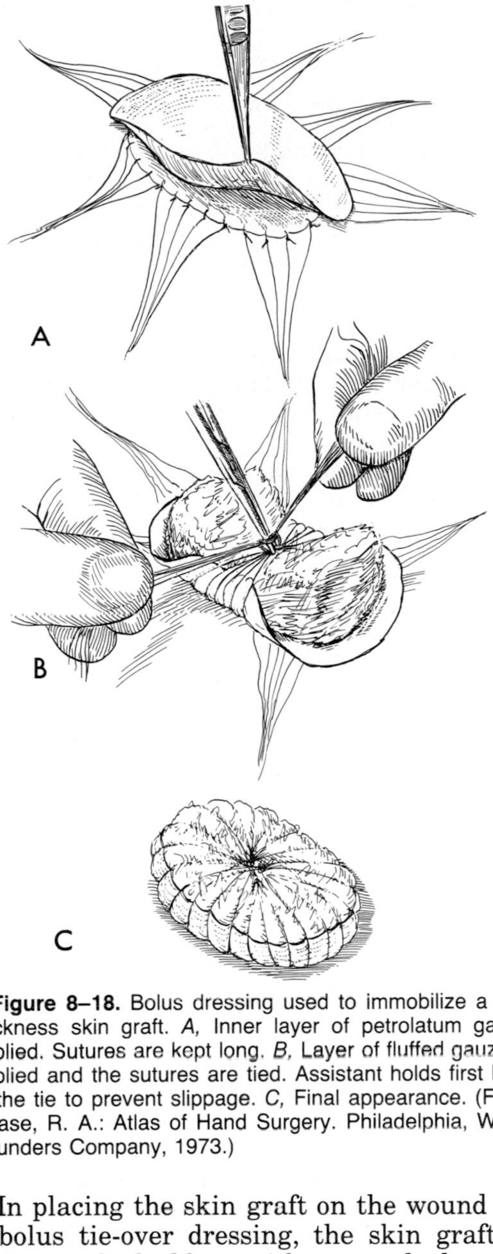

Figure 8–18. Bolus dressing used to immobilize a full-thickness skin graft. *A,* Inner layer of petrolatum gauze applied. Sutures are kept long. *B,* Layer of fluffed gauze is applied and the sutures are tied. Assistant holds first loop of the tie to prevent slippage. *C,* Final appearance. (From Chase, R. A.: Atlas of Hand Surgery. Philadelphia, W. B. Saunders Company, 1973.)

In placing the skin graft on the wound for a bolus tie-over dressing, the skin graft is laid over the bed but neither stretched excessively nor wrinkled. The graft is sutured using 4-0 or 5-0 silk, with sutures as close together as necessary, depending on the location. Facial sutures may be as close as 2 to 3 mm, whereas in other areas they may be as far apart as 1.5 to 2.5 cm. The sutures are tied over a piece of fine mesh, ointment impregnated gauze, covered with cotton sheeting or cotton balls (see Fig. 8–18). Care should be taken in placing the wadding material so that it is pressed down into any recesses to allow the graft to sit evenly on the wound. The tied sutures gently press the dressing down onto the skin graft, which in turn is pressed onto the wound bed. This maneuver immobilizes the graft on the wound and prevents hematoma collection. An outer dressing may be applied if desired.

Before the tie-over dressing is applied, the surgeon should ensure that there are no blood clots underneath the graft. These can be expressed by pressure, irrigated out with saline, or cleansed with small cotton-tipped applicators. This step before application of the dressing provides better adherence of the graft and improved survival rates.

The dressing is left in place for approximately seven days, at which time the sutures can be removed. *The temptation should be resisted to remove the dressing at two to three days to check the status of the graft.* The first dressing is the best and grafts do best if left intact. After removal of the dressing at seven days, small collections of seroma may be evacuated by cutting over the top of the graft.

The main object of the tie-over dressing is to ensure contact between the graft and the host bed. Such contact can also be achieved by using a *circumferential compression dressing* with an extremity skin graft. Polk (1966) has shown that the rate of graft adherence is greatest in the first eight hours, with a slower increase of adherence through the fourth day. The compression dressing ensures uniform pressure over the entire grafted area and the portion of the extremity distal to the grafted area. The extremity should be elevated to avoid edema in the limb. Plaster can also be incorporated into the dressing if necessary.

A variation of the bolus method of dressing is the skin graft inlay method (Fig. 8–19). The bolus dressing is often referred to as the Stent dressing, which has been derived from the skin graft inlay method. "Stent" is a trade name for a British dental compound used as the central material in a graft placed in the oral sulcus. A skin graft is wrapped around dental compound, the dermal side out. This combination of graft and dental compound can then be placed into the labial sulcus defect, where the graft will heal. Such grafts should also be splinted for six months to resist contraction. The skin graft outlay technique is similar but involves tying of sutures over the top of the combination of dental compound and skin graft (Fig. 8–20). This method allows placement of a large area of graft relative to the defect.

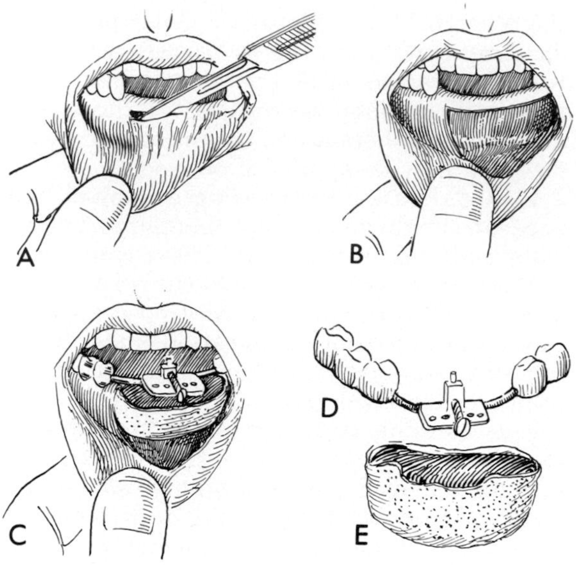

Figure 8–19. Skin graft inlay technique. *A*, The obliterated sulcus is incised. *B*, Resulting defect. *C*, Dental compound impression of the defect is covered with the skin graft and secured to a metal plate fitted to a dental splint. *D*, Metal plate attached to dental splint. *E*, Dental compound covered with skin graft (dermal side exposed).

Open Technique. On occasion, large skin grafts can be applied to the recipient site without an external dressing. This technique requires an ideal wound bed, without bleeding or fluid production, and a cooperative or sedated patient. The skin grafts can be sutured rapidly, using a running chromic catgut suture. In the immediate postoperative period, small collections of seroma or hematoma can be evacuated by incising over them and expressing the fluid. Limited motion may be allowed the patient. Bed cradles are used and the patient must be positioned so that the grafts are not disturbed. The graft usually is pink, adherent, and viable within 48 hours. Crusts appearing around the margin can be removed with forceps but may also be left in place to allow natural separation. In grafting by the open method, postoperative care is relatively simple as there are no dressings to change.

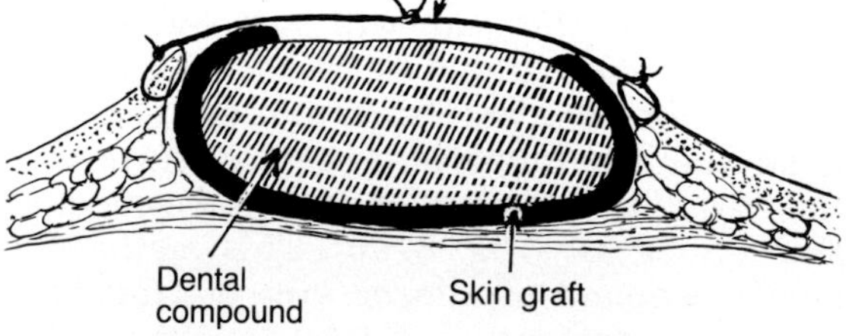

Figure 8–20. Skin graft outlay technique (cross section).

INITIAL HEALING

Skin Graft "Take." When a skin graft is cut, it turns pale as it is separated from its blood supply. Vessels within the graft constrict and squeeze out red blood cells. When the graft is placed on a wound, it slowly regains its former pink color as circulation returns. The graft survival on its new blood supply is a clinical "take." Pressure on the graft after three or four days should lead to blanching and immediate refilling of the blood vessels.

If the graft does not become revascularized, partial or complete necrosis develops. If the graft is thick, the upper portion of the graft may slough and yet deeper portions may remain, so watchful waiting is indicated.

The vascularization of skin grafts is discussed in detail later in this chapter under Biologic Behavior.

Causes of Failure. Ideally all skin grafts should "take." While some surgeons graft skin in the expectation that only a certain percentage of their grafts will survive, better success is achieved with the attitude that *all* should survive. If conditions are so unfavorable that skin graft success is exceedingly unlikely, it probably should not be done. The causes of graft failure are shown in Table 8–1.

Cellular Hyperplasia. Within the first two weeks after graft healing a pronounced *epidermal* hyperplasia occurs, manifested by surface scaling and crusting. Within the first week the thickness of the epidermis can increase seven- to eightfold. The hypertrophic epidermis has invasive characteristics at the edge of the graft; it can invade the surrounding dermis or granulation tissue, lifting a picture-frame rim of tissue around the healing graft (Gillman and associates, 1953). The tendency for graft epithelium to spread may

Table 8–1. Causes of Graft Failure

1. Inadequate graft bed (poor vascularity)
2. Hematoma
3. Movement
4. Infection
5. Technical errors such as placement over epithelizing wound, grafts cut too thick or too thin, or upside-down graft
6. Poor storage of grafts

be seen on the undersurface of a graft chronically elevated by serum (Littlewood, 1960). Since hair follicles and sebaceous sweat glands are exposed on the undersurface of a split-thickness graft, a chronic seroma may lead to epithelial growth underneath the graft and cause that portion of the graft to slough.

Dermal fibroblasts proliferate vigorously in healing skin grafts after an initial decrease of three days. By the seventh to eighth day there is a marked hyperplasia of fibroblasts as the graft begins to heal (Converse and Ballantyne, 1962). These fibroblasts are probably derived from local tissue and new blood vessels synthesize collagen within the skin graft to play a significant role in its eventual healing.

MATURATION

After the grafts have become vascularized and have "taken," they undergo changes that continue for many months, a remodeling process that has significant effects on the ultimate result of the skin graft.

Graft Contraction. Contractile fibroblasts, known as *myofibroblasts,* (see Chap. 5) contract open wounds (Guber and Rudolph, 1978). Skin grafting can affect this process, depending on the type of graft. Surgeons often speak of "skin graft contraction," but in fact what is seen is a combination of graft and wound contraction. Most likely it is the wound bed that contracts and the graft follows. Split-thickness skin grafts contract more where the wound is pliable and mobile (as on the axilla), and less where it is unyielding (as on the skull periosteum). On a similar wound, full-thickness grafts contract minimally, while split-thickness grafts contract significantly. Exceptionally thin split-thickness grafts (for example, the original Thiersch grafts composed largely of epidermis) contract as much as ungrafted wounds.

The contraction of a healing graft and wound is referred to as *secondary contraction.* In contrast, *primary contraction* refers to the immediate elastic recoil of a graft as it is cut. Primary contraction is greatest in full-thickness grafts and least in thin split-thickness grafts (Ragnell, 1953). *Secondary contraction* is clinically more important.

The *dermal* component of grafted skin appears to exert the main influence on wound (secondary) contraction (Rudolph, 1976). It has been said that the thicker the skin graft, the less does wound contraction occur, a statement that is not fully accurate. Very thick skin grafts obviously may slough and result in wound contraction. Many studies, in both humans and animals, indicate that it is not the absolute thickness of the graft that is important, but the *relative thickness of the entire skin* that is included. *The important factor is how much of the deep dermis is present.* Thus, Padgett (1939) used human split-thickness skin grafts that included three-fourths of the thickness of the full skin. Recipient wounds contracted little, almost as though they had been covered with full-thickness grafts.

In a highly significant study, Corps (1969) found that the relative proportion of the skin grafted is important in determining the amount of wound contracture. Taking 0.2 mm grafts from different areas in rats, Corps found that full-thickness ear grafts did not contract, whereas split-thickness grafts from the thick dorsal trunk skin contracted 75 per cent and split grafts from the thinner abdominal skin 60 per cent. Skin split-thickness grafts of identical thickness, when cut from thicker skin, contracted more than those cut from thinner areas. In studies by Klein and Rudolph (1972), rat abdominal full-thickness grafts of 0.010 inch contracted less than did thicker split-thickness grafts of 0.015 inch taken from the dorsal skin. Thus, the *relative thickness* of the skin graft was the most important factor in determining wound contraction.

Electron microscopic studies have shown that full-thickness skin grafts, which inhibit wound contraction most successfully, suppress the life cycle of the myofibroblast (Rudolph and associates, 1979). While identical numbers of myofibroblasts developed in rat granulating wounds, in wounds covered with split-thickness grafts, and in wounds covered with full-thickness grafts, the most rapid disappearance of the contractile myofibroblasts was in wounds covered with full-thickness grafts. Granulating wounds had the longest persistence of myofibroblasts, while split-thickness grafts with intermediate contraction had an intermediate time of myofibroblast survival.

In summary, the inhibitory effect of the full-thickness skin graft upon a contracting wound seems to be due to the inclusion of the full thickness of the deep dermis, and appears to work via suppression of the myofibroblast population.

Clinical prevention of graft contraction therefore means using full-thickness grafts whenever possible. If split-thickness grafts are essential to reduce wound contraction, they must be applied immediately to fresh wounds, as experimental studies have shown that split-thickness grafts applied to actively granulating wounds show little inhibition of contraction (Stone and Madden, 1974). The contraction of a wound covered by a split-thickness graft can be inhibited by splinting, which needs to be continued for four to six months to overcome the acute effect of the myofibroblasts.

Dermal Collagen Turnover. Since collagen is the main structural framework of the skin graft dermis, knowledge of its dynamics is important to an understanding of graft healing. Autoradiography using mature collagen labeled with radioactive hydrogen (in tritiated hydroxyproline) has been employed to study graft collagen turnover in rats (Zika, Rudolph, and Klein, 1973). These studies indicated uniform turnover of collagen in thin full-thickness skin grafts. However, in split-thickness grafts there was a greater collagen turnover underneath the epidermis, a finding suggesting that the epidermis might generate collagenase.

Quantitative isotopic studies by Klein and Rudolph (1972, 1974) have shown a massive turnover of collagen in skin grafts. In all types of skin grafts, 85 to 88 per cent of the original collagen was lost by 140 days. Full-thickness grafts had significant new collagen synthesis, more collagen being synthesized than was lost as the grafts grew with the animals. Split-thickness grafts, in contrast, lost surface area and never regained the total amount of collagen lost. Skin grafts from older animals had a slower collagen turnover, a trend not reversed by grafting old skin onto young syngeneic animals.

Other elements of connective tissue undergo turnover in the healing skin graft. Elastin filaments in the dermis begin to fragment by the seventh day and degenerate through 21 days; they begin to return after four to six weeks (Hinshaw and Miller, 1965). There is also an initial rise in mucopolysaccharide levels within the first three to four days, decreasing by the tenth postoperative day (Hilgert, 1963), data similar to the mucopolysaccharide changes observed in incised wounds.

Dermal/Epidermal Specificity. Human skin grafts transferred to new locations maintain their epidermal specificity. Thus, a split-thickness skin graft in the mouth continues to have squamous epithelium rather than mucous membrane. Studies in humans and animals have shown that epidermal specificity is in large part determined by the underlying dermis. Van Scott and Reinertson (1961) found that grafts with epidermis and dermis retain their own epithelial traits, whereas epidermis isolated from skin, mucous membrane, or basal cell epitheloma atrophies without its support dermis. Extensive animal studies by Billingham and Silvers (1963, 1967) suggested that the epidermis can be changed into another type if the underlying dermis is changed by means of recombination experiments.

Pigment Changes. A major problem with skin grafts is pigment mismatch. Full-thickness grafts maintain the best pigment match, and are thus preferred in areas such as the face. Facial full-thickness grafts from the postauricular or supraclavicular areas, however, may retain a permanent ruddy tone.

Split-thickness grafts often develop significantly dark pigmentation, particularly in darker-skinned patients. Skin grafts from the buttocks and abdomen applied to the face may produce a major pigment mismatch as the grafts develop a brownish-yellow hue. The best way to prevent hyperpigmentation is to use a well-matched, full-thickness graft (Rudolph, 1984). Although there is some debate in the literature, most plastic surgeons feel that sunshine should be avoided for the first six months by use of sun-blocking agents or clothing to prevent a long-lasting hyperpigmentation developing in a new skin graft. Serial dermabrasions (Mir y Mir, 1961) or chemical peel may reduce graft hyperpigmentation if it otherwise appears permanent.

Epithelial Appendages. *Hair* follicles undergo hyperplasia of the epithelium in the healing graft, a phenomenon observed in the other epithelial structures. If a full-thickness graft is transplanted with intact hair follicles, the skin often regrows hair in the same pattern as before. This is the basis for small plugs of hair-bearing skin being transplanted to the scalp to correct male pattern baldness (see Chap. 31) (Orentreich, 1959). Larger strips of skin can be used to replace missing eyebrows.

In a poorly healing graft, hair growth may be nonexistent, sporadic, or depigmented.

Split-thickness grafts rarely grow hair unless they are cut quite thick. Donor sites must be selected in children to avoid later unwanted hair growth, for example, in full-thickness groin donor sites.

Sweat glands ultimately resume function, with more complete function in full-thickness than in split-thickness grafts. Following nerve regeneration, sweating in the graft is dependent on the site to which it is transplanted rather than the site from which it came (Pontén, 1960).

Sebaceous glands are more preserved in full-thickness than in split-thickness grafts. Full-thickness grafts therefore tend to have a softer and more pliable appearance in their healed state. Because split-thickness grafts are cut horizontally through the dermis, there may be growth of sebaceous glands under the grafts, leading to multiple small milia that can be unroofed with a needletip. Both split-thickness grafts and their donor sites may scale and remain itchy and dry for many months because the lubricating sebaceous glands have been temporarily devitalized. Lubrication with bland ointment such as lanolin or cocoa butter helps to replace the lubricating function. Thicker split-thickness grafts and donor sites from thin grafts usually regain normal sebaceous gland function. Such function is independent of nerve return.

Durability and Growth. Graft durability is related to its thickness. Thick grafts have greater resistance to trauma, and thus full-thickness grafts are preferable in areas such as the fingertips. However, split-thickness grafts can provide excellent durability as long as they have a moderate thickness of dermis. Split-thickness grafting on the sole of the foot may be preferable to use of a flap with a fat layer that produces an unstable walking surface.

Full-thickness grafts grow successfully in children, whereas the growth of split-thickness grafts may be limited. Therefore, in a child's web-space hand contracture, a full-thickness rather than a split-thickness skin graft is preferable, to allow for later growth. If multiple split-thickness grafts are required, as for a major burn, serial split-thickness grafting may be needed as the child grows. Experimental studies in pigs (Baran and Horton, 1972) and rats (Klein and Rudolph, 1972) showed that full-thickness grafts enlarged as the animals grew, ultimately outgrowing their original area. In contrast, experimental split-thickness grafts in these animals did not grow beyond their original areas even if followed as long as five months.

Innervation of Skin Grafts. Once a skin graft is placed on a wound bed, sensation is regained as nerves regrow into the graft. In some areas, such as the fingertips, graft sensation return is particularly important. Full-thickness grafts appear to achieve better sensation than split-thickness grafts, although the rate of return of innervation is faster in split-thickness grafts.

Pontén (1960) found that touch and two-point discrimination were accurate indicators of reinnervation in humans. He reported that the sensory pattern of skin grafts becomes that of the recipient wound bed rather than that of the original graft donor site. Fitzgerald and associates (1967) reported that sensation in skin grafts returns from the margins toward the center. Using microscopy in pig skin grafts, they noted that nerves enter both the sides and the base of the grafts, and appear to follow empty neurolemma sheaths. There remains some debate whether ingrowing nerves totally follow the pattern of the old graft nerves or whether they make new paths. Probably some combination of the two mechanisms occurs. Studies by Adeymo and Wyburn (1957) showed that nerve fibers that do not link up with Schwann tube cells are able to penetrate only a short distance into the graft.

Terzis (1976) used electrophysiologic techniques in rabbit full-thickness skin grafts. She found that sensory mapping could be done, and that areas of high and low reinnervation return could be accurately outlined. After skin grafting, most of the incoming fibers conduct impulses at slow velocities, corresponding to the unmyelinated group of sensory fibers. With aging of the skin grafts, there is increasing myelinization as shown by faster conduction. This balance between myelinated and unmyelinated fibers may still be disrupted by 15 months. This electrophysiologic study correlates with the altered ratio of myelinated to unmyelinated fibers reported on electron microscopy of skin grafts. In most skin grafts there is usually some degree of permanent derangement of nerve regrowth, and this parallels the clinical observation.

Most patients with skin grafts do not obtain completely normal sensation, although they may have protective sensation. The recovery of sensation in humans can begin as early as one to two months after surgery, and may be abnormal during the first year or two. Pain may be more intense than in the surrounding skin, and touch, heat, and cold may be perceived as painful. Pain sensation develops most rapidly; those of touch, heat, and cold return later. The recipient site is important in determining the quality of sensation in skin grafts. Grafts placed on periosteum and muscle usually do not acquire satisfactory sensation.

DONOR SITE HEALING

Full-Thickness Grafts. These leave behind an open wound with no epithelial remnants. Most full-thickness grafts are cut so as to allow direct primary closure of the donor site after undermining (see Fig. 8–15). Rarely, split-thickness grafting of the full-thickness donor site can be done. The healing full-thickness donor wound is generally under sufficient tension for hematoma not to be a major problem, although a small drain can be placed for one to two days.

Split-Thickness Grafts. When a split-thickness skin graft is cut there is an immediate blood loss, measured by Robinson (1949) as 46 cc from a 4 × 8 inch area. After graft cutting, there is an initial blood loss at the donor site, followed by an inflammatory reaction with edema and exudation of protein. A scab of blood and fibrin soon forms over the surface of the wound. Within the first 24 hours, epithelium begins to grow from the epithelial remnants in the dermis such as hair follicles, sebaceous glands, and sweat glands. Epithelial migration also occurs at the wound margins. The more superficial a split-thickness graft is cut, the faster the donor site will heal (Converse and Robb-Smith, 1944). This may be as soon as seven days in a thin split-thickness graft. Donor sites from which thicker split grafts are cut may not heal for several weeks.

The process of epithelization may be visible on a healing donor site. With initial epithelium coverage the donor site may show small dark spots on the surface. Each of these represents an epithelial structure such as a hair follicle, sebaceous gland, or sweat gland producing epithelium. Since these are more mature structures, they have pigment that gradually spreads over the surface of the donor site.

An important consideration is that the new epithelium on a split-thickness donor site is not durably attached to the underlying dermis in the early stages. Tape removal can tear this fragile epithelium and must be guarded against. Epithelial healing is fastest in areas with multiple accessory skin structures such as the face, and less so in areas with scanty epithelial residual glands and hair follicles.

When a split-thickness graft is cut, the blood should first be absorbed with pads or sponges. A dressing is then applied of a single layer of nonadherent Xeroform gauze, followed by a layer of Telfa and bulky gauze on top of this. The next day the outer gauze and Telfa can be removed, leaving behind the Xeroform gauze, which can be allowed to air dry. A gentle heat lamp application speeds epithelization. In an area where external contamination is likely, a large pad can be placed and left in place for the expected time of healing. However, contamination must be guarded against and, if there is a suggestion of excess fluid output or infection, the outer dressing must be removed. Should infection occur, it is treated as it would be in other areas with topical dressings and soaks.

Split-thickness donor sites are painful and analgesia is often required. Some decrease in pain can be found with the application of artificial semipermeable membranes such as Biobrane or Opsite. The latter allows fluid pooling underneath, which is claimed to produce less pain for the patient. However, there is a risk of infection and this may have to be guarded against by making incisions in the dressing or by using suction catheters. These dressings are probably best used in the patient who has a low pain threshold, in whom comfort is a major factor, and who can be watched closely for the development of infection beneath the membrane. While some have claimed improved reduction of pain under allograft or xenograft, others have pointed out that immunologic sensitization and consequent inflammation may occur (Graham, 1969; Miller, 1974).

A risk in any split-thickness donor site, particularly a deep one, is the development of hypertrophic scar (see Chap. 21). This can be treated with injections of locally long-acting corticosteroids, such as Kenalog, and by careful attention to avoiding infection that might further damage the remaining deep dermis. Patients prone to keloid formation may have steroids injected judiciously under the donor site at the time of graft harvesting.

Multiple or serial thin split-thickness

grafts can be harvested from a donor area of thick dermis. Although the epithelium regenerates each time, the dermis does not and there is progressive thinning. Histologic studies have shown a significant amount of disorganized scar formation in the dermis after split-thickness skin harvesting. Fortunately the clinical appearance of a split-thickness donor site is usually superior to the histologic picture. However, patients must be warned that split-thickness graft harvesting, particularly of deeper grafts, may leave behind scars that are permanently visible. Split-thickness grafts taken from areas where previous harvesting has been done are possibly less likely to develop hyperpigmentation in the recipient area (Lopez-Mas and associates, 1972).

STORAGE

In storing any viable tissue, one must deal with the basic problem of controlling the destructive effects of hypoxic metabolism. A tissue removed from its blood supply dies unless the metabolic activity of the cell is decreased, or nutrients are provided to it (Rudolph, Fisher, and Ninnemann, 1979).

Autograft Banking. The simplest type of banking is that which occurs when a skin graft has been cut and yet cannot be used immediately because of inadequate bed hemostasis or suitability. Shepard (1972) has pointed out that a skin graft can be placed back on its donor site and harvested within five days to be used in the recipient area. This may cause pain and bleeding upon removal of the graft but is a useful clinical technique.

Skin grafts may also be stored for longer periods, away from the patient, by being refrigerated. Such grafts may be moistened in sterile saline with antibiotics as desired and then placed in a refrigerator, where they may retain viability as long as 21 days (Georgiade, Perschel, and Brown, 1956). Obviously the tissue should not be frozen or it will be completely nonvital because of cell death. This type of skin storage is most useful when excess skin is harvested in an operative procedure and conserved in case it should be needed later.

Long-term storage of autografts requires special techniques to protect against cell death. Freezing causes tissue death because of concentration within the cell, leaving behind a lethal concentration of salts. Protective agents such as glycerol bind water and protect against this type of injury. Control of the rate of freezing reduces the damage caused by intracellular ice crystals (Rudolph, Fisher, and Ninnemann, 1979).

Allograft Storage. Perhaps the most successful and commonly used storage technique for skin grafts is that of cadaver allografts. Specialized skin banks have been developed to store large amounts of cadaver skin for treatment of massive burns. Standardized techniques for graft preservation use glycerol and rapid freezing with liquid nitrogen. The treated allografts are thawed and used for temporary burn dressings to be changed every five days. Pigskin xenografts have also been used fresh or frozen for burn treatment.

Recently devised artificial membranes, composite grafts composed of shark cartilage glycosaminoglycans, bovine collagen, and autogenous epidermis tissue cultured cells (Burke and associates, 1981; Gallico and O'Connor, 1985) may make possible the growth of large sheets of tissue that will take on patients who have lost substantial areas of skin. Such techniques, if successful, may obviate the need for harvesting and tissue banking of allograft skin.

Nonliving Skin. Both pig and human skin have been lyophilized and freeze dried for use in treatment of patients with massive tissue loss. Current consensus is that frozen, fresh allograft is probably preferable to lyophilized, freeze-dried tissue. However, the latter can act as a burn dressing that may be useful if cadaver bank skin is not available.

The behavior of preserved skin is discussed in more detail later in the chapter under Biologic Behavior.

DERMAL OVERGRAFTING

Split-thickness skin grafts can be applied to a bed of dermis or scar tissue after removal of the surface epithelium. This was first described by Webster in 1954 and further developed by Hynes (1957) and Thompson (1960), who considered it a valuable addition to the plastic surgery armamentarium.

Principles of the Method. Hynes (1957) has shown that mature scars have a capillary circulation capable of vascularizing overlying skin grafts that become rapidly adherent. Studies by Thompson (1977) and Butcher and Hoover (1955) have shown the development of lymphatic circulation within the dermal overgraft, as manifested by rapid clearance of sterile technetium-99m and injected blue violet dye (Fig. 8–21). The application of a split-thickness graft with its normal dermis can restore the elastic *dermal pad* that is missing in scar. Dense scar often is relatively unyielding and inelastic, and the overlying epithelium may be easily stripped by trauma. The application of a thick split-thickness graft can reduce these problems.

Histologic Studies. Of necessity, overgrafting buries epidermal appendages such as hair follicles, sebaceous glands, and sweat glands. Such epithelial elements can lead to the development of microscopic epidermoid cysts, which Thompson (1960) has shown undergo dissolution within a year in most cases. Small cysts may develop that can be evacuated (Fig. 8–22). Thompson reported that elastic tissue is present in the dermis of the grafted skin, that hair follicles undergo epidermoid cyst formation and disintegration, that sebaceous glands persist as long as six weeks but then disappear, and that sweat gland elements functionally persist only if continuity is established between superficial and deep sweat gland function. The buried squamous epithelium produces keratin, which can form within small cysts. These generally rupture and incite an inflammatory reaction, eventually being replaced by granulation tissue and foreign body giant cells (Thompson, 1960).

Technique. The surface epidermis is removed either by dermabrasion or by dissection with a knife. Bleeding in the wound bed is controlled by pressure and careful electrocautery, as in any skin grafting procedure. Thompson (1977) recommends that the split-thickness graft be cut thickly and applied without tension to increase the bulk of the graft. Repeated grafting can be done in stages to augment the thickness of the dermis.

Indications. The most common indication for dermal overgrafting is in extensive unstable, contracted, depressed, pigmented, or hypertrophic scars that are matured. While such scars are often completely excised and replaced with skin grafts or flaps, dermal overgrafting may be of some benefit where these techniques are not available. Thick split-thickness grafts or laminated grafts may increase the capacity of the foot to bear weight.

Venous stasis ulcers can be overgrafted after an initial skin graft and appropriate vein ligation (Thompson, 1977) (Fig. 8–23). Thompson (1977) and Hynes (1956) also noted that dermal overgrafting could be used for correction of extensive pigmented nevi, although the risk of malignancy developing in giant hairy nevi would suggest that the pig-

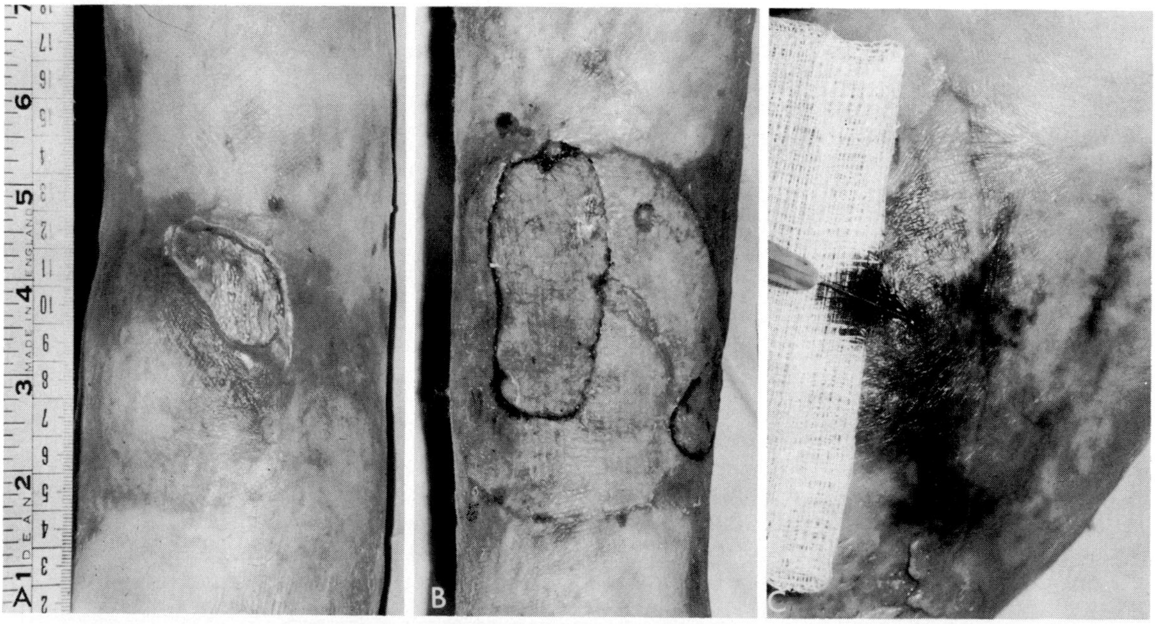

Figure 8–21. Dermal overgrafting technique. *A*, Unstable scar of the lower extremity. *B*, Following application of two layers of dermal onlay. *C*, Demonstration of dermal lymphatic plexus in the graft by patent blue violet dye. Note that the lymphatics are continuous with the surrounding tissue. (Courtesy of Mr. Noel Thompson.)

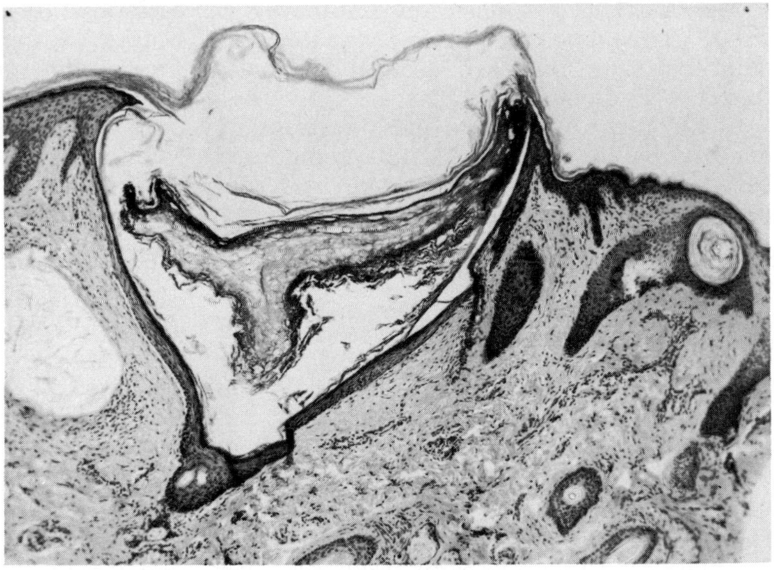

Figure 8–22. Microscopic section of epidermoid cyst at the graft surface following dermal overgrafting. (Courtesy of Mr. Noel Thompson.)

ment must be completely removed (which would not make overgrafting as likely to be useful). Chronic radiodermatitis in the past could be treated with dermal overgrafting (Thompson, 1977). However, studies by Rudolph (1984) have shown that skin grafting is not as useful with current radiotherapy techniques because of the deeper penetration of the beam; severe radiodermatitis now tends to be treated with more elaborate flap techniques. However, for relatively superficial chronic radiodermatitis, dermal overgrafting may still be of benefit.

BIOLOGIC BEHAVIOR

Transplantation of living tissues involves the surgical removal of viable cells from a donor area and subsequent transfer to a recipient site. Whether or not the transplanted cells survive and propagate a lineage of living cells in the recipient site depends on the following factors: (1) the accessibility of nutritive materials; (2) the resources for disposing of metabolic waste products; (3) the anatomic distinction between the tissue of the donor and recipient; and (4) the taxonomic and immunogenetic relationships between the donor and the recipient.

Because of its accessibility, skin has enjoyed considerable study as a transplantation

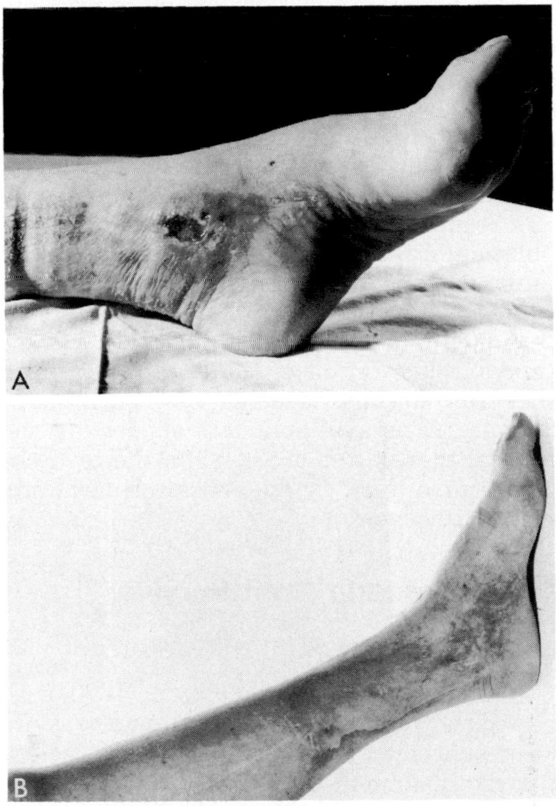

Figure 8–23. Dermal overgrafting for venous ulcers. *A,* Appearance of chronic venous ulcer of the medial malleolar area. *B,* Following serial application of dermal overgrafts. The perforating veins were also ligated. (Courtesy of Mr. Noel Thompson.)

model. Much of our basic understanding of tissue transplantation and the associated vascular changes has been derived primarily from the study of skin grafts.

At the time of surgical excision from its donor area, a graft of skin is completely severed from the surrounding skin and subjacent connective tissue layer; the circulation, lymphatic drainage, and nerve continuity are abruptly terminated.

It is recognized that the survival of a skin graft is dependent on rapidly acquiring a blood supply adequate for nutrition and for disposal of metabolic waste products. In the time interval between transplantation and the process of revascularization, survival of the axonic graft cells appears to be ensured by the absorption of fluid from the host (Converse and associates, 1957; 1969). This process of imbibition of exudate from the host bed, first noted by Hübscher in 1888 and Goldmann in 1890, and termed by them "plasmatische Zirkulation" (plasmatic circulation), appears to play an important role in ensuring an interim period of nourishment before the establishment of a definitive vasculature. However, it is not capable of indefinitely maintaining the survival of a skin graft, which eventually perishes if it does not become successfully vascularized.

The mode of vascularization of skin grafts is still a subject of debate. Revascularization has been attributed to one process or a combination of three: (1) direct connection of the graft and host vessels, referred to as "inosculation"; (2) ingrowth of host vessels into the endothelial channels of the graft; and (3) random penetration of the host vessels into the graft dermis, creating new endothelial channels. The available data supporting the roles of these three processes in the revascularization of various types of skin transplants will be reviewed.

Phases of Skin Graft Survival

SERUM IMBIBITION

Hübscher (1888) and Goldmann (1890) suggested that Thiersch grafts in human patients were nourished by fluid from the host before the establishment of new vascular and lymphatic channels in the graft. They termed this early process of fluid nourishment the "plasmatic circulation" of a graft. Using a modification of the Algire tissue chamber technique for evaluating skin grafts in mice, Conway, Stark, and Joslin (1951) observed a profuse flow of extracellular fluids from the surrounding area of the host into the transparent chamber during the first 24 hours. They stressed the importance of early plasmatic circulation, by which the grafts could be sustained during the first postoperative week.

Subsequent observations by Converse and associates (1957) on a series of skin xenografts removed from the rabbit and placed upon the chorioallantois of the chick embryo indicated a rapid fluid uptake in the graft. In this experiment the rabbit skin grafts were removed from the surface of the chorioallantoic membrane at time intervals varying from one to 20 hours after transplantation. These grafts were weighed before transplantation and again after being removed from the membrane by traction. A progressive weight increase with time was observed in 165 grafts: the average increase in graft weight was 10 per cent after one hour, and progressed steadily to 38.2 per cent after ten hours and 52 per cent after 20 hours. It has been suggested that a skin graft is capable of absorbing fluid from the host bed because of the spongelike structure of the dermis, which is canalized by innumerable spaces.

Most investigators have generally accepted Hübscher's original concept of plasmatic circulation as an important factor in the early nourishment of skin grafts before the restoration of an adequate blood supply. However, Clemmesen (1962; 1967) believed that the main role of the plasmatic circulation is not nutritional. He felt that it serves to prevent desiccation of the graft and to keep the graft vessels open. Henry and associates (1962), working with human skin grafts, reported that the donor skin derives its nutrition and oxygenation from the process of plasmatic circulation for the first two days after grafting. Thereafter, this type of nourishment is insufficient to maintain the viability of full-thickness grafts, unless it is supplemented by an adequate vascular supply.

More recently, Šmahel (1971; 1977) suggested that the existence, condition, and duration of the phase of plasmatic circulation depend on the following factors: (1) the graft thickness; (2) the length of time a recipient bed is allowed to remain open and heal before the graft is applied; and (3) the time lag between the excision of a skin graft from the donor site and its subsequent application to the recipient site.

Biochemical Studies. In a series of experimental studies involving biochemical determinations of skin autografts in the rat, Marckmann and Zachariae (1964) and Marckmann (1965a; 1965b; 1967) studied the response of the graft dermis to injury resulting from the transplantation procedure. During the first five critical days, the reaction of a graft to surgical trauma was reflected by edema and changes in the metabolic activity of sulfomucopolysaccharides and in the levels of hexosamine, hydroxyproline, uronic acid, and histamine. These authors assumed that the biochemical alterations in the graft were associated in part with the reduced blood supply, accompanied by changes in the metabolic equilibrium.

Psillakis and associates (1969), after transplanting auricular skin autografts in rabbits, measured water and electrolyte composition in the graft during the first five days. The findings indicated a significant increase in water content on the first day, lasting until the fifth day, whereas the sodium concentration, already significantly increased on the first day, showed a subsequent progressive diminution. In contrast, potassium content was significantly reduced during the first two days and increased considerably over the subsequent three days. As a consequence of injury, the graft dermis is rich in extracellular macromolecules capable of absorbing water and cations from the recipient site without direct vascular continuity with the host blood supply.

Vital Microscopic and Microangiographic Studies. Birch and Brånemark (1969) studied full-thickness scrotal skin autografts placed on the perichondrial recipient bed of an auricle in rabbits through a transparent ear chamber by vital microscopy. They observed graft edema immediately after grafting. The edema attained its maximum on the third postoperative day. The authors attributed the edema to ground substance depolymerization in the graft dermis, absorption of tissue fluids into the graft extracellular compartments, increased capillary pressure, and increased permeability in the inflamed host bed. The gradual subsidence of the graft edema is due to the improved hemodynamics that result from the reestablishment of the blood and lymphatic circulation. In a subsequent experiment using the same transplantation model as well as microangiography, Birch, Brånemark, and Lundskog (1969) reached similar conclusions concerning the graft edema.

Studies of Experimental Orthotopic Grafts. A study of plasmatic circulation under experimental conditions more closely approximating the events occurring in orthotopic grafting was undertaken by Converse, Uhlschmid, and Ballantyne (1969) in the rat. They found a 37.34 per cent weight gain in full-thickness autografts at 24 hours after transplantation, followed by a decrease in the relative weight increase to 25.69 per cent by 48 hours. After this drop, the average weight gain gradually increased again to 30.44 per cent by 96 hours and then steadily returned to its original weight by nine days. The authors suggested that the rise in weight between 48 and 72 hours coincided with the development of a stereomicroscopically visible blood circulation in the grafts. This weight gain was attributed to the filling of the graft vascular system and the inadequate venous and lymphatic drainage, probably the result of engorgement and interstitial edema. With improved venous drainage subsequent to the establishment of an arterial and venous network, the graft returned to its original weight by eight to nine days following transplantation. The negative values noted on the 11th day may well be attributed to improved venous and lymphatic drainage. The graft is first fixed to the host site by fibrin; thus, the fluid penetrating the graft is serum, not plasma. Consequently, it was proposed that the term "plasmatic circulation" be replaced by the term "phase of serum imbibition."

Using the cheek pouch of Syrian hamsters as the source of transparent skin grafts, Haller and associates (1964; 1966; 1967) attributed the early graft survival to the passive uptake of fluid and erythrocytes from the host bed into the preexisting graft vessels. They also termed this process the "phase of imbibition."

Intravenous Colloidal Carbon Suspension Studies. Kikuchi and Omori (1970) injected an intravenous colloidal carbon suspension at varying time intervals after full-thickness skin autografting. They reported that during the first two days after grafting the principal plasma leakage originated from the venules of the graft bed, although capillaries, terminal arterioles, and metarterioles were also leaking. This phenomenon at the graft-host junction was correlated with the phase of the so-called plasmatic circulation. However, on the third day a different pattern of carbon labeling, being more faint or even absent, appeared and possibly reflected the change to graft revascularization.

Studies on Color Changes in Skin Grafts. The graft when excised from the donor becomes chalk white and blanched. Within a few hours after grafting it takes on a pinkish hue, which progresses to a bright pink during the next few days. Douglas (1944) noted a faint pink tint in the graft as early as eight hours after grafting. McLaughlin (1954), studying the color changes in a composite graft of cartilage and skin that had been transferred from the ear to reconstruct the border of a nostril, described a change from blanched white to a more harmonious cutaneous coloration within six hours after grafting.

Hynes (1954) observed that the blood vessels in a freshly cut human skin graft varying from split thickness to full thickness are collapsed and empty. The graft vessels, probably as the result of separation from the donor site, undergo spasm, expelling most of the formed hemic elements through the severed ends of the vessels on the graft undersurface. Within 24 hours after transplantation, the graft vessels are again dilated. By 48 hours, the vessels are more distended and contain large numbers of erythrocytes. The exudate that accumulates at the line of demarcation between the graft and host tissues consists of plasma, erythrocytes, and polymorphonuclear leukocytes. This fluid exudate, after precipitating its fibrinogen in the form of fibrin on the surface of the host site, penetrates the overlying graft vessels as a fibrinogen-free suspension of erythrocytes, thereby nourishing the grafts and explaining the rapid color change that occurs within hours after transplantation.

Summary. The *phase of serum imbibition* may be described as a period during which the graft vessels fill with fibrinogen-free fluid and cells from the host bed. The term "circulation" is actually a misnomer, because the fluid absorbed by the graft from the host bed is passively trapped with the graft. Endothelial ingrowth from the host progresses until a definitive vasculature is established. The stagnant fluid absorbed by the graft during the early phase of serum imbibition is eventually drained by the newly established blood and lymphatic circulation. Clinically, skin grafts usually appear edematous and their surfaces are elevated above the surrounding host skin during the early postoperative period. Within a few days after grafting, however, the graft flattens and edema subsides. This observation reflects the establishment of a plasmatic and hemic flow and evacuation of the fluid initially trapped in the graft.

GRAFT REVASCULARIZATION

Autografts and Allografts

Controversy has existed over the method of graft acceptance and the mode of graft vascularization. Several research techniques have been developed to study the physiology of graft acceptance and vascularization.

Bert (1863) first noted an early connection between the blood vessels of the graft and host and employed the term "abouchement" to illustrate the mouth-to-mouth apposition of the vessels. In 1874 Thiersch, studying the histologic sections of experimental full-thickness skin grafts in man, used the term "inosculation" to signify the direct connection between graft and host vessels.

Garré (1889), studying human skin grafts, reported evidence of endothelial mitosis in the host bed 5½ hours after grafting, the presence of inflammatory cells in the grafts by 9 hours, and invasion of white cells into the donor vessels at 11 hours. He discounted the importance of the inosculatory process and described actual revascularization as an invasion of the graft by host capillary buds, which began on the third or fourth day, after most of the original graft vessels had become obliterated. Garré's conclusion coincided with those of Hübscher (1888) and Goldmann (1890). Jungengel (1891) and Enderlen (1897) also maintained that most of the preexisting graft vessels degenerated, but that some of the endothelial cells were able to survive and form new vessels that eventually connected with the ingrowing host vessels.

Braun (1899) believed that graft revascularization was achieved by a dual process of ingrowth of host vessels and anastomoses between the host and original graft vasculatures. Henle (1899), after injecting various dyes into rabbit recipients of full-thickness grafts, arrived at conclusions similar to those of Garré (1889), i.e., that there is early evidence of endothelial mitosis followed by rapid capillary ingrowth from the recipient site.

Most of the pioneer studies on the origin and development of the blood supply in skin grafts have been derived from experiments on split-thickness grafts during the years 1888–1897 (Enderlen, 1897; Garré, 1889; Goldmann, 1890; Hübscher, 1888; Jungengel, 1891). There were many subsequent reports concerning the process of vascularization in transplanted skin, but *no serious efforts* were made to study the nature of vascularization in skin of varying thicknesses.

Stereomicroscopic Studies. The technique of observing cutaneous blood vessels in skin in vivo was described by Lombard in 1911 and was developed by Lewis in 1927. The stereomicroscopic technique reported by Taylor and Lehrfeld (1953; 1955) for direct observation of the vascularization in rat skin grafts was modified for studies in man by Converse and Rapaport (1956). The stereomicroscopic appearance of autografts and allografts has been fully described, with particular attention to vascular changes, by Taylor and Lehrfeld (1953; 1955) in the rat and by Converse and Rapaport (1956) in man. These early changes may be summarized as follows: immediately after application of the graft to the recipient bed and during the subsequent 24 hours, the blood vessels of the grafts appear less filled with blood and are not readily detected when compared with those in the surrounding skin. On the first day after grafting, many vessels in the donor tissue show early evidence of distention and are rapidly filled with static blood. On the second day vessel distention continues, but blood circulation has not begun, although a sluggish flow of blood may occasionally be seen in the peripheral vessels. A slow flow of blood occurs in the graft vasculature on the third or fourth day and continues to improve until the fifth or sixth day. During subsequent days, a return of all blood vessels to normal caliber and circulation occurs in all *autografts*.

In *allografts*, the similarity persists only until the onset of the allograft rejection. This rejection reaction is heralded by increased distention in the vascular system, followed by the appearance of a sluggish circulation with clumped elements. Complete cessation of blood flow and vascular disruption in most skin allografts usually occur between seven and ten days after grafting.

Direct observation of the vessels in skin transplants by means of a dissecting microscope, as practiced by Converse and Rapaport (1956), has also been used by Ceppellini and associates (1966) for assessing vascularization and survival end points of human skin grafts. Although the use of skin stereomicroscopy is a useful tool for determining changes in the appearance and state of blood circulation in the grafted tissue from the time of transplantation to the rejection reaction, this direct method is not adequate for defining the actual source of the vascular supply or the mode of vascularization.

Histologic Studies. Henry and associates (1961; 1962), following their histologic studies in humans, attributed the vascularization of autografts and allografts of skin to the inosculation of the patent original capillaries in the deeper layers of the graft dermis with the capillary loops from the host bed. As a consequence of even a few initial vascular connections, the superficial graft capillaries, whose endothelial linings have degenerated during the first few postoperative days, are supplied with blood and become dilated. The authors infer that this feature persists until the superficial channels are reconstituted by endothelial cells growing along the existing vessels. Their histologic study showed no vascular connections between the donor and host skin for two days after transplantation; during this time, the superficial capillaries in the graft collapse and the endothelial cells degenerate, leaving the basement membrane intact. Although the graft vascular system appears dilated and engorged with static blood by the second or third day, the superficial vessels continue to demonstrate an intact basement membrane, with the endothelial nuclei either pyknotic or entirely absent; in the meantime the original vessels located in the deep dermal layers of the graft appear patent on histologic examination. The process of graft vascularization is completed on the sixth or seventh day.

Histochemical Studies. Until 1961, relatively few histochemical methods had been employed to evaluate the metabolic changes occurring in skin transplants (Scothorne and Tough, 1952; Scothorne and Scothorne, 1953; Thompson, 1962; Russell and Monaco, 1965); no efforts were made to define the mode of graft revascularization. In order to study this problem under experimental conditions that more closely approximated the events occurring in orthotopic grafting, autografts and allografts in mammalian recipients were studied by means of an enzyme-histochemical method (Converse and Ballantyne, 1962).

The reagents employed, neotetrazolium

chloride and reduced diphosphopyridine nucleotide (DPNH), indicate the presence of DPNH dehydrogenase (diaphorase) in fresh frozen sections (Antopol and associates, 1950). Histochemical sections of full-thickness skin autografts and allografts in rats have shown that the ingrowth of host capillaries into skin transplants is essential to establish the definitive vasculature of the graft. The structural differences between the preexisting graft and invading host blood vessels permit identification of the two types of vasculature. The process of graft revascularization by the host is very rapid; the host capillaries have penetrated through the demarcation line into the graft dermis by six hours and attain the dermoepidermal junction by 48 hours. The data in this study also indicate a progressive decline of enzymatic activity, accompanied by degenerative changes, in the original graft vasculature during the first four days after transplantation. In contrast to the vasculature of the surrounding host tissue, the vascular pattern in the graft is changed. The vessels are numerous, exhibit greater ramification and distention, and demonstrate a purposeful and parallel ingrowth in a perpendicular direction from the recipient bed to the dermoepidermal junction of the graft. The new vasculature progressively returns to a finer pattern during subsequent days. These findings appear to corroborate the stereomicroscopic observations of a progressive distention of the vessels and an increase in their number during the first postoperative days (Taylor and Lehrfeld, 1953; Converse and Rapaport, 1956; Ballantyne and Converse, 1957). Although these findings confirmed beyond a doubt that a rapid ingrowth of new vessels from the host occurs, it could not be inferred that inosculation does not take place.

Subsequent histochemical studies using various hydrolytic and oxidative enzymes in porcine split-thickness skin grafts were conducted by Wolff and Schellander (1965; 1966). They confirmed the enzymatic findings of Converse and Ballantyne (1962) and the original thesis of Garré (1889) that the definitive skin graft vasculature is formed by ingrowing host capillaries.

A divergent view suggested by Pedersen and associates (1970), working with skin autografts in rats, is that the histochemical methods of assessment employed by Converse and Ballantyne (1962), Converse, Filler, and Ballantyne (1965), and Wolff and Schellander (1965) are not reliable criteria of graft viability. This opinion is based on observations indicating a more distinct and intense enzymatic activity in grafts and skin from dead rats during the first three days compared with that of the healing skin grafts. Furthermore, the initial decline of the enzymatic activity in healing skin grafts within the first 24 hours and its subsequent return suggests the presence of a factor that temporarily inhibits the enzymatic activity at the time of wound healing.

Study of Early Filling of the Vessels. In 1925 Davis and Traut, using intracardiac injections of China ink in dogs, described the anastomosis of graft and host vessels, which began as early as 22 hours after application of the graft and persisted for up to 72 hours. They also stressed subsequent host capillary growth, occurring by the fourth day, and concluded that it is the decisive factor involved in establishing the definitive vascular system of the graft. Mir y Mir (1951), experimenting with postmortem dye injection into the canine aorta, considered the thickness of skin grafts an important factor controlling vascularization. According to Mir y Mir, the restoration of blood supply in the thin split-thickness skin grafts is achieved mainly by the establishment of direct vascular continuity between the respective vessels of the graft and host. The sequence of vascular changes in full-thickness skin grafts, as reported by this investigator, parallels that reported by Davis and Traut (1925): the vitality of such grafts is initially ensured by the direct vascular connections, followed in turn by extensive host vascular ingrowth. In his classic study, Medawar (1944) observed that the revascularization of skin grafts in the rabbit by the ingrowth of capillaries from the host site is achieved four days after grafting; the original graft vessels, which he termed "wound vessels," disappear between the fourth and eighth postoperative days.

Peer and Walker (1951) believed that the restoration of circulation in skin grafts is mainly achieved by direct connection between severed ends of blood vessels in the graft and host tissues, and they stressed the importance of early vascular anastomosis for survival of the centrally located cells in the grafted tissue.

Haller and associates (1964; 1966; 1967) studied the origin of the vasculature in skin grafts using the cheek pouch of Syrian hamsters. Being devoid of pigmentation and appendages, the skinlike tissue constituting the highly vascular cheek pouch is almost transparent. When grafted to genetically compatible hosts, it offers a window through which serial observation of the developing circulation can be made. The authors reported that following transplantation the blood vessels of the graft filled immediately, but no flow was observed before the fourth or fifth day. The pattern of blood vessels in the healed isografts was identical to those of the original graft vessels. The authors (1966; 1967) noted that when these vessels were blocked by previous injections of silicone rubber, the grafts became necrotic, which strongly suggested that the intrinsic vessels of the graft were utilized for its survival.

Study of Revascularization from the Host Bed Margins. Rees and associates (1968) inserted silicone rubber sheeting between a suprapannicular skin autograft and the host bed in rats. The insertion of the silicone rubber sheets failed to prevent the development of a blood supply in these small skin grafts. This finding strongly supports the concept that, while the vessels in the host bed may well be the main source of graft revascularization, the ingrowth of new vessels from the margins of the host bed can also play an important role in the vascularization of skin transplants.

Transparent Tissue Chamber Studies. The transparent tissue chamber has been frequently used as an experimental model for observing in vivo vascular changes in skin grafts, with particular attention to the revascularization process. However, it was not until 1951 that Conway, Stark, and Joslin first applied the chamber technique to evaluate the early physiologic phases of circulation in full-thickness skin grafts in the mouse. They found that the vascularization of skin *autografts* is achieved by capillary budding in the host site, followed by vascular ingrowth of capillary sprouts into the grafts. In 1952 Conway and associates, using a similar mouse chamber technique, and Ham (1952), who injected pigs with India ink suspensions, stated that skin *allografts* did not become vascularized, offering this finding as an example of allograft rejection. However, Taylor and Lehrfeld (1953), by means of direct skin stereomicroscopy, reported that allografts in rats are successfully vascularized before the rejection reaction; their finding that autografts and allografts are both vascularized was confirmed in man by Converse and Rapaport (1956). These findings are consistent with histologic evidence of the vascularization of skin allografts in man, as reported by Gibson and Medawar (1943) and McGregor (1955a,b). After injecting India ink and bromophenol blue into the circulatory system of rabbits, Scothorne and McGregor (1953) cited evidence of vascularization in allografts, but did not specify the actual mode. Subsequently, Conway and associates (1957) and Conway, Sedar, and Shannon (1957), accepting the criticisms of Scothorne and McGregor (1953) and Taylor and Lehrfeld (1953), modified their transparent apparatus and reported evidence of active blood circulation in murine skin allografts.

Further evidence of the effective restoration of blood circulation in allografts was reported by Edgerton and Edgerton (1955). In the mouse skin transparent chamber they noted vigorous vascular ingrowth from the host into the graft, filling the original graft vascular system with static blood as early as the second or third day. Subsequently, flow velocity, which is sluggish soon after the establishment of some vascular connections between the host and graft, progressively increased to a normal rate after the third or fourth postoperative day. The authors concluded that the vascular continuity between the original graft vessels and host vessels plays an important role in establishing a definitive vasculature with active circulation in the graft. A similar opinion was expressed by Kamrin (1960; 1961), who held that in rat autografts and allografts the ingrowth of capillary buds from the recipient site has achieved contact with the original graft vessels by the end of the fourth or beginning of the fifth day, as shown by the sudden emptying of the crenated (deformed) erythrocytes from the clotted graft vascular system and the replacement by normal host blood elements.

Injection Suspension Studies. Many investigative attempts have been made to define the actual source of new blood supply in orthotopic skin grafts by administering various dyes, colloidal suspensions, or radioactive substances into the animal vascular system. The conclusions of some authors, including Jungengel (1891), Enderlen (1897), Henle (1899), Davis and Traut (1925), Mir y

Mir (1951), and Ham (1952), have been described.

In 1957 Egdahl, Good, and Varco called attention to the disappearance of intradermally injected fluorescein during the early stages of vascularization in full-thickness rat allografts. They observed the disappearance of intradermal fluorescein as early as 12 hours before the onset of blood circulation, as shown by the direct skin stereomicroscopic method of Taylor and Lehrfeld (1953). The "removal of fluorescein test" and the capacity to develop localized Schwartzman phenomena in first set allografts are considered strong evidence of successful vascularization via direct connections between the vessels of the graft and those of the recipient.

After intravenous injections of the radioactive isotope ^{32}P into rabbits, Ohmori and Kurata (1960) noted the onset of blood circulation in full-thickness skin autografts and allografts on the fourth day after grafting. The velocity of the hemic flow is normal in autografts by the 29th day, whereas in allografts the flow diminishes by the sixth day and ceases on the ninth day. Later, Pihl and Weiber (1963) measured the impulse frequencies over the auricular full-thickness skin grafts in rabbits after intravenous administration of ^{32}P. The data indicate a progressive increase in the vascularization of autografts and allografts until maximal activity is attained by the fifth day. Subsequently, this activity gradually subsides in the autografts, persisting above the normal level noted in normal skin at 11 days, whereas in the allografts the values diminish with degeneration and the rejection reaction occurs.

Šmahel (1962; 1967) used intracardiac injections of a mixture of gelatin and India ink to study the vascularization of skin grafts in rats. He reported that during the first two days after grafting, the host capillaries form a rich, arcade-like network in the host bed. On the following day, endothelial sprouts originate from this dense network and invade the graft through the union line; on subsequent days, the host vessels link with the original vascular system of the graft. It has been implied by Šmahel (1962) that if the sprouting of the arcade-like network in the host bed does not develop, the definitive vasculature of the graft will not develop. According to Šmahel and Ganzoni (1970), the revascularization of the skin graft is largely dependent on the original graft vasculature. However, they were also convinced that under certain conditions the host vessels furnished the major definitive vasculature of the grafts. Šmahel and Clodius (1971) have stated that the degree of vascularization of the human skin graft is primarily dependent on the vascularity of the donor site, and secondly on the thickness of the graft.

Smith, Ringland, and Wilson (1964) injected silicone rubber at a high pressure into the vascular system of the rabbit hosts of auricular skin grafts between one and 30 days after grafting. Their histologic sections indicated, as had those of Converse and Ballantyne (1962), an early and profound sprouting of capillaries in the host bed underlying the graft, numerous sprouts growing in a parallel direction into the graft undersurface at between 48 hours and eight days.

Vital Microscopic and Microangiographic Studies. A modification of the mouse skin transparent chamber of Merwin and Algire (1956) was used by Zarem, Zweifach, and McGehee (1967) to evaluate the development of the microcirculation in full-thickness skin autografts in mice. Their microscopic findings indicate that endothelial budding arises from the small arteries and veins in the host bed rather than from the capillaries or arterioles and venules. The endothelial buds then progress along the original graft vessels, which serve as nonviable conduits, and develop into an immature plexus of thin-walled, irregular channels with an oscillatory or slow unidirectional flow. By the eighth postoperative day the immature plexus differentiates into arterioles, capillaries, and venules. On the basis of their observations, the authors conclude that the reestablishment of the graft vasculature occurs primarily as a vascular ingrowth from the host.

In a subsequent experiment, O'Donoghue and Zarem (1971), using the same chamber technique in mice, evaluated the differences in the angiogenic properties of fresh skin autografts, fresh skin allografts, lyophilized autografts, and freeze-thawed autografts. It was reported that despite a consistent difference in the angiogenic properties of various types of grafts, all grafts are capable of inducing hyperemia in the host beds and neovascularization, consisting of the formation of host vascular buds and the development of sausage-shaped vessels extending toward the graft. All grafts are effectively vascularized.

In both isografts and allografts, hyperemia is apparent on the third or fourth day after transplantation, neovascularization by the sixth day, and complete graft revascularization by the eighth day. The authors concluded that the original graft vasculature plays an important role in stimulating the vascular budding from the host site, either to form an anastomosis with the graft vessels or to penetrate the entire graft tissue.

Birch and Brånemark (1969), working with rabbits, placed a full-thickness scrotal skin autograft over a thin vascular bed of outer auricular perichondrium and employed the modified ear chamber of Brånemark and Lindström (1963) for vital microscopic evaluation. Immediately after surgery, the authors noted filling of most graft vessels. Between 24 and 28 hours after grafting, slow irregular blood circulation appeared in the original graft vessels. During the subsequent 24 hours most of the grafts had resumed normal circulation. Vascular proliferation was seen to begin soon after the development of circulation and to originate from the preexisting graft vessels; it reached a peak six to ten days after grafting. The investigators concluded that the blood flow noted in the graft depends on the vascular connection between the graft and recipient bed and on the host circulation.

In a subsequent experiment, Birch, Brånemark, and Lundskog (1969) repeated the procedure of transplanting rabbit scrotal skin autografts to the auricular host bed for microangiographic study and reached similar conclusions. The initial graft circulation appears to result from connections between vessels in the recipient bed and large dilated graft vessels. Between 48 and 72 hours after transplantation, capillaries in the host bed penetrate the lower layer of the graft; the small invading vessels are more numerous and penetrate deeper into the donor dermis at the extreme periphery of the graft. However, the capillary invasion does not account for the increased number of blood vessels seen in the superficial layers of the graft. Presumably, the new vessels observed in these layers originate from the preexisting graft vessels.

Another method of assessing the vascular condition and circulation in skin grafts was developed by Marckmann (1966). With a live rat positioned under a microscope and with a television screen amplifier for projection onto a monitor, it is possible to observe the condition of blood circulation in skin autografts and to obtain cinematographic and photographic records. Slow flow could be seen in some areas of the graft at two postoperative days; the flow velocity became normal by the seventh day.

In vivo microangiographic techniques were employed by Bellman and associates (1957; 1964) to define the vascular events in the full-thickness skin grafts removed from the auricle of the rabbit and then replaced on its bed. In one experiment (1957), all grafts were rotated 90 degrees before being replaced, and in another (1964) the grafts were not rotated but replaced with exact adaptation. After analyzing the results obtained from both experiments, the authors were unable to state definitely whether the original blood vessels of the transplanted skin participated in the establishment of the definitive vasculature of the graft; however, they wrote (1964) that "incorporation of graft vessels into the ambient vessel network is a function of the local hemodynamic status."

Assessment of Graft Revascularization by a Combination of Various Assay Methods. In an attempt to evaluate the source of blood supply in autologous and allogeneic transplants of mouse and rat skin, Rolle, Taylor, and Charipper (1959) utilized a combination of the following four methods of examination: direct skin microscopy, routine histologic methods, cardiac injections of India ink suspensions into the vascular system, and intravenous injections of a diffusible dye, bromophenol blue. They reported that many of the graft vessels, empty at the time of removal from the donor, begin to acquire stagnant blood and appear distended by 24 hours after surgery. At three days the blood circulation within the graft vasculature is restored, and it resumes the normal velocity of blood flow the following day; there is no histologic evidence of degenerative changes in the original graft vessels. Rolle, Taylor, and Charipper (1959) and Hildemann and Haas (1960) concluded that the definitive vasculature in the graft capable of supporting an active circulation appears to depend on the direct vascular continuity between the host and graft, not the growth of newly formed vessels from the host.

Ljungqvist and Almgård (1966) employed a combined stereomicroangiographic and histologic method at varying times after transplantation to determine the vascular changes in skin autografts and allografts on the auricles of rabbits. The results indicated that the ingrowth of precapillary and capillary vessels from the underlying host bed, first noted at two postoperative days, invades the graft and extends in a perpendicular and spiral fashion toward the dermoepidermal surface, replacing the degenerated graft vessels. These ingrowing vessels form the definitive vasculature of the graft. While there is some evidence of direct connection between the graft and host blood systems, the degenerative changes with thrombosis in the original graft vessels suggest that these vascular connections play only a minor and temporary role.

In 1974 Guthy, Billote, and Burke used daily gross and in vivo stereomicroscopic observations, coupled with histopathologic examination of skin biopsy specimens, to determine the sequence of events in full-thickness skin autografts and allografts in the guinea pig. Their data, collected on the fourth day, indicate minimal granulation tissue in the bed, graft-host coadaptation, and graft vascularization, as demonstrated by a pink color, blanching, and refilling upon application of digital pressure. These findings appear to corroborate the histologic data that numerous vascular buds originate from venules and precapillary arterioles in the recipient site, and form direct vascular continuity with preexisting graft vessels via temporary thin-walled vascular lakes, presumably of graft origin. At this time, the original graft and invading host vessels are engorged with red blood cells. Consequently, the authors considered that the ingrowing host vessels and subsequent anastomoses with the original graft vessels play an important role in establishing the definitive skin graft vasculature.

In 1975 Converse and associates evaluated the vascular patterns of suprapannicular skin autografts in the rat by the combined technique of direct skin stereomicroscopy, experimental separation of a graft from its bed, and supravital intracardiac injection of a contrast medium. As reported by the authors, the earliest stereomicroscopic evidence of an initial blood circulation, as represented by oscillatory or sluggish movements in the graft vessels at 48 hours, is in accord with concurrent observations of the filling of the graft vessels with India ink. Consequently, a delay of 48 hours must elapse for the proliferative host vessels to penetrate the fibrin layer and develop functioning links with the graft vasculature. With an increase in the number and size of the functioning anastomoses, accompanied by the gradual dissolution of thrombi, the grafts are completely revascularized between the fourth and fifth days after transplantation. These findings are correlated with complete filling of the graft vascular system with India ink and the stereomicroscopic appearance of brisk blood flow through the graft vessels.

Because only a few vascular anastomoses are found at five and six days, it was suggested that although numerous capillary sprouts of the host bed contact the graft vessels, only a few of them succeed in forming a functioning anastomosis. Furthermore, the presence of a few anastomoses, as evidenced by the injection method, coincides with the stereomicroscopic observation of a proportionally denser network of endothelial channels in the graft than in the adjacent host tissue. This has been interpreted as strong evidence that graft revascularization is achieved by a dual process of direct connection between the graft and host vasculatures and vascular ingrowth from the host site into the graft.

Split-Thickness Skin Grafts. It has been generally assumed that thin grafts of skin are revascularized more rapidly than thick grafts. The histologic appearance of thin and thick grafts shows that degenerative changes in the transplant depend on the rate of vascularization; the degenerative changes in the transplant appear to be inversely proportional to the rate of vascularization. The changes are less apparent in split-thickness grafts, because the invading blood vessels have a shorter distance to traverse through the entire thickness of donor dermis.

A study employing combined methods of vital skin microscopy and enzyme histochemistry with neotetrazolium chloride and reduced diphosphopyridine nucleotide (DPNH) as reagents was conducted in rats by Converse, Filler, and Ballantyne (1965). They attempted to define the actual source and development of the blood supply in split-thickness skin grafts that were removed, rotated 180 degrees, and immediately replaced on the dermal bed. Before beginning the experiment, the authors had presumed that the revascularization of a split-thickness skin graft transplanted to a suprapannicular bed would be more rapid than that of a full-thickness graft for two reasons: (1) the split-thickness graft is thinner, so that the invading vessels from the host have a shorter distance to travel; and (2) the suprapannicular host site contains a rich supply of vessels. The histochemical data, however, indicate that the new host capillaries originate as endothelial buds from deep-lying distended blood vessels in the upper epimysium of the panniculus carnosus, rather than from the host vessels in close proximity to the graft undersurface. In contrast to the vasculature noted in the surrounding host tissue, the vessels are numerous and show greater ramification and dilation. The complete revascularization with active circulation of the split-thickness graft occurs at the same rate as in the full-thickness graft on a suprapannicular bed.

In contrast to an early and rapid decrease of enzymatic activity in the vessels of full-thickness grafts placed on a suprapannicular bed (Converse and associates, 1965), the delayed and slower loss of activity in vessels in split-thickness grafts implies that the onset and rate of degenerative changes in the graft vessels vary with the thickness of the graft dermis. In thin grafts, nutrient fluids have a shorter distance to diffuse, and the thinner graft has fewer cellular elements requiring nourishment. As emphasized by Mir y Mir (1951), the rapidity of vascularization and the state of nutrition of the skin graft are controlled by the dermal thickness of the graft and the state of the host site. Woodruff (1960) supported the hypothesis of Mir y Mir that, in thin grafts, serum imbibition is adequate to maintain the viability of the grafted tissue for several days, and early vascularization is not essential; in thicker grafts, however, early or rapid vascularization is essential for survival.

As mentioned, Wolff and Schellander (1965; 1966), in somewhat similar enzyme histochemical studies, noted that the definitive vasculature of split-thickness skin grafts in pigs is formed entirely by the ingrowing capillaries from the host, and the original vessels degenerate. These investigators confirmed the histochemical studies of Converse and Ballantyne (1962) using full-thickness suprapannicular skin grafts in rats. Their findings also coincide with those of Converse and associates (1965) on split-thickness grafts in rats.

In 1964 Clemmesen injected India ink suspension into the vascular system of pigs under forced intracardiac pressure, and deduced from histologic examination that the revascularization of thin split-thickness skin autografts depends largely on the sinus-like channels between the vessels of the underlying host tissues and the graft vessels. He concluded that subsequently the sinus-like communications formed by the interstice in the fibrin network at the host-graft junction are transformed into thin-walled vessels, permitting the reestablishment of active hemal flow in the original graft vasculature. Various studies (stereomicroscopy, histology, or histochemistry) of the behavior and fate of skin transplants in animals, chick embryos, and man failed to confirm Clemmesen's findings of sinus-like channels at the host-graft junction. Presumably, excessive intracardiac pressure of the India ink injectant ruptured the newly formed blood vessels at the surface of the recipient areas or at the junction line between the host and graft bed, thus allowing the solution to form the ink-filled areas.

Summary. The present interpretation is that the early fillings of the graft endothelial spaces with serum-like fluid is accompanied by the infiltration of erythrocytes, as a result of the anastomosis of graft vessels with host vessels, coupled with the early ingrowth and penetration of host endothelium. These events may account for the pinkish tint that appears in human skin within the first 12 hours after transplantation. The color changes progress gradually to a cherry-red hue in vascularized grafts with the development of a blood circulation. The cyanotic color of more slowly revascularized grafts, which reflects poorly oxygenated hemoglobin, is due to incomplete or inadequate hemic flow caused by an embarrassed venous return or drainage from the graft. With time and improved circulation, the color progresses to a cherry-red hue.

Xenografts

The mode of vascularization and the morphology of vascular changes following the application of skin xenografts have not been extensively investigated. It has been generally held that, because skin transplanted between members of different species induces a more rapid and violent response than do allografts, the survival time of xenografts is too restricted to permit a successful reestablishment of blood circulation. According to Ribbert-Göttingen (1904), who transplanted skin from humans and guinea pigs to rabbits, xenografts were rejected within three days after transplantation. Loeb and Addison (1909; 1911) reported that skin xenografts interchanged between various animals eventually became necrotic after six to 11 days and sometimes even more rapidly. They did not provide information regarding either the vascularization or the vascular pattern of the xenografts.

In 1960 Woodruff stated that xenografts show little or no evidence of vascularization and that ischemia, rather than immunologic rejection, is responsible for the failure of these grafts. Indeed, for a long time most authorities agreed that xenografts invariably fail to receive a direct blood supply from the recipient before the onward rush of the rejection phenomenon. However, during the past two decades there have been indications in the literature that skin xenografts, particularly among certain rodents and between certain animal species, are capable of being revascularized from the host bed. There have also been reports of vessel distention, breakdown of the endothelial wall, blood clots, and focal hemorrhages in the dermis of a skin xenograft undergoing rejection, similar to those seen in allograft rejection.

Experiments with Chick Embryo as a Recipient Site. In 1917 Kiyono and Sueyasu were the first to report the transplantation of skin on the chorioallantoic membrane of the chick embryo, and to describe absorption of nutrient fluids by the graft from the embryonic tissue and the actual entry of avian blood vessels into the grafts. Goodpasture, Douglas, and Anderson (1938) reported the revascularization and growth of split-thickness human skin grafts transplanted to the chorioallantois of the chick embryo; the presence of nucleated chick red blood cells in the graft was considered presumptive evidence of vascular growth, an observation originally described by Murphy (1912) in malignant tumors transferred to avian membrane.

The chorionic capillaries penetrate the undersurface of the human skin dermis within 48 hours after grafting, and by three or four days the network of endothelial channels in the graft contains avian nucleated erythrocytes. Goodpasture, Douglas, and Anderson (1938) accepted the concept of the direct connection of host and graft vessels because their histologic sections indicate a mixture of human and chick erythrocytes. However, the authors implied that, while there is ample evidence favoring anastomoses between the vasculature of the human skin graft and that of avian membrane, their finding is not proof of active blood flow in the graft. The nourishment of the graft is primarily derived from the temporary vascular communication between the two vascular systems.

Further attempts to define the mode of vascularization of skin xenografts from man and various animal species transplanted to the surface of the chorioallantoic membrane were undertaken by Converse and associates (1958), who adopted the modified chick chorioallantoic method of Goodpasture, Douglas, and Anderson (1938). Differences in structure between the mammalian erythrocytes and the nucleated avian erythrocytes made it possible to determine that the definitive vasculature of the full-thickness skin xenografts of rabbit, rat, and bovine embryo is provided mainly by the host vascular ingrowth into the graft while the original vessels of the graft degenerate. When human skin of varying thickness is applied to the chorioallantois of the chick, the major definitive vasculature capable of supporting an active circulation between the graft and host is similarly derived from the progressive ingrowth of avian endothelial cells into the graft. There is also rapid deterioration of most of the original graft vessels. In addition, histologic studies by Ballantyne and Converse (1958) of composite grafts of skin and cartilage taken from the auricles of the rabbit and transferred to the chorionic membrane of chick embryos showed that the embryonal blood vessels make a tortuous course around the cartilage barrier, and eventually penetrate into the dermis above the cartilage. Meanwhile, most of the preexisting vessels in the auricular graft degenerate.

Stereomicroscopic Studies. Blood flow was observed in the vasculature of skin xenografts removed from the rabbit or mouse and transferred to a recipient rat by Egdahl, Good, and Varco (1957) and Egdahl, Varco, and Good (1958), whereas transplants from the rat, mouse, or guinea pig to the rabbit never became effectively vascularized nor adhered to the recipient site. According to the authors, who used the in vivo stereomicroscopic method and intradermal fluorescein as their criteria for circulation, donor skin of the mouse or rabbit placed on rat recipients is vascularized more slowly and has a shorter period of circulatory function than is usually seen in skin allografts. Blood flow in the xenografts is usually initiated on the fourth or fifth day after grafting, attains the maximal rate of circulation soon thereafter, continues at this velocity for only a few hours, and suddenly ceases on or around the sixth day.

Rolle, Taylor, and Charipper (1959) exchanged full-thickness skin grafts between mice and rats, and found that the early sequence of vascular events occurring in the xenografts is similar to that in autografts and allografts. As shown by stereomicroscopy, histology, and the injection of dyes, the onset and restoration of circulation as well as other vascular changes in xenografts prior to the rejection reaction are similar to those seen in allografts of mice or rats. The authors concluded that the blood supply in the xenografts is restored by the establishment of continuity between the host and graft vessels.

According to Ben-Hur, Solowey, and Rapaport (1969a), who combined daily gross and direct skin stereomicroscopic examinations with serial histologic studies to evaluate the physical condition and the status of blood flow in full-thickness skin xenografts, the response of mice to rat grafts was characterized by early mononuclear and polymorphonuclear infiltration of the xenografts, varying degrees of vascularization and circulation, and rapid epithelial degeneration of the graft epidermis and its appendages. Such grafts that had been successfully vascularized by the third day after transplantation showed an abrupt cessation of blood flow, thrombosis and hemorrhage on the third and fourth days. Other grafts that had failed to be vascularized showed the typical features of avascular white graft reaction, progressing into tan-colored eschars by the fifth to seventh days.

In contrast to the rat xenografts, most of the guinea pig grafts applied to mouse recipients were characterized by an absence of vascularization. There were a few instances, however, of an abortive attempt at vascular penetration into the graft base and a particularly prominent infiltration of mononuclear and fibroblast-like cells at the graft base. On the other hand, rabbit xenografts showed no evidence of vascularization or circulating blood for the first three days after surgery. At four days multiple vessels became filled with blood but did not manifest an active circulation.

The nature of the vascular response of guinea pig hosts to skin xenografts taken from the mouse, rat, and rabbit was studied by Ben-Hur, Solowey, and Rapaport (1969b). They found that the response reaction to the xenografts of all three species studied was basically a difference in intensity of the reaction. Unlike autograft and allograft controls, the rat xenografts were not vascularized and there was no vascular penetration from the host during the first few days after transplantation.

In a separate study, Ballantyne, Uhlschmid, and Converse (1969) transplanted full-thickness rabbit skin grafts to suprapannicular skin defects on the dorsum of rats. On the basis of daily gross and stereomicroscopic observations, they confirmed the findings of Egdahl, Varco, and Good (1958): tissue adhesion between the graft and host and the reestablishment of a definitive vasculature, in which brisk blood flow occurred in most grafts by three to four days after grafting. However, unlike most autografts and allografts, which normally assume a pinkish hue shortly after grafting, all xenografts appeared consistently pale, even with stereomicroscopic evidence of a rapid blood flow in the graft vessels.

Other Experimental Studies. The histologic and angiographic studies of Eastwood (1961) provided evidence that xenografts of pig skin applied to recipient rats are firmly adherent to the host bed, are successfully vascularized, and provide an effective cover for skin wound defects in the rat for an average of ten days. The grafts appear grossly unchanged for the same length of time before becoming dry and hard.

Bromberg, Song, and Mohn (1965) injected 5 per cent Evans blue dye into the femoral veins of recipient mice after porcine split-thickness skin grafts had been applied to defects of the lower extremity. Following sacrifice of the animals, histologic study failed to show any evidence of revascularization in the xenografts. In contrast, murine skin autografts and allografts demonstrated revascularization, even by the third day.

After transplanting porcine split-thickness skin grafts to mice, Pandya and Zarem (1974), using the transparent mouse chamber technique, noted that the host blood vessels in the near vicinity of transplants appeared slightly distended by the second day, but there was no demonstrable evidence of graft vascularization within 15 days after surgery.

With microangiographic techniques, Toranto, Salyer, and Myers (1974) demonstrated vascularization and viability of fresh full-thickness porcine skin xenografts on rabbit and rat recipient sites by the third and fourth days, respectively, but the authors did not define the actual process by which the grafts received their blood supply. On the other hand, in the human host they were unable to distinguish between xenograft vascularization and invasion at the graft-host interface by granulation tissue. At 14 days there was no evidence of vascularization or viability of any xenografts. Consequently, when porcine skin is used as a biologic dressing, the authors recommended removing the xenograft to minimize the risk of host sensitization.

Porcine skin xenografts have also been investigated for intraoral grafting. Kaspar and Laskin (1983) employed fresh split-thickness porcine skin grafts as biologic oral dressings in dogs after vestibuloplasty. Although the histologic appearance of the donor skin and wound sites was examined at frequent time intervals, detailed observations, with respect to the physiology of graft acceptance and vascularization, were not reported. It was noted that porcine skin is as effective as split-thickness grafts in limiting wound contraction, granulation tissue formation, and gross wound distortion in the oral cavity.

Summary. Diagnostic assay methods have been employed to assess the fate of orthotopic skin xenografts in their hosts, and have produced a variety of findings. In view of conflicting reports, the controversy regarding graft vascularization and the course of tissue morphology and vascular events in xenografts is not yet settled.

Indications for Allografts and Xenografts

ALLOGRAFTS

Autotransplantation of skin is widely used in reconstructive surgery and usually produces excellent results. However, when a patient has a loss of full-thickness skin coverage exceeding 30 per cent of body surface, autografts often are not available in sufficient quantity (Woodruff, 1960; Bromberg and Song, 1966; State and Peter, 1974). Temporary coverage can be obtained by skin allografts from volunteers, recently deceased patients, or the patient's relatives and friends and is often a life-saving measure. Réverdin recommended the use of skin allografts in 1872, and Brown and associates (1953) advocated their application as biologic dressings for extensive burn wounds and denuded areas.

As noted by Artz, Rittenbury, and Yarbrough (1972), skin allografts used as biologic dressings can serve several functions: (1) to clean granulating areas prior to autografting, (2) to protect open wounds from water and protein loss until autografts are available (Alsbjörn, 1984), (3) to decrease surface bacterial counts and pain at the site of an open wound, (4) to cover vital organs, and (5) to facilitate early motion of the affected part.

The initial vascularization of skin allografts before their ultimate immunologic rejection has already been reviewed. In order to avoid a rejection response, skin allografts applied as biologic dressings should be changed every two to three days.

The chief handicap in the use of skin allografts is availability. They can be obtained fresh, usually from relatives, and either used immediately or stored in the live state at temperatures near or above freezing. Large crops of allogeneic skin can also be obtained from disease free cadavers.

In burn patients the survival of skin allografts is prolonged (Rapaport and associates, 1964). Allergic responses of the delayed hypersensitivity type are also depressed by thermal injury (Casson and associates, 1966). Immunologic paralysis, antigen competition, and the chance sharing of histocompatibility antigens by randomly selected unrelated individuals are probably factors accounting for these phenomena following thermal injury.

The technique of alternating skin autografts and allografts for obtaining skin coverage for areas of extensive skin loss, such as occur in deep burns, was proposed by Mowlem (1952) and described by Jackson (1954) and Colson and associates (1959). The technique has been largely replaced by the application of skin allografts under which "seeds" of autografts are placed.

The Chinese (Burns Unit, 1973) reported remarkable improvement in survival rates after massive burns involving more than 70 per cent of body surface (third degree burns exceeding 50 per cent of body surface area). After early debridement of the eschars, minute skin autografts were introduced through holes in large sheets of cadaver skin and pig skin that covered the burn wounds. The allografts provided favorable wound conditions for spread and growth of the island autografts.

Skin allografts have also been recommended for coverage of second degree burns (Miller and associates, 1967; 1972). In addition to providing relief of pain and inhibition of evaporate and exudative water loss, skin allografts promote healing with an improved cosmetic result. However, Miller (1974) has cautioned against coverage of split-thickness skin donor sites with viable skin allografts, as rejection of the latter results in conversion of the donor site from a partial-thickness to a full-thickness defect.

XENOGRAFTS

Rogers and Converse (1958) used experimental fetal calf xenografts as biologic dressings in humans and observed a surprising lack of host reaction to the xenografts even after 12 to 17 days of graft retention. Bromberg, Song, and Mohn (1965) popularized the application of porcine xenografts as temporary biologic dressings. The functions of skin xenografts as biologic dressings are similar to those outlined in the above section on Allografts.

Burleson and Eiseman (1973) felt that the efficacy of biologic dressings could be attributed to their ability to adhere to tissue, and that the adherence was due to a fibrin-elastin biologic bonding system. The same authors (1972) demonstrated that the unique adherent qualities of porcine skin were responsible for its antibacterial effect. They (1973) also questioned the role of neomycin and povidone-iodine solution (Betadine), used in the commercial preparation of porcine xenografts, and speculated that these agents might be responsible for reducing surface bacterial counts.

While xenografts have been most extensively used in covering large burn wounds before autografting, the use of xenografts has also been extended to the temporary coverage of exposed vessels, tendons, leg ulcers, flap donor sites, and skin graft donor sites (Elliot and Hoehn, 1973; State and Peter, 1974).

Salisbury and coauthors (1973) have cautioned against the application of porcine skin as temporary biologic dressings of skin graft donor sites because the incorporation of porcine collagen in the subepithelial area of donor site may be detrimental. They found a significant incidence of donor site inflammation and delayed repair following the application of porcine xenografts.

Two cases of neomycin induced nephrotoxicity and ototoxicity following the application of commercially prepared porcine skin xenografts have been reported by Sugarbaker, Sabath, and Morgan (1974). Elevated neomycin blood levels were documented in both patients.

Behavior of Preserved Skin Grafts

It has long been recognized that an available and adequate source of preserved skin grafts is of major importance in reconstructive surgery, especially in the treatment of burn wounds. Preserved skin autografts are also useful in multiple stage reconstructive surgical procedures. Although eventually rejected by the host, they serve as a vital and often life-saving temporary cover, especially in the treatment of burns.

The prospect of covering extensive skin loss with fresh or preserved skin xenografts as temporary biologic dressings until permanent repair with autografts can be instituted has attracted investigators and surgeons during the past half-century. The application of bovine fetal skin (Silvetti and associates, 1957; Sokolic and associates, 1959) and pig skin (Eastwood, 1961; Song and associates, 1966) as temporary covers for large skin defects in humans has elicited considerable interest because they are readily available as commercial preparations. Apart from alleviating pain (Pandya and Zarem, 1974) and reducing bacterial counts in the granulation tissue (Eade, 1958; Song and associates, 1966; Switzer and associates, 1966), fetal calf and porcine skin xenografts have been of some use in enhancing the early appearance of healthy and highly vascular granulation tissue in the recipient bed (O'Donoghue and Zarem, 1971). Furthermore, these grafts do not provoke any significant immunologic reactions in the host (Pate, 1954; Rogers and associates, 1957; Sokolic and associates, 1959; Song and associates, 1966).

For many years the problem of developing satisfactory methods of preserving skin in the live state at temperatures near or above freezing, and storing it in the frozen state, has been a subject of considerable interest. Clinically, the freeze drying process consists of: (1) procurement of skin from patients, volunteers, or cadavers under sterile conditions; (2) rapid freezing of the tissue to low temperatures; (3) dehydration of skin from the frozen state; (4) long-term storage of the freeze dried grafts at room temperature; and (5) rehydration at the time of clinical application.

In his comprehensive review of approximately 200 reports, Perry (1966) discussed the advantages and difficulties associated with three methods of skin storage: (1) nutrient media refrigeration, (2) preservation of skin in the frozen state, and (3) freeze drying of skin for storage at room temperature.

STORAGE AT TEMPERATURES ABOVE FREEZING

Mammalian tissues, excised and kept at body or room temperature, become anoxemic and necrotic after a period of 48 hours; such changes can be retarded by oxygenation or by chilling. It would appear, therefore, that in order to keep isolated tissue viable, tissue metabolism of oxygen, nutrients, and waste products must be ensured and the rate of metabolism retarded by a decrease in temperature.

The simplest method of storing split-thickness skin grafts is to suture the grafts to the donor site. Shepard (1972) has shown that skin grafts can be stored without complications on their donor sites and transferred to a recipient site at the bedside without the need for an anesthetic for a period up to ten days. The technique lends itself to delayed grafting whenever hemostasis is incomplete or there is an avascular recipient bed.

Storage in Cryoprotective Medium by Refrigeration. Wentscher in 1903 was probably the first to report successful storage of skin by refrigeration. The grafts had been either wrapped with moistened gauze or immersed in saline solution and preserved at temperatures near 0°C for periods of seven or 12 days.

In 1944 Webster described his successful experiments with fresh human skin wrapped in Pliofilm, over which he placed several layers of vaseline gauze, which in turn was covered with two sterile towels for storage at approximately 4°C. He stated that, in a number of cases, such tissues had survived a storage period of three weeks when applied as autografts to suitable recipient sites.

Survival of autogenous human skin for longer periods was subsequently observed by Matthews (1945). He wrapped the tissue in a piece of tulle gras, surrounded it in turn with gauze tightly wrung out of saline solution, and kept the wrapped tissues in a screw-capped bottle in a refrigerator at 3° to 6°C. The rate of vascularization, the pattern of color changes, the texture and pliability, and the gross and histologic appearance of the refrigerated skin when applied as autografts after storage of three to eight weeks were similar to those of the freshly excised grafts.

Other investigators strove to determine the optimal conditions for survival of skin stored in a similar temperature. Hanks and Wallace (1949), experimenting with rabbit skin, cited the superiority of 19 per cent serum to mineral oil as a storage medium. Marrangoni (1950) and Allgöwer and Blocker (1952) also confirmed the superiority of dilute serum as a medium for the storage of rabbit and human skin grafts at refrigerator temperatures.

These experiments indicated that the optimal conditions for storage of skin grafts at temperatures above freezing include: (1) immersion in a medium consisting of 10 to 30 per cent serum in a balanced salt solution, (2) the presence of air, and (3) storage at a temperature of approximately 5°C. The viability of excised skin under these conditions may be sustained for at least one week, and at most for two months. The viability of the stored tissue progressively declines during the storage period, and prolonged storage introduces the risk of less than complete survival.

Modifications of dilute sera, physiologic solutions, or tissue culture media as well as other various protective agents for graft storage above 0°C were described by subsequent investigators (Hyatt and associates, 1952; Medawar, 1954; Pepper, 1954; Georgiade and associates, 1956; Perry and associates, 1957; Gresham, Perry, and Thompson, 1963; Raju and Grogan, 1969).

In 1983, Cram and Domayer reported that the viability of human split-thickness skin autografts can be maintained for up to 22 days by storing in a tissue culture medium (Roswell Park Memorial Institute 1640 [RPMI-1640]) at 4°C. The authors also cited the superiority of RPMI-1640 to saline as a storage medium. Hurst, Brown, and Murray

(1984), experimenting with rabbit scrotal skin grafts, stored autografts in various nutrient media at 4°C for up to 40 days before transplantation to rabbit ears. The best results were obtained with McCoy's solution plus 10 per cent serum and 80 mg gentamicin sulfate per liter as a storage medium for skin grafts.

Summary. Marrangoni (1950) recommended storage of skin autografts in 10 per cent serum in a standard refrigerator. Skin grafts can be wrapped in a saline soaked sponge and stored in a sterile Petri dish. As shown by Feller and DeWeese (1958), human skin covered with a small piece of sponge moistened with Hartman's solution and stored in a refrigerator at 4°C remains viable for up to 23 days. After 14 days of storage in saline, skin graft respiratory activity is halved (Lawrence, 1972). After 20 days skin cellular respiration ceases, and this effect corresponds with a progressive decrease in clinical viability of skin stored in a refrigerator at 3°C over a three week period (Georgiade and associates, 1956).

PRESERVATION BY FREEZING AND FREEZE DRYING

Injury to biologic systems preserved at low temperature has been attributed to the mechanical rupture and displacement of cytologic structures by growing ice crystals (Chambers and Hale, 1932) and to the forces of expansion and contraction accompanying temperature changes (Luyet and Gehenio, 1940). The failure to resume activities after freezing and drying has been attributed to changes in the concentration of electrolytes (Lovelock, 1953) by dehydration and the break-up of essential proteins and enzymes. These possibilities have been considered by investigators who have attempted to reduce mechanical distortions and physiologic changes within the cellular structures by treating the skin with dilute sera, physiologic media, or other protective agents before freezing and thawing.

Storage of Donor Skin in Frozen State. Early experimental evidence of the survival of mammalian skin was submitted by Mider and Morton in 1939: pieces of rat skin were frozen to −50°C and then grafted subcutaneously. Best results were obtained when the grafts were slowly frozen; the survival of some of the cells was evidenced by epithelial cyst formation and the presence of mitotic figures. Similar findings were observed in rat tissue frozen to −74°C, stored for 24 hours, thawed, and examined histologically ten days after transplantation. Briggs and Jund (1944) obtained successfully orthotopic transplantations of skin grafts in mice after the grafts were slowly frozen to −78.5°C, stored in dry ice for one to two days, and thawed. The successful application of frozen split-thickness autografts of human skin that had been frozen at −20°C to −25°C and stored below −15°C for one to six days was reported by Strumia and Hodge in 1945.

The discovery by Polge, Smith, and Parkes (1949) that treatment with glycerol solution offered considerable protection to spermatozoa against the injury of freezing gave impetus to research on the effects of protective treatment with glycerol and ethylene glycol to preserve skin (Billingham and Medawar, 1952; Keeley, Gomez, and Brown, 1952; Taylor and Gerstner, 1956). The action of glycerol protection against freezing was described by Lovelock (1953; 1954), who considered it a buffer against the harmful concentration of salt.

Stereomicroscopic observations were undertaken by Taylor, Gerstner, and Converse (1956) in order to follow the course of vascular changes in mammalian grafts preserved at temperatures below freezing. Revascularization was always delayed in frozen grafts, occurring as late as five to seven days after transplantation. In contrast, revascularization occurred within three days in untreated grafts. The effect of the various freezing and thawing treatments and of various cryoprotective agents on the viability and fate of the orthotopic skin grafts was correlated with the in vitro culture tests. The results were in agreement with the tissue culture experiments, showing a marked protective effect of pretreatment with glycerol and ethylene glycol.

Experimenting with full-thickness rat skin, Santoni-Rugiu (1962) observed that the rate of survival of deep frozen skin stored for 14 days at −70°C was 40 per cent. It was concluded that the reduced viability of deep frozen allografts is responsible for their superiority to fresh allografts when transferred to recipient animals. Using 15% glycerol in Ringer's solution as the cryoprotective medium, Bondoc and Burke (1971) observed that split-thickness skin taken from guinea pigs, live human donors, or cadavers within ten hours after death could be stored at −160°C with liquid nitrogen for up to six months. Their clinical and radiographic findings demonstrated no difference in the appearance of the graft vascularization and epidermal activity between the frozen, banked skin grafts and the freshly harvested grafts. In addition, Lawrence (1972) noted that the metabolic activity of guinea pig ear skin and human split-thickness skin grafts treated with 15% glycerol and stored in liquid nitrogen for periods of up to 28 days was 60 to 70 per cent of its original activity. These reports suggest that, for effective protection against freezing injury, freshly excised donor skin should be treated with a suitable protective medium, slowly frozen, and rapidly thawed.

Cryophylactic Action of Dimethyl Sulfoxide. The efficacy of dimethyl sulfoxide (DMSO) as a protective medium for skin storage at temperatures below freezing was evaluated by Lehr and associates (1964) and Barlyn, Berggren, and Lehr (1964). Segments of split-thickness skin removed from the rat abdomen were impregnated with various cryophylactic media for 20 to 30 minutes at room temperature, stored at 4° to 7°C over various periods of time, and then autografted. Preliminary findings indicated that under ideal conditions, glycerol and DMSO, in a concentration of 10% in either normal saline or serum, were comparable and seemed most effective in protecting grafts from the effects of the freezing and thawing process. Other observations showed that skin could be successfully transplanted after a storage period of seven days, and none survived when stored for 14 days.

Using gross and stereomicroscopic methods of observation, Berggren and Lehr (1965) reported that some human split-thickness autografts and allografts became effectively vascularized following treatment with 10 per cent dimethyl sulfoxide solution and storage in the frozen state for periods of up to 608 days. If the grafts were not viable, they indicated no evidence of vascularization and consequently became soft, white, and nonadherent.

In similar experiments with full-thickness skin autografts in the mouse, Sherman (1965) observed that both DMSO and glycerol protected tissues from injury by freezing and thawing. His technique consisted of immersing tissue segments in 5 per cent or 15 per cent volume solutions of glycerol or DMSO in Ringer's solution for one hour at 22°C. The tissue was subsequently frozen to −75°C at the rate of 1.3°C per minute, followed by thawing (in 22°C Ringer's solution at the rate of 180°C per minute) and transplantation. It was concluded that DMSO is at least as protective and toxic as glycerol, and that the 5 per cent solutions of DMSO and glycerol are less toxic and produce a greater freeze-thaw survival than the 15 per cent solutions.

On the other hand, from experience with guinea pig ear skin and split-thickness human skin stored in liquid nitrogen for two days, Lawrence (1972) reported that 15 per cent glycerol is superior to 15 per cent DMSO as a cryoprotective agent; the latter has been found to be more toxic after prolonged contact.

Other Experimental Studies. In 1970 Rappaport, Pepino, and Dietrick cited histologic similarities between the frozen irradiated and fresh refrigerated split-thickness porcine skin grafts placed on dogs, and observed no evidence of graft vascularization. Clinically, the porcine grafts provided an effective biologic dressing in the burn patient and an appreciable reduction in pain, particularly over second degree burns.

According to O'Donoghue and Zarem (1971), from direct examination of blood vessels within the mouse transparent chamber, the preserved isografts are capable of inducing hyperemia and neovascularization in the recipient bed and of becoming vascularized. Hyperemia appears in the host beds of the lyophilized grafts and the frozen thawed grafts by the fifth day after grafting; neovascularization occurs on the seventh and eighth days in respective beds. The vascularization of the grafts is completely achieved by the 10th and 11th days, respectively. It is of interest that lyophilized grafts seem to be more effective in inducing the host vascular budding and penetration into the lyophilized graft than are frozen thawed grafts. Similar results were reported by Rogers and Converse (1958) in an earlier study using fresh and freeze dried bovine embryo skin grafts transplanted to defects in man. With the same mouse chamber technique, Pandya and Zarem (1974) were unable to demonstrate vascularization in either vacuum dried or frozen xenografts of porcine split-thickness skin on mice during 15 days of observation.

Studies on Freeze Dried Skin Autografts and Allografts. Freeze drying nearly satisfies the requirements of a preservative method since it maintains most of the structural details of cells and presumably leaves many of the proteins and enzymes of the tissue intact. The process involves rapid freezing of the tissue by immersing it in liquid nitrogen or chilled isopentane. High speed freezing reduces the mechanical distortion of the microscopic structure caused by the slow growth of ice crystals in and between the cells. This tissue is subsequently kept frozen while water is removed from the solid state by sublimation. The dried tissue is usually sealed in a vacuum and stored at room temperature.

Billingham and Medawar (1952) made a quantitative study of the ability of rabbit skin to survive dehydration from the frozen state. Particular attention was given to calculating the water content of the skin at the completion of the drying process. Findings indicated that skin could not survive a state of dehydration in which the final overall water content was less than 25 per cent. Pretreatment of the tissue with glycerol solution did not increase the ability to withstand drying.

Buchanan and Lehman (1952) reported that freeze dried split-thickness skin grafts in the dog persist for only a short period of up to 22 days. Autografts and allografts dehydrated to within 36 to 41 per cent of their original weight endured for an approximately equal length of time.

Several subsequent studies indicating the lack of any significant immunologic reactions in the host in response to freeze dried skin allografts were reported by Sell, Hyatt, and Gresham (1962) in burned patients, Yukna and associates (1977) in humans, Yukna, Turner, and Robinson (1977) in guinea pigs, and Abbott and Hembree (1970) in mice.

Subsequently, freeze dried allogeneic skin grafts have been primarily used and studied in the oral environment (Gregory, Triplett, and Connole, 1983) as well as for the treatment of human mucogingival problems (Ouhayuon and associates, 1983).

Evaluation of Freeze Dried Skin Xenografts. Nonviable, freeze dried skin grafts removed from bovine embryos and placed on the chorioallantois of the chick embryo are readily penetrated by the membranous blood vessels, but at a reduced rate when compared with viable and untreated skin xenografts (Converse and associates, 1958). Rogers and Converse (1958) observed in histologic sections of fresh and freeze dried embryonic bovine skin applied to defects in man that endothelial buds from the host bed had grown into the graft; these disintegrated within ten days.

On the basis of combined gross, histologic, and angiographic examinations, Eastwood (1961) maintained that freeze dried grafts of pig skin are firmly adherent to the host bed of rats, with clear evidence of vascularization at seven to nine days, and provide an effective cover for an average of 14 days, compared with 21 days for freeze dried allografts of rat skin. Subsequently the porcine graft disintegrates, coinciding with the appearance of patches of superficial desquamation and discoloration.

Bromberg, Song, and Mohn (1965), working with freeze dried split-thickness pig skin grafts transplanted to mice, found no evidence of vascularization, although these grafts remained soft with a minimal inflammatory reaction for two weeks. Toranto, Salyer, and Myers (1974) were unable to distinguish vascularization of freeze dried porcine split-thickness skin grafts transplanted to humans and rats from the invasion of the graft-host interface by granulation tissue.

Summary. The findings appear to support the concept that the revascularization of frozen or freeze dried skin grafts applied to humans or animals is not entirely dependent on the viability of the original graft vasculature. As demonstrated in a study by Ballantyne and associates (1971), vascular ingrowth from the host site can occur readily, provided the pattern of tissue grafts after preservation at low temperature is not unduly disorganized. However, Bromberg, Song, and Mohn (1965), working with freeze dried split-thickness pig xenografts transplanted to mice, found no evidence of revascularization.

REFERENCES

Clinical Aspects

Adeymo, C., and Wyburn, G. M.: Innervation of skin grafts. Transplant. Bull., *4*:152, 1957.

Ballantyne, D. L., and Converse, J. M.: Experimental Skin Grafts and Transplantation Immunity: A Recapitulation. New York, Springer-Verlag, 1979.

Baran, N. K., and Horton, C. E.: Growth of skin grafts, flaps and scars in young minipigs. Plast. Reconstr. Surg., *50*:487, 1972.

Barker, D. E.: Vacutome, a new machine for obtaining split-thickness skin grafts. Plast. Reconstr. Surg., *3*:492, 1948.

Barker, D. E.: Skin thickness in the human. Plast. Reconstr. Surg., *7*:115, 1951.

Baronio, G.: Degli Innesti Animali. Milan, Stamperia e Fonderia del Genio, 1804.

Bennett, J. E., and Miller, S. R.: Evolution of the electrodermatome. Plast. Reconstr. Surg., *45*:131, 1970.

Billingham, R. E., and Silvers, W. K.: The origin and conservation of epidermal specificities. N. Engl. J. Med., *268*:477, 539, 1963.

Billingham, R. E., and Silvers, W. K.: Studies on the conservation of epidermal specificities of skin and certain mucosas in adult mammals. J. Exp. Med., *125*:429, 1967.

Blair, V. P., and Brown, J. B.: The use and uses of large split skin grafts of intermediate thickness. Surg. Gynecol. Obstet., *49*:82, 1929.

Braun-Falco, O.: The Pathology of Blister Formation. *In* Kopf, A. W., and Andrade, R. (Eds.): 1969 Year Book of Dermatology. Chicago, Year Book Medical Publishers, 1969.

Briggaman, R. A., and Wheeler, C. E., Jr.: Epidermal-dermal interactions in adult human skin: role of dermis in epidermal maintenance. J. Invest. Dermatol., *51*:454, 1968.

Bromberg, B. E., Song, I. C., and Mohn, M. P.: The use of pig skin as a temporary biological dressing. Plast. Reconstr. Surg., *36*:80, 1965.

Brown, J. B., Fryer, M. P., Randall, P., and Lu, M.: Postmortem homografts as "biological dressings" for extensive burns and denuded areas. Immediate and preserved homografts as life-saving procedures. Ann. Surg., *138*:618, 1953.

Brown, J. B., and McDowell, F.: Skin Grafting. 3rd Ed. Philadelphia, J. B. Lippincott Company, 1958.

Bünger, C.: Gelungener Versuch einer Nasenbildung aus einem völlig getrennten Hautstück aus dem Beine. J. d. Chir. Augenh., *4*:569, 1822.

Burke, J. F., Yannas, I. V., Quinby, W. C., Jr., et al.: Successful use of a physiologically acceptable artificial skin in the treatment of extensive burn injury. Ann. Surg., *194*:413, 1981.

Burleson, R., and Eiseman, B.: Nature of the bond between partial-thickness skin and wound granulations. Surgery, *72*:315, 1972.

Butcher, H. R., and Hoover, A. L.: Abnormalities of human superficial cutaneous lymphatics associated with stasis ulcers, lymphedema, scars and cutaneous autografts. Ann. Surg., *142*:633, 1955.

Chase, R. A.: Atlas of Hand Surgery. Philadelphia, W. B. Saunders Company, 1973, pp. 40–55, 166–167.

Clemmesen, T., and Ronhovde, D. A.: Restoration of the blood supply to human skin autografts. Scand. J. Plast. Reconstr. Surg., *2*:44, 1968.

Cohen, J.: Dermis, epidermis and dermal papillae interacting. Adv. Biol. Skin, *9*:1, 1969.

Converse, J. M., and Ballantyne, D. L., Jr.: Distribution of diphosphopyridine nucleotide diaphorase in rat skin autografts and homografts. Plast. Reconstr. Surg., *30*:415, 1962.

Converse, J. M., and Robb-Smith, A. H. T.: The healing of surface cutaneous wounds: its analogy with the healing of superficial burns. Ann. Surg., *120*:873, 1944.

Converse, J. M., Šmahel, J., Ballantyne, D. L., Jr., and Harper, A. D.: Inosculation of vessels of skin graft and host bed: a fortuitous encounter. Br. J. Plast. Surg., *28*:274, 1975.

Corps, B. V.: The effect of graft thickness, donor site and graft bed on graft shrinkage in the hooded rat. Br. J. Plast. Surg., *22*:125, 1969.

Creech, B. J., Devito, R. V., and Eade, G. G.: Viability of split-skin grafts from pigs following incubation on autologous blood or serum for various periods. Plast. Reconstr. Surg., *51*:572, 1973.

Cronin, T. D.: The use of a molded splint to prevent contracture after split skin grafting on the neck. Plast. Reconstr. Surg., *27*:7, 1961.

Davis, J. S., and Kitlowski, E. A.: The immediate contraction of cutaneous grafts and its cause. Arch. Surg., *23*:954, 1931.

Davis, J. S., and Kitlowski, E. A.: Regeneration of nerves in skin grafts and skin flaps. Am. J. Surg., *24*:501, 1934.

Donoff, R. B., and Grillo, H. C.: The effects of skin grafting on healing open wounds in rabbits. J. Surg. Res., *19*:163, 1975.

Doupe, J., and Sharp, M. E.: Studies in denervation: sebaceous secretion. J. Neurol. Psychiatr., *6*:133, 1943.

Eade, G. G.: The relationship between granulation tissue, bacteria and skin grafts in burned patients. Plast. Reconstr. Surg., *22*:42, 1958.

Edgerton, M. T., and Hansen, F. C.: Matching facial color with split-thickness skin grafts from adjacent areas. Plast. Reconstr. Surg., *25*:455, 1960.

Edlich, R. F., Prusak, M. P., Schmolka, I. R., and Edgerton, M. J.: The molecular basis for toxicity of surfactants in surgical wounds. J. Surg. Res., *14*:277, 1973.

Elliott, R. A., Jr., and Hoehn, J. G.: Use of commercial porcine skin for wound dressings. Plast. Reconstr. Surg., *52*:401, 1973.

Eriksson, G.: Studies in Regeneration and Autotransplantation of Epidermis in Man. Uppsala, Almqvist & Wiksell, 1972.

Fitzgerald, M. J., Martin, F., and Paletta, F. X.: Innervation of skin grafts. Surg. Gynecol. Obstet., *124*:808, 1967.

Flemming, W.: Zur Kenntniss der Regeneration der Epidermis beim Säugethier. Arch. f. Mikr. Anat., *23*:148, 1884.

Furnas, D. W.: Frost anesthesia for skin grafts. Plast. Reconstr. Surg., *35*:191, 1965.

Gabbiani, G., Hirschel, B. J., Ryan, G. B., Statkov, P. R., and Majno, G.: Granulation tissue as a contractile organ. A study of structure and function. J. Exp. Med., *135*:719, 1972.

Gallico, G. G., III, and O'Connor, N. E.: Cultured epithelium as a skin substitute. Clin. Plast. Surg., *12*:149, 1985.

Georgiade, N. G., Perschel, E., and Brown, I.: A clinical and experimental investigation of the preservation of skin. Plast. Reconstr. Surg., *17*:267, 1956.

Gillman, T., Penn, J., Bronks, D., and Roux, M.: Reactions of healing wounds and granulation tissue in man to auto-thiersch, autodermal and homodermal grafts. Br. J. Plast. Surg., *6*:153, 1953.

Gingrass, P., Grabb, W. C., and Gingrass, R. P.: Skin graft survival on avascular defects. Plast. Reconstr. Surg., *55*:65, 1975.

Goulian, D., Jr.: A new economical dermatome. Plast. Reconstr. Surg., *42*:85, 1968.

Graham, W. P., III: Allografting split-thickness skin donor sites. Surgery, *66*:460, 1969.

Guber, S., and Rudolph, R.: Collective review—the myofibroblast. Surg. Gynecol. Obstet., *146*:641, 1978.

Hagstrom, W. J., Jr., Nassos, T. P., Boswick, J. A., Jr., and Stuteville, O. H.: The importance of occlusive dressings in the treatment of mesh skin grafts. Plast. Reconstr. Surg., *38*:137, 1966.

Hamilton, J. B.: Patterned loss of hair in man: types and incidence. Ann. N.Y. Acad. Sci., *53*:708, 1951.

Hilgert, I.: Changes in the hydroxyproline and hexosamine content of grafts after transplantation. Folia Biol. (Praha), *9*:136, 1963.

Hinshaw, J. R., and Miller, E. R.: Histology of healing split-thickness, full-thickness autogenous skin grafts and donor sites. Arch. Surg., *91*:658, 1965.

Hutchison, J., Tough, J. S., and Wyburn, G. M.: Regeneration of sensation in grafted skin. Br. J. Plast. Surg., *2*:82, 1949.

Hynes, W.: The skin-dermis graft as an alternative to the direct or tubed flap. Br. J. Plast. Surg., *7*:97, 1954.

Hynes, W.: The treatment of pigmented moles by shaving and skin graft. Br. J. Plast. Surg., *9*:47, 1956.

Hynes, W.: The treatment of scars by shaving and skin graft. Br. J. Plast. Surg., *10*:1, 1957.

Hynes, W.: "Shaving" in plastic surgery with special reference to the treatment of chronic radiodermatitis. Br. J. Plast. Surg., *12*:43, 1959.

Jackson, D. M., and Stone, P. A.: Tangential excision and grafting of burns. The method, and a report of 50 consecutive cases. Br. J. Plast. Surg., *25*:416, 1972.

Keswani, R. K., and Goel, N. K.: Contraction and relaxation in split skin autografts—a human study. Indian J. Plast. Surg., *7*:46, 1974.

Kikuchi, I., and Omori, M.: Demonstration of leaking vessels under skin grafts. Plast. Reconstr. Surg., *45*:66, 1970.

Klein, L., and Rudolph, R.: ^{3}H-Collagen turnover in skin grafts. Surg. Gynecol. Obstet., *135*:49, 1972.

Klein, L., and Rudolph, R.: Turnover of soluble and insoluble ^{3}H-collagens in skin grafts. Surg. Gynecol. Obstet., *139*:883, 1974.

Krause, F.: Über die Transplantation grosser ungestielter Hautlappen. Verh. Dtsch. Ges. Chir., *22*:46, 1893.

Lawson, G.: On the transplantation of portions of skin for the closure of large granulating surfaces. Tr. Clin. Soc. Lond., *4*:49, 1871.

Le Fort, L.: Blépharoplastie par un lambeau complètement détaché du bras et reporté à la face; insuccès. Bull. Soc. Chir. Paris, *1*:39, 1872.

Lehman, J. A., Jr., and Saddawi, N.: Delayed open skin grafting. Br. J. Plast. Surg., *28*:46, 1975.

Littlewood, A. H. M.: Seroma: an unrecognised cause of failure of split-thickness skin grafts. Br. J. Plast. Surg., *13*:42, 1960.

Löfgren, L.: Recovery of nervous functions in skin transplants with special reference to the sympathetic functions. Acta Chir. Scand., *102*:229, 1951.

Lopez-Mas, J., Ortiz-Monasterio, F., Viale De Gonzales, M., and Olmedo, A.: Skin graft pigmentation. A new approach to prevention. Plast. Reconstr. Surg., *49*:18, 1972.

Majno, G., Gabbiani, G., Hirschel, B. J., Ryan, G. B., and Statkov, P. R.: Contraction of granulation tissue in vitro: similarity to smooth muscle. Science, *173*:548, 1971.

Marckmann, A.: Autologous skin grafts in the rat. Uptake of ^{35}S-sulfate. Proc. Soc. Exp. Biol. Med., *119*:557, 1965a.

Marckmann, A.: Autologous skin grafts in the rat. Biochemical analysis of mucopolysaccharides and hydroxyproline. Proc. Soc. Exp. Biol. Med., *119*:794, 1965b.

McGregor, I. A.: The regeneration of sympathetic activity in grafted skin as evidenced by sweating. Br. J. Plast. Surg., *3*:12, 1950.

Medawar, P. B.: The behaviour and fate of skin autografts and skin homografts in rabbits. J. Anat., *78*:176, 1944.

Medawar, P. B.: The micro-anatomy of mammalian skin. Q. J. Microscop. Sci., *94*:481, 1953.

Miller, T. A.: The deleterious effect of split-skin homograft coverage on split-skin donor sites. Plast. Reconstr. Surg., *53*:316, 1974.

Mir y Mir, L.: The problem of pigmentation in the cutaneous graft. Br. J. Plast. Surg., *14*:303, 1961.

Montagna, W.: The Structure and Function of Skin. 2nd Ed. New York, Academic Press, 1962.

Narjarian, J. S., Crane, J. T., and McCorkle, H. J.: An experimental study of the grafting of a suspension of skin particles. Surgery, *42*:218, 1957.

Ollier, L.: Sur les greffes cutanées ou autoplastiques. Bull. Acad. de Med. (Paris), *1*:243, 1872.

Orentreich, N.: Autografts in alopecias and other selected dermatological conditions. Ann. N.Y. Acad. Sci., *83*:463, 1959.

Padgett, E. C.: Calibrated intermediate skin grafts. Surg. Gynecol. Obstet., *69*:779, 1939.

Polk, H. C.: Adherence of thin skin grafts. Surg. Forum, *17*:487, 1966.

Pontén, B.: Grafted skin—observations on innervation and other qualities. Acta Chir. Scand. [Suppl.], *257*:1, 1960.

Ragnell, A.: The secondary contracting tendency of free skin grafts. Br. J. Plast. Surg., *5*:6, 1953.

Rees, T. D., and Casson, P. R.: The indications for cutaneous dermal overgrafting. Plast. Reconstr. Surg., *38*:522, 1966.

Réverdin, J. L.: De la greffe épidermique. Arch. Gen. de Med., *19*:276, 555, 703, 1872.

Robinson, D. W.: Blood loss from donor sites in skin grafting procedures. Surgery, *25*:105, 1949.

Robson, M. C., and Krizek, T. J.: Predicting skin graft survival. J. Trauma, *13*:213, 1973.

Rogers, B. O.: Historical development of free skin grafting. Surg. Clin. North Am., *39*:289, 1959.

Rudolph, R.: The effect of skin graft preparation on wound contraction. Surg. Gynecol. Obstet., *142*:49, 1976.

Rudolph, R.: Skin Grafting. *In* Goldwyn, R. M. (Ed.): The Unfavorable Result in Plastic Surgery: Avoidance and Treatment. 2nd Ed. Boston, Little, Brown & Company, 1984, pp. 143–149.

Rudolph, R., Earle, A. S., and Fratianné, R. B.: Reduction mammaplasty and other skin excisions as a source of homograft skin. Br. J. Plast. Surg., *28*:121, 1975.

Rudolph, R., Fisher, J. C., and Ninnemann, J. L.: Skin Grafting. Boston, Little, Brown & Company, 1979, pp. 1–205.

Rudolph, R., Guber, S., Suzuki, M., and Woodward, M.: The life cycle of the myofibroblast. Surg. Gynecol. Obstet., *145*:389, 1977.

Rudolph, R., Guber, S., and Woodward, M.: Inhibition of myofibroblasts by skin grafts. Plast. Reconstr. Surg., *63*:473, 1979.

Rudolph, R., and Klein, L.: Pathways of radioactive collagen loss from skin grafts. Surg. Gynecol. Obstet., *138*:55, 1974.

Rudolph, R., and Linnevold, R.: Rapid harvesting of precise split-thickness skin grafts in small animals. J. Invest. Dermatol., *57*:180, 1971.

Rudolph, R., and Milson, T.: Species differences in trypsin separation of epidermis and dermis. Plast. Reconstr. Surg., *58*:459, 1976.

Rudolph, R., and Noe, J. (Eds.): Chronic Problem Wounds. Boston, Little, Brown, & Company, 1983, pp. 1–8, 65–74, 87–94.

Rudolph, R., Suzuki, M., and Guber, S.: Free skin grafting in the pig. Br. J. Plast. Surg., *31*:227, 1978.

Rushmer, R. F., Buettner, K. J. K., Short, J. M., and Odland, G. F.: The skin. Science, *154*:343, 1966.

Sawhney, C. P., Subbaraju, G. V., and Chakravarti, R.

N.: Healing of donor sites of split skin graft. Br. J. Plast. Surg., *22*:359, 1969.

Scothorne, R. J., and Scothorne, A. W.: Histochemical studies on human skin autografts. J. Anat., *87*:22, 1953.

Scothorne, R. J., and Tough, J. S.: Histochemical studies of human skin autografts and homografts. Br. J. Plast. Surg., *5*:161, 1952.

Shepard, G. H.: The storage of split-skin grafts on their donor sites. Plast. Reconstr. Surg., *49*:115, 1972.

Šmahel, J., and Clodius, L.: The blood vessel system of free human skin grafts. Plast. Reconstr. Surg., *47*:61, 1971.

Southwood, W. F. W.: The thickness of the skin. Plast. Reconstr. Surg., *15*:423, 1955.

Stone, P. A., and Madden, J. W.: Effect of primary and delayed skin grafting on wound contraction. Surg. Forum, *25*:41, 1974.

Storey, W. F., and LeBlond, C. P.: Measurement of the rate of proliferation of epidermis and associated structures. Ann. N.Y. Acad. Sci., *53*:537, 1951.

Tanner, J. C., Jr., Vandeput, J., and Olley, J. F.: The mesh skin graft. Plast. Reconstr. Surg., *34*:287, 1964.

Tavis, M. J., Thornton, J. W., Harney, J. H., Danet, R. T., Woodroof, A., and Bartlett, R. H.: Mechanism of skin graft adherence: collagen, elastin and fibrin interactions. Surg. Forum, *28*:522, 1977.

Taylor, A. C., Gerstner, R., and Converse, J. M.: Preservation of skin grafts by refrigeration for reconstructive surgery. Plast. Reconstr. Surg., *18*:275, 1956.

Terzis, J. K.: Functional aspects of reinnervation of free skin grafts. Plast. Reconstr. Surg., *58*:142, 1976.

Thiersch, C.: Ueber die feineren anatomischen Veränderungen bei Aufheilung von Haut auf Granulationen. Verh. Dtsch. Ger. Chir., *3*:69, 1874.

Thiersch, C.: Ueber Hautverpflanzung. Verh. Dtsch. Ger. Chir., *5*:17, 1886.

Thompson, N.: A clinical and histological investigation into the fate of epithelial elements buried following the grafting of "shaved" skin surfaces. Br. J. Plast. Surg., *13*:219, 1960.

Thompson, N.: Dermal Overgrafting. *In* Converse, J. M. (Ed.): Reconstructive Plastic Surgery. 2nd Ed. Philadelphia, W. B. Saunders Company, 1977, pp. 183–188.

Thompson, N., and Ell, P. J.: Dermal overgrafting in the treatment of venous stasis ulcers. Plast. Reconstr. Surg., *54*:290, 1974.

Tsukada, S.: Studies on the pigmentation of skin grafts: the ultrastructure of epidermal melanocytes. Plast. Reconstr. Surg., *59*:98, 1977.

Unna, P. G.: Handbuch der Hautkrankheiten. Leipzig, F. C. W. Vogel, 1883.

Van Scott, E. J., and Reinertson, R. P.: The modulating influence of stromal environment on epithelial cells studied in human autotransplants. J. Invest. Dermatol., *36*:109, 1961.

Vecchione, T. R.: A technique for obtaining uniform split-thickness skin grafts. Arch. Surg., *109*:837, 1974.

Vecchione, T. R.: Hair growth as a late sequela in skin grafts from the groin. Br. J. Plast. Surg., *30*:52, 1977.

Webster, G. V., Peterson, R. A., and Stein, H. L.: Dermal overgrafting of the leg. J. Bone Joint Surg., *40A*:4,796, 1958.

Wexler, M. R., and Oneal, R. M.: Areolar sharing to reconstruct the absent nipple. Plast. Reconstr. Surg., *51*:176, 1973.

Wolfe, J. R.: A new method for performing plastic operations. Br. Med. J., *2*:360, 1875.

Wolff, K., and Schellander, F. G.: Enzyme-histochemical studies on the healing process of split skin grafts. I. Aminopeptidase, diphosphopyridine-nucleotide-diaphorase and succinic dehydrogenase in autografts. J. Invest. Dermatol., *45*:38, 1965.

Wolff, K., and Schellander, F. G.: Enzyme-histochemical studies on the healing process of split skin grafts. II. 5-Nucleotidase, adenosinetriphosphatase, acid and alkaline phosphatase in autografts. J. Invest. Dermatol., *46*:205, 1966.

Ye, R. C.: The relationship of pH of the granulation tissue and the take of the skin graft. Plast. Reconstr. Surg., *19*:213, 1957.

Zika, J., Rudolph, R., and Klein, L.: Autoradiographic distribution of collagen loss in skin grafts. Anat. Rec., *177*:377, 1973.

Biologic Behavior

Abbott, W. M., and Hembree, J. S.: Absence of antigenicity in freeze-dried skin allografts. Cryobiology, *6*:416, 1970.

Allgöwer, M., and Blocker, T. G., Jr.: Viability of skin in relation to various methods of storage. Tex. Rep. Biol. Med., *10*:3, 1952.

Alsbjörn, B.: In search of an ideal skin substitute. Scand. J. Plast. Reconstr. Surg., *18*:127, 1984.

Antopol, W., Glaubach, S., and Goldman, L.: The use of neotetrazolium as a tool in the study of active cell processes. Trans. N.Y. Acad. Sci., *12*:156, 1950.

Artz, C. P., Rittenbury, M. S., and Yarbrough, D. R., III: An appraisal of allografts and xenografts as biological dressings for wounds and burns. Ann. Surg., *175*:934, 1972.

Ballantyne, D. L., Jr., and Converse, J. M.: The relation of hair cycles to the survival time of suprapannicular and subpannicular skin homografts in rats. Ann. N.Y. Acad. Sci., *64*:958, 1957.

Ballantyne, D. L., Jr., and Converse, J. M.: Vascularization of composite auricular grafts transplanted to the chorio-allantois of the chick embryo. Transplant. Bull., *5*:373, 1958.

Ballantyne, D. L., Jr., Hawthorne, G. A., Rees, T. D., and Seidman, I.: An experimental evaluation of skin graft preservation with silicone fluid. Cryobiology, *8*:211, 1971.

Ballantyne, D. L., Jr., Uhlschmid, G. K., and Converse, J. M.: Massive rabbit skin xenografts in rats. Transplantation, *7*:274, 1969.

Barlyn, L. W., Berggren, R. B., and Lehr, H. B.: Frozen skin autografts protected by dimethyl sulfoxide. Surg. Forum, *15*:475, 1964.

Bellman, S., and Velander, E.: Vascular reaction following experimental transplantation of free full thickness skin grafts. *In* Transactions of the International Society of Plastic Surgeons, First Congress, Stockholm and Uppsala, 1955. Baltimore, Williams & Wilkins, 1957, p. 493.

Bellman, S., Velander, E., Frank, H. A., and Lambert, P. B.: Survival of arteries in experimental full-thickness skin autografts. Transplantation, *2*:167, 1964.

Ben-Hur, N., Solowey, A. C., and Rapaport, F. T.: The xenograft rejection phenomenon. I. Response of the mouse to rabbit, guinea pig and rat skin xenografts. Isr. J. Med. Sci., *5*:1, 1969a.

Ben-Hur, N., Solowey, A. C., and Rapaport, F. T.: The xenograft rejection phenomenon. II. Response of the guinea pig to mouse, rat and rabbit skin xenografts. Isr. J. Med. Sci., *5*:322, 1969b.

Berggren, R. B., and Lehr, H. B.: Clinical use of viable frozen human skin. J.A.M.A., *194*:129, 1965.

Bert, P.: De la Greffe Animale. Paris, J. B. Ballière et Fils, 1863.
Billingham, R. E., and Medawar, P. B.: The freezing, drying and storage of mammalian skin. Br. J. Exp. Biol., *29*:454, 1952.
Birch, J., and Brånemark, P.-I.: The vascularization of a free full thickness skin graft. I. A vital microscopic study. Scand. J. Plast. Reconstr. Surg., *3*:1, 1969.
Birch, J., Brånemark, P.-I., and Lundskog, J.: The vascularization of a free full thickness skin graft. II. A microangiographic study. Scand. J. Plast. Reconstr., *3*:11, 1969.
Bondoc, C. C., and Burke, J. F.: Clinical experience with viable frozen human skin and a frozen skin bank. Ann. Surg., *174*:371, 1971.
Brånemark, P.-I., and Lindström, J.: A modified rabbit's ear chamber. High-power, high-resolution studies in regenerated and preformed tissues. Anat. Rec., *145*:533, 1963.
Braun, W.: Klinisch-histologische Untersuchungen über die Anheilung ungestielter Hautlappen. Beitr. Klin. Chir., *25*:211, 1899.
Briggs, R., and Jund, L.: Successful grafting of frozen and thawed mouse skin. Anat. Rec., *89*:75, 1944.
Bromberg, B. E., and Song, I. C.: Skin substitutes, homo-, and heterografts. Am. J. Surg., *112*:28, 1966.
Bromberg, B. E., Song, I. C., and Mohn, M. P.: The use of pig skin as a temporary biological dressing. Plast. Reconstr. Surg., *36*:80, 1965.
Brown, J. B., Fryer, M. P., Randall, P., and Lu, M.: Postmortem homografts as "biological dressings" for extensive burns and denuded areas. Immediate and preserved homografts as life-saving procedures. Ann. Surg., *138*:618, 1953.
Buchanan, F. T., and Lehman, E. P.: An experimental study of preservation of skin grafts by the freeze-drying process. Surg. Forum, *2*:637, 1952.
Burleson, R., and Eiseman, B.: Nature of the bond between partial-thickness skin and wound granulations. Surgery, *72*:315, 1972.
Burleson, R., and Eiseman, B.: Mechanisms of antibacterial effect of biologic dressings. Ann. Surg., *177*:181, 1973.
Burns Unit, First Affiliated Hospital of Hou, Number 2 Unit, Chinese People's Liberation Army.: A review of the management of extensive third degree burns in 14 successive years. Chin. Med. J., *11*(Nov.):673, 1973.
Casson, P., Solowey, A. C., Converse, J. M., and Rapaport, F. T.: Delayed hypersensitivity status of burned patients. Surg. Forum, *17*:268, 1966.
Ceppellini, R., Curtoni, E. S., Mattiuz, P. L., Leigheb, G., Visetti, M., and Colombi, A.: Survival of test skin grafts in man: effect of genetic relationship and of blood groups incompatibility. Ann. N.Y. Acad. Sci., *129*:421, 1966.
Chambers, R., and Hale, H. P.: The formation of ice in protoplasm. Proc. R. Soc. Lond. [Biol.], *110*:336, 1932.
Clemmesen, T.: The early circulation in split skin grafts. Acta Chir. Scand., *124*:11, 1962.
Clemmesen, T.: The early circulation in split-skin grafts. Restoration of blood supply to split-skin autografts. Acta Chir. Scand., *127*:1, 1964.
Clemmesen, T.: Experimental studies on the healing of free skin autografts. Dan. Med. Bull., *14*[Suppl. II]:1, 1967.
Colson, P., Leclerq, P., Gangolphe, M., Houot, R., Janvier, H., and Prunieras, M.: Utilisation des homogreffes alternées avec des autogreffes dans le traitement des grand brules. II. Étude histo-biologique. Ann. Chir. Plast., *4*:177, 1959.
Converse, J. M., and Ballantyne, D. L., Jr.: Distribution of diphosphopyridine nucleotide diaphorase in rat skin autografts and homografts. Plast. Reconstr. Surg., *30*:415, 1962.
Converse, J. M., and Rapaport, F. T.: The vascularization of skin autografts and homografts; an experimental study in man. Ann. Surg., *143*:306, 1956.
Converse, J. M., Ballantyne, D. L., Jr., Rogers, B. O., and Raisbeck, A. P.: "Plasmatic circulation" in skin grafts. Transplant. Bull., *4*:154, 1957.
Converse, J. M., Ballantyne, D. L., Jr., Rogers, B. O., and Raisbeck, A. P.: A study of viable and non-viable skin grafts transplanted to the chorio-allantoic membrane of the chick embryo. Transplant. Bull., *5*:108, 1958.
Converse, J. M., Filler, M., and Ballantyne, D. L., Jr.: Vascularization of split-thickness skin autografts in the rat. Transplantation, *3*:22, 1965.
Converse, J. M., Šmahel, J., Ballantyne, D. L., Jr., and Harper, A. D.: Inosculation of vessels of skin graft and host bed: a fortuitous encounter. Br. J. Plast. Surg., *28*:274, 1975.
Converse, J. M., Uhlschmid, G. K., and Ballantyne, D. L., Jr.: "Plasmatic circulation" in skin grafts. The phase of serum imbibition. Plast. Reconstr. Surg., *43*:495, 1969.
Conway, H., Griffith, B. H., Shannon, J. E., Jr., and Findley, A.: Re-examination of the transparent chamber technique as applied to the study of circulation in autografts and homografts of the skin. Plast. Reconstr. Surg., *20*:103, 1957.
Conway, H., Joslin, D., Rees, T. D., and Stark, R. B.: Observations on the development of circulation in skin grafts. III. Morphologic changes observed in homologous skin grafts. Plast. Reconstr. Surg., *9*:557, 1952.
Conway, H., Sedar, J. D., and Shannon, J. E., Jr.: Re-evaluation of the transparent chamber technique in the study of the circulation in autografts and homografts of skin. Transplant. Bull., *4*:62, 1957.
Conway, H., Stark, R. B., and Joslin, D.: Observations on the development of circulation in skin grafts. II. The physiologic pattern of early circulation in autografts. Plast. Reconstr. Surg., *8*:312, 1951.
Cram, A. E., and Domayer, M. A.: Short-term preservation of human autografts. J. Trauma, *23*:872, 1983.
Davis, J. S., and Traut, H. F.: Origin and development of the blood supply of whole-thickness skin grafts. An experimental study. Ann. Surg., *82*:871, 1925.
Douglas, B.: The treatment of burns and other extensive wounds with special emphasis on the transparent jacket system. Surgery, *15*:96, 1944.
Eade, G. G.: The relationship between granulation tissue, bacteria, and skin grafts in burned patients. Plast. Reconstr. Surg., *22*:42, 1958.
Eastwood, D. S.: Observations on skin heterografts in rats. Br. J. Plast. Surg., *14*:160, 1961.
Edgerton, M. T., and Edgerton, P. J.: Vascularization of homografts. Transplant. Bull., *2*:98, 1955.
Egdahl, R. H., Good, R. A., and Varco, R. L.: Studies in homograft and heterograft survival. Surgery, *42*:228, 1957.
Egdahl, R. H., Varco, R. L., and Good, R. A.: Local reactions and lymph node response to skin heterografts between rabbits and rats. Int. Arch. Allergy Appl. Immunol., *13*:129, 1958.
Elliott, R. A., Jr. and Hoehn, J. G.: Use of commercial porcine skin for wound dressings. Plast. Reconstr. Surg., *52*:401, 1973.
Enderlen.: Histologische Untersuchungen über die Einheilung von Pfropfungen nach Thiersch and Krause. Dtsch. Z. Chir., *45*:453, 1897.

Feller, I., and DeWeese, M. S.: The use of stored cutaneous autografts in wound treatment. Surgery, *44*:540, 1958.

Garré, C.: Über die histologischen Vorgänge bei der Anheilung der Thiersch'-schen Transplantationen. Beitr. Klin. Chir., *4*:625, 1889.

Georgiade, N., Peschel, E., Georgiade, R., and Brown, I.: A clinical and experimental investigation of the preservation of skin. Plast. Reconstr. Surg., *17*:267, 1956.

Gibson, T., and Medawar, P. B.: The fate of skin homografts in man. J. Anat., *77*:299, 1943.

Goldmann, E. E.: Die künstliche Ueberhäutung offener Krebse durch Hauttransplantationen nach Thiersch. Zentralbl. Allg. Pathol., *1*:505, 1890.

Goodpasture, E. W., Douglas, B., and Anderson, K.: A study of human skin grafted upon the chorio-allantois of chick embryos. J. Exp. Med., *68*:891, 1938.

Gregory, E. W., Triplett, R. G., and Connole, P. W.: Comparison of fresh autogenous and freeze-dried allogeneic skin for mandibular vestibuloplasty. J. Oral Maxillofac. Surg., *41*:75, 1983.

Gresham, R. B., Perry, V. P., and Thompson, V. K.: Practical methods of short-term storage of homografts. Arch. Surg., *87*:417, 1963.

Guthy, E. A., Billote, J. B., and Burke, J. F.: Skin as an organ transplant. A critical re-evaluation of the allografts. Chir. Plast. (Berl.), *2*:263, 1974.

Haller, J. A., Jr., and Billingham, R. E.: Preliminary studies on the origin of the vasculature in free skin grafts. *In* Montagna, W., and Billingham, R. E. (Eds.): Advances in Biology of Skin. Vol. 5, Wound Healing. New York, MacMillan, 1964, p. 165.

Haller, J. A., Jr., and Billingham, R. E.: Studies of the origin of the vasculature in free skin grafts. Ann. Surg., *166*:896, 1967.

Haller, J. A., Jr., Rauenhorst, J., Adkins, J., and Billingham, R. E.: Origin of the vasculature in skin grafts. Surg. Forum, *17*:96, 1966.

Ham, A. W.: Some histophysiological problems peculiar to calcified tissues. J. Bone Joint Surg. [Am.], *34*:701, 1952.

Hanks, J. H., and Wallace, R. E.: Relation of oxygen and temperature in the preservation of tissues by refrigeration. Proc. Soc. Exp. Biol. Med., *71*:196, 1949.

Henle, A.: Klinische und experimentelle Beiträge zur Lehre von der Transplantation ungestielter Hautlappen. II. Experimenteller Teil. Beitr. Klin. Chir., *24*:615, 1899.

Henry, L., Marshall, D. C., Friedman, E. A., Dammin, G. J., and Merrill, J. P.: The rejection of skin homografts in the normal human subject. Part II. Histological findings. J. Clin. Invest., *41*:420, 1962.

Henry, L., Marshall, D. C., Friedman, E. A., Goldstein, D. P., and Dammin, G. J.: A histologic study of the human skin autograft. Am. J. Pathol., *39*:317, 1961.

Hildemann, W. H., and Haas, R.: Comparative studies of homotransplantation in fishes. J. Cell. Comp. Physiol., *55*:227, 1960.

Hübscher, C.: Beiträge zue Hautverpflanzung nach Thiersch. Beitr. Klin. Chir., *4*:395, 1888.

Hurst, L. N., Brown, D. H., and Murray, K. A.: Prolonged life and improved quality for stored skin grafts. Plast. Reconstr. Surg., *73*:105, 1984.

Hyatt, G. W., Turner, T. C., Bassett, C. A. L., Pate, J. W., and Sawyer, P. N.: New methods for preserving bone, skin and blood vessels. Postgrad. Med., *12*:239, 1952.

Hynes, W.: The early circulation in skin grafts with a consideration of methods to encourage their survival. Br. J. Plast. Surg., *6*:257, 1954.

Jackson, D.: A clinical study of the use of skin homografts for burns. Br. J. Plast. Surg., *7*:26, 1954.

Jungengel, M.: Die Hauttransplantation nach Thiersch. Verh. Phys. Med. Ges. Wurzb., *25*:1, 1891.

Kamrin, B. B.: Studies on the healing of successful homografts in albino rats. Ann. N.Y. Acad. Sci., *87*:323, 1960.

Kamrin, B. B.: Analysis of the union between host and graft in the albino rat. Plast. Reconstr. Surg., *28*:221, 1961.

Kaspar, D. W., and Laskin, D. M.: The effect of porcine skin and autogenous epithelial grafts on the contraction of experimental oral wounds. J. Oral Maxillofac. Surg., *41*:143, 1983.

Keeley, R. L. A., Gomez, A. C., and Brown, I. W., Jr.: An experimental study of the effects of freezing, partial dehydration, and ultra-rapid cooling on the survival of dog skin grafts. Plast. Reconstr. Surg., *9*:330, 1952.

Kikuchi, I., and Omori, M.: Demonstration of leaking vessels under skin grafts. Plast. Reconstr. Surg., *45*:66, 1970.

Kiyono, K., and Sueyasu, Y.: The experimental study in avian embryo after inoculation of tissues from various animals. I. Further classification of species for inoculation. Kyoto Igaku Zassi, *14*:68, 1917.

Lawrence, J. C.: Storage and skin metabolism. Br. J. Plast. Surg., *25*:440, 1972.

Lehr, H. B., Berggren, R. B., Lotke, P. A., and Coriell, L. L.: Permanent survival of preserved skin autografts. Surgery, *56*:742, 1964.

Lewis, T.: The Blood Vessels of the Human Skin and Their Responses. London, Shaw & Sons, 1927.

Ljungqvist, A., and Almgård, L. E.: The vascular reaction in the free skin allo- and autografts. A stereomicroangiographic and histological study in the rabbit. Acta Pathol. Microbiol. Scand., *68*:553, 1966.

Loeb, L., and Addison, W. H. F.: Beiträge zur Analyse des Gewebewachstums. 2. Transplantation der Haut des Meeschweinchens in Tiere verschiedener Spezies. Arch Entwickl. Organ., *27*:73, 1909.

Loeb, L., and Addison, W. H. F.: Beiträge zur Analyse des Gewebewachstums. 5. Ueber die Transplantation der Taubenhaut in die Taube und in andere Tierarten. Arch. Entwickl. Organ., *32*:44, 1911.

Lombard, W. P.: The blood pressure in the arterioles, capillaries, and small veins of the human skin. Am. J. Physiol., *29*:335, 1911–1912.

Lovelock, J. E.: The hemolysis of human red blood cells by freezing and thawing. Biochem. Biophys. Acta, *10*:414, 1953.

Lovelock, J. E.: Biophysical aspects of the freezing and thawing of living cells. Proc. R. Soc. Med., *47*:60, 1954.

Luyet, B. J., and Gehenio, P. M.: Life and death at low temperatures. Diodynamics (Monograph on General Physiology, No. 1), Normandy, MO, 1940.

Marckmann, A.: Autologous skin grafts in the rat. Uptake of ^{35}S-sulfate. Proc. Soc. Exp. Biol. Med., *119*:557, 1965a.

Marckmann, A.: Autologous skin grafts in the rat. Biochemical analysis of mucopolysaccharides and hydroxyproline. Proc. Soc. Exp. Biol. Med., *119*:794, 1965b.

Marckmann, A.: Autologous skin grafts in the rat: vital microscopic studies of the microcirculation. Angiology, *17*:475, 1966.

Marckmann, A.: Biology of skin autografts. Dan. Med. Bull., *14*:135, 1967.

Marckmann, A., and Zachariae, H.: Histamine in full-thickness skin autografts of rat. Proc. Soc. Exp. Biol. Med., *117*:705, 1964.

Markley, K., and Thornton, S. W. Skin graft prolongation caused by changes in grafting procedure. Transplantation, *16*:80, 1973.

Marrangoni, A. G.: An experimental study on refrigerated skin grafts stored in ten per cent homologous serum. Plast. Reconstr. Surg., *6*:425, 1950.

Matthews, D. N.: Storage of skin for autogenous grafts. Lancet, *1*:775, 1945.

McGregor, I. A.: The vascularization of human skin. Br. J. Plast. Surg., *7*:331, 1955a.

McGregor, I. A.: Vascularization of homografts of human skin. Transplant. Bull., *2*:11, 1955b.

McLaughlin, C. R.: Composite ear grafts and their blood supply. Br. J. Plast. Surg., *7*:274, 1954.

Medawar, P. B.: The behavior and fate of skin autografts and skin homografts in rabbits. J. Anat., *78*:176, 1944.

Medawar, P. B.: The storage of living skin. Proc. R. Soc. Med., *47*:62, 1954.

Merwin, R. M., and Algire, G. H.: The role of graft and host vessels in the vascularization of grafts of normal and neoplastic tissue. J. Natl. Cancer Inst., *17*:23, 1956.

Mider, G. B., and Morton, J. J.: The effect of freezing *in vitro* on some transplantable mammalian tumors and on normal rat skin. Am. J. Cancer, *35*:502, 1939.

Miller, T. A.: The deleterious effect of split skin homograft coverage on split-skin donor sites. Plast. Reconstr. Surg., *53*:316, 1974.

Miller, T. A., Switzer, W. E., Foley, F. D., and Moncrief, J. A.: Early homografting of second degree burns. Plast. Reconstr. Surg., *40*:117, 1967.

Miller, T. A., and White, W. L.: Healing of second degree burns. Comparison of effects of early application of homografts and coverage with tape. Plast. Reconstr. Surg., *49*:552, 1972.

Mir y Mir, L.: Biology of the skin graft. New aspects to consider in its revascularization. Plast. Reconstr. Surg., *8*:378, 1951.

Mowlem, R.: Skin homografts. Med. Illustrated, *6*:552, 1952.

Murphy, J. B.: Transplantability of malignant tumors to the embryos of a foreign species. J.A.M.A., *59*:874, 1912.

O'Donoghue, M. N., and Zarem, H. A.: Stimulation of neovascularization—comparative efficacy of fresh and preserved skin grafts. Plast. Reconstr. Surg., *48*:474, 1971.

Ohmori, S., and Kurata, K.: Experimental studies on the blood supply to various types of skin grafts in rabbits using isotope P^{32}. Plast. Reconstr. Surg., *25*:547, 1960.

Ouhayoun, J. P., Holzman, S., Etienne, D., Pierre, C., and Forest, N.: Freeze-dried skin allografts. A human clinical and histological study. J. Periodontol., *54*:463, 1983.

Pandya, N. J., and Zarem, H. A.: The absence of vascularization in porcine skin grafts on mice. Plast. Reconstr. Surg., *53*:211, 1974.

Pate, J. W.: Transplantation of preserved non-viable tissues. *In* Ciba Foundation Symposium on Preservation and Transplantation of Normal Tissues. Boston, Little, Brown & Company, 1954, p. 60.

Pederson, F. B., Matthiessen, M. E., and Garbarsch, C.: Enzyme histochemical studies on rat skin autografts. Scand. J. Plast. Reconstr. Surg., *4*:83, 1970.

Peer, L. A., and Walker, J. C.: The behavior of autogenous human tissue grafts. II. Plast. Reconstr. Surg., *7*:73, 1951.

Pepper, F. J.: Studies on the viability of mammalian skin autografts after storage at different temperatures. Br. J. Plast. Surg., *6*:250, 1954.

Perry, V. P.: A review of skin preservation. Cryobiology, *3*:109, 1966.

Perry, V. P., Evans, V. J., Young, J. M., Earle, W. R., and Hyatt, G. W.: Some recent studies with tissue culture as related to tissue transplantation. Transplant. Bull., *4*:28, 1957.

Pihl, B., and Weiber, A.: Studies of the vascularization of free full-thickness skin grafts with radioisotope techniques. Acta Chir. Scand., *125*:19, 1963.

Polge, C., Smith, A. U., and Parkes, A. S.: Revival of spermatozoa after vitrification and dehydration at low temperatures. Nature, *164*:666, 1949.

Psillakis, J. M., de Jorge, F. B., Villardo, R., Albano, A. de M., Martins, M., and Spina, V.: Water and electrolyte changes in autogenous skin grafts. Discussion of the so-called "plasmatic circulation." Plast. Reconstr. Surg., *43*:500, 1969.

Raju, S., and Grogan, J. B.: Effect of storage on skin allograft survival. Arch. Surg., *99*:100, 1969.

Rapaport, F. T., Converse, J. M., Horn, L., Ballantyne, D. L., Jr., and Mulholland, J. H.: Altered reactivity to skin homografts in severe thermal injury. Ann. Surg., *159*:390, 1964.

Rappaport, I., Pepino, A. T., and Dietrick, W.: Early use of xenografts as a biologic dressing in burn trauma. Am. J. Surg., *120*:144, 1970.

Rees, T. D., Ballantyne, D. L., Jr., Hawthorne, G. A., and Nathan, A.: Effects of Silastic sheet implants under simultaneous skin autografts in rats. Plast. Reconstr. Surg., *42*:339, 1968.

Réverdin, J. L.: De la greffe épidermique. Arch. Gen. Med., *19*:276, 1872.

Ribbert-Göttingen, H.: Ueber Transplantation auf Individuen anderer Gattung. Verh. Dtsch. Pathol. Ges., *8*:104, 1904.

Rogers, B. O., and Converse, J. M.: Bovine embryo skin zoografts as temporary biologic dressings for burns and other skin defects. Plast. Reconstr. Surg., *22*:471, 1958.

Rogers, B. O., Converse, J. M., and Silvetti, A. N.: Preliminary clinical studies on bovine embryo skin grafts. Transplant. Bull., *4*:24, 1957.

Rolle, G. K., Taylor, A. C., and Charipper, H. A.: A study of vascular changes in skin grafts in mice and their relationship to homograft breakdown. J. Cell. Comp. Physiol., *53*:215, 1959.

Russell, P. S., and Monaco, A. P.: The Biology of Tissue Transplantation. Boston, Little, Brown & Company, 1965.

Salisbury, R. E., Wilmore, D. W., Silverstein, P., and Pruitt, B. A., Jr.: Biological dressings for skin graft donor sites. Arch. Surg., *106*:705, 1973.

Santoni-Rugiu, P.: Compared studies on the viability of skin stored by different methods. Plast. Reconstr. Surg., *30*:586, 1962.

Scothorne, R. J., and McGregor, I. A.: The vascularization of autografts and homografts of rabbit skin. J. Anat., *87*:379, 1953.

Scothorne, R. J., and Scothorne, A. W.: Histochemical studies on human skin autografts. J. Anat., *87*:22, 1953.

Scothorne, R. J., and Tough, J. S.: Histochemical studies of human skin autografts and homografts. Br. J. Plast. Surg., *5*:161, 1952.

Sell, K. W., Hyatt, G. W., and Gresham, R. B.: The status of the freeze-dried skin homograft in the severely burned patient. *In* Artz, C. P. (Ed.): Research in Burns. Washington, DC, American Institute of Biological Sciences, and Philadelphia, F. A. Davis Company, 1962, pp. 351–356.

Shepard, G. H.: The storage of split-skin grafts on their donor sites. Clinical and experimental study. Plast. Reconstr. Surg., *49*:115, 1972.

Sherman, J. K.: Pretreatment with protective substances as a factor in freeze-thaw survival. Cryobiology, *1*:298, 1965.

Silvetti, A. N., Cotton, C., Bryne, R. J., Berrian, J. H., and Menendez, A. F.: Preliminary experimental studies of bovine embryo skin grafts. Transplant. Bull., *4*:25, 1957.

Šmahel, J.: Revascularization of a free skin autograft. Acta Chir. Plast., *4*:102, 1962.

Šmahel, J.: The revascularization of a free skin autograft. Acta Chir. Plast., *9*:76, 1967.

Šmahel, J.: Biology of the stage of plasmatic imbibition. Br. J. Plast. Surg., *24*:140, 1971.

Šmahel, J.: The healing of skin grafts. Clin. Plast. Surg., *4*:409, 1977.

Šmahel, J., and Clodius, L.: The blood vessel system of free human skin grafts. Plast. Reconstr. Surg., *47*:61, 1971.

Šmahel, J., and Ganzoni, N.: Contribution to the origin of the vasculature in free skin autografts. Br. J. Plast. Surg., *23*:322, 1970.

Smith, J. W., Ringland, J., and Wilson, R.: Vascularization of skin grafts. Surg. Forum, *15*:473, 1964.

Sokolic, I. H., Farpour, A., Ulin, A. W., and Howard, J.: The use of heterograft skin as a biological dressing. Surg. Forum, *10*:847, 1959.

Song, I. C., Bromberg, B. E., Mohn, M. P., and Koehnlein, E.: Heterografts as biological dressings for large skin wounds. Surgery, *59*:576, 1966.

State, D., and Peter, M. E.: Clinical use of porcine xenografts in conditions other than burns. Surg. Gynecol. Obstet., *138*:13, 1974.

Strumia, M. M., and Hodge, C. C.: Frozen human skin grafts. Ann. Surg., *121*:860, 1945.

Sugarbaker, P. H., Sabath, L. D., and Morgan, A. P.: Neomycin toxicity from porcine skin xenografts. Ann. Surg., *179*:183, 1974.

Switzer, W. E., Moncrief, J. A., Mills, W., Jr., Order, S. E., and Lindberg, R. B.: The use of canine heterografts in the therapy of thermal injury. J. Trauma, *6*:391, 1966.

Taylor, A. C., and Gerstner, R.: Tissue survival after exposure to low temperatures and the effectiveness of protective pretreatments. I. Evaluation by growth in tissue culture. J. Cell. Comp. Physiol., *46*:477, 1956.

Taylor, A. C., Gerstner, R., and Converse, J. M.: Preservation of skin grafts by refrigeration for reconstructive surgery. Plast. Reconstr. Surg., *18*:275, 1956.

Taylor, A. C., and Lehrfeld, J. W.: Determination of survival time of skin homografts in the rat by observations of vascular changes in the graft. Plast. Reconstr. Surg., *12*:423, 1953.

Taylor, A. C., and Lehrfeld, J. W.: Definition of survival time of homografts. Ann. N.Y. Acad. Sci., *59*:351, 1955.

Thompson, N.: The role of succinic dehydrogenase and sulfhydryl groups during epidermal rejection in skin homografts. A preliminary histochemical study in rats. Transplant. Bull., *30*:113, 1962.

Toranto, I. R., Salyer, K. E., and Myers, M. B.: Vascularization of porcine skin heterografts. Plast. Reconstr. Surg., *54*:195, 1974.

Wandall, J. H.: Healing of split skin autografts after storage in deuterated medium. Scand. J. Plast. Reconstr. Surg., *6*:36, 1972.

Webster, J. P.: Refrigerated skin grafts. Ann. Surg., *120*:431, 1944.

Wentscher, J.: Ein weiterer Beitrag zur Überlebensfähigkeit der menschlichen Epidermiszellen. Dtsch. Z. Chir., *70*:21, 1903.

Wolff, K., and Schellander, F. G.: Enzyme-histochemical studies on the healing process of split skin grafts. I. Aminopeptidase, diphosphopyridine-nucleotide-diaphorase and succinic dehydrogenase in autografts. J. Invest. Dermatol., *45*:38, 1965.

Wolff, K., and Schellander, F. G.: Enzyme-histochemical studies on the healing process of split skin grafts. II. 5-Nucleotidase, adenosinetriphosphatase, acid and alkaline phosphatase in autografts. J. Invest. Dermatol., *46*:205, 1966.

Woodruff, M. F. A.: The Transplantation of Tissues and Organs. Springfield, IL, Charles C. Thomas, 1960.

Yukna, R. A., Tow, H. D., Carroll, P. B., Vernino, A. R., and Bright, R. W.: Evaluation of the use of freeze-dried skin allografts in the treatment of human mucogingival problems. J. Periodontol., *48*:187, 1977.

Yukna, R. A., Turner, D. W., and Robinson, L. J.: Variable antigenicity of lyophilized allogeneic and lyophilized xenogeneic skin in guinea pigs. J. Periodont. Res., *12*:197, 1977.

Zarem, H. A., Zweifach, B. W., and McGehee, J. M.: Development of microcirculation in full thickness autogenous skin grafts in mice. Am. J. Physiol., *212*:1081, 1967.

9

Rollin K. Daniel
Carolyn L. Kerrigan

Principles and Physiology of Skin Flap Surgery

PRINCIPLES OF FLAP SURGERY

The defining characteristic of a skin flap is that its survival in the recipient bed is predicated upon a functioning intravascular circulation, in contrast to the dependent plasmatic imbibition of skin grafts. For a 50 year period from 1915 to 1965, the actual design of skin flaps was governed by a set of length-to-width ratios, varying from 5:1 for the face to 1:1 for the lower extremity. These rules evolved from empiric observations and became canons as the specialty of Plastic Surgery developed. Equally important was the distinction between a *local flap*, which could be easily advanced, pivoted, or interpolated and a *distant flap*, which could be either inset directly or tubed. In 1965, Bakamjian published his method of pharyngeal reconstruction employing a new flap of immense dimensions that did not require a delay procedure. The deltopectoral flap not only revolutionized head and neck reconstruction, but reintroduced the concept of arterial flaps as pioneered by Esser (Hacseker, 1983). The death knell for the restrictive arithmetic rules governing skin flap design was Milton's (1970) repudiation of the simplistic length-to-width ratio. On the basis of his work with arterial flaps and Daniel's investigation of random cutaneous flaps (Daniel, 1973, 1975a,b; Daniel and Williams, 1973), it was shown that increasing the width of a flap did *not* increase the surviving length. Rather, it was the incorporated blood supply that dictated the flap's surviving length. Thus freed from arithmetic restraints, a sudden surge occurred in the number and type of flaps available. McGregor and Jackson (1972) devised the groin flap supplied by the superficial circumflex iliac artery, and classified skin flaps as either random or axial. Daniel (Daniel, 1973,

1975a,b; Daniel and Williams, 1973) defined the blood supply to the skin as being from two types of arteries, either musculocutaneous or direct cutaneous arteries. As the design of skin flaps became increasingly determined by a knowledge of the cutaneous vascular anatomy, the times when the delay procedure was indicated and carried out became less frequent. Despite these advances, the entire spectrum of skin coverage was to be changed during the subsequent decade of microscopes and myocutaneous flaps.

From 1975 to 1985, the operating microscope revolutionized the method of flap movement, while the resurgence of myocutaneous flaps permanently altered flap composition. With the first report of a successful free flap by Daniel and Taylor (1973), skin flaps were effectively liberated from their restraining pedicle. Equally, the attendant waste of time and tissue that was a part of any tube flap migration was eliminated. Attention quickly focused on expanding the composition of free flaps with nerve, bone, tendon, and joints. Although myocutaneous flaps were originally conceived of as donor tissue for free flap transfers, their versatility, simplicity, and ubiquitousness led to their adoption as a local flap. Operative ease and development of new procedures, e.g., the latissimus dorsi flap for breast reconstruction, led to the rapid integration of myocutaneous flaps into all aspects of plastic surgery. The primary contributions of Vasconez, Bostwick and McCraw (1974), McCraw (1980), Mathes and Nahai (1979, 1982), Bostwick (1983), and Jurkiewicz and associates (1985) were critical.

This advance mandated a greater awareness of muscle anatomy and blood supply, especially the arcs of rotation (see Chap. 11). After this initial resistance was overcome, the work of Ger (1972, 1977) utilizing muscle transfers plus skin grafts was appreciated and quickly adopted. Muscle transfer plus a skin graft has evolved as a first option for coverage in the lower extremity, as it minimizes donor site deformity. Recently, new hybrid flaps have emerged, including expanded flaps in which greater flap size is achieved with minimal donor site morbidity, and fasciocutaneous flaps that combine the simplicity of random flaps with the vascularity of arterial flaps. This chapter attempts to integrate the rapidly changing field of skin flaps into a coherent set of principles.

Currently, three major trends appear to be evolving into the fundamental principles for the next decade. First, plastic surgeons are no longer restricted to skin flaps to provide skin replacement, but rather can utilize a wide array of operations to provide *soft tissue coverage.* Long-term follow-up by Nahai (1985) and sophisticated studies by May (May and Halls, 1985; May, Halls, and Simon, 1985) showed that a local muscle transfer plus a partial-thickness skin graft provides durable long-term coverage, and it is not necessary to replace full-thickness dermis and subcutaneous fat. Second, the number, type, and application of flaps continues to expand rapidly and the surgeon must remain open to *new techniques.* For example, the latissimus dorsi replaced the groin flap as the primary free flap donor site, yet the transverse abdominis myocutaneous flap has superseded the latissimus dorsi for breast reconstruction. Basic principles have also been altered: blood supply is now the critical design criterion for a flap, not arithmetic; the microscope has replaced the tube pedicle flap as the dominant method for distant flap transfer; and minimization of donor site morbidity has become of greater interest now that consistently reliable flaps have evolved. Third, the reconstruction of complex multitissue deformities, especially in the face, no longer involves the fabrication of a facsimile in numerous operations using several donor parts fused by scar tissue. Rather *en bloc composite reconstruction*, often employing microvascular anastomoses, has become the standard. It is this type of sophisticated composite replacement that is presaging the era of reconstructive transplantation surgery.

Classification

Any classification is merely a method of organization or clarification of one's thoughts on a particular subject. Although numerous systems are available, classification of skin flaps has evolved in three distinct groups: method of movement, blood supply, and composition (Table 9–1).

METHOD OF MOVEMENT

Skin flaps can be divided into local or distant flaps on the basis of the proximity of donor and recipient sites (Fig. 9–1). Local or adjacent flaps can be subdivided into advancement, pivot, and interpolation flaps. An *advancement* flap moves directly forward into

Table 9–1. Classification of Skin Flaps

Method of Movement
Local flaps
Advancement
Pivot
Interpolation
Pedicle
Subcutaneous
Distant flaps
Direct
Tube
Microvascular
Blood Supply
Musculocutaneous arteries
Random cutaneous
Myocutaneous
Septocutaneous arteries
Fasciocutaneous
Arterial
Composition
Cutaneous
Fasciocutaneous
Myocutaneous
Muscle ± skin
Osseocutaneous
Sensory

a defect without any lateral movement, the most common example being the V-Y advancement flap. In contrast, a *pivot* flap, either *transposition* or *rotation*, derives its name from the pivot point at the base of the flap as well as its arc of rotation whose radius is under the greatest tension. An *interpolation* flap is taken from a nearby but not immediately adjacent donor site, and transferred either above or below the intervening skin to the recipient defect. Even within local flaps there is a hierarchy of complexity. The advancement flap offers the economy of closing both the recipient and donor sites in the same procedure, whereas a pivot flap often requires either a skin graft or another flap to close the donor site. Even more complex is the interpolation flap whose donor site may be easily closed, but whose pedicle must either be skeletonized for subcutaneous passage, resulting in increased risk, or sectioned in stages when passed over the intervening skin, thereby necessitating additional operations. Flaps from a distance can be divided into direct, tube, or free. A *direct* flap allows approximation of the donor and recipient site, ranging from the easily executed thenar flap in which the index finger is brought down to the thenar prominence, to the more complicated cross leg flap. If the two sites cannot be approximated, the alternative is either a tube flap migration or a microvascular free flap transfer. A *tube* flap minimizes infection and contracture during its long migration. Alternatively, a *free* flap allows immediate and direct transfer of a large amount of tissue with its own permanent blood supply, albeit requiring greater technical expertise for the microvascular anastomoses. Rather than signifying a distinct type of flap, the term free or microvascular flap merely refers to a method of movement.

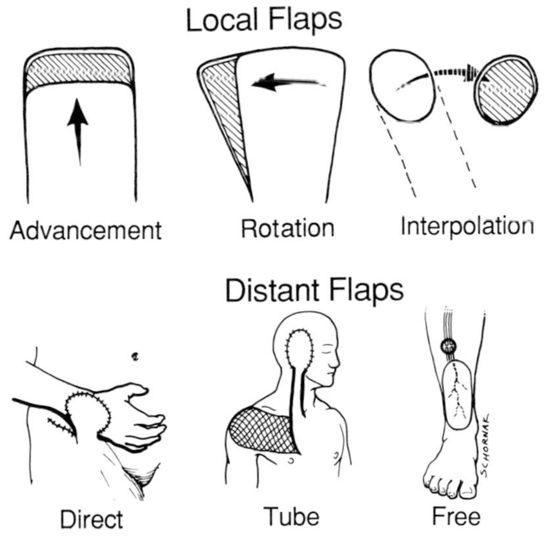

Figure 9–1. Classification of skin flaps by method of movement.

BLOOD SUPPLY

Although a simplistic division, the blood supply to the covering tissues may be subdivided into segmental, perforator, and cutaneous, the latter being composed of musculocutaneous and septocutaneous vessels (Fig. 9–2) (Daniel, 1975a,b). *Musculocutaneous* arteries are branches off the major vessels that supply muscle and then continue into the overlying dermal plexi. *Septocutaneous* arteries (previously referred to as direct cutaneous arteries) arise from either segmental or muscular vessels before passing through the fascial septa between muscles to supply both the enveloping fascia and the overlying skin.

Conceptually, musculocutaneous arteries nourish both random cutaneous and myocutaneous flaps. *A random cutaneous* flap is composed of skin and subcutaneous fat with multiple musculocutaneous arteries at its base. A *myocutaneous* flap is composed of skin, subcutaneous fat, and muscle with its blood supply coming from muscular arteries plus numerous terminal musculocutaneous

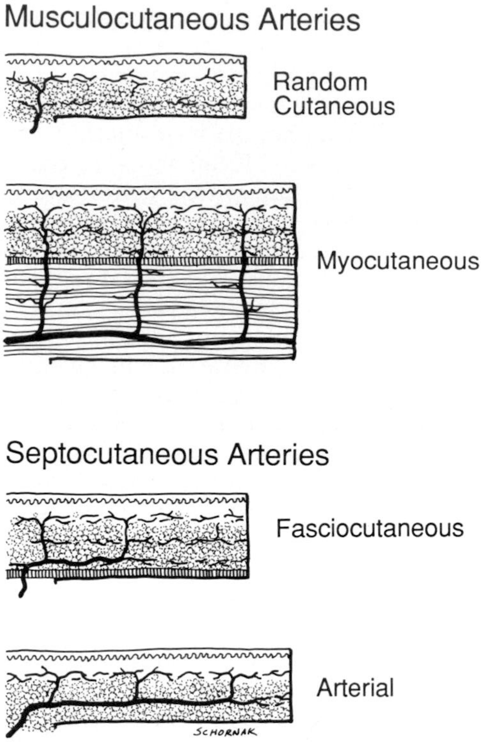

Figure 9–2. Classification of skin flaps by blood supply.

arteries. The critical factor that provides myocutaneous flaps with a greater reliability than random cutaneous flaps is the distinction between their anatomic and vascular bases. In a random cutaneous flap, the musculocutaneous arteries are located at the flap's anatomic base, whereas in a myocutaneous flap multiple musculocutaneous arteries are passing upward from the perfused muscle to the overlying skin. Thus, in a myocutaneous flap the vascular base is cantilevered far beyond the anatomic base, allowing greater length and reliability.

Septocutaneous arteries are a reflection of vascular embryology. Specifically, the cutaneous capillary plexi and underlying segmental arteries develop concurrently, but must join at a later date despite the intervening muscle mass. The connecting vessels are found in the dividing muscular septa and are labeled septocutaneous arteries. Surgically, one can achieve greater flap survival by incorporating fascia and aligning the *fasciocutaneous* flap on a distinct septocutaneous vessel. Septocutaneous arteries that course parallel to the skin and provide numerous side branches in a Christmas tree fashion can nourish large-sized *arterial* flaps. In contrast to the ubiquitous musculocutaneous arteries, these parallel vessels are few in number, but they are of great surgical importance. As in the groin and deltopectoral flaps, one can raise flaps of almost unlimited length with little regard for width or need for a delay procedure.

COMPOSITION

Although *compound* flaps have a long lineage, their application was infrequent until the introduction of myocutaneous flaps. For most defects, a simple skin flap usually sufficed. As defects became more complex and adjacent donor sites were compromised, the choice was broadened to include fasciocutaneous, myocutaneous, or muscle plus skin graft flaps (Fig. 9–3). Each flap must be considered on the basis of viability, surgical dissection, and donor site morbidity. Muscle flaps with skin grafts have the least donor site morbidity but require greater surgical dissection, and their viability may be compromised in the severely traumatized limb. Myocutaneous flaps are usually highly reliable and require moderate surgical expertise, but they leave a significant donor site defor-

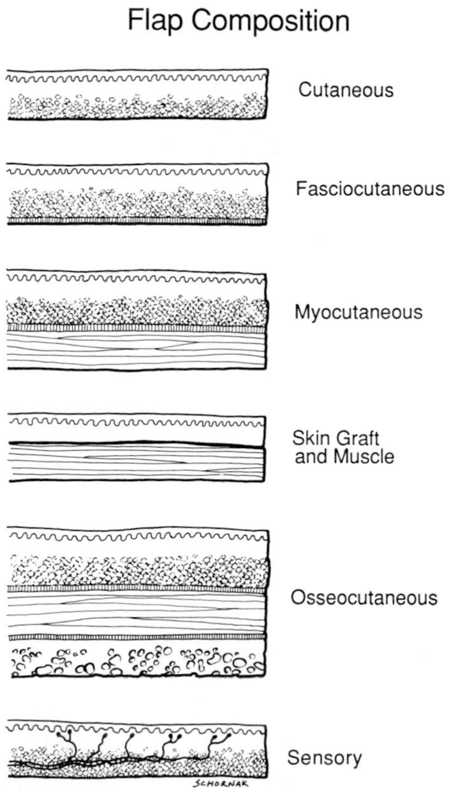

Figure 9–3. Classification of skin flaps by composition.

mity, especially in the lower extremity. Fasciocutaneous flaps generally fall between a random cutaneous and a myocutaneous flap. They have a greater viability than random cutaneous flaps but less than a myocutaneous flap, while requiring greater anatomic knowledge and surgical finesse. Unfortunately, the donor site deformity they involve is often unacceptable. As beautifully demonstrated by Swartz and associates (1986), *composite* flaps are of value in complex cases requiring en bloc reconstruction, especially in the head and neck region. These flaps are often composed of skin, muscle, and bone plus the intervening subcutaneous fat and fascia all isolated on a single pedicle. Classic examples include the pectoralis major flap incorporating a skin paddle plus rib for mandibular reconstruction, or the osseocutaneous groin flap on the deep circumflex iliac artery for lower extremity reconstruction. These flaps allow single-stage reconstruction plus a permanent blood supply, usually through a major segmental or muscular artery. *Specialized* flaps are rarely used but are of great elegance. Sensory flaps can be either pedicled or free, the digital island flaps of the hand or first web space of the foot being utilized most frequently. In these cases, terminal septocutaneous arteries of the extremities supply the flap, and venous drainage occurs through paired venae comitantes. Functional muscle transfers, with repair of the motor nerve and preservation of the correct resting tension, represent a significant sophistication over the standard muscle flap.

Soft Tissue Coverage

Numerous choices exist for closing any wound, so the surgical challenge is that of selecting the *optimal method.* It is necessary to balance multiple factors, including recipient site requirements, donor site morbidity, operative complexity, and patient factors. Wounds may be divided into single, compound, composite, and complex tissue defects. As might occur in the facial region, resection of a large skin cancer often causes a single tissue defect (skin), whereas removal of an intraoral squamous cell tumor can produce a compound defect (oral lining and bone), a composite defect (oral lining, bone, skin), or even a complex defect (oral and nasal lining, three-dimensional maxillary bone loss, skin, and subcutaneous tissue). In extensive wounds, exact replacement is neither possible nor mandatory. Major skin loss around the knee can be treated with a small flap to cover the open joint and large skin grafts applied to the surrounding muscle; total flap coverage is rarely necessary. It is in the hand and facial regions that the greatest creative challenge arises of achieving optimal function and esthetic reconstruction.

Limiting donor site morbidity is emphasized in the aphorism "Never rob Peter to pay Paul unless Peter can afford it." Certainly, documented cases exist in which donor site morbidity exceeds the original recipient site problem, necessitating a second flap to reconstruct the donor site. During the era of tube pedicle flaps, it was acceptable to place the donor site scar beneath clothing, but with more active leisure life styles concern for donor site deformity is of greater significance. Perhaps the best example of this heightened awareness is with myocutaneous flaps below the knee. Owing to the poverty of viable flaps in the lower extremity, the gastrocnemius myocutaneous flap was readily accepted and widely utilized. The flap survived and the wound was closed, but the donor site was often worse than the original defect. Thus, muscle flaps with their simple linear scar, or the gracilis free flap with its incision hidden in the medial thigh, have reduced the frequency of myocutaneous flaps in the lower extremity. Numerous donor site complications are often overlooked while one concentrates on the successful flap transfer. With greater assurance of flap viability, minimization of donor site morbidity has increased dramatically.

For a given wound, there is a *hierarchy* of closure techniques based on operative complexity (Table 9–2, Fig. 9–4). This progression is important in considering *all the options* available for a specific defect. As characterized by a standard distribution curve, each operative procedure has its own safe characteristic range of application that is affected by local conditions. For example, the soleus muscle flap is ideal for defects in the middle third of the leg, but falters when it is either extended beyond its range of application to the lower third or inappropriately selected in a severely traumatized limb. To evaluate the coverage of a middle third defect of the lower limb, one might follow this scenario: (1) the size of the defect precludes suture closure; (2) a compound tibial fracture is present in the base of the

Table 9–2. Soft Tissue Coverage

Primary closure
Secondary closure
Delayed closure
Secondary healing
Skin graft
Split-thickness
Full-thickness
Local flap
Random cutaneous
Fasciocutaneous
Muscle ± STSG
Myocutaneous
Distant flap
Adjacent area
Tube transfer
Free flap
Specialized flap
Sensory
Osseocutaneous
Compound
Composite

wound, and neither secondary healing nor skin graft closure is desirable; (3) extensive soft tissue trauma precludes a local random cutaneous or fasciocutaneous flap, and an arterialized dorsalis pedis flap is not tenable; and (4) muscle flaps of soleus plus flexor digitorum longus would be ideal, but severe trauma may necessitate a free latissimus dorsi muscle flap with a skin graft. Throughout, numerous alternatives and modifications

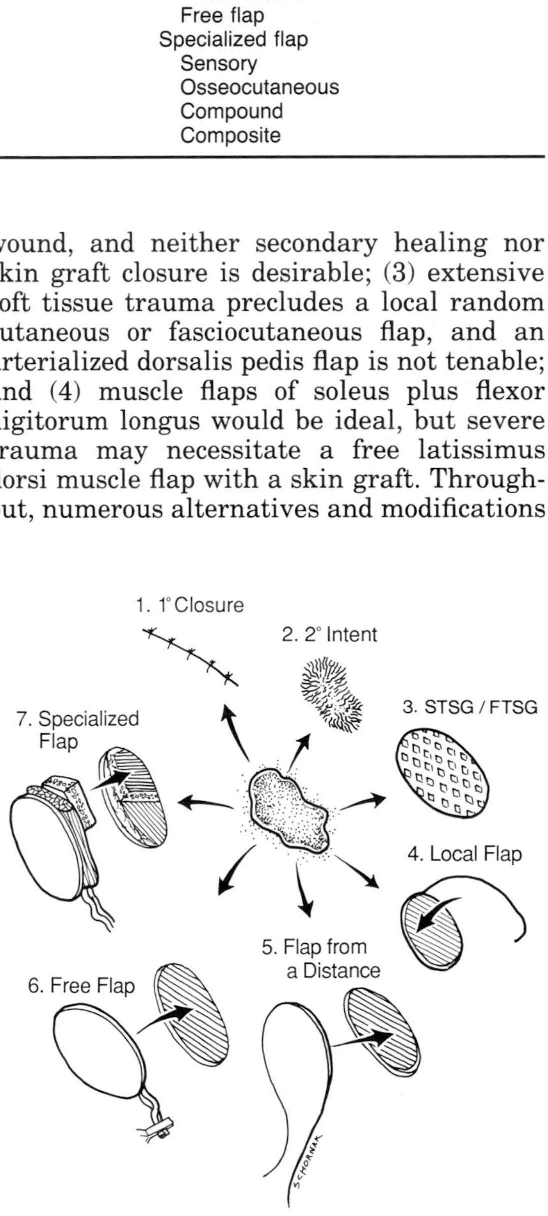

Figure 9–4. Principal techniques of wound closure, progressing in complexity clockwise.

are considered as one searches for the optimal solution.

Patient factors are gaining importance in view of the increased number of procedures available and the cases of litigation over informed consent. For example, closure of a pressure sore in a paraplegic must take into account the timing of the occurrence of the condition (early or late after spinal cord transection), patient cooperation, the likelihood of recurrence, previous surgical procedures, and the long-term outlook. Certainly, the unmotivated depressed patient with multiple pressure sores occurring soon after spinal cord transection requires a local random cutaneous flap to achieve closure without compromising the future surgical options of muscle or myocutaneous flaps. In contrast, the active working paraplegic who develops a single pressure sore several years after spinal cord injury requires optimal coverage with a myocutaneous flap that will allow rapid return to a supportive environment. Patient factors are numerous, including patients' occupation and avocation, mobility or immobility, age (young or elderly), and so forth.

Macrocirculation

Any discussion of the cutaneous blood supply must be viewed from an anatomic, physiologic, and surgical vantage. Anatomic classification of the vasculature attempts to organize a very disparate system. The surgeon is imposing principles and perspective onto a cutaneous region supplied by numerous types of blood vessels. Under normal circumstances, these blood vessels are dynamically changing their individual distribution patterns, depending on physiologic conditions. It must be remembered that the creation of a skin flap markedly reduces the blood flow to the skin, renders it dependent on only a few blood vessels, and is exceedingly traumatic. The following discussion describes the embryology and anatomy of the cutaneous vessels and plexuses.

EMBRYOLOGY

Numerous investigations of the cutaneous blood supply throughout the body are currently being reported, usually with auras of discovery and attributed significance, yet anatomy is the final reflection of a dynamic embryologic process. Central to an understanding of this evolution is the recognition that vascular development is occurring simultaneously at the major vessels and in the skin. In the 5 mm human embryo the primary vessels are the dorsal and ventral aorta. Dorsally, 30 rows of segmental branches occur whose ventral rami become the intercostal-lumbar arteries. Ventrally, longitudinal anastomoses exist between parallel rows, which become the internal mammary-epigastric system (Fig. 9–5). In describing the definitive vessels, Arey (1974) noted at least 13 different developmental patterns, including direct sprouting, parallel fusion, and cross anastomosis. For example, the blood supply to the posterior portion of the lower limb is derived by "longitudinal annexation" in which a middle portion of the primitive sciatic artery is inserted between the stem of the femoral artery and a more distal portion of the femoral artery, thus producing the definitive femoropopliteal–posterior tibial system. While this type of active recombination of primordial vessels is occurring, the cutaneous circulation is being derived from vasodermal cells. The process of angiogenesis occurs in sequential stages, with a provisional temporary plexus in which preferential channels develop followed by atrophy of the unused parts.

Thus, major embryologic changes are occurring on three levels: (1) the deep distribution system of primary vessels, which are in continuity with the aorta and are achieving their final definitive configuration; (2) the intervening muscle mass, which is undergoing numerous recombinations and migrations; and (3) the various plexuses of the cutaneous vasculature, which are responding to external factors. As noted by Schäfer (1975), differentiation of the fascial vascular network begins from a fetal vascular network in the second half of intrauterine life, but the final pathway is not determined until the perinatal period. From an embryologic view, it is proposed that the following four factors govern the vascularity of any organ: (1) the size of a vessel lumen is determined by the rate of blood flow, (2) the length of a vessel is governed by longitudinal tension (a factor recently confirmed by skin expansion experiments), (3) the vessel wall thickness is dependent on blood pressure, and (4) increased capillary pressure results in the formation of new capillaries.

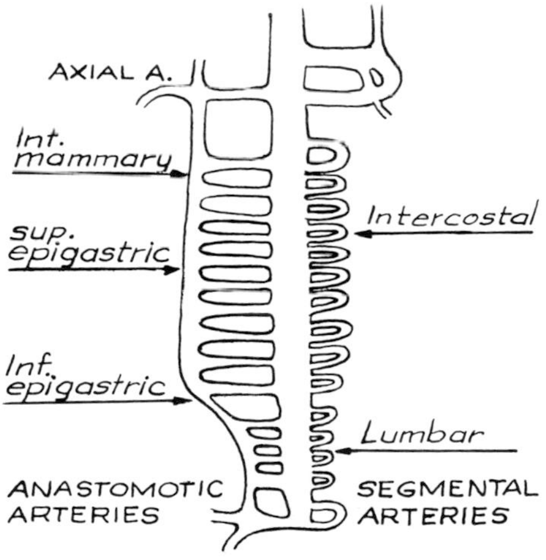

Figure 9–5. Vascular anatomy of a 5 mm human embryo. (From Daniel, R. K., and Williams, H. B.: The free transfer of skin flaps by microvascular anastomoses. An experimental study and a reappraisal. Plast. Reconstr. Surg., *52*:16, 1973. Copyright 1973, The Williams & Wilkins Company, Baltimore.)

ANATOMY

In view of the surgical advances of the past two decades, which required new anatomic studies, a complete reappraisal of the entire blood supply to the skin is warranted. An attempt will be made to reconcile the priority of anatomists' terminology with the proprietary interests of surgeons to produce a more accurate and accommodative description. The blood supply throughout the body may be perceived as existing on three levels: internal, muscular, and cutaneous. The *internal system* consists of the body's main distributing vessels, which are a continuation of the aorta in regard to perfusion pressure. The next level is the *muscular system*, which provides nutritional blood supply to the muscles. The third level consists of the *cutaneous circulation*, which can be subdivided into fascia, subcutaneous tissue, and skin. On the basis of detailed investigations, the third level can be subdivided into five distinct plexuses supplied by two types of arteries with variable regional patterns (Fig. 9–6). An example of this tertiary progression is seen over the upper thigh where the femoral artery (internal) distributes blood to the extremity by providing numerous muscular branches, including the lateral femoral circumflex (muscular), which has a descending branch that penetrates the septum to supply the overlying skin (septocutaneous).

Internal System. The aorta is the body's primary vessel and its numerous branches

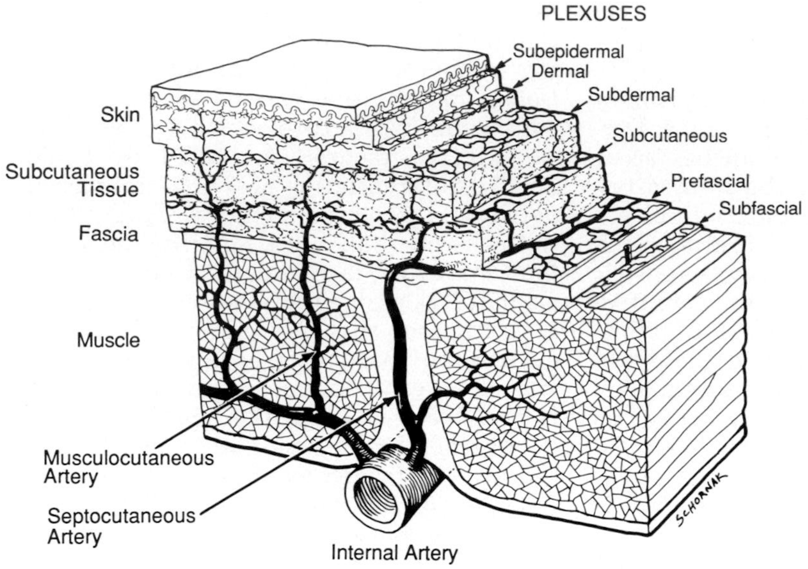

Figure 9–6. The cutaneous macrocirculation.

distribute blood throughout the body. As subsequent divisions and terminal trunks are reached, use of major arteries for flap perfusion becomes possible, including the dorsalis pedis and radial forearm flaps. As one moves peripherally, the need to include overlying muscle, tendon, or nerve decreases, but the risk of having to reconstruct the essential artery increases as collateral flow is reduced. The intercostal flap is the classic internal artery flap where all intervening tissue between the skin paddle and the underlying intercostal artery is sacrificed to ensure preservation of the essential cutaneous artery (Fig. 9–7) (Kerrigan and Daniel, 1979). In contrast, dissection by Timmons (1986) showed that a thin gossamer connection between the overlying skin and internal artery allows the radial forearm flap to survive. This distinction emphasizes the difference between flaps of the trunk, with their large flat muscles having numerous musculocutaneous arteries, and the distal extremities, with their longitudinal muscular mass having a plethora of septocutaneous arteries.

Muscular System. The blood supply to a specific muscle probably reflects its embryologic formation. Although a myomeric arrangement persists in certain areas, most muscles are derived from one of the following six patterns: migration (latissimus dorsi), fusion (rectus abdominis), longitudinal splitting (trapezius), tangential splitting (transversus abdominis), a change in direction, or degeneration. The rectus abdominis represents the fusion of multiple myomeres while both its segmental blood supply from the intercostal arteries and the longitudinally aligned epigastric arteries are retained. This muscle and its overlying skin can be incorporated into either an intercostal or a rectus abdominis flap. Mathes and Nahai (1979) classified the blood supply to muscle into the following five

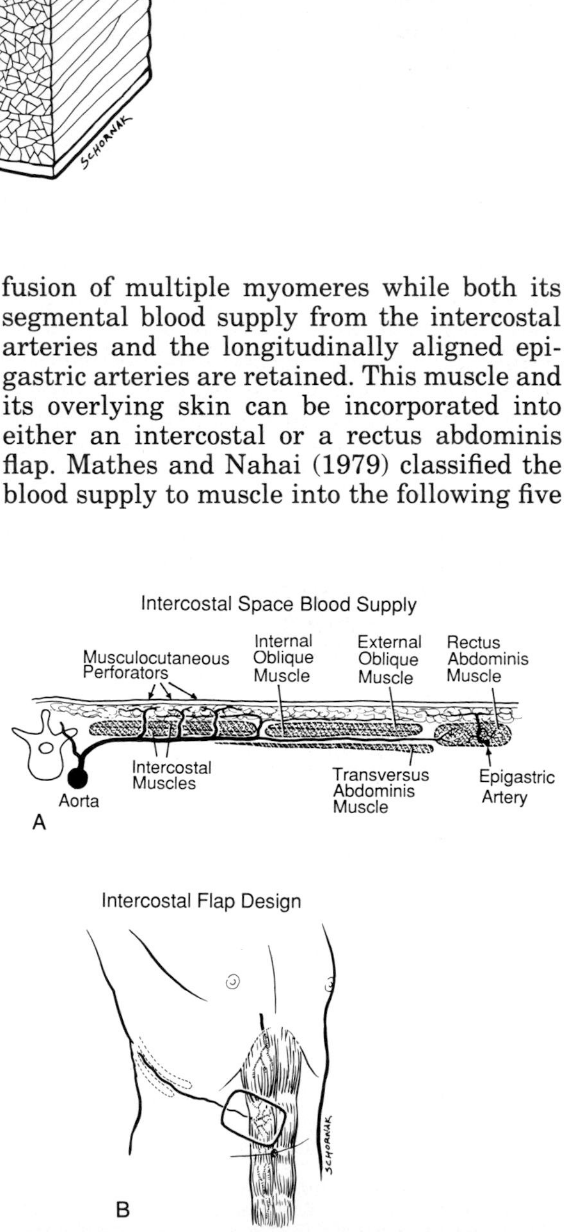

Figure 9–7. The internal vascular system typified by the intercostal flap. *A*,, The vascular supply to an interspace. *B*, The clinical design of the flap.

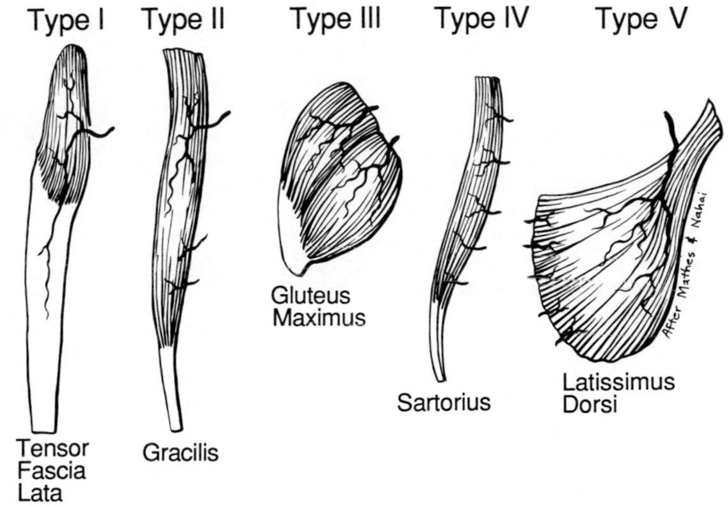

Figure 9–8. Classification of muscles by the type of blood supply (after Mathes and Nahai, 1979).

types: Type I, one vascular pedicle (tensor fascia lata); Type II, dominant pedicle and minor pedicle(s) (gracilis); Type III, two dominant pedicles (gluteus maximus); Type IV, segmental vascular pedicles (sartorius); and Type V, one dominant pedicle and secondary segmental pedicles (latissimus dorsi) (Fig. 9–8). The important clinical correlation is that Type III muscles may not survive transposition on one vascular pedicle, while only one-third of a Type IV muscle may survive reduction onto a single vascular pedicle. An important factor in skin flap design is the musculocutaneous artery, specifically what percentage of branches of the supplying artery terminate within the muscle and how many continue upward into the overlying skin. Although a precise figure is unavailable, one can speculate that at least one-third of the supplying musculocutaneous arteries will continue upward through the fascia into the overlying skin, while two-thirds will terminate in the muscle itself.

Cutaneous System. The cutaneous system exists on three anatomic levels (fascia, subcutaneous fat, and skin) and is made up of five recognizable vascular plexuses (fascial, subcutaneous, cutaneous, dermal, and subepidermal) supplied by two types of cutaneous arteries (musculocutaneous and septocutaneous) (Fig. 9–9). If the supplying arteries are visualized in a vertical plane, their distribution is best conceived of as a stacked series of interconnected horizontal networks or plexuses. Any discussion of terminology must begin with Spalteholz (1893), who classified cutaneous arteries into two types: pure and mixed. As summarized by Moretti (1968):

The "pure" cutaneous arteries are direct branches from the large arterial trunks (the superficial epigastric artery) that come directly to the skin and

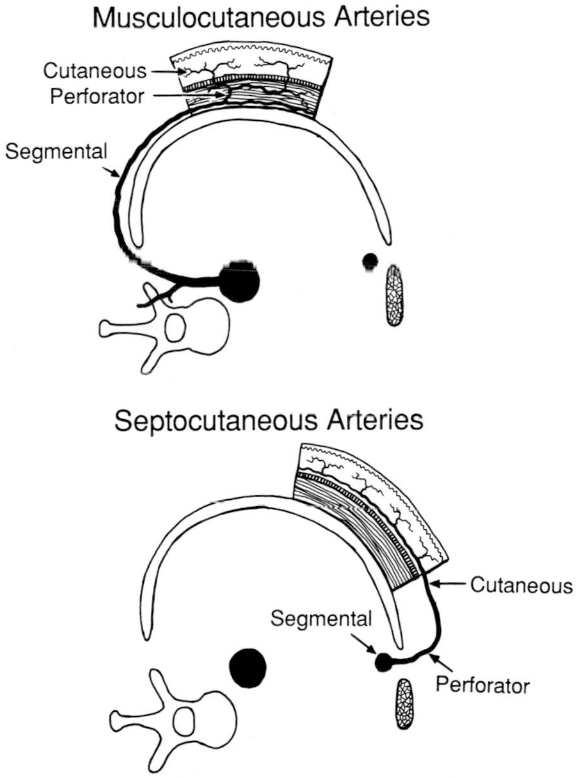

Figure 9–9. The differences between musculocutaneous and septocutaneous vessels.

divide and subdivide themselves . . . these vessels usually come from the connective intermuscular spaces and move into the subcutaneous tissues which they traverse in a direction oblique or parallel to the surface.

The "mixed" cutaneous arteries, before reaching the skin, provide larger or smaller branches for other organs and especially for the muscles (musculocutaneous artery) . . . they come out from the fibers in a direction perpendicular to their surface, then cross with a slight loop, the muscular fascia, and thereafter enter directly into the skin.

Thus, the original discussion of the anatomy and hemodynamics of the cutaneous circulation and their influence on skin flap design incorporated the classic anatomic terminology: musculocutaneous and direct cutaneous. In light of recent anatomic studies and the growing emphasis on fasciocutaneous flaps, *it would appear prudent to substitute the term septocutaneous for direct cutaneous,* since the former reflects Spalteholz's emphasis on passage through the intermuscular septa.

Initially, these two types of vessels were distinguished as to their location, size, course, distribution, and dominance: a distinction that has become blurred by greater knowledge. It appears that both types of vessels are present throughout the body. Musculocutaneous arteries are prevalent over the torso; septocutaneous arteries predominate in the extremities, especially in the more distal areas. A spectrum exists for septocutaneous arteries, ranging from the relatively short cutaneous scapular artery (4 cm) to the long superficial circumflex iliac artery (SCIA) (10 cm) supplying the groin flap (Fig. 9–10). The size and number of muscle branches vary from minor (superficial circumflex iliac) to major (descending lateral femoral circumflex), while the course within the septum may be short (SCIA) or long (scapular). Continuation beneath the fascia may be long (superficial circumflex iliac), while continuation within the skin can be extensive (anterior thoracic perforans). As noted by Timmons (1986), the orientation of the vessels varies with the amount of fat; the greater the volume of fat, the more perpendicular and separated are the fascial vessels, while thin skin gives the impression of a richer vascular network. Each of these distinguishing characteristics influences the design of a specific skin flap, and illustrates the difficulty of classifying the blood supply to the skin.

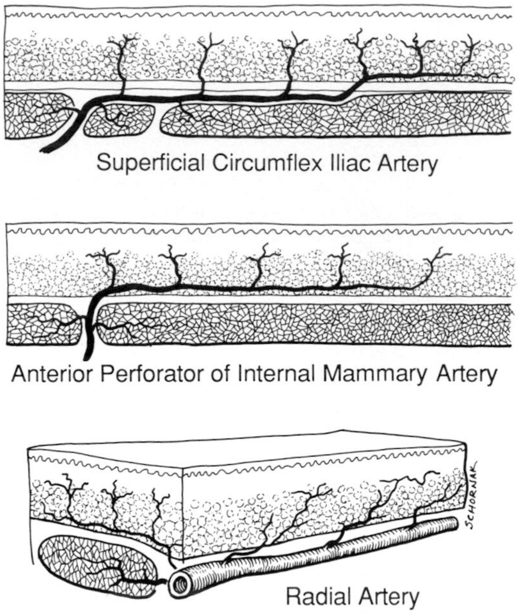

Figure 9–10. The spectrum of septocutaneous arteries.

Fascial Plexus. As noted by Salmon (1936), confirmed by the injection studies of Cormack and Lamberty (1984), and clinically applied by Ponten (1981) and Tolhurst, Haeseker, and Zeeman (1983), significant vascular plexuses are associated with muscle fascia, especially in the extremities (Fig. 9–11). The composition and blood supply of fascia was detailed by Lang (1962) and Schäfer (1975). The former described a basic diagonal network composed of two layers in the lower limb, and a more circular and longitudinal orientation in the upper extremity. Schäfer's detailed studies of the blood supply to fascia and subcutaneous tissues reveal an angioarchitecture that has three layers and three sources. Although blood vessels can be found within the fascia itself, including capillaries, there is little metabolic demand to warrant a robust internal circulation. Instead, the vascular plexuses are located below (subfascial) and above (prefascial) the fascia itself. The subfascial plexus is relatively minor and incapable of sustaining a fascial flap. It consists primarily of a few branches to adjacent areolar and fibrous tissue with minor distribution, the one exception being tensor fascia lata. In contrast, the prefascial plexus is considered the dominant distribution system (fascial plexus) whose development varies between regions, as noted by Cormack and Lamberty (1984). The blood supply to these plexuses is

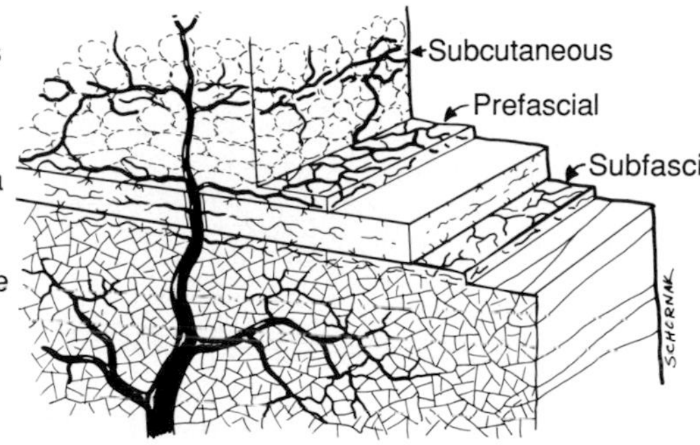

Figure 9–11. The fascial vascular plexuses.

from numerous sources and not merely the "fasciocutaneous" arteries proposed by some studies. These origins include the septocutaneous arteries that pass along the interconnecting muscular septum to interconnect with the plexuses, plus the adjacent musculocutaneous arteries and retrograde flow from the overlying subcutaneous plexuses. A separate fasciocutaneous artery is not recognized. As noted by Spalteholz (1893), each cutaneous artery, whether musculocutaneous or septocutaneous, pierces the fascia through distinct openings and then provides three to five radiating branches, which lie directly in the fascia and anastomose with each other. The dominant blood supply is from both types of cutaneous arteries that penetrate the fascia, while the dominant distribution is along the prefascial plexus. Is there an axiality and a regional distribution for the fascial plexuses? From an extensive number of injection studies, Cormack and Lamberty (1984) implied that a reciprocal relationship exists between the development of the musculocutaneous and septocutaneous blood supply and their associated fascial plexuses. Specifically, the musculocutaneous system is most prevalent along the broad flat muscles of the torso, whereas the septocutaneous fascial system is well developed in the longer, thinner muscles of the extremities. Thus, the contribution of the fascial plexuses would be minimal in an axillary flap, but of great significance in a forearm flap.

Subcutaneous Plexus. As noted originally by Spalteholz (1893), confirmed by Pearl and Johnson (1983) and clinically applied by Marty and associates (1984), a significant network exists at the level of the superficial fascia that splits the subcutaneous fat into a superficial (dense) and deep (loose) layer (Fig. 9–12). This fascial plane corresponds phylogenetically to the panniculus carnosus muscle, whose vestigial remnants in man include the platysma muscle and Scarpa's fascia. Within this fascia, a horizontal-linear vascular plexus of arteries and veins exists that varies according to body regions, being more developed over the torso than in the lower extremity. Spalteholz (1893) emphasized this regional variation as well as the reciprocal relationship between the subcutaneous and dermal plexuses—the former being dominant over the torso. As noted by Marty and associates (1984), one can design a subcutaneous flap of the upper extremity for closure of significant defects without incorporating the deep fascia, thus clearly distinguishing it from a fasciocutaneous flap. Of particular importance are the major supplying arteries, both musculocutaneous and septocutaneous, which give branches to form this plexus, and the numerous smaller side branches that nourish the overlying cutaneous plexus.

Subdermal Plexus. The subdermal or cutaneous plexus has long been considered the primary blood supply to skin: "it is the wide meshworks, as well as the strong muscular vessels of the 'cutaneous' arterial and venous networks, which in man have the task of distributing the blood suitably to the various parts of the skin" (Moretti, 1968). This plexus is considered by Moretti (1968) to be the junction between the deep reticular portion of the dermis and the underlying subcutaneous fat (Fig. 9–12). It is the level that corresponds with "dermal bleeding" at the edge of a skin flap. From here, numerous arterioles run upward through the lower dermis in an oblique or vertical direction to the overlying dermal plexus, while others pass downward to supply adipose tissue and var-

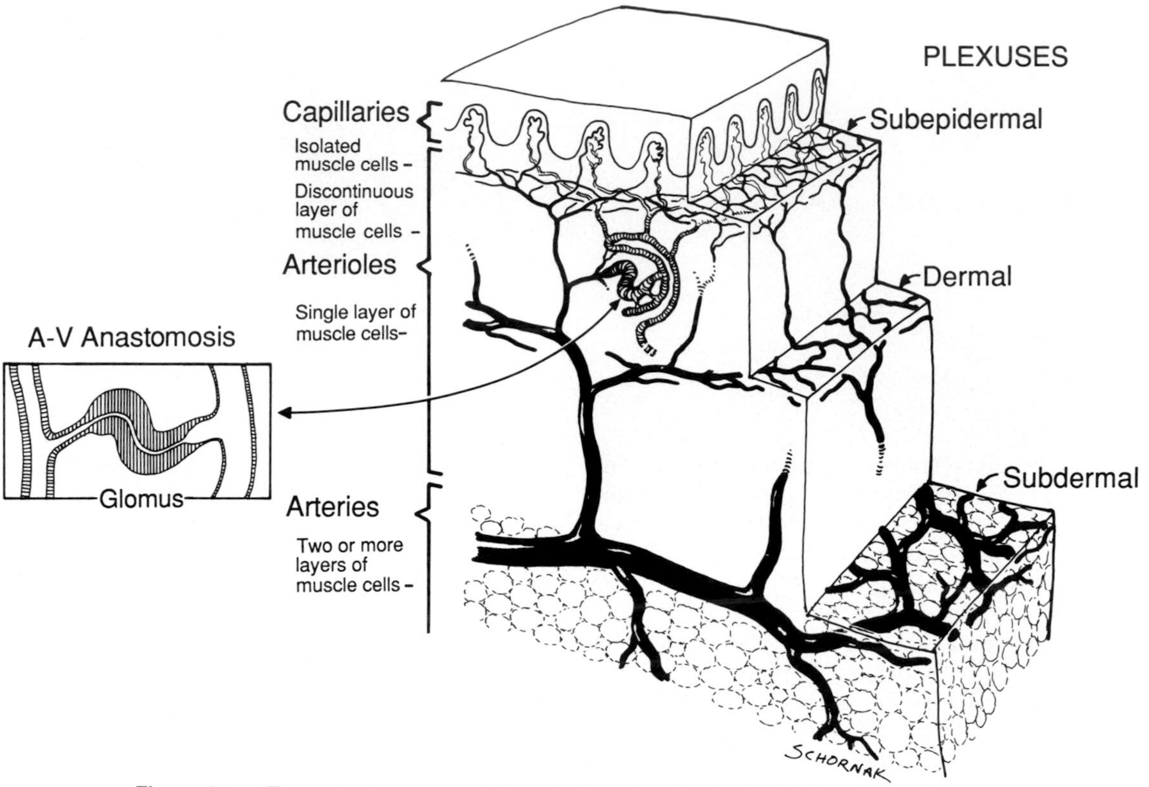

Figure 9–12. The subcutaneous, subdermal, dermal, and subepidermal vascular plexuses.

ious glands. From the subdermal plexus, numerous candelabra arteries ascend through the reticular dermis, communicating with one another to form arched anastomoses.

Dermal and Subepidermal Plexuses. These plexuses provide the true skin circulation, as they are in close proximity and their vast quantity provides a surface area far greater than all other plexuses combined. They are present from the lower limits of the dermal papillary ridge to the dermoepidermal line (Fig. 9–12). The arterial system is rapidly arborizing and a transition occurs from artery (cutaneous) to arteriole (dermal) to capillary (subepidermal). As one progresses upward, the following changes occur in structure and function: the *subdermal plexus* has a continuous arterial muscular wall and primary distribution function, to the *dermal plexus* with its arterioles having isolated muscular elements and primary thermoregulating function, to the *subepidermal plexus* with its capillaries having no muscular coverage and primary nutritive function. It has been proposed that 70 per cent of the blood utilized in thermoregulation is contained within this "external vascular belt." Equally important is the perifollicular vascular network, which varies with the growth and evolution of hairs and sweat glands. Despite the density of capillaries (150/mm^2), skin is far less vascularized than muscle (2000/mm^2), approximately 1:7, while on a functional level only 4.5 per cent of total blood is in skin compared with 13.2 per cent in muscle. Only 1 to 20 per cent of cutaneous blood flow is for nutrition; the rest has pressure and thermoregulatory functions.

Regional Patterns. From the early injection studies of Manchot (Morain, 1983) and the clinical investigations of McGregor and Morgan (1973) and Taylor and Palmer (1987), it is obvious that the skin can be divided into multiple regions (see also Chap. 10) on the basis of the distribution patterns of significant cutaneous arteries (Fig. 9–13). But are these captive territories and what is their significance for the plastic surgeon? Our understanding of the cutaneous blood supply indicates that the skin is vastly overperfused as regards its nutritional requirements. A skin flap is perfused through numerous types of vessels and plexuses. The ability to raise myocutaneous flaps provides an entirely new

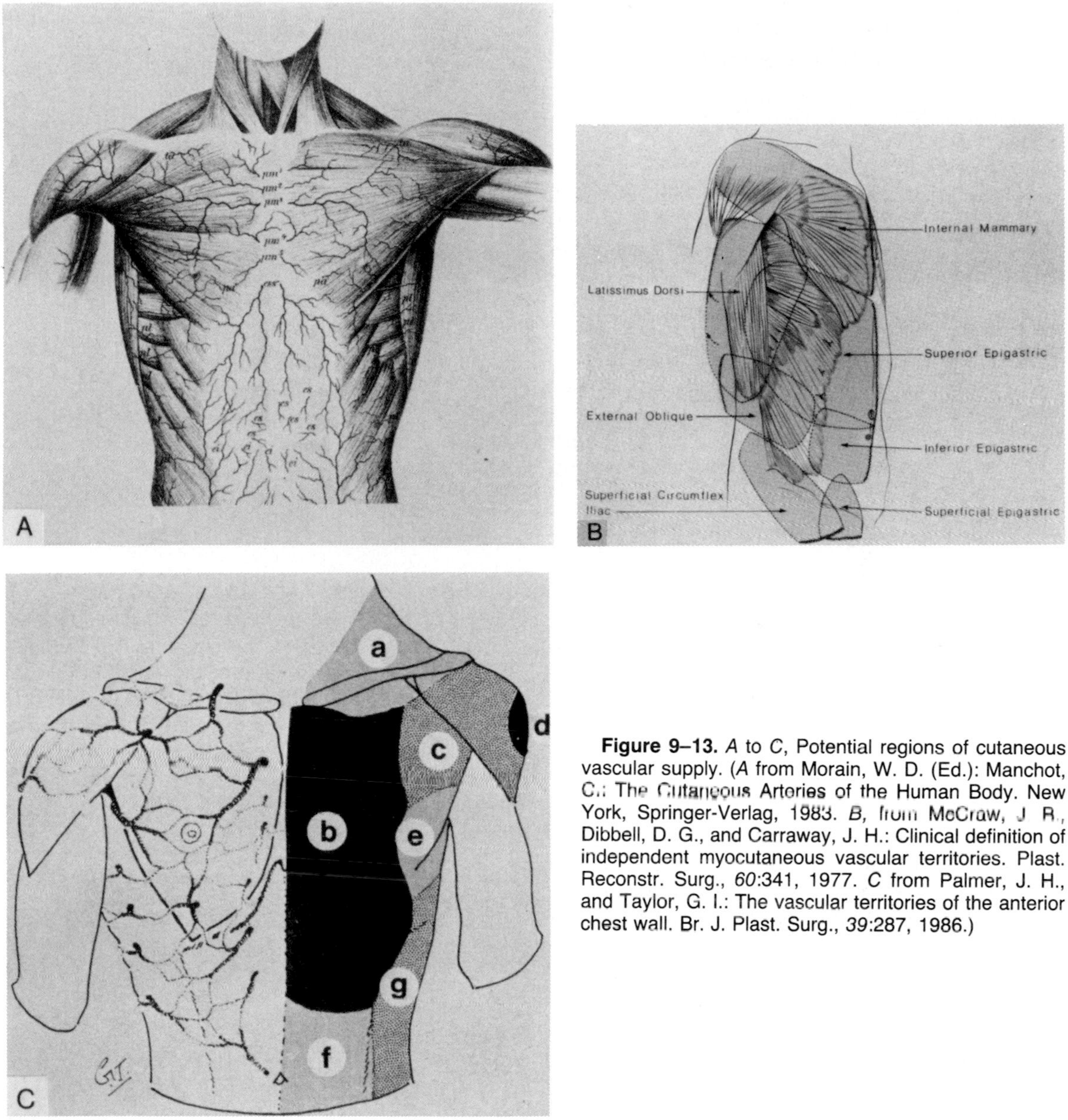

Figure 9–13. *A* to *C*, Potential regions of cutaneous vascular supply. (*A* from Morain, W. D. (Ed.): Manchot, C.: The Cutaneous Arteries of the Human Body. New York, Springer-Verlag, 1983. *B*, from McCraw, J. B., Dibbell, D. G., and Carraway, J. H.: Clinical definition of independent myocutaneous vascular territories. Plast. Reconstr. Surg., *60*:341, 1977. *C* from Palmer, J. H., and Taylor, G. I.: The vascular territories of the anterior chest wall. Br. J. Plast. Surg., *39*:287, 1986.)

set of principles to govern skin blood supply. Thus, an initial infatuation with the cutaneous maps of Manchot (Morain, 1983) has given way to a greater in-depth knowledge of specific arteries, alternative composition, and ultimately selection of a donor site irrespective of a specific blood supply. In the future, the optimal donor site will be selected, and then its requisite blood supply for surviving tissue transfer will be analyzed.

Types of Flaps

In the past two decades, the number and variability of flaps have increased dramatically. No longer are recipient site requirements compromised by the available donor sites. The reliability of flaps has been improved by greater understanding of blood supply, and the time of transfer lessened by microsurgical techniques. These advances now require that the plastic surgeon have a large repertoire of operations, an in-depth understanding of the blood supply to the skin, and greater clinical skills.

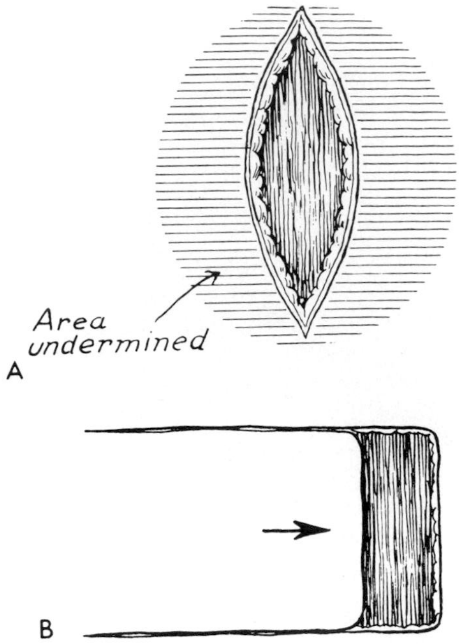

Figure 9–14. Advancement flap. *A,* The simplest advancement flap is that produced by the closure of a defect after undermining of the skin, facilitating linear closure of the defect. *B,* Example of a straight advancement flap. (From Kazanjian and Converse.)

RANDOM CUTANEOUS FLAPS

Random cutaneous flaps are characterized by their *blood supply*, from either musculocutaneous or septocutaneous vessels whose anatomic and vascular bases coincide. These flaps can be subdivided according to their method of movement: advancement, pivot, or interpolation.

Advancement Flaps. An advancement flap moves directly forward into a defect without any lateral movement (Fig. 9–14). These flaps were first employed by Celsus in ancient Rome and later popularized as rectangular sliding flaps by French surgeons in the first half of the nineteenth century (Converse, 1977). Their execution is facilitated whenever a relative skin excess exists, such as in older patients, or whenever skin elasticity is greatest, such as in the very young.

The usual advancement flap is rectangular and is oriented to benefit from the skin elasticity and regional blood supply. The flap should be perpendicular to the lines of minimal tension, with as much consideration as possible given to camouflaging the incisions. The presence of known septocutaneous arteries, especially in the lower extremity, should influence the initial orientation and extent of undermining. The overall shape of the flap can be altered to gain additional movement. When the flap is advanced, a fold of skin forms on each side of the base of the pedicle. Burow devised a method of excising triangles of skin from the adjacent base, thus gaining advancement (Converse, 1977). Alternatively, the base can be made more angular or curved, or small Z-plasties can be added to it (Fig. 9–15).

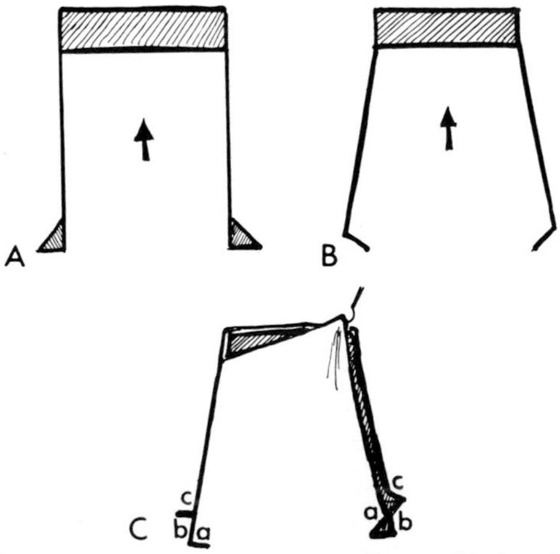

Figure 9–15. An advancement flap modified with (*A*), Burow's triangles, (*B*), counterincision at the base, and (*C*), Z-plasty at the base.

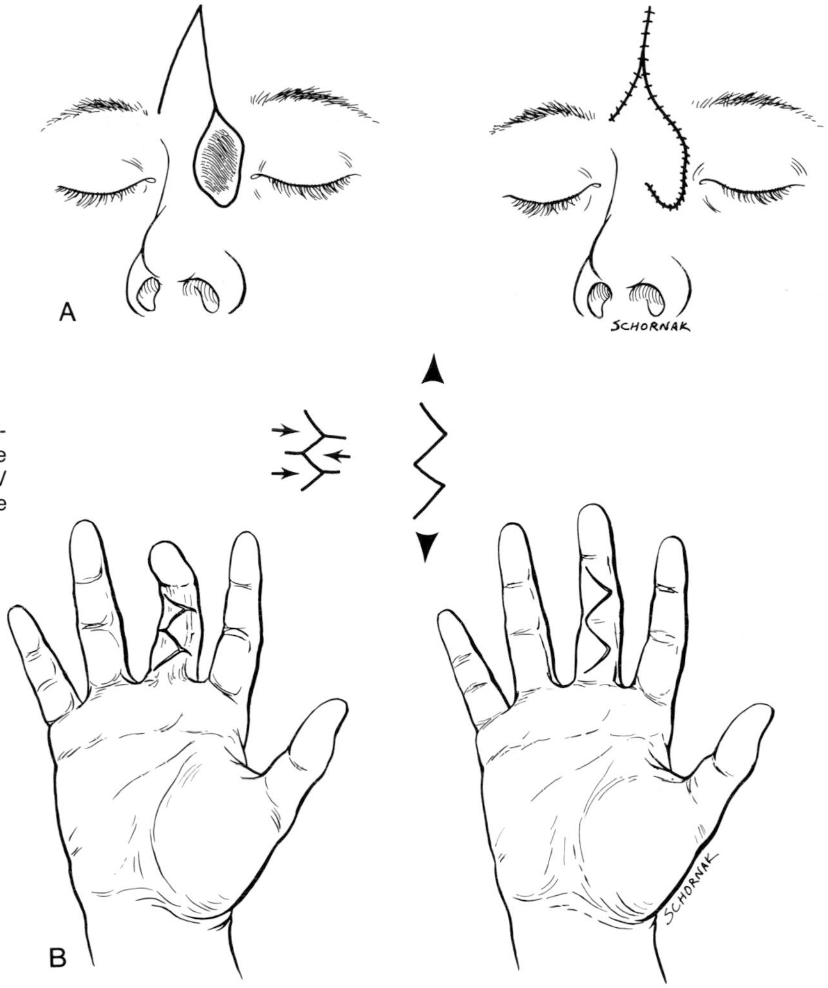

Figure 9–16. *A*, A V-Y advancement flap from the glabella to the medial canthal region. *B*, The Y-V advancement principle used in the digit.

Both the V-Y and Y-V advancement flaps are modifications of this method of movement. The V-Y principle is used both in small flaps such as in columellar advancement and glabellar flaps (Fig. 9–16*A*) and in large flaps such as the V-Y hamstring myocutaneous flap. The Y-V advancement can be used to interrupt contractures and gain length, such as in mild cases of Dupuytren's contracture (Fig. 9–16*B*).

Two variations on the advancement flap principle are the bipedicle advancement flap and the staged procedure. Bipedicle flaps, especially in the scalp or lower extremities, can be viewed horizontally as advancement flaps or vertically as transposition flaps that require a skin graft to cover the donor site. Bipedicle flaps are rarely done except in cleft palate repair, since the technique doubles the donor site morbidity, is more extensive, and often increases the risk. A two stage advancement flap provides the requisite skin at the recipient site initially, but requires a second stage to divide the pedicle and to skin graft the donor site. This technique is much less commonly employed than previously, although one example, the thenar flap, remains quite useful for fingertip reconstruction.

Pivot Flaps. A pivot flap, either transposition or rotation, derives its name from the pivot point at the base of the flap as well as its arc of rotation whose radius is under the greatest tension.

A *transposition* flap is usually a rectangular or square flap located immediately adjacent to the defect (Fig. 9–17). In design it is critical that the flap should extend beyond the defect. This maneuver ensures adequate flap length after its transposition. Additional length can be gained by a back cut away

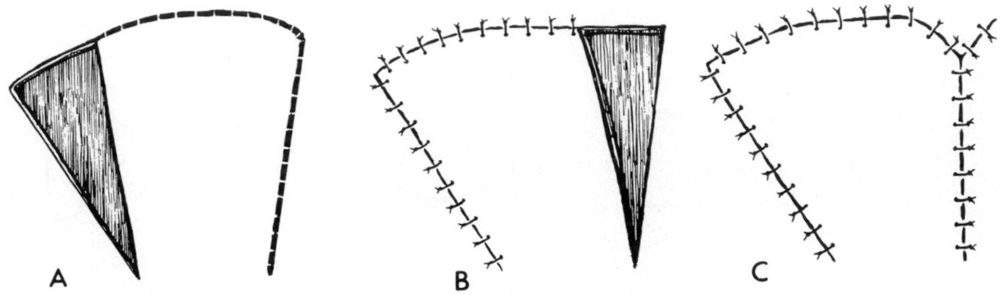

Figure 9–17. Transposition flap. *A,* Design of the transposition flap. *B,* Transposition of the flap with the resulting donor defect. *C,* Closure of the secondary defect by the V-Y advancement principle.

from, or into, the base of the flap, the latter carrying a risk of reducing the flap's blood supply. Closure of the donor site may be by either a skin graft or another skin flap. The latter method is best exemplified by the bilobed flap of Zimany (1953) or the multiple flaps of Limberg (1946) (Fig. 9–18).

A *rotation* flap is a semicircular flap that rotates about a pivot point to fill the defect (Fig. 9–19). To ensure primary closure, it is essential that the flap be quite large, often with a circumference five to eight times the width of the defect. It is located along appropriate skin tension lines. The use of back cuts into or away from the base, as well as Burow's triangle from the lateral aspect of the base, can be considered (Converse, 1977)(Fig. 9–20). Alternatively, one can close the donor site with either a skin graft or another flap.

Interpolation Flaps. An interpolation flap is taken from a nearby, but not immediately adjacent, donor site and transposed either above or below the intervening skin to the recipient defect (Fig. 9–21). This type of flap can be subdivided according to its pedicle's composition (cutaneous, subcutaneous, or island) (Fig. 9–22) as well as the number of stages. Typical examples include the median forehead flap, which can be transposed as a cutaneous flap over the intervening skin to reconstruct the nasal tip or isolated on the supraorbital vessels as an island flap to be passed beneath the intervening skin. The cutaneous interpolation flap requires two

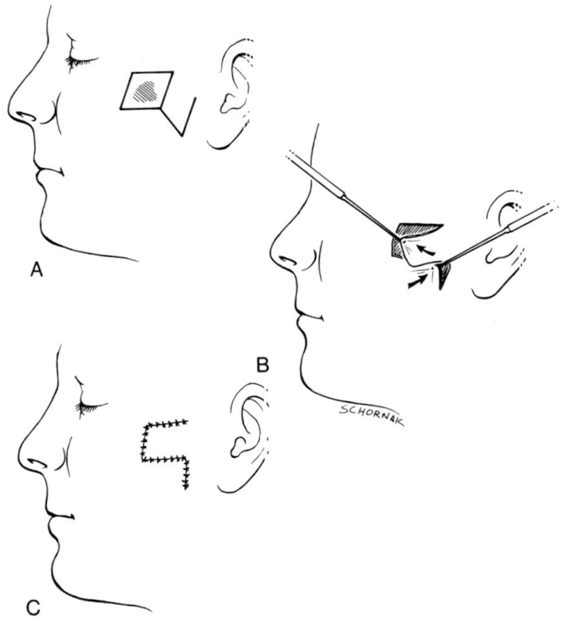

Figure 9–18. Transposition flap using the Limberg design. *A,* Creation of the rhomboid defect with flap design, with attention paid to the minimal skin tension lines and the lines of maximal extensibility. *B,* Elevation and transposition of the flap. *C,* Closure of both recipient and donor defects.

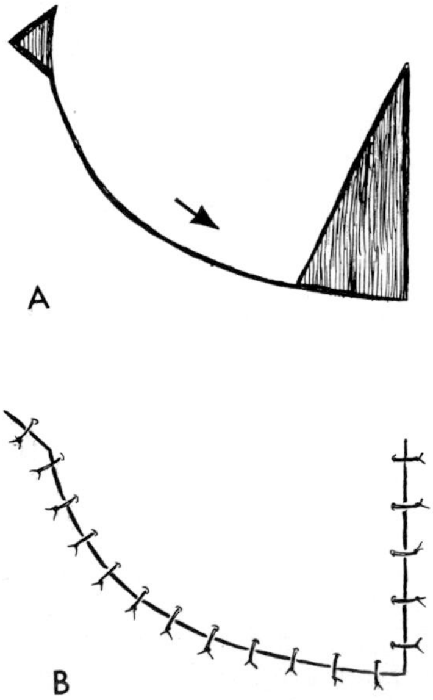

Figure 9–19. A standard rotation flap with excision of a Burow's triangle at the base to facilitate closure.

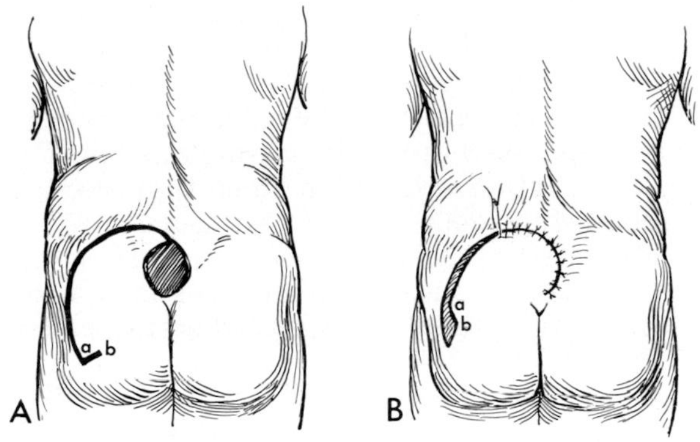

Figure 9–20. Rotation flap to cover a sacral pressure sore. Note the back cut into the base of the flap.

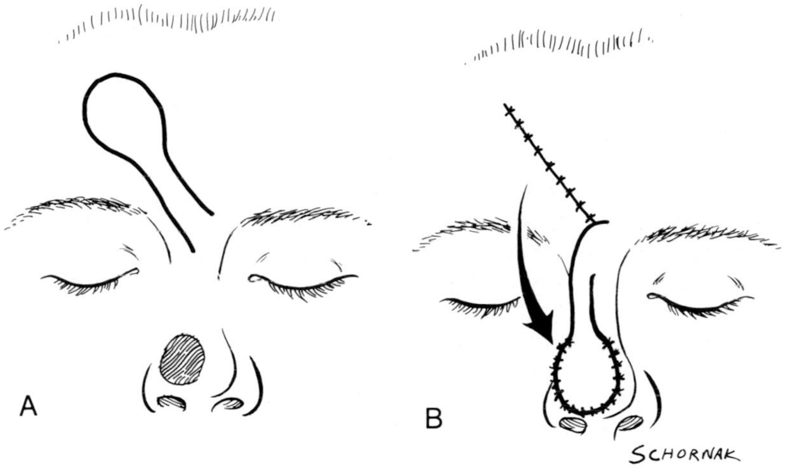

Figure 9–21. Interpolation flap requiring two stages for completion of the reconstruction: (*A*), design of flap and (*B*), flap elevation and insetting. The second stage involves division and discarding of the flap pedicle.

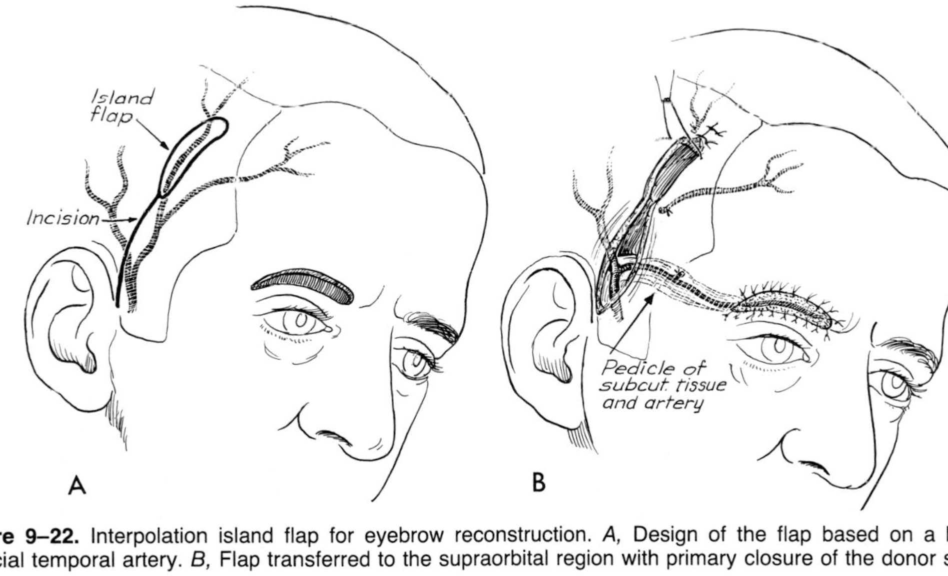

Figure 9–22. Interpolation island flap for eyebrow reconstruction. *A,* Design of the flap based on a branch of the superficial temporal artery. *B,* Flap transferred to the supraorbital region with primary closure of the donor site.

stages but is more reliable than the island version, which offers more elegance but greater risk. Barron and Emmett (1965) popularized the concept of the subcutaneous pedicle flap taken from the nasolabial fold for reconstruction of the nose. In certain cases, a second-stage defatting may be necessary.

As noted, random cutaneous flaps offer the advantages of ideal color match and composition, since they are often adjacent to the defect. Their size and flexible orientation frequently ensure survival. When the recipient site is of small size and in the face, the alternative is a full-thickness skin graft. By comparison, a flap offers superior color match, better composition, economy of donor site, and greater reliability. However, as the size increases and applications extend beyond the face, the alternative becomes the entire spectrum of flaps.

The principal disadvantages are donor site morbidity, vascular compromise, limited composition, and unreliability as size increases. The classical methods of achieving greater surviving length by increasing width (length-to-width ratio) or a delay procedure have given way to designing a flap with an augmented blood supply, i.e., either an arterial or a myocutaneous flap. Thus, the use of random cutaneous flaps to cover large defects has decreased dramatically, but their value in closing smaller facial defects remains. As demonstrated by Feldman (1987), the value of random cutaneous flaps in reconstructing the burned face is without peer. It behooves every plastic surgeon to master their fundamental principles.

ARTERIAL CUTANEOUS FLAPS

The applications of axial or arterial flaps were codified by Esser (Haeseker, 1983) and Webster (1937), applied to the torso by Bakamjian (1965), and mastered by McGregor and Jackson (1972). In view of their initial application on the face, these flaps were considered arterial flaps since they were designed to include a specific artery within their pedicle. Venous drainage was through an associated subcutaneous vein, paired venae comitantes, or the subdermal plexuses. As reviewed by Haeseker (1983), Esser devised numerous arterial and island flaps to reconstruct a multitude of war casualties. In 1965, Bakamjian dramatically altered conventional concepts of skin flap design by demonstrating that a medially based deltopectoral flap of impressive length could be raised without regard for the length-to-width ratio or the need for a delay procedure (Fig. 9–23). Rather than following arithmetic guidelines, he based the flap on the anterior thoracic perforators and incorporated the lateral cutaneous branches into the flap's pedicle. In essence, the vascular base that coincides with the termination of the supplying arteries into the cutaneous plexuses was cantilevered far beyond the anatomic base that marks the entry point of the arteries into the flap (Fig. 9–24). Subsequently, McGregor and Jackson (1972) used this principle to discover the groin flap based on the superficial circumflex iliac artery (Fig. 9–25).

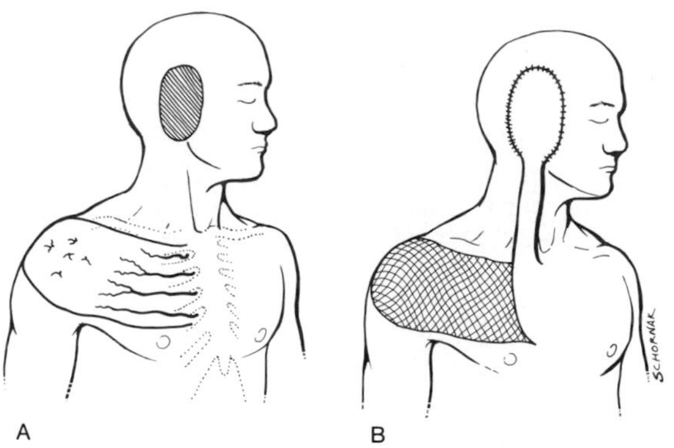

Figure 9–23. Bakamjian's deltopectoral flap. *A,* Design and vascular supply to the flap. *B,* Transposition of the flap to a cheek and ear defect with skin grafting of the donor defect.

In 1973, the introduction of free flap transfers by microvascular anastomoses led to an explosive interest in arterial flaps as donor sites, and numerous anatomic studies were initiated (Fig. 9–26). Initial efforts concentrated on the easily transferred groin, dorsalis pedis, and superficial temporal flaps, as long vascular pedicles were easily obtained. Rigid classifications and lists of direct cutaneous arteries appeared that totally ignored the shorter but more ubiquitous septocutaneous arteries. It was only with the subsequent development of myocutaneous flaps, muscle flaps, and fasciocutaneous flaps that the entire spectrum of septocutaneous arteries was appreciated. Septocutaneous arteries are branches of major arteries that pass throughout the intermuscular septum, often providing branches to the adjacent muscles, before supplying the cutaneous circulation. As noted by Song, Chen, and Song (1984),

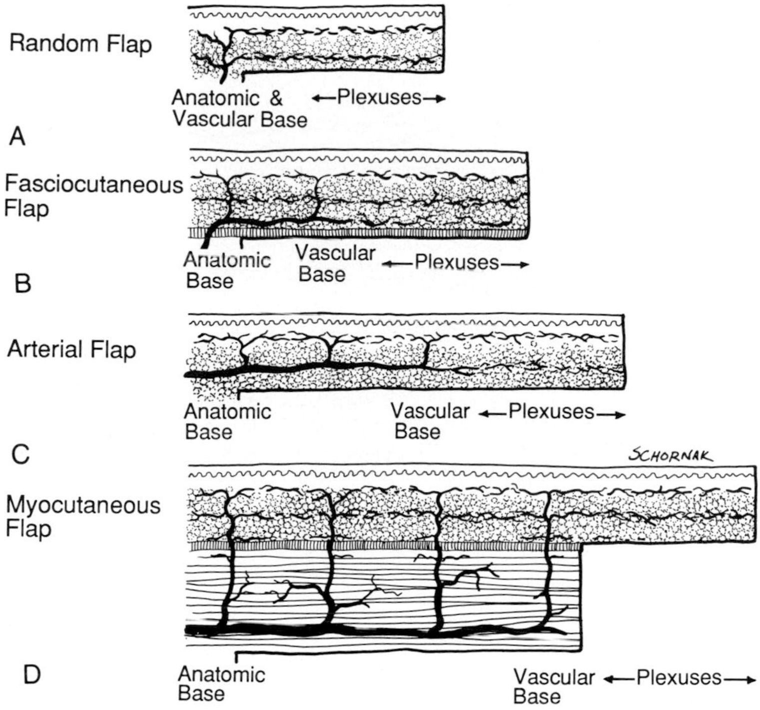

Figure 9–24. The cantilever principle. *A,* In a random flap the anatomic and vascular bases coincide. *B* to *D,* In fasciocutaneous, arterial, and myocutaneous flaps the anatomic and vascular bases may be at different locations.

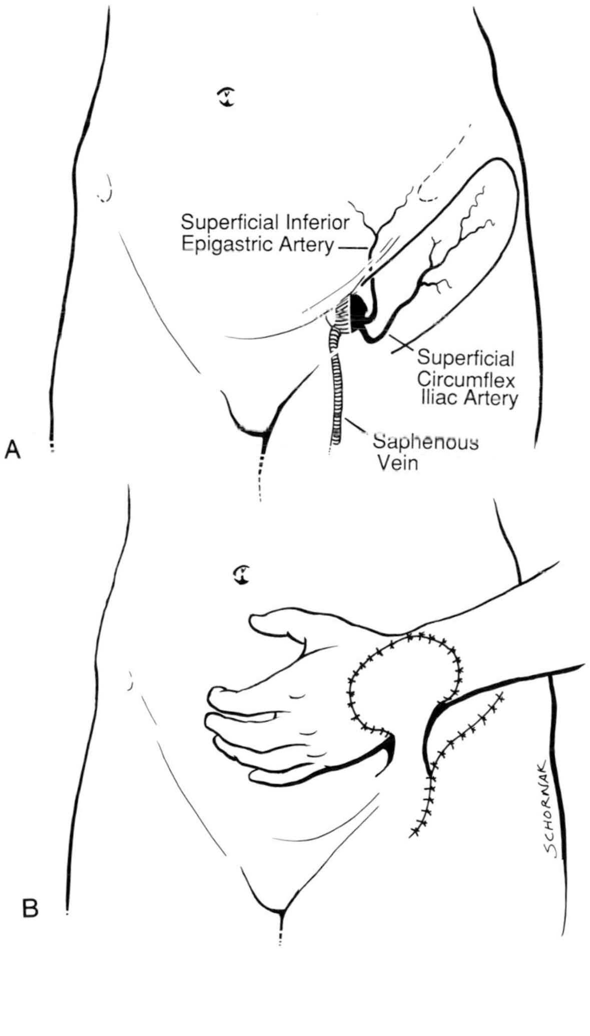

Figure 9–25. The groin flap. *A,* Key anatomic landmarks with design and vascular supply illustrated. *B,* Transfer of the flap to cover a distant hand defect with tubing of the intervening pedicle.

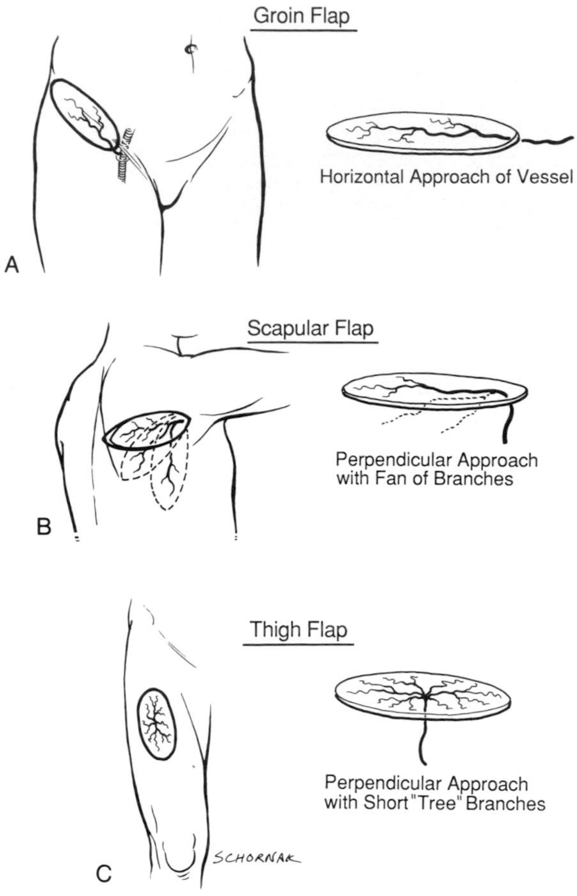

Figure 9–26. The vascular patterns of arterial flaps. *A,* The horizontal or parallel approach of the vessel, as exemplified by the groin flap. *B,* The perpendicular approach with long terminal branches permitting choice of a multitude of flap orientations, as exemplified by the scapular/parascapular flaps. *C,* The perpendicular approach with short terminal branches, as exemplified by the anteromedial thigh flap.

Nakajima, Fujino, and Adachi (1986), and Carriquiry, Aparecida Costa, and Vasconez (1985), design of skin flaps on these vessels begins with localization of the vessel's penetration point through the fascia, while the length of its vascular pedicle is gained by retrograde dissection with stripping of small muscular branches until a major muscle artery of sufficient diameter for microanastomoses is found. With this approach, Song, Chen, and Song (1984) devised three free thigh flaps, including the anterolateral (descending branch of the lateral femoral circumflex artery), anteromedial (innominate descending artery), and posterior (third perforator of the profundus femoris). Song, Chen, and Song (1984) clearly stated that in the three flaps the septocutaneous artery "does not present an axial distribution but divides into several branches which join the vascular plexus above the deep fascia . . . the cutaneous artery can provide blood to a large area of skin." Thus, arterial flaps can be designed on the basis of their cutaneous distribution plus the desired type of pedicle. If an attached pedicle flap is required, a vessel of maximal length is required, whereas for a free flap the vascular pedicle can be obtained by retrograde dissection along the intermuscular septum.

The principles governing the use of arterial flaps can best be illustrated by the groin and scapular flaps (Fig. 9–26). The first step in the execution of a groin flap is to outline the expected course of the superficial circumflex iliac artery, from its origin on the femoral artery to its termination beyond the anterior superior iliac spine. This course corresponds with the flap axis, which parallels the inguinal ligament for the standard groin flap, but parallels the artery for free flaps as it permits incorporation of the adjacent superficial inferior epigastric artery. The proximal portion represents the arterial pedicle, and the skin beyond the anterior superior iliac spine represents the random plexus portion. Maximal width is rarely a consideration, but maximal length is often a necessity. Width is determined by the recipient site requirement and the mandatory inclusion of the essential artery, with allowance for anatomic variations. Minimal width is not significant, because as width decreases one converts the arterial flap to an island flap. Owing to the deep location of the essential artery, a full thickness of subcutaneous fat is essential in the proximal portion. The surviving length of the flap is related to the length of the artery (approximately 12 cm) plus a relatively fixed random cutaneous length (approximately 15 to 20 cm). Elevation of the flap is begun by incision on all sides except the base, and it continues proximal to the anterior superior iliac spine. At that point, the inferior incision is continued medially and the sartorius muscle fascia is incised. For most upper extremity defects, retrograde dissection to within 5 cm of the femoral artery suffices. When used as a free flap, the artery is traced back to its origin and the associated veins are carefully preserved.

As originally described by Dos Santos (1984) and perfected by Gilbert and Teot (1982), the scapular flap is supplied by the cutaneous scapular artery, which is a terminal branch of the circumflex scapular artery. The lateral third of the flap overlaps the triangular space, which is the point of penetration of the cutaneous artery. The flap is usually of limited size (15 × 10 cm) and oriented in a transverse direction over the inferior two-thirds of the scapula. The dissection is begun along the superior border and continued toward the triangular space where the loose areolar tissue containing the artery is located. The circumferential incision is completed and the flap elevated in the loose areolar plane between the subcutaneous tissue and the fascia of the infraspinatus muscle. Following complete elevation, the vascular pedicle is dissected in a retrograde fashion through the triangular space back to the circumflex scapular artery, and even to the subscapular artery if necessary.

As noted by Dos Santos (1984), the cutaneous scapular artery averages 4 cm in length with an external diameter of 1.5 to 2.5 mm; it passes horizontally along the scapula toward the vertebral midline, and provides several muscular branches. The scapular flap is designed to overlay the artery and it can have its axis oriented in a fan-shaped manner, thus confirming that axial orientation is not critical. From numerous experiments, it is obvious that most cutaneous arteries have a circular perfusion pattern due probably to a Christmas tree–like branching pattern in which the proximal branches are longer than the distal ones. The flap can be raised without muscle fascia. The scapular flap is an arterial flap whose pedicle is purely vascular and perpendicular to the flap itself, in contrast to the standard groin flap where the pedicle is linearly oriented within the flap. This distinction is reflected in clinical usage in which the scapular flap is applied almost exclusively as a free flap donor site, whereas the standard groin flap is most often employed as a pedicle flap. In addition, the scapular flap probably presaged the septocutaneous flaps of the thigh, which are truly a pure cutaneous flap whose vascular pedicle is dissected out between muscles.

In summary, arterial cutaneous flaps are supplied by septocutaneous arteries. The critical characteristic is their design on a specific vessel, which allows the vascular base to be cantilevered far beyond the anatomic base. A broad spectrum (Fig. 9–26) exists from the long linear *groin flap*, with its arterial pedicle continuing into a random portion, to the *scapular flap*, with its distinct arterial flap plus a perpendicular island vascular pedicle, to the *anterior thigh flap*, with its cutaneous flap attached to a septocutaneous artery. All these flaps require an in-depth knowledge of the cutaneous arteries and skilled dissection techniques, but offer greater dimension and reliability in return.

FASCIOCUTANEOUS FLAPS

As pioneered by Ponten (1981), championed by Tolhurst, Haeseker, and Zeeman (1983), and investigated by Cormack and Lamberty (1984), the fasciocutaneous flap requires incorporation of deep fascia into a skin flap to gain an improved vascularity (Fig. 9–27). In 1981, Ponten presented 23 fasciocutaneous flaps used to cover lower extremity defects, with excellent results in 17 and partial loss in three. Haertsch (1981) subsequently noted that the fascia of the lower extremity is richly associated with a vascular plexus, which indicates that the preferred dissection plane is deep to fascia rather than superficial to it as classically described. Tolhurst, Haeseker, and Zeeman (1983) presented their clinical experience with fasciocutaneous flaps throughout the body, and this was followed by in-depth dissection studies by numerous authors. Concurrently, Song, Chen, and Song (1984) intro-

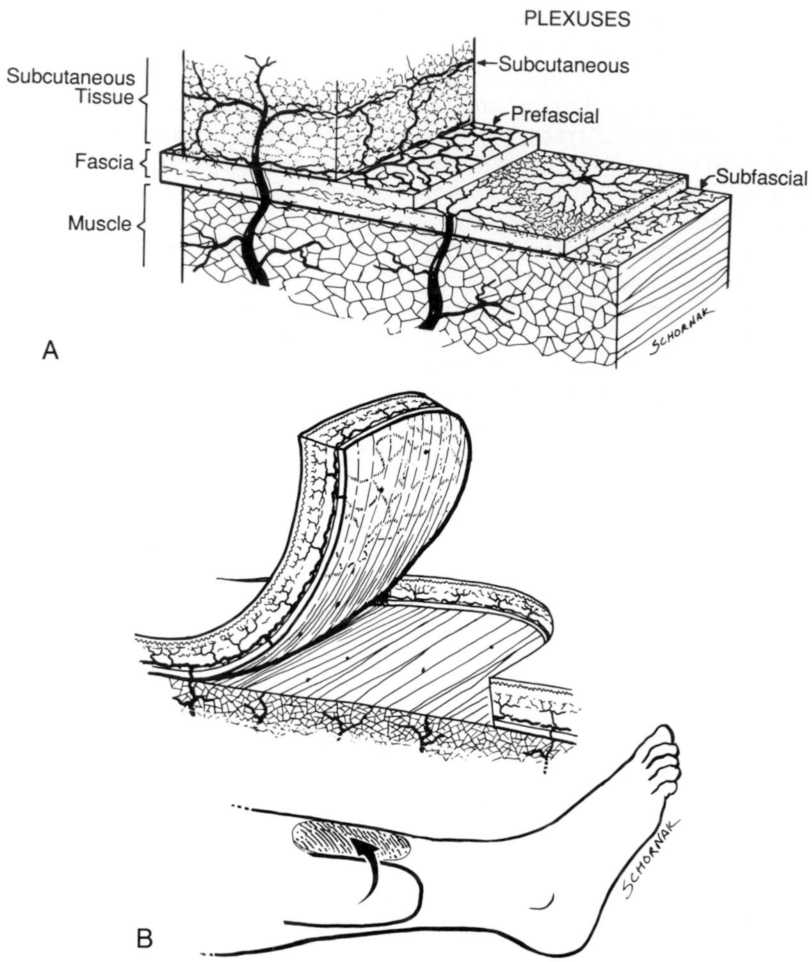

Figure 9–27. Fasciocutaneous flaps. *A,* Fascial blood supply. *B,* Flap composition.

duced the radial forearm flap, which was quickly accepted as a fasciocutaneous free flap, and later as an island flap capable of surviving on a retrograde venous flow. These rapid advances culminated in the anatomic studies of Cormack and Lamberty (1984), who presented injection studies of fasciocutaneous vessels throughout the body and proposed a classification of fasciocutaneous flaps. From this evolution, it would appear worthwhile to answer the following four questions: (1) are there distinct fasciocutaneous vessels?, (2) is there a rich vascular supply to fascia?, (3) does inclusion of fascia translate into increased surviving length?, and (4) where do fasciocutaneous flaps fit in the pantheon of flaps?

From a detailed review of the literature, it is evident that fasciocutaneous arteries are merely a part of the cutaneous artery spectrum. These vessels represent branches from major arteries that penetrate the intermuscular septum before providing branches to fascia and the overlying subcutaneous tissue. To date, investigators have not reported vessels that terminate in the fascia or that run longitudinally within the fascia itself. The sole exception is the tensor fascia lata, which embryologically consists of a fusion of two fascial layers, thereby sandwiching the descending branch of the lateral femoral circumflex. From the work of Schäfer (1975), it is obvious that fascia varies considerably in its composition, organization, and distribution throughout the body. As previously discussed, fascia has a limited intrinsic capillary system, but has well-developed extrinsic associated plexuses more on its superficial surface than on its deep surface. Cormack and Lamberty (1984) attempted to place an axiality onto the direction of the supplying arteries associated with the plexus. However, since fascia is most highly developed over the extremities, which in turn are longitudinal structures, it is difficult to accept an inherent axial orientation. However, inclusion of the associated vascular plexuses rather than the fascia itself is what gives a greater surviving length to these flaps. In experimental studies, Tolhurst, Haeseker, and Zeeman (1983), and later Thomson and Kerrigan (1987a), demonstrated a 15 per cent greater surviving length in flaps including the fascia than in those without it. McCraw (1980) and later Haertsch (1981) emphasized the importance of raising bipedicle flaps beneath the fascia rather than above to close anterior tibial defects.

What are the characteristics of fasciocutaneous flaps and where do they fit in clinical application? Fasciocutaneous flaps undoubtedly represent a significant advance in flap design and have provided a strong stimulus for an understanding of the soft tissue circulation. To the original requirement of Ponten that the entire flap be raised beneath the fascia has now been added the concept of increased vascularity through specific supplying vessels. Despite the classification of Cormack and Lamberty (1984), it appears that a similar vascular spectrum exists for fasciocutaneous flaps as for cutaneous flaps. For example, the "super-flap" of Ponten (1981) in the lower extremity and several upper arm flaps are based on multiple perforators occurring along the intermuscular septum. Next, one can isolate a major extremity artery (radial) and nourish the flap via numerous small septocutaneous branches. Fasciocutaneous flaps can ultimately be designed on a single septocutaneous perforator whose location and distribution are known (saphenous artery flap). As greater vascularity is achieved, the closer one gets to an arterial flap nourished by a septocutaneous artery, the less difference there is between it and an arterial cutaneous flap. For example, the parascapular flap has been raised both as a cutaneous and a fasciocutaneous flap based on the same artery with comparable success rates.

The ultimate fasciocutaneous flap is the radial forearm flap, which was developed by Yang and associates (1981) and perfected by Song, Chen, and Song (1984) (Fig. 9–28). Initially, the flap was designed as a free flap centered over the radial artery, drained by the cephalic vein, and used for reconstruction of burned neck contractures. From their experience with 31 consecutive successful free

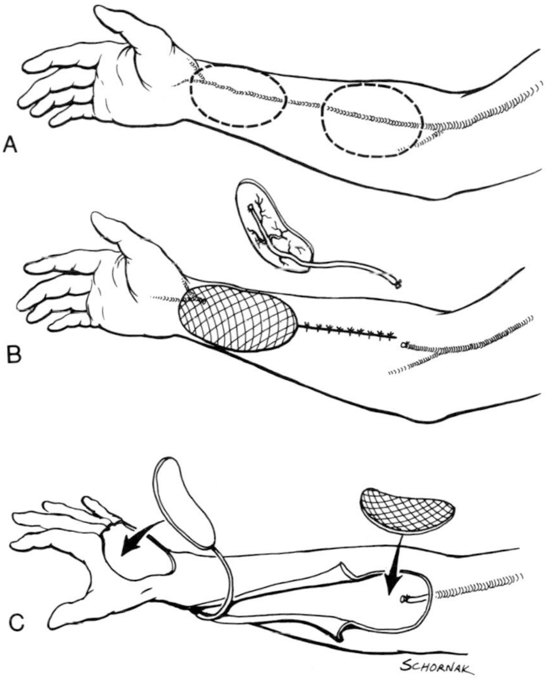

Figure 9–28. The radial forearm fasciocutaneous flap. *A*, Essential anatomy with potential donor sites. *B*, The flap elevated as a free flap. *C*, The flap employed as a reverse forearm flap. The crosshatching indicates skin grafting of the donor site.

flaps, it was apparent to the authors that a reliable flap was available that could be of extreme dimensions, from the distal one-third of the arm to the wrist, while incorporating almost the entire circumference. Central to survival was preservation of the numerous septocutaneous branches of the radial artery and inclusion of the deep fascia. On the basis of injection studies, Manchot (Morain, 1983) divided the forearm into seven vascular regions, which Cormack and Lamberty (1984) later reduced to four principal regions: (1) the radial artery with its inferior cubital artery plus septocutaneous arteries between the brachioradialis and pronator teres in the proximal third, plus branches between the brachioradialis and flexor carpi radialis in the distal two-thirds; (2) the ulnar artery; (3) the posterior interosseus artery; and (4) the anterior interosseus artery. Timmons (1986) divided the septocutaneous branches of the radial artery into three groups: a proximal portion off the radial recurrent artery, branches off the proximal artery, and those from the distal half. It is interesting to note that at the level of the fascia the proximal vessels tend to be oriented longitudinally, while the distal vessels appear transversely.

With transfers to the contralateral hand and oral cavity, smaller segments of skin measuring 10 × 10 cm were commonly isolated in the distal one-third of the forearm. Incorporation of the adjacent radius and cutaneous nerves broadens the flap's flexibility, leading to osseocutaneous and neurovascular flaps. The radial forearm flap has been rapidly accepted owing to its numerous advantages, which include ease of dissection, thin skin, variable composition, a long vascular pedicle with vessels of large diameter, and the feasibility of a two-team approach. Although it was initially considered a rather heretical decision to sacrifice the radial artery and include the deep fascia, these principles had previously been established with the dorsalis pedis flap in which requisite septocutaneous arteries are even more delicate and their blood supply more tenuous. However, the true value and ultimate affront to basic principles came with the description of the distally based island radial forearm flap with its retrograde venous drainage (Stock, Muhlbauer, and Biemer, 1981). This design placed the flap in a different location (middle to proximal forearm rather than distal), on an alternative arterial supply (more proximal septocutaneous arteries perfused via the ulnar artery–deep palmar arch), and with an uncertain retrograde venous drainage (the paired venae comitantes rather than the cephalic vein). Although retrograde blood flow through an artery is easily accepted, how does it occur through the veins? Initially, it was assumed that the venae comitantes did not have valves. Lin, Lal, and Chiu (1984) proposed an anatomic explanation that it was possible because of a "crossover pattern" of communicating branches between the two venae comitantes and a "bypass pattern" of collateral branches on each vein. However, subsequent dissections confirmed the presence of valves. In contrast, Timmons (1986) provided a physiologic explanation that three factors are required: denervation, blood in the vein proximal and distal to the valve, and venous blood pressure higher proximal to the valve than distal to it.

Two important variations of the fasciocutaneous concept are the "fascial" and "fascio-fat" flaps. As pioneered and utilized by Brent and associates (1985), temporal fascia can provide a highly vascularized bed for skin grafts, either locally for ear reconstruction or distally as a free flap (Fig. 9–29). Subsequently, Walton, Matory, and Petry (1985) designed a posterior calf fascial free flap and demonstrated its flexibility in six cases. Although originally described as a fasciocutaneous flap, it can be isolated as a fascial or fascio-fat flap supplied by a dominant septocutaneous artery arising from either the sural or the popliteal artery. Flaps as large as 17 × 22 cm can be raised and transferred as free flaps, usually to the hand. The inclusion of subcutaneous fat provides excellent coverage for exposed tendons and bones, thus facilitating future reconstruction. As the overlying skin is not incorporated, donor site morbidity is acceptable. These variations provide a highly vascularized bed that is exceedingly thin and allows ideal skin coverage. However, fascia is not as resistant to infection as muscle, and monitoring of the flap is exceedingly difficult.

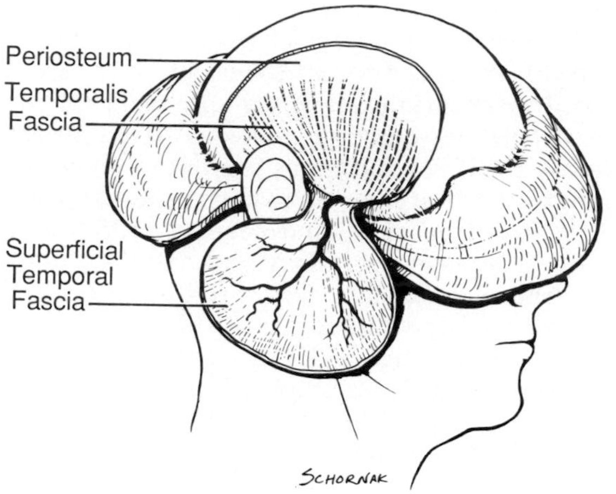

Figure 9–29. Anatomy of the temporalis fascial flap. The fascial flap may be used for local defects such as those of the ear or as a free flap with skin graft coverage where thin tissue is required. The donor site can be closed primarily with minimal residual morbidity.

Fasciocutaneous flaps, whether of the upper or lower extremity, have certain distinct advantages. As noted by Tolhurst, Haeseker, and Zeeman (1983), the flaps are very simple to raise, are quick to execute, and have a high reliability. On the basis of experimental studies, it is reasonable to accept that a fasciocutaneous flap has a 15 to 20 per cent increased surviving length over comparable random cutaneous flaps. Since most flap deaths are usually partial and amount to only a few distal centimeters, it would appear prudent to use a fasciocutaneous flap whenever a large random cutaneous flap is required, especially in the lower extremity. However, the donor site of most fasciocutaneous flaps is significant and can often be justified only when the alternatives are limited. Certainly, a local muscle flap with skin graft would be preferred to a fasciocutaneous flap in the lower extremity in most cases. For a segmental mandibular defect, a free osseocutaneous iliac crest flap might be the first choice for a young girl, but a radial forearm flap more suitable for an older patient.

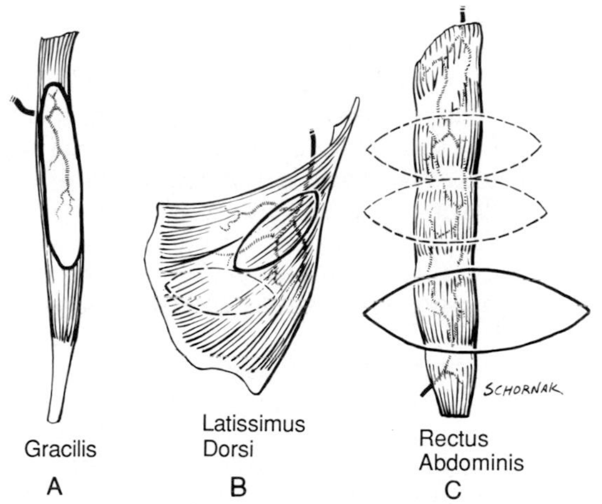

Figure 9–30. Three patterns of skin island design as related to myocutaneous flaps. *A,* The gracilis myocutaneous flap with a small skin island limited to the proximal portion of a narrow muscle pedicle. *B,* The latissimus dorsi myocutaneous flap with a small skin island over a very large muscle. *C,* The rectus abdominis myocutaneous flap with a huge skin island over a relatively narrow muscle.

MYOCUTANEOUS FLAPS

As conceived by Owens (1955), perfected by McCraw (1980) and Orticochea (1983), and championed by Mathes and Nahai (1982), myocutaneous flaps have revolutionized soft tissue coverage. Originally, a myocutaneous flap was perceived as a composite soft tissue flap in which the skin portion provided wound closure while the muscle mass merely served as a carrier for the essential blood supply. However, additional clinical experience demonstrated that the muscle provides bulk for dead space closure, and its high vascularity helps to control infection. Critical to the use of myocutaneous flaps are the following four questions: (1) what is the anatomic and physiologic interrelationship between the blood supply to muscle and the overlying skin within a myocutaneous flap?, (2) how are the cutaneous and myocutaneous territories reconciled?, (3) what are the different types of myocutaneous flaps?, and (4) where do myocutaneous flaps fit in the hierarchy of flaps?

The initial experience with myocutaneous flaps involved closure of difficult wounds, employing the muscle as a pedicle to nourish the essential skin flap. Myocutaneous flaps combined the cantilevered vascular base of the arterial flap with the perfusion characteristics of a random cutaneous flap. Specifically, the survival pattern of a myocutaneous flap is determined by the musculocutaneous arteries that emerge from the underlying muscle. For example, the proximal two-thirds of the gracilis muscle can survive on a single dominant neurovascular bundle while the distal third undergoes necrosis (Fig. 9–30). Therefore, design of a gracilis myocutaneous flap can safely incorporate the skin overlying the proximal two-thirds perfused by the musculocutaneous perforators, while the associated distal third would have to be considered a random portion nourished via the cutaneous plexuses or even delayed if necessary. Thus, the critical first step in the design of a myocutaneous flap is to know the blood supply to the muscle, its internal segmentation, and the location of the essential neurovascular pedicle. Once outlined, the requisite amount of overlying skin is determined by donor site requirement and marked over the muscle as influenced by pedicle length and arcs of rotation. The quintessential myocutaneous flap is the latissimus dorsi. The introduction of this flap by Bostwick (1983) renewed interest in breast reconstruction, since it restored a breast in a single operation. The latissimus dorsi muscle can be isolated in its virtual entirety on the thoracodorsal artery, while the skin portion can be oriented in virtually any direction, the only size restriction being primary closure of the donor site. From a hemodynamic perspective, the flap does not challenge the relationship between the muscle and overlying skin, as the muscle is extremely large and well vascularized, whereas the skin required is comparatively small and usually overlies the muscle directly without a random portion. However, the same cannot be said for its successor in breast reconstruction, the rectus abdominis myocutaneous flap (Fig. 9–30).

In 1977, Drever reported the first rectus abdominis myocutaneous flap, which was a vertical island flap nourished by paraumbilical perforators off the vascular axis formed by the superior and inferior epigastric vessels (Fig. 9–31). This clinical triumph stood in direct defiance of conventional wisdom, which stated that "one can never elevate more than half of this muscle and still maintain viability of the distal end." Drever (1977) correctly concluded that the two epigastric arteries arborize within the muscle to form physiologically a single longitudinal vascular axis that can support the entire rectus muscle. In addition, numerous perforators were present, allowing design of a myocutaneous flap that could incorporate skin as far caudad as the pubic level and could be totally isolated as an island flap. Robbins (1981) applied this technique to breast reconstruction, which offered several advantages over the latissimus dorsi flap, including elimination of the breast prosthesis and of the need to modify the contralateral breast. These flaps were vertically oriented island flaps that directly overlay the rectus muscle and resulted in a paramedian incision. In order to minimize the scar and to increase the flap's bulk, Hartrampf, Scheflan, and Black (1982) devised the transverse rectus abdominis myocutaneous flap. Although a simple change in orientation, this modification required a radical reassessment of the blood supply to the lower abdominal wall.

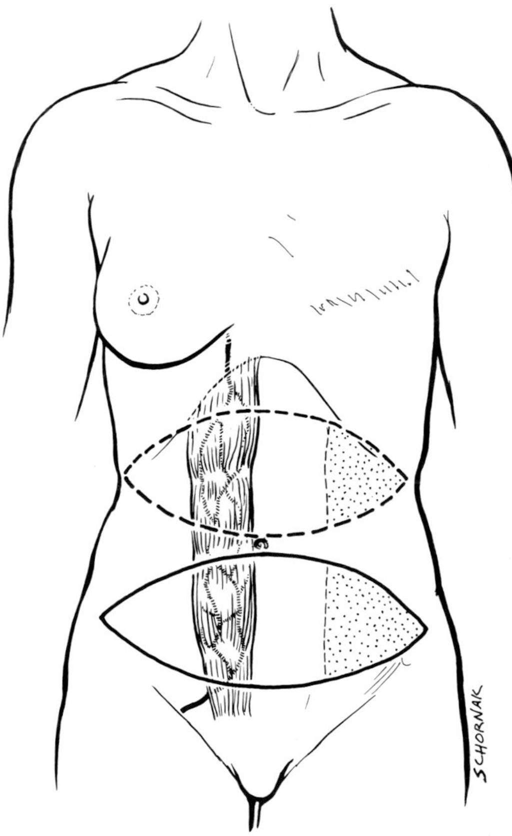

Figure 9–31. The rectus abdominis myocutaneous flap as utilized for breast reconstruction. The drawing illustrates the potential location of skin islands, the stippled zones denoting endangered blood supply.

As noted by Hartrampf, Scheflan, and Black (1982), the vast majority of perforators through the anterior rectus sheath occur in the paraumbilical area and can supply a variety of transverse flaps. The blood supply to the lower abdominal skin is derived from five sources: (1) the deep epigastric system (superior and inferior), (2) the superficial epigastric system, (3) the intercostal system (T10 to T11), (4) the external pudendal system, and (5) the superficial circumflex iliac system. However, isolation of a transverse island flap onto a single rectus abdominis muscle eliminates the last four sources completely and reduces the deep epigastric system to a single superior source. Further, the flap is raised above the fascia, except where it overlies the muscle, thus eliminating distribution within the fascial plexus. It should be noted that the higher the transverse axis, the greater is the flap's survival. This is virtually complete when the flap is located above the umbilicus, but a significant loss occurs when it is below the umbilicus. At its common inferior location, the elliptic flap is divided into four zones: (1) that overlying the rectus pedicle, (2) that overlying the contralateral rectus, (3) the distal ipsilateral portion, and (4) the distal contralateral portion. In most cases one-half of the most distal contralateral portion is so poorly perfused as to require removal intraoperatively. Since the abdominal ellipse is to be excised to permit a bikini-line closure, this flap offers a rare clinical opportunity to determine maximal surviving patterns. It must be remembered that many of these flaps measure 30 × 14 cm with only a 6 cm wide transverse strip of underlying muscle. Thus, the transverse rectus abdominis myocutaneous flap represents a unique progression in myocutaneous flaps of the torso.

How does one reconcile the cutaneous regions defined by Manchot (Morain, 1983) and Salmon (1936) with the myocutaneous territories proposed by McCraw (1980)? The former divide the skin into multiple regions on the basis of the distribution pattern of the significant cutaneous arteries, whereas the latter emphasizes the perfusion of the essential neurovascular hila of the underlying muscle, which produces a captive cutaneous territory. Obviously, both concepts are correct and merely represent a surgical declaration based on clinical necessity rather than on an anatomic and hemodynamic reality. The skin receives its blood supply from diverse and changing sources. The skin is made dependent on only a single source by the surgeon, who transects all others when a flap is created. A typical example of this regionality is the anterior thoracic skin, which can be used in myriad configurations, depending on the specific objectives of the surgeon (Fig. 9–32). The pectoral skin can be incorporated into (1) a thoracoacromial flap (random cutaneous) for coverage of degloving hand injuries, (2) a deltopectoral flap (arterial cutaneous) for reconstruction of a postresection defect of the jaw, or (3) a laterally based pectoral flap (myocutaneous) for restoration of a sternal defect. In each example, the blood supply to the flap is different, yet the skin component is the same. The blood supply will be altered and reoriented to a greater or lesser degree, depending on the design selected.

It is tempting to assume that a specific myocutaneous flap is the same under all conditions, but vascularity and risk, as well as technical demands, can vary considerably. The medial gastrocnemius flap can be utilized in a variable manner (Fig. 9–33). The medial gastrocnemius muscle has a single dominant pedicle, the medial sural artery arising from the popliteal artery. The standard flap is outlined between the tibia and posterior midline, with a skin-fascial extension to within 5 cm of the medial malleolus, and a proximal base at the level of the medial condyle of the femur. It can be raised as a myocutaneous flap incised on three sides, as a skin island and pedicle muscle, or as a completely isolated island flap. The standard medial gastrocnemius flap can easily cover tibial defects in the proximal one-third of the leg. To cover an open knee joint it may be necessary to cut the skin base, whereas coverage of the distal one-third of the femur may require section of the muscle origin. Each step in this progression offers greater movement, but necessitates increased surgical finesse and produces a greater risk due to a decreased number of supplying vessels. Proximal transection of the skin and deep fascia undoubtedly interrupts the subcutaneous venous system and any axial septocutaneous arteries, thereby rendering the flap totally dependent on the musculocutaneous perforators. Division of the muscle origin eliminates any additional nondominant neurovascular hila or intercommunicating vessels from adjacent muscles as well as the periosteal blood supply, which can be considerable. Thus, the design of a myocutaneous flap is as important as the choice of a specific flap.

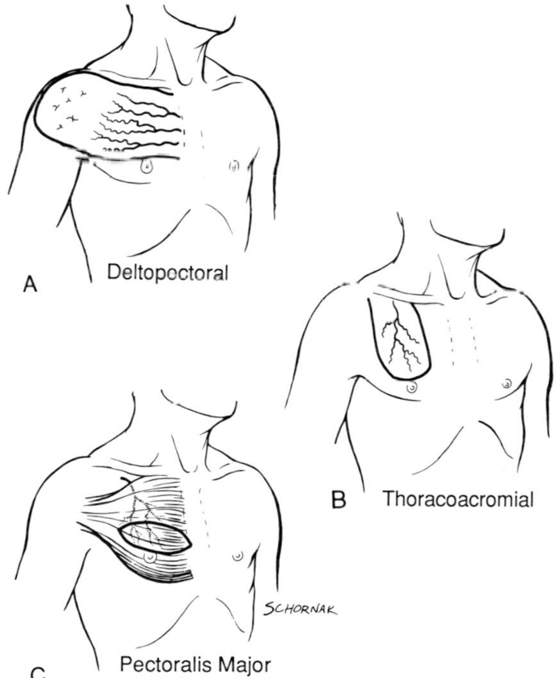

Figure 9–32. Potential flaps from the same prepectoral skin. *A,* An arterial deltopectoral flap. *B,* A random thoracoacromial flap. *C,* A pectoralis major myocutaneous flap.

MUSCLE FLAPS

In contrast to the plurality of parenthood for other methods of soft tissue coverage, muscle flaps are associated with the work of one individual: Ralph Ger. Over a six year period from 1966 to 1972, Ger (1972, 1977) formulated the principles, established the operative procedures, and demonstrated a wide range of applications for muscle flaps. His contribution was extrapolated to plastic surgery by Vasconez, Bostwick, and McCraw (1974), McCraw (1980), Arnold and Mixter (1983), and others. However, the value of muscle flaps plus skin grafts was soon lost in the rush to embrace local and free myocutaneous flaps. These new procedures appeared to be a more elegant solution to coverage problems. The myocutaneous flap retained

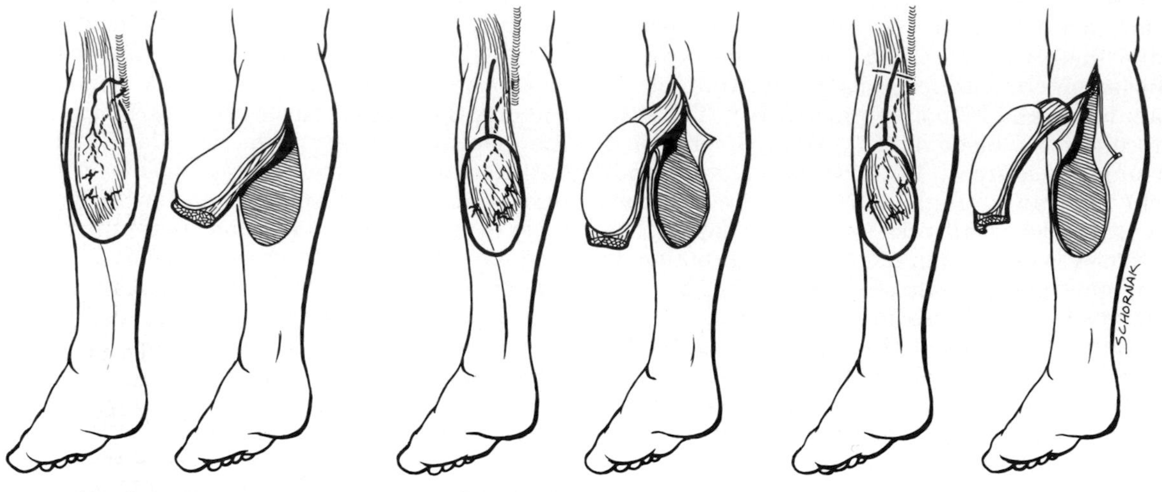

Figure 9–33. Three ways to use a medial gastrocnemius myocutaneous flap. *A,* A pedicle flap with both skin and muscle tethered at their bases. *B,* An island skin and pedicle muscle flap giving improved rotation over *A. C,* An island flap of skin and muscle being attached by only a vascular pedicle, thus providing the greatest arc of rotation and freedom of movement.

full-thickness skin with subcutaneous fat as thick padding, in contrast to a thin split-thickness skin graft over a muscle flap. The free myocutaneous flap could provide maximal tissue in areas where muscle tissue was limited, especially the distal one-third of the lower extremity. Within the past few years, muscle flaps plus skin grafts have reemerged as a dominant form of soft tissue coverage as the limitations of local and free myocutaneous flaps have been documented. The logical use of a muscle flap plus a skin graft requires answers to the following four questions: (1) what are the principles of muscle flaps?, (2) what is the blood supply to muscle?, (3) what is the functional cost of their transfer?, and (4) what is their role in the management of chronic wounds?

As previously discussed, the blood supply to muscle may be classified according to the number and dominance of the vascular hila as well as the muscle's ability to survive on a surgically reduced blood supply. In most instances, the blood supply is more than adequate to ensure that the entire muscle will survive. This is evidenced by the frequency and success of the latissimus dorsi (Type V), gluteus maximus (Type III), and gastrocnemius (Type I) muscle flaps. Problems arise when muscles are transferred that have numerous pedicles (Type IV) or are rendered dependent on a minor pedicle following severance of the dominant pedicle (Type II). The distally based soleus flap was devised out of desperation as a method of covering defects in the perimalleolar area. The dominant proximal pedicle is severed and the muscle is perfused via minor distal branches from the posterior tibial artery. The latter vessels are small, inconsistent, and often damaged by previous trauma, resulting in a failure rate of over 25 per cent. In dealing with muscle flaps, it is mandatory that the blood supply to, distribution within, and survival on a surgically reduced number of pedicles be clearly understood for each individual muscle.

Selection of a muscle flap must meet certain technical criteria: (1) the ability to transpose the muscle to the wound; (2) an adequate size of the muscle belly, both for its pedicle and flap portions; (3) the location, constancy, and adequacy of the vascular pedicle; (4) accessibility; and (5) limited functional loss. In most cases, a readily adjacent muscle of adequate size is selected for wound coverage. This ease of transposition is evidenced in defects of the upper third of the lower extremity where the medial belly of the gastrocnemius muscle is preferred to the lateral belly. The medial unit is larger with a greater arc of rotation, whereas the rotation of the lateral unit is restricted by the fibula and the intervening anterior compartment. The muscle belly may be small but can be expanded by longitudinal cuts in the deep fascia. The arc of rotation is determined by the penetration point of the dominant vascular hila plus the degree of mobilization. For example, the vascular pedicle enters the soleus muscle in its middle third in a perpendicular fashion, whereas it enters the medial gastrocnemius muscle in its proximal third in a longitudinal direction. Therefore, the pivot point of the gastrocnemius muscle can be dramatically altered by the extent of dissection. The muscle's reach may be restricted to the upper third of the tibia, but with detachment of its origin the muscle will reach the knee, whereas complete isolation onto the sural vessels permits coverage of the distal femur. Increased mobility entails increased risk and a progressive reduction in blood supply. The interplay of transposition, size, and vascularity in selecting muscles for flap coverage is demonstrated by the pectoralis major muscle for closure of sternal dehiscences (Fig. 9–34). The pectoralis major is classified as a Type V muscle having one dominant pedicle (thoracoacromial) and multiple secondary segmental pedicles (anterior thoracic perforators). In its initial applications, the thoracic origin and humeral insertion were divided, rendering it dependent on the dominant thoracoacromial pedicle. The muscle belly was dragged medially into the sternal defect. Subsequently, surgeons realized that basing the flap medially on the anterior thoracic perforators alone provided both easier transposition and greater size while maintaining adequate blood supply. Familiarity with both techniques is essential, since the internal mammary artery may be compromised by previous bypass surgery, peristernal wiring, or debridement. The medially based flap was further refined by Nahai and associates (1982). The muscle is divided vertically just medial to the thoracoacromial pedicle. The lateral portion with its retained vascular supply and motor innervation is sutured to the pectoralis minor to preserve the anterior axillary fold, while the medial portion is turned over into the sternal defect. Often it is necessary to subdivide one of the pectoral muscle bellies into multiple segments to provide coverage of the distal defect. Thus, surgeons have progressed from isolation of the muscle on its dominant pedicle to isolation on its secondary pedicles to even a single segmental pedicle.

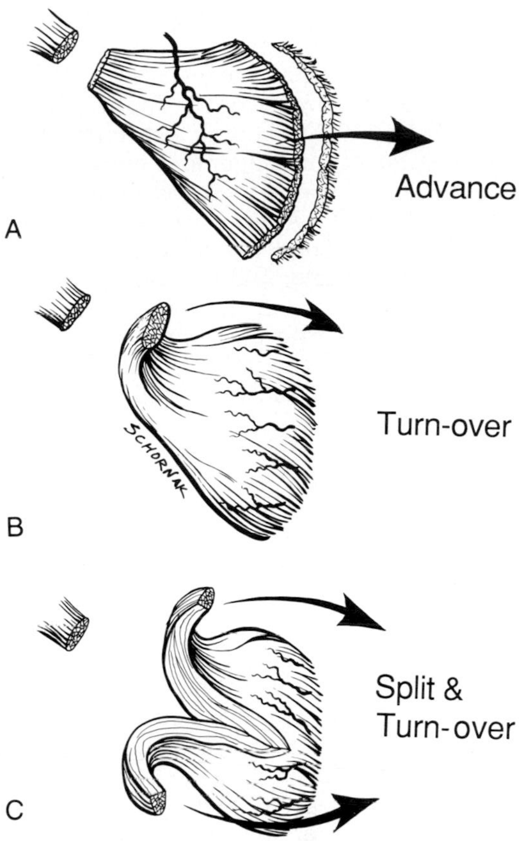

Figure 9–34. Three applications of the pectoralis major muscle flap. *A,* As an advancement flap based on the thoracoacromial blood supply. *B,* As a turn-over flap based on the internal mammary perforators. *C,* As a split mammary system. In all examples the humeral insertion was divided.

In his original publications, Ger (1972) emphasized the highly vascular nature of muscle flaps both for ensuring their own viability and for providing the wound with a permanent blood supply to promote fracture healing and to control infection. In 1977, Ger reported his experience with muscle flaps in the management of lower extremity compound trauma cases. His 43 patients were divided into the following groups: (1) delayed closure up to 30 days after injury (22); (2) secondary closure after initial failure (4); and (3) chronic osteomyelitis (17). With the use of muscle flaps and delayed skin grafting, all open wounds were successfully closed, both the acute injuries and the long-standing cases of chronic osteomyelitis. Subsequently, Mathes, Alpert, and Chang (1982) and May, Gallico, and Lukash (1982) confirmed the value of muscle flaps, whether pedicled or transferred, to control osteomyelitis. Mathes, Alpert, and Chang (1982) compared bacterial counts and oxygen tension beneath paired random cutaneous and myocutaneous flaps. The myocutaneous flaps demonstrated a greater resistance to intradermal necrosis as well as a lower bacterial count, but a higher oxygen level. Godina (1979, 1986) established the principles for the management of chronic osteomyelitis: (1) extensive resection of scarred surrounding soft tissue, (2) radical debridement of necrotic bone, (3) coverage with well-vascularized muscle, and (4) end to side vascular anastomoses. On the basis of over 400 cases, a success rate exceeding 95 per cent was obtained and the value of muscle coverage as a means of controlling chronic infection was established.

Whenever a muscle is sacrificed, the question of functional loss arises. In most instances, multiple synergistic muscles offer adequate compensation. Problems arise in the fully mobile patient in whom diminished knee extension may occur from transfer of the rectus femoris, or loss of hip extension if the entire gluteus maximus is utilized. Certain muscles can be employed if their tendon is tenodesed to an adjacent muscle to ensure functional preservation. The degree of flexibility and adjustments that exist in the musculoskeletal system is readily demonstrated in breast reconstruction. If a radical mastectomy has been done, the pectoralis major muscle is obviously removed, the pectoralis minor may be partially denervated, and the latissimus dorsi muscle may be utilized for reconstruction. A functional deficit would seem inevitable. As documented by Bostwick (1983), long-term evaluation of patients having latissimus dorsi myocutaneous flap breast reconstruction confirms that shoulder and upper extremity function remain within the normal range. This question is further debated in evaluating the extent of abdominal wall weakness following transverse rectus abdominis flap transfer. Despite claims to the contrary by others, both Drever (1977) and Dinner, Labandter, and Dowden (1982) reinforced the abdominal wall with Marlex mesh. Long-term studies are required to determine the degree of functional compromise, if any.

What are the early and long-term results of muscle flaps plus skin grafts? During the first year after transfer, muscle atrophy is significant, ranging from 25 to 50 per cent. Daniel and Faibisoff (1982) demonstrated that dramatic atrophy occurred in myocutaneous flaps transposed for closure of pressure sores. Although primary closure and padding over the bony prominence was achieved, long-term follow-up indicated that significant muscle atrophy occurred, thus precluding any preventive advantages. However, Ger (1977) and Mathes and Nahai (1982) demonstrated stable skin coverage over the anterior tibial region six to eight years after muscle flaps with skin grafting. Perhaps the greatest challenge is found over the weight-bearing area of the foot, especially where sensation is limited. May, Halls, and Simon (1985) demonstrated in a scientifically convincing fashion that muscle flaps with skin grafts can provide long-term durable coverage for the sole of the foot. Utilizing footprint force-plate analysis in nine patients, they clearly demonstrated that patients bear weight in a normal fashion and that breakdown did not occur over a two year period. Equally important, patients were able to wear normal shoes and continue heavy work.

Ultimately, one must compare and contrast muscle flaps with myocutaneous flaps. When an esthetic skin match or substantial soft tissue is required, as is often the case in breast reconstruction, a myocutaneous flap is the first choice. In other cases, especially in the lower extremity, a myocutaneous flap offers greater size than the comparable muscle flap. However, long-term follow-up indicates that the donor site of myocutaneous flaps in the lower extremity is frequently unacceptable, while that of muscle flaps involves a simple incision. The proved durability of muscle plus skin graft no longer justifies the selection of a myocutaneous flap. As regards the lower extremity, muscle has replaced myocutaneous flaps for both local and free flap transfer; the circle is now complete and muscle flaps have returned to a position of preeminence.

SPECIALIZED FLAPS

Specialized flaps include sensory neurovascular, osseocutaneous, and en bloc flaps. Each of these procedures is predicated upon isolation of the tissue onto a functioning intravascular circulation, which can either be pedicled as an island flap or transferred as a free flap.

Sensate Flaps. The first specialized flaps were neurovascular flaps of the digit as pioneered by Littler (1960) (Fig. 9–35). The principal application was in cases requiring resurfacing of the thumb using an area of skin from a digit, isolated on an island neu-

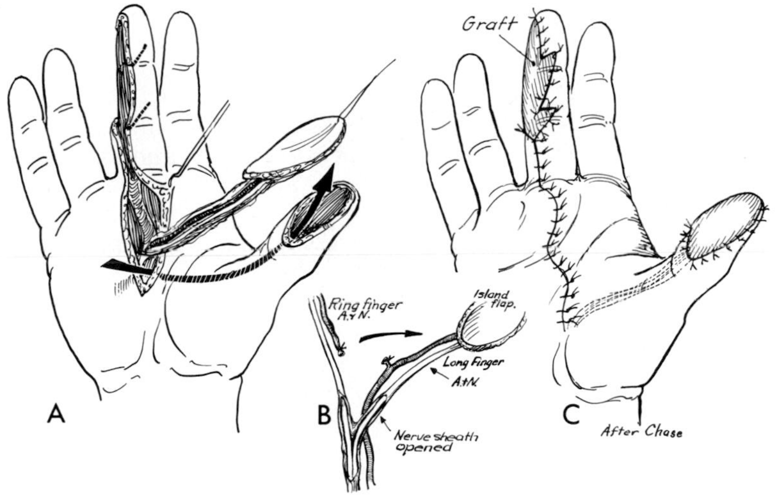

Figure 9–35. The neurovascular island flap (Littler). *A,* An island of skin raised on its neurovascular pedicle. *B,* Mobilization of the flap. *C,* The flap sutured into the recipient defect with skin graft closure of the donor site. (From Chase, R. A.: Atlas of Hand Surgery. Philadelphia, W. B. Saunders Company, 1973.)

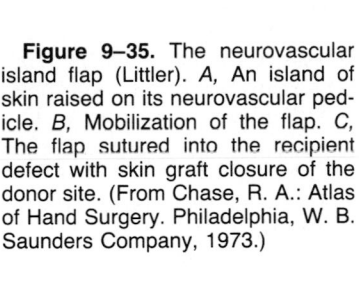

rovascular bundle. Although sensory skin could be restored, the patient's ability to localize sensation as coming from the thumb was often compromised and referred to the donor digit. With the advent of microscopes and myocutaneous flaps, both cutaneous and myocutaneous neurovascular free flaps were developed. As devised experimentally and performed clinically by Daniel, Terzis, and Midgley (1976), the following principles were established for neurovascular free flaps: (1) vascular distribution and sensory innervation must overlap, (2) it must be possible to isolate the flap on an anastomosable vascular pedicle, (3) the nerve supplying the flap should be identifiable and anastomosable, (4) the quality of sensation is appropriate for the defect, and (5) donor site morbidity is acceptable. Clinical confirmation came with the free dorsalis pedis flap, which proved that reinnervation did occur and correct localization was possible. This principle has been extended to the wrap-around flap of the great toe for resurfacing the thumb. This flap has the distinct advantages of providing a low two-point discrimination (6 to 8 mm), durable soft tissue coverage, and an optional fingernail. At the present time, the radial forearm flap is utilized in severe degloving injuries of the upper extremity, sensation being provided by the lateral cutaneous nerve of the forearm. Kerrigan and Daniel (1979) explored neurovascular flaps of the torso based on the intercostal system. It was demonstrated experimentally that a single intercostal neurovascular bundle can support a flap five interspaces wide, which would exceed the ability for primary donor site closure. These flaps were used to provide both soft tissue coverage and sensation over the sacrum in selected paraplegics. The sensate flaps have proved especially valuable in young children with spina bifida who develop pressure sores over the lumbar kyphoses. On the basis of initial and long-term studies of the tensor fascia lata neurovascular free flap (Nahai, 1980), the need for cutaneous sensate coverage over the weight-bearing areas of the foot is infrequent at best.

Osseocutaneous Flaps. The osseocutaneous flap, as originally devised by Blair (1912), extended by Snyder and associates (1970), and perfected by Taylor, Miller, and Ham (1975), has proved valuable in managing difficult cases. Blair (1912) incorporated portions of the clavicle in a cervical neck flap, while Snyder and associates (1970) carefully preserved its periosteal attachments to ensure a vascularized bone graft for composite mandibular reconstruction. However, it was Taylor's (1982) introduction of the free fibular operation and the osseocutaneous groin flap that dramatically expanded the application of osseocutaneous flaps to all body regions (Fig. 9–36). The rim of the iliac crest was elevated with the overlying groin flap, which was transferred to the lower extremity for single-stage repair of compound defects. The distinct value of this flap in mandibular defects was proved by Taylor (1982) with the introduction of the deep circumflex iliac perfusion system. The critical questions for all osseocutaneous flaps are whether the osteocytes are really kept alive and whether their

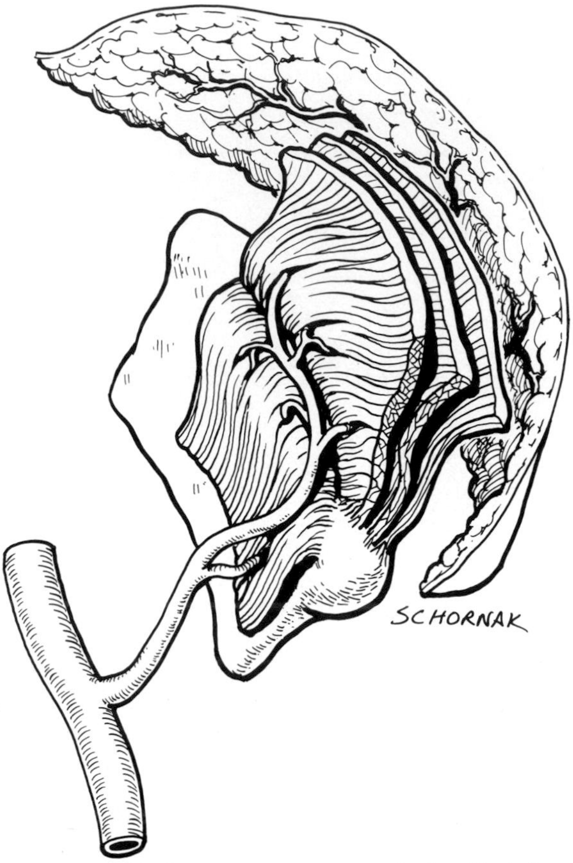

Figure 9–36. The osseocutaneous groin flap (Taylor).

preservation makes a difference. On the basis of the experimental work of Östrup and Fredrickson (1974) and Weiland, Phillips, and Randolph (1984), it is evident that a revascularized autograft has a higher rate of union, shows earlier evidence of bony hypertrophy, and has greater mechanical strength than a comparable nonvascularized bone graft. A vascularized osseocutaneous flap provides the best possible recipient bed for the most viable bone graft, resulting in the lowest rate of infection and nonunion, a fact proved experimentally and observed clinically.

Composite Flaps. En bloc reconstruction in a single operation has long been a goal of plastic surgeons. Initially, surgeons used multiple flaps and tissue grafts to restore the defect. For example, a shotgun blast to the face would be treated with a local flap for oral lining, a rib graft to replace bone, and a deltopectoral flap for skin coverage. Unfortunately, infection and necrosis often resulted. The concept of single en bloc reconstruction utilizing free tissue transfers for severe facial injuries was pioneered by Daniel (1978), perfected by Taylor (1982), and expanded by Swartz and associates (1986) (Fig. 9–37). Composite tissue loss of oral lining, bone framework, subcutaneous soft tissue, and skin coverage was replaced initially with osseocutaneous flaps from the groin and more recently from the forearm and scapula. The distinct advantages of the scapular flap include (1) multiple skin paddles of varying thickness for both internal and external lining, (2) optional inclusion of additional soft tissue (latissimus dorsi muscle), and (3) complementary bone architecture. In a combined series of 26 patients, Swartz and associates (1986) reported a 100 per cent success rate for the scapular flap when used to reconstruct composite defects of the maxilla (five) and mandible (21). Thus, composite flaps have extended the range of facial reconstruction by including a permanent blood supply that promotes rapid, infection-free wound healing and, if meticulously planned, three-dimensional results rarely achieved with conventional methods.

Complications

Complications resulting in partial or complete loss of a flap are all too common (Table 9–3). Perioperative decision making is the critical factor affecting the fate of a flap. It is imperative that the general health of the patient be assessed and factors such as hypertension, malnutrition, anemia, and infection be addressed preoperatively. The detri-

Table 9–3. Causes of Flap Complications

Preoperative
Poor flap design
Underestimation of recipient requirements
Premorbid condition of patient
Intraoperative
Technical errors
Design errors
Poor choice of recipient vessels
Judgmental errors
Postoperative
Extrinsic
Pedicle kinking/pressure
Infection
Vascular thromboses
Intrinsic
Distal ischemia

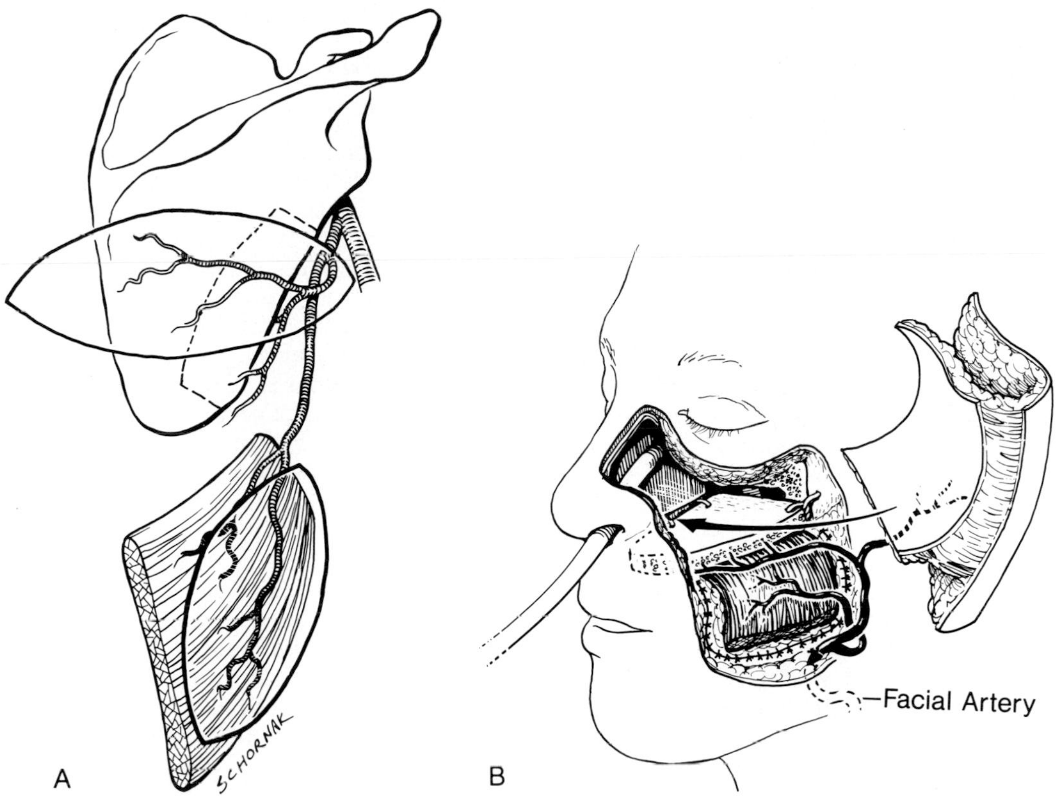

Figure 9–37. Composite scapular flap reconstruction of a facial defect. *A,* The composite skin flap, bone flap, and muscle flap with a common pedicle. *B,* Midfacial reconstruction with three-dimensional use of a composite tissue transfer.

mental effects of smoking must be recognized and, if appropriate, the habit discontinued.

Preoperatively, the surgeon outlines the recipient site requirements, selects the optimal flap, and defines the operative sequence. The size of the defect is frequently underestimated, resulting in an inadequate or inappropriate flap. Radiation necrosis of the chest wall is often greater than anticipated, producing a defect that expands centripetally from the central ulcer through adjacent scar until healthy bleeding skin is encountered beyond the radiation port. If one had planned an adjacent rotation flap, failure would probably ensue irrespective of the flap's dimensions—tissue should have been transferred from a distance, preferably including well-vascularized muscle. Selection of a specific flap should be based on its inherent range of application as well as its restrictions. Traumatic injuries of the lower extremity provide the greatest challenge for choosing the optimal flap. Within the context of the traumatized lower extremity, local flaps offer conceptual simplicity, but the actual risk is great, since failure often occurs when ideal local conditions do not exist. In contrast, the free flap is a complicated, technically demanding operation, but one quite capable of providing adequate coverage. Local flaps are often justified on the basis of simplicity, not on efficacy or a risk-reward ratio. The operative design must be adapted for each individual patient, otherwise failure can ensue. Breast reconstruction employing a transverse rectus abdominis flap illustrates these problems. Flap designs are determined initially by recipient site requirements and secondarily by donor site realities. The donor site restrictions affect both the pedicle and the flap. The epigastric blood supply may have been compromised by previous surgery (abdominal or thoracic) and by severe radiation, thus obliging one to choose the ipsilateral side rather than the contralateral. The abdominal wall may be crisscrossed by numerous scars, forcing one to alter the flap's placement, orientation, and size.

Intraoperatively, technical execution and judgmental decisions often determine the types of complications. Technical errors appear to be inversely proportional to the flap's inherent complexity. Execution of most local flaps is relatively straightforward, but their design may be quite complex. For example, in a Limberg flap the longitudinal axis of the rhomboid excision must be placed parallel to the line of minimal skin tension; if perpendicular, the design will result in immobile flaps. The incising, elevation, and transposition of the flap are relatively simple. As one progresses to fasciocutaneous and arterial flaps, the design of the flaps remains critical, while isolation on its essential vessel can be demanding. Conversion to an island flap requires maximal technical finesse. Free flaps offer the ultimate challenge, since they are technically demanding and require flawless decision making. In any free flap, selection of the recipient vessel remains a critical factor. Unless the artery has a strong pulsatile flow and the vein is scar free with a wide diameter, the operation is destined to fail. Following the anastomoses, the flap must be well perfused as evidenced by bleeding on incision. Unquestionably, postoperative complications are confirmations of both intraoperative suspicions and judgmental errors. As detailed by Lidman and Daniel (1981), anastomotic suture errors are virtually nonexistent in free flap transfers; the problem rather is selection of the recipient vessels.

Postoperatively, flap complications can be divided into extrinsic and intrinsic problems. The most common extrinsic complications include (1) dressing or positioning errors, (2) tension or kinking of the flap's pedicle, (3) wound problems, and (4) nonfunctioning vascular anastomoses. Tracheostomy tapes have been tied across the base of a pectoral flap, or patients have been allowed to roll on their flaps. Equally disastrous is compression of a flap's pedicle as a result of either surgical or nursing errors. Wound problems include hematoma, which can prevent venous drainage from a free flap. A delayed complete flap loss can occur owing to infection resulting from inadequate debridement. In contrast, partial flap loss is due to intrinsic factors causing distal flap ischemia, which will be discussed in depth. At the present time, intrinsic flap failure is best avoided by designing a flap with a robust vascular supply and minimizing all potential extrinsic factors.

FLAP PHYSIOLOGY

Microcirculation

ANATOMY

The microcirculation is composed of the smallest vessels in the circulatory system and it defies absolute classification. From a functional viewpoint, the microcirculation is composed of vessels responsible for the exchange of nutrients and waste as well as local regulation of blood flow. These vessels include the arterioles, capillaries, venules, and arteriovenous anastomoses. The cutaneous vessels are arranged in several plexuses as previously described. The arteriolar network functions as the primary regulator of blood flow to the tissues. Sympathetic innervation is directed primarily to the arterioles, precapillary sphincters, and arteriovenous anastomoses. The capillaries have a diameter of 4 to 10 μm and the cutaneous microvessels have very thick walls, 2 to 3 μm. The capillary density of skin is 16 to 55/mm^2, which is relatively low compared with the density of skeletal muscles (1000 to 2000/mm^2). Arteriovenous anastomoses or shunts are highly specialized vessels that enable blood to bypass the capillary bed. Their thick wall is composed of vascular smooth muscle with a rich sympathetic innervation.

Normal total blood flow in skin is approximately 20 ml per min per 100 gm. This rate increases greatly with heating or acute sympathetic blockage. The increased flow occurs chiefly through the arteriovenous anastomoses, bypassing the nutrient capillary bed.

In order to understand the hemodynamic events taking place in a skin flap, it is important to have a basic knowledge of the normal regulatory factors affecting blood flow in the skin (Fig. 9–38). The regulation of blood flow occurs at both systemic and local levels. Thermoregulation, the skin's primary function, is systemically regulated by the sympathetic nervous system. Local control of blood flow in the skin, or "autoregulation," plays an additional minor role in determining flow in normal intact skin.

PHYSIOLOGY

Systemic Control of Cutaneous Blood Flow

Neural Regulation. The most important system of circulatory control in skin is neural

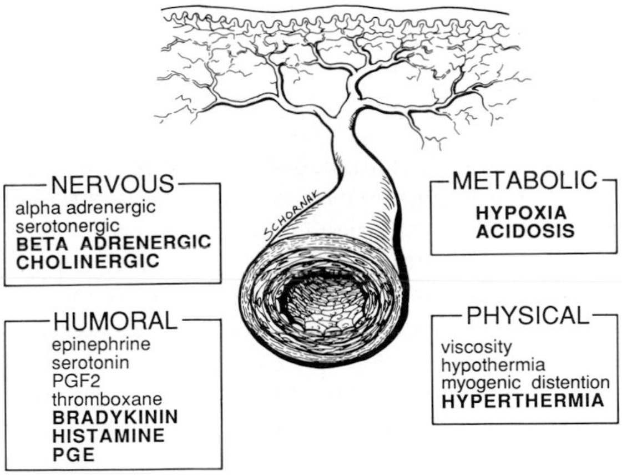

Figure 9–38. Physiologic factors playing a role in the regulation of the cutaneous microcirculation.

regulation, which consists predominantly of sympathetic vasoconstrictor fibers. In addition to the fibers, several types of receptors are present on the vessel walls. Alpha-adrenergic receptors with a vasoconstricting influence are by far the most common in skin. Beta-adrenergic receptors with a vasodilating influence and serotonergic receptors with a vasoconstricting influence are located primarily at the arteriovenous anastomoses. Withdrawal of sympathetic tone causes a profound vasodilatation, particularly in the arteriovenous anastomoses. An increase in sympathetic adrenergic tone leads to vasoconstriction and a decrease in skin blood flow.

Humoral Regulation. Epinephrine and norepinephrine can both act directly on alpha-adrenergic receptors in the cutaneous vessels to cause vasoconstriction. Serotonin is also a vasoconstrictor, whereas histamine and bradykinin are known vasodilators. Several arachidonic acid metabolites, prostaglandins, and thromboxanes have opposing effects on the microcirculation. Thromboxane A_2 is a potent vasoconstrictor, as is PGF_2 alpha. PGE_1 is a vasodilator and prostacyclin (PGI_2) is a potent vasodilator as well as an inhibitor of platelet aggregation. Additional arachidonic acid metabolites, the leukotrienes (LTC_4, LTD_4), have also been shown to increase skin microcirculatory flow.

Local Control of Cutaneous Blood Flow

Metabolic Regulation. Autoregulation of blood flow is not as prominent in the skin as it is in other organs in which the metabolic requirements are greater. Metabolic factors act primarily as vasodilators. An increase in pCO_2 (hypercapnia), decrease in pO_2 (hypoxia), decrease in pH (acidosis), and interstitial potassium all cause vasodilatation.

Physical Regulation. An increase in perfusion pressure causes distention in an isolated cutaneous vessel, thus triggering vasoconstriction. This myogenic reflex acts as a regulatory response to maintain capillary flow at a constant level independent of arterial pressure. Local hypothermia causes a decrease in blood flow and initiates an increase in flow. Rheologic factors such as blood viscosity have been shown to have an effect on flow rates only in grossly pathologic conditions of circulatory deficiency, such as severe ischemia.

In summary, the regulation of cutaneous blood flow is predominantly performed by sympathetic vasoconstrictor fibers. The major function of skin is to act as a thermoregulatory organ, and under normal conditions, other regulatory factors are of only minor importance.

Pathophysiologic Changes

When a skin flap is elevated, profound changes take place and the fine equilibrium that had regulated blood flow is completely disrupted. The flap is in a state of vascular imbalance. Of prime importance in this initial stage is the functional loss of sympathetic innervation and the insult of ischemia. The unit of skin is no longer a thermoregulatory organ but an isolated tissue struggling for survival by reestablishing a new hemodynamic equilibrium with the assistance of humoral, metabolic, and physical mechanisms. For the skin flap to survive, an adequate nutrient circulation must be ensured and the damages of ischemia minimized. This must be accomplished within the first eight to 12 hours postoperatively or the damage becomes irreversible (Kerrigan and Daniel, 1982a,b).

An understanding of the pathophysiology is centered on two interrelated clinical phenomena. First, the all too often observed complication of distal flap necrosis. Why does this happen and can it be prevented or treated? Second, the miraculous benefit that the delay procedure has on increasing flap survival. How does it work and is there any way to mimic it without an operation? These two issues can be addressed by examining the research data on the anatomic, hemodynamic, and metabolic changes in both acute and delayed flaps.

ANATOMIC CHANGES

Findings from early anatomic studies showed that after skin flap elevation there is an increase in the size and number of the small arteries of the subdermal plexus as well as a longitudinal reorientation, and an increase in the size of the dermal venous channels. It was also speculated that these vessels were toneless, dilated, and unable to respond to local changes. Further studies using in vitro and in vivo microangiographic techniques showed that there is no establishment of new longitudinal vessels but instead a dilatation of preexisting anastomoses between transversely lying vessels. There is also an increase in the number of vessels at the base of the flap, a condition that persists for approximately two or three weeks and appears to result from an inflammatory reaction induced by surgical trauma. Pang and associates (1986a), measuring angiogenesis in experimental pig flaps, showed that there is no increase in the density of blood vessels as measured by morphometry comparing acute and delayed flaps for up to two weeks. The ingrowth of new vessels from the surrounding tissue begins four to five days postoperatively, followed by anastomosis with preexisting vessels in the flap (Serafin, Shearing, and Georgiade, 1977).

Changes in the autonomic innervation of the flaps have also been documented for both acute and delayed flaps. Palmer (1970) used a histofluorescent catecholamine staining technique to assess the presence or absence of sympathetic transmitters in acute rat skin flaps. Disappearance of catecholamines began 18 hours after surgical incision and was complete by 30 hours. Reaccumulation of the catecholamines, signaling reinnervation, began four to eight weeks postoperatively. Quantitative levels of norepinephrine have been measured in the acute rat flap (Jurell and Hjemdahl, 1981) and delayed pig flank flaps (Cutting and associates, 1982). In rats, norepinephrine depletion occurred mainly between six and 24 hours postoperatively (Fig. 9–39*A*). In delayed pig flaps a decrease in norepinephrine concentration was evident by two hours postoperatively, but this gradually returned to normal by ten days (Fig. 9–39*B*). The delayed pig skin flaps do not lose their sympathetic innervation but rather demonstrate a transient discharge and depletion of neurotransmitter. Because of the dermatome design of pig flank flaps in addition to its bipedicle connection, in contrast to the longitudinal design of a unipedicle rat flap, the sympathetic terminals are less likely to be severed. However, the severance and/or disturbance of the sympathetic nerve causes a spontaneous discharge of vasoconstricting neurotransmitters. In the acute situation, these have a profound effect on the hemodynamics of the microvasculature.

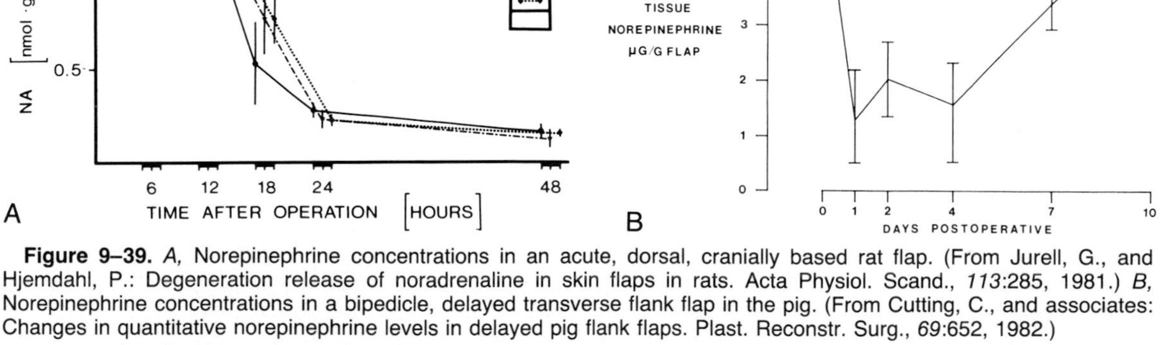

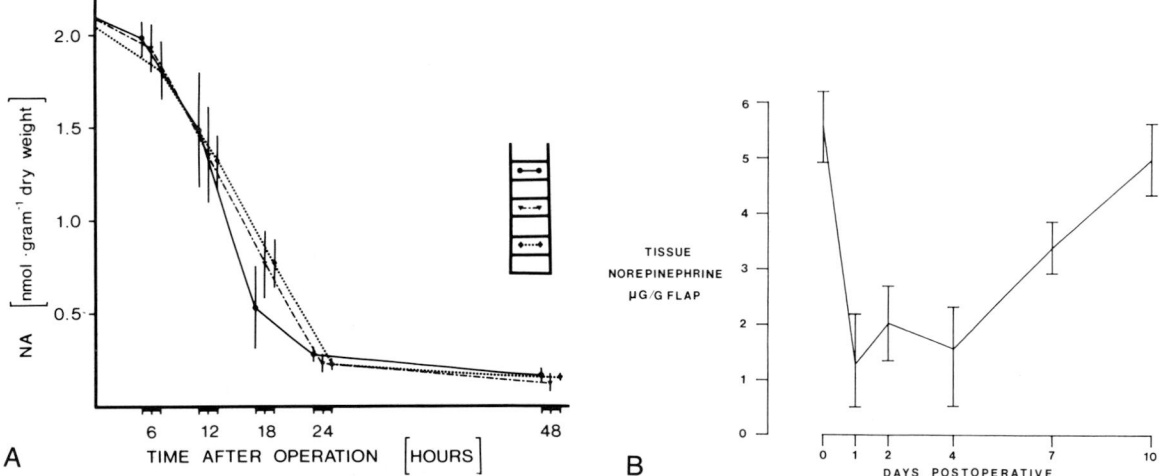

Figure 9–39. *A,* Norepinephrine concentrations in an acute, dorsal, cranially based rat flap. (From Jurell, G., and Hjemdahl, P.: Degeneration release of noradrenaline in skin flaps in rats. Acta Physiol. Scand., *113*:285, 1981.) *B,* Norepinephrine concentrations in a bipedicle, delayed transverse flank flap in the pig. (From Cutting, C., and associates: Changes in quantitative norepinephrine levels in delayed pig flank flaps. Plast. Reconstr. Surg., *69*:652, 1982.)

HEMODYNAMIC CHANGES

Changes in skin flap blood flow have been studied largely by means of radioactive isotopes and microspheres. The first most sophisticated and thorough studies were carried out in rats by Palmer, Jurell, and Norberg (1972) using xenon clearance from the site of intracutaneous injection as a measure of capillary blood flow. Changes of flow were documented in primary flaps, both arterial and random, and bipedicle delayed flaps. Flow at the base of a pedicle flap remained at 100 per cent of control, but flow at the tip of the flap decreased to 18 per cent on the first postoperative day. The flow gradually increased to 65 per cent in the first week and 75 to 90 per cent in two weeks (Fig. 9–40*A*). Bipedicle flaps showed increased flow at the arterial end up to 135 per cent of control, decreased flow to 70 per cent centrally, and 100 per cent flow at the cutaneous end. Within 30 days the flows had returned to approximately normal levels. Similar changes in blood flow have since been documented using the microsphere technique in acute dog flaps (Nathanson and Jackson, 1975) and in bipedicle delayed pig flaps (Guba and Callahan, 1979).

Until the 1980's the most popular concept of the changes in delayed skin flaps was that proposed by Reinisch (1974). Following observations of warm temperature in the distal, nonfluorescent, and doomed end of pig skin flaps, he postulated that non-nutritive blood flow was occurring through arteriovenous shunts. Reinisch carried out additional experiments with radioactive red blood cells, dynamic scans, and radioactive microspheres to confirm the hypothesis. He concluded that the delay procedure works by maintaining

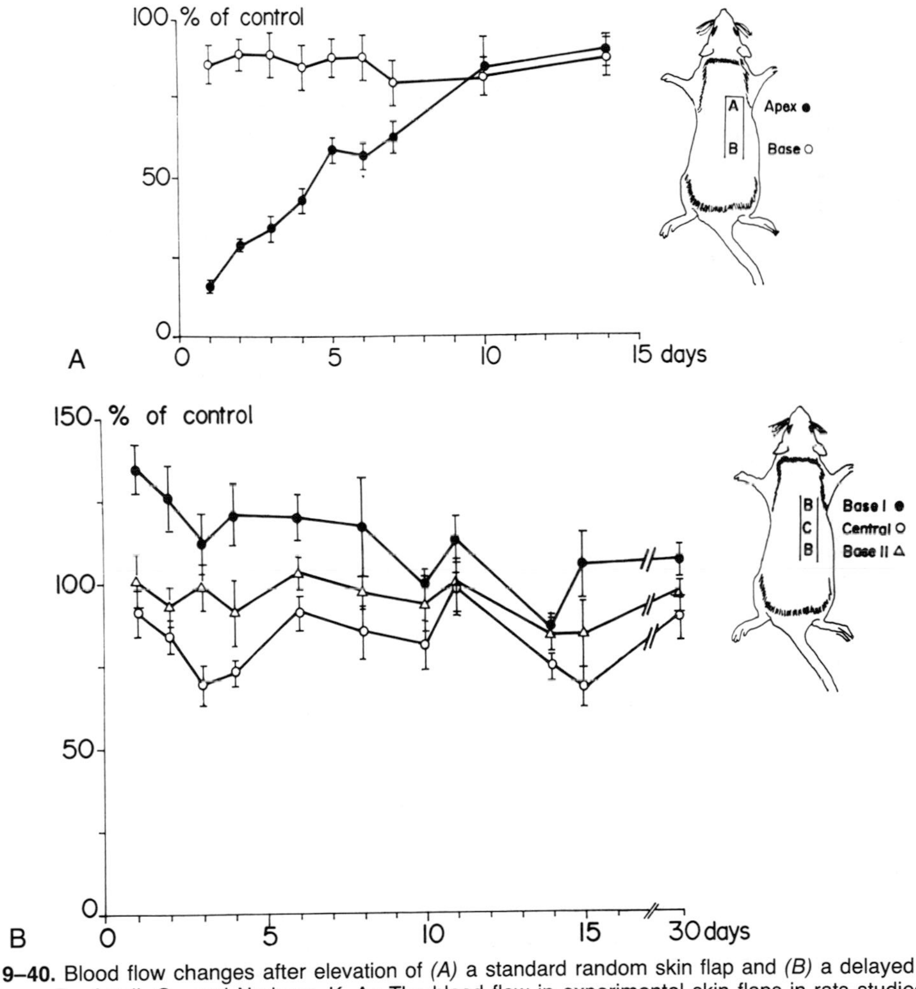

Figure 9–40. Blood flow changes after elevation of *(A)* a standard random skin flap and *(B)* a delayed bipedicle flap. (From Palmer, B., Jurell, G., and Norberg, K.-A.: The blood flow in experimental skin flaps in rats studied by means of the 133 Xenon clearance method. Scand. J. Plast. Reconstr. Surg., 6:6, 1972.)

adequate nutrient and non-nutrient flow until the dilated arteriovenous shunts spontaneously constrict. Since Reinisch's data were obtained from single (acute) and bipedicle (delayed) flaps, it was implied that the distal portion of an acute skin flap fails because of inappropriate non-nutrient flow through arteriovenous shunts.

Subsequent publications questioned the validity of the arteriovenous shunt concept. None directly addressed the problem of acute skin flap failure, and thus each study has its limitations in clarifying the problem. Prather and associates (1979) assessed various methods of predicting skin flap viability. Their results with radioactive red blood cells were strikingly different from Reinisch's, and they concluded that the distal, nonfluorescent end of the flap was virtually nonperfused. Sasaki and Pang (1980) evaluated hemodynamic changes in acute rat flaps. Low total blood flow, nutrient flow, and arteriovenous shunt flow were found in the early postoperative period (six hours). By 12 to 24 hours a pattern of steadily increasing flow, both nutrient and arteriovenous, was observed. Pearl (1981) suggested a "unifying theory" of the delay phenomenon and performed experimental studies in rat abdominal flaps to support his proposal. These focused on the "hyperadrenergic" state that results immediately after sympathectomy secondary to the obligatory discharge of vasoconstricting neurotransmitters. Delayed flaps have adequate blood flow to survive this early stage of vasoconstriction, whereas acute flaps do not.

Kerrigan (1983) undertook to address directly the issue of arteriovenous shunt flow in acute skin flaps with the pig as an experimental model. Using radioactive microspheres, she measured total flow by 50 μm spheres and nutrient flow by 15 μm spheres. Her data showed that in acutely elevated flaps, arterial insufficiency was the prime cause of distal flap failure (Fig. 9–41). She found no evidence of arteriovenous shunt flow in the distal, destined to die portion of a flap, a finding determined by lack of fluorescein dye penetration. This work was corroborated by the findings of Pang and associates (1986b) and has been extended to include delayed flaps. In no type of flap, acute or delay, was there significant change in the percentage of shunt flow or evidence of shunt flow in the distal ischemic portion of the flap.

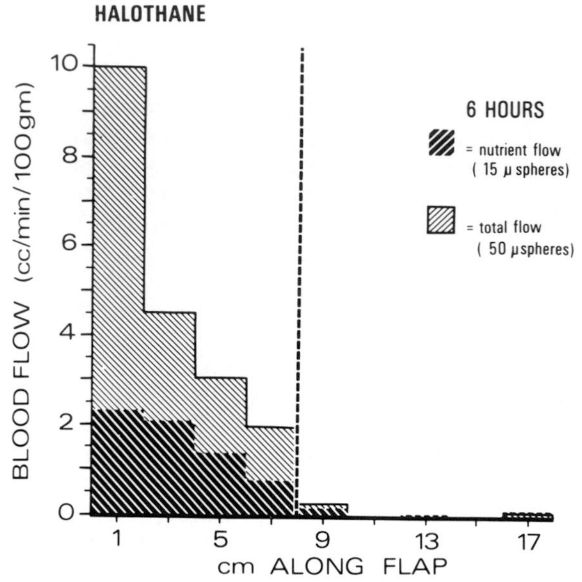

Figure 9–41. Flow rates in a 6 hour old acutely elevated pig flap (From Kerrigan, C. L.: Skin flap failure: pathophysiology. Plast. Reconstr. Surg., *72*:766, 1983.)

METABOLIC CHANGES

The ischemic insult occurring secondary to flap elevation creates havoc at the local metabolic level. Tissues with an inadequate oxygen supply switch to anaerobic metabolism. In acutely elevated flaps, designed to have a distal zone of severe ischemia, O_2, glucose, and adenosine triphosphate (ATP) fall dramatically as one progresses distally along the flap. As expected, CO_2 and lactate simultaneously rise.

The tissue glucose level and its utilization also undergo changes in ischemic flaps. Glucose consumption in ischemic distal but viable flaps is at a maximum by three days and has recovered by seven days. Lactate production is also increased, and tissue glycogen and glucose content is significantly decreased (Cohen, Harmon, and Phizackerley, 1983; Im and associates, 1983). Cyclic AMP falls in the acute stages, but in viable portions of the flap it increases markedly after 12 hours (Jurell and Fredholm, 1981). This effect may reflect a period of increased metabolic activity.

In the ischemic portions of island, free, or delayed flaps there is increased anaerobic metabolism, and subsequently the production of toxic superoxide radicals is elevated (Manson and associates, 1983; Im and Hoopes, 1985). These radicals are a by-product of xanthine metabolism and are detrimental to flap survival. Im and Hoopes (1985) measured endogenous levels of superoxide dismutase (SOD), an enzyme that plays a key role in defending against free radical toxicity, in both acute and delayed rat flaps. The delayed flaps exhibited normal levels of SOD, whereas the distal portions of the acute flaps had a decrease in SOD levels. It has been shown that, if superoxide radical production is blocked with allopurinol or is neutralized with exogenous SOD (Im and associates, 1985), the viability of ischemic tissues may be improved. The importance of these mediators of tissue injury in any ischemic organ must not be underestimated (Angel and associates, 1987).

Many of the metabolic changes alter the rheologic properties of blood at the microcirculatory level, and thus affect skin viability. Experimental studies have shown both an increase in flap blood flow with decreasing viscosity (Awwad and associates, 1983) and an increase in flap survival length with anemia (Gatti and associates, 1982) and protein depletion (Ruberg and Falcone, 1978). Fibrinolysis is also dramatically altered, with a decrease in fibrinolytic activity 24 hours after reperfusion of ischemic skin flaps (Cherry and associates, 1975), and the same finding has been noted in the distal flap with marginal ischemia (Cherry, 1987).

With local ischemia, there are changes in platelet aggregation and arachidonic acid pathways. Prostacyclin and thromboxane production is altered. In delayed flaps, prostacyclin levels are maximally elevated on the seventh postoperative day (Hauben and Zijlstra, 1984). In acute flaps, the venous effluent is found to contain a significant elevation of thromboxanes (Balkovich and Edstrom, 1984).

To summarize the pathophysiologic events in an acute flap, one should consider a flap that is created too large for its supporting blood supply (Fig. 9–42). During its elevation, cutaneous blood vessels and sympathetic nerves are severed. This results in a dramatic alteration in flow. During the first 18 hours flow decreases secondary to lowered perfusion pressure and release of sympathetic vasoconstrictors. In the distal flap where flow is inadequate during the first 12 hours, irreversible ischemia will result in flap necrosis. As ischemia becomes evident, many metabolic vasodilators (CO_2, lactate, prostaglandins, histamine, etc.) act in concert to in-

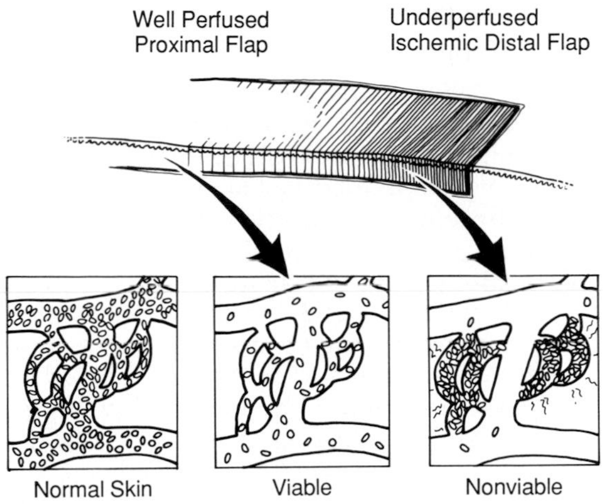

Figure 9–42. The pathophysiologic changes in an acutely elevated skin flap.

crease flow gradually. With depletion of sympathetic vasoconstrictors there is further increase in flow from 12 to 48 hours postoperatively. Only the proximal flap benefits from these effects, as any improvements after 12 hours cannot reverse the ischemic damage in the distal flap. A new equilibrium is soon reached, and wound healing in the periphery and flap bed progress. By four to five days, in a healthy bed, there are adequate collateral connections to support the flap without its original primary blood supply.

In the delayed flap vessels are severed, but to a lesser extent than with a fully elevated acute flap. The sympathetic nerves are also cut but perhaps not completely, depending on the orientation of the flap. In the first 12 hours postoperatively, there is an increase in flow as the metabolic vasodilators can take advantage of the adequate perfusion pressure. In the ensuing 12 to 48 hours more sympathetic neurotransmitters are depleted, local metabolites are released, and flow continues to increase until it reaches a steady state. At a later date, when the flap undergoes its second stage of transfer, there is once again a severance of cutaneous blood vessels but no further release of sympathetic neurotransmitters, since these have already been depleted by the initial delay procedure. Unfortunately, this is a somewhat simplistic explanation for the delay phenomenon, as there is experimental evidence that delay can be successful in denervated skin (May and Piliero, 1979). Thus, there is continued interest in the experimental investigation of the pathophysiology of skin flap failure and the delay phenomenon.

Pharmacology

In the 1950's and 1960's, skin flap research focused on finding an explanation for the delay phenomenon. With the evolution and increasing sophistication of flap design, the delay procedure is rarely used except indirectly in soft tissue expansion. However, a significant number of acute skin flaps show signs of ischemia and impending failure. If the delay phenomenon were fully understood, perhaps this information could be used to create an immediate chemical delay in the threatened flap. Thus, pharmacologic studies have been designed not only to salvage the flap failing from intrinsic causes but also to test hypotheses about the delay phenomenon and improve our understanding of the pathophysiology of intrinsic skin flap failure.

Since 1960, over 100 experimental studies have been published in the English medical literature employing over 75 different agents specifically trying either to mimic delay or to improve the survival area of an acute flap. In addition, there have been many unpublished studies in which no beneficial effect was found. Of the 75 different agents tried, only 30 have been investigated by more than one researcher and only 14 by more than two researchers.

With the multitude of studies and conflicting results, all reports must be read critically. A common problem has been inadequate sample size. Haeck, Spira, and Divine (1984) demonstrated that to show a 10 per cent difference with 80 per cent confidence using the standard rat dorsal flap based cephalad, 249 rats are needed per group. If a 25 per cent increase is deemed significant, 40 animals per group are needed. The average study uses 10 animals per group! Using the same statistical analysis but changing the flap model to the rat epigastric flap, the authors noted that only 19 animals would be required to show a 25 per cent beneficial effect with 80 per cent confidence. In addition to small sample sizes, the effect of the agent used is often not measured or documented. Changes in blood flow, serum levels, or dose-response curves are not usually reported. In many studies the control groups are inadequate. The ultimate clinical goal is to treat the endangered acute flap, and therefore an effective *postoperative* regimen is needed. The following section summarizes the available pharmacologic data by considering agents according to their mechanism of action.

AXON BLOCKERS

The autonomic nervous system can be blocked at a variety of levels. Agents affecting the ganglion or axon itself will be discussed separately from the receptor blockers. Agents tested by several investigators include reserpine, dopamine, and guanethidine. Several other sympatholytic agents acting proximal to the receptor have been used experimentally: trimethaphan, bretylium, alpha-methyl-*p*-tyrosine, cocaine, pheniprazine, and desipramine. Information on the latter agents is too sparse to permit comment.

Reserpine. Reserpine depletes intraneuronal stores of norepinephrine, thus blocking the action of the sympathetic nerve terminals. However, the sympathetic *receptors* remain functional. On the theory that delay in part works because of sympathectomy, several researchers administered reserpine preoperatively to rats, using doses from 0.6 to 5 mg per kg. In some studies (Jurell and Jonsson, 1976; Cutting, Koss, and Robson, 1976; Morain and associates, 1983; Hendel, Lilien, and Buncke, 1983a,b) there was an increase in flap survival, whereas in another there was not (Kennedy, Pistone, and Miller, 1979). In one pig study (Kerrigan and Daniel, 1982b), reserpine was administered postoperatively but no beneficial effect was demonstrated. Reserpine may be useful preoperatively but there are no data to support a therapeutic benefit postoperatively. This agent has been of more benefit in testing the hypothesis of delay more than in the treatment of the failing flap.

Dopamine. Dopamine is an adrenergic axon blocker that at appropriate doses destroys the nerve terminal. Several studies reveal its beneficial effects when given preoperatively (Reinisch, 1974; Wexler and associates, 1975; Jurell and Jonsson, 1976), whereas others under the same conditions show no benefits (Smith and associates, 1980). Like reserpine, this agent, if helpful at all, is beneficial if given preoperatively.

Guanethidine. Guanethidine interferes with the adrenergic terminal by blocking release of the neurotransmitter and may also have a weak effect on the beta-adrenergic receptors. All experimental studies involve preoperative treatment and again conflicting results are noted (Jurell and Jonsson, 1976; Finseth and Adelberg, 1978; Aarts, 1980; Hendel, Lilien, and Buncke, 1983a,b). As with the other adrenergic neuron blockers, clinical application is unlikely to be successful unless guanethidine is given preoperatively.

RECEPTOR BLOCKERS

Sympathetic receptors in the peripheral vasculature can be divided into alpha receptors and beta receptors. The beta receptors can be further divided into $beta_1$ and $beta_2$ receptors. Stimulation of alpha receptors causes vasoconstriction, whereas stimulation of beta receptors causes vasodilatation. In skin, the alpha receptors are predominant; in muscle, the beta receptors are more important. Aims in flap research have been to block alpha receptors and stimulate beta receptors. Many of the pharmacologic agents that have been developed have more than one action, but they are grouped for the purpose of this chapter according to their primary mode of action. The alpha receptor blockers that have been tested include phenoxybenzamine, phentolamine, tolazoline, and thymoxamine. Agents active at the beta receptor include epinephrine, isoproterenol, metaproterenol, terbutaline, isoxsuprine, and propranolol.

If our current understanding of skin flap pathophysiology is correct, this group of drugs theoretically would have the most significant effect on flap survival. However, inconsistent results abound in the literature. Only the five most frequently tested agents will be discussed: phenoxybenzamine, phentolamine, propranolol, isoxsuprine, and chlorpromazine.

Phenoxybenzamine. Phenoxybenzamine was one of the first drugs used to treat the failing flap. It has been used most extensively in the rat, only one pig study having been reported (Kerrigan and Daniel, 1982b). Several studies described an increase in survival when the drug was administered preoperatively (Myers and Cherry, 1968; Wexler and associates, 1975; Finseth and Adelberg, 1978; Monteiro, Santamore, and Nemir, 1986; Hendel, Lilien, and Buncke, 1983a,b; Barlev and associates, 1983; Goshen, Wexler, and Peled, 1985), but in others there was no beneficial effect noted (Smith and associates, 1980; Griffiths and associates, 1981; Kerrigan and Daniel, 1982b). As previously emphasized, most studies had an inadequate number of animals for meaningful statistical analysis within the range of improvement.

Phentolamine. Phentolamine is also an alpha-adrenergic receptor blocker with additional actions as a direct smooth muscle relaxant. Eight investigators used this agent in rats, all but one using the dorsal flap model. Dosages ranged from 1 to 20 mg per kg. An increase in skin flap survival was shown in many of the studies (Norberg and Palmer, 1969; Palmer, 1972; Wexler and associates, 1975; Jonsson and associates, 1975; Toomey, Conayer, and Ogura, 1979; Barlev and associates, 1983) and a decrease in survival was observed in one (Smith and associates, 1980). One study applied topical phentolamine and demonstrated improved survival (Goshen, Wexler, and Peled, 1985). However, the base used in the control group was different from any of the treatment groups, so that the validity of the conclusions was in question.

Propranolol. Propranolol is a nonselective beta-adrenergic blocker that has been used in several rat studies and one pig study. The study groups are all small and the data once again conflicting. Increased survival was found in two rat studies (Jonsson and associates, 1975; Barlev and associates, 1983) and no benefit in others (Smith and associates, 1980; Griffiths and associates, 1981). Similar studies in the pig did not confirm any beneficial effects (Wray and Young, 1984).

Isoxsuprine. Isoxsuprine is the most controversial vasodilator that has been used experimentally to treat the failing skin flap. Seventeen reports can be reviewed in the literature in several different rat and pig flap models, but not all are cited here. In skin flap models most of the studies show no increase in flap survival (Cherry, 1979; Sasaki and Harii, 1980; Smith and associates, 1980; Griffiths and associates, 1981; Kinkead, Zook, and Card, 1981; Griffiths and Humphries, 1981; Blomain and associates, 1982; Kerrigan and Daniel, 1982b; Wray and Young, 1984; Neligan and associates, 1985; Pang and associates, 1985), whereas several do show an increase (Finseth and Adelberg, 1978; Finseth and Adelberg, 1979; Hillelson and associates, 1980). In myocutaneous flap or muscle survival, five demonstrate an improvement (Finseth and Zimmerman, 1979; Finseth and Adelberg, 1979; Finseth, Zimmerman, and Liggins, 1979; Cherry, 1979; Kerrigan and Daniel, 1984) and two show no effect (Neligan and associates, 1985; Pang and associates, 1985). These studies utilized a variety of doses and dosing schedules. In the few studies that actually measured the effect of isoxsuprine on flow, the flow in the control and the proximal flap was increased, whereas flow in the distal flap was not (Neligan and associates, 1985; Pang and associates, 1985). The use of isoxsuprine to treat the clinical failing flap cannot be justified on the basis of these experimental studies.

Chlorpromazine. Chlorpromazine is a phenothiazine that is widely used, primarily for its antipsychotic effects. It has a series of complex actions on the cardiovascular system because it acts both centrally and peripherally. It causes alpha-adrenergic blockade, it may act as a direct vasodilator, and it has mild antagonistic effects at histamine and serotonin receptors. This agent has been used in acute dorsal rat flaps. One investigator pretreated animals for two weeks and the other pretreated them for 20 minutes. The former found no beneficial effect (Toomey, Conoyer, and Ogura, 1979) whereas the latter noted an increase in flap survival (Bibi, Ferder, and Strauch, 1986). As in every other study, small group sizes were used and the effects on flow were not well documented. Further investigation is necessary if chlorpromazine is to be seriously considered for clinical use.

DIRECT SMOOTH MUSCLE RELAXANTS

If flap necrosis occurs because of persistent relative vasoconstriction, any vasodilator, if it can compete with the constricting elements, ought to increase flap survival. Agents whose predominant mode of action is smooth muscle relaxation include hydralazine, nitroglycerin, diazoxide, dimethyl sulfoxide and a variety of calcium channel blockers.

Hydralazine. Hydralazine is a direct smooth muscle relaxant whose effect on skin flap survival has been tested by three groups of investigators (Finseth and Adelberg, 1978; Toomey, Conoyer, and Ogura, 1979; Hendel, Lilien, and Buncke, 1983a,b). All used the rat but with different flap models. The study of Hendel, Lilien, and Buncke (1983a,b) is the most detailed and includes dose-response curves. These authors concluded that at low doses hydralazine can be effective at increasing skin flap survival, but it is unclear from their report whether preoperative treatment is necessary. This drug would need further testing in a variety of animal models before it could be recommended for clinical applications.

Nitroglycerin. Nitroglycerin is a direct-acting vascular smooth muscle relaxant with a greater effect on the venous system than on the arterial system. Several investigators postulate that flap failure is more a problem of venous congestion than of arterial failure, although experimental data suggest otherwise (Kerrigan and Daniel, 1983b). Perhaps on this basis nitroglycerin would be beneficial to the failing skin flap. Five groups of researchers investigated this drug in two animals (rat and pig) using four different flap models (Blomain and associates, 1982; Rohrich, Cherry, and Spira, 1984; Nichter, Sobieski, and Edgerton, 1985; Gatti and associates, 1986; Waters and associates, 1986). In all studies but one the nitroglycerin was administered topically; in the one study it was given as a continuous intravenous infusion. In the studies that demonstrated increased survival, increases were in the range of 30 per cent over controls. In the one study in which no increase was found, one of the placebo groups showed increased survival (Nichter, Sobieski, and Edgerton, 1985)! To date, the literature cannot support the use of topical or intravenous nitroglycerin to treat the failing skin flap.

Dimethyl Sulfoxide. Dimethyl sulfoxide (DMSO) is a drug with a multitude of actions. It was one of the first agents to be used on the failing skin flap (Adamson and associates, 1966, 1967; Ketchum and associates, 1967; Arturson and Khanna, 1970; Myers and Cherry, 1968; Koehnlein and Lemperle, 1970). Most studies have used topical DMSO but one report described intraperitoneal administration (Grossman and associates, 1983). Results are conflicting and in no studies was the effect on blood flow measured. DMSO cannot be recommended for clinical use.

Calcium Channel Blockers. Regulation of Ca^{++} channels across cell membranes can be dramatically altered by ischemic states, and such agents can interfere with vascular responsiveness. It has been suggested that inhibition of calcium entry into cells may prolong ischemic tolerance and limit vascular spasm. Many investigators have tried a variety of calcium channel blockers in ischemic skin flaps in the hope that survival would be increased. The results have been disappointing and most studies have never been published (Myers, 1986; Myers and Valencia, 1986). It appears that the systemic effects of the drugs become intolerable before any beneficial increase in cutaneous flow can be detected (Miller and associates, 1985).

Prostaglandins and Blockers. A variety of local metabolic substances dramatically alter cutaneous blood flow. There have been isolated attempts at increasing flap survival with histamine (Ketchum and associates, 1967; Milton and Corbett, 1969) and bradykinin, but most research has focused on prostaglandins and other metabolites of arachidonic acid. As with the sympathetic nervous system, the metabolites of arachidonic acid have both vasodilatory and vasoconstricting properties. In addition, the compounds interfere with platelet function. PGE compounds and PGI_2 are potent vasodilators, whereas PGF compounds and thromboxane are vasoconstrictors.

Experiments in rats, rabbits, and pigs with both PGE_1 and PGI_2 (prostacyclin) have consistently shown an improvement in skin flap survival or an increase in cutaneous blood flow (Nozaki and associates, 1981; Emerson and Sykes, 1981; Morain and associates, 1983; Reus and associates, 1984; Knight and associates, 1985; Zachary and associates, 1986). The agents have an extremely short half-life, are unstable, and have to be given by continuous intravenous or intra-arterial infusion. Further research has thus focused on blocking the formation of arachidonic acid metabolites.

Agents interfering with arachidonic acid metabolism include indomethacin, ibuprofen, and imidazole. *Indomethacin* is a potent inhibitor of cyclooxygenase and also inhibits the motility of polymorphonuclear leukocytes. It has been effective at increasing rat skin flap survival (Sasaki and Pang, 1981; Pang and Sasaki, 1981) but not rabbit flap blood flow (Knight and associates, 1985). *Ibuprofen*, a proprionic acid derivative, inhibits both cyclooxygenase and lipoperoxidase, thus blocking two pathways of arachidonic acid. In rat studies it has effectively increased flow and flap survival (Sasaki and Pang, 1981; Nichter, Sobieski, and Edgerton, 1986). *Imidazole* and its derivatives are selective thromboxane synthesis inhibitors. In theory, their use would decrease vasoconstricting and platelet aggregation effects and thus tip the balance in favor of increased cutaneous flow. However, no such beneficial effects have been demonstrated on skin flap survival (Kay and Green, 1986). Although this group of drugs has exciting possibilities, it has not been adequately tested in the research laboratory to justify clinical application.

ALTERING RHEOLOGY OF BLOOD

Many attempts have been made to improve skin flap blood flow by agents known to alter the rheology of blood. Most have been inadequately tested; they include ancrod, xanthinol niacinate (Complamin), low molecular weight dextran, dicumoral, dipyridamole, heparin, hyaluronidase, and streptokinase; protein depletion has also been tried. Two treatments have, however, been tested more thoroughly.

Pentoxifylline. Pentoxifylline is a vasoactive drug derived from xanthine. Its mechanism of action is not fully understood but is thought to include smooth muscle relaxation, improved flexibility of red blood cells, and promotion of platelet deaggregation. Its use in rats as preoperative treatment can increase flap survival (Takayanagi and Ogawa, 1980; Monteiro, Santamore, and Nemir, 1986). However, further documentation must be carried out in the rat and other animal species before clinical use can be recommended.

Anemia. Several investigators have rendered animals anemic in the hope that the hemodynamics will improve. Increased flap survival is found to be inversely correlated with the hematocrit (Earle, Fratianne, and Nunez, 1974; Gatti and associates, 1982; Ramasastry and associates, 1985). Information gained is useful to an understanding of the pathophysiology of skin flap failure, but this is not a treatment technique that is feasible in the human patient. However, the data suggest that a slightly low hematocrit in the postoperative course need not be aggressively corrected by transfusion.

INCREASING TOLERANCE TO ISCHEMIA

Steroids. Steroids have been used in an attempt to salvage the failing flap, because of their membrane-stabilizing properties. The latter theoretically might increase tissue tolerance to ischemia. If the tolerance could be supported for a few days, any spontaneous increase in blood flow would be of benefit to the relatively ischemic portion of the flap. Five studies have described the use of a variety of steroids: methylprednisolone (Mendelson and Woods, 1978; Nakatsuka and associates, 1985), prednisolone (Mes, 1980), and dexamethasone (Nancarrow, 1981; Hendel, Lilien, and Buncke, 1983a, b). The most careful study (Nakatsuka and associates, 1985) cannot substantiate the claims of other researchers. The literature does not provide adequate data to support the use of steroids in the failing skin flap.

Superoxide Radical Scavengers or Blockers. It has been established that the generation of free radicals in ischemic tissue is detrimental to survival of that tissue (Granger, Hollwarth, and Parks, 1986). If free radical production can be blocked or if the radicals can be scavenged, tissue damage should be minimized. Most free radicals are generated by xanthine oxidase. Their production can be blocked by *allopurinol*, a well-known xanthine oxidase inhibitor, and skin flap survival increased by preoperative treatment (Mes, 1980; Im and associates, 1985; Angel and associates, 1987). *Superoxide dismutase* (SOD) is one of the key enzymes in protecting against free radical toxicity, and it is dramatically decreased in the distal ischemic end of acute skin flaps (Im and Hoopes, 1985); it has been used by researchers in rat abdominal flaps (Im and associates, 1985; Zimmerman, Sasaki, and Khattab, 1987; Huang and associates, 1987) to increase flap tolerance to ischemia. Deferoxamine, an iron chelating agent and free radical scavenger, has also been utilized to treat the ischemic skin flap. Two rat studies using different skin flap models (Angel and associates, 1986; Huang and associates, 1987) have both demonstrated an increase in flap survival area. The mechanism of these benefits was explored by Angel and associates (1987) who demonstrated a decrease in malonyldialdehyde, a compound resulting from free radical metabolism.

This class of agents minimizes free radical generation and toxicity and has exciting possibilities for further research efforts in additional laboratories and animal models.

Hyperbaric Oxygen. One of the most promising early techniques for the treatment of postoperative ischemic acute flaps involved the use of hyperbaric oxygen. "Successful" clinical cases have been reported (Perrins, 1966), and experimental studies carried out in the rat and rabbit have demonstrated a beneficial effect from hyperbaric oxygen (Arturson and Khanna, 1970; Jurell and Kaijser, 1973; Champion, McSherry, and Goulian, 1967; McFarlane and Wermuth, 1966; Tan and associates, 1984). However, work in the pig has been disappointing (Kernahan and Zingg, 1965; Perrins, 1972). The equipment required for hyperbaric treatment is extremely cumbersome and involves some risk to the patient unless the therapy is administered by a well-trained team. Uncontrolled clinical cases plus negative results in pig studies call the validity of this technique into question. In addition, if it were truly effective, why have there been no further reports of its clinical use in the last 20 years?

Miscellaneous Agents. A variety of other therapies have been used to treat the failing flap and are described in isolated reports whose results are difficult to interpret. They include silver sulfadiazine, moist environment, hematoma, diapulse, direct current, ultrasound, formic acid, low power laser irradiation, and stress.

Tests of Skin Flap Circulation/Monitors

The ability to monitor the status of flap perfusion or its viability is of paramount importance in the prevention, recognition, and treatment of complications. Numerous tests, both subjective and objective, are available to aid this endeavor (Table 9–4). When delay procedures and tube flaps were commonly used, their goal was to help the surgeon decide if the flap was ready for division or transfer. With the widespread use of free tissue transfers and large arterial flaps or myocutaneous flaps, monitors are required that signal extrinsic complications such as vascular thrombosis, or intrinsic complications such as distal flap ischemia.

As so many tests are available, it is important to evaluate critically their optimal applications and recognize their limitations. Several important factors must be considered. First, is the monitor to be used for clinical or research purposes? In clinical practice relative flows suffice, whereas in the research laboratory quantitative values are often required. Second, is flow at one point on the flap an adequate reflection of total flap perfusion, or do several points or the whole flap need to be assessed? In free flaps, one point usually suffices because an "all or none" phenomenon is to be detected. In local flaps, the whole unit must be assessed differentially to

Table 9–4. Monitors of Flap Perfusion

Test	Setting	Uses	Number of Sites	Repeat-ability	Time to Perform	Comments
Color	Clinical	Skin flaps, I&E	Infinite	Infinite	Seconds	Not a reliable test
Capillary blanching	Clinical	Skin flaps, I&E	Infinite	Infinite	Seconds	Not very reliable, needs experience to interpret
Warmth	Clinical	Skin flaps, I&E	Infinite	Infinite	Seconds	Much too subjective to be of clinical use
Stab wound bleeding	Clinical	Skin and muscle flaps, E	Infinite	Infinite	Seconds	Useful subjective measure, especially in free flaps
pH	Clinical and research	Skin and buried flaps, I&E	One site	Infinite	Minutes	Has been disappointing, although possibilities for buried tissue transfers still exist
$tcpO_2$	Clinical and research	Skin flaps, E	One site	Infinite	20–30 min	Has been disappointing and most have abandoned its use
Laser Doppler	Clinical and research	Skin and buried flaps, I&E	One site	Infinite	Continuous	Most promising test currently available for clinical use; implantable probes recently developed
Photoplethys-mography	Clinical	Skin flap, I&E	One site	Infinite	Minutes	Disappointing results, although some modifications have improved its use
Surface temperature	Clinical and research	Skin flaps, E	Multiple sites, continuous	Infinite	Minutes	Most widely used test for monitoring free flaps but must be interpreted by experienced persons
Differential thermometry	Clinical and research	Skin and buried flaps, E	One site	Infinite	Continuous	Current standard for buried tissue transfers, although not widely used
Fluorescein	Clinical and research	Skin flaps, I&E	Whole flap	Every 8 hr	30 min	Currently the best test available for intrinsic failure
Dermofluorometry	Clinical and research	Skin flaps, I&E	One site, or more sequentially	Infinite	20–30 min	Relatively inexpensive instrumentation for very useful information
Clearance (H, Tc, Xe, etc.)	Clinical and research	Skin and ?buried flaps, I&E	One site, or more sequentially	Infinite	30–60 min	Particularly useful for research laboratory; equipment may be cumbersome for clinical use
Radioactive microspheres	Research	All flaps, I&E	Infinite	3 times	Hours	Golden standard for laboratory; test takes seconds to perform but data analysis takes hours
Electromagnetic flowmetry	Research	All island flaps, E	One site	Infinite	Continuous	Technically demanding but gives excellent measure of total flap flow; cannot differentiate nutrient from total flow

I = intrinsic failure; E = extrinsic complications.

detect areas of distal ischemia. Third, how long does it take to do the test, is it repeatable, and how long does it take to respond to changes in flow? Some tests take seconds to perform and others take minutes or even hours. Certain tests cannot be repeated more than once and others may take hours to respond to the changes in vascular perfusion. Fourth, does the test provide intermittent or continuous monitoring of the flap? Finally, can the technique be applied to buried free tissue transfers?

SUBJECTIVE TESTS

Subjective tests aid the *experienced* surgeon to evaluate the status of a skin flap's circulation. Tests commonly used include observation of color, capillary blanching and refill, warmth, and bleeding from stab wounds.

Color. Skin color may be a very deceptive index of flap perfusion. As it is so variable, a simple observation tells us nothing. Comparing a free flap taken from the back, which has not been sun exposed, with its site of transfer, the leg, which has been sun exposed, one notes that the flap appears pale and underperfused. A "blue" flap is usually a late change of severe ischemia in a random flap or venous failure in a free flap. Thus, color as an indicator is of limited clinical use (Acland, 1976).

Capillary Blanching. Blanching of a skin flap by gentle pressure, with subsequent observation of capillary refill, is a widely used test. Unfortunately, it has been shown that even a free flap, totally isolated from the body, may demonstrate this phenomenon. In pale skin, it may be impossible to visualize the blanching, and thus a negative test may be misinterpreted to indicate arterial failure when in fact the flap is well perfused. In hyperemic skin, the response may be a useful way of confirming other subjective or objective tests. Taken in the appropriate context and interpreted by experienced personnel, blanching may be a helpful index of perfusion.

Warmth. Subjective assessment of flap temperature is not a reliable way to assess flap perfusion.

Bleeding from Stab Wounds. Bleeding from stab wounds in the flap is a useful test of skin flap perfusion (Kerrigan and Daniel, 1983b). The test is usually made with an 18 gauge needle or a No. 11 scalpel blade; the absence of bleeding from the stab wound indicates arterial failure. Delayed bleeding of bright red blood signifies some degree of arterial spasm. Brisk, bright red bleeding can be interpreted as normal arterial perfusion or perhaps some degree of hyperemia. Cyanotic bleeding that promptly clears to bright red blood indicates some degree of venous congestion. The test can be used routinely on flaps to assess extrinsic complications, but it is not particularly useful in detecting intrinsic failure.

OBJECTIVE TESTS

Objective tests must be used as an adjunct to clinical judgment. Their major benefit is that they alert the surgeon to a potential problem long before subjective signs become evident. The surgeon must then decide how to respond to the objective changes in the context of the overall clinical picture.

Metabolic Tests. The two metabolic tests most frequently used for monitoring skin flap perfusion are for pH and transcutaneous pO_2. Tissue pH can be measured by implantation of an electrode and continuous monitoring of the trends (Glinz and Clodius, 1972; Dickson and Sharpe, 1985). Transcutaneous pO_2 is measured by placing a heated electrode on the skin surface and also measuring trends (Serafin and associates, 1981; Smith and associates, 1983; Achauer and Black, 1984). The major disadvantage of both these techniques is the expense of the equipment involved. Although initially used with great enthusiasm, the transcutaneous pO_2 is now rarely made for flap monitoring. Tissue pH testing is still being investigated for its possible application to monitoring of buried tissue transfers.

Photoelectric Tests. For assessing blood flow, the Doppler effect has been used in two different ways. *Ultrasound* Doppler uses reflected sound to pick up large subcutaneous pulsatile arteries. *Laser* Doppler (LD) measures the frequency shift of light rather than sound reflection. The laser light has limited penetration and thus measures flow to a depth of only 1.5 mm. LD has become a popular research and clinical monitor used with varied enthusiasm and success. The LD readings measure voltage and provide a relative but not absolute measure of flow rates, although efforts to generate a true flow rate are being made. This technique may provide the most useful index of flow in the monitoring of free flaps for extrinsic complications. The technique is noninvasive. It can be used continuously (thus giving trends), but it is expensive. Some experience is required to allow accurate interpretation of changing signals. Refinements in both laser and ultrasound Dopplers have permitted fabrication of small implantable probes, which are now being investigated experimentally for their ability to detect microvascular thromboses in buried free tissue transfers (Jones and Mayou, 1982; Svensson and associates, 1985).

Photoplethysmography has been available since the 1940's and the instrumentation has undergone several modifications (Harrison and associates, 1983). This technique measures fluid volume by detecting variations in light absorption by the skin. As with laser Doppler, flow in the tissues to a depth of only 1 to 1.5 mm may be detected. In extrinsic complications with arterial failure, the wave form disappears, and in venous failure the wave form patterns require experience to interpret. For detecting intrinsic flap failure, the photoplethysmograph has been disappointing. However, Bardach and associates (1979) modified the signal interpretation and believed this change gives a reasonably good prediction of the survival-necrosis interface. Current equipment is limited to measurement of one site at a time. Other plethysmographic techniques, such as impedance plethysmography, have not been adapted for use in skin flaps.

Temperature Tests. Several types of temperature tests have been made to monitor skin flaps and free tissue transfers. They include surface temperature, differential thermometry, temperature clearance, and thermography. Only the first two will be discussed. Temperature can be measured by a thermistor or a thermocouple. The thermocouple is a more sensitive and precise instrument that measures a voltage differential between two wires of different metals. Thermistors are semiconductors that have a lowered resistance at higher temperature. Thermistors are less precise than thermocouples but they provide adequate information for most types of monitoring.

Surface Temperature. Skin surface temperature is easily measured and requires relatively inexpensive equipment. To provide an effective monitor, several guidelines must be followed: the patient's core temperature should be recorded, extraneous light-heat sources should be avoided, dressings should not cover the flap, and room temperature and air currents must remain constant. If the patient is moved one should expect a transient change in the temperature reading. Surface temperature is the current standard for monitoring extrinsic complications. Used as a relative index, it has proved a dependable and useful clinical tool. For the evaluation of intrinsic flap failures, it is inadequate.

Differential Thermometry. There is a need for a reliable objective technique to monitor vascular patency in buried free tissue transfers. The only technique that has any significant clinical data to support its use is that of differential thermometry (May and Halls, 1985). Thermocouple probes are sutured both proximal and distal to the arterial anastomoses, and their temperature difference is recorded. These are monitored on a continuous basis, and any difference greater than 3° C is judged to be significant. Time must be invested in learning to interpret this test accurately; if not, many false alarms are called and may cause greater harassment to the surgeon than no monitor at all.

Vital Dye. When vital dyes are administered systemically, they stain skin that is adequately perfused. Several dyes have been used, including fluorescein, Disulphine Blue, and vital green. Fluorescein is the only one used clinically at the present time and may be employed two different ways. When administered intravenously, peak serum concentrations occur at 20 minutes, which is the usual time for observation of the flap by Wood's lamp illumination. At a dosage of 1.5 mg per kg, this test may be used to monitor both extrinsic and intrinsic flap failure (McCraw, Myers, and Shanklin, 1977). The major disadvantages are that the test tends to underestimate flap survival and can be repeated only every eight hours. The reason for underestimation of flap survival can best be understood if one remembers the dynamic nature of skin flap circulation and the fact that skin blood flow tends to increase with the time after flap elevation. Thus, fluorescein given one hour after flap elevation will assess flap circulation at that time. Any subsequent increase in flow within the next 12 hours will contribute to the increase in flap survival, but it will not have been measured by the early postoperative dye test. A few reported cases of anaphylactic reactions to fluorescein are in the literature, but the most common adverse reaction seen clinically is nausea. This can be minimized by slow intravenous administration.

The second method of using fluorescein requires a smaller dose of 0.15 mg per kg. Tissue fluorescence at this level is not detectable by the human eye, but an instrument has been developed, the dermofluorometer, to quantitate these levels (Silverman and associates, 1980; Graham and associates, 1983). This test has the advantage of providing an objective measure of skin flap circulation, and it may be repeated as often as needed, although it takes about 30 minutes to complete. An index relating fluorescein levels in the flap to control skin is then calculated. Clinically an index of greater than 30 per cent is considered to be safe. In the authors' experimental work, it was shown that, if the test is done early postoperatively, an index as low as 8 per cent may be acceptable (Thomson, 1988). This is again a reflection of the dynamic nature of skin flap circulation. The technique is equally applicable in dark-skinned individuals and, as mentioned previously, it can be used to detect both intrinsic and extrinsic complications.

Quantitative Tests. Absolute quantitative tests are used primarily for research purposes and they provide a measure of nutrient blood flow in ml per min per gm of tissue. They tend to be more time consuming to perform and require expensive instrumentation or equipment. It may also take some time for data analysis before the measured flow rate is known.

Clearance Tests. The principle of all clearance tests is the same. A substance, which can be objectively measured, is introduced into the tissue of concern, and over a period of time the disappearance of this substance is measured. The speed of disappearance or clearance reflects flow rates. Several radioactive tracers have been employed, including Xe133 (Palmer, Jurell, and Norberg, 1972), Na22, Kr85, and Tc99 (Young and Hopewell, 1983). Hydrogen ion is the only nonradioactive substance used in the same quantitative way (Glogovac, Bitz, and Whiteside, 1982). With the use of the radioactive isotopes, a small amount of substance is injected intradermally or placed in a small sealed chamber over the skin. Radioactivity of the isotope is measured over a period of time, thus generating a clearance curve. High local concentrations of hydrogen ion can be achieved in two ways. Traditionally, the animal or patient inhales a 5 per cent concentration of hydrogen gas until the tissues are saturated, as measured by stable electrical activity in the skin. More recently a technique has been devised to generate hydrogen ion electrochemically at the site of a skin electrode, thus obviating the need for tissue saturation by inhalation of hydrogen gas (Suzuki and associates, 1985). In both cases, after delivery of hydrogen ion has peaked, its clearance over time is used to calculate an index of flow. These tests frequently sample only one point at a time and take one to two hours to perform, as stabilization is required and clearance curves often need to be followed for 30 minutes or longer. Data must also be analyzed, and unless a computer is directly connected to the monitoring equipment this may take several hours to days to accomplish.

Radioactive Microspheres. Radioactive microspheres can be used to measure blood flow in experimental situations only (Pang, Neligan, and Nakatsuka, 1984). Small spheres, usually 15 μm in size, are available, tagged with a variety of radioactive isotopes. They are administered to the experimental animal via the left ventricle, and thus embolize peripheral tissues in direct proportion to their blood flow. Samples of tissue are counted for radioactivity and compared with an organ with known flow rates, so as to calculate flow rates of the tissue in question. The study can be repeated only three times, otherwise peripheral embolization begins to interfere with normal hemodynamics. Fifteen μm spheres reflect nutrient flow, but larger spheres are available if data regarding shunt flow or total flow is needed. The radioactive microspheres are the current optimal technique for quantitative measures of blood flow in the research laboratory.

Electromagnetic Flowmetry. This technique is designed for experimental use only and requires a small probe capable of setting up an electrical field across a vessel lumen (Acland and Schwartz, 1981). Blood flow in the vessel interferes with the electrical field and can be translated into precise flow rates. The technique is demanding if it is to be reliable and reproducible data are to be generated, but it is the only method that provides immediate, continuous, and quantitative measurements of total flow. The disadvantage of this technique is that it measures total flow in the flap and can differentiate neither between nutrient and shunt flow nor between flow in the proximal flap and flow in the distal flap. However, it does provide crucial experimental information about flow to free flaps.

Miscellaneous Tests. Several other tests of interest should be mentioned, as they provide additional tools for studying the cutaneous microcirculation or buried tissue transfers. Vital capillary microscopy employs a microscope and video camera to observe and record the dynamic changes occurring within a vascular bed. Special tissue preparation is required for application of this technique. Microangiography, electroarteriography, and interstitial fluid pressure measurements have also been used to study cutaneous microcirculation.

In summary, monitors of skin circulation are used for many reasons. A thorough understanding of the benefits and limitations of all available tests is imperative for their use and interpretation. The two most widely needed clinical applications at present are the monitoring of free tissue transfers and the assessment of an acute skin flap for a distal zone of ischemia. For the former, if a skin flap has been utilized, surface temperature is the monitor of choice; if a buried tissue is to be monitored, differential thermometry with thermocouple probes is the standard, although it is not widely used. For the latter, the fluorescein dye test remains the best available monitor. In the research laboratory, radioactive microspheres are the golden standard. Future research will concentrate on improving techniques available to the clinician, with special emphasis on the monitoring of buried free tissue transfers.

REFERENCES

Aarts, H. R.: Regional intravascular sympathetic blockade for better results in flap surgery: an experimental study of free flaps, island flaps and pedicle flaps in the rabbit ear. Plast. Reconstr. Surg., *66*:690, 1980.

Achauer, B. M., and Black, K. S.: Transcutaneous oxygen and flaps. Plast. Reconstr. Surg., *74*:721, 1984.

Acland, R. D.: A method of eliminating errors in the perception of skin colour. Br. J. Plast. Surg., *29*:97, 1976.

Acland, R. D., and Schwartz, K. S.: Electromagnetic flowmetry: additional data (letter). Plast. Reconstr. Surg., *67*:565, 1981.

Adamson, J. E., Horton, C. E., Crawford, H. H., and Ayers, W. T.: The effects of dimethyl sulfoxide on the experimental pedicle flap: a preliminary report. Plast. Reconstr. Surg., *37*:105, 1966.

Adamson, J. E., Horton, C. E., Crawford, H. H., and Ayers, W. T.: Studies on the action of dimethyl sulfoxide on the experimental pedicle flap. Plast. Reconstr. Surg., *39*:142, 1967.

Angel, M. F., Narayanan, K., Swartz, W. M., Ramasastry, S. S., Kuhns, D. B., et al.: Deferoxamine increases skin flap survival: additional evidence of free radical involvement in ischaemic flap surgery. Br. J. Plast. Surg., *39*:469, 1986.

Angel, M. F., Ramasastry, S. S., Swartz, W. M., Basford, R. E., and Futrell, J. W.: Free radicals: basic concepts concerning their chemistry, pathophysiology, and relevance to plastic surgery. Plast. Reconstr. Surg., *79*:990, 1987.

Arey, L. B.: The vascular system. *In* Developmental Anatomy. Philadelphia, W. B. Saunders Company, 1974, p. 695.

Arnold, P. G., and Mixter, R. C.: Making the most of the gastrocnemius muscles. Plast. Reconstr. Surg., *72*:38, 1983.

Arturson, G., and Khanna, N. N.: The effects of hyperbaric oxygen, dimethyl sulfoxide and Complamin on the survival of experimental skin flaps. Scand. J. Plast. Reconstr. Surg., *4*:8, 1970.

Awwad, A. M., White, R. J., Lowe, G. D. O., and Forbes, C. D.: The effect of blood viscosity on blood flow in the experimental saphenous flap model. Br. J. Plast. Surg., *36*:383, 1983.

Bakamjian, V. Y.: A two stage method for pharyngoesophageal reconstruction with a primary pectoral skin flap. Plast. Reconstr. Surg., *36*:173, 1965.

Balkovich, M., and Edstrom, L.: Skin flap: prostacyclin and thromboxane. Paper presented at Plastic Surgery Research Council 29th Annual Meeting, Detroit, MI, 1984.

Bardach, J., Voots, R. J., McCabe, B. F., and Hsu, M. M.: Photoplethysmography in the prediction of experimental flap survival. Ann. Otol., *88*:673, 1979.

Barlev, A., Peled, I. J., Bergmann, F., and Wexler, M. R.: Improvement of skin flap survival by local injections of Regitine and propranolol. An experimental study in the rat. Isr. J. Med. Sci., *19*:108, 1983.

Barron, J. N., and Emmett, A. J.: Subcutaneous pedicle flaps. Br. J. Plast. Surg., *18*:51, 1965.

Bibi, R., Ferder, M., and Strauch, B.: Prevention of flap necrosis by chlorpromazine. Plast. Reconstr. Surg., *77*:954, 1986.

Blair, V. P.: Surgery and Diseases of the Mouth and Jaws. St. Louis, C. V. Mosby Company, 1912.

Blomain, E. W., Manders, E. K., Saggers, G., Davis, T. S., and Graham, W. P.: Topical nitroglycerin ointment enhances the survival of skin flaps. Surg. Forum, *33*:594, 1982.

Bostwick, J.: Aesthetic and Reconstructive Breast Surgery. St. Louis, C. V. Mosby Company, 1983.

Brent, B., Upton, J., Acland, R. D., Shaw, W. W., Finseth, F. J., et al.: Experience with the temporoparietal fascial free flap. Plast. Reconstr. Surg., *76*:177, 1985.

Carriquiry, C., Aparecida Costa, M., and Vasconez, L. O.: An anatomic study of the septocutaneous vessels of the leg. Plast. Reconstr. Surg., *76*:354, 1985.

Champion, W. M., McSherry, C. K., and Goulian, D.: Effect of hyperbaric oxygen on the survival of pedicled skin flaps. J. Surg. Res., *7*:583, 1967.

Cherry, G. W.: The differing effects of isoxsuprine on muscle flap and skin flap survival in the pig. Plast. Reconstr. Surg., *64*:670, 1979.

Cherry, G. W.: Personal communication, 1987.
Cherry, G. W., Ellis, J. P., Kanan, M. W., and Ryan, T. J.: Tissue fibrinolytic activity in skin following ischaemia. Bibl. Anat., *13*:294, 1975.
Cohen, B. E., Harmon, C. S., and Phizackerley, P. J. R.: Glucose metabolism in experimental skin. Plast. Reconstr. Surg., *71*:79, 1983.
Converse, J. M.: Introduction to plastic surgery. *In* Reconstructive Plastic Surgery. Philadelphia, W. B. Saunders Company, 1977, pp. 3–68.
Cormack, G. C., and Lamberty, B. G. H.: A classification of fascio-cutaneous flaps according to their patterns of vascularisation. Br. J. Plast. Surg., *37*:80, 1984.
Cutting, C., Bumsted, R., Bardach, J., Mooney, M., and Johnson, S.: Changes in quantitative norepinephrine levels in delayed pig flank flaps. Plast. Reconstr. Surg., *69*:652, 1982.
Cutting, C. B., Koss, N., and Robson, M. C.: Pharmacology and flap physiology. Surg. Forum, *27*:563, 1976.
Daniel, R. K.: Direct transfer of skin flaps by microvascular anastomoses. Montreal, McGill University (Thesis), 1973.
Daniel, R. K.: The anatomical and hemodynamic characteristics of the cutaneous circulation and their influence on skin flap design. *In* Grabb, W. C., and Myers, M. B. (Eds.): Skin Flaps. Boston, Little, Brown & Company, 1975a, pp. 111–134.
Daniel, R. K.: Toward an anatomical and hemodynamic classification of skin flaps. Plast. Reconstr. Surg., *56*:330, 1975b.
Daniel, R. K.: Mandibular reconstruction with free tissue transfers: an overview. Ann. Plast. Surg., *1*:346, 1978.
Daniel, R. K., and Faibisoff, B.: Muscle coverage of pressure points: the role of myocutaneous flaps. Ann. Plast. Surg., *8*:446, 1982.
Daniel, R. K., and Kerrigan, C. L.: Skin flaps: an anatomical and hemodynamic approach. Clin. Plast. Surg., *6*:181, 1979.
Daniel, R. K., and Taylor, G. I.: Distant transfer of an island flap by microvascular anastomoses: a clinical technique. Plast. Reconstr. Surg., *52*:111, 1973.
Daniel, R. K., Terzis, J., and Midgley, R. D.: Restoration of sensation to an anesthetic hand by a free neurovascular flap from the foot. Plast. Reconstr. Surg., *57*:275, 1976.
Daniel, R. K., and Williams, H. B.: The free transfer of skin flaps by microvascular anastomoses: an experimental study and a reappraisal. Plast. Reconstr. Surg., *52*:16, 1973.
Dickson, M. G., and Sharpe, D. T.: Continuous subcutaneous tissue pH measurement as a monitor of blood flow in skin flaps: an experimental study. Br. J. Plast. Surg., *38*:39, 1985.
Dinner, M. I., Labandter, H. P., and Dowden, R. V.: The role of the rectus abdominis myocutaneous flap in breast reconstruction. Plast. Reconstr. Surg., *69*:209, 1982.
Dos Santos, L. F.: The vascular anatomy and dissection of the free scapular flap. Plast. Reconstr. Surg., *73*:599, 1984.
Drever, J. M.: The epigastric island flap. Plast. Reconstr. Surg., *59*:343, 1977.
Earle, A. S., Fratianne, R. B., and Nunez, R. D.: The relationship of hematocrit levels to skin flap survival in the dog. Plast. Reconstr. Surg., *54*:341, 1974.
Emerson, D. J. M., and Sykes, P. J.: The effect of prostacyclin on experimental random pattern flaps in the rat. Br. J. Plast. Surg., *34*:264, 1981.
Feldman, J.: Facial resurfacing: the single-sheet concept. *In* Brent, B. (Ed.): The Artistry of Reconstructive Surgery. St. Louis, C. V. Mosby Company, 1987.
Finseth, F. J., and Adelberg, M. G.: Prevention of skin flap necrosis by a course of treatment with vasodilator drugs. Plast. Reconstr. Surg., *61*:738, 1978.
Finseth, F., and Adelberg, M. G.: Experimental work with isoxsuprine for prevention of skin flap necrosis and for treatment of the failing flap. Plast. Reconstr. Surg., *63*:94, 1979.
Finseth, F. J., and Zimmerman, J.: Prevention of necrosis in island myocutaneous flaps in the pig by treatment with isoxsuprine. Plast. Reconstr. Surg., *64*:536, 1979.
Finseth, F. J., Zimmerman, J., and Liggins, D.: Prevention of muscle necrosis in an experimental neurovascular island muscle flap by a vasodilator drug—isoxsuprine. Plast. Reconstr. Surg., *63*:774, 1979.
Gatti, J. E., Brousseau, D. A., Silverman, D. G., and LaRossa, D.: Intravenous nitroglycerin as a means of improving ischemic tissue hemodynamics and survival. Ann. Plast. Surg., *16*:521, 1986.
Gatti, J. E., LaRossa, D., Neff, S. R., and Silverman, D. G.: Altered skin flap survival and fluorescein kinetics with hemodilution. Surgery, *92*:200, 1982.
Ger, R.: Current Problems in Surgery. Chicago, Year Book Medical Publishers, 1972, p. 3.
Ger, R.: Muscle transposition for treatment and prevention of chronic post-traumatic osteomyelitis of the tibia. J. Bone Joint Surg., *59A*:784, 1977.
Gilbert, A., and Teot, L.: The free scapular flap. Plast. Reconstr. Surg., *69*:601, 1982.
Glinz, W., and Clodius, L.: Measurement of tissue pH for predicting viability in pedicle flaps: experimental studies in pigs. Br. J. Plast. Surg., *25*:111, 1972.
Glogovac, S. V., Bitz, D. M., and Whiteside, L. A.: Hydrogen washout technique in monitoring vascular status after replantation surgery. J. Hand Surg., *7*:601, 1982.
Godina, M.: Preferential use of end-to-side arterial anastomoses in free flap transfers. Plast. Reconstr. Surg., *64*:673, 1979.
Godina, M.: Early microsurgical reconstruction of complex trauma of the extremities. Plast. Reconstr. Surg., *78*:285, 1986.
Goshen, J., Wexler, M. R., and Peled, I. J.: The use of two alpha blocking agents, phenoxybenzamine and phentolamine, in ointment and injection form to improve skin flap survival in rats. Ann. Plast. Surg., *15*:431, 1985.
Graham, B. H., Walton, R. L., Elings, V. B., and Lewis, F. R.: Surface quantification of injected fluorescein as a predictor of flap viability. Plast. Reconstr. Surg., *71*:826, 1983.
Granger, D. N., Hollwarth, M. E., and Parks, D. A.: Ischemia-reperfusion injury: role of oxygen-derived free radicals. Acta Physiol. Scand. (Suppl.), *548*:47, 1986.
Griffiths, R. W., Hobby, J. A. E., Humphries, N. L., and Trengove-Jones, G.: The influence of postoperative pharmacological vasodilator agents on the pattern of necrosis in a standardised rat skin flap. Br. J. Plast. Surg., *34*:441, 1981.
Griffiths, R. W., and Humphries, N. L.: Isoxsuprine and the rat abdominal pedicle flap: a controlled study. Br. J. Plast. Surg., *34*:446, 1981.
Grossman, J. A. I., McGonagle, B. A., Dowden, R. V., and Dinner, M. I.: The effect of hyaluronidase and

dimethyl sulfoxide (DMSO) on experimental skin flap survival. Ann. Plast. Surg., *11*:223, 1983.

Guba, A. M., Jr., and Callahan, J.: Nutrient blood flow in delayed axial pattern skin flaps in pigs. Plast. Reconstr. Surg., *64*:372, 1979.

Haeck, P. C., Spira, M., and Divine, G.: Sampling errors in the use of the rat dorsal skin flap: how many rats are enough? Surg. Forum, *35*:572, 1984.

Haertsch, P.: The surgical plane in the leg. Br. J. Plast. Surg., *34*:464, 1981.

Haeseker, B.: Dr. J. F. S. Esser and his influence on the development of plastic and reconstructive surgery. Doctoral thesis. Erasmus Universiteit, Rotterdam, Netherlands, 1983.

Harrison, D. H., Girling, M., Mott, G., and Eng, T.: Methods of assessing the viability of free flap transfer during the postoperative period. Clin. Plast. Surg., *10*:21, 1983.

Hartrampf, C. R., Jr., Scheflan, M., and Black, P. W.: Breast reconstruction with a transverse abdominal island flap. Plast. Reconstr. Surg., *69*:216, 1982.

Hauben, D. J., and Zijlstra, F. J.: Prostacyclin formation in delayed pig flank flaps. Ann. Plast. Surg., *13*:304, 1984.

Hendel, P. M., Lilien, D. L., and Buncke, H. J.: A study of the pharmacologic control of blood flow to acute skin flaps using xenon washout. Part I. Plast. Reconstr. Surg., *71*:387, 1983a.

Hendel, P. M., Lilien, D. L., and Buncke, H. J.: A study of the pharmacologic control of blood flow to delayed skin flaps using xenon washout. Part II. Plast. Reconstr. Surg., *71*:399, 1983b.

Hillelson, R. L., Glowacki, J., Healey, N. A., and Mulliken, J. B.: A microangiographic study of hematoma-associated flap necrosis and salvage with isoxsuprine. Plast. Reconstr. Surg., *66*:528, 1980.

Huang, L., Privalle, C. T., Serafin, D., and Klitzman, B.: Increased survival of skin flaps by scavengers of superoxide radical. FASEB J., *1*:129, 1987.

Im, M. J., and Hoopes, J. E.: Increased superoxide dismutase (SOD) activities in delayed skin flaps. Fed. Proc., *44*:1272, 1985.

Im, M. J., Manson, P. N., Bulkley, G. B., and Hoopes, J. E.: Effects of superoxide dismutase and allopurinol on the survival of acute island skin flaps. Ann. Surg., *201*:357, 1985.

Im, M. J., Su, C-T., Hoopes, J. E., and Anthenelli, R. M.: Skin-flap metabolism in rats: oxygen consumption and lactate production. Plast. Reconstr. Surg., *71*:685, 1983.

Jones, B. M., and Mayou, B. J.: The laser Doppler flowmeter for microvascular monitoring: a preliminary report. Br. J. Plast. Surg., *35*:147, 1982.

Jonsson, C. E., Jurell, G., Nylen, B., and Pandeya, N.: Effect of phentolamine and propranolol on the survival of experimental skin flaps. Scand. J. Plast. Reconstr. Surg., *9*:98, 1975.

Jurell, G., and Fredholm, B. B.: Early changes in ATP and cyclic AMP levels in experimental critical skin flaps. Acta. Physiol. Scand., *113*:33, 1981.

Jurell, G., and Hjemdahl, P.: Degeneration release of noradrenaline in skin flaps in rats. Acta Physiol. Scand., *113*:285, 1981.

Jurell, G., and Jonsson, C. E.: Increased survival of experimental skin flaps in rats following treatment with antiadrenergic drugs. Scand. J. Plast. Reconstr. Surg., *10*:169, 1976.

Jurell, G., and Kaijser, L.: The influence of varying pressure and duration of treatment with hyperbaric oxygen on the survival of skin flaps. Scand. J. Plast. Reconstr. Surg., *7*:25, 1973.

Jurkiewicz, M. J., Bostwick, J., III, Hester, T. R., Bishop, J. B., and Craver, J.: Infected median sternotomy wound. Successful treatment by muscle flap. Ann. Surg., *191*:738, 1985.

Kay, S., and Green, C.: The effect of a novel thromboxane synthetase inhibitor dazmegrel (UK38485) on random pattern skin flaps in the rat. Br. J. Plast. Surg., *39*:361, 1986.

Kennedy, T. J., Pistone, G., and Miller, S. H.: The effect of reserpine on microcirculatory flow in rat flaps. Plast. Reconstr. Surg., *63*:101, 1979.

Kernahan, D. A., and Zingg, W.: The effect of hyperbaric oxygen on the survival of experimental skin flaps. Plast. Reconstr. Surg., *36*:19, 1965.

Kerrigan, C. L.: Skin flap failure: pathophysiology. Plast. Reconstr. Surg., *72*:766, 1983.

Kerrigan, C. L., and Daniel, R. K.: The intercostal flap: an anatomical and hemodynamic approach. Ann. Plast. Surg., *2*:411, 1979.

Kerrigan, C. L., and Daniel, R. K.: Critical ischemia time and the failing skin flap. Plast. Reconstr. Surg., *69*:986, 1982a.

Kerrigan, C. L., and Daniel, R. K.: Pharmacologic treatment of the failing skin flap. Plast. Reconstr. Surg., *70*:541, 1982b.

Kerrigan, C. L., and Daniel, R. K.: The etiology of skin flap failure. *In* Williams, H. B. (Ed.): Transactions of the 8th International Congress of Plastic and Reconstructive Surgery. Montreal, 1983a, pp. 48–50.

Kerrigan, C. L., and Daniel, R. K.: Monitoring acute skin-flap failure. Plast. Reconstr. Surg., *71*:519, 1983b.

Kerrigan, C. L., and Daniel, R. K.: Skin flap research: a candid view. Ann. Plast. Surg., *13*:383, 1984.

Ketchum, L. D., Ellis, S. S., Robinson, D. W., and Masters, F. W.: Vascular augmentation of pedicled tissue by combined histamine iontophoresis and hypertensive perfusion. Plast. Reconstr. Surg. *39*:138, 1967.

Kinkead, L. R., Zook, E. G., and Card, E.: Vasoactive drugs and skin flap survival in the pig. Paper presented at the 26th Annual Plast. Surg. Res. Council Meeting. Springfield, IL, 1981.

Knight, K. R., Crabb, D. J. M., Niall, M., Angus, J. A., Martin, T. J., and O'Brien, B. M.: Pharmacologic modification of blood flow in the rabbit microvasculature with prostacyclin and related drugs. Plast. Reconstr. Surg., *75*:692, 1985.

Koehnlein, H. E., and Lemperle, G.: Experimental studies on the effect of dimethyl sulfoxide on pedicle flaps. Surgery, *67*:672, 1970.

Lang, J.: Über die Textur und die Vascularisation der Fascien. Acta Anat., *48*:61, 1962.

Lidman, D., and Daniel, R. K.: Evaluation of clinical microvascular anastomoses—reasons for failure. Ann. Plast. Surg., *6*:215, 1981.

Limberg, A. A.: Matematicheskie Osnovuy Mestnoy Plastiki Na Poverchnosti Chelovecheskogo Tela. Medgiz, 1946.

Lin, S-D., Lai, C-S., and Chiu, C-C.: Venous drainage in the reverse forearm flap. Plast. Reconstr. Surg., *74*:508, 1984.

Littler, J. W.: Neurovascular skin island transfer in reconstructive hand surgery. Trans. Intl. Soc. Plast. Surg., *2*:175, 1960.

Manson, P. N., Anthenelli, R. M., Im, M. J., Bulkley, G. B., and Hoopes, J. E.: The role of oxygen-free radicals in ischemic tissue injury in island skin flaps. Ann. Surg., *198*:87, 1983.

Marty, F. M., Montandon, D., Gumener, R., and Zbrodowski, A.: The use of subcutaneous tissue flaps in the repair of soft tissue defects of the forearm and hand: an experimental and clinical study of a new technique. Br. J. Plast. Surg., *37*:95, 1984.

Mathes, S. J., Alpert, B. S., and Chang, N.: Use of the muscle flap in chronic osteomyelitis: experimental and clinical correlation. Plast. Reconstr. Surg., *69*:815, 1982.

Mathes, S. J., and Nahai, F.: Clinical Atlas of Muscle and Musculocutaneous Flaps. St. Louis, C. V. Mosby Company, 1979.

Mathes, S. J., and Nahai, F.: Vascular anatomy of muscle: classification and application. *In* Clinical Applications for Muscle and Musculocutaneous Flaps. St. Louis, C. V. Mosby Company, 1982, pp. 16–94.

May, J. W., Jr., Gallico, G. G., III, and Lukash, F. N.: Microvascular transfer of free tissue for closure of bone wounds of the distal lower extremity. N. Engl. J. Med., *306*:253, 1982.

May, J. W., Jr., and Halls, M. J.: Thermocouple probe monitoring for free tissue transfer, replantation, and revascularization procedures. Clin. Plast. Surg., *12*:197, 1985.

May, J. W., Jr., Halls, M. J., and Simon, S. R.: Free microvascular muscle flaps with skin graft reconstruction of extensive defects of the foot: a clinical and gait analysis study. Plast. Reconstr. Surg., *75*:627, 1985.

May, J. W., Jr., and Piliero, C. R.: The surgical delay phenomenon in denervated rabbit abdominal skin. Paper presented at the 24th Annual Meeting, Plastic Surgery Research Council, Dallas, TX, 1979.

McCraw, J. B.: The recent history of myocutaneous flaps. Clin. Plast. Surg., 7:3, 1980.

McCraw, J. B., Myers, B., and Shanklin, K. D.: The value of fluorescein in predicting the viability of arterialized flaps. Plast. Reconstr. Surg., *60*:710, 1977.

McFarlane, R. M., and Wermuth, R. E.: The use of hyperbaric oxygen to prevent necrosis in experimental pedicle flaps and composite skin grafts. Plast. Reconstr. Surg., *37*:422, 1966.

McGregor, I. A., and Jackson, I. T.: The groin flap. Br. J. Plast. Surg., *25*:3, 1972.

McGregor, I. A., and Morgan, C.: Axial and random pattern flaps. Br. J. Plast. Surg., *26*:202, 1973.

Mendelson, B. C., and Woods, J. E.: Effect of corticosteroids on the surviving length of skin flaps in pigs. Br. J. Plast. Surg., *31*:293, 1978.

Mes, L. G. B.: Improving flap survival by sustaining cell metabolism within ischemic cells: a study using rabbits. Plast. Reconstr. Surg., *65*:56, 1980.

Miller, A. P., Falcone, R. E., Nappi, J., and Redmon, H. A.: The lack of effect of nifedipine on failing skin flaps. J. Dermatol. Surg. Oncol., *11*:612, 1985.

Milton, S. H.: Pedicled skin-flaps: the fallacy of the length-width ratio. Br. J. Surg., *57*:502, 1970.

Milton, S. H., and Corbett, J. L.: Failure to increase the survival of experimental flaps by histamine and hypertension. Plast. Reconstr. Surg., *43*:235, 1969.

Monteiro, D. T., Santamore, W. P., and Nemir, P., Jr.: The influence of pentoxifylline on skin-flap survival. Plast. Reconstr. Surg., *77*:277, 1986.

Morain, W. D. (Ed.): Manchot, C.: The Cutaneous Arteries of the Human Body. New York, Springer-Verlag, 1983.

Morain, W. D., Pettit, R. J., Rothkopf, D. M., and Coombs, D. W.: Augmentation of surviving flap area by intraarterial vasodilators administered through implantable pumps. Ann. Plast. Surg., *11*:46, 1983.

Moretti, G.: The blood vessels of the skin. *In* Gans, O., and Steigleder, G. K. (Eds.): Handbuch der Haut und Geschlechtskrankheiten. Vol. 1/1. Berlin, Heidelberg, Springer-Verlag, 1968, pp. 491–623.

Myers, B.: The minimal requirement of circulation for survival of undelayed and delayed flaps in rats. (Discussion). Plast. Reconstr. Surg., *78*:227, 1986.

Myers, M. B., and Cherry, G. Enhancement of survival in devascularized pedicles by the use of phenoxybenzamine. Plast. Reconstr. Surg., *41*:254, 1968.

Myers, B., and Valencia, S.: Augmentation of vascularity—measured with the flash fluorometer—and survival in rat flaps from nitrendipine. 31st Annual Meeting of the Plastic Surgery Research Council, Norfolk, VA, 1986, p. 67.

Nahai, F.: The tensor fascia lata flap. Clin. Plast. Surg., *7*:51, 1980.

Nahai, F.: Discussion: Free microvascular muscle flaps with skin graft reconstruction of extensive defects of the foot: a clinical and gait analysis study. Plast. Reconstr. Surg., *75*:640, 1985.

Nahai, F., Morales, L., Bone, D. K., and Bostwick, J., III: Pectoralis major muscle turnover flaps for closure of the infected sternotomy wound with preservation of form and function. Plast. Reconstr. Surg., *70*:471, 1982.

Nakajima, H., Fujino, T., and Adachi, S.: A new concept of vascular supply to the skin and classification of skin flaps according to their vascularization. Ann. Plast. Surg., *16*:1, 1986.

Nakatsuka, T., Pang, C. Y., Neligan, P., Lindsay, W. K., and Zuker, R. M.: Effect of glucocorticoid treatment on skin capillary blood flow and viability in cutaneous and myocutaneous flaps in the pig. Plast. Reconstr. Surg., *76*:374, 1985.

Nancarrow, J. D.: Augmentation of island flaps by preoperative cell membrane stabilisation: an experimental study in rats. Br. J. Plast. Surg., *34*:212, 1981.

Nathanson, S. E., and Jackson, R. T.: Blood flow measurements in skin flaps. Arch. Otolaryngol., *101*:354, 1975.

Neligan, P., Pang, C. Y., Nakatsuka, T., Lindsay, W. K., and Thomson, H. G.: Pharmacologic action of isoxsuprine in cutaneous and myocutaneous flaps. Plast. Reconstr. Surg., *75*:373, 1985.

Nichter, L. S., Sobieski, M. W., and Edgerton, M. T.: Efficacy of topical nitroglycerin for random-pattern skin-flap salvage. Plast. Reconstr. Surg., *75*:847, 1985.

Nichter, L. S., Sobieski, M. W., and Edgerton, M. T.: Augmentation of critical skin flap survival following ibuprofen therapy. Ann. Plast. Surg., *16*:305, 1986.

Norberg, K.-A., and Palmer, B.: Improvement of blood circulation in experimental skin flaps by phentolamine. Eur. J. Pharmacol., *8*:36, 1969.

Nozaki, M., Hayashi, M., Hirayama, T., and Huang, T. T.: The use of prostaglandin E in both experimental animals and patients to enhance the skin flap survival. Plast. Surg. Forum, *4*:237, 1981.

Orticochea, M.: History of the discovery of the musculocutaneous flap method as a universal and immediate substitute for the method of delay. Br. J. Plast. Surg., *36*:524, 1983.

Östrup, L. T., and Fredrickson, J. M.: Distant transfer of a free living bone graft by microvascular anastomoses. Plast. Reconstr. Surg., *54*:274, 1974.

Owens, N.: A compound neck pedicle designed for the

repair of massive facial defects. Plast. Reconstr. Surg., *15*:369, 1955.

Palmer, B.: Sympathetic denervation and reinnervation of cutaneous blood vessels following surgery. Scand. J. Plast. Reconstr. Surg., *4*:93, 1970.

Palmer, B. The influence of stress on the survival of experimental skin flaps. Scand. J. Plast. Reconstr. Surg., *6*:110, 1972.

Palmer, B., Jurell, G., and Norberg, K.-A.: The blood flow in experimental skin flaps in rats studied by means of the 133 Xenon clearance method. Scand. J. Plast. Reconstr. Surg., *6*:6, 1972.

Pang, C. Y., Forrest, C. R., Neligan, P. C., and Lindsay, W. K.: Augmentation of blood flow in delayed random skin flaps in the pig: effect of length of delay period and angiogenesis. Plast. Reconstr. Surg., *78*:68, 1986a.

Pang, C. Y., Neligan, P. C., Forrest, C. R., Nakatsuka, T., and Sasaki, G. H.: Hemodynamics and vascular sensitivity to circulating norepinephrine in normal skin and delayed and acute random skin flaps in the pig. Plast. Reconstr. Surg., *78*:75, 1986b.

Pang, C. Y., Neligan, P. C., and Nakatsuka, T.: Assessment of microsphere technique for measurement of capillary blood flow in random skin flaps in pigs. Plast. Reconstr. Surg., *74*:513, 1984.

Pang, C. Y., Neligan, P. C., Nakatsuka, T., and Sasaki, G. H.: Pharmacologic manipulation of the microcirculation in cutaneous and myocutaneous flaps in pigs. Clin. Plast. Surg., *12*:173, 1985.

Pang, C. Y., and Sasaki, G. H.: Potential use of prostaglandin synthetase inhibitors in augmentation of skin flap viability. Paper presented at the 26th Annual Plast. Surg. Res. Council Meeting. Springfield, IL, 1981.

Pearl, R. M.: A unifying theory of the delay phenomenon—recovery from the hyperadrenergic state. Ann. Plast. Surg., 7:102, 1981.

Pearl, R. M., and Johnson, D.: The vascular supply to the skin: an anatomical and physiological reappraisal—Part II. Ann. Plast. Surg., *11*:196, 1983.

Perrins, D. J. D.: Hyperbaric oxygenation of ischemic skin flaps and pedicles. 3rd International Conference on Hyperbaric Medicine, Natl. Acad. Sci., Washington, DC, 1966, p. 613.

Perrins, D. J. D.: Hyperbaric Oxygen and Wound Healing. Thesis submitted to Cambridge University for Doctor of Medicine, 1972.

Ponten, B.: The fasciocutaneous flap: its use in soft tissue defects of the lower leg. Br. J. Plast. Surg., *34*:215, 1981.

Prather, A., Blackburn, J. P., Williams, T. R., and Lynn, J. A.: Evaluation of tests for predicting the viability of axial pattern skin flaps in the pig. Plast. Reconstr. Surg., *63*:250, 1979.

Ramasastry, S. S., Waterman, P., Angel, M. F., and Futrell, J. W.: Effect of Fluosol-DA (20%) on skin flap survival in rats. Ann. Plast. Surg., *15*:436, 1985.

Reinisch, J. F.: The pathophysiology of skin flap circulation. The delay phenomenon. Plast. Reconstr. Surg., *54*:585, 1974.

Reus, W. F., Murphy, R. C., Heggers, J. P., Robson, M. C., and McCauley, R. L.: Effect of intraarterial prostacyclin on survival of skin flaps in the pig: biphasic response. Ann. Plast. Surg., *13*:29, 1984.

Robbins, T. H.: Post-mastectomy breast reconstruction using a rectus abdominis musculocutaneous island flap. Br. J. Plast. Surg., *34*:286, 1981.

Rohrich, R. J., Cherry, G. W., and Spira, M.: Enhancement of skin-flap survival using nitroglycerin ointment. Plast. Reconstr. Surg., *73*:943, 1984.

Ruberg, R. L., and Falcone, R. E.: Effect of protein depletion on the surviving length in experimental skin flaps. Plast. Reconstr. Surg., *61*:581, 1978.

Salmon, M.: Arteres de la Peau. Paris, Masson et Cie., 1936.

Sasaki, A., and Harii, K.: Lack of effect of isoxsuprine on experimental random flaps in the rat. Plast. Reconstr. Surg., *66*:105, 1980.

Sasaki, G. H., and Pang, C. Y.: Hemodynamics and viability of acute neurovascular island skin flaps in rats. Plast. Reconstr. Surg., *65*:152, 1980.

Sasaki, G. H., and Pang, C. Y.: Experimental evidence for involvement of prostaglandins in viability of acute skin flaps: effects on viability and mode of action. Plast. Reconstr. Surg., *67*:335, 1981.

Schäfer, K.: Das subcutane Gefäbetasystem (untere Extremität): Mikropräparatorische Untersuchungen. Gegenbaurs Morphol. Jahrb., *121*:492, 1975.

Serafin, D., Lesesne, C. B., Mullen, R. Y., and Georgiade, N. G.: Transcutaneous pO_2 monitoring for assessing viability and predicting survival of skin flaps: experimental and clinical correlations. J. Microsurg., *2*:165, 1981.

Serafin, D., Shearing, C., and Georgiade, N. G.: The vascularization of free flaps. Plast. Reconstr. Surg., *60*:233, 1977.

Silverman, D. G., LaRossa, D. D., Barlow, C. H., Bering, T. G., Popky, L. M., and Smith, T. C.: Quantification of tissue fluorescein delivery and prediction of flap viability with the fiberoptic dermofluorometer. Plast. Reconstr. Surg., *66*:545, 1980.

Smith, A. R., Sonneveld, G. J., Kort, W. J., and van der Meulen, J. C.: Clinical application of transcutaneous oxygen measurements in replantation surgery and free tissue transfer. J. Hand. Surg., *8*:139, 1983.

Smith, G., Kraemer, B., Young, L., Wray, R. C., and Weeks, P. M.: Pharmacologic enhancement of skin island flap survival. Surg. Forum, *31*:562, 1980.

Snyder, C. C., Bateman, J. M., Davis, C. W., and Warden, G. D.: Mandibulo-facial restoration with live osteocutaneous flaps. Plast. Reconstr. Surg., *45*:14, 1970.

Song, Y. G., Chen, G. Z., and Song, Y. L.: The free thigh flap: a new free flap concept based on the septocutaneous artery. Br. J. Plast. Surg., *37*:149, 1984.

Spalteholz, W.: Die Vertheilung der Blutgefässe in der Haut. Arch. Anat. Entwcklngsgesch., *1*:1, 1893.

Stock, W., Muhlbauer, W., and Biemer, E.: Der neurovaskulare Unterarm-Insel-Lappon. Z. Plast. Chir., *5*:158, 1981.

Suzuki, S., Isshiki, N., Ogawa, Y., Ohtsuka, M., Nose, K., and Nishimura, R.: Measurement of cutaneous blood flow by clearance of hydrogen gas generated by electrolysis. Ann. Plast. Surg., *15*:183, 1985.

Svensson, H., Svedman, P., Holmberg, J., and Wieslander, J. B.: Detecting changes of arterial and venous blood flow in flaps. Ann. Plast. Surg., *15*:35, 1985.

Swartz, W. M., Banis, J. B., Newton, E. D., Ramasastry, S. S., Jones, N. F., and Acland, R.: The osteocutaneous scapular flap for mandibular and maxillary reconstruction. Plast. Reconstr. Surg., *77*:530, 1986.

Takayanagi, S., and Ogawa, Y.: Effects of pentoxifylline on flap survival. Plast. Reconstr. Surg., *65*:763, 1980.

Tan, C. M., Im, M. J., Myers, R. A. M., and Hoopes, J. E.: Effects of hyperbaric oxygen and hyperbaric air on the survival of island skin flaps. Plast. Reconstr. Surg., *73*:27, 1984.

Taylor, G. I.: Reconstruction of the mandible with free composite iliac bone grafts. Ann. Plast. Surg., *9*:361, 1982.

Taylor, G. I., Miller, G. D. H., and Ham, F. J.: The free vascularized bone graft: a clinical extension of microvascular techniques. Plast. Reconstr. Surg., *55*:533, 1975.

Taylor, G. I., and Palmer, J. H.: The vascular territories (angiosomes) of the body: experimental study and clinical applications. Br. J. Plast. Surg., *40*:113, 1987.

Thomson, J. G., and Kerrigan, C. L.: Fasciocutaneous flaps: an experimental model in the pig. Plast. Reconstr. Surg. (accepted for publication, 1987).

Thomson, J. G.: Surgical Flaps: A New Model and Assessment of Anesthetic and Monitoring Technique. M. Sc. Thesis. McGill University, Montreal, 1988.

Timmons, M. J.: The vascular basis of the radial forearm flap. Plast. Reconstr. Surg., *77*:80, 1986.

Tolhurst, D. E., Haeseker, B., and Zeeman, R. J.: The development of the fasciocutaneous flap and its clinical applications. Plast. Reconstr. Surg., *71*:597, 1983.

Toomey, J. M., Conoyer, J. M., and Ogura, J. H.: Vasodilating agents in augmentation of skin flap survival. Otolaryngol. Head Neck Surg., *87*:757, 1979.

Vasconez, L. O., Bostwick, J., III, and McCraw, J.: Coverage of exposed bone by muscle transposition and skin grafting. Plast. Reconstr. Surg., *53*:526, 1974.

Walton, R. L., Matory, W. E., Jr., and Petry, J. J.: The posterior calf fascial free flap. Plast. Reconstr. Surg., *76*:914, 1985.

Waters, L. W., Pearl, R. M., MacAulay, R., and Arnstein, D.: Pharmacologic augmentation of skin flap survival. Plast. Surg. Forum, *9*:267, 1986.

Webster, J. P.: Thoraco-epigastric tubed pedicles. Surg. Clin. North Am., *17*:145, 1937.

Weiland, A. J., Phillips, T. W., and Randolph, M. A.: Bone grafts: a radiologic, histologic, and biomechanical model comparing autografts, allografts, and free vascularized bone grafts. Plast. Reconstr. Surg., *74*:368, 1984.

Wexler, M. R., Kalisman, M., Yeschua, R., and Neuman, Z.: The effect of phenoxybenzamine, phentolamine and 6-hydroxydopamine on skin flap survival in rats. J. Surg. Res., *19*:83, 1975.

Wray, R. C., Jr., and Young, V. L.: Drug treatment and flap survival. Plast. Reconstr. Surg., *73*:939, 1984.

Yang, G., Chen, B., Gao, Y., Liu, X., Li, J., et al.: Forearm free skin flap transplantation. Natl. Med. J. China, *61*:139, 1981.

Young, C. M. A., and Hopewell, J. W.: The isotope clearance technique for measuring skin blood flow. Br. J. Plast. Surg., *36*:222, 1983.

Zachary, L. S., Heggers, J. P., Robson, M. C., and Murphy, R.: Combined prostacyclin and thromboxane synthetase inhibitor UK 38485 in flap survival. Ann. Plast. Surg., *17*:112, 1986.

Zimany, A.: The bi-lobed flap. Plast. Reconstr. Surg., *11*:423, 1953.

Zimmerman, T. J., Sasaki, G. H., and Khattab, S.: Improved ischemic island skin flap survival with continuous intra-arterial infusion of adenosine triphosphate–magnesium chloride and superoxide dismutase: a rat model. Ann. Plast. Surg., *18*:218, 1987.

10

G. Ian Taylor
John H. Palmer
Douglas McManamny

The Vascular Territories of the Body (Angiosomes) and Their Clinical Applications

In recent years there has been an intensive reappraisal of the anatomy of the vasculature of the skin and deeper tissues. This anatomic revolution has been catalyzed by the evolution of the microvascular free flap, the revival of the musculocutaneous flap, and the introduction of the fasciocutaneous flap. There has been an explosion of newly described flaps together with new nomenclature, new classifications of flaps, and attempts to define the vessels on which they are based. It was previously stated (Converse, 1977) that "there is no simple and all-encompassing system which is suitable for classifying skin flaps. It is now generally agreed that the anatomical vascular basis of the flap provides the most accurate approach for classification." The veracity of this statement has been borne out with the passage of time.

HISTORICAL BACKGROUND

Plastic surgery evolved as a specialty in Europe and North America to restore the mutilated victims of the two World Wars. With artistic flair and geometric precision, tissues were advanced and rotated. They were transposed locally and dispatched to distant sites on limb carriers, only to be rebuffed on occasion by necrosis. Gillies often lamented that "plastic surgery is a constant battle between blood supply and beauty" (Gillies and Millard, 1957). Gradually, rigid length-breadth flap ratios were calculated for different regions of the body, because most of the flaps were designed without a precise knowledge of the vessels on which they were based.

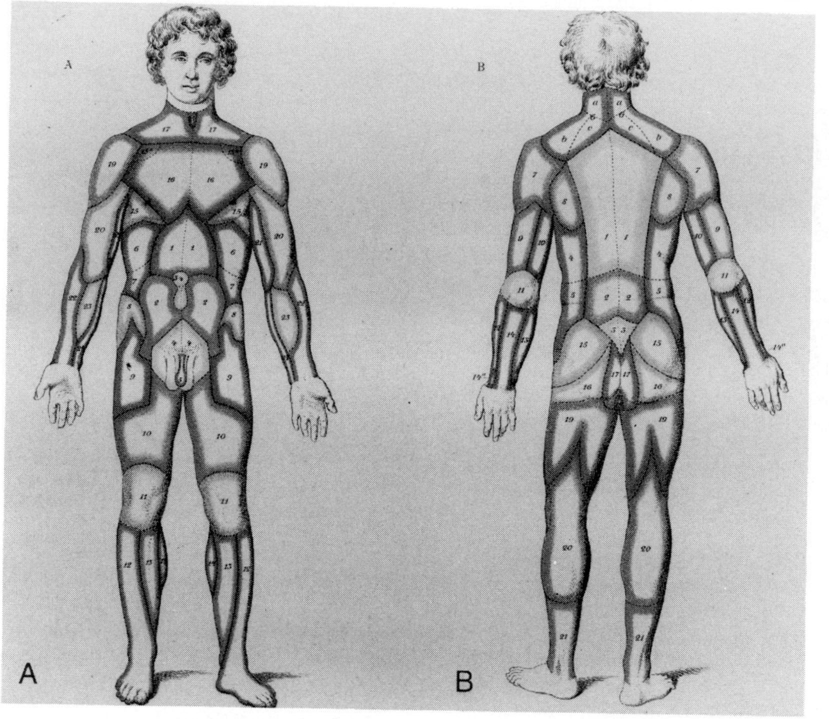

Figure 10–1 *See legend on opposite page*

This anatomic information was available but hidden in texts in foreign languages. In 1889 Manchot performed the first examination of the cutaneous vascular territories. His treatise, *Die Hautarterien des Menschlichen Körpers, The Skin Arteries of the Body,* was published in German and has finally been made available in English (1983). Manchot identified the cutaneous perforators, assigned them to their underlying source vessels, and charted the cutaneous vascular territories of the body (Fig. 10–1). He did not have the advantage of radiography since Roentgen was not to make his discovery until several years later; nevertheless the accuracy of Manchot's work has mostly stood the test of time.

In 1893 Spalteholz published an important paper on the origin, course, and distribution of the cutaneous perforators, studied in different regions of adult and neonatal cadavers. He injected into the arteries gelatin to which were added various pigments. The soft tissues were fixed in alcohol and subtracted in xylol, and the resulting vascular network was embedded in Canada balsam. Spalteholz's main study concentrated on the detailed circulation of the skin. He made an important distinction between *direct* cutaneous vessels, whose main purpose was to supply the skin, and *indirect* cutaneous vessels, which were terminal branches of vessels supplying the deeper organs, especially the muscles. A detailed account of this work was published by Timmons (1985) in a review of the landmarks in the anatomic study of the skin's blood supply.

The next major study was performed by Salmon, a French anatomist and surgeon in the 1930's (1936a,b). Manchot had defined approximately 40 cutaneous territories that excluded the head, neck, hands, and feet. Salmon knew of Manchot's studies and set out to reappraise his work. Aided by radiography, he was able to delineate the smaller radicles of the cutaneous circulation, and charted over 80 territories encompassing the entire body (Fig. 10–2). Salmon noted the interconnections that exist between perforators, and his observation of the density and size of the vessels in different regions of the body led him to define what he called the hypervascular and hypovascular zones. His

Figure 10–1. Overview of the cutaneous arterial territories as defined by Carl Manchot, 1889.

Illustration A:

1. Cutaneous territory of the superficial superior epigastric artery.
2. Cutaneous territory of the superficial inferior epigastric artery.
3. Cutaneous territory of the superior and inferior epigastric arteries.
4. Cutaneous territory of the external pudendal arteries.
5. Cutaneous territory of the dorsal penile arteries.
6. Cutaneous territory of the perforating branches from the intercostal arteries.
7. Cutaneous territory of the perforating branches from the lumbar arteries.
8. Cutaneous territory of the superficial circumflex iliac artery.
9. Cutaneous territory of the profunda femoris artery (circumflex femoral arteries).
10. Cutaneous territory of the femoral artery.
11. Cutaneous territory of the superficial genicular rete.
12. Cutaneous territory of the anterior tibial artery.
13. Cutaneous territory of the posterior tibial artery.
14. Cutaneous territory of the popliteal artery (sural arteries)
15. Cutaneous territory of the thoracic arteries.

15a. Cutaneous territory of the thoracoacromial artery.

16. Cutaneous territory of the perforating branches of the internal mammary artery.
17. Cutaneous territory of the thyrocervical trunk.
18. Cutaneous territory of the superior thyroid artery.
19. Cutaneous territory of the subcutaneous anterior deltoid artery.
20. Cutaneous territory of the brachial artery.
21. Cutaneous territory of the superior ulnar collateral artery.
22. Cutaneous territory of the radial artery.
23. Cutaneous territory of the median artery.
24. Cutaneous territory of the ulnar artery.

Illustration B:

1. Cutaneous territory of the dorsal branches from the intercostal arteries.
2. Cutaneous territory of the dorsal branches of the lumbar arteries.
3. Cutaneous territory of the dorsal branches from the sacral arteries.
4. Cutaneous territory of the posterior perforating branches of the intercostal arteries.
5. Cutaneous territory of the posterior perforating branches of the lumbar arteries.
6. Cutaneous territory of the thyrocervical trunk.
   a. Of the superficial artery.
   b. Of the transverse sacpular artery.
   c. Of the transverse cervical artery.
7. Cutaneous territory of the subcutaneous posterior deltoid artery.
8. Cutaneous territory of the superficial circumflex scapular artery.
9. Cutaneous territory of the inferior radial collateral artery.
10. Cutaneous territory of the superior ulnar collateral artery.
11. Cutaneous territory of the cubital rete.
12. Cutaneous territory of the radial artery.
13. Cutaneous territory of the ulnar artery.
14. Cutaneous territory of the external and internal interosseous artery.
15. Cutaneous territory of the superior gluteal artery.
16. Cutaneous territory of the inferior gluteal artery.
17. Cutaneous territory of the internal pudendal artery.
18. Cutaneous territory of the obturator artery.
19. Cutaneous territory of the perforating branches of the profunda femoris artery.
20. Cutaneous territory of the popliteal artery.
21. Cutaneous territory of the anterior and posterior tibial artery.

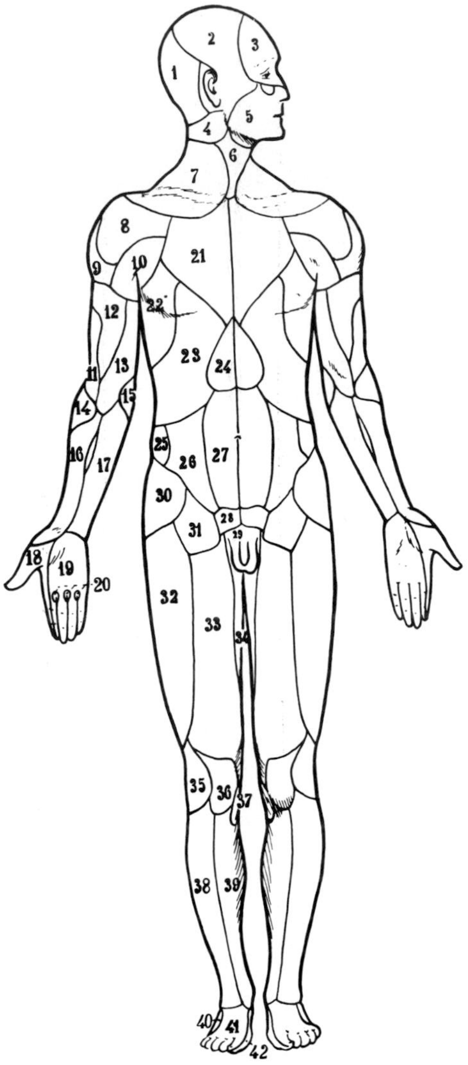

Figure 10–2. The cutaneous territories as defined by Salmon, 1936.

Left, Summary of the cutaneous arterial territories of the ventral surface of the body.

1. Occipital artery.
2. Superficial temporal artery.
3. Ophthalmic artery.
4. Sternocleidomastoid artery.
5. Facial artery.
6. Thyroid arteries.
7. Transverse cervical and suprascapular arteries.
8. Deltoid branch of the acromiothoracic trunk.
9. Circumflex humeral arteries.
10. Small thoracic branches of the acromiothoracic trunk.
11. Profunda brachii artery.
12. Brachial artery (muscular branches).
13. Brachial artery (direct branches).
14. Epicondylar arteries.
15. Epitrochlear arteries.
16. Radial artery.
17. Ulnar artery.
18. Deep palmar arch.
19. Superficial palmar arch.
20. Anterior interosseous artery.
21. Internal mammary artery.
22. External mammary (lateral thoracic) and subscapular arteries.
23. Intercostal arteries.
24. Superficial superior epigastric artery.
25. Lumbar arteries.
26. Inferior superficial epigastric artery.
27. Deep epigastric artery.
28. External superior pudendal artery.
29. External inferior pudendal artery.
30. Superficial circumflex iliac artery.
31. Femoral artery.
32. Artery to the vastus lateralis muscle.
33. Superficial femoral artery.
34. Artery to the adductor muscles.
35. Lateral articular branches.
36. Medial articular branches.
37. Genus descendens artery.
38. Anterior tibial artery.
39. Posterior tibial artery.
40. Peroneal artery.
41. Dorsalis pedis artery.
42. Medial plantar artery.

work has become available in English (Taylor and Tempest, 1988).

In 1975 another important study, published in German by Schäfer, focused on the lower extremity. The venous plexus was investigated as well as the arterial network. Scribtol and an ink-serum mixture were injected into the lower limbs of adults and into the entire circulation of fetal and neonatal cadavers. Schäfer concluded that most cutaneous arteries emerged in rows from the intermuscular septa or occasionally from the intramuscular septa. In addition, he highlighted the two systems of perforating veins: the *venae communicantes,* large veins that pierce the deep fascia and connect the superficial venous plexus to the deep venous system, and the *venae comitantes,* small, usually paired veins that accompany the cutaneous arterial perforators.

Early in this century advances on the clinical front gave significance to the work of these great anatomists. In 1906, Tansini reported a latissimus dorsi flap supplied by the thoracodorsal artery. In 1919 Davis published *Plastic Surgery* and introduced many of the chapters with illustrations from Manchot's book. In 1921 Blair described a forehead flap based on the superficial temporal vessels and in 1929 Esser published *Artery Flaps*. In 1937

Figure 10–2. *Continued*

Right, Summary of the cutaneous arterial territories of the dorsal surface of the body.

1. Superficial temporal artery.
2. Occipital artery.
3. Posterior auricular artery.
4. Deep cervical artery.
5. Sternocleidomastoid arteries.
6. Deep branch of the transverse cervical artery.
7. Suprascapular artery.
8. Dorsospinal branch of the intercostal artery.
9. Subscapular artery.
10. Posterior circumflex humeral artery.
11. Brachial artery (medial collateral branches).
12. Profunda brachii artery.
13. Posterior recurrent ulnar artery.
14. Radial recurrent ulnar artery.
15. Ulnar artery.
16. Posterior interosseous artery.
17. Anterior interosseous artery.
18. Dorsal branch of the ulnar artery.
19. Dorsal carpal artery.
20. Posterior interosseous arteries.
21. Deep palmar arch.
22. Digital arteries.
23. Intercostal arteries (perforating branches).
24. Lumbar arteries (dorsospinal branches).
25. Lumbar arteries (perforating branches).
26. Superficial circumflex iliac artery.
27. Superior gluteal artery.
28. Internal pudendal artery.
29. Inferior gluteal artery.
30. Artery to the adductor muscles.
31. Artery accompanying the sciatic nerve.
32. and 33. Perforating arteries.
34. Popliteal artery.
35. Gastrocnemius arteries.
36. Small saphenous artery.
37. Posterior tibial artery.
38. Peroneal artery.
39. Dorsalis pedis artery.
40. Lateral plantar artery.

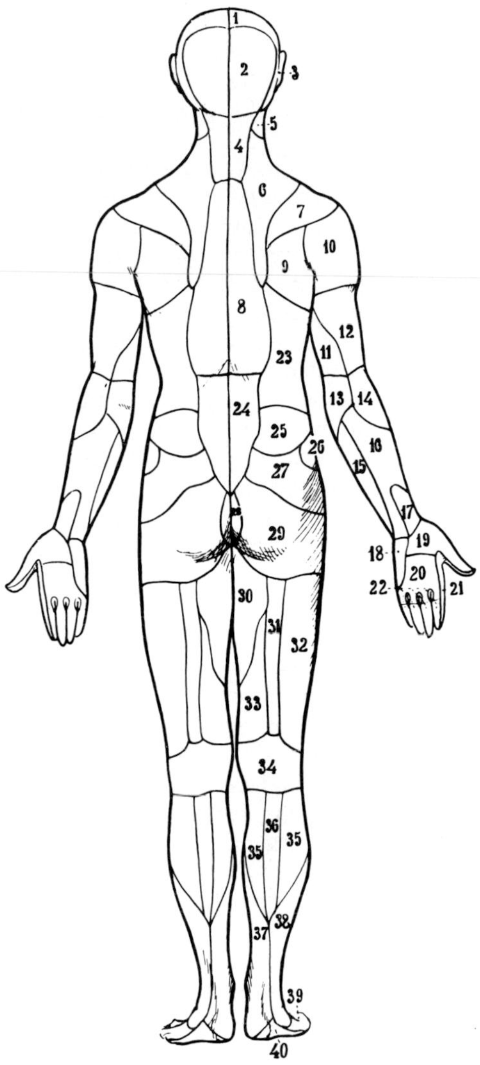

Webster again cited the work of Manchot when he described a long, bipedicled thoracoepigastric flap based on named arteries that extended from the groin to the axilla. Shaw and Payne (1946) utilized the clinical information available in wartime to provide one-stage direct flaps for hand reconstruction. In 1965 Bakamjian drew attention to the long paramedian perforators of the internal thoracic system.

The 1970's witnessed the beginning of the "anatomic revolution." McGregor and Morgan (1973) differentiated between large flaps based on a known axial blood supply and those based on random vessels in the area. Daniel and Williams (1973) reappraised the work of Manchot and others, and classified the cutaneous arteries into direct cutaneous and musculocutaneous vessels.

Studies on the free flap by Taylor and Daniel and Daniel and Taylor were published in 1973 and in the same year the musculocutaneous flap was revived by McCraw (McCraw and Dibbell, 1977; McCraw, Dibbell, and Carraway, 1977; McCraw, 1980). Both procedures demanded a precise knowledge of the cutaneous vasculature. In the search for new donor sites for tissue transfer, surgeons returned to the dissection room. Many new and exciting techniques were developed. However, there was a tendency for the techniques to neglect the esthetic side of plastic surgery. The results could sometimes be what McDowell (1979) described as "globs and blobs."

To escape from the hamburger of muscle and skin, surgeons soon rediscovered that blood vessels follow fascial planes. In the 1980's a new model emerged—the fasciocutaneous flap (Pontén, 1981). With this development there has been an explosion of new terms and new classifications of the cutaneous circulation. The thesaurus of flaps now includes a bewildering array of terms such as axial, random, direct cutaneous, musculocutaneous, fasciocutaneous, supercutaneous, and septocutaneous. Indeed, there has been an attempt to classify flaps into no less than ten types and subtypes based on the origin of the cutaneous perforators (Nakajima, Fujino, and Adachi, 1986).

In many ways these terms are simply different expressions of the basic cutaneous architecture that Manchot and Salmon wrote about 100 and 50 years ago, respectively. A reappraisal of their work is timely, especially in view of the modern concepts of flap surgery. The reawakened interest in cutaneous anatomy has encouraged workers to explore new methods of investigating the circulation both in vivo and in vitro. The use of fluorescein by McGregor and Morgan (1973) and prostaglandin E by Nakajima, Maruyama, and Koda (1981) has increased an understanding of the manner in which individual vascular territories relate dynamically to the neighboring territories when their anastomoses are intact.

It would be difficult to improve on the radiographs produced by Salmon using lead oxide, but attempts at simplifying his mixture have produced satisfactory results (Rees and Taylor, 1986; Crosthwaite, Taylor, and Palmer, 1987). Improved radiographic film has assisted the imaging of small blood vessels.

The relationship of vessel size to vascular territory has been correlated by Cormack and Lamberty (1986b) using digitizing tablets linked to a microcomputer. These workers also discussed in detail the axiality of vessels in the fasciocutaneous system. Cormack and Lamberty (1986a) published a book, *The Arterial Anatomy of Skin Flaps,* which contains a concise appraisal of the history, anatomy, and clinical aspects of skin flap surgery.

In our department the authors have performed over 2000 fresh cadaver studies, investigating various regions, tissues, and combinations of tissues. More recently this has extended to an investigation of the entire integument and underlying deep structures in a series of total body studies (Taylor and Palmer, 1987).

The results of this work, considered in conjunction with that of other workers, especially Manchot and Salmon, provide the basis for the remainder of this chapter.

BASIC RESEARCH

A brief account of the authors' work is essential in order to understand how we defined the vascular territories of the body, how we arrived at the angiosome concept, and how we explain where our studies overlap or vary from those of previous workers. An *angiosome* (from the Greek *angeion,* meaning vessel, and somite, meaning segment or sector of the body, derived from *soma,* body) is defined as a composite block of tissue supplied by a named source artery. The source arteries (segmental or distributing arteries) that supply these blocks of tissue are responsible for the supply of the skin and the underlying deep structures. When pieced together like a jigsaw puzzle, they constitute the three-dimensional vascular territories of the body.

The investigations were conducted in fresh cadavers. They involved dissection, ink injection, and radiographic studies using either barium sulfate or a mixture containing lead oxide. In each case the anatomic studies were problem oriented and designed to provide a surgical solution to the patient's needs.

The investigations initially involved an analysis of various regions of the body to define possible donor sites for free skin flap transfer (Taylor and Daniel, 1975). The studies subsequently focused on other tissues and included the anatomic basis for the transfer of bone (Taylor, Miller, and Ham, 1975), nerve (Taylor and Ham, 1976), and certain muscles (Taylor, Corlett, and Boyd, 1983, 1984). Encouraged by the success of some of the resulting clinical procedures, the authors expanded the research to investigate *composite* units of tissue, supplied by a single vascular system. Units of skin and tendon (Taylor and Townsend, 1979), muscle with nerve (Taylor, 1978), and skin, muscle, and bone (Taylor and Watson, 1978; Taylor, Townsend, and Corlett, 1979a,b) were analyzed. *It was from this work that the angiosome concept germinated.* Various regions including the anterior abdominal wall (Taylor and Corlett, 1981; Boyd, Taylor, and Corlett, 1984; Taylor, Corlett, and Boyd, 1984), the anterior thorax (Reid and Taylor, 1984; Palmer and Taylor, 1986), the lower limb, and the upper limb were then studied. The results added strength to the angiosome concept of the blood supply and revealed the interconnections that exist at all levels between adjacent vascular territories, a relationship that is evident throughout the body (Taylor, 1983).

Since commencing the total body studies we have performed dissection and radiographic analysis of eight whole bodies plus two amputated upper limbs and four amputated lower limbs. The injected substance (modified from Salmon's original mixture) contained lead oxide, gelatin, and a preservative (Crosthwaite, Taylor, and Palmer, 1987).

The integument (skin and subcutaneous tissue) was removed and the sites of emergence of the dominant cutaneous perforators (0.5 mm or greater) were identified on the surface of the deep fascia with lead beads. The integument was removed in each subject to provide as wide an expanse of tissue for study as possible. The subjects were chosen and the incisions were planned to provide a comparison between sexes and to obtain anterior, posterior, lateral, "bird's eye," and "worm's eye" views of the cutaneous vasculature. Previous workers, including Salmon, had made topographic boundary incisions to remove areas of skin, particularly in the lines of the groins, axillae, neck, and limb joints. These junctional regions are of great clinical importance and for this reason the incisions were designed to retain their continuity wherever possible.

The integument was radiographed and a montage of the entire cutaneous circulation was constructed in "plan view" (Figs. 10–3, 10–4). Although Manchot and Salmon described the origin and course of the cutaneous arteries, and Salmon (1936b) made a separate study of the individual muscles, neither worker illustrated the course of the arteries between the deep tissues and the skin. Therefore, the skin and subcutaneous tissues were cut into parallel strips and placed on their side and radiographs were taken to provide "elevation views" of the vessels in different regions of the body (Fig. 10–5).

The deep tissues were also radiographed (Fig. 10–6) and the cutaneous perforators were traced to their underlying source arteries and color coded. The results were averaged from each study and plotted on a diagram of the body (Fig. 10–9). Finally, in one subject the integument was not removed; instead, cross sections of the limbs and the torso were made at 5 cm intervals to retain in continuity the vessels between the deep tissues and the skin (Fig. 10–7).

In this way a three-dimensional picture of the arterial framework of the body was constructed. The precise origin, course, and distribution of the vessels supplying the deep tissues and the skin were identified. With this information the vascular territory of each named source artery (distributing or segmental artery) was plotted in the deep tissues and in the integument, and compared (Fig. 10–8). The results were averaged and correlated with a series of regional ink injections studies in another 50 fresh cadavers. This study provided a definitive picture of the angiosomes of the body (Fig. 10–10), drawn with the underlying muscles and depicting their vascular territories as well as those of the overlying skin.

ANATOMIC CONCEPTS

The following concepts provide an overview of the blood supply to the integument and to the deep tissues. They are fundamental to the mapping of the vascular territories and to the planning of incisions and flaps. They help to explain the anatomic variations that exist between the vessels of different regions of the body, and allow for a better understanding of the various classifications of the cutaneous blood supply that have appeared in the literature. Finally, they provide the basis for interpreting many physiologic and pathologic processes, including the delay phenomenon and the necrosis line of flaps.

Vessels Follow the Connective Tissue Framework of the Body

This concept is fundamental to the design of flaps in general and to fasciocutaneous and septocutaneous flaps in particular. The connective tissue framework of the body is a continuous syncytium, like the walls of a

Text continued on page 344

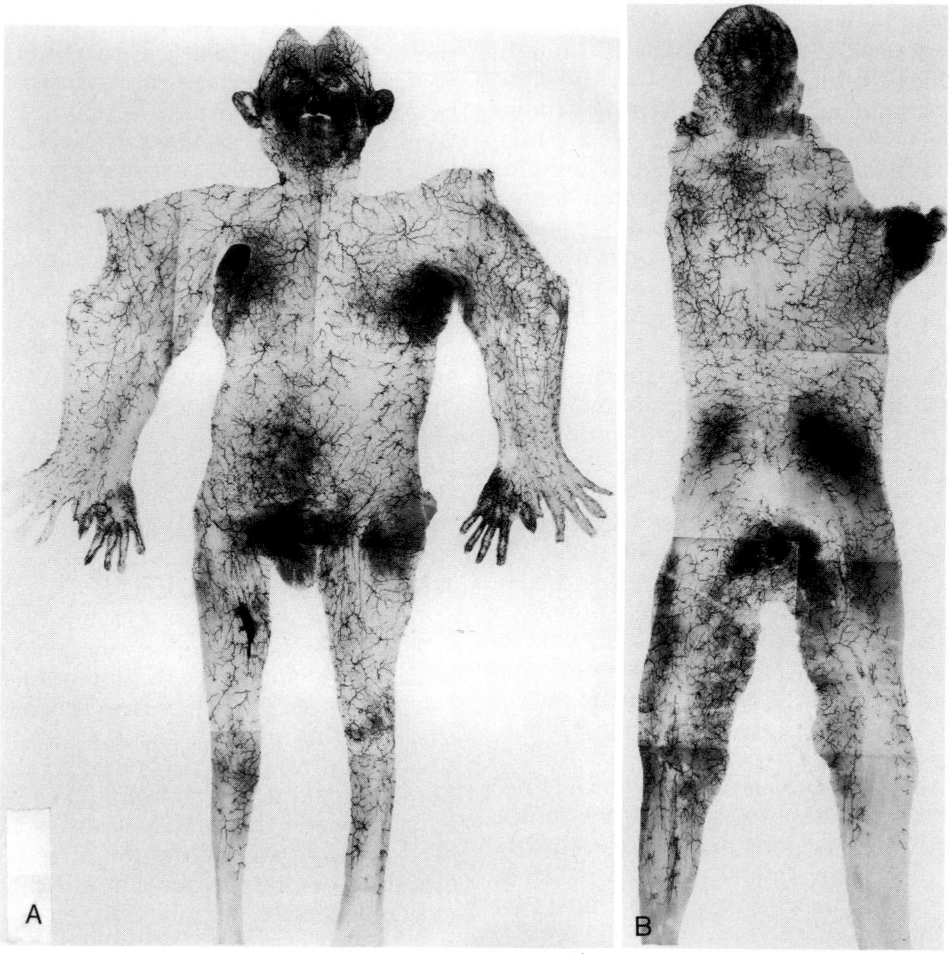

Figure 10–3. One of the montages of the cutaneous circulation demonstrating the continuous network of arteries and arterioles, and their origin, size, orientation, and density in different regions of the body. Several pressure areas on the back did not perfuse in this subject. Note the large perforators in the head, neck, torso, and proximal limbs compared with the small, closely packed perforators in the forearms and legs. Note also the long axial vessels radiating from the groins and popliteal fossae. (From Br. J. Plast. Surg.)

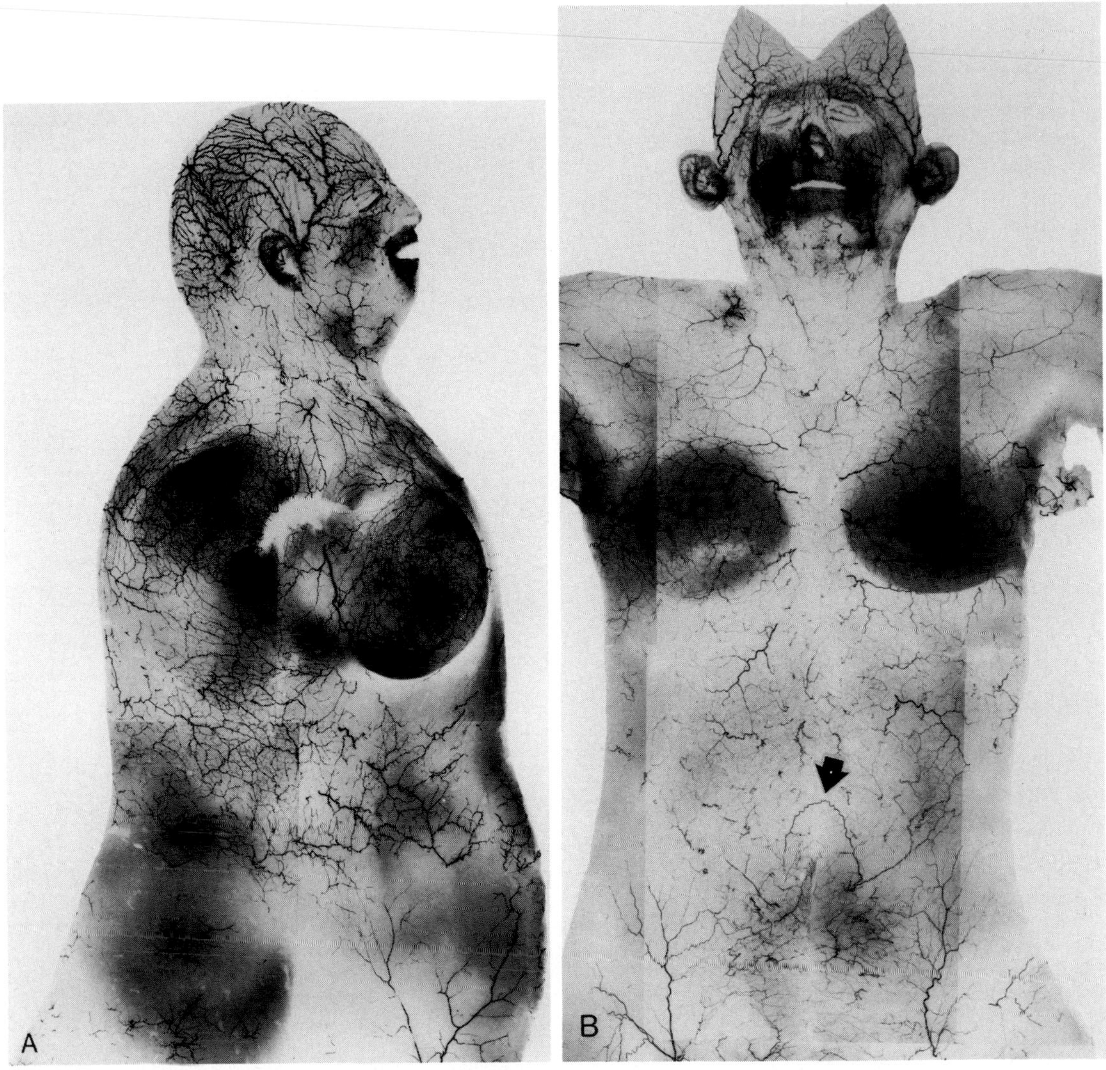

Figure 10–4. Lateral view of one female subject *(A)* and anterior view of another *(B)*. The arm has been removed in *A*. Note the network of large vessels that sweep laterally from the ventral and dorsal midlines, ascend from the groins, descend from the shoulder girdle, and converge on the summits of the scalp and the breasts. This demonstrates the principle that vessels radiate from fixed concave zones and radiate to mobile convex areas. A lower midline scar interrupts the vessels in *B* with compensatory opening of a large choke vessel above the umbilicus *(arrow)* to reestablish the flow across the midline. (From Br. J. Plast. Surg.)

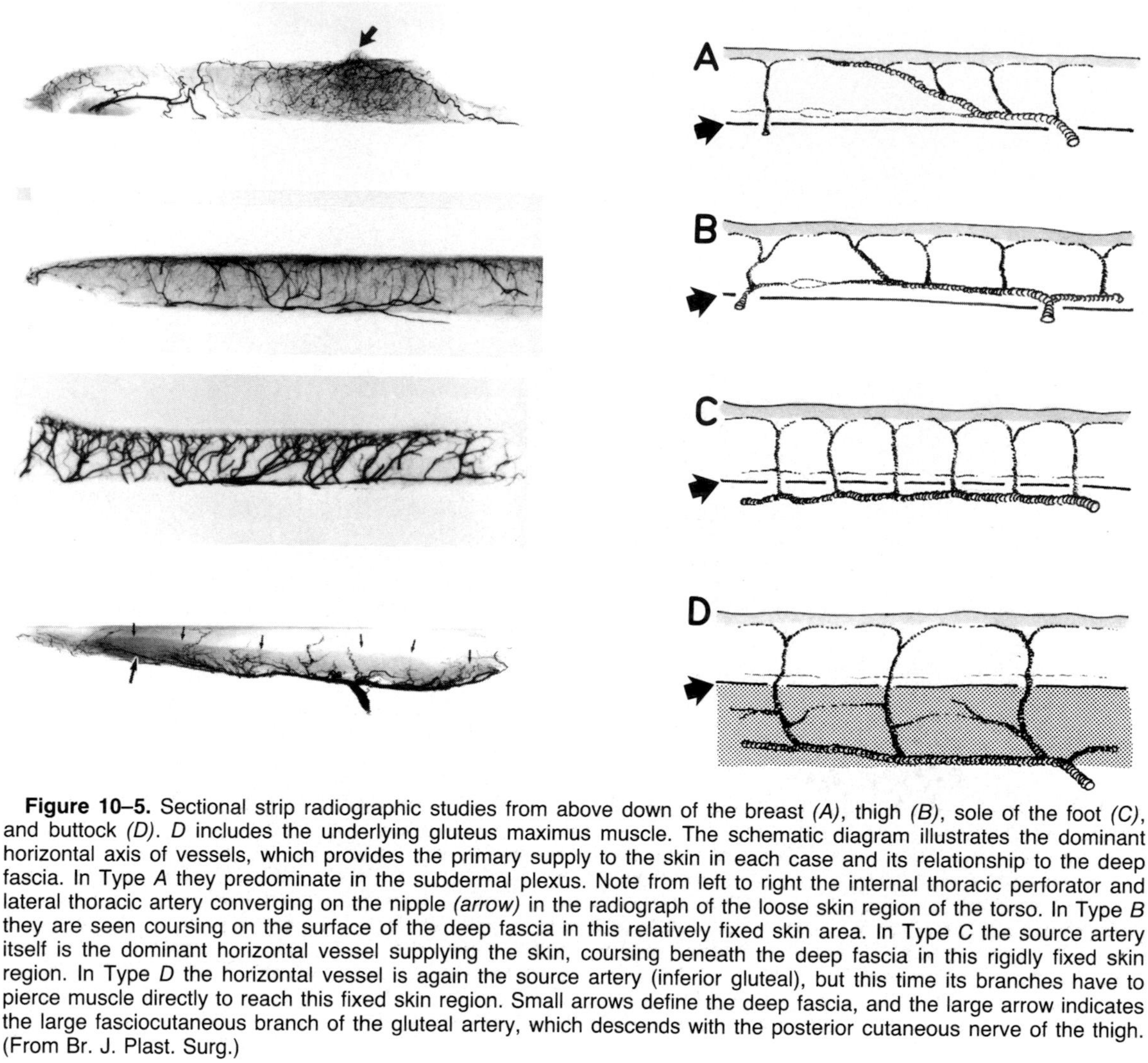

Figure 10–5. Sectional strip radiographic studies from above down of the breast *(A)*, thigh *(B)*, sole of the foot *(C)*, and buttock *(D)*. *D* includes the underlying gluteus maximus muscle. The schematic diagram illustrates the dominant horizontal axis of vessels, which provides the primary supply to the skin in each case and its relationship to the deep fascia. In Type *A* they predominate in the subdermal plexus. Note from left to right the internal thoracic perforator and lateral thoracic artery converging on the nipple *(arrow)* in the radiograph of the loose skin region of the torso. In Type *B* they are seen coursing on the surface of the deep fascia in this relatively fixed skin area. In Type *C* the source artery itself is the dominant horizontal vessel supplying the skin, coursing beneath the deep fascia in this rigidly fixed skin region. In Type *D* the horizontal vessel is again the source artery (inferior gluteal), but this time its branches have to pierce muscle directly to reach this fixed skin region. Small arrows define the deep fascia, and the large arrow indicates the large fasciocutaneous branch of the gluteal artery, which descends with the posterior cutaneous nerve of the thigh. (From Br. J. Plast. Surg.)

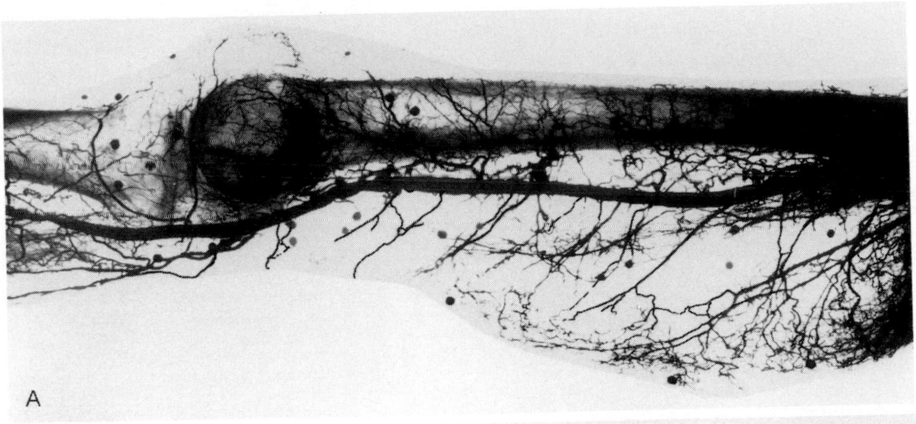

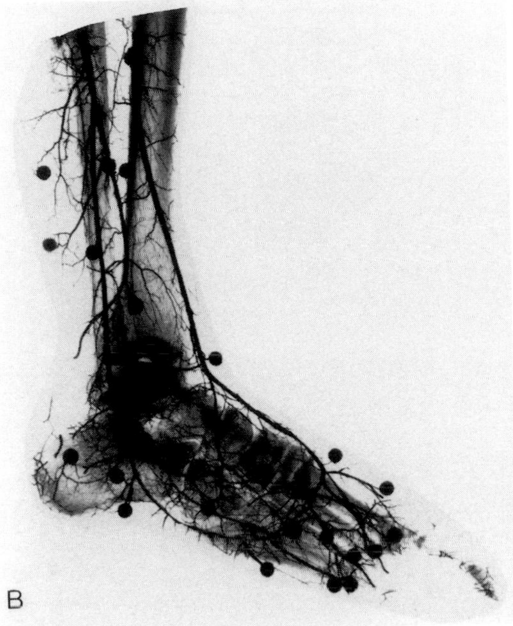

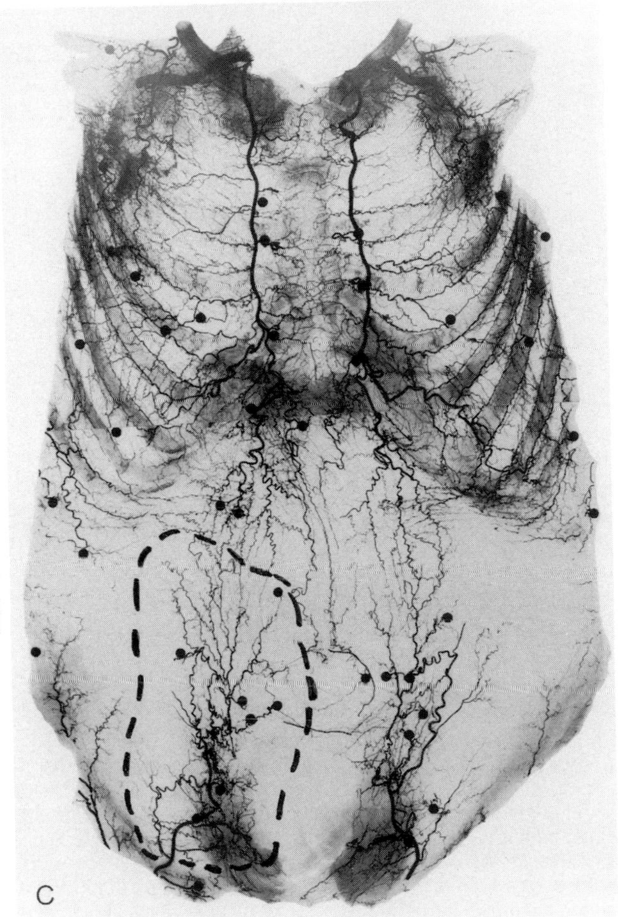

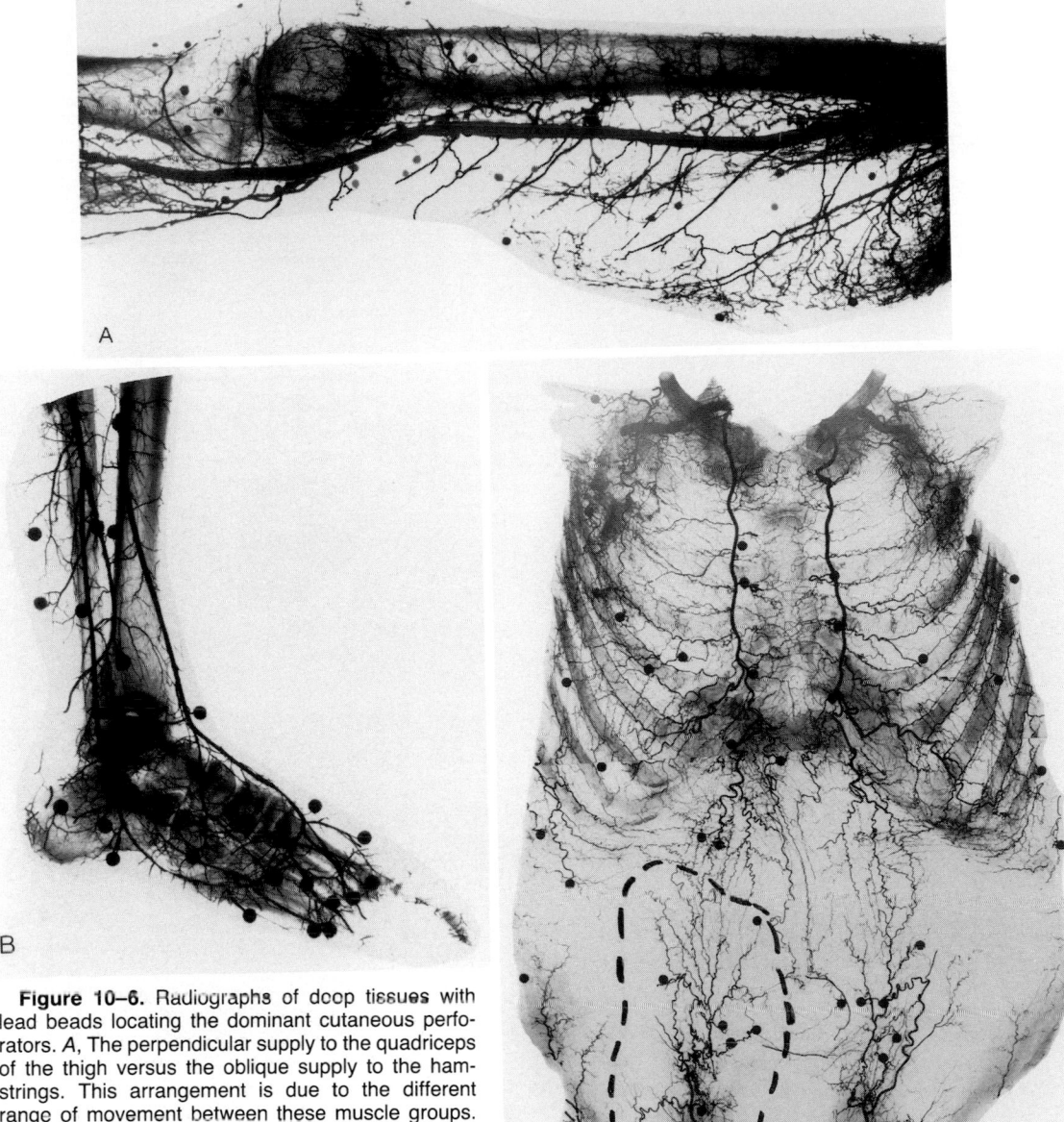

Figure 10–6. Radiographs of deep tissues with lead beads locating the dominant cutaneous perforators. *A*, The perpendicular supply to the quadriceps of the thigh versus the oblique supply to the hamstrings. This arrangement is due to the different range of movement between these muscle groups. *B*, The continuous arch formed between the anterior and posterior tibial arteries. *C*, The choke vessels above the umbilicus that connect the internal thoracic-superior epigastric arteries with the deep inferior systems to establish the ventral railroad between the clavicles and the groins. Branches of these systems radiate laterally to connect in approximately the midclavicular line from above down with the acromiothoracic, lateral thoracic, posterior intercostals, lumbar, and ascending branches of the deep circumflex iliac arteries. The territory of one DIEA (deep inferior epigastric artery) is defined. (From Br. J. Plast. Surg.)

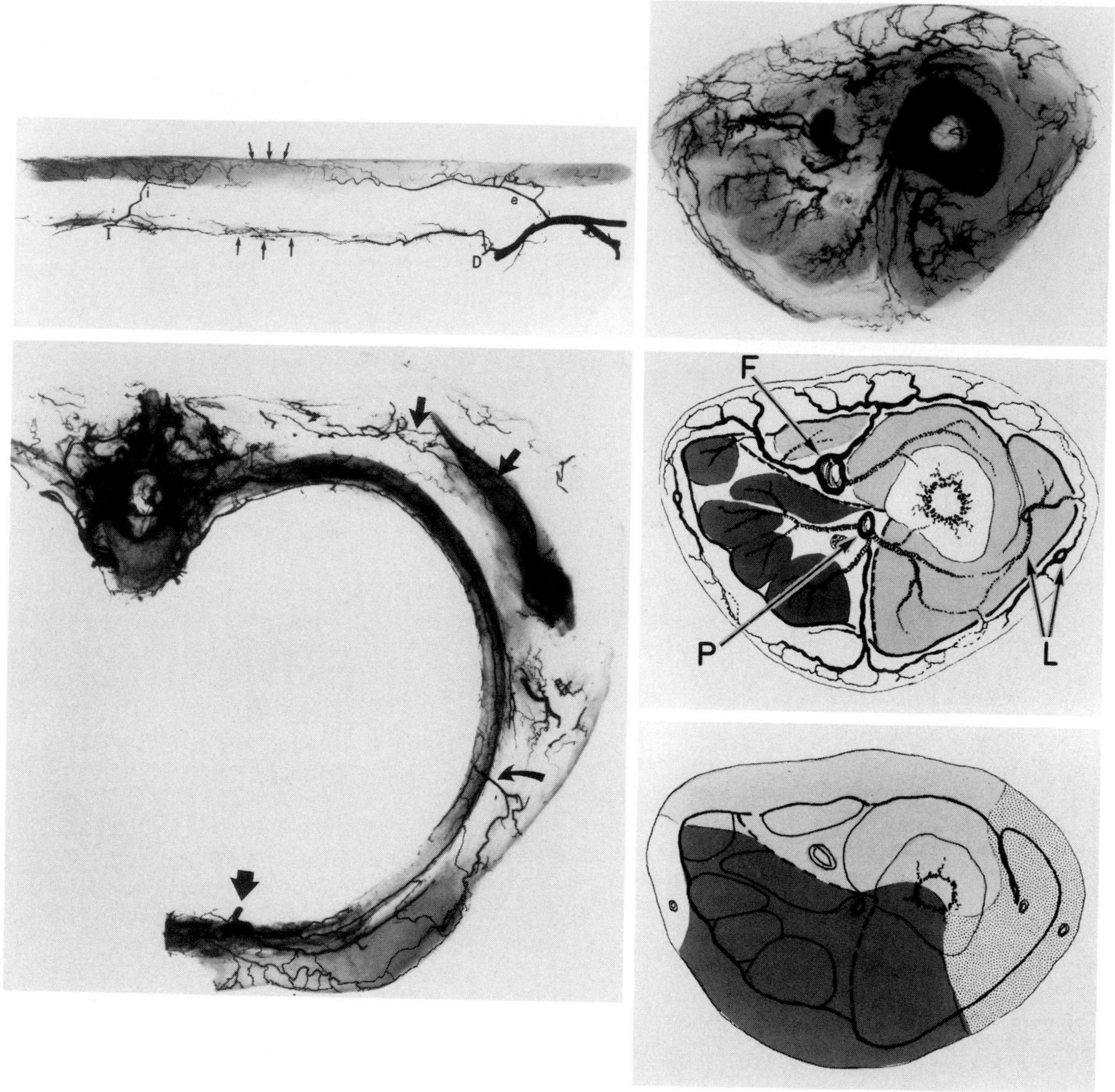

Figure 10–7. Sectional studies selected from the abdomen, thorax, and thigh revealing the course of the cutaneous and muscular branches derived from the source arteries in the deep tissues. *Top left*, The section is taken obliquely along the intercostal-femoral artery axis showing two angiosomes linked by choke vessels at corresponding levels in the integument and deep tissues *(arrows)*. The cutaneous *(i)* and muscular branches of the posterior intercostal *(I)* angiosome connect with the superficial inferior epigastric *(e)* and ascending branch of the deep circumflex iliac artery *(D)*. The source artery on the right is the external iliac–femoral artery trunk. *Bottom left*, The internal thoracic artery *(arrow)* with its anterior intercostal muscular and cutaneous branches, which sweep laterally to meet the posterior intercostal artery and its lateral cutaneous perforator *(arrow)*. Posteriorly, branches of the posterior intercostal artery anastomose with the circumflex scapular artery at this level *(arrows)*. *Top and center right*, The dominant cutaneous perforators that arise from the superficial femoral *(F)*, profunda *(P)*, and descending branch of the lateral circumflex femoral *(L)* arteries. They reach the skin via the intermuscular septa. *Bottom right*, The angiosomes of the three source arteries that supply the skin, muscle, and bone (compare with Fig. 10–8). (From Br. J. Plast. Surg.)

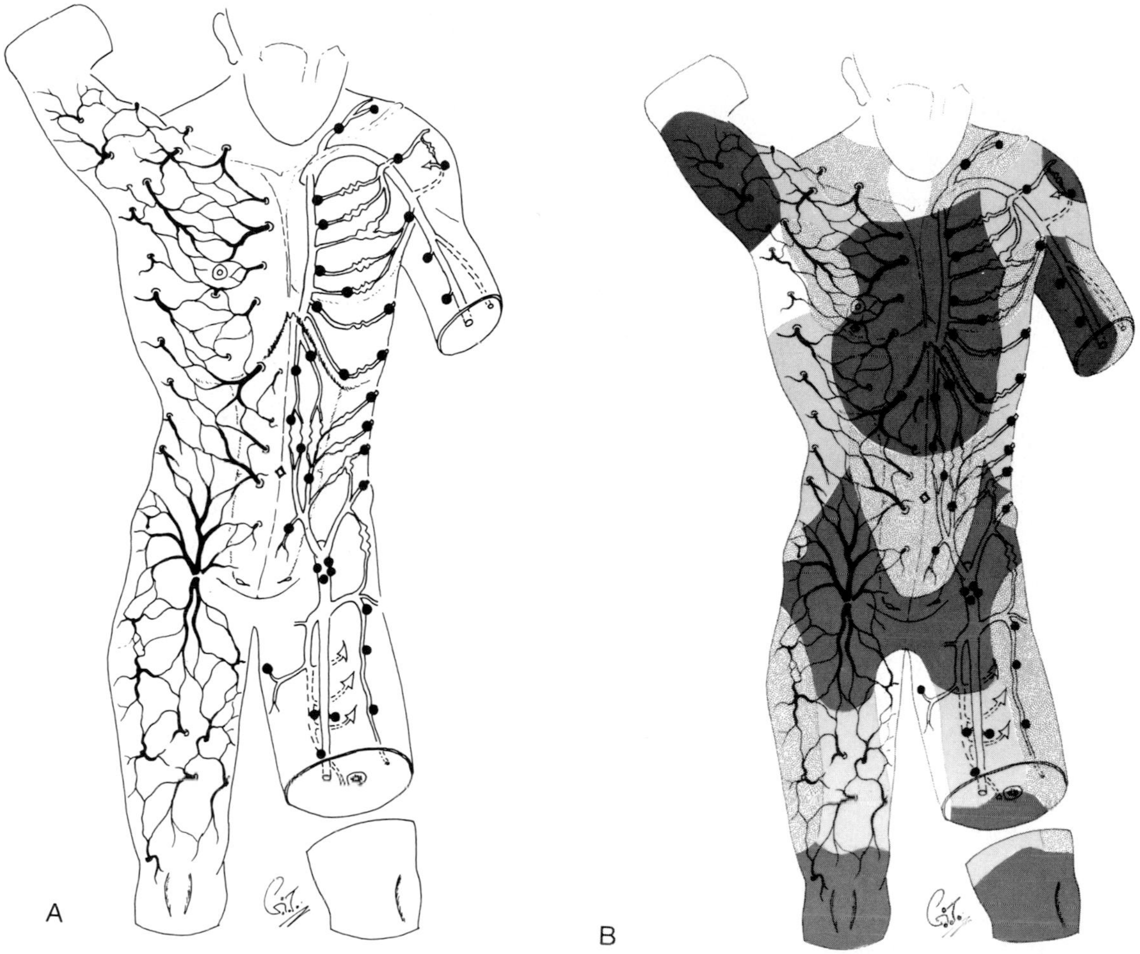

Figure 10–8. The technique by which the angiosomes were defined. *A*, The cutaneous perforators with their choke connections are depicted on the left. The origin of the perforators from their underlying source arteries and their muscular branches is shown on the right. *B*, The vascular territories of each source artery are illustrated in the integument *(left)* and deep tissues *(right)* by lines drawn through the choke connecting vessels. Note that the territories correspond in these two layers and how they appear as sectors in the limbs. (From Br. J. Plast. Surg.)

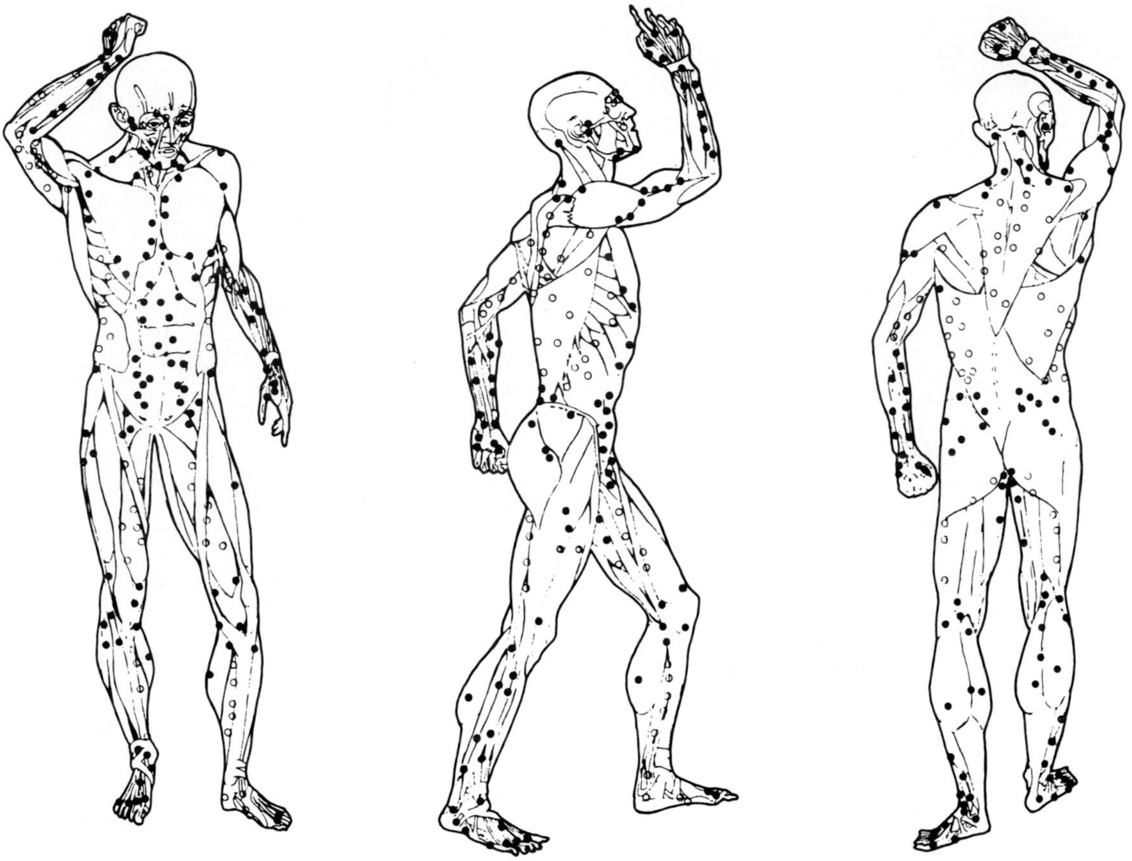

Figure 10–9. The dominant cutaneous perforators emerging from the deep fascia that identify their corresponding source arteries in the deep layers (compare with Fig. 10–10). Note their relationship to the intermuscular and intramuscular septa. This result was averaged from all the studies. (From Br. J. Plast. Surg.)

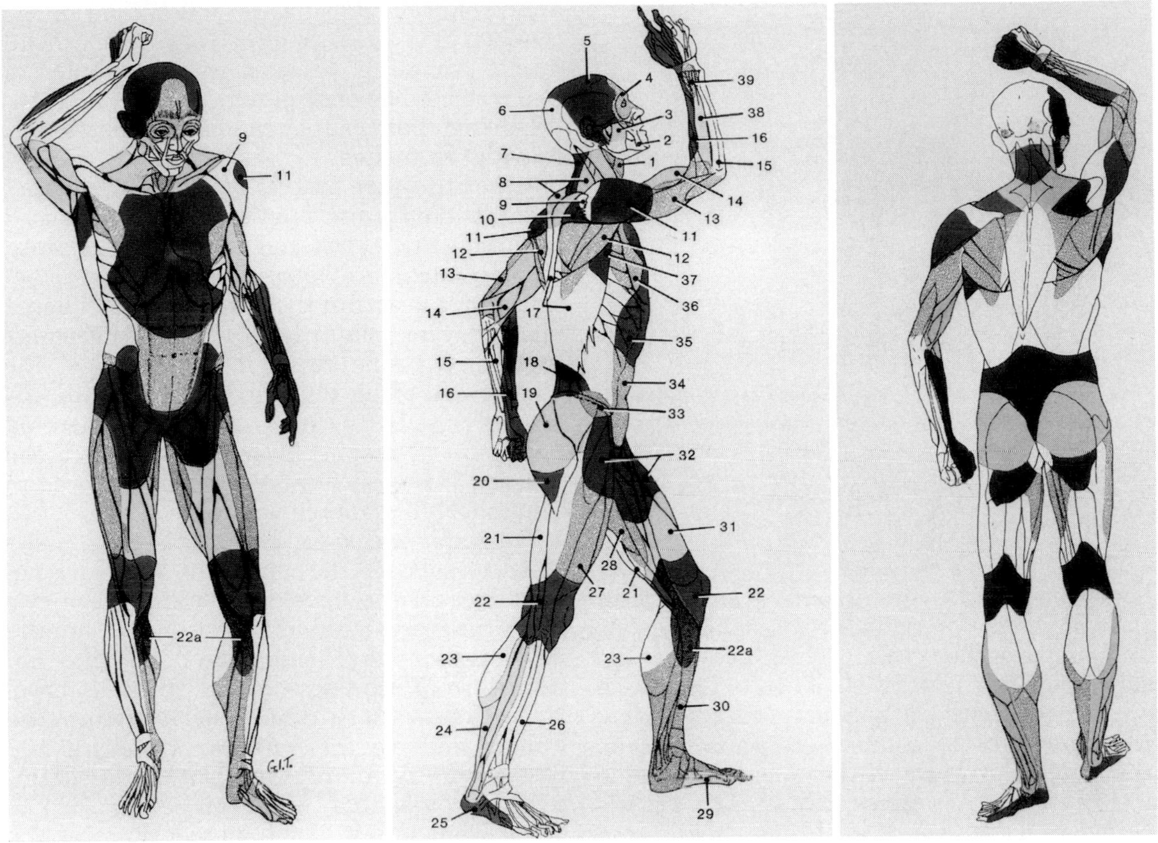

Figure 10–10. The angiosomes of the source arteries of the body shaded to correspond with Figure 10–9. They are: (1) thyroid, (2) facial, (3) buccal (internal maxillary), (4) ophthalmic, (5) superficial temporal, (6) occipital, (7) deep cervical, (8) transverse cervical, (9) acromiothoracic, (10) suprascapular, (11) posterior circumflex humeral, (12) circumflex scapular, (13) profunda brachii, (14) brachial, (15) ulnar, (16) radial, (17) posterior intercostals, (18) lumbar, (19) superior gluteal, (20) inferior gluteal, (21) profunda femoris, (22) popliteal, (22a) descending genicular (saphenous), (23) sural, (24) peroneal, (25) lateral plantar, (26) anterior tibial, (27) lateral femoral circumflex, (28) adductor (profunda), (29) medial plantar, (30) posterior tibial, (31) superficial femoral, (32) common femoral, (33) deep circumflex iliac, (34) deep inferior epigastric, (35) internal thoracic, (36) lateral thoracic, (37) thoracodorsal, (38) posterior interosseous, (39) anterior interosseous, and (40) internal pudendal.

Note: This figure represents the territories of the skin and of each muscle. (From Br. J. Plast. Surg.)

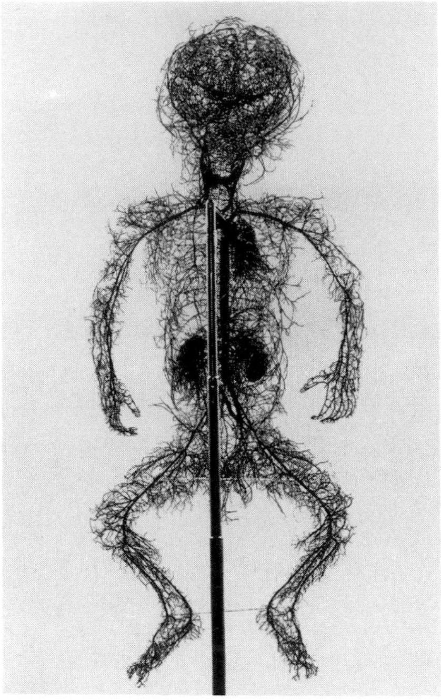

Figure 10–11. Tompsett's corrosion cast of the arteries in a stillborn baby. Note how the major vessels relate to the bony skeleton of the body. (Reproduced by permission from the Department of Anatomy, Royal College of Surgeons of England.) (From Br. J. Plast. Surg.)

honeycomb, calcified in some areas to form the bony skeleton, which houses, permeates, and supports the specialized tissues. The vessels follow this framework down to the microscopic level as if for support and protection. In general, if the connective tissue is rigid, they hug its surface; if the connective tissue is loose, they travel within it. The vessels occasionally travel in a fibrous sheath or a bony canal, but this tunnel always contains loose areolar tissue. *Gray's Anatomy* (Williams and Warwick, 1980) stated the reason for this: to allow the veins to dilate and the arteries to pulsate.

The pattern is well illustrated if the arterial network is traced from the heart to the periphery. The major arteries are closely related to the bones of the axial skeleton (Fig. 10–11). Their branches at first follow the intermuscular septa. In the deep tissues they penetrate the muscles, usually on their deep surface, the tendons, the bones, the nerves, and the deep fat deposits. As the vessels divide and subdivide within the specialized tissues, their branches again follow the connective tissue framework to reflect the architecture of the tissue in question. The arterial framework is beautifully illustrated in the corrosion cast studies of Last and Tompsett (1962).

The cutaneous perforators exhibit the same pattern. They arise from their source artery (*segmental* or *distributing* artery) or one of its muscular branches, and follow the intermuscular or intramuscular septa toward the surface. They pierce the deep fascia, branch, and ramify on its surface, and ascend in the connective tissue framework of the superficial fascia, traveling between the fat lobules to reach the subdermal plexus.

During their course the cutaneous vessels provide branches to the adjacent tissues, whether they are muscle, nerve, bone, fascia, or fat. If the connective tissues are condensed to form thick septa and sheets, the vessels, as mentioned previously, usually travel beside and not within these structures. When a muscle gains origin from the intermuscular septum, e.g., in the thigh and the leg, the vessels are often found coursing within the muscle close by the septum, but not plastered against it. These facts are important to the surgeon if the perforators are to be traced to the underlying source vessels.

The explanation for the coexistence of the blood vessels and the connective tissue framework lies in the developing human embryo. Unfortunately, many of the studies of human development have been based on data obtained from the developing chick embryo. Nevertheless, it is known that within the human embryo the vascular system is the first tissue to differentiate in the mesoderm, and the connective tissue can be regarded as being what is left of the mesoderm after the specialized tissues have developed from it (Johnston, Davies, and Davies, 1958). It is reasonable to speculate that, if the specialized tissues such as muscle, nerve, and fat have developed within this mesh of connective tissue and vessels, this could explain why vessels have become captured within, and compressed between, the specialized tissues. It would explain why they follow the intermuscular septa, the intramuscular septa, the deep fascia, and the connective tissue septa of the superficial fascia to reach the skin. As mobility develops between tissue planes, presumably some of the interconnections between vessels would have been lost, with a compensatory enlargement of vessels arising from fixed tissue sites.

Vessels Radiate from Fixed to Mobile Areas

Few vessels cross mobile tissue planes. Instead, they cross where tissues are anchored and radiate parallel to the plane of mobility, often for long distances. This pattern is seen typically where muscles piston beneath the deep fascia, where the integument glides above it, or where the deep fascia (e.g., the galea) is mobile over bone.

The cutaneous vessels pierce and emerge from the outer layer of the deep fascia near where it is anchored, either to its deep septa or to bone. The overlying integument is fixed also to the deep fascia at these sites. The fixed skin regions are seen easily in a well-muscled individual as grooves and valleys: around the perimeter of muscles, especially where they interdigitate; over well-developed intermuscular septa; over the flexor surface of joints; adjacent to the dorsal and ventral midline of the body; around the base of the skull; and in the region of some bony prominences.

From the grooves and valleys in the deep fascia the vessels flow toward the convexities of the body surface, branching within the integument. The wider the distance between the concavities and the higher the summit, the longer is the vessel. This pattern is well demonstrated in the blood supply to the integument of the scalp, nose, ears, breasts, and genitalia; the extensor surface of the joints; and the bulging surface of muscles (see Fig. 10–4).

Where the skin is relatively fixed to the deep fascia over a wide area, e.g., in the scalp and many areas of the limbs, the vessels remain close to the surface of the deep fascia for a considerable distance. In the loose-skinned areas of the body, especially over the pectoralis major muscle, the iliac fossa, and the extensor surface of joints, the vessels course for a short distance adjacent to the deep fascia. Soon they are plastered to the undersurface of the subcutaneous layer by a thin glistening sheet of fascia, and they then pierce the fat obliquely to reach the subdermal plexus, where they travel for long distances.

It follows that where there is mobility between tissue planes over a wide area, large flaps are available for transfer. They will be fed by sizable vessels that enter the tissue from around its fixed perimeter. The clinical applications of this concept are discussed later in this chapter.

Vessels "Hitchhike" with Nerves

It is well known that in the deep tissues the vessels and nerves course together as neurovascular bundles. The pattern is seen also, however, in the superficial layers, especially where a cutaneous nerve courses on the surface of the deep fascia. An artery may accompany the nerve for a considerable distance, often connecting with its neighbor in chain-link fashion to provide the basis for an axially oriented neurovascular flap (Fig. 10–12).

The cutaneous vessels and the nerve are occasionally in juxtaposition; in other situations they course parallel to each other but at a distance. When the cutaneous nerve crosses a fixed skin site, it frequently "picks up" its next vascular companion.

There are numerous instances throughout the body where this pattern of distribution of nerves and vessels exists to supply the integument: the supraorbital, infraorbital, and occipital neurovascular bundles in the head; the supraclavicular nerves collecting branches of the suprascapular and supraclavicular vessels as they cross the clavicle onto the chest; the intercostal neurovascular bundles on the torso; and the cutaneous nerves of the arm, forearm, thigh, leg, and digits, which are accompanied by long named or unnamed vessels or a chain-linked system of vessels. Indeed, many of the fasciocutaneous flaps designed in the leg are in fact neurovascular

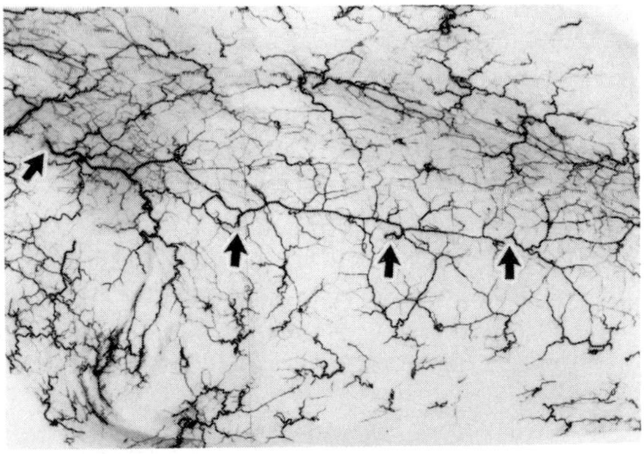

Figure 10–12. Chain-link system of arteries *(arrows)* that accompany the lateral cutaneous nerve of the arm without change in caliber. Compare with Figure 10–3, front view, right arm. (From Br. J. Plast. Surg.)

flaps that incorporate the saphenous or sural systems.

Vessel Size and Orientation Are the Product of Tissue Growth and Differentiation

Two centuries ago John Hunter (1794) suggested that at some stage of fetal development, and certainly at birth, there are a fixed number of arteries in the body. This has been the authors' impression when comparing the number of cutaneous perforators encountered while raising the same flap in a child and in an adult.

If this concept is correct, it provides a plausible explanation for the density and morphology of the cutaneous arteries in different regions of the body. It explains why vessels radiate from concavities and converge on convexities, and why the vessels in some areas are small and close together, while in others they are large and spaced well apart.

There are numerous examples to support this hypothesis (Fig. 10–13). The sternomastoid and trapezius muscles split from the same somite (Patten, 1968). The trapezius "drags" its supplying transverse cervical artery (and nerve) across the root of the neck to the back, together with a large band of skin that it nourishes. Manchot (1889) suggested that the long course and the direction of the superficial superior and inferior epigastric arteries is brought about by the extension of the fetal torso. If one remembers that the cutaneous perforators pierce the deep fascia at fixed points and that they all interconnect, this would explain why, as the brain and skull expand, the scalp vessels hypertrophy and are stretched from the base of the calvarium toward its vertex. Similarly, this could explain why large vessels converge on the nipple from all directions as the breast develops. This pattern is seen also in the limbs. Growth of the long bones would stretch the vessels apart and therefore make clear why vessels radiate in all directions from the flexor surface of the joints.

Where skin becomes mobile over the deep fascia, certain vessel connections are lost in these areas. One would expect compensatory hypertrophy of the remaining vessels, and indeed this is so. In mobile skin areas, large vessels are seen in the integument arising from fixed points around the perimeter and running parallel to the skin surface for long distances. Perforators of the internal thoracic system and the cutaneous branches that radiate from the groin are excellent examples.

The primitive cutaneous perforators in the fetus branch in all directions after piercing the deep fascia, and have a stellate appearance. This pattern is retained into adulthood in many regions of the body. When a perforator departs from this pattern and becomes oriented in one direction, it highlights the differential increase in growth that has occurred along that axis or the influence of a developing cutaneous nerve. Where small perforators are clustered close together, this pattern suggests that by comparison the growth and hypertrophy in the area is less than at those sites where the perforators are large and spaced well apart. This is well demonstrated by comparing the perforators in the proximal and distal regions of the limbs (see Figs. 10–3, 10–26 to 10–34).

Arteries (and Veins) Interconnect to Form a Continuous Three-dimensional Network of Vascular Arcades

This is evident in each tissue whether it is the integument, muscle, nerve, or bone. The arteries do not supply discrete areas with occasional anastomoses. Instead, their branches are linked with each other and with the branches of neighboring vessels to form arches. The "keystones" in these arcades are formed sometimes by true anastomoses without change in caliber. More commonly they are represented by reduced caliber *choke* arteries and arterioles. The perimeter of *choke* or anastomotic vessels defines the anatomic territory of each artery (Fig. 10–14). Thus, each tissue is supplied by a series of linked arterial territories, some small and some large.

The concept is three-dimensional and was documented by Hunter in 1794. He quoted the vascular arcades in the hands and the feet as examples, and stated that the arcades are smaller and occur more frequently as the arteries become more distal (see Figs. 10–6, 10–27). Thus, like a Roman aqueduct, the arterial framework consists of tiers of vascular arcades that commence from the aorta and become progressively smaller as the cap-

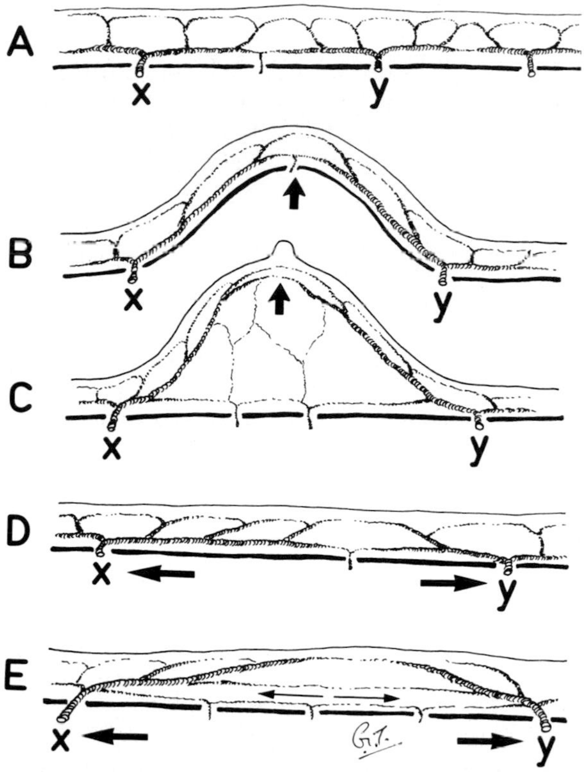

Figure 10–13. Diagram showing how the size and course of the direct cutaneous perforators X and Y, which emerge from fixed points in the deep fascia, could be modified by growth either before or after birth. In *A* the perforators, which are fixed in number and position, form a major connecting network on the surface of the deep fascia in the "resting stage." In *B* they are stretched with the deep fascia by the expansion of underlying tissues—e.g., the scalp vessels as the brain and skull expand during fetal development. In *C*, as the breast develops within the integument, the vessels are displaced toward the dermis and lengthened as they converge on the nipple. In *D* they are stretched apart in the limbs as the long bones grow, but they still retain their original relationship to the deep fascia. In *E* the vessels are again stretched apart by growth, but the mobile relationship between the undersurface of the integument and the deep fascia is responsible for their oblique course. This pattern is characteristic of the loose skin areas of the torso. (From Br. J. Plast. Surg.)

illary bed is approached. In general the large arcades are formed by the segmental or distributing source arteries, e.g., the intercostal, radial, ulnar, and deep epigastric arteries, which course between the tissues. Successive tiers of arcades are formed by the arteries, arterioles, and capillaries that supply those tissues.

The arterial arcades in the bowel mesentery are a classic example (Fig. 10–15). They are smaller and more numerous as they approach the intestine. The basic pattern exists

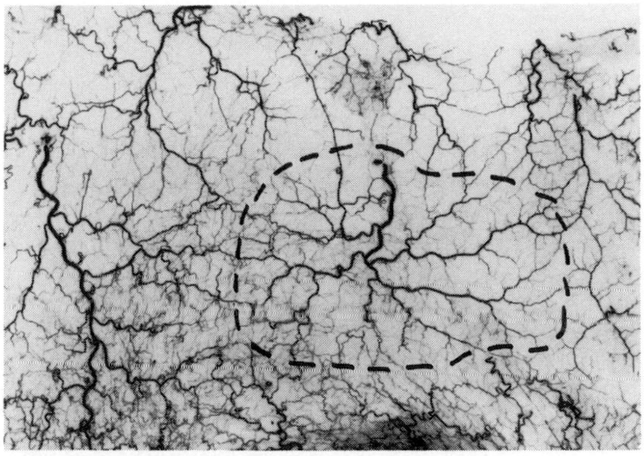

Figure 10–14. Dotted line drawn through choke connecting vessels of a large acromiothoracic perforator to define its anatomic territory. Compare with Figure 10–3, left side of chest. (From Br. J. Plast. Surg.)

in all tissues and is modified by the morphology and function of that tissue. Even during tissue repair the pattern of vascular arcades is reproduced in granulation tissue. Undoubtedly there are many reasons for the interconnections that exist between arteries, but almost certainly one of these is to allow the equilibration of pressure across the arcades before the capillary bed is perfused.

Comparison of the vascular architecture in humans with that of other animals and other species reveals a similar arrangement of arcades. In the loose-skinned animals the arcades in the integument are stretched over long distances (Fig. 10–16). In the wings of insects and in the leaves of plants the "veins" assume a pattern of interconnecting arcades similar to those of the intestinal mesentery (Fig. 10–17).

Thus, the blood supply of the integument consists of a three-dimensional mesh of vessels that spans the body like a national road map of interconnecting roadways and subways. The meshwork is composed of a series of linked vascular territories, fed at fixed skin points by arteries that pierce the deep fascia. When a flap is elevated, a series of arterial territories is captured in succession by the vessels in the base of the flap. The authors' experimental animal studies reveal that when a flap is delayed, the choke arteries linking adjacent vessels dilate (Fig. 10–18).

ANGIOSOME CONCEPT

When the authors defined the anatomic territory of a source artery in the integument

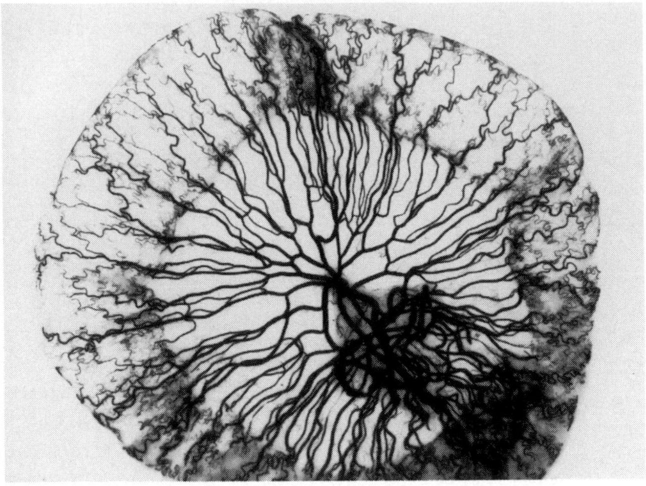

Figure 10–15. The interconnecting arcades of the small intestine. (From Br. J. Plast. Surg.)

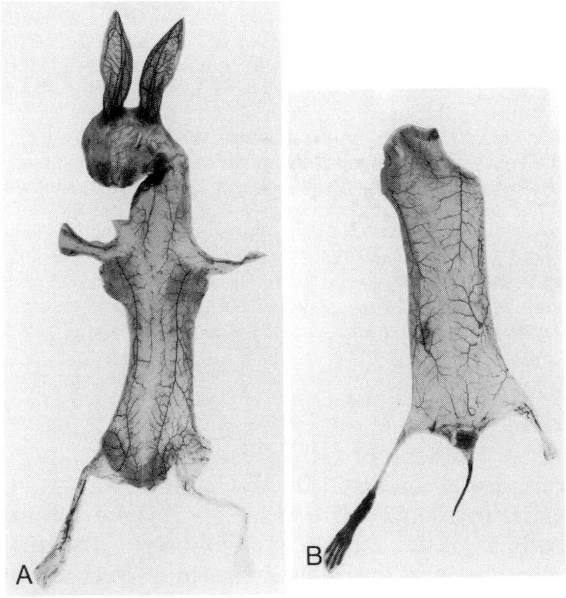

Figure 10–16. The cutaneous blood supply of the rabbit. Note the large, long vessels that course in the loose-skinned area of the torso, their choke connections, and their origins from the fixed skin areas of the axillae and the groins. (From Br. J. Plast. Surg.)

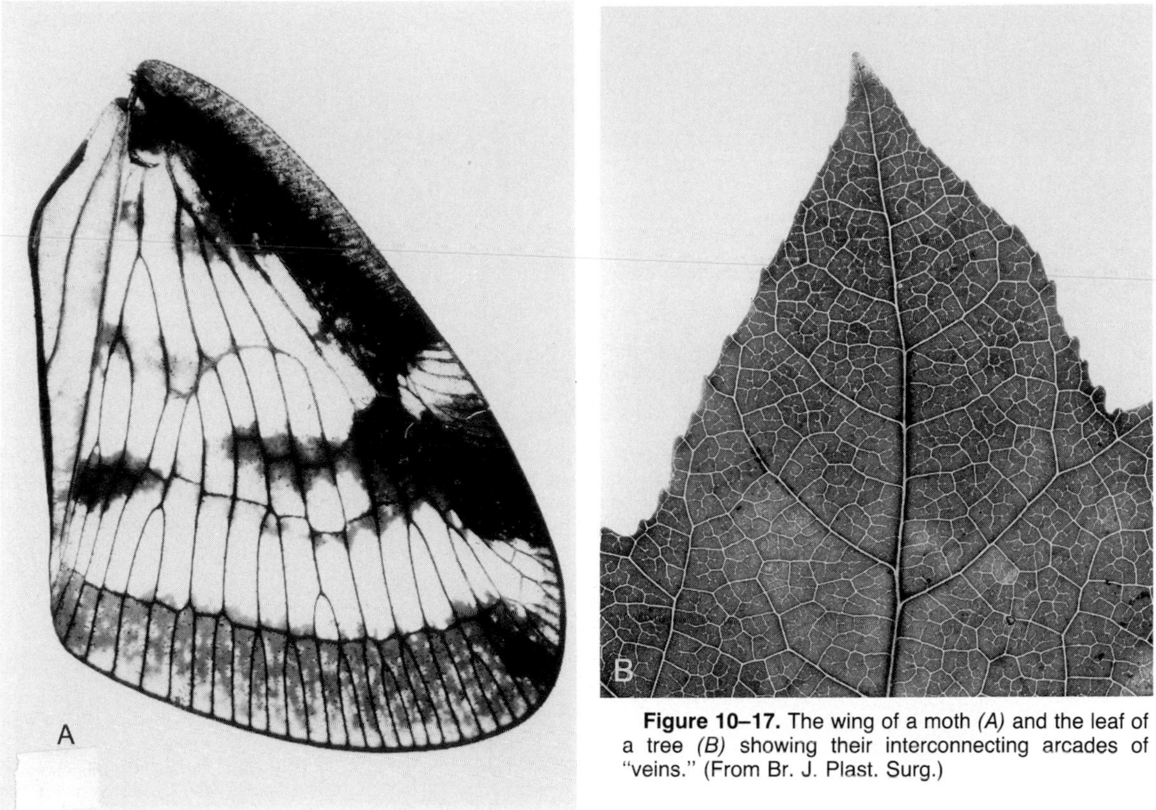

Figure 10–17. The wing of a moth *(A)* and the leaf of a tree *(B)* showing their interconnecting arcades of "veins." (From Br. J. Plast. Surg.)

and compared it with its deep tissue counterpart, it was observed that the perimeter of these two territories often coincided (see Fig. 10–8). In other words, each source artery supplying a composite of muscle, nerve, and bone was usually responsible for the nourishment of its overlying area of skin. In some regions the integument is supplied in this way by few large cutaneous vessels (e.g., in the scalp and groin); in other areas the source artery provides multiple small branches (e.g., in the forearm and sole of the foot).

The authors named the composite segments of tissue *angiosomes,* and these are illustrated in Figure 10–10. Forty are described, but many can be subdivided into smaller segments to correspond with Salmon's chart of over 80 skin territories. When one considers the anatomic territories in the light of clinical experience, it can be seen that in most cases when a flap is based on the vessels of one angiosome, the corresponding tissue or tissues of the adjacent angiosome can be "captured" with safety. Necrosis tends to occur in a flap, whether it is skin, muscle, or bone, when an attempt is made to capture the next or subsequent angiosome. This presumably is due to the pressure gradient that must occur as blood flows across the choke vessels that link adjacent arterial territories. The more choke systems there are in a flap, the less pressure is available for flow at the distal end.

Although the boundaries of the angiosomes are illustrated as lines, they represent the middle of choke zones. They outline the composite vascular territories of the integument *and* the deep structures such as muscles, nerves, bones, and peritoneum, which can be designed as a flap on each source artery. Where a tissue crosses a series of angiosomes it receives a segmental blood supply from the source artery of each angiosome.

Examination of Figures 10–10 and 10–19 shows that some muscles, such as the thenar muscles, are contained wholly within one angiosome. Many span two angiosomes, e.g., the rectus abdominis and gluteus maximus muscles. However, most span more than two angiosomes, e.g., the latissimus dorsi, pector-

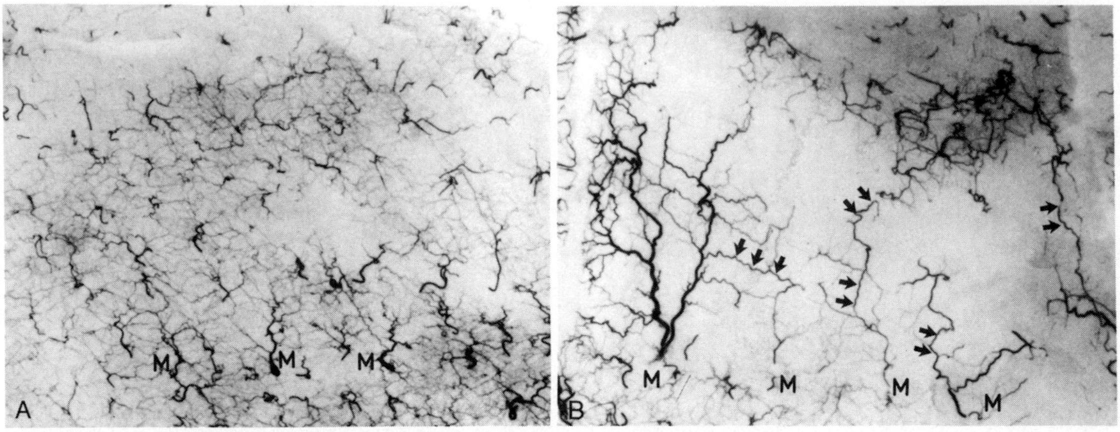

Figure 10–18. Radiographs of corresponding regions of the abdominal integument of a pig nourished by the internal mammary system. A skin flap has been delayed on the right side for one week. Specimens were obtained after sacrificing the animal and total body arterial injection. Note the significant enlargement of the internal mammary perforators *(M)*, and in particular their choke connections *(arrows)* on the delayed side.

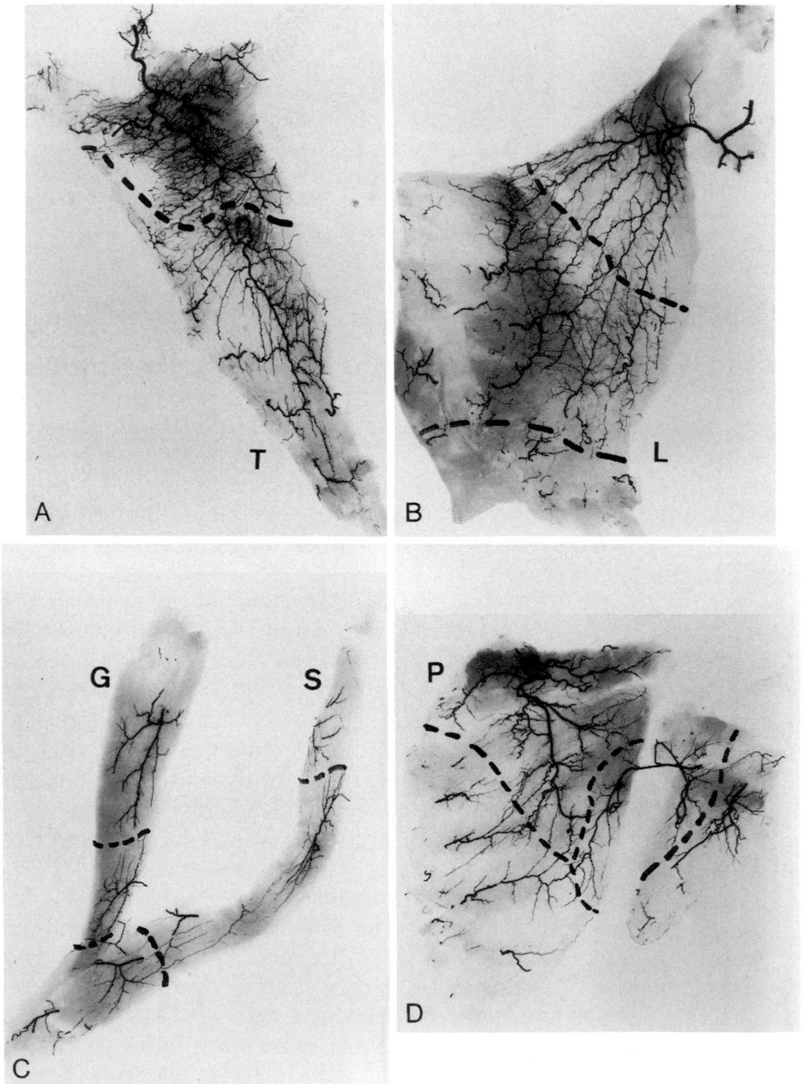

Figure 10–19. Radiographs of the trapezius *(T)*, latissimus dorsi *(L)*, gracilis *(G)*, sartorius *(S)*, pectoralis major *(P)*, and pectoralis minor muscles with their vascular territories defined. Each muscle traverses several angiosomes and receives a contribution from the respective source arteries. The trapezius is supplied by the transverse cervical *(above)* and posterior intercostals *(below)*; the latissimus dorsi by the thoracodorsal *(upper)*, posterior intercostal *(middle)*, and lumbar *(lower)* vessels; the gracilis by the adductor (profunda), superficial femoral, and descending genicular arteries; and the sartorius by the common femoral (superficial circumflex iliac artery branch), superficial femoral, and descending genicular vessels; the pectoralis major receives contributions from the internal thoracic *(left)*, acromiothoracic *(right)*, and lateral thoracic *(below right)*; and the pectoralis minor from the last two angiosomes. Compare with Figure 10–10. (From Br. J. Plast. Surg.).

alis major, and sartorius muscles. Where multiple angiosomes are traversed, the vascular contributions from each source artery are linked within the muscle usually by choke vessels (see Figs. 10–6, 10–19). The choke vessels often exhibit a characteristic corkscrew appearance.

A knowledge of the number and size of the chain-linked territories within each muscle is fundamental to flap design and has been discussed in detail by many workers (McCraw and Dibbell, 1977; McCraw, Dibbell, and Carraway, 1977; Mathes and Nahai, 1979, 1982; McCraw and Arnold, 1986). It is one of the factors that explains the reliability of some musculocutaneous flaps and the uncertainty of others. For example, the skin paddle of the latissimus dorsi flap usually spans the primary territory of the thoracodorsal artery and extends onto the intercostal territory (see Figs. 10–10, 10–19). The skin paddle of the pectoralis major flap is nourished by the captured perforators of the internal thoracic artery, not the pectoral artery, when it is designed in the parasternal and submammary regions. In the case of the lower transverse rectus abdominis (TRAM), flap viability is taken to the limit. In this flap the cutaneous paddle is placed over the captured perforators of the deep *inferior* epigastric system when the skin paddle is designed below the umbilicus (see Figs. 10–8, 10–10). If the skin paddle is extended laterally beyond the muscle, tertiary skin territories are borrowed. On the ipsilateral side the third territory is that of the superficial inferior epigastric artery. However, before this territory can be captured on the contralateral side the territory of the opposite deep inferior epigastric artery and its choke connections must be traversed. It is no wonder that problems of flap viability often arise in the latter instance.

Another factor highlighted in 1987 by Carramenha e Costa and associates is the importance of the venous drainage. They demonstrated the existence of choke veins within the rectus abdominis muscle that connect the deep superior and inferior epigastric systems in the same way as their arterial counterparts. They showed that, in addition, the venae comitantes of the deep superior and inferior epigastric arteries have valves that direct flow in opposite directions. Therefore, because the superficial veins are disconnected in a TRAM flap, the venous drainage is thrust on the deep system. Blood must flow first against the valves of the deep inferior epigastric veins and across the choke veins within the muscle to reach the deep superior epigastric veins at the base of the flap (see Fig. 10–23). It is likely that this situation exists in the musculocutaneous flaps where the skin paddle is designed in the territory of an adjacent captured angiosome. This factor may be just as important as, indeed more important than, the arterial supply. It is highlighted by the clinical observation that when necrosis is impending in part of a musculocutaneous flap, that portion of the flap occasionally becomes blue and turgid, not pale and flaccid. Since venae comitantes accompany the cutaneous arteries, it is quite likely that, on the basis of the deep venous system, the body can be charted into venous territories.

The angiosome concept extends beyond the integument and muscle. For example, the iliac crest is nourished by at least five vessels that interconnect within the bone. These are the superficial and deep circumflex iliac arteries, the superior gluteal artery, the ascending branch of the lateral circumflex femoral artery, and the iliolumbar artery. Nearly all of these have been utilized in pedicled or free bone flap transfer. Similarly the fibula can be transferred on either the peroneal or the anterior tibial vessels (Taylor and associates, 1985), and the rib on the anterior or posterior intercostal vessels.

There is a close correlation between the angiosomes and the neurologic dermatomes in many areas of the torso and the head. In the extremities this is less evident where the angiosomes appear as sectors (see Figs. 10–7, 10–8). Occasionally the angiosome concept is clouded by nomenclature:

1. *The territory of the superficial temporal artery*. This fan-shaped territory overlies a similar territory supplied by the deep temporal vessels. This in turn overlies a comparable territory in the dura supplied by the middle meningeal artery. The latter two groups of arteries are derived from the internal maxillary artery, but all three are derived directly or indirectly from the terminal bifurcation of the external carotid system. In other words, the angiosome is the composite block of integument, muscle, pericranium, bone, and dura supplied by the distal part of the external carotid artery—the terminal external carotid artery angiosome (Fig. 10–20).

2. *The territory of the superficial inferior*

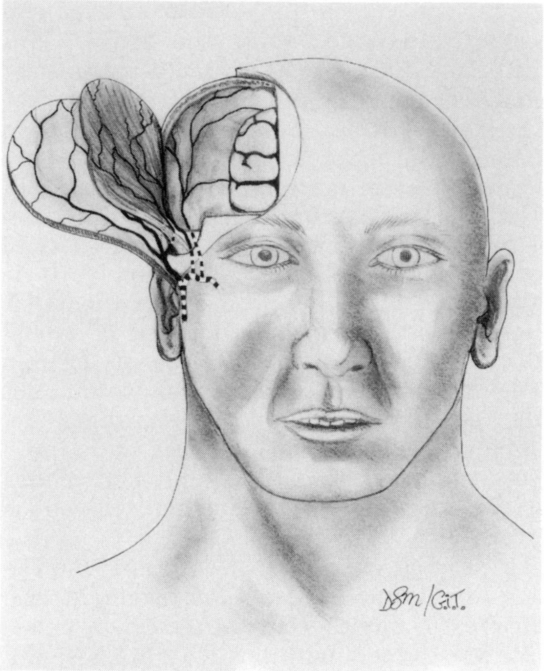

Figure 10–20. View of the terminal external carotid angiosome, which provides three successive fan-shaped strata of vessels to the superficial and deep tissues. From within out they are provided by the middle meningeal, the deep temporal (arising from the internal maxillary), and the superficial temporal arteries.

epigastric artery (SIEA). The common femoral angiosome (see Fig. 10–10) can be subdivided into smaller angiosomes. The ascending branch of the deep circumflex iliac artery (DCIA) is the deep tissue counterpart of the SIEA (see Fig. 10–7). The continuation of the DCIA is the counterpart of the superficial circumflex iliac artery (SCIA). Unfortunately the deep vessels arise from the terminal part of the external iliac artery, and the cutaneous perforators arise from the beginning of the common femoral artery. Terminology again obscures the angiosome concept.

CLASSIFICATION OF CUTANEOUS ARTERIES

Many attempts have been made to classify the cutaneous arteries. Terms such as *musculocutaneous* and *septocutaneous* relate the origin of the arteries to the deep tissues *before* they perforate the outer sheath of deep fascia. *Axial* and *random* pertain to the size and orientation of the vessels *after* they pierce the enveloping sheath and give significance to their importance in skin flap design. *Direct* and *indirect* relate to the origin of the perforators from their source arteries.

The authors prefer the last classification, described originally by Spalteholz (1893). It implies that some vessels have a dominant role in the supply to the integument and others are supplementary (Fig. 10–21). Without doubt this is the case, as demonstrated by the authors' total body studies. The terms *direct* and *indirect* embrace the other classifications and allow for the variable origin and course of the cutaneous perforators, even within the same individual. For example, in most cases a large direct perforator arises from the deltoid or acromial branch of the acromiothoracic axis in the region of the deltopectoral groove (see Figs. 10–3, 10–12, 10–28 to 10–30). The artery may emerge between the deltoid and pectoralis major muscles as a "septocutaneous" artery, or may pierce either muscle near its perimeter as a "musculocutaneous" artery. Thereafter it has a definite "axial" course downward and laterally across the chest and shoulder.

Direct Cutaneous Arteries

These arteries constitute the *primary* cutaneous supply. Whether they follow the intermuscular septa, or pierce muscles en route, their main destination is the skin. They are usually large and spaced well apart in the head, neck, torso, arms, and thighs, especially in the mobile skin areas. In the forearms and legs they are smaller and more numerous, except where they accompany cutaneous nerves. In the palms of the hands and the soles of the feet, perhaps the most fixed skin areas of the body, their density is at a maximum (see Figs. 10–3, 10–4, 10–27 to 10–34). In each case they supply branches to the nearby tissues during their course to the skin.

Indirect Cutaneous Arteries

The indirect vessels constitute the *secondary* cutaneous supply. They emerge from the deep fascia as terminal "spent" branches of arteries whose main purpose is to supply the muscles and other deep tissues. They reinforce and interconnect with the primary supply to the skin. They are sparse where the muscle pistons beneath the deep fascia, and are plentiful where the muscle is fixed to that structure. This explains the security of some musculocutaneous flaps, e.g., the latissimus dorsi, and the treachery of others, e.g., the gracilis.

The above is a broad classification and embraces a range of vessels. The origin, course, and distribution of the cutaneous arteries depend to a large extent on the proximity of the source artery to the undersurface of the deep fascia. The *direct* cutaneous vessels may arise:

1. From the source artery as it courses just beneath the deep fascia: e.g., the superior ulnar collateral artery, the superficial inferior epigastric artery, and the cutaneous perforators of the transverse cervical, radial, and plantar arteries.
2. As a direct continuation of the source artery: e.g., the cutaneous branches of the internal and external carotid vessels, such as the supratrochlear and the superficial temporal arteries.
3. From a deeply situated source artery, or one of its branches to a muscle. They follow the intermuscular septa to the surface: e.g., the cutaneous branch or branches of the circumflex scapular and lateral circumflex femoral vessels.
4. From the source artery as it courses on the undersurface of a muscle. A single large vessel or a number of vessels are given off, each piercing the muscle vertically or obliquely to reach and penetrate the deep fascia: e.g., the cutaneous perforators of the internal thoracic artery, the intercostal vessels, the deep inferior epigastric artery, and the gluteal vessels.

VENOUS DRAINAGE OF INTEGUMENT

The skin and subcutaneous tissues are drained by a dual system of vessels, a large capacitance subdermal network and a system of smaller venae comitantes that accompany the cutaneous arteries. To a large extent they are interdependent, but both communicate with the deep venous system and their flow is directed by valves. When the valves become incompetent, the former appear on the surface as long, tortuous varicosities, whereas the latter have a stellate appearance. Generally, flow is directed from the superficial to the deep veins, but in some areas, e.g., the palms of the hands and soles of the feet, the reverse may apply.

There are many gaps in our knowledge about the venous drainage of the integument and its relationship to that of the deep tissues. Most studies deal with isolated regions of the body. Schäfer (1975) described the situation in the lower limb and his findings have been combined with those of Carramenha e Costa and associates (1987) in Figure 10–22. This schematic illustration highlights the anatomy of the perforating veins and their importance in the design of island skin flaps.

The perforating veins may be venae communicantes or venae comitantes.

Venae Communicantes

These are large veins that connect the subcutaneous network with the deep veins and may or may not be accompanied by cutaneous arteries.

Venae Comitantes

These are small veins that accompany the cutaneous arteries as a countercurrent heat-conserving mechanism. They may drain into the deep system directly, or indirectly via the venae communicantes or the veins within the muscles. They are responsible mainly for draining the deeper layers of the subcutaneous fat (Schäfer, 1975).

The venous drainage of a flap may be anatomically *favorable* or *unfavorable,* depending on the presence or absence of valves in the region, the orientation of the valves, the connections with the deep veins, and (last but not least) the design of the flap.

There are no valves in the scalp veins, as shown in Figure 10–25. The veins in this region form a rich interconnecting network; hence, flaps designed in this region have a favorable drainage, regardless of the siting of the base and the axis of the flap.

In the limbs and the torso, the superficial and deep veins have valves that direct flow, as shown in Figure 10–22. Problems may arise with an island skin flap when the superficial veins are disconnected and the venous drainage is diverted via the venae comitantes and the venae communicantes to the deep veins. The *anatomic* obstructions to flow may be a diminutive deep venous system,

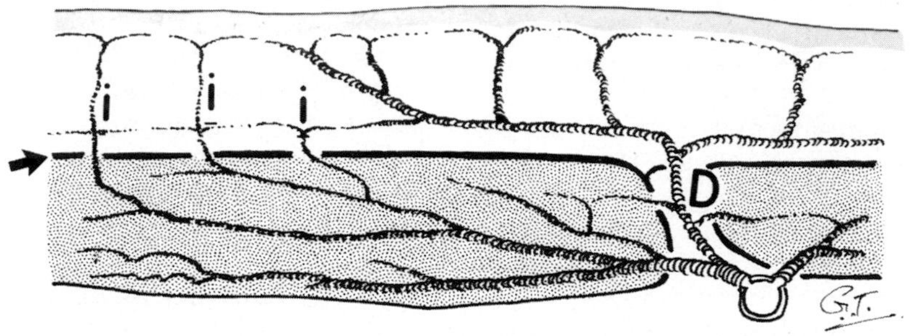

Figure 10–21. A source artery with direct and indirect cutaneous perforators. The direct vessel *(D)* courses in the intermuscular septum to reach the integument, supplying muscle and other deep tissues en route. The smaller indirect perforators *(i)* arise as terminal twigs of large arteries to the muscles. Both systems communicate within the connective tissue framework of the muscles, on the surface of the deep fascia *(arrow)* and within the integument to form a continuous three-dimensional network of vessels. (From Br. J. Plast. Surg.)

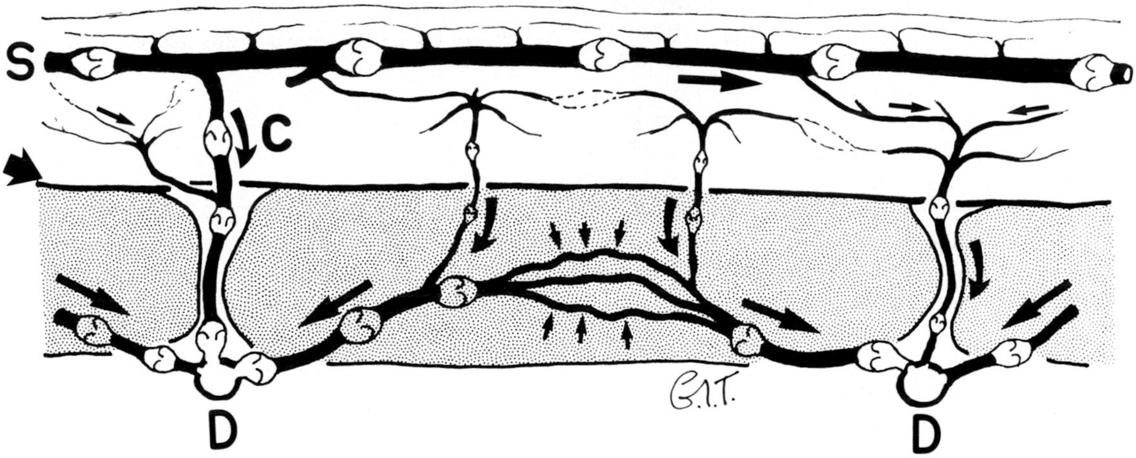

Figure 10–22. Composite diagram of the integument and underlying muscle *(shaded)* illustrating the superficial *(S)* and deep *(D)* venous systems with their interconnections. A large vena communicans *(C)* connects these systems, and the alternative pathways of 4 venae comitantes are shown. Note the choke system of veins within the muscle *(small arrows)* and the diverging direction of flow of the muscular veins as determined by the orientation of their valves. (From Taylor, G. I., Crock, J. G., and Caddy, C. D.: The venous territories (venosomes) of the body. Plast. Reconstr. Surg., in press.)

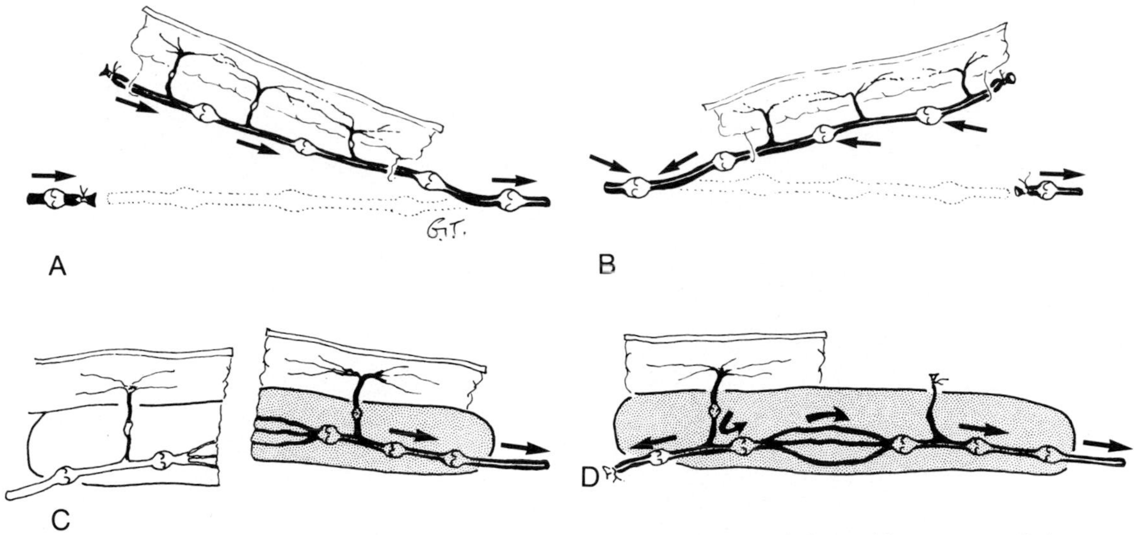

Figure 10–23. Diagram of *anatomically* favorable *(left)* and unfavorable *(right)* flaps with respect to their venous drainage. In *A* and *C* the venous drainage is along normal anatomic pathways. In *B* and *D* the direction of flow is against the valves of the deep veins, and in the latter case the venous drainage must negotiate also a system of choke veins within the muscle. (From Br. J. Plast. Surg.)

e.g., when an island neurovascular flap is raised from a digit; when there is unidirectional flow of the valves as in a distally based radial forearm flap; and when the venous flow is diverted through a system of choke veins, e.g., when the skin paddle of a musculocutaneous flap is based distally in a captured angiosome.

Some of the anatomically favorable and unfavorable island flaps are shown in Figure 10–23. Although in clinical practice the venous drainage can adapt to surmount most of these obstacles, it may be as important as the arterial network in terms of flap viability.

REGIONAL ANATOMY OF CUTANEOUS ARTERIES

The perforator mapping studies revealed that an average of 374 cutaneous arteries of 0.5 mm or greater supplied the cutis of the 40 angiosomes mapped in Figure 10–10. These were *direct* cutaneous arteries and collectively provided the primary supply to most of the integument. In most cases they pierced the deep fascia between muscles, or emerged from the muscles close to their attachment to bone or to fibrous septa. With experience the authors have found that a knowledge of the likely sites of emergence of these vessels gives precision to flap design. In a lean individual many of the points of emergence of the perforators can be identified with the Doppler ultrasonic probe. If a line is drawn between two such loci, and particularly if the integument is mobile between them, a safe flap can be planned along such an axis. The applied anatomy of the dominant vessels in each region of the body will be discussed briefly.

The Head

This region is supplied by an abundance of arteries that interconnect to form a rich network (Figs. 10–24, 10–25). It is an area par excellence that illustrates all the above basic principles of supply to the integument. The cutaneous vessels radiate from fixed points, either from bony foramina or from sites where the deep fascia is attached to bone. Frequently they are accompanied by cutaneous nerves. They radiate from concavities and grooves, especially around the base of the skull, the orbital margins, the lower border of the mandible, the nasolabial grooves, and the pre- and postauricular regions. Their branches converge on the convexities of the ears, nose, lips, and chin and the apex of the skull. They connect across the midline with their opposite artery to form vascular arches. The versatility of flaps that defy the conventional length-breadth ratios attests to the rich

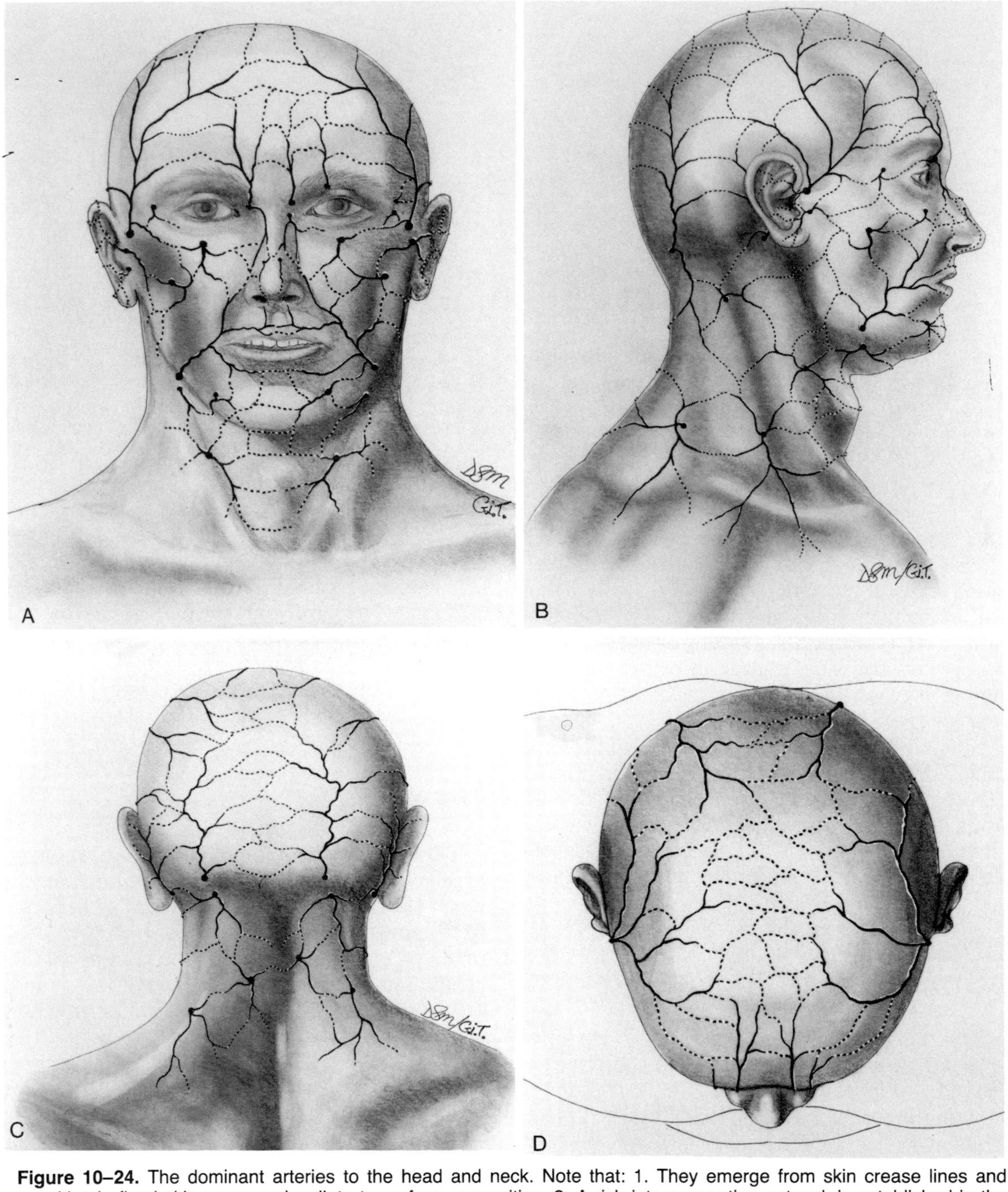

Figure 10–24. The dominant arteries to the head and neck. Note that: 1. They emerge from skin crease lines and concavities in fixed skin areas and radiate to surface convexities. 2. A rich interconnecting network is established in the midline of the scalp, face, and neck. 3. The vertical supraorbital and supratrochlear network intercepts and interconnects the superficial temporal pathways from each side in the forehead. 4. Flaps can be based in almost any direction because of the rich radiating networks of vessels. (From Taylor, G. I.: The Angiosomes of the Body. To be published by Churchill Livingstone.)

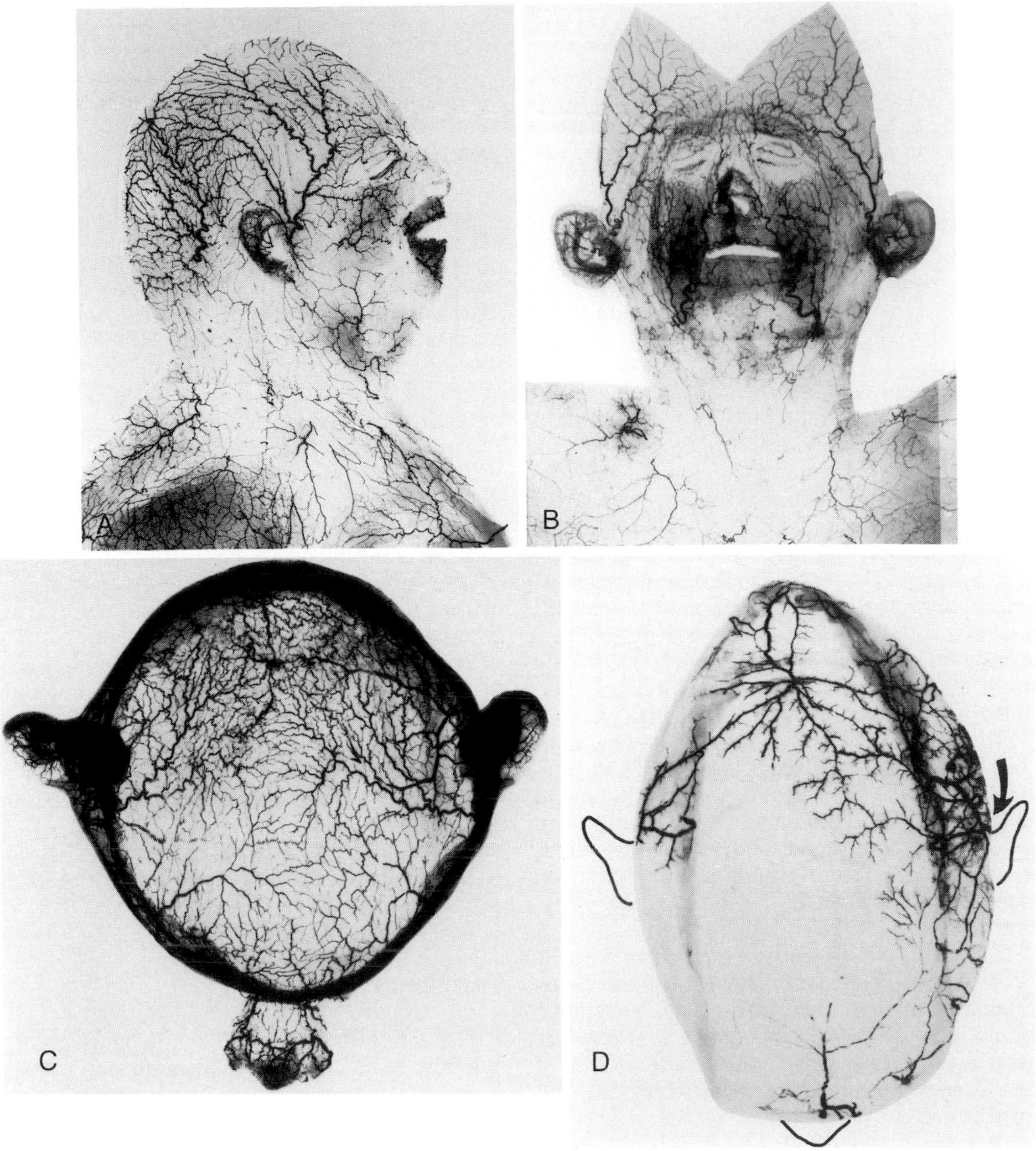

Figure 10–25. Radiographs of the arterial framework of the head and neck *(A, B, and C)* and the venous plexus of the scalp *(D)*. The vessels often interconnect without change in caliber, especially in the scalp; the facial arteries are well developed in *B* but are represented by several smaller vessels in *A*. The venous network in *D* has been established by injecting a single vein *(arrow)*, revealing the absence of valves in the scalp veins. (*D*, Courtesy of Dr. Prahlad Kolhe.) (From Br. J. Plast. Surg.)

blood supply of this region. The arteries are intimately related to the muscles of facial expression, muscles that belong to the panniculus carnosus.

Most of the integument of the head is supplied by branches of the *external* carotid system. The exception is a masklike area that surrounds the eyes and covers the central forehead and upper two-thirds of the nose. Arteries to this region arise from the ophthalmic branch of the *internal* carotid system and their distribution is similar to the ophthalmic division of the trigeminal nerve. The largest branches, the dorsal nasal, supratrochlear, and supraorbital arteries, emerge from the concavity of the inner canthus and their branches radiate to supply the eyelids, the central forehead, and the dorsum of the nose.

The branches of the external carotid system are well known and pierce the deep fascia along a curved loop around the base of the skull (occipital, posterior auricular, and superficial temporal arteries), along the lower border of the mandible (facial and submental arteries), from the groove in front of the parotid gland (buccal arteries), and from foramina in the maxilla and mandible (the infraorbital and mental vessels). The latter three arteries are by comparison relatively small and are derived from the internal maxillary branch of the external carotid system.

The pattern of distribution of the branches of these arteries reflects the growth and development of the underlying skull, facial bones, nose, lips, and ears. The branches form arcades to cover the convexities of these structures, and their course and distribution is well described in the anatomic texts. However, certain points should be highlighted.

1. There is a rich midline network of vessels in the forehead and nose, provided by branches of the internal carotid systems, which link the facial and superficial temporal arteries of either side as an arcade.

2. The superficial temporal artery may bifurcate or trifurcate. In the latter situation a large branch crosses the forehead just above the eyebrow. This vessel has an inverse relation with the supratrochlear and supraorbital arteries to satisfy the law of equilibrium, so that, when the supratrochlear and supraorbital arteries are small, this branch of the superficial temporal artery is large, and vice versa.

3. There is an extremely rich lattice of vessels in the face and scalp that provide connections between the branches of each artery and between their neighboring vessels. Often the connections are by reduced caliber choke arteries, but frequently they are true anastomoses without change in caliber. The latter pattern is particularly well developed in the scalp.

4. The scalp vessels course in close relation to the surface of the galea (deep fascia) and send numerous radiating branches to the subdermal plexus.

APPLIED ANATOMY

Many versatile flaps are available, especially those designed on the named branches to the face and scalp. Space does not permit a detailed account, but several points are worthy of comment.

1. The forehead flap is usually a reliable procedure. However, when the flap crosses the midline toward the opposite temple, its distal end is sometimes poorly perfused. A dominant supply from the supraorbital and supratrochlear systems, which intercepts the pathway of the diminutive frontal branches of the superficial temporal arteries, plus a system of reduced caliber choke vessels, accounts for this.

2. Successful replantation of the scalp has been achieved by reanastomosis of a single artery and vein. This highlights the rich interconnections that exist between the vessels supplying this area.

3. The frequent recurrence of a hemangioma after ligation or embolization of its major supplying arteries attests to the rich network of interconnecting vessels that supply the face and the scalp.

The Neck

The integument of the neck is bound firmly over the trapezius muscles posteriorly, to the base of the skull and the lower border of the mandible superiorly, and to the clavicle and manubrium inferiorly. Between these fixed skin zones the integument is mobile, except for its linear attachment to the cricoid cartilage (producing the transverse skin crease below the submental triangles) and to the anterior and posterior borders of the sternocleidomastoid muscles.

The fixed skin zones mark the sites of emergence of the major cutaneous perforators. They pierce the cervical fascia and branch in stellate fashion to form a rich plexus across the neck that overflows onto the neighboring chest, shoulder, and back. The branches are intimately related to the undersurface and substance of the platysma muscle, which they perforate to supply the subdermal plexus. They arise:

1. Superiorly from the occipital artery, the upper sternomastoid branch of that artery (emerging behind the muscle), the submandibular (glandular) branch of the facial artery, and the submental artery.
2. Inferiorly from the transverse cervical and/or the suprascapular artery—branches that emerge in the supraclavicular fossa.
3. Anteriorly from the superior thyroid artery, emerging in the groove in front of the sternomastoid muscle just below the hyoid bone, and from the transverse cervical artery, emerging from the groove behind the above muscle.
4. Posteriorly by a descending branch of the occipital artery and by direct cutaneous perforators of the muscular branches of the deep cervical and transverse cervical arteries. These vessels emerge from the surface of the trapezius muscle and from a position in front of its anterior border.

The origin of the above vessels is subject to considerable variation and the resulting network is reinforced by smaller arteries. A rich anastomosis is formed across the midline anteriorly.

APPLIED ANATOMY

The above vessels form a rich network within the platysma muscle and in the subdermal plexus. This accounts for the viability of the various flaps raised during block dissections of the neck, whether they include the platysma muscle or not. The pattern of supply provides also for the versatility of the platysma musculocutaneous flap. It also explains the problems that may be encountered with the skin paddle of the sternocleidomastoid musculocutaneous flap, since the direct perforators in the lower neck emerge from the deep fascia beside the muscle and not from its surface.

The Upper Limb

The direct (dominant) perforators of each angiosome arise from the source arteries or their muscular branches. They follow usually the intermuscular septa, but may pierce the muscle bellies. They emerge from the deep fascia around the perimeter of muscles or between their tendons. In the shoulder and arm the vessels are large and spaced well apart. Except where they travel with cutaneous nerves, the vessels become smaller and more numerous in the forearm and reach a maximum density in the palm of the hand. They radiate from the concavities of the intermuscular grooves, the axilla, the antecubital fossa, the palm of the hand, and the flexor surfaces of the interphalangeal joints. They converge on the bulging surfaces of muscles, especially the biceps and triceps, the summits of the shoulder, the elbow joint, the extensor surfaces of the metacarpophalangeal and interphalangeal joints, and the tips of the digits (Figs. 10–26, 10–27).

The Shoulder. The vessels arise superiorly from the transverse cervical and suprascapular arteries, anteriorly from the deltoid artery or its acromial branch, inferiorly from the profunda brachii, and posteriorly from the posterior circumflex humeral artery. They pierce the deep fascia around the perimeter of the deltoid muscle and form a rich network over the shoulder tip.

The Arm. The vessels arise medially from the brachial artery, its muscular branches, or the ulnar collateral arteries. Laterally they arise from the profunda brachii or its descending branches. They emerge in rows from the deep fascia over the medial and lateral intermuscular septa. Their branches radiate anteriorly and posteriorly to form a rich network over the biceps and triceps muscles, and longitudinally to accompany the cutaneous nerves.

The Forearm. The dominant supply is by longitudinal rows of perforators that arise from the distal brachial artery, the radial and ulnar recurrent vessels, the radial and ulnar arteries, and the anterior and posterior interosseous arteries—either from these vessels or from their muscular branches.

In the proximal forearm the direct cutaneous perforators may emerge between the muscles or may perforate the muscles directly. Their branches may be long and may accompany the cutaneous nerves of the forearm. In the distal aspect the perforators emerge between the muscles or between their tendons, and in general are smaller and closer together as they approach the wrist. Their branches radiate to form a rich network on the surface of the deep fascia.

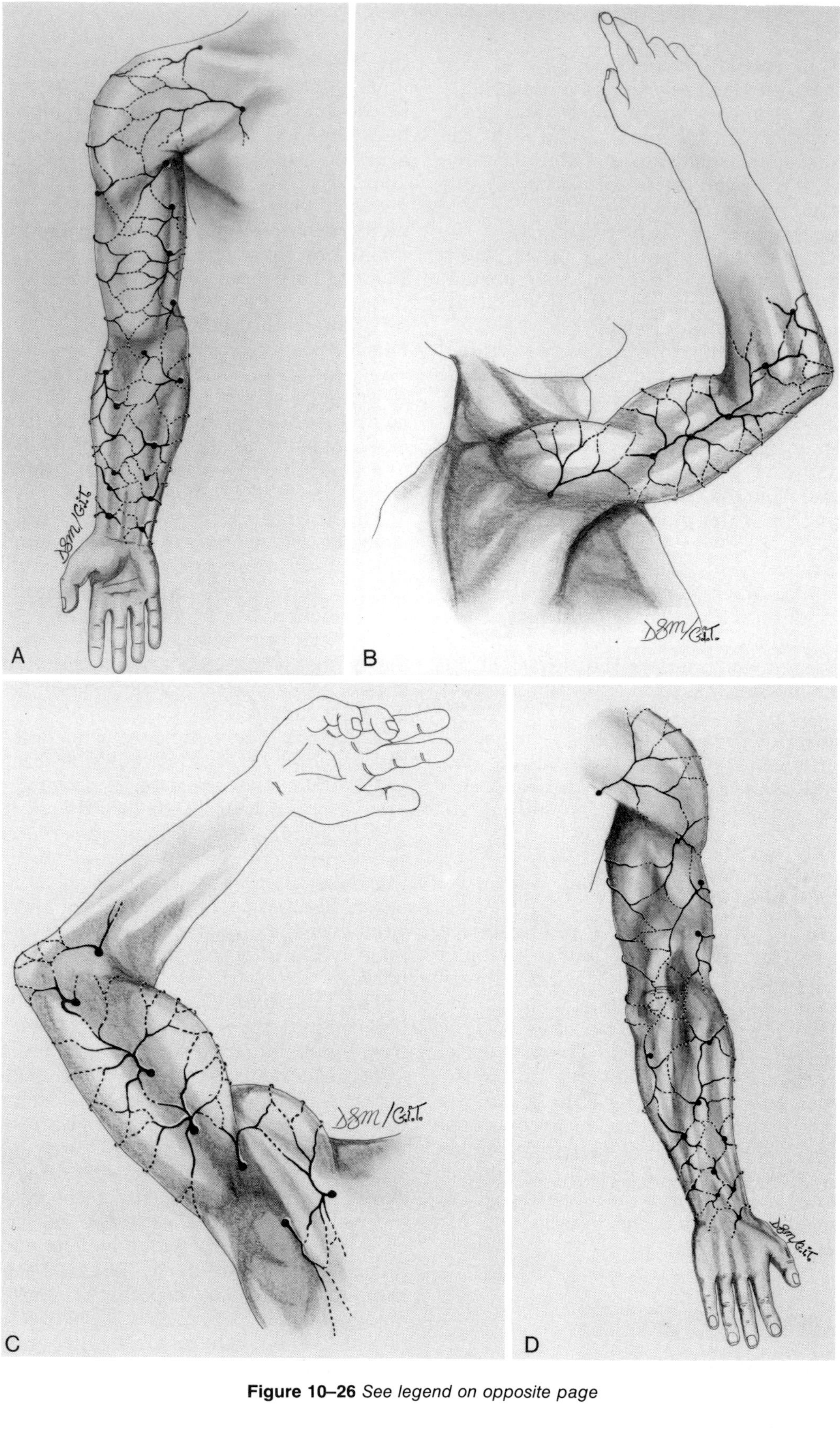

Figure 10–26 *See legend on opposite page*

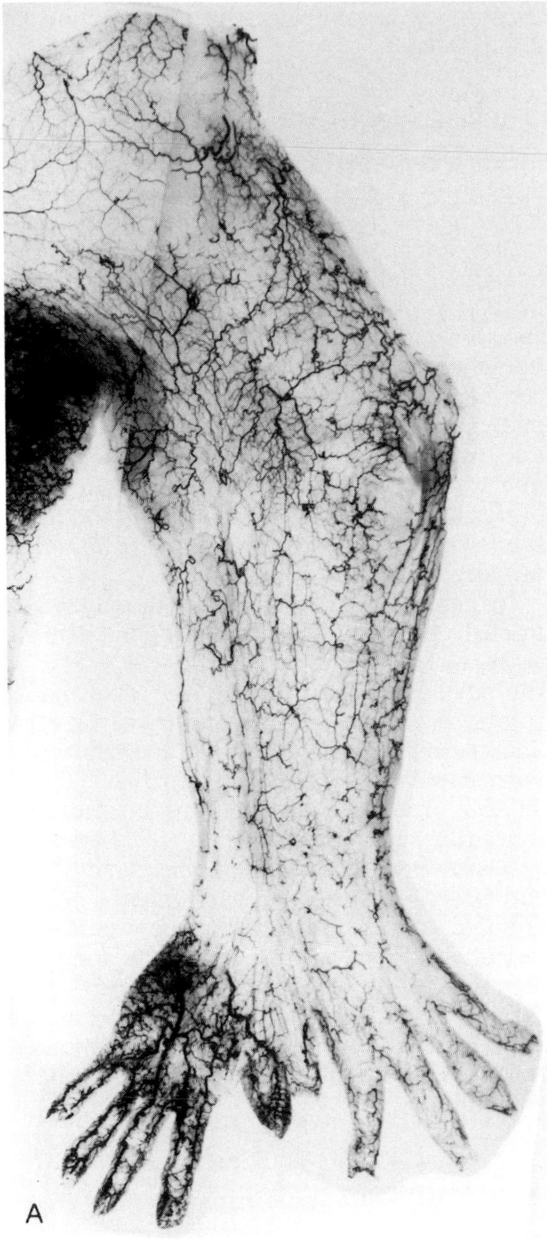
A

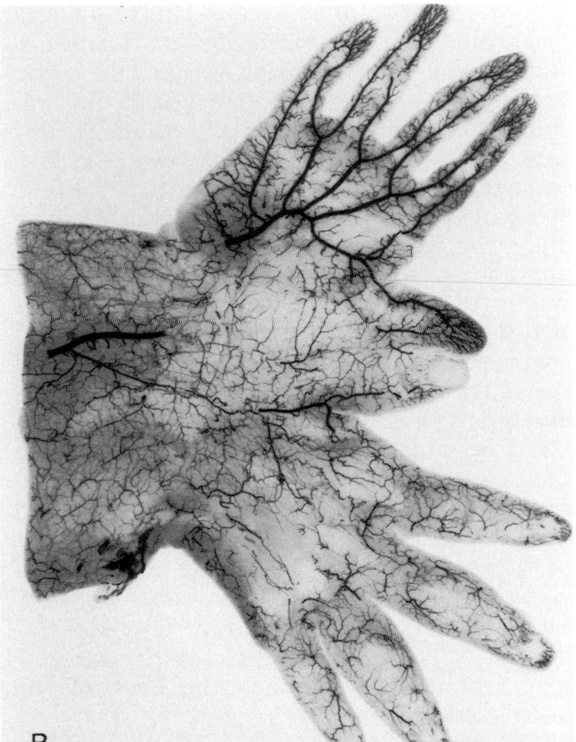
B

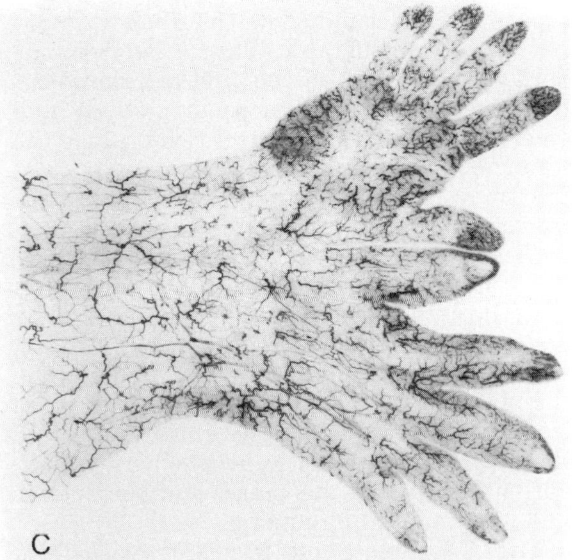
C

Figure 10–27. Radiographs of the integument of the upper limb and hand. The skin has been incised along the ulnar border in *A.* It has been removed with the deep fascia in *B* and without it in *C.* Note (1) the size and density of perforators in different regions of the limb, and especially compare them in the volar and dorsal aspects of the hand, and (2) the convergence of vessels over the dorsum of the joints of the thumb and fingers. (From Br. J. Plast. Surg.)

Figure 10–26. The cutaneous arterial network of the upper limb. Note that: 1. Perforators emerge around the perimeter of the deltoid and converge on the shoulder tip. 2. The longitudinal rows of perforators in the arm and forearm are usually in the region of the intermuscular septa. 3. The density of perforators increases toward the periphery as their size decreases. 4. The rich network of vessels converging over the olecranon and muscle bellies of the biceps and triceps. 5. The longitudinal orientation of vessels that parallel the cutaneous nerves. (From Taylor, G. I.: The Angiosomes of the Body. To be published by Churchill Livingstone.)

Anteriorly the vessels pierce the deep fascia most constantly in certain sites: on the medial side of the biceps tendon—from the distal brachial artery; from the surface of the brachioradialis muscle—from the radial recurrent artery; in the groove between the brachioradialis and flexor carpi radialis structures—arising from the radial artery; and from the surface of the flexor carpi ulnaris muscle, or the groove between it and the flexor digitorum sublimis—as perforators of the ulnar artery.

Posteriorly the vessels again emerge in rows. They pierce the deep fascia in the following sites: on the lateral side of the extensor carpi ulnaris muscle or its tendon—from the posterior radial recurrent and the posterior interosseous arteries; between the ulna and the flexor carpi ulnaris muscle—as a posterior branch of the ulnar artery; and between the tendons of the wrist extensors. The latter vessels arise from the anterior interosseous artery, and pierce the interosseous membrane to reach the back of the distal forearm.

The Hand. On the dorsum of the hand the vessels generally are larger and more widely separated to accommodate the relative laxity of the skin in this area. They arise from the dorsal metacarpal vessels and the radial artery in the intermetacarpal grooves and emerge between the extensor tendons. On the ulnar side a large vessel arises usually from the ulnar artery at the wrist and accompanies the dorsal branch of the ulnar nerve.

On the palmar aspect the vessels are short and numerous and accompany the septa that bind the skin to the palmar aponeurosis. They are smaller where the skin is rigidly fixed in the center of the palm, and larger over the thenar and hypothenar eminences. They arise from the underlying arteries and either pierce the aponeurosis, emerge between its prolongations, or pierce the muscles of the thenar and hypothenar eminences.

The Fingers. Short branches arise from the volar surface of the digital arteries in abundant numbers to accompany the fibrous septa. Dorsal branches arise proximally from the dorsal metacarpal arteries and radiate over the back of the proximal phalanges. Beyond this the dorsal branches are derived from the volar digital arteries. They radiate distally around the phalanges to the dorsum, and their branches converge from all directions to form networks in the loose skin over the dorsum of each interphalangeal and metacarpophalangeal joint.

In the pulp of the digits the density of branches is at a maximum where they again accompany the fibrous septa and form a vascular sponge.

APPLIED ANATOMY

Since the dominant cutaneous perforators supplying the shoulder, arm, and proximal forearm are sizable and spaced well apart, large flaps are available. Because their branches radiate in all directions, flaps can be based proximally or distally. Their axes can be orientated longitudinally, transversely, or obliquely, especially along the course of the cutaneous nerves. The same principles apply in the distal forearm, hand, and fingers. However, since the perforators and their territories are smaller, the design of large flaps usually incorporates the underlying source artery: e.g., the radial, ulnar, and digital vessel flaps.

In general, skin flaps should include the underlying deep fascia, since a dominant network is formed between the perforators on the surface of the fascia. The integument is relatively mobile over the bellies of the biceps and triceps muscles, and the perforators are vulnerable to degloving injuries as they emerge from the medial and lateral intermuscular septa.

A knowledge of the branches derived from the source arteries of each angiosome has enabled the design of many new cutaneous, musculocutaneous, and composite flaps from the upper limb for local and distant transfer. This information also provides a basis for explaining the patterns of tissue necrosis encountered in such conditions as Volkmann's ischemia.

The Trunk

The blood supply to the integument and the deeper layers of the anterior thorax, the abdomen, and the back reflects the embryologic growth, differentiation, and migration of the tissues in the area. To a large extent it is segmental and follows the pattern of the neurologic dermatomes.

The walls of the torso consist of an inner musculoskeletal barrel superimposed upon which is an outer layer of shoulder girdle muscles. The inner "barrel" of vertebrae, ribs, sternum, intercostal muscles, sacrospinalis muscle mass, and muscles of the abdominal wall are supplied segmentally by the posterior intercostal and lumbar vessels that link anteriorly with corresponding branches of the paired internal thoracic–deep epigastric systems. They form a series of lateral arches extending from the thoracic inlet to the groin. The paired internal thoracic–deep epigastric systems similarly form longitudinal ventral arches between the subclavian and external iliac vessels. Perforators arise from the longitudinal and transverse arches, particularly in the paravertebral region, in the midaxillary line, and adjacent to the ventral midline.

The shoulder girdle muscles have migrated downward onto the thorax from the cervical and upper thoracic myotomes. They are accompanied by their neurovascular pedicles that arise in the neck and in the axilla to lie outside the plane of the inner musculoskeletal barrel. The neurovascular pedicles of the trapezius, latissimus dorsi, rotator cuff, pectoralis major, and serratus anterior muscles all follow this pattern. When the migrating muscles flow onto the chest wall, they receive in sequence secondary and tertiary vascular territories from the perforators of the deep arcades (the intercostal, internal thoracic, and deep epigastric systems) as these vessels pass through the muscles en route to the skin.

The above pattern of development and supply to the deep tissues determines the site of origin of the cutaneous perforators. The following factors influence the size and orientation of these vessels:

1. The extension of the fetus.
2. The expansion of the abdominal and thoracic cavities.
3. The closure of the abdominal wall at the umbilicus.
4. The loose skin areas that develop over the torso, especially over the pectoralis major muscles and the anterolateral abdominal wall.
5. The development of the breast in the female.

In the limbs the direct perforators tend to emerge from the deep fascia in longitudinal rows between muscles, but in the torso they are grouped in broader bands or clusters. They pierce the fascia at fixed skin sites. They flow onto the torso from the neck, axillae, and groins or emerge from the deeper tissues after piercing the muscles and their aponeurotic tendons and sheaths, or appear between the muscles, especially where they interdigitate.

The muscles of the torso are generally wide and flat and this has some bearing on the arrangement of the perforators. The muscle attachments are often broad, and when the perforators pierce them they usually do so close to the muscle attachments. This is in keeping with the concept that vessels hug fixed tissue regions.

The vessels are often large. They interconnect and radiate to span mobile skin areas, traveling frequently for very long distances. The location of these dominant cutaneous perforators in relation to their respective angiosomes, their sites of emergence from the deep fascia, and their subsequent course and interconnections are shown in Figures 10–3, 10–4, 10–8 to 10–10, 10–28 to 10–31. Many of these vessels have been described in detail elsewhere. They emerge from the deep fascia and arise *usually:*

1. *Anteriorly.*
   a. From the supraclavicular fossa as branches of the transverse cervical or suprascapular arteries that flow over the clavicle onto the chest with the supraclavicular nerves.
   b. From the parasternal region as perforators of the internal thoracic artery. They pierce the pectoralis major muscle near its insertion. One vessel usually dominates. It is oriented toward the nipple and emerges in most cases from the second or third intercostal space. It plays a major role in the supply of the breast (see Figs. 10–3, 10–4, 10–29, 10–30).
   c. From the inframammary crease as perforators of the anterior intercostal branches of the internal thoracic artery. They emerge usually from the fourth or fifth intercostal space and are large in the female breast.
   d. From just below the costal margin as a large cutaneous branch of the deep superior epigastric artery, which arises usually from the lateral division of that artery and is named the *superficial* superior epigastric artery; it courses downward and laterally.
   e. As a band of perforators that emerge from the anterior rectus sheath or appear along its lateral border. In the

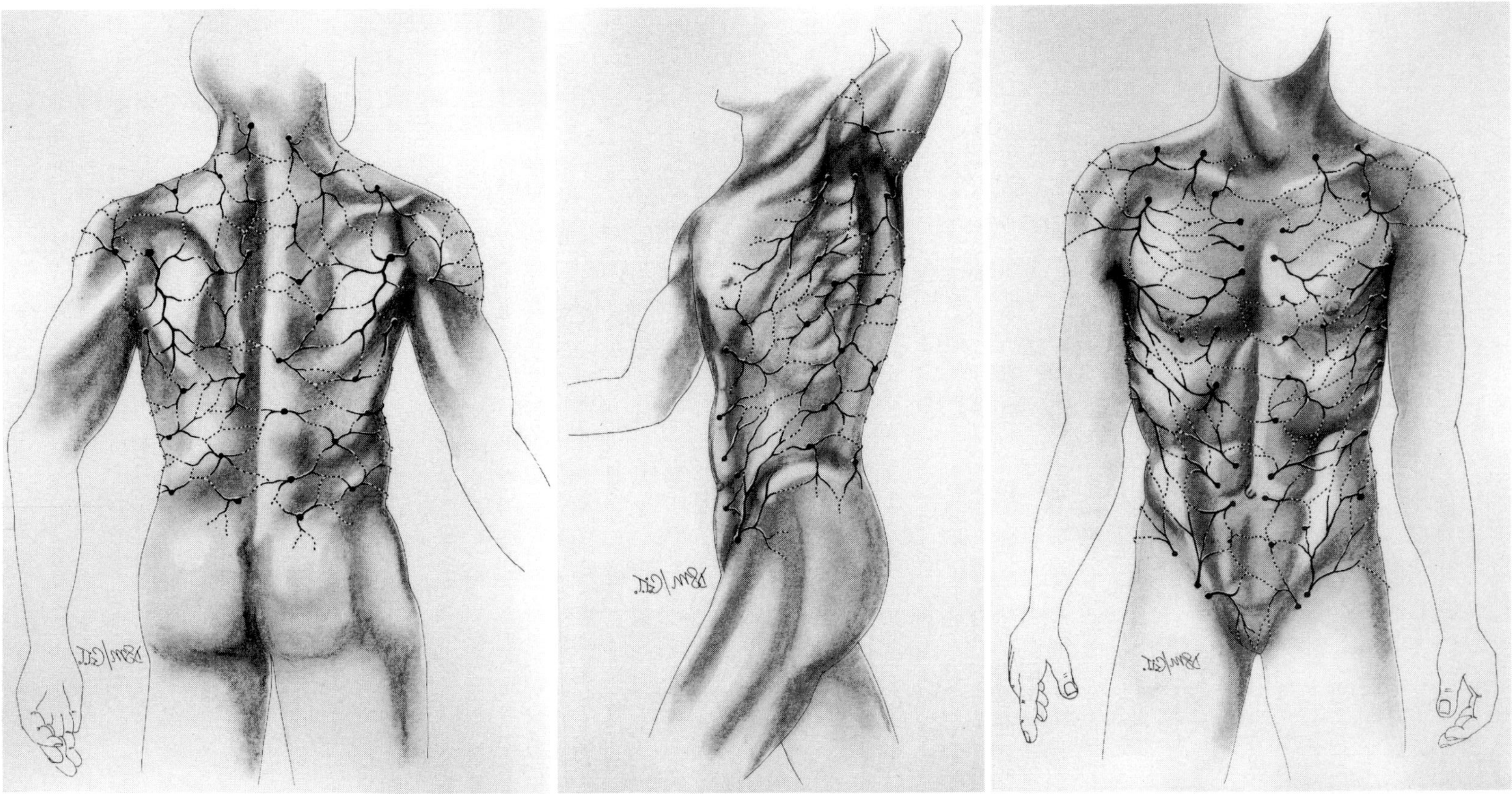

Figure 10–28. The arterial network of the skin of the trunk. Note (1) the overflow of vessels onto the trunk from the neck, axillae, and groins; (2) the bands of perforators that emerge from the fixed skin regions and the large perforators that appear from the second or third intercostal space, the costal margin, the paraumbilical region, the groin, and the axilla and near the lateral border of the scapula; and (3) the rich interconnecting network of vessels in the loose skin areas, especially over the pectoral muscles and iliac fossae and back of the scapula. (From Taylor, G. I.: The Angiosomes of the Body. To be published by Churchill Livingstone.)

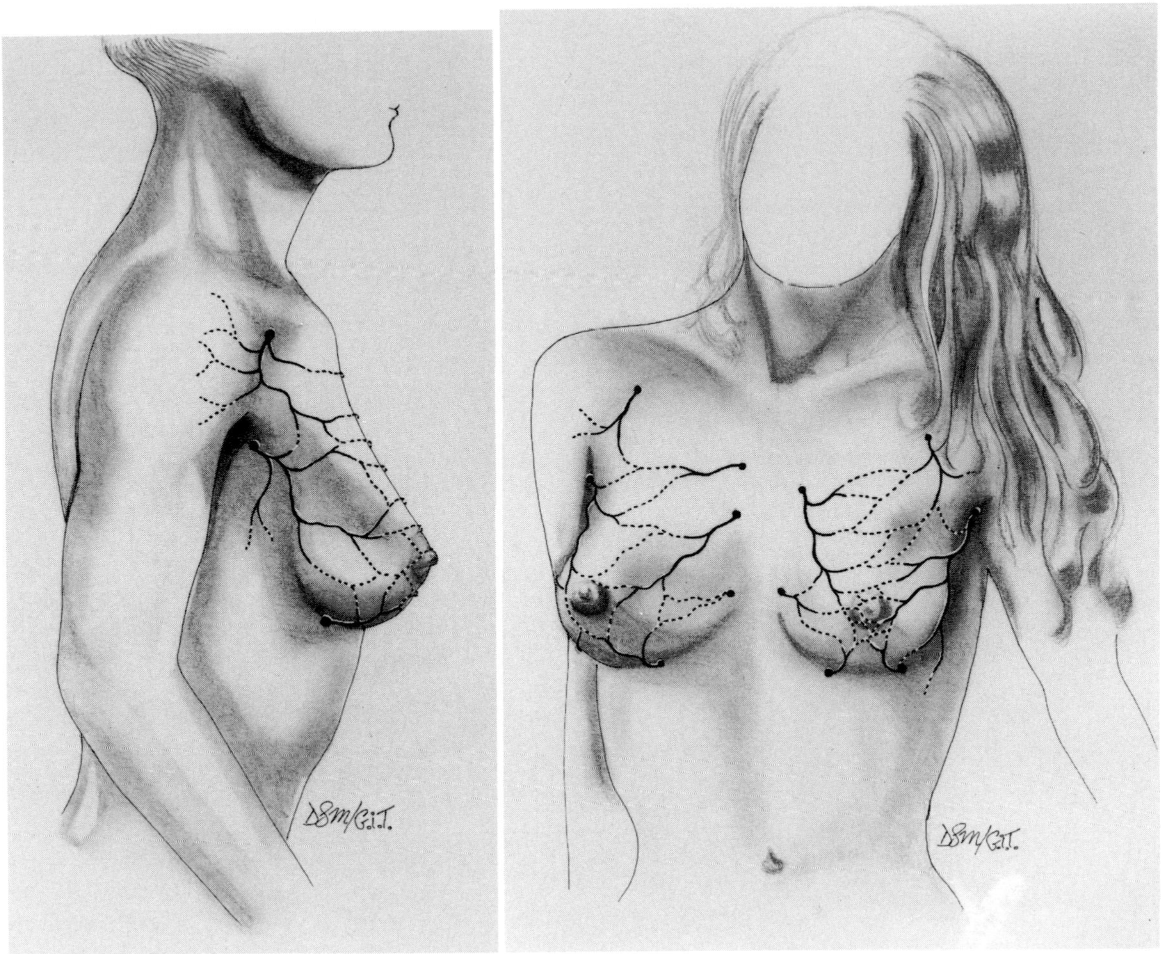

Figure 10–29. The dominant arteries supplying the breast. They emerge particularly from the axilla, from the second or third intercostal space, and in the region of the inframammary groove. They converge to form a rich network in the nipple-areola area. (From Taylor, G. I.: The Angiosomes of the Body. To be published by Churchill Livingstone.)

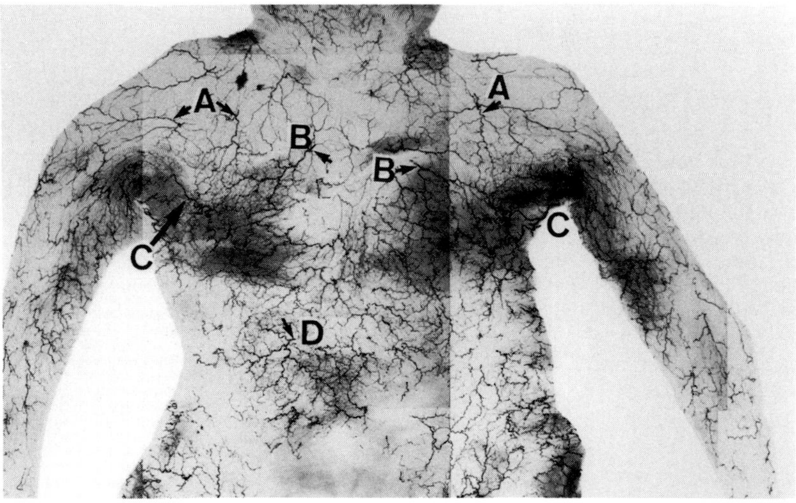

Figure 10–30. Radiograph of the anterior chest and shoulders. Note the large perforators of the acromiothoracic axis *(A)* and the internal thoracic *(B)*, lateral thoracic *(C)*, and deep superior epigastric *(D)* arteries. (From Br. J. Plast. Surg.)

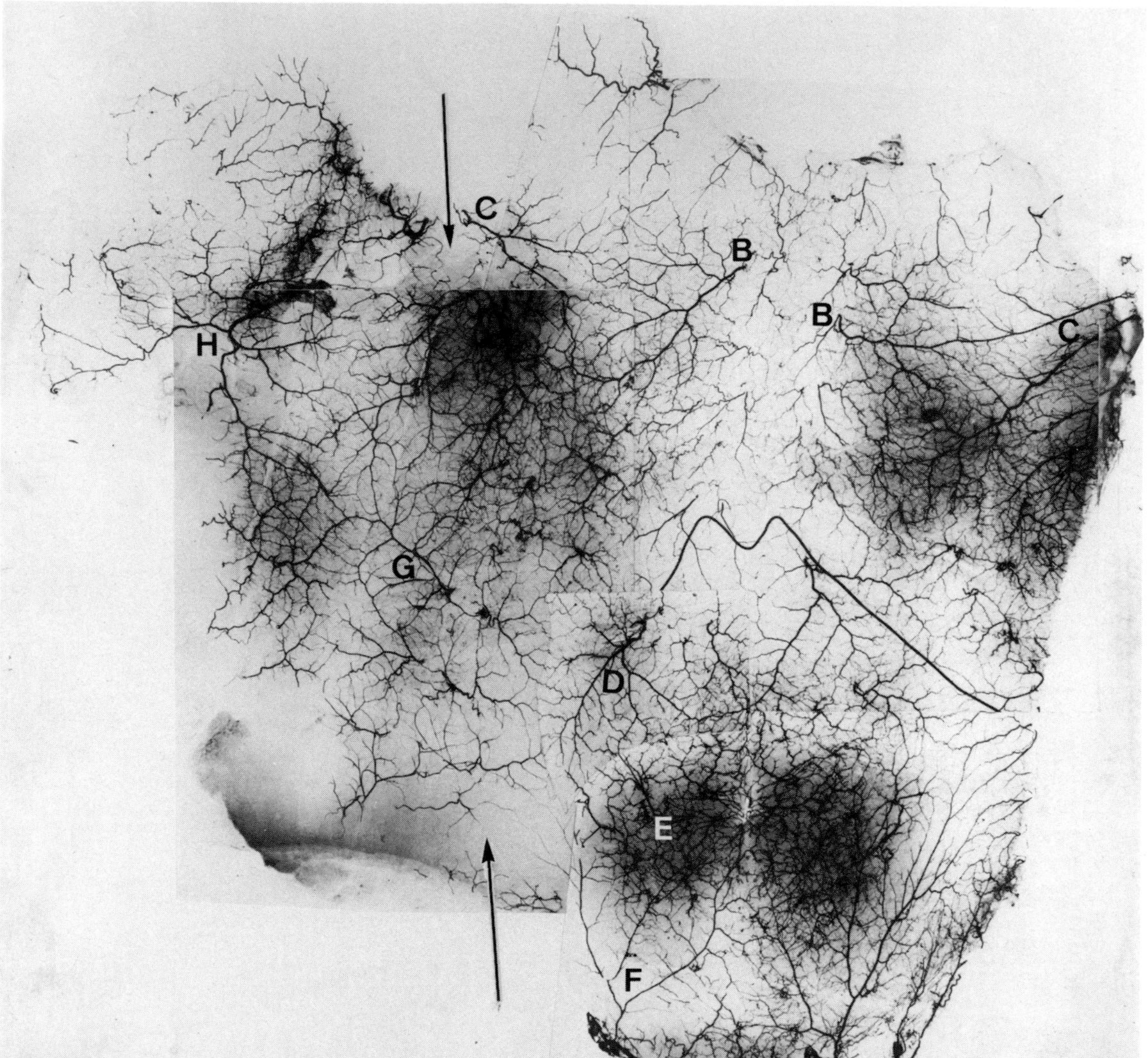

Figure 10–31. Radiograph of the integument of the trunk from the dorsal midline to the left midaxillary line. The costal margin and right midaxillary line *(arrows)* of the subject are indicated. Note (1) the oblique pathway of vessels extending from the groin to the scapula, established by the branches and choke connections of the large superficial inferior epigastric *(F)*, paraumbilical *(E)*, superficial superior epigastric *(D)*, intercostal *(G)*, and circumflex scapular *(H)* perforators—other perforators are labeled as in Figure 10–30; and (2) the rich midline crossover in the abdomen compared with the diminutive connections across the sternum in this male subject. (From Br. J. Plast. Surg.)

epigastrium they arise from the deep *superior* epigastric artery and below this from the deep *inferior* system. The largest perforators are clustered around the umbilicus. They are continuations of the main branches of the deep inferior epigastric artery. They radiate in all directions, but predominantly upward and laterally parallel to the ribs.

f. From the groin as the external pudendal, superficial inferior epigastric, and superficial circumflex iliac branches of the common femoral artery. They radiate from their origin, as described by McGregor and Jackson (1972), "like the spokes of a wheel." They are, however, subject to considerable variation (Taylor and Daniel, 1975).

2. *Laterally.*
   a. From the deltopectoral groove as a large branch of the deltoid artery or its acromial branch.
   b. From the axilla as a large vessel, sometimes referred to as the *superficial thoracic artery,* which courses toward the nipple. Its origin is variable and it may arise from the lateral thoracic artery or thoracodorsal artery or directly from the axillary artery. It is a major vessel supplying the female breast and links constantly in the nipple region with the dominant perforator of the internal thoracic artery (see Figs. 10–3, 10–4, 10–29 to 10–31).
   c. From between the digitations and interdigitations of the serratus anterior, external oblique, and latissimus dorsi muscles. These perforators are subdivisions of the lateral branches of the posterior intercostal arteries. They radiate in all directions but have a dominant axis parallel to the ribs.
   d. From the region of the iliac crest as perforators of the deep circumflex iliac artery. These are usually small *indirect* perforators but occasionally are large, especially if the superficial circumflex iliac artery is small. This is another example of "the law of equilibrium."
3. *Posteriorly.*
   The skin is firmly attached to the deep fascia over most regions of the back and especially over the dorsal midline. It is relatively mobile over the shoulder girdle and the lumbar fascia. A rich network of large vessels supplies this region derived from the transverse cervical, circumflex scapular, thoracodorsal, posterior intercostal, and lumbar vessels (see Figs. 10–3, 10–4, 10–9, 10–28, 10–30).
   a. The transverse cervical perforators emerge from the trapezius muscle above the spine of the scapula and flow downward onto the back.
   b. The circumflex scapular artery, the largest branch of the subscapular vessel, provides a large perforator that emerges from the triangular space between the teres major, the teres minor, and the long head of the triceps muscle. It may be very long and may reach as far as the twelfth rib. Its general direction is downward and medially roughly parallel to the fibers of the latissimus dorsi muscle. It branches medially and laterally as it descends. One of its upper medial branches is usually large and constant.
   c. The thoracodorsal artery provides a number of perforators that emerge from the latissimus dorsi muscle laterally.
   d. The posterior intercostal vessels provide the dominant supply to the skin of the back. Their perforators pierce the muscles that have migrated from the cervical region, namely, the trapezius and latissimus dorsi muscles. They provide a major contribution to each of these muscles and then appear from their surface as a broad band of vessels in the paravertebral region, and a band that fans laterally over the lower region of the back. One of the perforators provides a large descending muscular branch that links with the deep branch of the transverse cervical artery to supply the lower half of the trapezius muscle (see Fig. 10–19).
   e. The lumbar arteries provide large perforators that emerge above the iliac crest to supply the lower back.

APPLIED ANATOMY

A multitude of flaps have been designed on the direct cutaneous vessels supplying the torso. In fact, in this region it is almost impossible to design a flap that is not based on a major perforator. There are many mobile skin areas, as gauged by the "pinch test," between the fixed skin zones. It is in these mobile regions that large vessels course for long distances parallel to the skin surface, for example, in the iliac fossa. Here the vessels are separated from the deep fascia by loose areolar tissue as they rapidly approach the subdermal plexus.

In most cases it is not necessary to include the deep fascia with cutaneous flaps; indeed, it may be technically difficult to do so. The deep fascia is sometimes poorly understood by some authors in their description of flaps in this region. In most areas the deep fascia is firmly attached to the deep tissues. Its structure varies considerably by comparison with its counterpart in the limbs. It forms the perimysium of the muscles, the external oblique aponeurosis, the lumbar fascia, and the rectus sheath and it is continued between muscles to form septa, clefts, and tendinous intersections.

It is impossible to give an account of the plethora of flaps on the trunk that are available to the surgeon. However, the following points have been chosen as examples to illustrate the importance of the vascular anatomy in this area:

1. The vertical zone of perforators that emerge in the paravertebral region, the midaxillary line, and the area adjacent to the ventral midline provide the basis for a large number of long transverse or oblique flaps (see Fig. 10–35).

2. The centripetal arrangement of perforators that converge on the nipple from around the perimeter of the breast accounts for the versatility and variety of the various breast reduction procedures (see Fig. 10–29).

3. With careful planning, large vascular territories can be captured in succession from adjacent angiosomes to provide very long flaps. For example, the deltopectoral flap captures the territory of the acromiothoracic perforator(s) on the internal thoracic vessels. If the flap is extended beyond the shoulder tip with a delay, it borrows another large territory—the large perforator of the posterior circumflex humeral angiosome. The long thoracoepigastric tube pedicle of Webster (1937) consists of three substantial territories, each supplied by large perforators—the superficial inferior epigastric, the large perforators of the posterior intercostals, and the lateral thoracic. The skin paddle of the extended deep inferior epigastric flap captures the lateral intercostal branches of the posterior intercostal arteries on the large paraumbilical perforators of the deep inferior system. In each case, choke vessels connect the arteries of adjacent territories.

4. In many cases the skin paddle of a musculocutaneous flap is supplied by perforators of an adjacent angiosome, captured by choke connections between the muscular arteries. When the skin paddle of a pectoralis major flap is placed laterally over the muscle, it is supplied by indirect perforators of the pectoral artery. When it is designed medially in the parasternal region or in the inframammary crease, it is supplied by the captured direct and indirect perforators of the internal thoracic artery.

The Lower Limb

The arrangement of the vessels is similar to that of the upper extremity. The dominant direct perforators emerge from the deep fascia around the perimeter of the gluteus maximus, radiate from the groin and popliteal fossa, and emerge in longitudinal rows in the grooves between the muscles. They converge on the convexities over the muscles, especially the gluteus maximus, quadriceps group, and gastrocnemius, and over the prominences of the knee and back of the Achilles tendon. They are large and spaced well apart in the proximal limb and, except where they accompany cutaneous nerves, the direct cutaneous arteries become progressively smaller and more numerous toward the periphery (Figs. 10–32 to 10–34). Their maximal density is in the sole of the foot. In most areas they course for considerable distances in the loose areolar layer on the surface of the deep fascia, where they interconnect to form a rich network.

The Buttock. This is a fixed skin region where the integument is well padded with fat lobules and bound firmly to the deep fascia over the gluteus maximus by numerous septa, similar to the palms of the hands and soles of the feet. The skin is bound around the perimeter of the gluteus muscle, especially over the natal cleft, gluteal fold, iliac crest, and iliotibial tract. Large perforators appear around this perimeter and form a plexus over the summit of the muscle. They are reinforced by direct and indirect perforators of the superior and inferior gluteal arteries that emerge from the intramuscular septa of the gluteus maximus. The versatility of large cutaneous and musculocutaneous flaps designed in this area attests to its abundant blood supply.

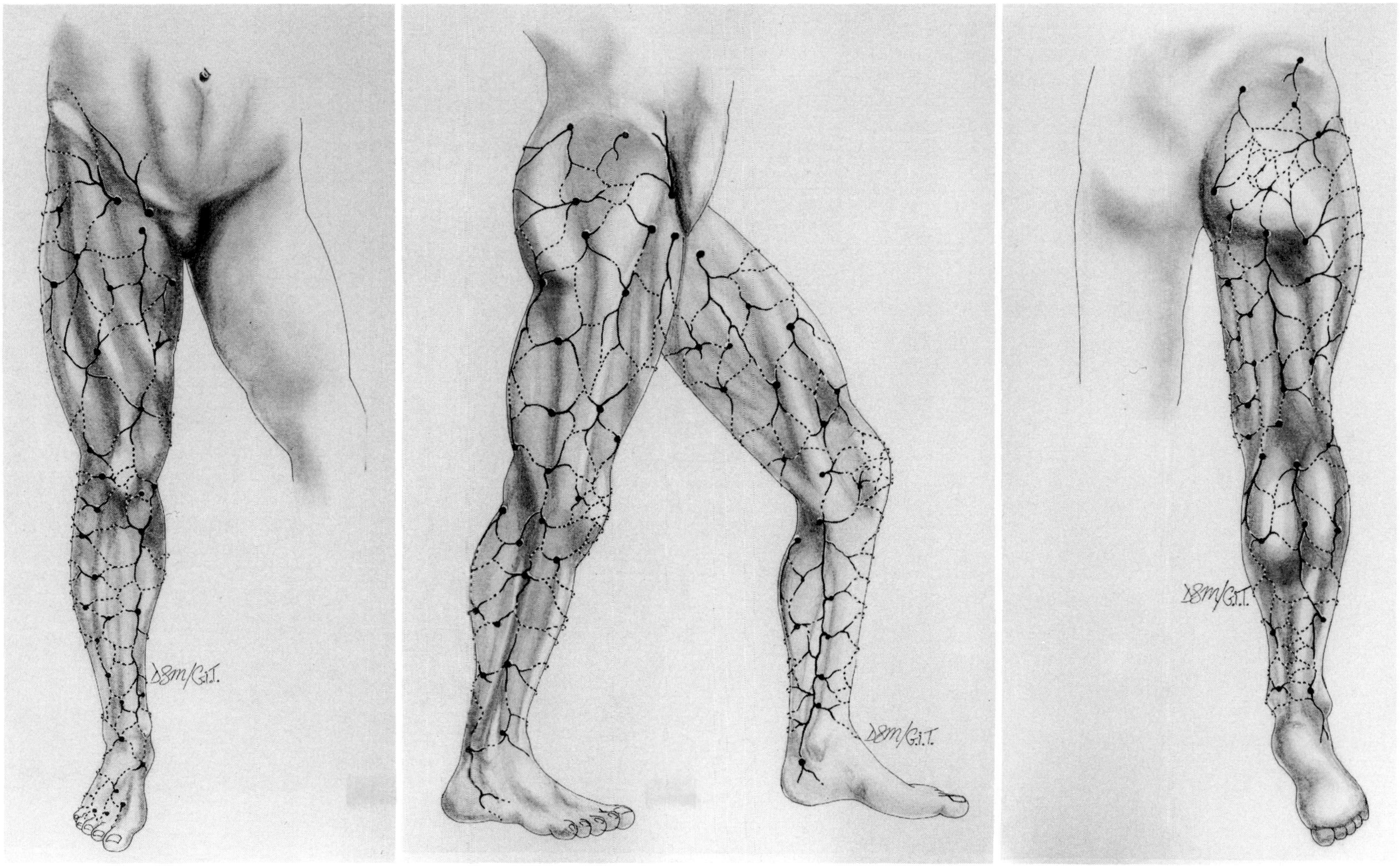

Figure 10–32. The arterial network of the lower limbs. Note (1) the emergence of perforators around the perimeter of the buttock and in longitudinal rows between the muscles or beside the tibia; (2) the radiation of vessels from the groin and the popliteal fossa; (3) the convergence of vessels to form rich networks over the gluteus maximus, vastus lateralis, gastrocnemius muscle, the patella, and the tendo Achillis; and (4) the dominant axis of vessels that parallel the medial or intermediate cutaneous nerve of the thigh, the posterior cutaneous nerve of the thigh, and the saphenous and sural nerves. (From Br. J. Plast. Surg.)

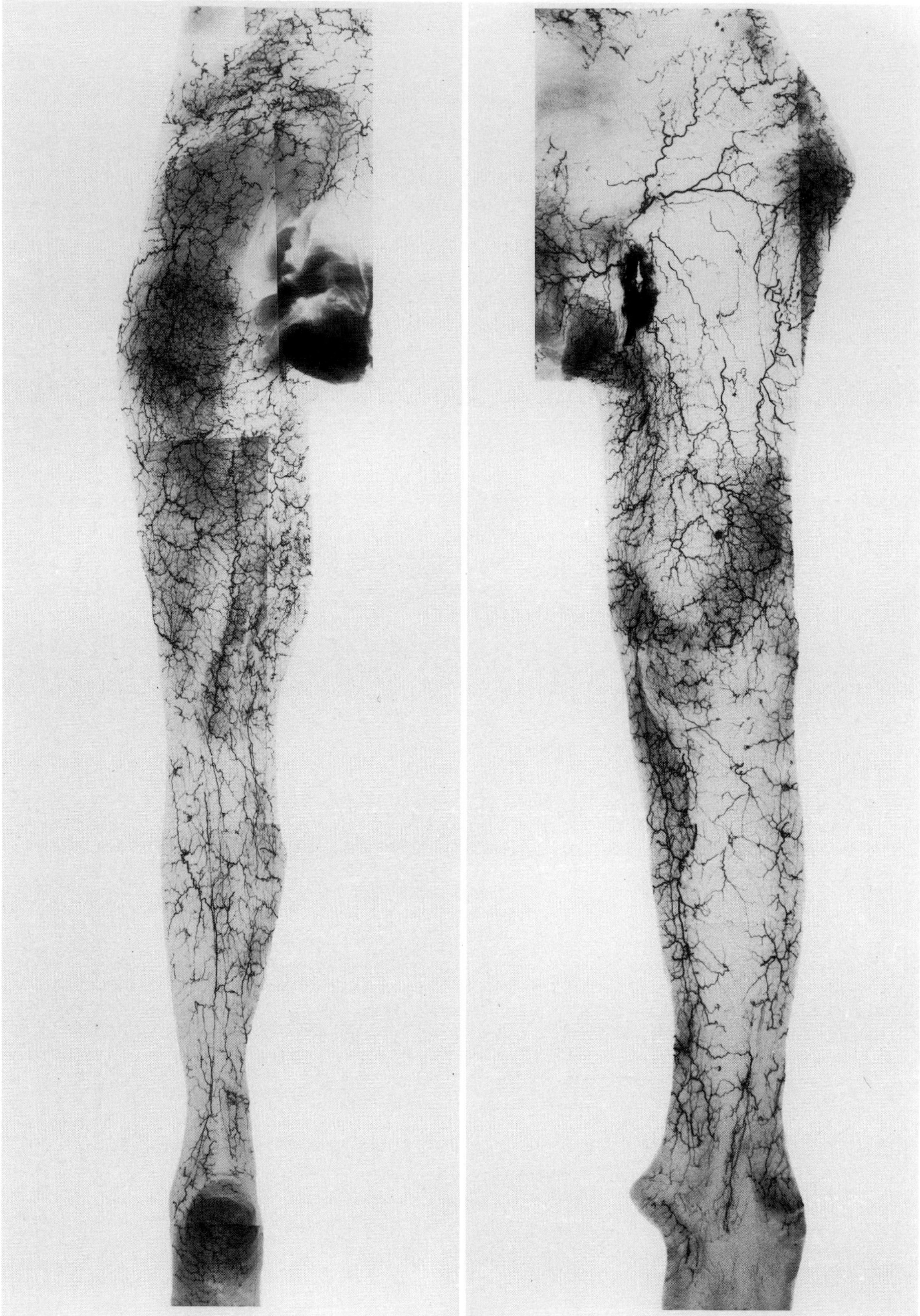

Figure 10–33. Radiographs of the integument of the anterior *(left)* and posterior *(right)* aspects of the lower limb, excluding the forefoot. Note the position and size of vessels compared with Figure 10–32, the poor network of vessels over the subcutaneous surface of the tibia, and the well-established vertical pathways of vessels that accompany the cutaneous nerves in this subject. (From Br. J. Plast. Surg.)

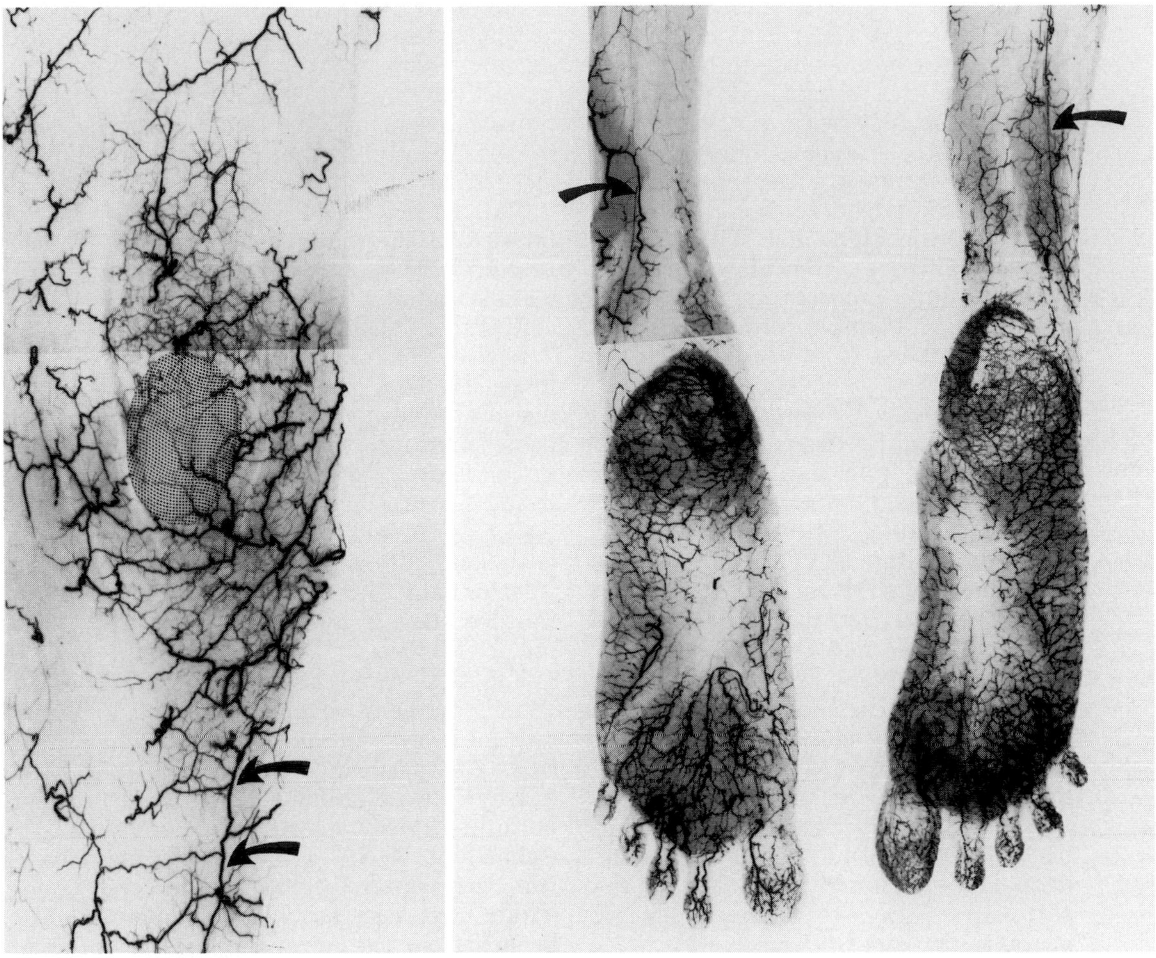

Figure 10–34. Radiograph of the skin over the front of the knee *(left)* and the soles of the feet *(right)*. Note the convergence of vessels over the patella *(shaded)*; the profusion of small vessels in this fixed skin region of the feet; and the longitudinal orientation of vessels that accompany the cutaneous nerves *(arrows)*. (From Br. J. Plast. Surg.)

The perforators that emerge around the perimeter of the muscle arise:

1. Above from the lumbar vessels, especially the fourth.
2. Medially from the internal pudendal and sacral arteries.
3. Below from the inferior gluteal.
4. Laterally from the superior gluteal. They are reinforced by terminal branches of the superficial circumflex iliac artery.

The Thigh. The dominant supply to this region is by the cartwheel of vessels that emerge from the groin and by longitudinal rows of vessels that emerge between the muscles, particularly in relation to the well-defined intermuscular septa (see Figs. 10–32, 10–33). Although several large vessels arise from the common and superficial femoral vessels, most can be traced to the profunda, lateral femoral circumflex, and other unnamed muscular branches as they course between the muscles of the thigh. The muscular branches of the common and superficial femoral arteries are subject to considerable variation. Nevertheless, the sites of emergence of their cutaneous perforators from the deep fascia, their numbers, and their subsequent course and distribution are relatively constant. The largest perforators pierce the deep fascia and emerge:

1. *Anteriorly.*
   a. From the femoral triangle as a radiating cobweb of arteries, derived from the common femoral artery or sometimes from the beginning of the profunda artery. They fan to supply the lower abdomen, upper thigh, and genitalia. They are the superficial external pu-

dendal, the superficial inferior epigastric (SIEA), the superficial circumflex iliac (SCIA), and a large unnamed artery, sometimes duplicated, which descends vertically with the medial or intermediate cutaneous nerves of the thigh. These arteries frequently have a common origin from the femoral artery, especially the SIEA and SCIA (Taylor and Daniel, 1975). They pierce the deep fascia, usually around the perimeter of the femoral triangle, after supplying small branches to the adjacent deep tissues.

   b. In vertical rows: between the vastus lateralis and rectus femoris muscles—arising from the lateral femoral circumflex artery and particularly its long descending branch. They also emerge on either side of the sartorius muscle—derived from the superficial femoral artery or its muscular branches to the vastus medialis and adductor brevis muscles. The lowest of the latter row of vessels, the saphenous artery, is a branch of the descending genicular artery, just after the genicular vessel arises from the terminal part of the superficial femoral artery. It accompanies the saphenous nerve and pierces the deep fascia behind the tendon of the sartorius at the level of the upper end of the tibia.

2. *Posteriorly.*
   a. From the gluteal fold emerging at the lower border of the gluteus maximus muscle. They are derived from the inferior gluteal artery and radiate to the thigh as well as to the buttock. A large branch often descends to form a chain-link system of vessels that accompanies the posterior cutaneous nerve of the thigh (see Figs. 10–32, 10–33).
   b. In a vertical row between the vastus lateralis and the biceps femoris, derived from the profunda femoris artery.
   c. From the upper apex of the popliteal fossa as a perforator that arises from the popliteal artery and ascends in the midline of the thigh.
3. *Medially.* In vertical rows between the adductor muscles and along the anterior and posterior borders of the gracilis muscle. The perforators are derived from the muscular branches of the profunda artery, especially the large unnamed branches to the adductor muscles.

The above vessels represent the dominant supply to the integument of the thigh. Other large vessels may emerge between the hamstring muscles or from the surface of muscles, especially the lower end of the rectus femoris, vastus medialis, and sartorius muscles.

The Knee. This is an important region because of the many incisions that are used to gain access to the knee joint. In general, vessels radiate from the popliteal fossa and converge on the kneecap.

Few vessels pierce the roof of the popliteal fossa. Instead, they emerge from the deep fascia around its perimeter and radiate to the posterior thigh, the calf, and the front of the knee. They arise posteriorly in the midline from the proximal and distal ends of the popliteal artery or its muscular (sural) branches, laterally from the superior and inferior genicular arteries, and medially from the descending genicular artery and its saphenous branch.

The skin over the patella is mobile, and vessels converge over its surface to form a rich network. In addition to contributions from the perforators described above, this network is established by further rows of perforators that pierce the deep fascia on either side of the patella. They are derived from the medial, lateral, and descending genicular arteries, as well as a substantial branch from the anterior tibial or its recurrent genicular branch.

The Leg. The attachments and various modifications of the deep fascia in this surgically important region play a major role in determining the pattern of the cutaneous perforators. In the leg the deep fascia is a very rigid stocking attached proximally to the head of the tibia and fibula, the margins of the patella, the tendons of the hamstring muscles medially and laterally, and the ligamentum patellae. It becomes the periosteum of the subcutaneous surface of the tibia. It is modified distally to form the extensor retinaculae, and it is lashed to the fibula by its anterior and posterior intermuscular septa.

Thus, the deep tissues are segregated into three compartments: (1) a large posterior compartment between the tibia and the posterior intermuscular septum where the gastrocnemius and soleus muscles are mobile beneath the deep fascia; (2) a peroneal compartment between the anterior and posterior intermuscular septa where the muscles attach to the septa but glide beneath the outer layer of the deep fascia; and (3) a narrow anterior compartment where the muscles are wedged between, and attach to, the tibia and the anterior intermuscular septum.

The direct perforators emerge from the deep fascia in longitudinal rows in close relation to the subcutaneous borders of the tibia and the intermuscular septa, from the popliteal fossa and from the surface of the gastrocnemius muscle. They branch in stellate form and interconnect on the surface of the deep fascia over the bulges of the muscles. Their branches are well developed in relation to the saphenous and sural nerves, where they course longitudinally for longer distances and interconnect in chain-link fashion, often without change in caliber. They arise:

1. From the popliteal artery or its sural branches to the gastrocnemius muscle. These vessels emerge in the midline between the heads of the gastrocnemius or pierce the muscle directly, especially near its perimeter. In the midline they accompany the sural nerve and short saphenous vein. The largest of these, the small saphenous artery, arises usually from the medial sural artery.

2. As the saphenous branch of the descending genicular artery. This vessel emerges behind the tendon of the sartorius and descends with the saphenous nerve and long saphenous vein for a variable distance.

3. From the anterior tibial artery. Proximally the perforators are larger; they arise usually from the muscular arteries and emerge beside the tibia or from between the sandwiched muscles. Distally they are smaller; they arise from the anterior tibial artery and emerge between the extensor tendons.

4. From the peroneal artery. The major perforators are of considerable size, usually four or five in number, and emerge in relation to the posterior intermuscular septum. Proximally they tend to pierce the muscles of the soleus and peroneus longus, close to the septum, whereas distally they usually hug the septum and emerge between the flexor hallucis longus and peroneus brevis. A large perforator emerges usually on the lateral side of the Achilles tendon above the ankle joint, and sends proximal and distal branches to accompany the sural nerve and its lateral branch.

5. From the posterior tibial artery. This vessel provides a row of six or seven perforators that emerge behind the tibia and connect with the saphenous branch of the descending genicular artery. They supply the medial side of the calf and form a chain-link system of vessels to accompany the saphenous nerve. Their origin is from the muscular branches to the soleus and the tibialis posterior. The branches radiate anteriorly over the periosteum of the subcutaneous surface of the tibia and posteriorly over the bulge of the calf muscles.

The Ankle and the Foot. Except for the extensor digitorum brevis, there is no muscle around the ankle or on the dorsum of the foot. The source arteries and their branches are closely related to bone and their arrangement is subject to considerable anatomic variation. The cutaneous branches in general are small, sparse, and vulnerable to trauma.

The ankle region is supplied by small branches of the anterior tibial artery, the medial and lateral malleolar arteries, the posterior tibial artery, and the posterior terminal branch of the peroneal artery. The last-named may descend for a considerable distance along the lateral side of the ankle and heel.

The dorsum of the foot receives branches from the dorsalis pedis artery, its tarsal branches, and especially its first dorsal metatarsal branch. These emerge from around the extensor hallucis longus tendon and the belly of the extensor digitorum brevis muscle. Perforators are sparse laterally, as is the arterial network.

The sole of the foot, by contrast, receives a rich blood supply from numerous perforators that arise from the medial and lateral plantar arteries, especially on either side of the flexor digitorum brevis muscle. They exhibit the same pattern as the perforators in the palm of the hand, and hug the fibrous septa that bind the skin to the plantar aponeurosis.

The perforators are long near the heel and become progressively shorter toward the toes. They pass vertically toward the skin and then branch medially and laterally to form a rich network, especially in the "footprint" area of the sole. In the region of the apex of the concavity of the sole, the perforators are small and less numerous.

APPLIED ANATOMY

Much attention has been focused on the anatomy of the arteries and veins in the lower limb, especially in relation to incisions around the groin and knee and the design of local and distant flaps to provide tissue for free transfer. Examples follow:

Incisions. During a groin dissection the hub of large radiating perforators is disconnected from the superficial femoral artery. The perforators with which they link around their perimeter are at a considerable distance. It is well known that flaps raised in this dissection are at best tenuous. For this reason a vertical or gently curved incision, centered over the femoral artery, is favored by most surgeons. Wide zigzag incisions or Z-plasties are avoided since they frequently result in extensive flap necrosis.

Bilateral parapatellar incisions place the skin over the knee cap in jeopardy, especially when they are curved toward the midline at each end. This is because vessels arise from around the perimeter of the patella and radiate to converge in the loose skin over its surface. *Anatomically* the safest incisions are those designed vertically or transversely over the center of the patella, or broad flaps that circumnavigate this bone and are based superiorly, medially, or laterally.

Local Flaps. The rigid length-breadth ratios have been abandoned in many areas owing to a precise knowledge of the underlying vasculature. Flaps that include the deep fascia and especially those designed along the course of cutaneous nerves have extended flap dimensions. Many are now based distally; they are possible because the perforators radiate in all directions and are well developed where they accompany these nerves.

Cross Leg Flaps. The conventional, medially based, transverse cross leg flap is nourished usually by the perforators of the posterior tibial artery that emerge behind the subcutaneous border of the tibia. However, long oblique or vertical flaps designed on the saphenous chain-link system of vessels, or the sural vessels, have increased the versatility of this procedure.

Island Flaps. The inclusion of the underlying source artery has, in select cases, extended the use of local flaps and provided donor sites for free transfer: e.g., the dorsalis pedis and peroneal artery flaps. The inclusion of other tissues within the same or adjacent angiosome, such as muscle, tendon, or bone, has also expanded the surgeon's armamentarium. For example, the underlying extensor tendons can be included with the dorsalis pedis flap, and the fibula can be transferred with skin, designed on either the peroneal or anterior tibial artery. The latter is possible since the fibula is overlapped by these two angiosomes.

Degloving Injuries. The lower limb is prone to trauma, and the perforators are subject to damage from shearing forces as they emerge from the deep fascia. Similarly, their branches are vulnerable as they depart from the surface of the deep fascia after coursing on its surface. These problems are prevalent, particularly over the subcutaneous surface of the tibia and around the ankle joint. The deep fascia is rigid as it becomes the periosteum of the bone; the vessels are easily torn; the network is not well developed; and trauma to these areas is common.

CLINICAL APPLICATIONS

The anatomic information outlined in this chapter represents an attempt to correlate the efforts of many workers, especially those of Manchot (1889) and Salmon (1936a,b). It aims to provide some concepts to aid in the design of flaps and incisions, simplify nomenclature, and stimulate further research. Although much is now known about the arterial framework of the body, there are still many gaps in our knowledge of the anatomy of the venous system. Some of the applications of the anatomic information will be considered briefly, since the details are covered in other chapters.

Axes of Skin Flaps

The arterial atlas of the integument details the origin, course, size, density, and interconnections of the cutaneous perforators. It therefore provides for the logical planning of the base and the axis of a flap. It is obvious from the above studies that there are many more axial flaps available for transfer than have been described to date. Several of these are included in Figure 10–35 with known flaps.

The cross sectional studies confirm the reason for including the outer layer of the deep fascia with flaps raised in the scalp and in the extremities, because in these situations the vessels hug the fascia for considerable distances. If a flap is designed along the course of a cutaneous nerve, such as the saphenous or the sural nerves, long, safe flaps can and have been elevated. Pontén's (1981) original flaps were designed in this way and

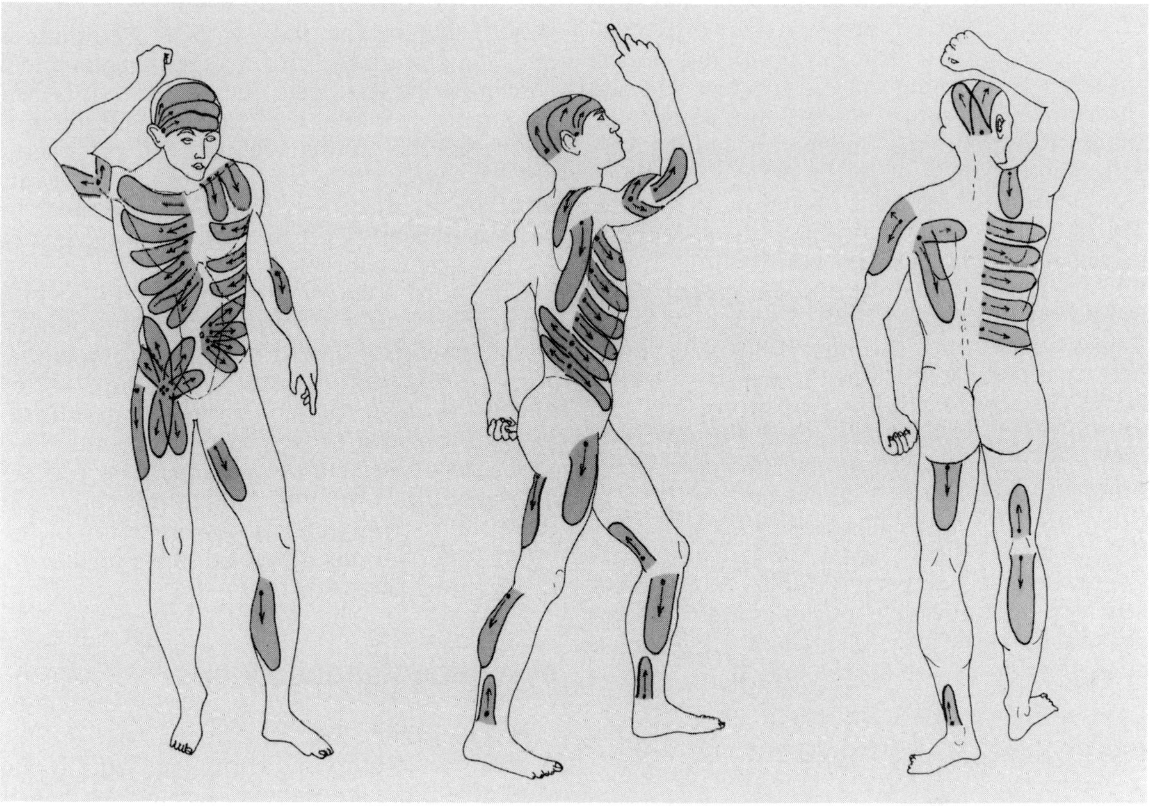

Figure 10–35. Some of the large axial cutaneous flaps that have been used, or are available, as defined by radiographic studies of the integument. In the scalp and the limbs they should include the deep fascia. (From Br. J. Plast. Surg.)

the saphenous neurovascular flap was planned in a similar manner (Acland and associates, 1981).

In the loose-skinned areas of the torso, it is unnecessary to include the deep fascia as the cutaneous arteries course at an early stage within the integument. They frequently correspond with the course of a cutaneous nerve (Badran, El-Helaly, and Safe, 1984). Comparing the above radiographic studies and illustrations of the vessels in the integument with the course of the cutaneous nerves, as depicted in *Grant's Atlas of Anatomy* (Anderson, 1958), a remarkable resemblance in orientation of the cutaneous arteries and nerves is evident.

Finally, since the large cutaneous vessels emerge from the deep fascia predominantly around the perimeter of muscles, the Doppler probe is a useful aid to locate the perforators in lean individuals. If a line is drawn to join two such perforators, and the skin between is mobile, a safe flap can be planned along this axis. This is of particular use on the torso and especially on the back.

Skin Flap Dimensions

Since the blood supply of the integument has been shown to be a continuous system of linked vascular territories, the survival length of a skin flap must depend on:

1. The caliber and length of the dominant vessel upon which the flap is based.
2. The caliber and span of the adjacent captured artery or arteries.
3. The caliber and length of the connecting choke vessels.
4. An adequate venous return.

If the arterial perforators are large and widely separated, the territory of each is large and a long flap can be raised with safety. The flaps are characteristic of the loose-skinned areas of the torso and of the scalp. Conversely, if the perforators are diminutive and close together, the territory of each is small. The viable length of the flap is short unless the underlying source vessel is included in the design. This is evident in the fixed skin area of the sole of the foot.

If very large flaps are required or if vessels of a large caliber are necessary for microvascular anastomoses, the requirements can be satisfied by chasing the perforators via the intermuscular septa or the intramuscular septa to include the underlying source vessels. The intelligent use of a delay also allows safe capture of adjacent vascular territories. Many studies of the septocutaneous vessels have been made and have resulted in various flap designs (Shanahan and Gingrass, 1979; Song and associates, 1982; Carriquiry, Aparecida Costa, and Vasconez, 1985). The above principles are outlined in Figure 10–5, which highlights the dominant axis of vessels that course parallel to the skin surface in different areas of the body. However, the concept of septocutaneous vessels is not original and is illustrated by many of the early anatomists (Quain and Wilson, 1842; Anderson, 1958). Cormack and Lamberty (1986a) have added much to the knowledge of the anatomy of the cutaneous perforators and have suggested a classification of fasciocutaneous flaps.

Fasciocutaneous Flaps

It is interesting how these flaps have evolved. In many ways the plastic surgeon has historically come full circle. The senior author was taught by Sir Benjamin Rank, as a dictum from Sir Harold Gillies, always to take the deep fascia with a skin flap in the extremities, especially in the lower limb. The precise vascular basis, however, was not known.

We then labored through many bulky musculocutaneous flaps, some of which have been major contributions. However, we now know why the flaps are safer in the limbs when the deep fascia is included. Nevertheless, too much emphasis has been placed on the intrinsic value of the blood supply of the deep fascia. Every experienced surgeon knows that, when the deep fascia is exposed, it desiccates, sloughs, and granulates with reluctance. Our studies show that the dominant vessels course adjacent to the surface of the deep fascia, not within it. With care they can be dissected free. Inclusion of the deep fascia with the overlying integument simply avoids such a tedious dissection. It also preserves the adjacent subfascial course of arteries in some situations.

The term "fasciocutaneous" flap is the subject of much debate. Pontén (1981) included the outer layer of the deep fascia in his description of the flap. It is a well-defined sheet in the limbs but in certain regions it is continued as the periosteum of the tibia, the ligaments of joints, the external oblique aponeurosis, the lumbar fascia, and the rectus sheath—to cite just a few examples where its structure is modified. Therefore one must be careful in applying the term fasciocutaneous to these regions.

One must also remember that there is a superficial fascia, stuffed with fat pellets, which connects the dermis to the deep fascia. It is more appropriate to name flaps raised above the deep fascia *superficial fasciocutaneous flaps,* and those that include the deep fascia *deep fasciocutaneous flaps*. The authors are reluctant to suggest new terminology, but it would certainly clarify the structure of the many new "fasciocutaneous" flaps appearing in the literature.

Musculocutaneous Flaps

It is apparent from the above studies that in many situations the cutaneous paddle of a musculocutaneous flap is supplied by small indirect perforators. Where the skin and deep fascia are firmly bound to the underlying muscle, e.g., the gluteus maximus and latissimus dorsi muscles, the blood supply to the skin is ensured. At each fixed site over the muscle vessels emerge, some large and some small, to supply the integument. However, where the muscle is mobile beneath the deep fascia, e.g., the gracilis muscle, the cutaneous supply is at best tenuous.

In general, musculocutaneous flaps can be raised safely if the skin paddle is placed over the perforators of the feeding artery or those in the adjacent muscular territory. Attempts to capture territories beyond that in either muscle or skin, without previous delay, frequently result in vascular insufficiency. This situation may prevail, for reasons already outlined, in the pectoralis major and the lower transverse rectus abdominis (TRAM) flaps.

Composite Flaps

A knowledge of the supply of all the tissues that constitute each angiosome provides the basis for the transfer of composite units of skin, muscle, nerve, tendon, and bone supplied by a single arteriovenous system. This knowledge has been applied extensively in free composite tissue transfer.

The vessels within the angiosome interconnect between the various layers. This type of interconnection is well illustrated with the transfer of composite tissue from the groin region. The direct cutaneous perforators of the SCIA interconnect with the indirect perforators of the DCIA. When a composite osteocutaneous flap is based on the deep system, the perforators of the DCIA capture the territory of the SCIA to perfuse the skin (Taylor, Townsend, and Corlett, 1979a). When the superficial system is utilized, the reverse applies to perfuse the anterior segment of iliac crest and the attached muscles (Taylor and Watson, 1978).

Hypervascular and Hypovascular Planes

These have been referred to in considerable detail by Salmon (1936a). The fixed skin areas of the body, which mark the sites of emergence of the dominant cutaneous perforators, constitute the hypervascular zones. Where the skin is mobile over the deep fascia or skull, or where muscles slide freely beneath the deep fascia, few small vessels cross these gliding planes. These are the hypovascular planes that are often used by surgeons to minimize blood loss. The placement of a breast prosthesis beneath the mammary gland or the pectoralis major muscle takes clinical advantage of this fact.

Acknowledgement: Most of the illustrations in this chapter are reproduced from the British Journal of Plastic Surgery. All of the illustrations except Figure 10–22 have been or will be published by Churchill Livingstone, Edinburgh.

REFERENCES

Acland, R. D., Schusterman, M., Godina, M., Eder, E., Taylor, G. I., and Carlisle, I. R.: The saphenous neurovascular free flap. Plast. Reconstr. Surg., *67*:763, 1981.

Anderson, J. E. (Ed.): Grant's Atlas of Anatomy. 7th Ed. Baltimore, Williams & Wilkins Company, 1958.

Badran, H. A., El-Helaly, M. S., and Safe, I.: The lateral intercostal neurovascular free flap. Plast. Reconstr. Surg., *73*:17, 1984.

Bakamjian, V. Y.: A two stage method for pharyngoesophageal reconstruction with a primary pectoral skin flap. Plast. Reconstr. Surg., *36*:173, 1965.

Blair, V. P.: The delayed transfer of long pedicle flaps in plastic surgery (face). Surg. Gynecol. Obstet., *33*:261, 1921.

Boyd, J. B., Taylor, G. I., and Corlett, R. J.: The vascular territories of the superior epigastric and the deep inferior epigastric systems. Plast. Reconstr. Surg., *73*:1, 1984.

Carramenha e Costa, M. A., Carriquiry, C., Vasconez, L. O., Grotting, J. C., Herrera, R. H., and Windle, B. H.: An anatomic study of the venous drainage of the transverse rectus abdominis musculocutaneous flap. Plast. Reconstr. Surg., *79*:208, 1987.

Carriquiry, C., Aparecida Costa, M., and Vasconez, L. O.: An anatomic study of the septocutaneous vessels of the leg. Plast. Reconstr. Surg., *76*:354, 1985.

Converse, J. M. (Ed.): Reconstructive Plastic Surgery. 2nd Ed. Philadelphia, W. B. Saunders Company, 1977, p. 193.

Cormack, G. C., and Lamberty, B. G. H.: A classification of fascio-cutaneous flaps according to their patterns of vascularisation. Br. J. Plast. Surg., *37*:80, 1984.

Cormack, G. C., and Lamberty, B. G. H.: The Arterial Anatomy of Skin Flaps. Edinburgh, Churchill Livingstone, 1986a.

Cormack, G. C., and Lamberty, B. G. H.: Measurement of geometric parameters in plastic surgery research: use of the departmental microcomputer. Br. J. Plast. Surg., *39*:307, 1986b.

Crock, H. V.: The Blood Supply of the Lower Limb Bones in Man. Edinburgh, E. & S. Livingstone, 1967.

Crosthwaite, G. L., Taylor, G. I., and Palmer, J. H.: A new radio-opaque injection technique for tissue preservation. Br. J. Plast. Surg., *40*:113, 1987.

Daniel, R. K., and Taylor, G. I.: Distant transfer of an island flap by microvascular anastomoses. Plast. Reconstr. Surg., *52*:111, 1973.

Daniel, R. K., and Williams, H. B.: The free transfer of skin flaps by microvascular anastomoses. Plast. Reconstr. Surg., *52*:16, 1973.

Davis, J. S.: Plastic Surgery, Its Principles and Practice. Philadelphia, P. Blakiston, Son and Company, 1919.

Esser, J. F. S.: Artery Flaps. Antwerp, De Vos-van Kleef, 1929.

Gillies, H. D., and Millard, D. R.: The Principles and Art of Plastic Surgery. Boston, Little, Brown & Company, 1957.

Hunter, J.: A Treatise on the Blood, Inflammation and Gunshot Wounds. London, John Richardson, 1794.

Johnston, T. B., Davies, I. E. S., and Davies, F. (Eds.): Gray's Anatomy. 32nd Ed. London, Longmans, 1958.

Last, R. J., and Tompsett, D. H.: Corrosion cast of the blood vessels of stillborn babies. Acta Anat., *51*:338, 1962.

Manchot, C.: Die Hautarterien des Menschlichen Körpers. Leipzig, F. C. W. Vogel, 1889.

Manchot, C.: The Cutaneous Arteries of the Human Body. Translated by Ristic, J., and Morain, W. D. New York, Springer-Verlag, 1983.

Mathes, S. J., and Nahai, F.: Clinical Atlas of Muscle and Musculocutaneous Flaps. St. Louis, C. V. Mosby Company, 1979.

Mathes, S. J., and Nahai, F.: Clinical Applications for Muscle and Musculocutaneous Flaps. St. Louis, C. V. Mosby Company, 1982.

McCraw, J. B.: The recent history of myocutaneous flaps. Clin. Plast. Surg., *7*:3, 1980.

McCraw, J. B., and Arnold, P. G.: McCraw and Arnold's Atlas of Muscle and Musculocutaneous Flaps. Norfolk, VA, Hampton Press, 1986.

McCraw, J. B., and Dibbell, D. G.: Experimental defini-

tion of independent myocutaneous vascular territories. Plast. Reconstr. Surg., *60*:212, 1977.
McCraw, J. B., Dibbell, D. G., and Carraway, J. H.: Clinical definition of independent myocutaneous vascular territories. Plast. Reconstr. Surg., *60*:341, 1977.
McDowell, F.: Logs vs. harpsichords, blobby flaps vs. finished results. Plast. Reconstr. Surg., *64*:249, 1979.
McGregor, I. A., and Jackson, I. T.: The groin flap. Br. J. Plast. Surg., *25*:3, 1972.
McGregor, I. A., and Morgan, G.: Axial and random pattern flaps. Br. J. Plast. Surg., *26*:202, 1973.
Nakajima, H., Fujino, T., and Adachi, S.: A new concept of vascular supply to the skin and classification of skin flaps according to their vascularization. Ann. Plast. Surg., *16*:1, 1986.
Nakajima, H., Maruyama, Y., and Koda, E.: The definition of vascular skin territories with prostaglandin E1—the anterior chest, abdomen and thigh-inguinal region. Br. J. Plast. Surg., *34*:258, 1981.
Palmer, J. H., and Taylor, G. I.: The vascular territories of the anterior chest wall. Br. J. Plast. Surg., *39*:287, 1986.
Patten, B. M.: Human Embryology. 3rd Ed. New York, Blakiston Division, McGraw-Hill Book Company, 1968.
Pontén, B.: The fasciocutaneous flap: its use in soft tissue defects of the lower leg. Br. J. Plast. Surg., *34*:215, 1981.
Quain, J., and Wilson, E.: A Series of Anatomical Plates in Lithography. Vol. 2. London, Taylor & Walton, 1842.
Rees, M. J. W., and Taylor, G. I.: A simplified lead oxide cadaver injection technique. Plast. Reconstr. Surg., *77*:141, 1986.
Reid, C. D., and Taylor, G. I.: The vascular territory of the acromiothoracic axis. Br. J. Plast. Surg., *37*:194, 1984.
Ryan, T. J.: *In* Jarret, A. (Ed.): The Physiology and Pathophysiology of the Skin. Vol. 2. London, Academic Press, 1973.
Salmon, M.: Artères de la Peau. Paris, Masson et Cie, 1936a.
Salmon, M.: Artères des Muscles des Membres et du Tronc. Paris, Masson et Cie, 1936b.
Schäfer, K.: Das subcutane Gefäss-System (untere Extremität). Mikropräparatorische Untersuchungen. Gegenbaurs Morphol. Jahrb., *121*:492, 1975.
Shanahan, R. E., and Gingrass, R. P.: Medial plantar sensory flap for coverage of heel defects. Plast. Reconstr. Surg., *64*:295, 1979.
Shaw, D. T., and Payne, R. L., Jr.: One-stage tubed abdominal flaps; single pedicle tubes. Surg. Gynecol. Obstet., *83*:205, 1946.
Song, R., Gao, Y., Song, Y., Yu, Y., and Song, Y.: The forearm flap. Clin. Plast. Surg., *9*:21, 1982.
Spalteholz, W.: Die Vertheilung der Blutgefässe in der Haut. Arch. Anat. Entwcklngs-gesch. (Leipz.), *1*:54, 1893.
Tansini, I.: Sopra il mio nuovo processo di amputazione della mammella. (Coverage of the anterior chest wall following mastectomy.) Gazz. Med. Ital., *57*:141, 1906.
Taylor, G. I.: Nerve grafting with simultaneous microvascular reconstruction. Clin. Orthop., *133*:56, 1978.
Taylor, G. I.: Foreword. *In* Manchot, C.: The Cutaneous Arteries of the Human Body. Translated by Risic, J., and Morain, W. D. New York, Springer-Verlag, 1983.
Taylor, G. I., and Corlett, R. J.: The vascular territories of the body and their relation to tissue transfer. Plast. Surg. Forum, *4*:113, 1981.
Taylor, G. I., Corlett, R. J., and Boyd, J. B.: The extended deep inferior epigastric flap: a clinical technique. Plast. Reconstr. Surg., *72*:751, 1983.
Taylor, G. I., Corlett, R. J., and Boyd, J. B.: The versatile deep inferior epigastric (inferior rectus abdominis) flap. Br. J. Plast. Surg., *37*:330, 1984.
Taylor, G. I., and Daniel, R. K.: The free flap: composite tissue transfer by vascular anastomosis. Aust. N. Z. J. Surg., *43*:1, 1973.
Taylor, G. I., and Daniel, R. K.: The anatomy of several free flap donor sites. Plast. Reconstr. Surg., *56*:243, 1975.
Taylor, G. I., and Ham, F. J.: The free vascularized nerve graft. Plast. Reconstr. Surg., *57*:413, 1976.
Taylor, G. I., Miller, G. D. H., and Ham, F. J.: The free vascularized bone graft. Plast. Reconstr. Surg., *55*:533, 1975.
Taylor, G. I., and Palmer, J. H.: The vascular territories (angiosomes) of the body: experimental study and clinical applications. Br. J. Plast. Surg., *40*:113, 1987.
Taylor, G. I., and Tempest, M.: Salmon's Arteries of the Skin. Edinburgh, Churchill Livingstone, 1988.
Taylor, G. I., and Townsend, P. L.: Composite free flap and tendon transfer: an anatomical study and a clinical technique. Br. J. Plast. Surg., *32*:170, 1979.
Taylor, G. I., Townsend, P. L., and Corlett, R. J.: Superiority of the deep circumflex iliac vessels as the supply for free groin flaps: experimental work. Plast. Reconstr. Surg., *64*:595, 1979a.
Taylor, G. I., Townsend, P. L., and Corlett, R. J.: Superiority of the deep circumflex iliac vessels as the supply for free groin flaps: clinical work. Plast. Reconstr. Surg., *64*:745, 1979b.
Taylor, G. I., and Watson, N.: One stage repair of compound leg defects with revascularized flaps of groin skin and iliac bone. Plast. Reconstr. Surg., *61*:494, 1978.
Taylor, G. I., Wilson, K., Rees, M. J., and Corlett, R. J.: The dual blood supply of the fibula. Presented at the VIIth Congress of the International Society of Microsurgery, Paris, 1985.
Timmons, M. J.: Landmarks in the anatomical study of the blood supply of the skin. Br. J. Plast. Surg., *38*:197, 1985.
Webster, J. P.: Thoraco-epigastric tubed pedicles. Surg. Clin. North Am., *17*:145, 1937.
Williams, P., and Warwick, R.: Gray's Anatomy. 36th Ed. Edinburgh, Churchill Livingstone, 1980.

11

Stephen J. Mathes
Issa Eshima

The Principles of Muscle and Musculocutaneous Flaps

The reconstructive surgeon today possesses a formidable armamentarium of reconstructive techniques. The muscle flap, the musculocutaneous flap, the fasciocutaneous flap, and the various techniques of microvascular composite tissue transplantation have made possible major advances in the field of plastic and reconstructive surgery. By applying a precise knowledge of the anatomy of skin, muscle, bone, and fascia in planning reconstructive procedures, the surgeon has the ability to restore form and function in congenital and acquired defects in most topographic regions.

Recent modifications and refinements in flap design offer considerable variety and versatility in the techniques available for use in reconstructive surgery. By applying the principles of flap design and technique, it is possible greatly to simplify the approach to the surgical defect. Coverage, form, and function are the three most important factors in determining a successful outcome. Through careful analysis of every individual surgical defect, the most appropriate method of reconstruction can be selected.

The surgical defect must be covered by reliable and durable tissues. Whether it is an exposed carotid artery or a chronically infected open bone, stable coverage is essential.

Restoring form is vital to the success of any reconstructive procedure. When utilizing the muscle or musculocutaneous flap, the plastic surgeon must strive to restore form at the recipient site and simultaneously avoid donor site deformity. Reconstructing a breast after mastectomy with a rectus abdominis musculocutaneous flap, for example, cannot be considered a success if the mound does not resemble a breast, or a hernia develops in the abdominal wall.

In transposing or transplanting a muscle from one site to another, the reconstructive surgeon must realize the effect on function. If the selected muscle has synergistic muscles that can compensate for this loss, or if the selected muscle serves no purpose in its present state (e.g., hamstrings in a paraplegic patient), the use of such a muscle does not produce a functional deficit. On the other hand, if a particular muscle is vital to a specific function (e.g., the gluteus maximus in an ambulatory patient), it is recommended that either a segment of muscle with preserved function be used or an entirely different muscle be selected.

The selection of the most appropriate technique can be difficult. A "reconstructive ladder" should be used to place the particular problem into perspective (Fig. 11–1). The surgeon should consider the simplest appropriate surgical technique first for any given defect. One can then proceed "up the ladder" as required until the most satisfactory method of reconstruction is found.

CLASSIFICATION OF MUSCLE FLAPS

In 1981 Mathes and Nahai described a classification system in which muscles are categorized on the anatomic relationships between a muscle and its vascular pedicles: (1) the regional source of the pedicle entering the muscle, (2) the number and size of the pedicle, (3) the location of the pedicle with respect to the muscle's origin and insertion, and (4) the angiographic patterns of the intramuscular vessels.

The classification system enables the surgeon to categorize the various muscle and musculocutaneous flaps into distinctly different, clinically applicable groups based on the vascular anatomy. For example, only certain muscles can be safely elevated based on their secondary vascular pedicles; by categorizing these muscles as such, flap selection and application are facilitated. Through this system of muscle classification, it is evident that the clinical utility of each muscle is largely dependent on its vascular anatomy (Mathes and Nahai, 1979, 1981, 1982; Cormack and Lamberty, 1986).

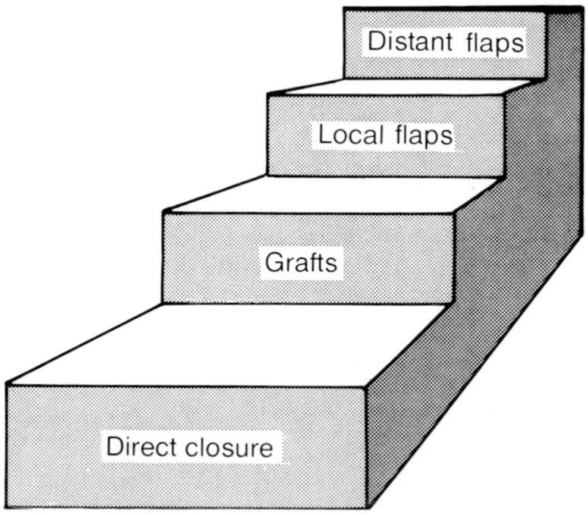

Figure 11–1. Reconstructive ladder: from simple to more complex techniques.

There are five different vascular patterns in which the various muscles are categorized (Fig. 11–2).

Type I: One Vascular Pedicle. Muscles in this group possess a single vascular pedicle, and include the medial gastrocnemius, lateral gastrocnemius, rectus femoris, and tensor fascia lata.

Type II: Dominant Vascular Pedicles and Minor Vascular Pedicles. Muscles in this group possess both dominant and smaller minor vascular pedicles. The large pedicles can sustain the entire muscle, permitting safe ligation of the smaller pedicles. Members include the abductor digiti minimi, abductor hallucis, biceps femoris, flexor digitorum brevis, gracilis, peroneus longus, peroneus brevis, platysma, semitendinosus, soleus, sternocleidomastoid, trapezius, and vastus lateralis.

Type III: Two Dominant Pedicles. Muscles in this group possess two large vascular pedicles from separate vascular sources. The entire muscle often survives on the basis of only one of the paired pedicles. The muscle may also be split, allowing the use of only part of the muscle as a muscle or musculocutaneous flap. Members of this group include the gluteus maximus, rectus abdominis, serratus anterior, semimembranosus, and temporalis.

Type IV: Segmental Vascular Pedicles. Muscles in this group possess multiple segmental vascular pedicles entering the course of the muscle belly. Each pedicle provides circulation to a segment of the muscle. Division of more than two to three of the pedicles results in distal muscle necrosis. Members include the extensor digitorum longus, extensor hallucis longus, flexor digitorum longus, flexor hallucis longus, sartorius, and tibialis anterior.

Type V: One Dominant Vascular Pedicle and Secondary Segmental Vascular Pedicles. Muscles in this group have one large dominant vascular pedicle near the insertion of the muscle with several segmental pedicles near the origin. The internal vasculature can be supplied by either the dominant

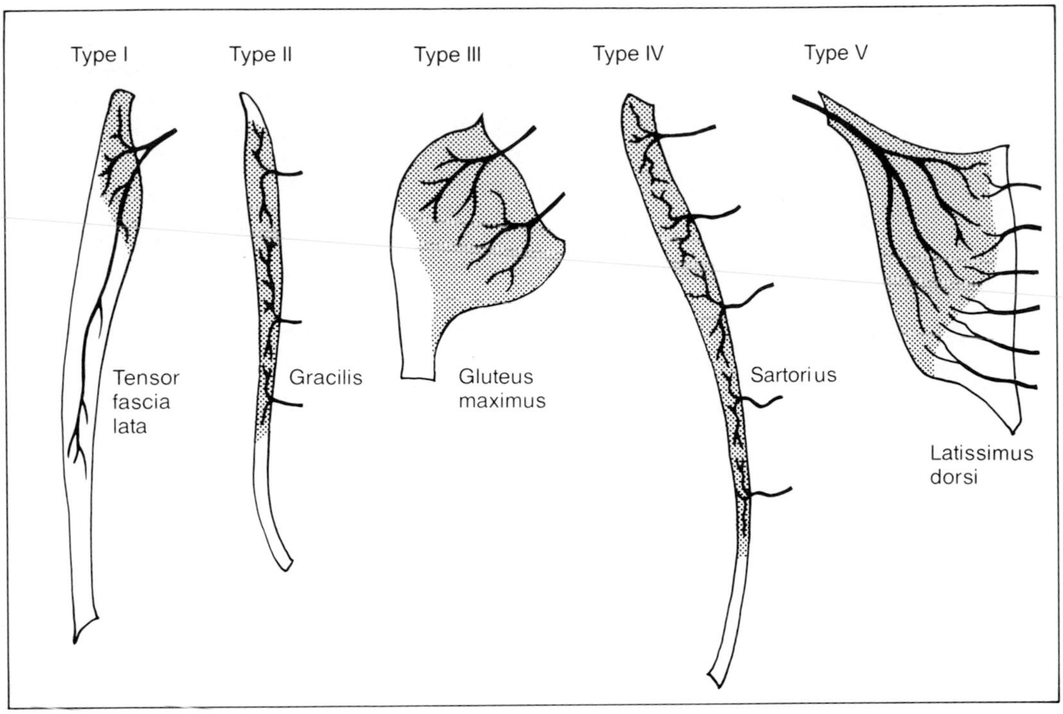

Figure 11–2. Patterns of vascular anatomy of muscle: Type I, one vascular pedicle; Type II, dominant pedicle(s) and minor pedicle(s); Type III, two dominant pedicles; Type IV, segmental vascular pedicles; Type V, one major pedicle and secondary segmental pedicles. (From Mathes, S. J., and Nahai, F.: Classification of the vascular anatomy of muscles: experimental and clinical correlation. Plast. Reconstr. Surg., *67*:177, 1981.)

or the segmental pedicles, and therefore the muscle may be elevated as a flap on either vascular system. Members include the pectoralis major and latissimus dorsi.

PREDICTION OF ARC OF ROTATION

The arc of rotation of a muscle is determined by (1) the extent of elevation of the muscle from its anatomic bed and (2) the ability of the muscle to reach adjacent areas without devascularization. The measurement of muscle mobility is dependent on the number of vascular pedicles and the location of the dominant vascular pedicle relative to the muscle's origin and insertion (Fig. 11–3).

In general, the arc of rotation is inversely proportional to the number of vascular pedicles. If a muscle has a large number of pedicles, it usually has a limited arc of rotation. Type IV muscles, such as the sartorius and tibialis anterior, are examples of muscles with multiple segmental vascular pedicles and limited arcs of rotation. Similarly, the location of the dominant vascular pedicle relative to the muscle's origin and insertion greatly determines the arc of rotation. In general, the closer the dominant vascular pedicle is to either the origin or insertion of the muscle, the greater is the arc of rotation. For example, a Type V muscle, such as the pectoralis major, has its major vascular pedicle near its insertion, and correspondingly has a wide arc of rotation.

Some muscles have a safe dual arc of rotation. Type III muscles are an example of muscles that can be rotated on either of the two large vascular pedicles. Similarly, Type V muscles have a dual arc of rotation. Type V muscles can also be transposed either on the secondary segmental pedicles or on the major vascular pedicle. The degree of transposition of a flap based on its secondary segmental vascular pedicles is defined as its *reverse arc of rotation.*

PREDICTION OF SKIN TERRITORY

The successful use of the overlying skin in a musculocutaneous flap is dependent on the skin's blood supply. Recent advances in the anatomic study of the cutaneous vascular

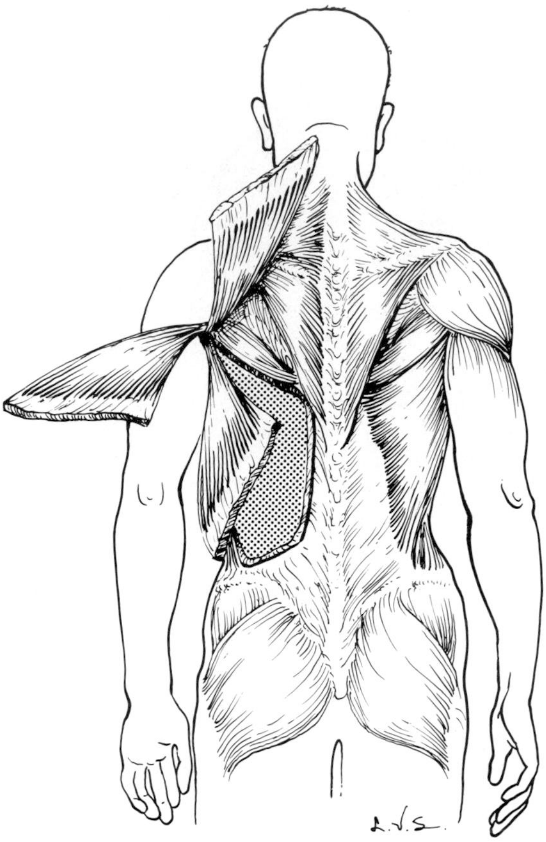

Figure 11–3. Arc of muscle rotation (latissimus dorsi).

system have revealed three distinct vascular patterns supplying the skin (see also Chaps. 9, 10): (1) direct cutaneous vessels, specific vessels in the subcutaneous fat running parallel to the skin surface; (2) musculocutaneous perforators, vessels arising from underlying muscle; and (3) fasciocutaneous vessels, specific vessels arising from regional vasculature and extending through intermuscular spaces into the overlying fascia.

The major blood supply to skin is subject to regional variation. Skin overlying the broad, flat muscles of the trunk (e.g., the latissimus dorsi) is largely dependent on the musculocutaneous perforating arteries. Skin overlying the thin, narrow muscles (e.g., the gracilis) are largely dependent on the fasciocutaneous perforating vessels.

Each musculocutaneous perforating artery nourishes a certain territory of skin. There can be much overlap, depending on the complexity of the skin's interconnecting vascular system. By appreciating this vascular system, the surgeon can safely design the skin territory for the flap.

All muscles, with the exception of the Type I group, require the division of vascular pedicles for flap transposition. Muscles with Type II or Type IV patterns require division of minor or segmental pedicles for flap elevation. This maneuver can jeopardize the corresponding skin territories. Type III muscles have two large vascular pedicles arising from separate vascular sources. The entire skin overlying the muscle often survives on either of the two pedicles. Type V muscles are the most useful because the skin islands can be based on either the proximal dominant pedicle or the secondary segmental pedicles. Type I muscles are especially useful in that the blood supply generally supports all the overlying skin.

In general, each superficial muscle supplies the skin lying directly over it, and the skin territory may be safely extended 3 to 4 cm beyond the borders of the underlying muscle. The additional skin is supported by various anastomotic networks in the subcutaneous tissues. In certain cases, there appears to be a degree of axiality in the musculocutaneous perforators that anastomoses with the cutaneous vessels. This anatomic arrangement enables an even larger territory of skin to be safely elevated. For example, in the extended deep inferior epigastric musculocutaneous flap described by Taylor, Corlett, and Boyd in 1983, certain paraumbilical musculocutaneous perforators from the inferior epigastric artery course superolaterally in the line of the intercostal spaces, anastomosing with the lateral cutaneous branches of the intercostal system. This arrangement enables the skin island to extend over the costal margin toward the tip of the scapula. Gottlieb and associates (1986) stated that the skin island of this flap can extend as far as the posterior axillary line, certainly a considerable distance from the borders of the underlying muscle. As modifications and refinements in the musculocutaneous flap continue, it is certain that various other extended skin territories, supported by the intricate anastomoses of the cutaneous, musculocutaneous, and fasciocutaneous systems, will be discovered.

DESIGN OF DISTALLY BASED FLAPS

Certain muscles can be elevated on minor or secondary segmental pedicles. Division of the dominant vascular pedicle and transposition of the muscle, distally based on the lesser pedicle, can be successfully performed. However, because the lesser pedicles may vary in size and location, the distally based flap is not entirely reliable. Prior delay of the muscle by selective division of the dominant vascular pedicle may improve the chances of flap survival (Mathes, Nahai, and Vasconez, 1978). The transposition of only a portion of the muscle based on a minor pedicle is, however, more reliable.

REFINEMENTS IN MUSCLE AND MUSCULOCUTANEOUS FLAPS

There has been considerable progress in the clinical application of muscle and musculocutaneous flaps over the past 15 years. Countless modifications and refinements in both technique and design have been described in the continuing quest for the optimal result in reconstructive surgery.

Techniques of splitting the muscle to preserve tissue and function have been described. For example, in the reconstruction of the cervical esophagus, the latissimus dorsi musculocutaneous flap can be split into two skin paddles that can be used for lining and skin coverage (Mathes and Nahai, 1981, 1982; Tobin and associates, 1981a,b; Matsunaga and associates, 1983). Splitting the pectoralis major muscle into segments has been performed when the segmental transfer of a single intercostal portion of the pectoralis muscle, based on a single medial perforating branch of the internal thoracic artery, is required for chest wall and neck reconstruction (Morain, Colen, and Hutchings, 1985). The concept of segmental transposition of muscle allows transplantation of independent neuromuscular units (segments of muscle innervated by a single nerve fascicle) (Manktelow and Zuker, 1984).

The preservation of function can be extremely important when nonexpendable muscles are used as flaps. The techniques of function preservation generally involve transposing part of the muscle without completely interrupting the origin or insertion of the muscle. For example, the transposition of the superior half of the gluteus maximus muscle for sacral coverage in the ambulatory patient can be performed without loss of thigh extension or hip stability because the remainder of the gluteus maximus is functionally intact (Mathes and Nahai, 1980; Parry and Mathes, 1982).

The development of combination flaps (e.g., the musculocutaneous-fasciocutaneous flap, the musculocutaneous-axial pattern flap, and combined muscle flaps sharing a single vascular pedicle flap) is useful in treatment of the extensive defect. The latissimus dorsi combined with a scapular flap is one example of a combination flap. Another example is the gluteal thigh flap, which is an inferior gluteal musculocutaneous flap with a posterior fasciocutaneous extension (Hurwitz, 1980; Hurwitz, Swartz, and Mathes, 1981; Stevenson and associates, 1987). The combination of various tissues has given these flaps added bulk as well as added length. Furthermore, the more subtle characteristics (e.g., texture) of each tissue component enable the surgeon to tailor the flap precisely to the specifications of the individual defect.

The development of specialized tissue flaps has provided the surgeon with the ability to restore sensation, motor function, and bony structure in the surgical defect. Using such complex tissues as innervated muscle, omentum, intestine, joint, digit, iliac crest, and various long bones, the innovative surgeon can produce, in the words of McDowell (1979), "a few harpsichords, rather than so many logs—recognizable, new, artistic and fully acceptable noses, cheeks, chins, necks, legs and arms rather than indistinguishable globs and blobs of transported tissue in those areas."

ADVANTAGES AND DISADVANTAGES OF MUSCLE AND MUSCULOCUTANEOUS FLAPS

Selection of the most appropriate reconstructive method can be difficult. Careful consideration must be given to all the possible methods of repair, and the advantages and disadvantages of each technique must be weighed accordingly.

The advantages of muscle or musculocutaneous flaps include the following: (1) they have a rich blood supply with distinct vascular pedicle(s); (2) the vascular pedicle is often located outside the surgical defect owing to the arc of rotation and the length of the muscle—the location of the vascular pedicle can be important, particularly for wounds with an extensive zone of injury beyond the actual wound (i.e., after radiation, trauma); (3) the muscle provides bulk for deep, extensive defects and protective padding for exposed vital structures (e.g., tendons, nerves, vessels, bones, and prostheses); (4) a muscle is malleable and can be manipulated (e.g., folded on itself) to produce a desired shape or volume; (5) well-vascularized muscle is resistant to bacterial inoculation and infection (Chang and Mathes, 1982); (6) reconstruction using muscle or musculocutaneous flaps is often a one stage procedure; (7) restoration of function (motor/sensory) is possible using certain flaps; and (8) the reliability and availability of muscle and musculocutaneous flaps make them an excellent alternative means of reconstruction when the method of choice for a particular defect is unavailable or inadequate.

The disadvantages of muscle and musculocutaneous flaps include the following: (1) the donor defect may lose some degree of function—e.g., the use of the rectus abdominis muscle below the arcuate line may structurally weaken the abdominal wall and result in hernia formation; (2) the donor defect may be esthetically unacceptable to the patient; (3) muscle or musculocutaneous flaps may provide excessive bulk, leaving an esthetically unacceptable result; (4) muscle or musculocutaneous flaps may eventually atrophy and fail to provide adequate coverage; and finally (5) the loss of muscle and musculocutaneous flaps may result in a larger deformity.

SELECTION OF SPECIFIC MUSCLE AND MUSCULOCUTANEOUS FLAPS

After the decision has been made to use a muscle or musculocutaneous flap, the reconstructive surgeon must choose a specific muscle. Certain factors can assist the selection:

1. The muscle ideally should be adjacent to the defect.

2. The muscle should be of sufficient size and bulk to cover the defect. It is important to note that one should make the final design of the flap after the defect has been completely debrided. The defect, once debrided, is often much larger and deeper than anticipated. By making the final design of the flap after the debridement, costly errors in inadequate coverage can be avoided. Atrophy of the muscle must also be anticipated if the origin, insertion, or motor nerve of the muscle are disrupted.

3. The muscle should be expendable. There often are synergistic muscles that can compensate for the loss of the selected muscle in order that function at the donor site is not impaired. However, if no synergistic muscle groups are available, either techniques to preserve muscle function (e.g., muscle splitting) should be employed or an entirely different muscle should be used.

4. The status of the vascular pedicle that will sustain the proposed flap must be known preoperatively. Selective arteriography can be helpful when previous surgery has been performed in proximity to the vascular pedicle or when muscle paralysis is noted on examination. Earlier division of the motor nerve may also include ligation of the vascular pedicle. Examples of clinical situations when arteriography is particularly helpful include the evaluation of the sural artery (gastrocnemius) after knee surgery, of the transverse cervical artery (trapezius) after neck and shoulder surgery, and of the thoracodorsal artery (latissimus dorsi) after axillary surgery (Fisher, Bostwick, and Powell, 1983).

5. The donor defect must be carefully considered. Some patients do not accept the use of a skin graft at the donor site, and certain muscles are more likely than others to require grafts for closure. Likewise, some patients prefer one scar site to another (e.g., the abdominal scar of the transverse rectus abdominis musculocutaneous flap versus the back scar of the latissimus dorsi flap in breast reconstruction).

6. The cutaneous territory of the proposed flap must be of sufficient size and of acceptable texture.

7. If restoration of sensation or motor function is necessary, only a select number of muscle or musculocutaneous flaps are available. The tensor fascia lata flap is an example of a neurosensory flap (Mathes and Buchanan, 1979; Nahai, Hill, and Hester, 1979; Nahai, 1980).

8. Osteomusculocutaneous flaps are available for defects in need of vascularized bone. Examples of such flaps include the trapezius flap with vascularized clavicle and scapular spine (Panje and Cutting, 1980; Shapiro, 1981; Bem and O'Hare, 1986) and the pectoralis major flap with vascularized rib (Cuono and Ariyan, 1980).

REGIONAL APPLICATION OF MUSCLE AND MUSCULOCUTANEOUS FLAPS

Head and Neck

Local: 1. Temporalis
2. Sternocleidomastoid
3. Platysma

Distant: 1. Pectoralis major
2. Trapezius
3. Latissimus dorsi
4. Microvascular transplantation

In 1983, at the 29th Annual Meeting of the Society of Head and Neck Sugeons, Conley stated: "A great advance came about five years ago with the introduction of the regional myocutaneous flaps. They are now the most important flaps in the armamentarium of the head and neck surgeon."

Radical ablative surgery can produce massive defects. Many of the simpler defects can be adequately treated with skin grafts and local scalp flaps, but for the more complicated defect the muscle and musculocutaneous flaps play a major role. Defects following extirpative surgery in the head and neck are now immediately reconstructed with distant muscle and musculocutaneous flaps.

The primary applications of the muscle or musculocutaneous flap in head and neck reconstruction include (1) provision of tissue bulk for a significant defect (e.g., after hemimandibulectomy), (2) protective coverage for vital structures (e.g., the carotid artery), (3) provision of skin for intraoral lining and coverage, and (4) provision of skin for skull, facial, and neck defects.

The local muscle and musculocutaneous flaps for head and neck reconstruction include the temporalis, sternocleidomastoid, and platysma flaps.

The *temporalis* muscle is a Type III, fan-shaped, bipenniform muscle. Transposition of the muscle as a turnover flap is especially useful for coverage of the orbit, superior maxilla, and ear.

The *sternocleidomastoid* is a Type II muscle, first described in head and neck reconstruction by Owens (1955). Since then, Bakamjian (1963), Littlewood (1967), O'Brien (1970), and Ariyan (1979a, 1980) have made significant contributions to the development of this musculocutaneous flap.

The sternocleidomastoid flap has been most commonly used for intraoral and pharyngeal reconstruction (Ariyan, 1979a; Parkash, Ramakrishman, and Ananthakrishnan, 1980; Larson and Goepfert, 1982; Alvarez, Escamilla, and Carranza, 1983). Furthermore, as a carrier for the vascularized clavicle (segmental), the sternocleidomastoid flap can be applied in mandibular reconstruction (Siemssen, Kirkby, and O'Connor, 1978; Alvarez, Escamilla, and Carranza, 1983). Other uses include augmentation of soft tissue defects of the upper neck and jaw, protective coverage of major vessels, and closure of pharyngocutaneous fistulas (Littlewood, 1967; Conley, 1972; Larson and Goepfert, 1982). Of all the musculocutaneous flaps used for head and neck reconstruction, however, the sternocleidomastoid flap is considered the least reliable. With a reported 20 per cent failure rate, a 30 per cent complication rate, and in one series a reported 50 per cent incidence of partial epithelial loss of the skin paddle, the sternocleidomastoid musculocutaneous flap should be used only in select cases (Ariyan, 1979a; Larson and Goepfert, 1982; Cormack and Lamberty, 1986).

The *platysma* is a Type II, thin, broad, sheetlike muscle extending over the entire anterior and lateral aspects of the neck. Its use as a musculocutaneous island flap was probably first described in 1887 by Gersuny, who employed it in reconstructing a full-thickness defect of the cheek. The platysma musculocutaneous flap is particularly useful for intraoral, lip, lower midface, and anterior neck reconstruction. Its unique advantages include thinness, pliability, regionality, skin texture, color match, and even the capability of providing sensation and animation (Hurwitz and Kerber, 1981; Coleman, Nahai, and Mathes, 1982; Coleman and associates, 1983; Hurwitz, Rabson, and Futrell, 1983; Nieto, Gallego, and Cortes, 1983; Georgiade, Riefkohl, and Georgiade, 1985). One series reported a 42 per cent incidence of minor complications; most of the problems were attributed to improper selection and technique (Coleman and associates, 1983). Owing to the thinness of the platysma muscle, the reconstructive surgeon must be particularly careful to avoid disrupting the muscle fibers during the dissection and creating undue tension at the vascular pedicle on transposition of the flap.

The distant muscle and musculocutaneous

flaps in head and neck reconstruction include the pectoralis major, trapezius, and latissimus dorsi flaps and several flaps requiring microvascular transplantation.

The *pectoralis major* is a Type V, large, broad muscle, described in 1968 by Hueston and McConchie as part of a compound deltopectoral flap. In 1977 Brown, Fleming, and Jurkiewicz described the use of the pectoralis major as a flap for mediastinal coverage. In 1979 Ariyan (1979b) introduced the pectoralis major musculocutaneous flap and its application in head and neck reconstruction (Fig. 11–4). In the ensuing years, the pectoralis major musculocutaneous flap (see also Chap. 70) has proved more valuable than the deltopectoral flap, and it has supplanted the latter skin fascial flap as the primary flap in head and neck reconstruction. The deltopectoral flap, however, is an excellent choice for thin defects of the middle and lower thirds of the face and neck.

The most common applications of the pectoralis major musculocutaneous flap in head and neck reconstruction include the following: (1) for external resurfacing of the skin of the face and neck, (2) for intraoral and pharyngeal lining, (3) for carrying vascularized rib and skin in mandibular reconstruction, and (4) for reconstruction of the esophagus (Maruyama, Nakajima, and Fujino, 1980; Withers and associates, 1981; Ryan, Krementz, and Cardona-Loya, 1981; Baek, Lawson, and Biller, 1981, 1982; Ariyan, 1983; Neifeld and associates, 1983; Morgan, Sargent, and Hoopes, 1984; Lam, Wei, and Siu, 1984; Kudo and associates, 1985; Rees and associates, 1986). The pectoralis major musculocutaneous flap is one of the most versatile flaps used in head and neck reconstruction (Fig. 11–5).

The *trapezius* muscle is less widely used than the pectoralis major muscle, yet its superior location and wide anterior arc of rotation make it a valuable musculocutaneous (Type II) flap (McCraw, Dibbell, and Carraway, 1977; Mathes and Nahai, 1979; McCraw, Magee, and Kalwaic, 1979; Demergasso and

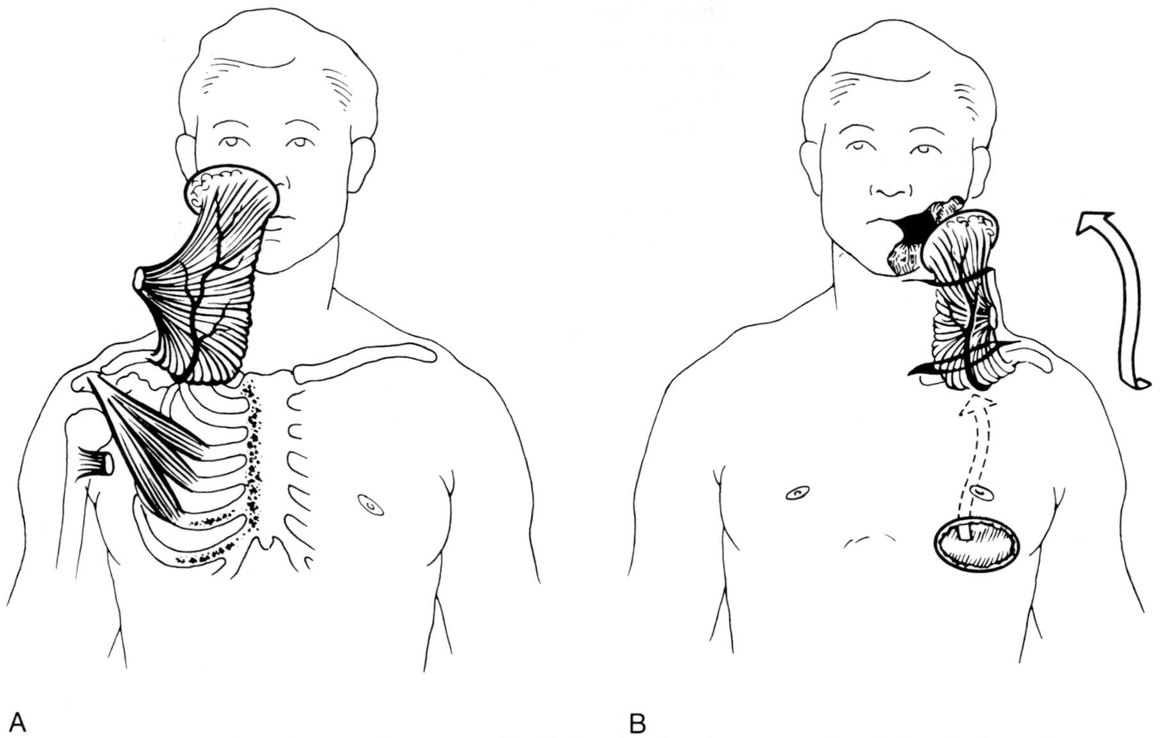

A B

Figure 11–4. Pectoralis major musculocutaneous flap for head and neck reconstruction. *A,* Standard arc of rotation for coverage of lower and midface defects. Note that isolating the vascular pedicle would produce an extended arc of rotation that would provide coverage for the upper one-third of the face and temporal skull defects. *B,* Reconstruction of oral cavity defects. Note that the skin island and anterior surface of the muscle rotate into the oral cavity after the flap is transposed from the chest to the head. (From Stark, R. B.: Plastic Surgery of the Head and Neck. New York, Churchill Livingstone, 1987, pp. 950, 952.)

Piazza, 1979). Modifications in design have enabled the trapezius muscle to be used as distinctly different upper and lower musculocutaneous flaps (Mathes and Nahai, 1982; Cormack and Lamberty, 1986). The various clinical applications of the trapezius musculocutaneous flap include (1) lower facial reconstruction, especially the ear and parotid regions; (2) lateral upper face and scalp repair; (3) anterior and posterior neck reconstruction; (4) orbital reconstruction using an extended flap (Baek and associates, 1980; Yoshimura, Maruyama, and Takeuchi, 1981; Shapiro, 1981; Rosen, 1985); and (5) pharyngoesophageal reconstruction (Guillamondegui and Larson, 1981; Miyamoto, Hattori, and Nosoh, 1984). The trapezius muscle can also be used as an osteomusculocutaneous flap incorporating either the lateral aspect of the clavicle or the spine of the scapula. The incorporated vascularized bone is particularly useful for reconstruction of the mandible (Dufresne and associates, 1987; Panje and Cutting, 1980; Shapiro, 1981; Bem and O'Hare, 1986).

The *latissimus dorsi* is a Type V muscle originally described as a superiorly based flap by Tansini in 1895 (Tansini, 1896a). Since that time, there have been various modifications and refinements of the flap (Olivari, 1976; Mendelson and Masson, 1977; McCraw, Penix, and Baker, 1978; Bostwick and associates, 1979). The flap is perhaps not as versatile as the pectoralis major musculocutaneous flap in head and neck reconstruction, yet certain qualities such as the hair-free skin and the donor site scar make the latissimus dorsi an invaluable alternative to the pectoralis major musculocutaneous flap.

The latissimus dorsi musculocutaneous flap in head and neck reconstruction is indicated for the replacement of large amounts of vascularized tissues when previous irradiation or surgery preclude the use of other more convenient flaps. Since Quillen, Shearin, and Georgiade in 1978 reported the use of the latissimus dorsi as a transposed island flap to cover the left side of the mandible and neck after excision of a tumor, various other clinical applications of the muscle have been described. The reports of Watson and Lendrum (1981), Watson (1982), and Watson and associates (1982) have been instrumental in the application of the latissimus dorsi musculocutaneous flap in intraoral and pharyngeal reconstruction. In 1981 Mathes and Nahai and Tobin and associates (1981a,b) described the split latissimus dorsi musculocutaneous flap, which, as a single branched flap, provides both skin coverage and lining. This flap has been particularly useful in intraoral and pharyngeal reconstruction. Barton, Spicer, and Byrd (1983) reported the use of the latissimus dorsi musculocutaneous flap in 60 cases involving reconstruction of the retromolar trigone, pharyngeal wall, floor of the mouth, segmental esophagus, temporozygomatic region, and cheek. In these particularly difficult regions there was a 6.7 per cent incidence of total flap failure and a 1.6 per cent incidence of partial sloughing. Overall, the most common uses of the latissimus dorsi musculocutaneous flap in head and neck surgery include reconstructive defects of the posterior neck, shoulder, anterior neck, lower face, occipital scalp, and intraoral-pharyngoesophageal regions (Quillen, 1979; Krishna and Green, 1980; Bostwick, 1982; Watson and associates, 1982; Barton, Spicer, and Byrd, 1983; Matsunaga and associates, 1983).

The use of microvascular tissue transplantation in head and neck reconstruction has made a significant contribution in the past decade. The microvascular transplantation of fasciocutaneous flaps and gastrointestinal segments has been particularly successful. Various microvascular muscle transplants have also been useful in the restoration of facial function and contour.

Breast

Local:	1. Pectoralis major
Distant:	1. Latissimus dorsi
	2. Rectus abdominis
	3. Microvascular transplantation

Muscle and musculocutaneous flaps have made a tremendous impact on breast reconstruction (see also Chap. 79), converting a procedure that typically had poor results to one that provides an acceptable breast mound in terms of shape and symmetry (Cooper, Webster, and Bell, 1984; Kincaid, 1984).

The modified radical mastectomy, preserving the pectoralis muscle, has largely replaced the classic radical mastectomy as the treatment of choice for breast cancer. Additional tissue-preserving techniques such as the "lumpectomy" have also gained in popularity. The change in approach has resulted in a smaller defect and a greater amount of local tissue available for use in reconstruc-

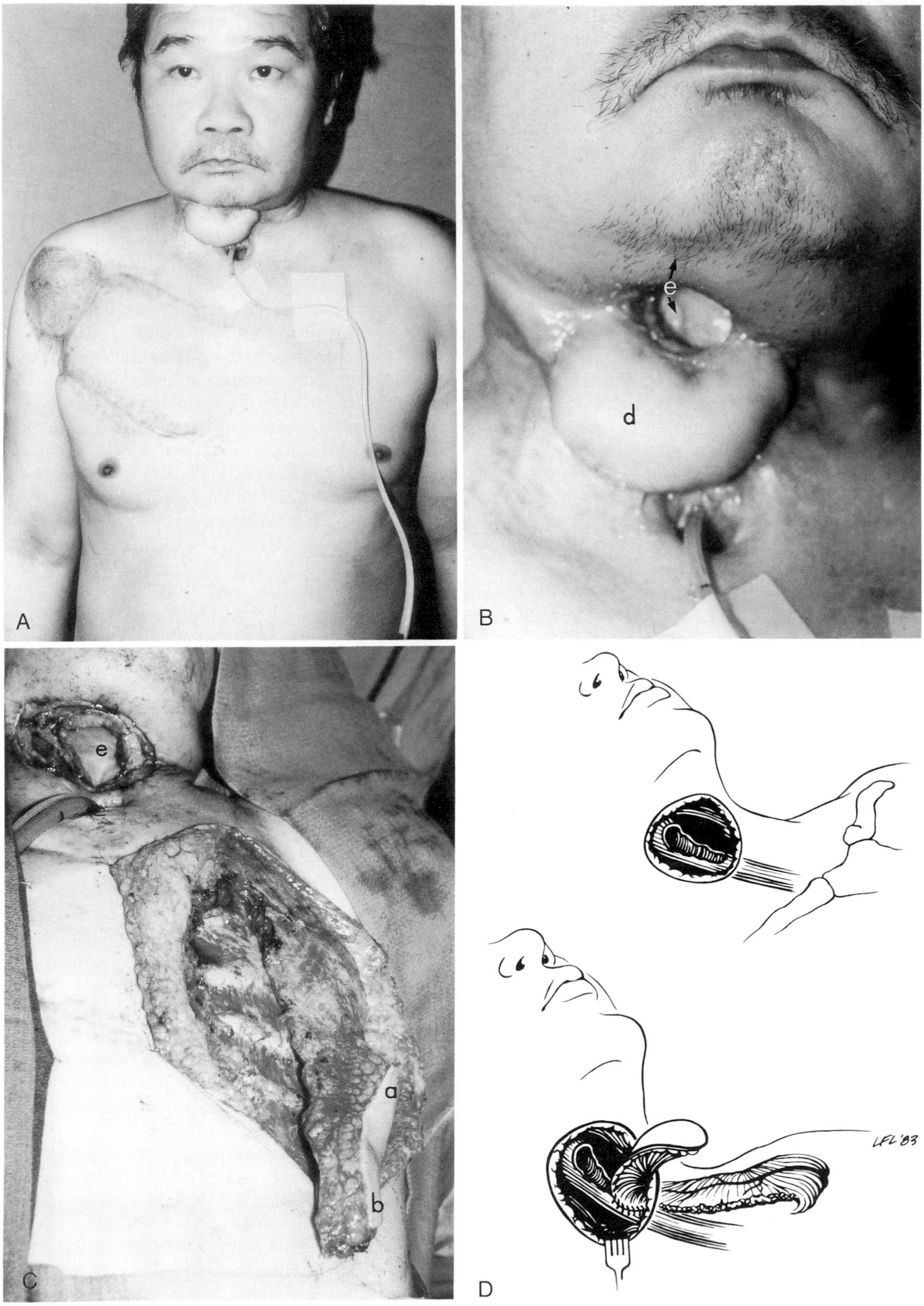

Figure 11–5 *See legend on opposite page*

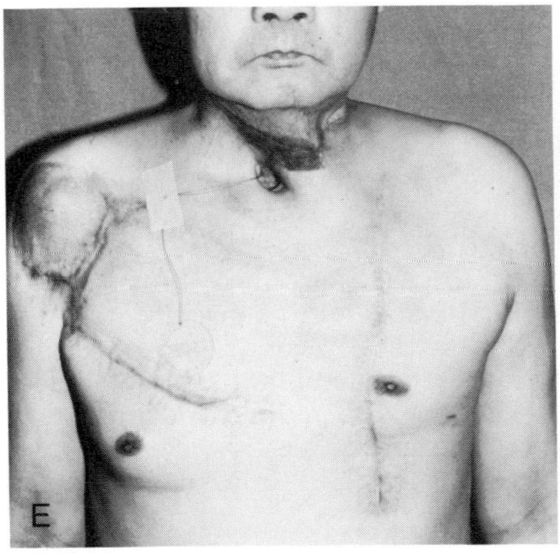

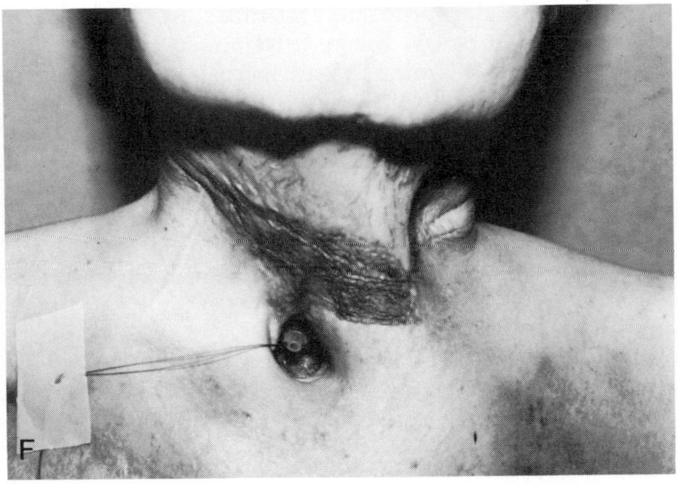

Figure 11–5. Pectoralis major musculocutaneous flap for reconstruction of a pharyngoesophageal fistula in a patient presenting with radiation necrosis and failed deltopectoral flap. *A,* Preoperative view. The patient had recurrent squamous cell carcinoma of the larynx after primary radiation therapy, which necessitated laryngectomy. Complications secondary to poor wound healing resulted in right-sided carotid rupture and necrosis of the anterior cervical esophageal wall. *B,* The deltopectoral flap failed to provide stable coverage. Site of deltopectoral flap inset (d). Anterior wall defect of the pharynx-cervical esophagus extending to the site of the tracheostomy (e). *C,* Deltopectoral flap excised. Pharyngeal-cervical esophageal defect debrided (e). Left pectoralis major musculocutaneous flap elevated with distal vertical skin island. Superior aspect of skin island (a). Inferior aspect (b). *D,* After flap transposition to the neck, the skin island was inset in the defect with the superior edge of the skin island sutured to the esophagus at the level of the trachea, and the inferior portion (b) was placed into the superior aspect of the pharyngeal defect. *E,* One month after reconstructive surgery, the patient demonstrated normal pharyngeal-esophageal continuity. *F,* Close-up view demonstrating stable coverage provided by skin grafts on the exposed deep surface of the pectoralis major muscle. (From Stark, R. B.: Plastic Surgery of the Head and Neck. New York, Churchill Livingstone, 1987, pp. 958–960.)

tion. Various techniques employing local tissues, such as thoracic advancement flaps (Ryan, 1982), dermal fat pedicle flaps (Longacre, 1956; Scuderi and Campus, 1982), contralateral abdominomammary flaps (De la Plaza, 1981; Millard, 1981), and direct flaps using abdominal lipectomy tissue (Marshall, Anstee, and Stapleton, 1981), can be useful in breast reconstruction. The temporary tissue expander introduced by Radovan (1978, 1982) is particularly helpful for patients who do not have an adequate amount of local tissue available for reconstruction.

The local muscles available in breast reconstruction are the pectoralis major and serratus anterior. For patients who undergo prosthetic implant insertion, these muscles are of primary importance. The submuscular (subpectoral or subserratus-pectoral) placement of a prosthetic implant is the most common reconstructive technique for patients with an intact pectoralis major muscle and adequate overlying skin. It is generally believed that submuscular placement of an implant is clinically superior to subcutaneous placement in that there is a softer more natural contour, a lower risk of implant exposure or extrusion, and a smaller incidence of capsular contracture (Woods, Irons, and Arnold, 1980; Apfelberg and associates, 1981; Gruber and associates, 1981). Another local muscle that can assist in implant coverage is the pectoralis minor. If it remains intact after mastectomy, the pectoralis minor flap is particularly useful for patients with a thin or underdeveloped pectoralis major muscle or for those who have undergone an extensive axillary node dissection (Manstein and associates, 1985). This muscle provides additional coverage for the prosthetic implant.

The distant muscles available in breast reconstruction include the latissimus dorsi, the rectus abdominis, and various muscles that require microvascular transplantation, such as the gluteus maximus. Distant musculocutaneous flaps are usually indicated for patients with inadequate local tissue, unacceptable overlying skin, or radiation damage.

The *latissimus dorsi* is a distant muscle used in breast reconstruction. Tansini described the earliest version of the latissimus dorsi flap (1896a,b). Since then, this muscle has become one of the most versatile flaps in plastic and reconstructive surgery (Schneider, Hill, and Brown, 1977). Bostwick and associates (1979), Bostwick and Scheflan (1980), and Bostwick, Vasconez, and Jurkiewicz (1978) described the various applications of latissimus dorsi muscle and musculocutaneous flaps in breast reconstruction. A 2 per cent incidence of minor skin necrosis and a zero incidence of total flap loss has been reported in a review of over 200 patients (Bostwick, Vasconez, and Jurkiewicz, 1978). The major drawback in using the latissimus dorsi for breast reconstruction is that a prosthetic implant is usually required to provide adequate projection; the musculocutaneous flap by itself is generally too thin (Fig. 11–6).

The *rectus abdominis* is a Type III muscle that commonly supplies a generous amount of abdominal fat and overlying skin. As a musculocutaneous flap it has proved to be one of the most valuable techniques in breast reconstruction today. Variations in flap design have produced different types of rectus abdominis musculocutaneous flaps (e.g., vertical, transverse, bipedicled, superiorly based, inferiorly based, and so forth). Mathes and Bostwick (1977), Robbins (1979, 1981), and Drever (1981, 1983) described the vertically oriented rectus abdominis musculocutaneous flap, which, like the latissimus flap, generally requires a prosthetic implant to provide adequate projection. The main disadvantage of the vertically oriented rectus abdominis flap, compared with the latissimus dorsi flap, is

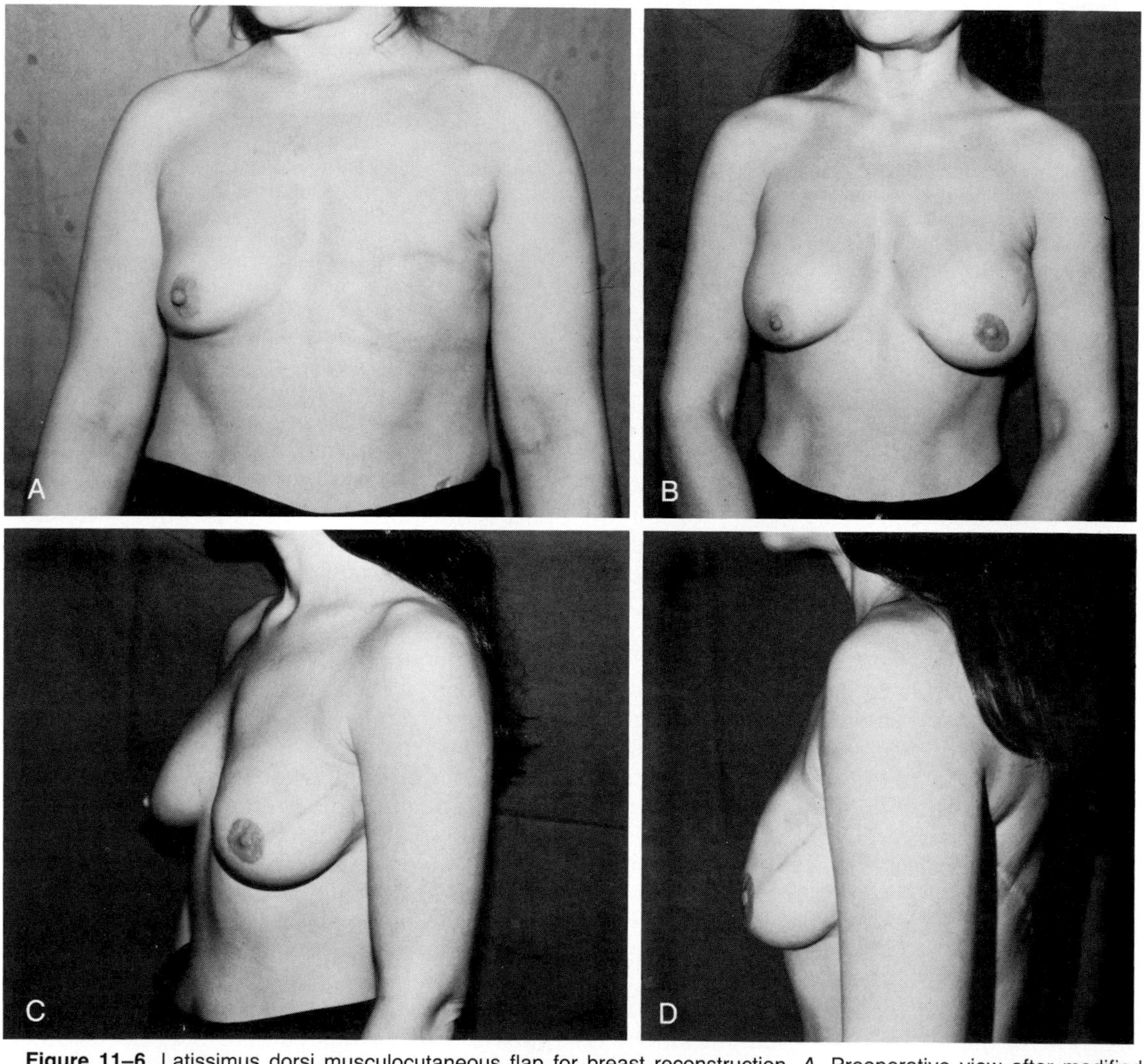

Figure 11–6. Latissimus dorsi musculocutaneous flap for breast reconstruction. *A*, Preoperative view after modified radical mastectomy for breast carcinoma. *B*, Postoperative view after breast reconstruction utilizing a latissimus dorsi musculocutaneous flap with silicone gel implant. The nipple was reconstructed with a full-thickness skin graft. *C*, Oblique view. *D*, Lateral view. Note the donor site scar.

the depressed, paramedian abdominal scar at the donor site. In 1982 Hartrampf, Scheflan, and Black described a technique that changed the entire approach to breast reconstruction. By alignment of the skin island in a transverse direction, between the umbilicus and pelvis, the rectus abdominis musculocutaneous flap provided skin and soft tissue for breast reconstruction, and left an improved contour on the abdomen. The transverse rectus abdominis musculocutaneous (TRAM) flap is considered the musculocutaneous flap of choice for breast reconstruction (Fig. 11–7).

The indications for using the TRAM flap in breast reconstruction include (1) a patient in need of additional soft tissue and overlying skin who has a moderate amount of lower abdominal tissues; (2) a patient who prefers autogenous tissue reconstruction without the use of a prosthetic implant; (3) a patient who prefers an abdominal donor scar rather than a back scar; and (4) a patient who has had an unacceptable result after undergoing other reconstructive methods (Dinner, Labandter, and Dowden, 1982; Dinner, Dowden, and Scheflan, 1983; Scheflan and Dinner, 1983a,b).

The relative contraindications for using the TRAM flap include (1) an extremely thin patient who has little lower abdominal tissue, (2) a nulliparous patient in her child-bearing years, (3) a patient with a history of abdominal wall herniation, (4) an extremely obese patient, (5) a heavy smoker, (6) a patient who has previously undergone irradiation to the chest wall (along the course of the internal mammary artery), and (7) a patient with lower abdominal scars.

The advantages of the TRAM flap include the following: (1) it provides sufficient bulk so that a prosthetic implant usually is not required, (2) the suprapubic horizontal donor site scar is esthetically acceptable, (3) transposition of the flap can be performed with the patient in a single operative position, (4) the quality of the skin is generally better than that of the latissimus dorsi flap, and (5) a simultaneous abdominoplasty is accomplished. The major disadvantage of the TRAM flap is that there is a risk of abdominal hernia formation.

The rectus abdominis muscle plays a vital role in flexing the vertebral column and supporting the abdominal wall. It also assists in defecation and urination. Using the rectus abdominis muscle as a muscle or musculocutaneous flap disrupts the integrity of the rectus sheath. Above the arcuate line, the strength of the posterior rectus sheath is comparable with that of the anterior sheath; therefore, the use of the superior half of the rectus abdominis does not significantly weaken the abdominal wall. However, below the arcuate line, the posterior sheath consists of only transversalis fascia and is extremely weak. By removing the anterior rectus sheath below the arcuate line, one may therefore seriously jeopardize the integrity of the lower abdominal wall. In an attempt to minimize the risk of hernia formation, several surgical techniques appear useful. Closing the abdominal wall in a direct, anatomic, multilayered fashion and centralizing the remaining abdominal musculature are the most important maneuvers to reestablish abdominal wall integrity. In dissecting the rectus abdominis muscle during flap mobilization, one should avoid violating the linea alba and the linea semilunaris. One should also preserve margins of the anterior sheath both laterally and medially to facilitate subsequent anterior sheath repair. The use of the contralateral anterior rectus sheath as a turnover flap may occasionally be helpful. Utilizing a muscle-sparing technique in the dissection of the vascular pedicle may preserve additional tissue that may help to buttress the abdominal wall. Relaxing incisions can be used to mobilize local tissues to ensure closure. Autogenous grafts (e.g., deepithelized skin, upper anterior rectus fascia, and so forth) may also be useful. Prolene mesh may occasionally be necessary, especially for the donor defects resulting from bilateral rectus abdominis flaps. Most unilateral defects can be closed primarily. In a large series of patients who underwent breast reconstruction with the TRAM flap, Hartrampf (1984) reported a 1.2 per cent incidence of hernia formation.

The long-term effects of the loss of one or both rectus abdominis muscles are not known at this time. Clearly the incidence of problems such as back pain, spinal curvature abnormalities, constipation, and complications of pregnancy needs to be studied. One case report (Brandner and Bunkis, 1987) described uneventful pregnancies in women who had previously undergone a rectus abdominis musculocutaneous flap. In one patient the abdominal wall was described as being weak and attenuated at the time of delivery. Many factors must be considered before selecting

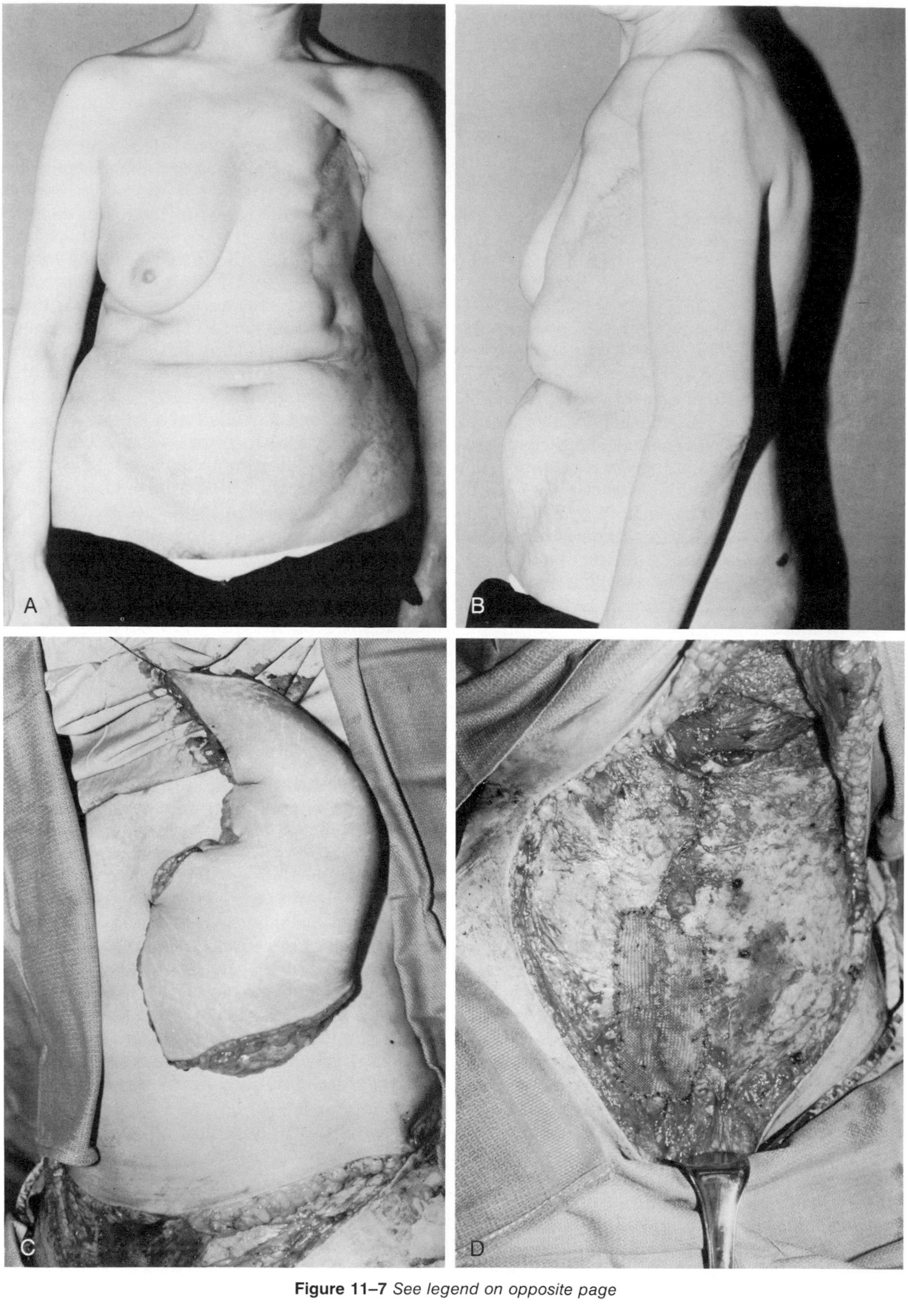

Figure 11–7 *See legend on opposite page*

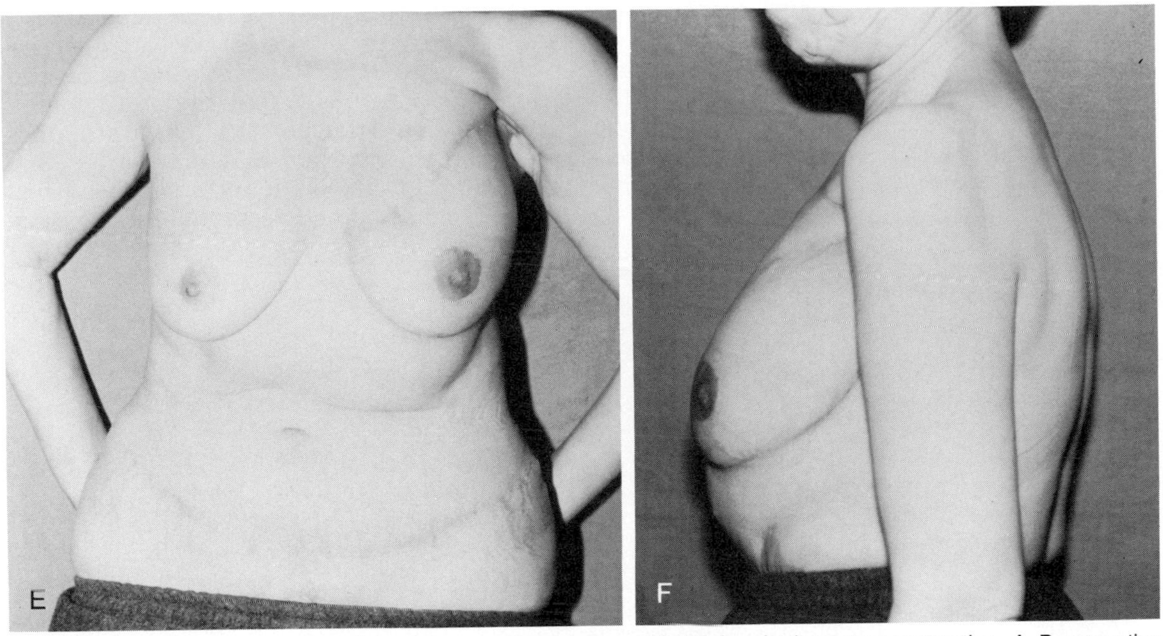

Figure 11–7. Transverse rectus abdominis musculocutaneous (TRAM) flap for breast reconstruction. *A,* Preoperative frontal view after left radical mastectomy and adjuvant radiotherapy. *B,* Preoperative lateral view. *C,* TRAM flap before insetting. Note the donor site at the bottom. *D,* Prolene mesh is utilized to reinforce the anterior fascial closure. Note that the point of rotation of the rectus muscle is at the left costal margin. *E,* Postoperative frontal view. *F,* Postoperative lateral view.

the rectus abdominis muscle as a flap. At present, the morbidity rate of this particular musculocutaneous flap appears to be acceptably low.

Reconstruction of the breast using *microvascular* composite tissue transplantation is rarely necessary thanks to the success of tissue expansion and the transverse rectus abdominis musculocutaneous flap. Several reports, however, have demonstrated acceptable results in patients who for one reason or another could not undergo the above methods of breast reconstruction. Fujino, Harashina, and Aoyagi (1975) described the technique of microvascular tissue transplantation of the gluteus maximus muscle for breast reconstruction. Subsequently, Shaw (1983) reported the use of a superior gluteal muscle and Serafin, Voci, and Georgiade (1982) described the microvascular transplantation of several flaps for breast reconstruction including the groin, latissimus dorsi, tensor fascia lata, and gluteus maximus. Microsurgical techniques can also be used in certain situations to assist in the transposition of a flap. An excellent example is the microvascular anastomosis of the inferior pedicle of the TRAM flap to the appropriate recipient vessels in the axilla when the circulation of the TRAM flap via the superior pedicle is in question (Harashina and associates, 1987).

Mediastinum

Local: 1. Pectoralis major
Distant: 1. Rectus abdominis
2. Latissimus dorsi

The typical patient who requires reconstruction of the mediastinum is the individual who suffers the complication of an infected median sternotomy wound. Although the incidence of such a complication is low, the morbidity and mortality rates can be significant. The treatment of the infected sternotomy wound depends on the extent of the infection and the amount of tissue necrosis. In the past, muscle flap coverage was generally reserved for wounds recalcitrant to "standard" therapy (e.g., debridement, closed tube irrigation). However, it now appears that early muscle flap transposition may decrease morbidity (lower hospitalization costs, shorter length of stay, and so forth), and therefore the use of the muscle flap should always be considered earlier rather than later for the treatment of extensive median sternotomy wounds.

The preferred local muscle flap for mediastinal coverage is the *pectoralis major* (Fig. 11–8). Jurkiewicz and associates (1980) described the use of the pectoralis major muscle flap to obliterate the sternal—mediastinal dead space.

The pectoralis major can be mobilized in several ways. The muscle can be transposed either on the dominant thoracoacromial pedicle or as a turnover flap on the segmental secondary vascular pedicles (perforating vessels from the internal mammary artery and vein) (Fig. 11–9). Nahai and associates (1982) described a modified technique of the turn-

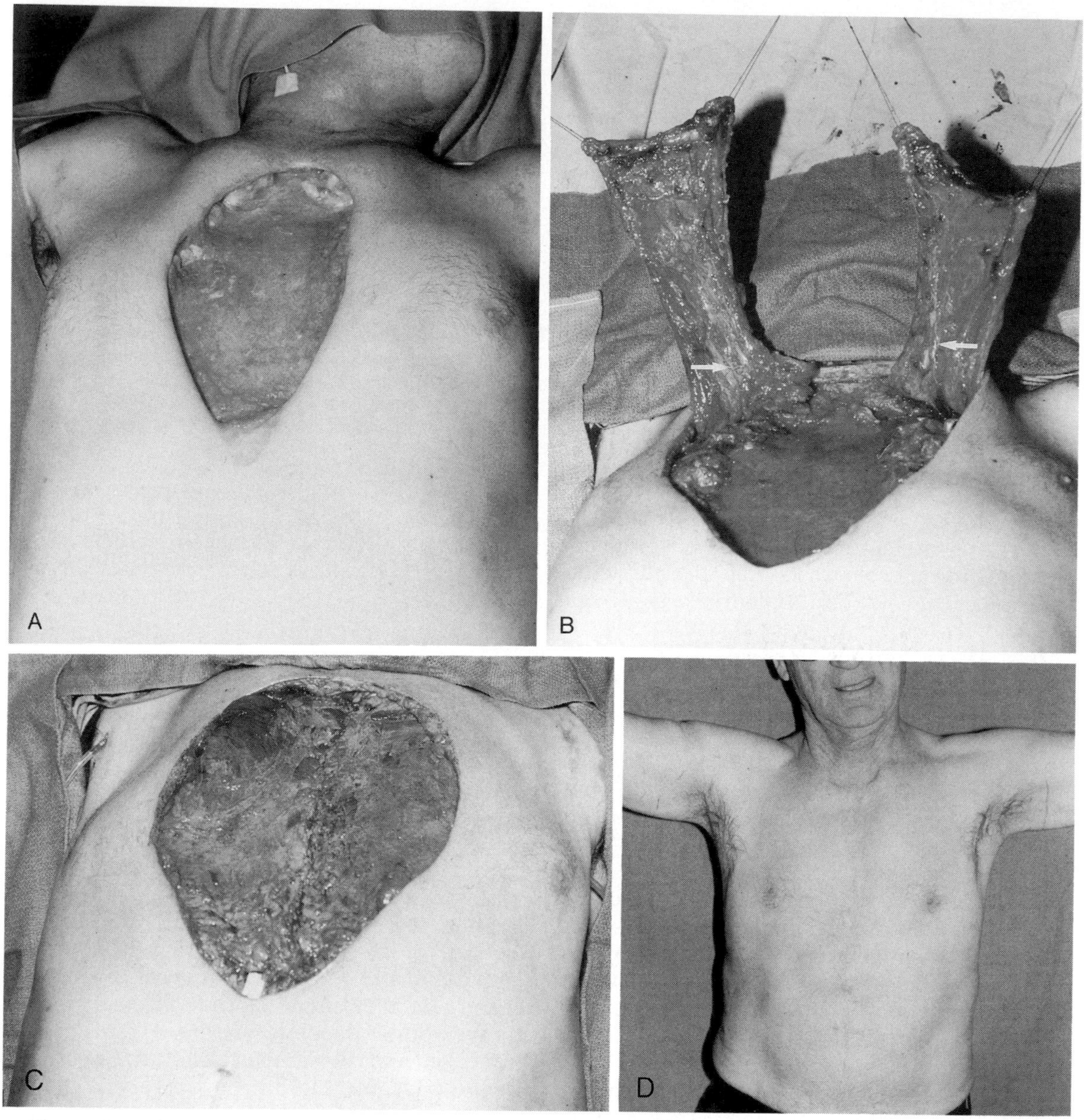

Figure 11–8. Bilateral pectoralis major muscle flaps for mediastinal reconstruction. Flap rotation was based on the major vascular pedicle—Type V muscle. *A,* Chronic mediastinal wound infection 14 months after a myocardial revascularization procedure. *B,* Wound debridement included removal of bilateral costal cartilages and the medial third of both clavicles. The bilateral pectoralis major muscle flaps were elevated for wound coverage. Arrows indicate the site of the vascular pedicle (thoracoacromial artery). *C,* Bilateral pectoralis major muscle flaps provide coverage at the site of the mediastinal and cartilage debridement. *D,* Appearance two years postoperatively. The patient has stable chest wall coverage without recurrent infection. (From Mathes, S.: Muscle flaps and thoracic problems: coverage of a chronic and infected mediastinal wound. *In* Kittle, C. F. (Ed.): Current Controversies in Thoracic Surgery. Philadelphia, W. B. Saunders Company, 1986, p. 246.)

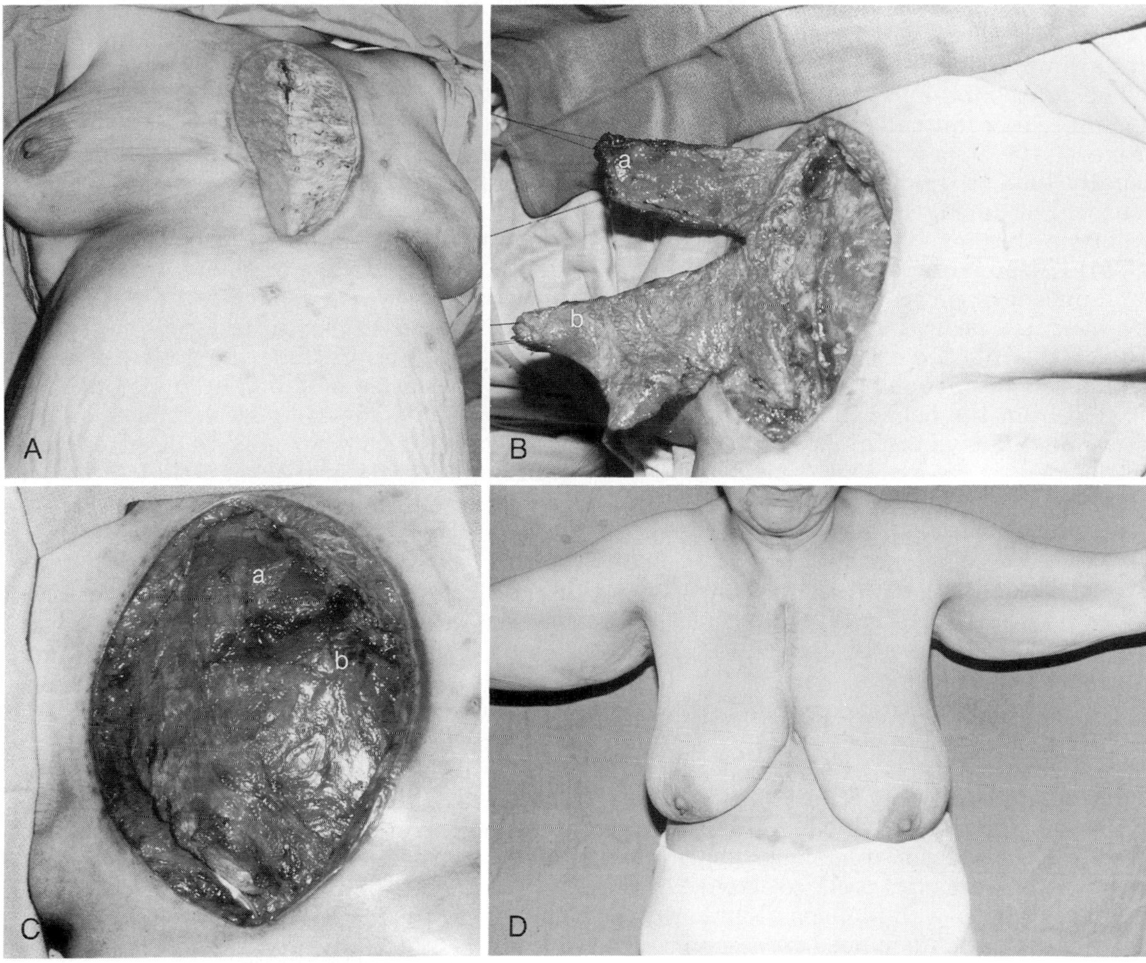

Figure 11–9. Pectoralis major muscle flap for coverage of a mediastinal defect. The flap rotation was based on the segmental secondary vascular pedicles—Type V muscle. *A*, Diabetic patient with an anterior mediastinal infection after a coronary artery bypass graft (left internal mammary artery). *B*, After complete debridement of the left sternum and partial debridement of the right sternum, the right pectoralis major muscle was elevated on the segmental vascular pedicles from the right internal mammary artery. The muscle was split at the fourth intercostal space into two flaps (a and b). *C*, Flap a was placed into the superior anterior mediastinum. Flap b completed coverage of the inferior mediastinal defect. *D*, Six month postoperative view.

over flap that preserves the lateral one-third of the muscle based on the dominant vascular pedicle and its motor nerves; the advantage of this technique is that it preserves the anterior axillary fold.

Depending on the size of the defect, the surgeon can use one or both pectoralis major muscles. If additional coverage is necessary, the rectus abdominis muscle can be used along with the pectoralis major muscles to cover the inferior aspect of the wound. Used as either a muscle or a musculocutaneous flap (Neale and associates, 1981), the rectus abdominis muscle is a reliable and successful source for inferior mediastinal coverage. It is important to note, however, that the superior epigastric artery is a branch of the internal mammary artery, which may be injured during the debridement of the wound. Furthermore, with the increasing use of the internal mammary artery in coronary artery bypass procedures, this vessel often is not available. Collateral circulation to the internal mammary vessels via the intercostal branches is abundant, however, and studies are currently under way to document whether or not a rectus abdominis muscle/musculocutaneous flap can be safely mobilized and transposed primarily on this collateral system (Neale and associates, 1981).

The *omentum* is an alternative available source of tissue transfer for mediastinal reconstruction. In view of the risk of exposing the peritoneum to a contaminated field, however, the omentum is generally reserved for patients in whom the pectoralis major muscles are unavailable.

The *latissimus dorsi* provides an alternative muscle or musculocutaneous flap for coverage of the upper mediastinum. Its use is usually indicated when the pectoralis major is absent or damaged by previous incisions or radiation therapy (Tizian, Borst, and Berger, 1985). The advantage of using the latissimus dorsi muscle or musculocutaneous flap is that the vascular pedicle and the donor site are outside the infected area. The disadvantages include the inconvenience of obtaining a muscle flap from the back, and the fact that the latissimus dorsi muscle may be too thin for the deeper, more extensive mediastinal defects.

Chest Wall and Pulmonary Cavity

Local: 1. Pectoralis major
2. Latissimus dorsi
3. Serratus anterior

Distant: 1. Rectus abdominis

Reconstruction of the chest wall can be a challenging endeavor (see Chap. 76). Ablative surgery for neoplasm, infection, radiation necrosis, and trauma can produce extensive full-thickness chest wall defects. Furthermore, many of the patients in need of reconstruction have previously undergone some form of chemotherapy, high dose irradiation, or hyperthermia treatment for their primary disease. Wound healing can therefore be severely compromised at the time of reconstruction.

In the past, methods of chest wall reconstruction consisted of various random and tube flaps that often required several stages before completion. Today, the reconstruction of the chest wall is successfully accomplished without the need for delay or the staging of procedures.

The pectoralis major and latissimus dorsi muscle and musculocutaneous flaps are the ones most commonly used in chest wall reconstruction. Larson and McMurtrey (1984) stated that the *pectoralis major* musculocutaneous flap is the flap of choice for defects of the lower neck and upper third of the sternum, while the latissimus dorsi musculocutaneous flap is preferred for wounds of the anterior chest wall that require removal of two or three ribs and resection of less than 8 cm of skin. In these authors' series of 53 flaps in 50 patients, the musculocutaneous flap alone provided adequate support and stability; fascia, ribs, and prosthetic material (e.g., Marlex mesh) were not necessary for support.

The use of the *latissimus dorsi* flap in a patient who had previously undergone a thoracotomy raises questions regarding the safety and reliability of ipsilateral flap transposition. Scheflan, Bostwick, and Nahai (1982) reported that a standard anterolateral thoracotomy, which separates the latissimus dorsi into an upper third and lower two-thirds, does not preclude the subsequent use of the muscle as a flap. The upper third of the latissimus dorsi muscle, based on the thoracodorsal pedicle, may be used to cover superior anterolateral chest wall defects. The lower two-thirds of the muscle, based on its secondary pedicles from the paraspinal perforators, can be used as a reverse latissimus dorsi flap with or without the overlying skin to cover inferolateral and posterior chest wall defects. Reports by McCraw, Penix, and Baker (1978) and by Bostwick and associates (1980) were instrumental in the development of the reverse latissimus dorsi flap.

Latissimus dorsi muscle and musculocutaneous flaps have proved invaluable in the treatment of other chest wall and pulmonary cavity disorders: Poland's syndrome (Ohmori and Takada, 1980; Amoroso and Angelats, 1981; Hester and Bostwick, 1982), spina bifida defects (McCraw, Penix, and Baker, 1978; Blaiklock, Demetriou, and Rayner, 1981; Scheflan, Mehrhof, and Ward, 1984; Moore, Dreyer, and Bevin, 1984; McCraw and associates, 1987), and diaphragmatic hernias (Bianchi, Doig, and Cohen, 1983).

The *serratus anterior* muscle can also be useful as a local muscle flap for chest wall and pulmonary cavity reconstruction. Arnold, Pairolero, and Waldorf (1984) described its use in reconstructing the chest wall, closing bronchopleural fistulas, and reinforcing tracheal reconstructions.

The *rectus abdominis* muscle provides a distant muscle or musculocutaneous flap for chest wall reconstruction. Larson and McMurtrey (1984) stated that the rectus abdominis musculocutaneous flap is particularly useful for large chest wall defects. The availability of the flap, however, is dependent on the status of the internal mammary arteries. Miyamoto and associates (1986) favored the rectus abdominis musculocutaneous flap over the latissimus dorsi in chest wall reconstruction because of its convenience (the patient's position does not have to be changed intraoperatively), and because of the ease of elevation of the rectus abdominis muscle and subsequent closure of the donor wound. The major disadvantage of using the rectus abdominis muscle as a flap is the risk of abdominal hernia formation at the donor site.

Abdomen

Local: 1. Rectus abdominis
2. External oblique

Distant: 1. Latissimus dorsi
2. Rectus femoris
3. Tensor fascia lata

In reconstructing abdominal wall defects, the surgical objective is to provide soft tissue coverage and to reestablish abdominal wall integrity (see Chap. 76).

The two available local flaps are the rectus abdominis and the external oblique. The *rectus abdominis* muscle or musculocutaneous flap is the flap of choice for unilateral abdominal defects. In 1977 Mathes and Bostwick described the use of the rectus abdominis musculocutaneous flap for reconstruction of an abdominal wall defect. Parkash and Ramakrishnan (1980) reported the use of a rectus abdominis musculocutaneous island flap for coverage of an extensive radionecrotic abdominal wall ulcer that had been resistant to conservative therapy. Upon debridement of the ulcer, it was noted that the defect measured 12.5 × 9.5 cm and extended as deeply as the rectus abdominis sheath. The contralateral rectus abdominis muscle was used as a flap and the postoperative course was uneventful. Taylor, Corlett, and Boyd (1983) described the extended deep inferior epigastric flap, which consists of an inferiorly based rectus abdominis musculocutaneous flap with a superolateral fasciocutaneous extension. With this larger skin territory, extensive defects of the abdomen, as well as those of the groin and thigh, have been successfully treated (Irons, 1983; Giampapa and associates, 1984; Logan and Mathes, 1984; Taylor, Corlett, and Boyd, 1984; Gottlieb and associates, 1986).

The *external oblique* musculocutaneous flap is an alternative local flap, useful for reconstructing small, full-thickness upper abdominal wall defects (Hershey and Butcher, 1964; Hodgkinson and Arnold, 1980).

The distant muscle and musculocutaneous flaps used in abdominal wall reconstruction include the latissimus dorsi, tensor fascia lata, and rectus femoris flaps. Transposition of the *latissimus dorsi* musculocutaneous flap is a reliable technique (Bostwick, 1982) that is particularly useful for superolateral abdominal wall defects.

The use of the *tensor fascia lata* as a musculocutaneous and musculofascial flap is indicated in the reconstruction of the abdominal wall. Reports by Hill, Nahai, and Vasconez (1978), Nahai, Hill, and Hester (1979), and Nahai (1980) have been instrumental in the development of the many clinical applications of this flap. The unique qualities of the tensor fascia lata flap include the relatively generous amount of vascularized fascia and skin and the low donor site morbidity. The tensor fascia lata flap is the one of choice for lower abdominal wall reconstruction (Nahai, Hill, and Hester, 1979; Withers and associates, 1980; White and associates, 1981; O'Hare and Leonard, 1982; Caffee, 1983).

The *rectus femoris* musculocutaneous flap is a dependable alternative flap for abdominal wall reconstruction (Ger and Duboys, 1983). However, it tends to be bulkier than the tensor fascia lata flap and has greater donor site morbidity. Knee extension may also be adversely affected with the use of this flap (Caffee, 1983). In certain instances, however, the rectus femoris flap with its well-vascularized muscle is preferred to the tensor fascia lata flap. The use of the rectus femoris flap to treat a radionecrotic ulcer involving the lower abdominal properitoneal region is a prime example (Mathes and Hurwitz, 1986).

Groin and Perineum

Local: 1. Sartorius

Distant: 1. Gracilis
2. Tensor fascia lata
3. Rectus femoris
4. Rectus abdominis
5. Gluteus maximus

Reconstruction of the groin and perineum is often indicated for defects due to trauma and ablative surgery. These wounds can be extensive and, owing to their proximity to the anus and urethra, are susceptible to fecal and urinary contamination. Vascular prosthetic grafts in the trauma patient and adjunctive radiation therapy in the cancer patient serve only to compound the problems.

The *sartorius* is a Type IV muscle with multiple segmental vascular pedicles that limit its arc of rotation. The division of one or two of the most proximal pedicles, however, enables the superior aspect of the sartorius muscle to be transposed medially into the groin. The technique is useful for coverage of exposed femoral vessels and prosthetic vascular grafts.

The *gracilis* is a Type II muscle that has both an anterior and a posterior arc of rotation. Anteriorly, the muscle can be used for groin and perineal reconstruction, while posteriorly, ischial and perirectal defects can be reconstructed. Other common uses of the gracilis muscle and musculocutaneous flap include the reconstruction of the vagina, penis, scrotum, and anal sphincter (Fig. 11–10) (McCraw and associates, 1976; Ben-Hur and associates, 1980; Heckler and associates, 1980; Westfall and Keller, 1981; Woods and Beart, 1983; Ramos, Andrews, and Ferreira, 1984; Nakajima, Naide, and Kami, 1984).

The *tensor fascia lata* is particularly useful for groin and perineal reconstruction. It can be used as either a musculocutaneous or a musculofascial flap and is considered the flap of choice for coverage of the groin. Wounds involving an exposed prosthetic vascular graft are an exception where direct coverage with muscle rather than fascia is preferred. A sartorius, rectus femoris, rectus abdominis, or vastus lateralis flap is preferable in this situation. The tensor fascia lata is also used in vulvar reconstruction and recurrent inguinal hernia reconstruction (Nahai, Hill, and Hester, 1979; Nahai, 1980).

The *rectus femoris* is useful for coverage of the groin and perineum. It is a large, bulky muscle that has an arc of rotation similar to

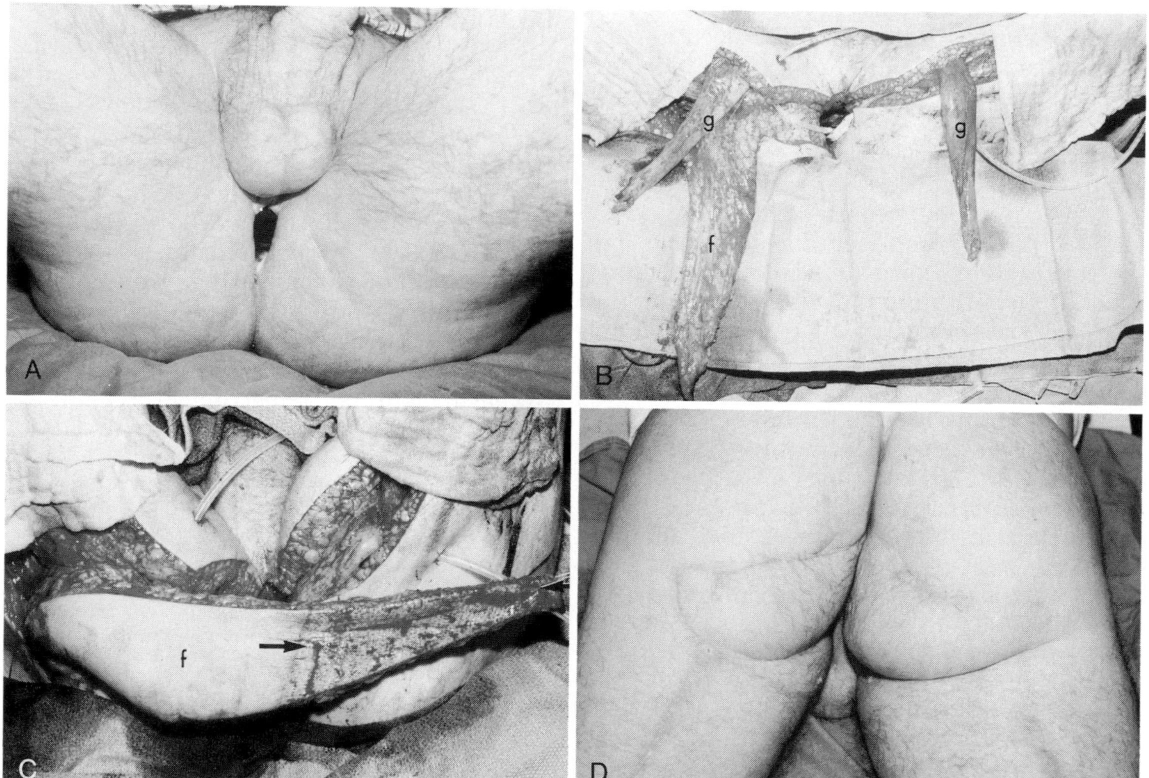

Figure 11–10. Bilateral gracilis and gluteal thigh flaps for reconstruction of a radiation defect of the perineum. *A,* Necrotic lesion of the perineum and sacral cavity after radiation therapy and abdominoperineal resection for carcinoma of the rectum. The wound extended from the perineum into the pelvic cavity at the level of the peritoneal reflection. *B,* Bilateral gracilis (g) and gluteal thigh (f) fasciocutaneous flaps elevated for wound coverage. *C,* After deepithelization of the distal half of both gluteal thigh flaps, which were used to fill the pelvic cavity and provide skin coverage. (Arrows denote the site of flap deepithelization; f, skin surface of the gluteal thigh flap.) *D,* Stable wound coverage one year after repair. The flap donor sites were closed primarily. (From Mathes, S. J., and Hurwitz, D. J.: Repair of chronic radiation wounds of the pelvis. World J. Surg., *10*:274, 1986.)

that of the tensor fascia lata. Despite its reliability and desirable muscle bulk, however, this muscle is generally used as an alternative flap in the ambulatory patient. This is because the rectus femoris is not an entirely expendable muscle (Nahai, Hill, and Hester, 1979).

The *rectus abdominis* muscle based on its inferior pedicle provides a reliable flap for defects of the anterior pelvis and groin (Logan and Mathes, 1984; Ishii and associates, 1985; Mathes and Hurwitz, 1986). Its wide arc of rotation and abundant blood supply via the inferior epigastric vessels make it an excellent reconstructive flap for this region.

The *gluteus maximus* muscle provides stable coverage for pelvic and perineal defects. Its large mass is particularly useful for obliterating pelvic dead space and covering perineal wounds; it is also useful for rectal sphincter reconstruction (Maruyama, Nakajima, and Kodaira, 1980; Hentz, 1982; Maruyama and Nakajima, 1983; Ramirez, Hurwitz, and Futrell, 1984; Orgel and Kucan, 1985). Hurwitz (1980; Hurwitz, Swartz, and Mathes, 1981; Hurwitz and Walton, 1982) described the gluteal thigh flap, which includes the inferior part of the gluteus maximus muscle and a large cutaneous territory of the posterior thigh that is supplied by the descending branch of the inferior gluteal artery. The compound gluteus maximus musculocutaneous and fasciocutaneous flap is particularly useful for reconstructing deep perineal and pelvic defects.

Lower Extremity

Local: 1. Gastrocnemius
2. Soleus

Distant: 1. Microvascular transplantation
2. Cross leg flaps

The reconstruction of the lower extremity has been particularly challenging to the reconstructive surgeon (see also Chap. 82). Defects including exposed joints or prostheses, infected bone, and fractures are common. Furthermore, the availability of adequate soft tissue for coverage is limited, particularly in the lower third of the leg.

There are two local sources of muscle or musculocutaneous flaps available for reconstruction of the leg: the gastrocnemius and the soleus. Use of distant flaps involves the microvascular transplantation of various muscles such as the gracilis, latissimus dorsi, serratus anterior, and rectus abdominis. Cross leg flaps are also available but have generally been supplanted by either local muscle flaps or microvascular composite tissue transplantation techniques.

The *gastrocnemius* is a Type I muscle, consisting of a medial and a lateral head. Each head has a wide arc of rotation based on its single vascular pedicle. The gastrocnemius muscle or musculocutaneous flap is the flap of choice for coverage of the knee and for coverage of exposed bone, including fractures involving the upper third of the leg. Defects of the middle third of the leg can also be reconstructed with the gastrocnemius muscle (McCraw, Fishman, and Sharzer, 1978; Salibian and Menick, 1982; Linton, 1982; Arnold and Mixter, 1983; Cheng and associates, 1984; Ersek, Abell, and Calhoun, 1984; Malawer and Price, 1984; Salibian, Rogers, and Lamb, 1984).

The *soleus* muscle flap is the local source of choice for reconstructing most defects involving the middle third of the leg. Defects of the upper third of the leg can be reached by the soleus, but this maneuver requires extensive mobilization of the muscle. In the lower third of the leg, the soleus muscle can be used as either a proximally or distally based flap (Fig. 11–11). In this particular region, however, the soleus muscle flap is generally used for the smaller defects. Microvascular transplantation is the method of choice for the larger defects.

The soleus muscle is the prime ankle plantar flexor and it serves to stabilize the ankle in ambulation by opposing dorsiflexion (Simon and associates, 1978). Owing to compensatory mechanisms, the use of the soleus muscle as a flap does not impair function at the donor site. Function-preserving techniques such as muscle splitting (Vaca and Garramone, 1983; Tobin, 1985), however, are recommended if the soleus is used in a patient who does not have functional medial and lateral gatrocnemius muscles.

Microvascular transplantation has made a significant impact on reconstruction of the lower leg. Extensive defects are successfully reconstructed by using muscles such as the latissimus dorsi, gracilis, serratus, and rectus abdominis. In certain individuals, microvascular transplantation is not possible. For such patients, alternative methods of reconstruction include the use of random or fasciocutaneous cross leg flaps. Following the recogni-

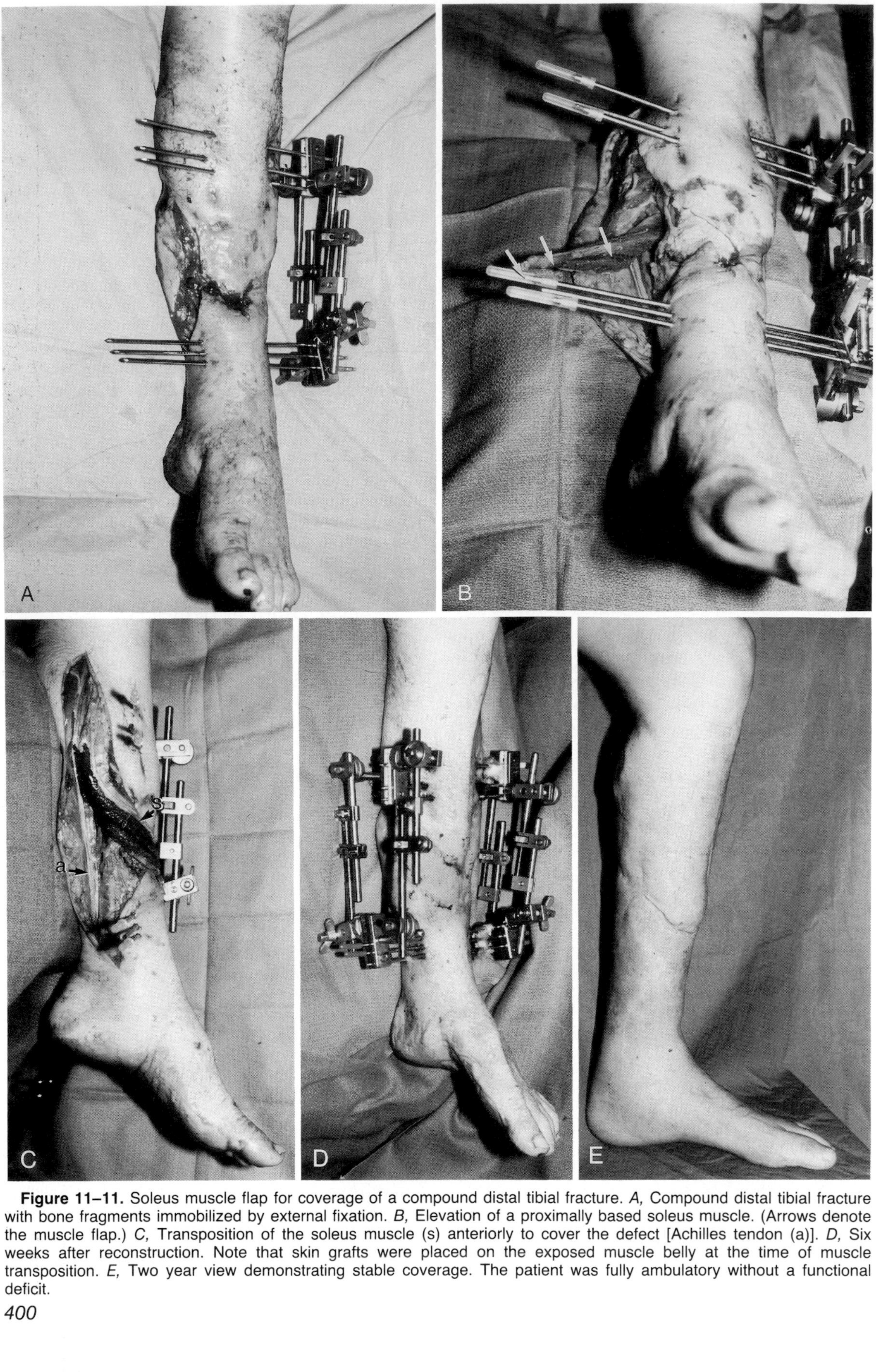

Figure 11–11. Soleus muscle flap for coverage of a compound distal tibial fracture. *A,* Compound distal tibial fracture with bone fragments immobilized by external fixation. *B,* Elevation of a proximally based soleus muscle. (Arrows denote the muscle flap.) *C,* Transposition of the soleus muscle (s) anteriorly to cover the defect [Achilles tendon (a)]. *D,* Six weeks after reconstruction. Note that skin grafts were placed on the exposed muscle belly at the time of muscle transposition. *E,* Two year view demonstrating stable coverage. The patient was fully ambulatory without a functional deficit.

tion of the skin-fascial circulation, various local fasciocutaneous flaps have been identified and are of definite clinical utility. The musculocutaneous gastrocnemius cross leg flap is another means of reconstruction, but it tends to be bulky. Furthermore, the donor site defect is large and in most cases is unacceptable.

Foot

Local: 1. Flexor digitorum brevis
2. Abductor hallucis
3. Abductor digiti minimi

Distant: 1. Microvascular transplantation
2. Cross foot flaps

Defects of the foot are most often due to trauma or the long-standing effects of certain underlying systemic disorders such as diabetes mellitus and peripheral vascular disease. These wounds can be extremely difficult to treat and often are best left uncovered until the underlying disease is treated (e.g., by revascularization). For some patients with severe, irreversible underlying systemic disease, local conservative wound care may be the only appropriate form of therapy.

When reconstruction is necessary, several issues must be addressed: the size of the defect and the patient's vascular, neurosensory, and weight-bearing status. For small defects, skin grafts are often the procedure of choice provided that there is adequate protective soft tissue within the bed of the defect. For small defects involving weight-bearing areas, axial innervated skin flaps and fasciocutaneous flaps have been successful in providing stable coverage.

For the deeper, more extensive foot defect, the use of a muscle or musculocutaneous flap is usually necessary. The local muscles available for use as flaps include the flexor digitorum brevis, the abductor hallucis, and the abductor digiti minimi. These muscles are small and are inadequate for the larger defect. The use of distant muscle (i.e., in microvascular transplantation) is usually necessary for coverage of any major wound (Fig. 11–12).

The anatomy of the *flexor digitorum brevis* muscle for use as a flap was demonstrated in 1974 by Mathes, McCraw, and Vasconez, and this muscle was used clinically to cover a calcaneal defect by Vasconez, Bostwick, and McCraw (1974). In 1980 Hartrampf, Scheflan, and Bostwick described a modification of this technique, using the muscle as an island flap that increased the arc of rotation. As an island flap based on the lateral plantar artery, the flexor digitorum brevis muscle reaches the malleolus and can cover the entire posterosuperior aspect of the heel pad (Hartrampf, Scheflan, and Bostwick, 1980). The authors recommended that the patency of both the dorsalis pedis and the tibialis posterior artery should be confirmed before the lateral plantar artery is divided. In patients who have occluded either the dorsalis pedis or the tibialis posterior artery, the lateral plantar artery serves as a vital conduit of collateral flow.

The *retrograde lateral plantar artery* flap was described by Reiffel and McCarthy in 1980. The flap is fashioned by dividing the lateral plantar vessels proximally; the plantar fascia and the flexor digitorum brevis muscle can be elevated as a flap based on distal retrograde flow. This flap is particularly useful for coverage of medial and lateral metatarsal head defects.

The *abductor hallucis* is a Type II muscle with branches of the medial plantar artery as its dominant vascular pedicle. Based on the latter, the abductor hallucis can be elevated as a muscle or musculocutaneous flap, and it can reach defects just inferior to the medial malleolus as well as defects of the proximal medial aspect of the dorsum of the foot. Like the lateral plantar artery, the medial plantar artery should not be divided if either the dorsalis pedis or the posterior tibial artery is occluded.

The *abductor digiti minimi* is a Type II muscle with branches of the lateral plantar artery as its dominant vascular pedicle. This small muscle based on its dominant pedicle can reach defects adjacent to the lateral malleolus. Because of its size, however, the flap is limited in its ability to provide adequate coverage for the larger defect. In 1985 Yoshimura, Nakajima, and Kami, using the concept originally described by Reiffel and McCarthy (1980), reported the use of a distally based abductor digiti minimi muscle flap. Based on the communication between the lateral plantar artery and the plantar arch, this distally based muscle flap can be used to cover small tissue defects of the distal half of the foot.

For extensive foot defects, microvascular transplantation is the procedure of choice. The gracilis, serratus, and latissimus dorsi

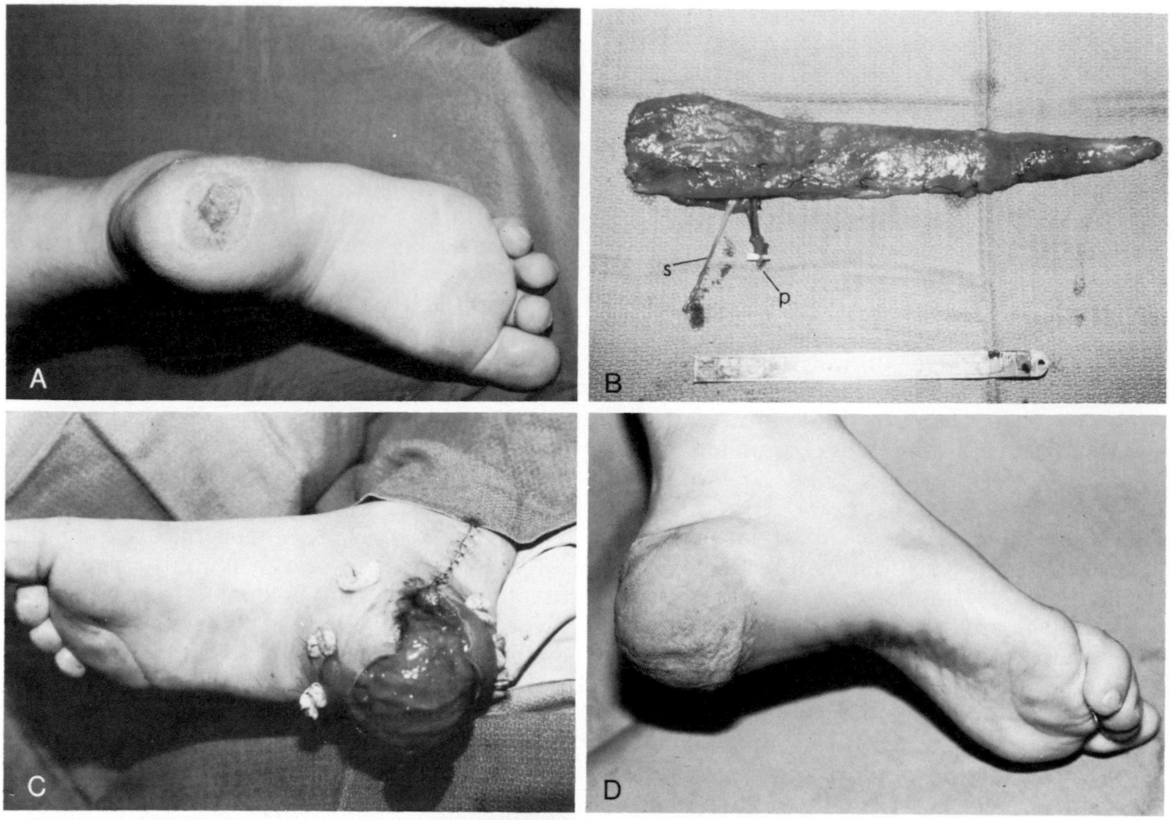

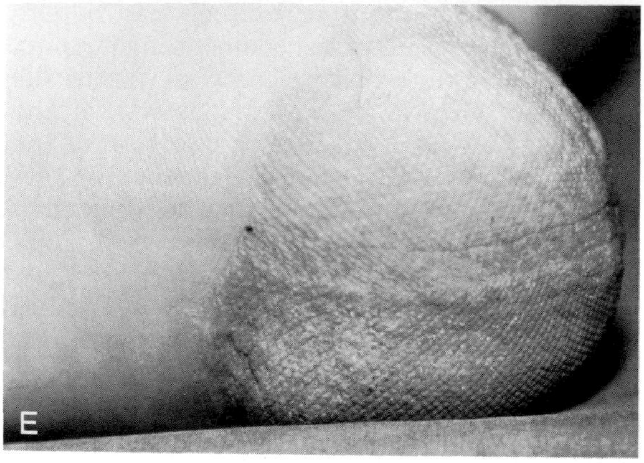

Figure 11–12. Microvascular transplantation of the gracilis muscle for foot reconstruction. *A,* Post-traumatic defect on the plantar surface of the right heel with exposed calcaneus. Attempts at local wound care and skin grafting were unsuccessful. *B,* Gracilis muscle prepared for microvascular transplantation. p, Medial femoral circumflex artery and paired venae comitantes; s, obturator nerve. *C,* Gracilis muscle after revascularization by microvascular repair of the pedicle end to side with the posterior tibial vessels. *D,* Two year postoperative view. The combination of muscle flap with skin graft provided satisfactory contour with the adjacent plantar foot surface. *E,* Close-up view of the reconstructed heel demonstrating stable coverage in a fully ambulatory patient. (From Stevenson, T. R., and Mathes, S. J.: Management of foot injuries with free-muscle flaps. Plast. Reconstr. Surg., *78*:665, 1986.)

muscles have been particularly successful sources for reconstruction of these defects. Alternative methods include the use of cross leg and cross foot flaps.

Pressure Sores

Local: 1. Gluteus maximus
Distant: 1. Tensor fascia lata
2. Gracilis
3. Hamstrings

The *gluteus maximus* is the local muscle used for the surgical treatment of pressure sores (see Chap. 77). It is a Type III muscle and it provides the flap of choice for reconstructing deep sacral and ischial pressure sores (Fig. 11–13). Function-preserving techniques such as bilateral advancement flaps using only the superior halves of the gluteus maximus for sacral coverage (Parry and Mathes, 1982; Fisher and associates, 1983; Vaca and Garramone, 1983; Ramirez, Orlando, and Hurwitz, 1984) are recommended for the ambulatory patient. Variations in technique, involving the sliding gluteus maximus flap (Scheflan, Nahai, and Bostwick, 1981; Ramirez, Orlando, and Hurwitz, 1984) and the transposition gluteus maximus flap (Scheflan, Nahai, and Bostwick, 1981), have been described. The sliding flap is indicated for small sacral defects, whereas the transposition flap (unilateral or bilateral) is generally appropriate for larger defects because it has a greater range of coverage. For extensive pressure sores, the gluteal thigh flap has also been useful (Hurwitz, 1980; Hurwitz, Swartz, and Mathes, 1981; Hurwitz and Walton, 1982).

The three distant muscles used in the reconstruction of pressure sores are the tensor fascia lata, the gracilis, and the hamstrings. The *tensor fascia lata* (TFL) is a Type I muscle that provides the flap of choice for reconstructing trochanteric pressure sores (Withers and associates, 1980; Scheflan, 1981). It is also a reliable alternative flap for ischial defects because of the following advantages: (1) there is relatively low donor site morbidity, especially in an ambulatory patient; (2) the flap provides vascularized, durable fascia; and (3) the flap can provide sensibility in certain instances.

Nahai, Hill, and Hester (1979) and Nahai (1980) described the use of the innervated tensor fascia lata flap, based on the lateral femoral cutaneous nerve (L2–L3), for reconstruction of ischial defects. They reported

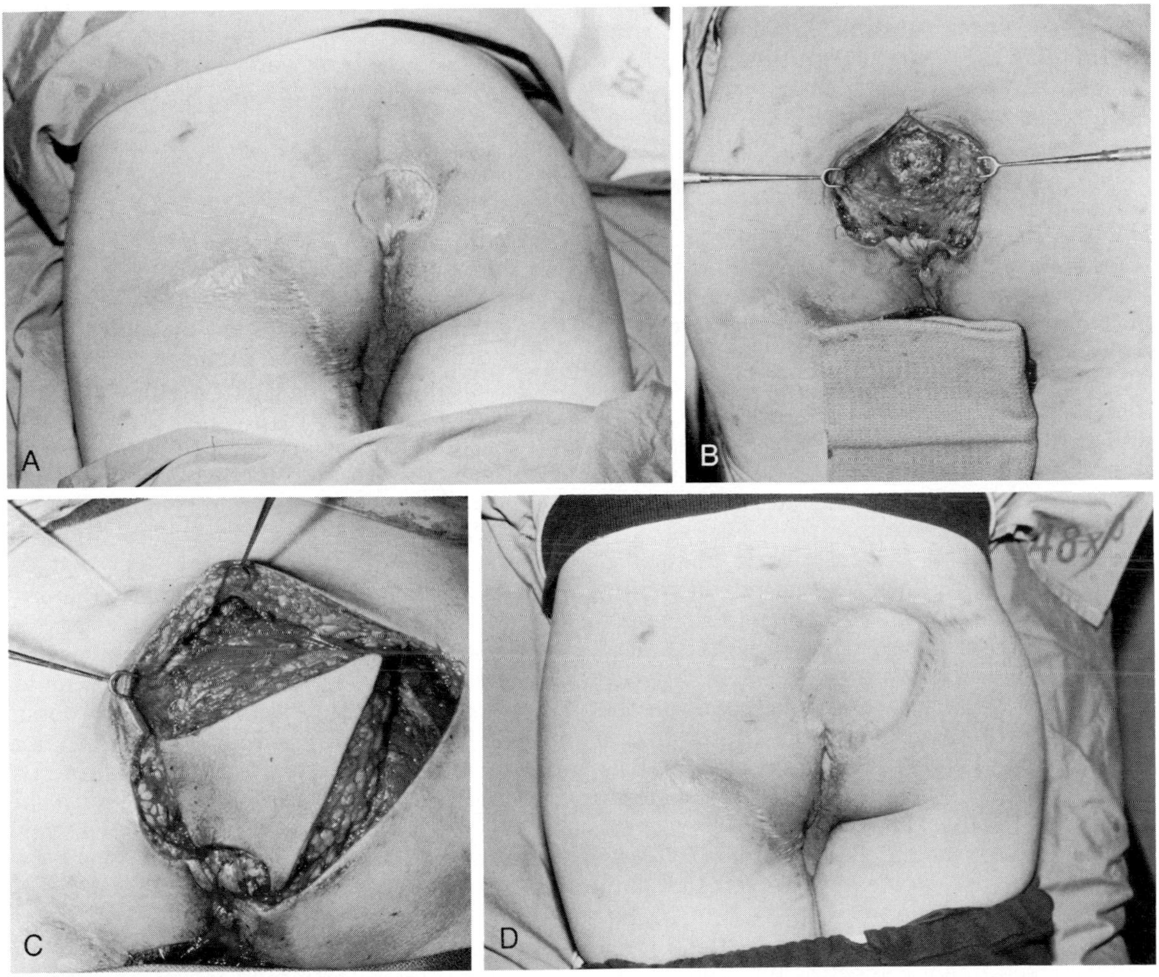

Figure 11–13. Gluteus maximus musculocutaneous flap for treatment of a sacral pressure sore. *A,* Preoperative view of a sacral pressure sore in a quadriplegic patient. *B,* Wound debridement included excision of the sinus and the infected outer table of the sacrum. *C,* Right superior gluteus maximus musculocutaneous flap elevated and based on the superior gluteal artery and veins. The muscle origin and superior half-insertion are incised to permit flap transposition into the sacral defect. The donor site is closed directly after V-Y advancement of the muscle flap. *D,* Six month postoperative view demonstrating stable wound coverage at the site of the sacral pressure sore.

successful protective sensibility without recurrence of pressure ulceration in paraplegic patients with lesions below the L3 level.

Cochran, Edstrom, and Dibbell (1981) reported a series of nine paraplegic patients in whom the innervated tensor fascia lata flap was used for the reconstruction of ischial pressure sores. A total of ten innervated TFL flaps were attempted and nine of these were successful; one flap upon elevation lost its distal perfusion and could not be used. Of the nine flaps completed, all maintained sensibility postoperatively and there were no reported recurrent ulcers during six to 24 months of follow-up.

The major disadvantage of the tensor fascia lata flap is its relative thinness, a problem for the deeper pressure sore. In 1981 Scheflan described a technique to increase the bulk of the tensor fascia lata flap. By deepithelizing the distal aspect of the flap and folding the inferior portion of the flap underneath, part of the flap gains bulk. Used as a "sandwich," the modified flap can usually fill the deeper defect.

Modifications in the design of the tensor fascia lata flap have been described in attempts to minimize the donor site morbidity. Problems such as dog ears, excessive tension at wound closure, skin necrosis at certain wound margins, and the need for skin grafts have prompted techniques such as the use of a bilobed tensor fascia lata flap (Lynch, 1981) and the V-Y retroposition tensor fascia lata flap (Lewis, Cunningham, and Hugo, 1981). These modifications appear to facilitate closure in certain instances.

The *gracilis* is a Type II muscle, the use of which as a musculocutaneous flap was first described by Orticochea in 1972. In the treatment of pressure sores, the gracilis is used primarily to repair the ischial defect. Utilization of the gracilis does not preclude the future use of the gluteus maximus or the posterior thigh flap if the ulcer recurs. The muscle can be elevated with the patient prone, but the distal muscle should be located before the skin island is incised, in order to ensure the correct localization of the skin overlying the muscle.

The *hamstrings*, consisting of the biceps femoris, semimembranosus and semitendinosus, are a group of muscles of the posterior thigh that share a common origin, the ischial tuberosity. (The biceps femoris also has a short head originating from the linea aspera of the femur.) As a group, these muscles are extremely useful in the reconstruction of ischial pressure sores. Used as a transposition flap, depending on the size of the defect, one or more of the hamstring muscles can provide ischial coverage. Hurteau and associates (1981) described V-Y advancement of the hamstring musculocutaneous flap for coverage of the ischial pressure sore. A triangular island of skin overlying the hamstring muscles is designed with the base of the triangle at the inferior margin of the ischial defect. The hamstring muscles are divided distal to the skin island, and the entire muscle group is mobilized superiorly. The origins of the hamstring muscles are detached from the ischium, thus enabling further advancement, and the flap is sutured into place. The donor site is closed primarily. In these authors' series of ten patients in whom this technique was employed, there were no reported complications and there were no reported recurrences during a follow-up of three to 15 months.

MANAGEMENT OF THE PATIENT

In general, the management of a patient undergoing a muscle or musculocutaneous flap technique is not unlike that of any other surgical patient. The basic principles of proper nutrition, hydration, wound care, and attention to underlying medical problems apply to the care of such a patient. However, certain factors unique to the care of the patient undergoing muscle or musculocutaneous flap transposition deserve special mention.

Preoperative education is of particular importance for these patients. Expectations of operative outcome may differ considerably between surgeon and patient. For example, the patient may not realize that the donor scar will be situated transversely or that a skin graft may be required for closure. By thoroughly discussing the procedure with the patient preoperatively, the surgeon can avoid these misunderstandings.

A complete physical examination can provide valuable information. Evidence of previous incisions, muscle atrophy, neuropathic disorders, and so forth may assist the surgeon in selecting the most appropriate muscle or musculocutaneous flap. Additional diagnostic measures (e.g., selective arteriography) may be indicated, depending on the physical findings.

The design of the flap has an impact on future procedures if the defect should recur or require revisions. The operation chosen should therefore not preclude the future use of other flaps if at all possible. This is particularly important for the care of the paraplegic patient with recurrent pressure sores.

The technique of handling of tissues is important in muscle and musculocutaneous flap transposition. The vascular pedicle is subject to spasm and injury if manipulated incorrectly. Hemostasis also is obviously essential. Intramuscular hematomas or excessive electrocauterization of the minor pedicles may result in muscle flap necrosis. Suction catheters should be used to avoid postoperative fluid collections, and perioperative antibiotics are indicated in selected patients to minimize the risk of infection. Patients with contaminated or infected wounds should always receive antibiotic therapy.

The accurate assessment of vascular flow and tissue perfusion is vital to the care of patients undergoing muscle or musculocutaneous flap transposition. Assessment of skin color, tissue turgor, temperature, capillary refill, and oxygen tension is useful in checking flap viability (see Chap. 9). The use of Doppler and intravenous fluoroscein studies is helpful in patients in whom the clinical findings are equivocal.

In the postoperative period, the maintenance of proper positioning, temporary immobilization, and proper dressing of the wound are vital. Flap positioning is dependent on the adequacy of the vascular pedicle(s) and the cardiovascular volume status of the patient. Flap dependency may impede venous outflow and thus cause venous congestion. Excessive elevation of the flap can hinder arterial inflow. In general, slight elevation of the flap is helpful in the postoperative period to prevent edema and venous congestion. Immobilization of the flap prevents undue stress and tension at the vascular pedicle and at the incision sites. Immobilization also promotes hemostasis. The ideal dressing is one that is never constricting and is easily removable for inspection of the flap. At the appropriate time, mobilization of the patient is encouraged to minimize the risk of postoperative morbidity (e.g., atelectasis, pneumonia, pulmonary embolism, and so forth). Physical therapy and rehabilitation are also helpful.

COMPLICATIONS

Most of the complications seen in surgery can be attributed to an error made in one of the following three areas: judgment, technique, and patient management. In muscle or musculocutaneous flap transposition, the complications most commonly seen include seroma, hematoma, superficial skin necrosis, wound separation, inadequate coverage of the defect, infection, and loss of flap (partial/complete). By analyzing these complications in relation to judgment, technique, and patient management, the surgeon should be able to understand the cause of each complication and learn how to prevent it.

Errors in surgical judgment are usually due to (1) inadequate preparation, (2) inadequate flap design, and (3) inadequate knowledge of anatomy.

Inadequate preparation is characterized by proceeding with a reconstructive procedure without having sufficient resources to perform the operation. For example, a surgeon may be asked to evaluate an elderly patient who has an extensive nonhealing ulcer involving the distal third of the leg. The surgeon recommends microvascular transplantation of a muscle flap, yet foregoes a preoperative arteriogram even though the patient is elderly and shows clinical evidence of peripheral vascular disease. Intraoperatively, adequate recipient vessels cannot be found and the flap is therefore aborted. Clearly, if an integral component of the operation is suspect, appropriate diagnostic measures must be undertaken preoperatively.

Inadequate flap design is usually due to the surgeon's failure to account for every aspect of the surgical defect. For example, if a flap is designed and elevated before the wound is actually debrided, one may be left with a large defect and an inadequately small flap. It is always best to make the final designs of the flap after the wound is debrided.

Inadequate knowledge of the anatomy may result in flap failure. It is obvious that injuring the vascular pedicles can compromise the integrity of the flap, and it is also important to realize that surgical dissection is not the only mode of pedicle injury. A surgeon can indirectly injure a pedicle by using a flap whose vascular pedicle is within the zone of injury, as in defects involving infection and radiation necrosis. Vascular pedicles within this environment may be subject to compromise. In a distally based flap, for example, the minor pedicle is usually close to the defect. The pedicle may therefore be affected by the underlying cause of the defect (infection, radiation injury, and so on). This is one of the reasons why the distally based flap is generally less reliable than the muscle flap based on its dominant, major, or segmental secondary vascular pedicles. Through an appreciation of these subtle anatomic differences, proper flap selection and safe flap transposition are virtually assured. It behooves the surgeon to know the precise anatomy of the muscle or musculocutaneous flap and to appreciate the relative importance of each vascular pedicle.

Surgical technique is an obvious determinant of surgical complications. The handling of tissue, particularly the vascular pedicles, is of utmost importance to the success of the flap. Subject to spasm, kinking, shearing, and twisting, blood vessels can clearly be injured at any stage of the operation. Some preventive measures include the placement of temporary sutures between the skin of the flap and the underlying muscle or fascia to prevent shearing of the musculocutaneous perforating vessels. Other techniques include avoiding the skeletonization of the vascular pedicle unless absolutely necessary to avoid spasm and injury. Lastly, in flaps that are tunneled beneath skin bridges, it is important to avoid a tourniquet effect produced by a constrictive skin bridge.

Errors in patient management are a common cause of surgical complications. For patients undergoing a muscle or musculocutaneous flap transposition, the most common errors of management include (1) inadequate attention to underlying medical problems, (2) inadequate assessment of intravascular volume status, and (3) inadequate surveillance of flap viability and perfusion.

The safety and reliability of the muscle or musculocutaneous flap have been repeatedly demonstrated. Such success now encourages refinement where, in certain cases, a complex procedure may be more appropriate than a simple one; i.e., the quality of the result may at times take precedence over the conventional technique. For example, in the reconstruction of a defect involving the lower leg, the soleus and gastrocnemius provide reliable and safe closure. However, the esthetic and functional results may be unacceptable to some patients. In circumstances such as this, a more sophisticated technique (e.g., microvascular transplantation) is appropriate and should be the procedure of choice.

Major microvascular centers currently report microvascular tissue transplantation success rates of 90 to 95 per cent, equivalent to the success rates for standard transposition techniques. With such acceptable results, microvascular tissue transplantation is clearly indicated as the procedure of choice for certain defects. The quality of the result is far greater than the risk involved.

REFERENCES

Alvarez, G. E., Escamilla, J. T., and Carranza, A.: The split sternocleidomastoid myocutaneous flap. Br. J. Plast. Surg., *36*:183, 1983.

Amoroso, P. J., and Angelats, J.: Latissimus dorsi myocutaneous flap in Poland syndrome. Ann. Plast. Surg., *6*:287, 1981.

Apfelberg, D. B., Laub, D. R., Maser, M. R., and Lash, H.: Submuscular breast reconstruction—indications and techniques. Ann. Plast. Surg., *7*:213, 1981.

Ariyan, S.: One stage reconstruction for defects of the mouth using a sternomastoid myocutaneous flap. Plast. Reconstr. Surg., *63*:618, 1979a.

Ariyan, S.: The pectoralis major myocutaneous flap. Plast. Reconstr. Surg., *63*:73, 1979b.

Ariyan, S.: The sternocleidomastoid myocutaneous flap. Laryngoscope, *90*:676, 1980.

Ariyan, S.: The pectoralis major for single-stage reconstruction of the difficult wounds of the orbit and pharyngoesophagus. Plast. Reconstr. Surg., *72*:468, 1983.

Arnold, P. G., and Mixter, R. C.: Making the most of the gastrocnemius muscles. Plast. Reconstr. Surg., *72*:38, 1983.

Arnold, P. G., Pairolero, P. C., and Waldorf, J. C.: The serratus anterior muscle: intrathoracic and extrathoracic utilization. Plast. Reconstr. Surg., *73*:240, 1984.

Baek, S., Biller, H. F., Krespi, Y. P., and Lawson, W.: The lower trapezius island myocutaneous flap. Ann. Plast. Surg., *5*:108, 1980.

Baek, S., Lawson, W., and Biller, H. F.: Reconstruction of hypopharynx and cervical esophagus with pectoralis major island myocutaneous flap. Ann. Plast. Surg., *7*:18, 1981.

Baek, S., Lawson, W., and Biller, H. F.: An analysis of 133 pectoralis major myocutaneous flaps. Plast. Reconstr. Surg., *69*:460, 1982.

Bakamjian, V.: A technique for primary reconstruction of the palate after radical maxillectomy for cancer. Plast. Reconstr. Surg., *31*:103, 1963.

Barton, F. E., Jr., Spicer, T. E., and Byrd, H. S.: Head and neck reconstruction with the latissimus dorsi myocutaneous flap: anatomic observations and report of 60 cases. Plast. Reconstr. Surg., *71*:199, 1983.

Bashir, A. H.: Inferiorly-based gastrocnemius muscle flap in the treatment of war wounds of the middle and lower third of the leg. Br. J. Plast. Surg., *36*:307, 1983.

Bem, C., and O'Hare, P. M.: Case report: reconstruction of the mandible using scapular spine pedicled upon trapezius muscle; description of the posterior approach to the transverse cervical vessels. Br. J. Plast. Surg., *39*:473, 1986.

Ben-Hur, N., Gilai, A., Golan, J., Sagher, U., and Issac, M.: Reconstruction of the anal sphincter by gracilis muscle transfer: the value of electromyography in the preoperative assessment and postoperative management of the patient. Br. J. Plast. Surg., *33*:156, 1980.

Bertotti, J. A.: Trapezius-musculocutaneous island flap in the repair of major head and neck cancer. Plast. Reconstr. Surg., *65*:16, 1980.

Bianchi, A., Doig, C. M., and Cohen, S. J.: The reverse latissimus dorsi flap for congenital diaphragmatic hernia repair. J. Pediatr. Surg., *18*:560, 1983.

Blaiklock, C. R., Demetriou, E. L., and Rayner, C. R. W.: The use of a latissimus dorsi myocutaneous flap in the repair of spinal defects in spina bifida. Br. J. Plast. Surg., *34*:358, 1981.

Bostwick, J., III: Latissimus dorsi flap: current applications. Ann. Plast. Surg., *9*:377, 1982.

Bostwick, J., III, Nahai, F., Wallace, J. G., and Vasconez, L. O.: Sixty latissimus dorsi flaps. Plast. Reconstr. Surg., *63*:31, 1979.

Bostwick, J., III, and Scheflan, M.: The latissimus dorsi musculocutaneous flap: a one-stage breast reconstruction. Clin. Plast. Surg., *7*:71, 1980.

Bostwick, J., III, Scheflan, M., Nahai, F., and Jurkiewicz, M.: The "reverse" latissimus dorsi muscle and musculocutaneous flap: anatomical and clinical considerations. Plast. Reconstr. Surg., *65*:395, 1980.

Bostwick, J., III, Vasconez, L. O., and Jurkiewicz, M. J.: Breast reconstruction after a radical mastectomy. Plast. Reconstr. Surg., *61*:682, 1978.

Boyd, J. B., Taylor, G. I., and Corlett, R. J.: The vascular territories of the superior and deep inferior epigastric systems. Plast. Reconstr. Surg., *73*:1, 1984.

Brandner, M. D., and Bunkis, J.: Shotgun blast injuries to the groin: reconstruction using the rectus abdominis flap. Ann. Plast. Surg., *18*:541, 1987.

Brown, R. G., Fleming, W. H., and Jurkiewicz, M. J.: An island flap for the pectoralis major muscle. Br. J. Plast. Surg., *30*:161, 1977.

Buchanan, D. L., and Agris, J.: Gluteal plication closure of sacral pressure ulcers. Plast. Reconstr. Surg., *72*:49, 1983.

Caffee, H. H.: Reconstruction of the abdominal wall by variations of the tensor fasciae latae flap. Plast. Reconstr. Surg., *71*:348, 1983.

Chang, N., and Mathes, S. J.: Comparison of the effect of bacterial inoculation in musculocutaneous and random-pattern flaps. Plast. Reconstr. Surg., *70*:1, 1982.

Cheng, H. H., Rong, G. W., Yin, T. C., Wang, H. Y., and Jiao, Y. C.: Coverage of wounds in the distal lower leg by advancement of an enlarged medial gastrocnemius skin flap. Plast. Reconstr. Surg., *73*:671, 1984.

Cochran, J. H., Jr., Edstrom, L. E., and Dibbell, D. G.: Usefulness of the innervated tensor fascia lata flap in paraplegic patients. Ann. Plast. Surg., *7*:286, 1981.

Coleman, J. J., III, Jurkiewicz, M. J., Nahai, F., and Mathes, S. J.: The platysma musculocutaneous flap: experience with 24 cases. Plast. Reconstr. Surg., *72*:315, 1983.

Coleman, J. J., III, Nahai, F., and Mathes, S. J.: The platysma musculocutaneous flap: clinical and anatomic considerations in head and neck reconstruction. Am. J. Surg., *144*:477, 1982.

Conley, J.: Use of composite flaps containing bone for major repairs in the head and neck. Plast. Reconstr. Surg., *49*:522, 1972.

Conley, J.: Changes in head and neck surgery. Am. J. Surg., *146*:425, 1983.

Cooper, G. G., Webster, M. H. C., and Bell, G.: The results of breast reconstruction following mastectomy. Br. J. Plast. Surg., *37*:369, 1984.

Cormack, G. C., and Lamberty, B. G. H.: The Arterial Anatomy of Skin Flaps. Edinburgh, Churchill Livingstone, 1986, pp. 87–97, 232, 266–270, 334, 405, 422, 430–436.

Cuono, C. B., and Ariyan, S.: Immediate reconstruction of a composite mandibular defect with a regional osteomusculocutaneous flap. Plast. Reconstr. Surg., *65*:477, 1980.

De la Plaza, R.: Postmastectomy reconstruction by a contralateral abdominomammary flap. Ann. Plast. Surg., *6*:97, 1981.

Demergasso, F., and Piazza, M. V.: Trapezius myocutaneous flap in reconstructive surgery for head and neck cancer: an original technique. Am. J. Surg., *138*:533, 1979.

Dinner, M. I., Dowden, R. V., and Scheflan, M.: Refinements in the use of the transverse abdominal island flap for postmastectomy reconstruction. Ann. Plast. Surg., *11*:362, 1983.

Dinner, M. I., Labandter, H. P., and Dowden, R. V.: The role of the rectus abdominis myocutaneous flap in breast reconstruction. Plast. Reconstr. Surg., *69*:209, 1982.

Drever, J. M.: Total breast reconstruction. Ann. Plast. Surg., *7*:54, 1981.

Drever, J. M.: The lower abdominal transverse rectus abdominis myocutaneous flap for breast reconstruction. Ann. Plast. Surg., *10*:179, 1983.

Dufresne, C., Cutting, C., Valauri, F., Klein, M., Colen, S., and McCarthy, J. G.: Reconstruction of mandibular and floor of mouth defects using the trapezius osteomyocutaneous flap. Plast. Reconstr. Surg., *79*:687, 1987.

Ersek, R. A., Abell, J. M., Jr., and Calhoun, J. H.: The island pedicle rotation advancement gastrocnemius musculocutaneous flap for complex coverage of the popliteal fossa. Ann. Plast. Surg., *12*:533, 1984.

Fisher, J., Arnold, P. G., Waldorf, J., and Woods, J. E.: The gluteus maximus musculocutaneous V-Y advancement flap for large sacral defects. Ann. Plast. Surg., *11*:517, 1983.

Fisher, J., Bostwick, J., III, and Powell, R. W.: Latissimus dorsi blood supply after thoracodorsal vessel division: the serratus collateral. Plast. Reconstr. Surg., *72*:502, 1983.

Fujino, T., Harashina, T., and Aoyagi, T.: Reconstruction for aplasia of the breast and pectoral region by microvascular transfer of a free flap from the buttock. Plast. Reconstr. Surg., *56*:178, 1975.

Georgiade, G., Riefkohl, R., and Georgiade, N.: A flap for moderate-sized oral defects. Ann. Plast. Surg., *14*:55, 1985.

Ger, R., and Duboys, E.: The prevention and repair of large abdominal-wall defects by muscle transposition: a preliminary communication. Plast. Reconstr. Surg., *72*:170, 1983.

Gersuny, R.: Plastischer Ersatz der Mangenscheimhunt. Zentralbl. Chir., *14*:706, 1887.

Giampapa, V., Keller, A., Shaw, W. W., and Colen, S. R.: Pelvic floor reconstruction using the rectus abdominis muscle flap. Ann. Plast. Surg., *13*:56, 1984.

Gottlieb, M. E., Chandrasekhar, B., Terz, J. J., and

Sherman, R.: Clinical applications of the extended deep inferior epigastric flap. Plast. Reconstr. Surg., *78*:782, 1986.

Gruber, R. P., Kahn, R. A., Lash, H., Maser, M. R., Apfelberg, D. B., and Laub, D. R.: Breast reconstruction following mastectomy: a comparison of submuscular and subcutaneous techniques. Plast. Reconstr. Surg., *67*:312, 1981.

Guillamondegui, O. M., and Larson, D. L.: The lateral trapezius musculocutaneous flap: its use in head and neck reconstruction. Plast. Reconstr. Surg., *67*:143, 1981.

Harashina, T., Sone, K., Inoue, T., Fukuzumi, S., and Enomoto, K.: Augmentation of circulation of pedicled transverse rectus abdominis musculocutaneous flaps by microvascular surgery. Br. J. Plast. Surg., *40*:367, 1987.

Hartrampf, C. R., Jr.: Abdominal wall competence in transverse abdominal island flap operations. Ann. Plast. Surg., *12*:139, 1984.

Hartrampf, C. R., Jr., Scheflan, M., and Black, P. W.: Breast reconstruction with a transverse abdominal island flap. Plast. Reconstr. Surg., *69*:216, 1982.

Hartrampf, C. R., Jr., Scheflan, M., and Bostwick, J., III: The flexor digitorum brevis muscle island pedicle flap: a new dimension in heel reconstruction. Plast. Reconstr. Surg., *66*:264, 1980.

Heckler, F. R., Aldrige, J. E., Jr., Songcharoen, S., and Jabaley, M. E.: Muscle flaps and musculocutaneous flaps in the repair of urinary fistulas. Plast. Reconstr. Surg., *66*:94, 1980.

Hentz, V. R.: Construction of a rectal sphincter using the origin of the gluteus maximus muscle. Plast. Reconstr. Surg., *70*:82, 1982.

Hershey, F. B., and Butcher, H. R., Jr.: Repair of defects after partial resection of the abdominal wall. Am. J. Surg., *107*:586, 1964.

Hester, T. R., Jr., and Bostwick, J., III: Poland's syndrome: correction with latissimus muscle transposition. Plast. Reconstr. Surg., *69*:226, 1982.

Hill, H. L., Nahai, F., and Vasconez, L. O.: The tensor fascia lata myocutaneous free flap. Plast. Reconstr. Surg., *61*:517, 1978.

Hodgkinson, D. J., and Arnold, P. G.: Chest-wall reconstruction using the external oblique muscle. Br. J. Plast. Surg., *33*:216, 1980.

Hueston, J. T., and McConchie, H. A.: A compound pectoral flap. Aust. N.Z. J. Surg., *38*:61, 1968.

Hurteau, J. E., Bostwick, J., Nahai, F., Hester, R., and Jurkiewicz, M. J.: V-Y advancement of hamstring musculocutaneous flap for coverage of ischial pressure sores. Plast. Reconstr. Surg., *68*:539, 1981.

Hurwitz, D. J.: Closure of a large defect of the pelvic cavity by an extended compound myocutaneous flap based on the inferior gluteal artery. Br. J. Plast. Surg., *33*:256, 1980.

Hurwitz, D. J., and Kerber, C. W.: Hemodynamic considerations in the treatment of arteriovenous malformations of the face and scalp. Plast. Reconstr. Surg., *67*:421, 1981.

Hurwitz, D. J., Rabson, J. A., and Futrell, J. W.: The anatomic basis for the platysma skin flap. Plast. Reconstr. Surg., *72*:302, 1983.

Hurwitz, D. J., Swartz, W. M., and Mathes, S. J.: The gluteal thigh flap: a reliable sensate flap for the closure of buttock and perineal wounds. Plast. Reconstr. Surg., *68*:521, 1981.

Hurwitz, D. J., and Walton, R. L.: Closure of chronic wounds of the perineal and sacral regions using the gluteal thigh flap. Ann. Plast. Surg., *8*:375, 1982.

Irons, G. B.: Rectus abdominis muscle flaps for closure of osteomyelitis hip defects. Ann. Plast. Surg., *11*:469, 1983.

Ishii, C. H., Jr., Bostwick, J., III, Raine, T. J., Coleman, J. J., III, and Hester, T. R.: Double-pedicle transverse rectus abdominis myocutaneous flap for unilateral breast and chest-wall reconstruction. Plast. Reconstr. Surg., *76*:901, 1985.

Jarrett, J. R., Cutler, R. G., and Teal, D. F.: Subcutaneous mastectomy in small, large, or ptotic breasts with immediate submuscular placement of the implants. Plast. Reconstr. Surg., *62*:702, 1978.

Jurkiewicz, M. J., Bostwick, J., III, Hester, T. R., Bishop, J. B., and Craver, J.: Infected median sternotomy wound: successful treatment by muscle flap. Ann. Surg., *191*:738, 1980.

Kincaid, S. B.: Breast reconstruction: a review. Ann. Plast. Surg., *12*:431, 1984.

Krishna, B. V., and Green, M. F.: Extended role of latissimus dorsi myocutaneous flap in reconstruction of the neck. Br. J. Plast. Surg., *33*:233, 1980.

Kudo, K., Miyasawa, M., Fujioka, Y., and Sasaki, J.: Immediate repair of mandibular defects following surgery for carcinoma of the lower alveolus and gingiva using the pectoralis major osteomyocutaneous flap. J. Maxillofac. Surg., *13*:116, 1985.

Laitung, J. K. G., and Peck, F.: Shoulder function following the loss of the latissimus dorsi muscle. Br. J. Plast. Surg., *38*:375, 1985.

Lam, K. H., Wei, W. I., and Siu, K. F.: The pectoralis major costomyocutaneous flap for mandibular reconstruction. Plast. Reconstr. Surg., *73*:904, 1984.

Larson, D. L., and Goepfert, H.: Limitations of the sternocleidomastoid musculocutaneous flap in head and neck cancer reconstruction. Plast. Reconstr. Surg., *70*:328, 1982.

Larson, D. L., and McMurtrey, M. J.: Musculocutaneous flap reconstruction of chest-wall defects: an experience with 50 patients. Plast. Reconstr. Surg., *73*:734, 1984.

Lewis, V. L., Jr., Cunningham, B. L., and Hugo, N. E.: The tensor fascia lata V-Y retroposition flap. Ann. Plast. Surg., *6*:34, 1981.

Linton, P. C.: The combined medial and lateral gastrocnemius musculocutaneous V-Y island advancement flap. Plast. Reconstr. Surg., *70*:490, 1982.

Littlewood, M.: Compound skin and sternomastoid flaps for repair in extensive carcinoma of the head and neck. Br. J. Plast. Surg., *20*:403, 1967.

Logan, S. E., and Mathes, S. J.: The use of a rectus abdominis myocutaneous flap to reconstruct a groin defect. Br. J. Plast. Surg., *37*:351, 1984.

Longacre, J. J.: Correction of the hypoplastic breast with special reference to reconstruction of the "nipple-type breast" with local dermo-fat flaps. Plast. Reconstr. Surg., *14*:431, 1956.

Lynch, S. M.: The bilobed tensor fascia lata myocutaneous flap. Plast. Reconstr. Surg., *67*:796, 1981.

Malawer, M. M., and Price, W. M.: Gastrocnemius transposition flap in conjunction with limb-sparing surgery for primary bone sarcomas around the knee. Plast. Reconstr. Surg., *73*:741, 1984.

Manktelow, R. T., and Zuker, R. M.: Muscle transplantation by fascicular territory. Plast. Reconstr. Surg., *73*:751, 1984.

Manstein, C. H., Manstein, G., Somers, R. G., and Barswick, W. J.: Use of pectoralis minor muscle in im-

mediate reconstruction of the breast. Plast. Reconstr. Surg., *76*:566, 1985.
Marshall, D. R., Anstee, E. J., and Stapleton, M. J.: Postmastectomy breast reconstruction using a direct flap from an abdominal lipectomy. Br. J. Plast. Surg., *34*:280, 1981.
Maruyama, Y., and Nakajima, H.: One-stage reconstruction of a massive buttock and sacroperineal defect with multiple myocutaneous flaps. Br. J. Plast. Surg., *36*:116, 1983.
Maruyama, Y., Nakajima, H., and Fujino, T.: A dynamic reconstruction of a facial defect with a pectoralis major myocutaneous flap. Br. J. Plast. Surg., *33*:145, 1980.
Maruyama, Y., Nakajima, H., and Kodaira, S.: Primary reconstruction of perineal defect with a bilobed myocutaneous flap: case report. Br. J. Plast. Surg., *33*:440, 1980.
Mathes, S. J., and Bostwick, J., III: A rectus abdominis myocutaneous flap to reconstruct abdominal wall defects. Br. J. Plast. Surg., *30*:282, 1977.
Mathes, S. J., and Buchanan, R. T.: Tensor fascia lata: neurosensory musculocutaneous free flap. Br. J. Plast. Surg., *32*:184, 1979.
Mathes, S. J., and Hurwitz, D. J.: Repair of chronic radiation wounds of the pelvis. World J. Surg., *10*:269, 1986.
Mathes, S. J., McCraw, J. B., and Vasconez, L. O.: Muscle transposition flaps for coverage of lower extremity defects: anatomical considerations. Surg. Clin. North Am., *54*:1337, 1974.
Mathes, S. J., and Nahai, F.: Clinical Atlas of Muscle and Musculocutaneous Flaps. St. Louis, MO, C. V. Mosby Company, 1979.
Mathes, S. J., and Nahai, F.: Muscle flap transposition with function preservation. Plast. Reconstr. Surg., *66*:242, 1980.
Mathes, S. J., and Nahai, F.: Classification of the vascular anatomy of muscles: experimental and clinical correlation. Plast. Reconstr. Surg., *67*:177, 1981.
Mathes, S. J., and Nahai, F.: Clinical Application for Muscle and Musculocutaneous Flaps. St. Louis, MO, C. V. Mosby Company, 1982.
Mathes, S. J., Nahai, F., and Vasconez, L. O.: Myocutaneous free flap transfer: anatomical and experimental consideration. Plast. Reconstr. Surg., *62*:162, 1978.
Matsunaga, W., Ebihara, S., Ono, I., et al.: Reconstruction of the cervical esophagus by means of a latissimus dorsi myocutaneous flap. Jpn. J. Plast. Reconstr. Surg., *26*:98, 1983.
McCraw, J. B., Dibbell, D. G., and Carraway, J. H.: Clinical definition of independent myocutaneous vascular territories. Plast. Reconstr. Surg., *60*:341, 1977.
McCraw, J. B., Fishman, J. H., and Sharzer, L. A.: The versatile gastrocnemius myocutaneous flap. Plast. Reconstr. Surg., *62*:15, 1978.
McCraw, J. B., Magee, W. P., Jr., and Kalwaic, H.: Uses of the trapezius and sternomastoid myocutaneous flaps in head and neck reconstruction. Plast. Reconstr. Surg., *63*:49, 1979.
McCraw, J. B., Massey, F. M., Shanklin, K. D., and Horton, C. E.: Vaginal reconstruction with gracilis myocutaneous flaps. Plast. Reconstr. Surg., *58*:176, 1976.
McCraw, J. B., Penix, J. O., and Baker, J. W.: Repair of major defects of the chest wall and spine with the latissimus dorsi myocutaneous flap. Plast. Reconstr. Surg., *62*:197, 1978.
McCraw, J. B., Penix, J. O., Freeman, B. G., Vincent, M. P., and Wirth, F. H.: Soft-tissue repair of myelomeningocele defects using bilateral latissimus dorsi and trapezius musculocutaneous flaps. Ann. Plast. Surg., *18*:147, 1987.
McDowell, F.: Logs vs. harpsichords, blobby flaps vs. finished results (editorial). Plast. Reconstr. Surg., *64*:249, 1979.
Mendelson, B. C., and Masson, J. K.: Treatment of chronic radiation injury over the shoulder with a latissimus dorsi myocutaneous flap. Plast. Reconstr. Surg., *60*:681, 1977.
Millard, D. R., Jr.: Reconstruction mammaplasty using an economical flap from the opposite breast. Ann. Plast. Surg., *6*:374, 1981.
Miyamoto, Y., Hattori, T., Niimoto, M., and Toge, T.: Reconstruction of full-thickness chest wall defects using rectus abdominis musculocutaneous flap: a report of fifteen cases. Ann. Plast. Surg., *16*:90, 1986.
Miyamoto, Y., Hattori, T., and Nosoh, Y.: One-stage antethoracic reconstruction of the thoracic oesophagus using myocutaneous flaps. Br. J. Plast. Surg., *37*:577, 1984.
Moore, T. S., Dreyer, T. M., and Bevin, B. G.: Closure of large spina bifida cystica defects with bilateral bipedicled musculocutaneous flaps. Plast. Reconstr. Surg., *73*:288, 1984.
Morain, W. D., Colen, L. B., and Hutchings, J. C.: The segmental pectoralis major muscle flap: a function preserving procedure. Plast. Reconstr. Surg., *75*:825, 1985.
Morgan, R. F., Sargent, L. A., and Hoopes, J. E.: Midfacial and total nasal reconstruction with bilateral pectoralis major myocutaneous flaps. Plast. Reconstr. Surg., *73*:824, 1984.
Nahai, F.: The tensor fascia lata flap. Clin. Plast. Surg., *7*:51, 1980.
Nahai, F., Hill, H. L., and Hester, T. R.: Experiences with the tensor fascia lata flap. Plast. Reconstr. Surg., *63*:788, 1979.
Nahai, F., Morales, L., Jr., Bone, D. K., and Bostwick, J., III: Pectoralis major muscle turnover flaps for closure of the infected sternotomy wound with preservation of form and function. Plast. Reconstr. Surg., *70*:471, 1982.
Nakajima, T., Naide, Y., and Kami, T.: Repair of a prostatomembranous urethral stricture with a gracilis myocutaneous flap. Br. J. Plast. Surg., *37*:539, 1984.
Neale, H. W., Kreilein, J. G., Schreiber, J. T., and Gregory, R. O.: Complete sternectomy for chronic osteomyelitis with reconstruction using a rectus abdominis myocutaneous island flap. Ann. Plast. Surg., *6*:305, 1981.
Neifeld, J. P., Merritt, W. A., Theogoraj, S. D., and Parker, G. A.: Tubed pectoralis major musculocutaneous flaps for cervical esophageal replacement. Ann. Plast. Surg., *11*:24, 1983.
Nieto, C. S., Gallego, L. L., and Cortes, J. C. G.: Reconstruction of the posterior wall of the pharynx using a myocutaneous platysma flap. Br. J. Plast. Surg., *36*:36, 1983.
O'Brien, B.: A muscle-skin pedicle for total reconstruction of the lower lip. Plast. Reconstr. Surg., *45*:395, 1970.
O'Hare, P. M., and Leonard, A. G.: Reconstruction of major abdominal wall defects using the tensor fasciae latae myocutaneous flap. Br. J. Plast. Surg., *35*:361, 1982.
Ohmori, K., and Takada, H.: Correction of Poland's

pectoralis major muscle anomaly with latissimus dorsi musculocutaneous flaps. Plast. Reconstr. Surg., *65*:400, 1980.

Olivari, N.: The latissimus flap. Br. J. Plast. Surg., *29*:126, 1976.

Orgel, M. G., and Kucan, J. O.: A double-split gluteus maximus muscle flap for reconstruction of the rectal sphincter. Plast. Reconstr. Surg., *75*:62, 1985.

Orticochea, M.: The musculocutaneous flap method: an immediate and heroic substitute for the method of delay. Br. J. Plast. Surg., *25*:106, 1972.

Owens, N.: A compound neck pedicle designed for the repair of massive facial defects: formation, development, and application. Plast. Reconstr. Surg., *15*:369, 1955.

Panje, W., and Cutting, C.: Trapezius osteomyocutaneous island flap for reconstruction of the anterior floor of the mouth and mandible. Head Neck Surg., *3*:66, 1980.

Parkash, S., and Ramakrishnan, K.: A myocutaneous island flap in the treatment of a chronic radionecrotic ulcer of the abdominal wall. Br. J. Plast. Surg., *33*:138, 1980.

Parkash, S., Ramakrishnan, K., and Ananthakrishnan, N.: Sternomastoid based island flap for lining after resection of oral carcinomas. Br. J. Plast. Surg., *33*:115, 1980.

Parry, S. W., and Mathes, S. J.: Bilateral gluteus maximus myocutaneous advancement flaps: sacral coverage for ambulatory patients. Ann. Plast. Surg., *8*:443, 1982.

Quillen, C. G.: Latissimus dorsi myocutaneous flaps in head and neck reconstruction. Plast. Reconstr. Surg., *63*:664, 1979.

Quillen, C. G., Shearin, J. C., Jr., and Georgiade, N. G.: Use of the latissimus dorsi myocutaneous island flap for reconstruction in the head and neck area. Plast. Reconstr. Surg., *62*:113, 1978.

Radovan, C.: Reconstruction of the breast after radical mastectomy using temporary expander. ASPRS Plast. Surg. Forum, *1*:41, 1978.

Radovan, C.: Breast reconstruction after mastectomy using the temporary expander. Plast. Reconstr. Surg., *69*:195, 1982.

Ramirez, O. M., Hurwitz, D. J., and Futrell, J. W.: The expansive gluteus maximus flap. Plast. Reconstr. Surg., *74*:757, 1984.

Ramirez, O. M., Orlando, J. C., and Hurwitz, D. J.: The sliding gluteus maximus myocutaneous flap: its relevance in ambulatory patients. Plast. Reconstr. Surg., *74*:68, 1984.

Ramos, R. R., Andrews, J. M., and Ferreira, L. M.: A gracilis myocutaneous flap for reconstruction of the scrotum. Br. J. Plast. Surg., *37*:171, 1984.

Rees, R. S., Ivey, G. L., Shack, R. B., Franklin, J. O., and Lynch, J. B.: Pectoralis major musculocutaneous flaps: long-term follow-up of hypopharyngeal reconstruction. Plast. Reconstr. Surg., *77*:586, 1986.

Reiffel, R. S., and McCarthy, J. G.: Coverage of heel and sole defects: a new subfascial arterialized flap. Plast. Reconstr. Surg., *66*:250, 1980.

Robbins, T. H.: Rectus abdominis myocutaneous flap for breast reconstruction. Aust. N.Z. J. Surg., *49*:527, 1979.

Robbins, T. H.: Post-mastectomy breast reconstruction using a rectus abdominis musculocutaneous island flap. Br. J. Plast. Surg., *34*:286, 1981.

Rosen, H. M.: The extended trapezius musculocutaneous flap for cranio-orbital facial reconstruction. Plast. Reconstr. Surg., *75*:318, 1985.

Ryan, J. J.: A lower thoracic advancement flap in breast reconstruction after mastectomy. Plast. Reconstr. Surg., *70*:153, 1982.

Ryan, R. F., Krementz, E. T., and Cardona-Loya, O.: One stage cervical esophageal and pharyngeal reconstruction for a fourth primary cancer. Plast. Reconstr. Surg., *67*:224, 1981.

Salibian, A. H., and Menick, F. J.: Bipedicle gastrocnemius musculocutaneous flap for defects of the distal one-third of the leg. Plast. Reconstr. Surg., *70*:17, 1982.

Salibian, A. H., Rogers, F. R., and Lamb, R. C.: Microvascular gastrocnemius muscle transfer in the distal leg using saphenous vein grafts. Plast. Reconstr. Surg., *73*:302, 1984.

Scheflan, M.: The tensor fascia lata: variations on a theme. Plast. Reconstr. Surg., *68*:59, 1981.

Scheflan, M., Bostwick, J., III, and Nahai, F.: Chest wall reconstruction—management of the difficult chest wound. Ann. Plast. Surg., *8*:122, 1982.

Scheflan, M., and Dinner, M. I.: The transverse abdominal island flap. Part I: Indications, contraindications, results and complications. Ann. Plast. Surg., *10*:24, 1983a.

Scheflan, M., and Dinner, M. I.: The transverse abdominal island flap. Part II: Surgical technique. Ann. Plast. Surg., *10*:120, 1983b.

Scheflan, M., Mehrhof, A. I., Jr., and Ward, J. D.: Meningomyelocele closure with distally based latissimus dorsi flap. Plast. Reconstr. Surg., *73*:956, 1984.

Scheflan, M., Nahai, F., and Bostwick, J., III: Gluteus maximus island musculocutaneous flap for closure of sacral and ischial ulcers. Plast. Reconstr. Surg., *68*:533, 1981.

Schneider, W. J., Hill, L. H., and Brown, R. G.: Latissimus dorsi myocutaneous flap for breast reconstruction. Br. J. Plast. Surg., *30*:277, 1977.

Scuderi, N., and Campus, G.: Breast reconstruction with dermofat flaps after subcutaneous mastectomy. Ann. Plast. Surg., *9*:139, 1982.

Serafin, D., Voci, V. E., and Georgiade, N. G.: Microsurgical composite tissue transplantation: indications and technical considerations in breast reconstruction following mastectomy. Plast. Reconstr. Surg., *70*:24, 1982.

Shapiro, M. J.: The use of trapezius myocutaneous flaps in the reconstruction of head and neck defects. Arch. Otolaryngol., *107*:333, 1981.

Shaw, W. W.: Breast reconstruction by superior gluteal microvascular free flaps without silicone implants. Plast. Reconstr. Surg., *72*:490, 1983.

Siemssen, S. O., Kirkby, B., and O'Connor, T. P. F.: Immediate reconstruction of a resected segment of the lower jaw using a compound flap of clavicle and sternomastoid muscle. Plast. Reconstr. Surg., *61*:724, 1978.

Simon, S. R., Mann, R. A., Hagy, J. L., and Larsen, L. J.: Role of the posterior calf muscles in normal gait. J. Bone Joint Surg., *60A*:465, 1978.

Stevenson, T. R., Grekin, R. C., Friedman, R. J., and Zucker, S. E.: Squamous cell carcinoma of the perineum: management with Mohs' surgical excision and gluteal thigh flap. Ann. Plast. Surg., *18*:248, 1987.

Tansini, I.: Nuovo processo per l'amputazione della mammella per cancro. Riforma Med., *12*:3, 1896a.

Tansini, I.: Sopra il niro nuovo progresso di amputazione della mammella. Riforma Med., *12*:757, 906, 1896b.

Taylor, G. I., Corlett, R., and Boyd, J. B.: The extended deep inferior epigastric flap: a clinical technique. Plast. Reconstr. Surg., *72*:751, 1983.

Taylor, G. I., Corlett, R. J., and Boyd, J. B.: The versatile deep inferior epigastric (inferior rectus abdominis) flap. Br. J. Plast. Surg., *37*:330, 1984.

Tizian, C., Borst, H. G., and Berger, A.: Treatment of total sternal necrosis using the latissimus dorsi muscle flap. Plast. Reconstr. Surg., *76*:703, 1985.

Tobin, G. R.: Hemisoleus and reversed hemisoleus flaps. Plast. Reconstr. Surg., *76*:87, 1985.

Tobin, G. R., Moberg, A. W., DuBou, R. H., Weiner, L. J., and Bland, K. I.: The split latissimus dorsi myocutaneous flap. Ann. Plast. Surg., *7*:272, 1981a.

Tobin, G. R., Schusterman, M. A., Peterson, G. H., Nichols, G., and Bland, K. I.: Intramuscular neurovascular anatomy of the latissimus dorsi: the basis for splitting the flap. Plast. Reconstr. Surg., *67*:637, 1981b.

Vaca, F. J., and Garramone, R.: Hemimuscular transfer of the soleus muscle. Cir. Plast. Argent., *7*:12, 1983.

Vasconez, L. O., Bostwick, J., III, and McGraw, J.: Coverage of exposed bone by muscle transposition and skin grafting. Plast. Reconstr. Surg., *53*:526, 1974.

Watson, J. S.: The use of the latissimus dorsi island flap for intra-oral reconstruction. Br. J. Plast. Surg., *35*:408, 1982.

Watson, J. S., and Lendrum, J.: One stage pharyngeal reconstruction using a compound latissimus dorsi island flap. Br. J. Plast. Surg., *34*:87, 1981.

Watson, J. S., Robertson, G. A., Lendrum, J., Stranc, M. F., and Pohl, M. J.: Pharyngeal reconstruction using the latissimus dorsi myocutaneous flap. Br. J. Plast. Surg., *35*:401, 1982.

Wei, F. C., Chen, H. C., Chuang, C. C., and Noordhoff, M. S.: Fibular osteoseptocutaneous flap: anatomic study and clinical application. Plast. Reconstr. Surg., *78*:191, 1986.

Westfall, C. T., and Keller, H. B.: Scrotal reconstruction utilizing bilateral gracilis myocutaneous flaps. Plast. Reconstr. Surg., *68*:945, 1981.

White, D. N., Pearl, R. M., Laub, D. R., and De Fiebre, B. K.: Tensor fascia lata myocutaneous flap in lower abdominal wall reconstruction. Ann. Plast. Surg., *7*:155, 1981.

Withers, E. H., Franklin, J. D., Madden, J. J., Jr., and Lynch, J. B.: Further experience with the tensor fascia lata musculocutaneous flap. Ann. Plast. Surg., *4*:31, 1980.

Withers, E. H., Franklin, J. D., Madden, J. J., and Lynch, J. B.: Immediate reconstruction of the pharynx and cervical esophagus with the pectoralis major myocutaneous flap following laryngopharyngectomy. Plast. Reconstr. Surg., *68*:898, 1981.

Woods, J. E., and Beart, R. W., Jr.: Reconstruction of nonhealing perineal wounds with gracilis muscle flaps. Ann. Plast. Surg., *11*:513, 1983.

Woods, J. E., Irons, G. B., Jr., and Arnold, P. G.: The case for submuscular implantation of prostheses in reconstructive breast surgery. Ann. Plast. Surg., *5*:115, 1980.

Yoshimura, Y., Maruyama, Y., and Takeuchi, S.: The use of lower trapezius myocutaneous island flaps in head and neck reconstruction. Br. J. Plast. Surg., *34*:334, 1981.

Yoshimura, Y., Nakajima, T., and Kami, T.: Distally based abductor digiti minimi muscle flap. Ann. Plast. Surg., *14*:375, 1985.

12

Bernard M. O'Brien
Wayne A. Morrison
Graham J. Gumley

Principles and Techniques of Microvascular Surgery

THE OPERATING MICROSCOPE

Microsurgery literally means surgery in which a microscope is used. The modern operating microscope, with its refined optics and wide range of magnification, enables a surgeon to carry out procedures not possible with conventional nonmicroscopic techniques. The skills of the surgeon are also augmented by fine instrumentation and microsutures, which not only minimize trauma to small structures but enable these to be repaired with a precision not previously attainable. The operating microscope is essential for precision surgery on structures 3 mm or less in diameter.

The compound microscope was invented in 1590 by Zacharia Janssen and was used for centuries with frequent modification in the fields of microbiology, histology, and pathology. It was not until 1921 that the operating microscope was first used experimentally by Nylen in Sweden, who operated on labyrinthine fistulas and carried out fenestrations in rabbits, using a magnification of 10 to 15 ×. A monocular microscope was designed with a magnification of up to 235 × (Nylen, 1954, 1972). In 1921 Nylen used a primitive binocular microscope in a case of chronic otitis and several cases with pseudofistula symptoms. In 1922 his chief, Holmgren, introduced a Zeiss binocular microscope to otology. Microsurgery in otolaryngology then progressed slowly over the next three decades, but in the early 1950's more rapid progress led to a higher degree of sophistication that is routine today.

In 1946 Perritt (1950), in the United States, commenced the use of the microscope in ophthalmic surgery. There followed the successful experiments of Jacobson and Suarez (1960) in microvascular surgery and the application of the microscope to peripheral nerve surgery (Smith, 1964; Kurze, 1964; Michon and Masse, 1964), to plastic and reconstructive surgery (Buncke and Schulz, 1965), to experimental organ transplantation (Fisher, 1965), and to neurosurgery (Donaghy and Yasargil, 1967).

The value of magnification can be illustrated by comparison of the naked eye view of an artery, diameter 0.8 mm, repaired with microtechniques using a nylon microsuture, and a simple household pin adjacent to the vessel, with the same vessel seen at 6 and 20 × magnification through the operating microscope (Fig. 12–1).

The operating microscope does have certain disadvantages because of its bulk, restricted mobility, small operative area, and limited depth of focus. These aspects are of little significance when the surgery demands higher magnification, and these disadvantages have also been reduced by the newer microscope models. A serviceable microscope should possess strong, even, and cold lighting of a wide-angle field with magnification ranging from 6 to 40 ×. A foot-operated control panel alters magnification and focus and has the capacity to move the microscope approximately 3 cm horizontally in any direction (XY plotter). Some models are so maneuverable by sterile handles that the XY plotter is not necessary. The head of the microscope should tilt in all planes to provide access in all clinical situations. The assistant's binocular system should view the same operating field as the surgeon and the optics should provide a satisfactory depth of focus. For teaching and recording purposes the microscope should be capable of carrying an observation tube, as well as still, movie, or television cameras. Microscope stands need to be as light as possible yet sufficiently heavy to carry the microscope head and its accessories. Ceiling suspensions (Fig. 12–2) have many merits in eliminating cumbersome stands and avoiding storage problems. Ceiling tracks enable the microscope to be moved to the side of the operating room when not in use. Ceiling suspensions do have the disadvantage that microsurgery is restricted to the one operating room. An additional microscope on a floor stand overcomes this problem and, in addition, is available for replantation cases and for two simultaneous microsurgical operations.

Ceiling mounts are best introduced during the construction of an operating room, to avoid construction problems and interference with the operating theater (Hoerenz, 1980). Operating room lights can be incorporated in the ceiling mount.

The microscope must be free of vibration,

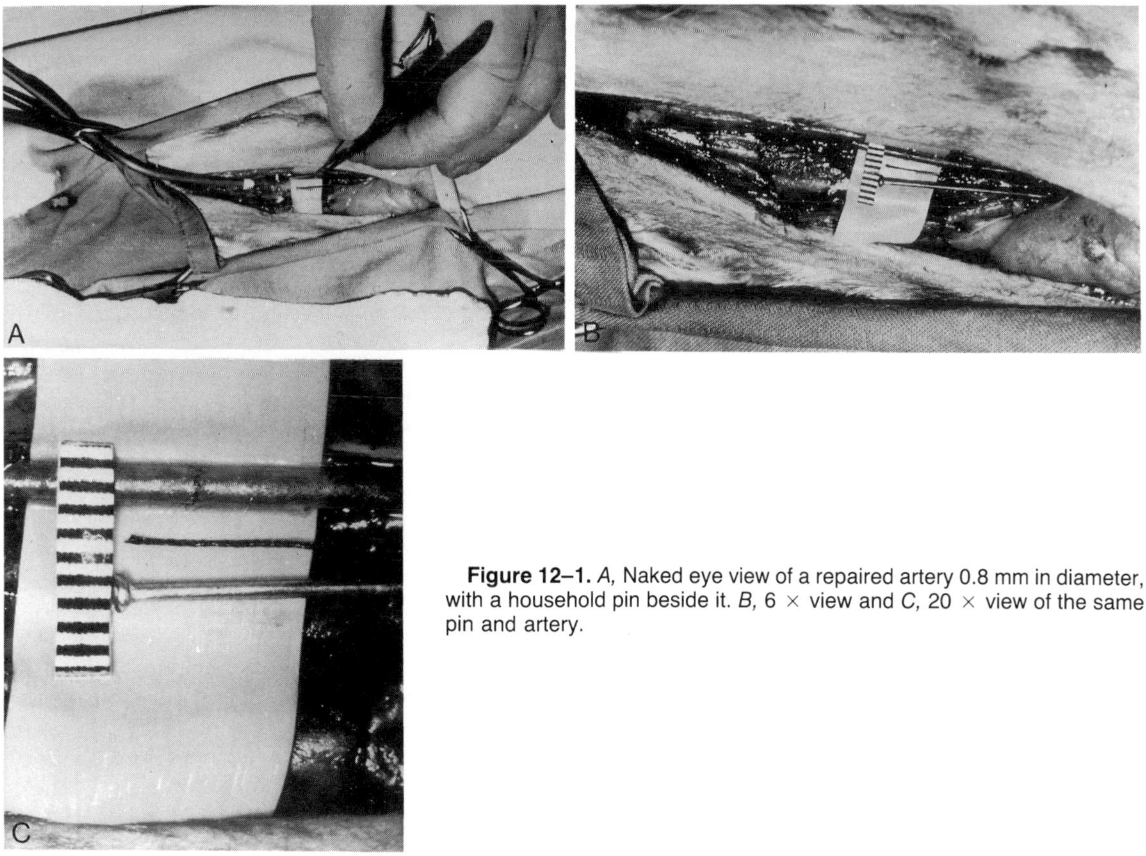

Figure 12–1. *A,* Naked eye view of a repaired artery 0.8 mm in diameter, with a household pin beside it. *B,* 6 × view and *C,* 20 × view of the same pin and artery.

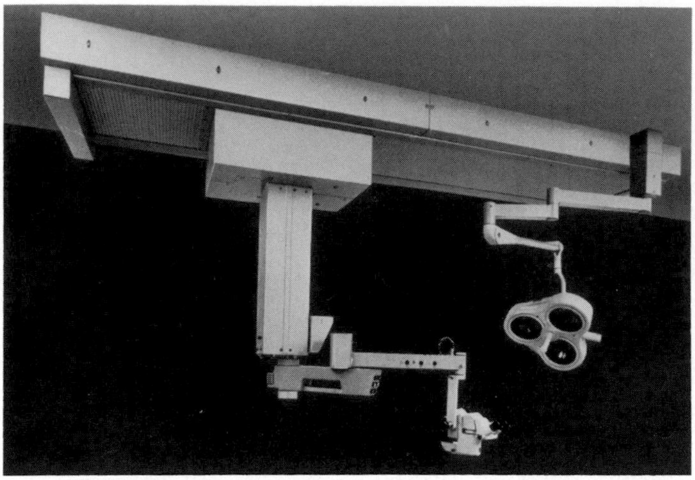

Figure 12–2. Ceiling mount microscope attached to a rail.

as this effect is increased with magnification. The head and eye of the surgeon should be relatively immobile, to achieve satisfactory precision, and likewise the operating field should possess little or no movement. Interchangeable lenses should be available but a focal length of 200 mm is the one most commonly used.

Preoperative Preparation of Microscope

The lens and oculars should be thoroughly cleaned before use. The position of the microscope stand is selected first and the microscope brake is applied in this site. For surgery on the upper limb, head and neck, thorax, or upper abdomen, the stand is usually placed at the head of the operating table. This position allows the microscope complex to be centered over the operating field without full extension of the overhead couplings, especially when heavy accessories are in place. The surgeon should select his own position carefully to provide ready access to the operative field. Knobs should be lightly tightened to a degree that just allows the microscope head to be moved. Lighting of the microscope, both internal and external, is checked before the surgery is begun. A third binocular system (if available) for the nurse or second assistant is placed on the correct side of the beam splitter, and the observer tube or other photographic equipment on the opposite side of the beam splitter. The beam splitter and stereo beam splitter reduce the light intensity available so that the monocular observation tube and the third binocular system attached to the beam splitter receive light through only one-half of the lens system.

The interpupillary distance is selected in order that both images are fused precisely. The eyepieces with a range of +9 to −9 are adjusted for each individual eye after pushing them into their sockets, and the setting is fixed into position by a locking device for each calibration or by tape. A mobile inclined binocular tube is now available with an interpupillary distance, which can be changed easily with knobs that have sterile covers. The eyepieces need to provide as wide an operative field as possible, particularly for surgeons who wear spectacles, which automatically narrow the field as the eyes are placed further away. An ocular micrometer in the eyepiece of the nondominant eye is an accurate method of measuring the size of the vessel. Focusing is tested at high power for each eye in turn and, as the microscope is zoomed from high magnification to the lowest magnification, each eye is opened in turn, ensuring that the focusing remains sharp throughout the range. Once these adjustments have been made, the microscope complex is swung away from the operative area.

Complete sterile covers are not available for all types of microscope, but, with the assistance of a scout nurse, warm sterile rubber caps can be placed over the various knobs. With care, surgeons can avoid touching unsterile sections of the microscope during surgery.

Photography

The magnification of the microscope should be adjusted so that the object of interest is as large as possible. A frequent mistake is to have the magnification too low. If the object of interest is a vessel or nerve, it is frequently best to have it running parallel with the long axis of the rectangular picture frame (Acland, 1977).

The depth of focus is limited in the operating microscope and it is difficult to bring into focus all the features of interest in the scene. The depth of focus is dependent on the magnification setting and on the stop setting of the photographic adapter. The higher the magnification, the smaller is the depth of focus. The larger the aperture (i.e., the f stop number is low), the smaller is the depth of focus (Acland, 1977).

The focal length of the microscope objective is printed on the frame of the lens and corresponds to the distance between the lens and the operative site. The oculars normally used are 12.5 × magnification. For photographic purposes, hairlines in the left or nondominant ocular are used for focusing. The focusing cannot be judged by looking down the camera view finder. The eyepiece must be adjusted so that the hairline is in sharp focus and the object to be photographed is brought into sharp focus by means of the foot pedal. With a 200 mm focal length objective, and a bright background, adequate color photographs are obtained with a shutter speed of 1/30 second at film speed ASA 64 and an f number of 16 set on the photo adaptor. To photograph a dull object, the lens is opened to f14. For faster film the lens is closed to f32 at low magnification with bright light and f22 in duller conditions. An electronic flash is the only suitable source of light, and turning off the fiberoptic has been found to be an advantage.

The diameter (D) of the operative field is calculated from the formula $D = 200/V$ (V is ocular magnification). Special adaptors are required for both cine and television purposes and are inserted into the beam splitter.

Television

Many television cameras are available but, despite the claims of the manufacturers, the authors have not yet found a design that gives an image of the highest quality. Such resolution would be advantageous for teaching purposes.

Maintenance

The microscope requires regular maintenance and careful handling. Its storage area should not be remote from the operating room. It should always be wheeled with folded couplings to avoid damage. The appropriate caps should be in place to prevent dust from entering the internal mechanism. It is essential for the surgical, nursing, and orderly staff to be familiar with the workings of the microscope. Loose particles, especially dust, can be blown away by a small rubber bulb, or removed by a brush made of fine hair. A lens soiled during an operation can be cleaned with cotton-wool applicators moistened with distilled water. The external surface of the microscope should be washed regularly with clean linen cloth that has been dipped in mild soap and water. Spare bulbs for the illuminating system should always be available.

Fiberoptic cables should never be bent too sharply, as this could lead to a fracturing of the thin glass fibers within the cable, which reduces the illumination level (Hoerenz, 1981).

MAGNIFYING LOUPES

Magnifying loupes are occasionally more practical than a microscope, particularly for microdissection. Preliminary dissection is often performed with magnifying loupes until the stage is reached at which only the operating microscope can provide the necessary resolution and control.

Loupes with high magnification have too small a field of vision with a restricted depth of focus. It is difficult for the surgeon to keep his head immobile for any lengthy period. Lightweight models that incorporate a head light may overcome some of these problems, although at this level of magnification the operating microscope is more practical.

MICROINSTRUMENTATION

Little advantage can be obtained from operative microscopy without adequate minia-

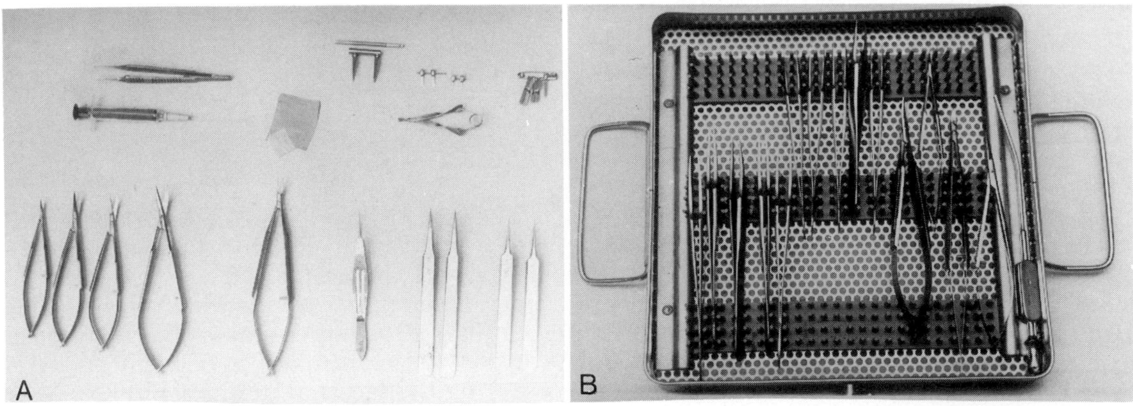

Figure 12–3. *A,* Basic microvascular instrument set. *Front row, left to right:* Vanass scissors; curved and straight Westcott scissors; microneedleholder; forceps, including jeweler's forceps nos. 2 and 5. *Top row,* Toothed forceps and 2 ml syringe, green plastic sheeting for background, double adjustable microvascular clamp with cylindric key (Henderson, O'Brien), small double adjustable microvascular clamps (Kleinert and Kutz) with applicator, and various single soft clamps on a safety pin. *B,* Microsurgical instruments mounted on a sterile instrument tray.

turization of instruments and sutures. Fine instruments have been available for many years from surgical instrument makers and jewelers, but many others specially designed for the purpose have been developed during research on vascular, lymphatic, and neural microsurgery. Experience has shown that microinstruments need only be simple, glare free, and few in number (Fig. 12–3). They require careful maintenance, and their fine pointed tips need protection by silicone or rubber tubes during storage. Their efficient design and use constitute one of the many important ergonomic aspects of microsurgery, which include tremor, visual acuity, the study of the forces applied by the operator, and surgical time and motion planning.

Nontoothed forceps should be of good quality and resistant to staining and rusting. The tips should be fine, smooth, and uniform with the jaws meeting precisely. Care should be taken that they do not become magnetized. Once damaged, the forceps should be discarded immediately, since they are still relatively inexpensive. The attachment of a rounded handle is an aid in holding forceps (Lendvay, 1973).

Scissors should be spring operated with delicate sharp blades of pencil length, approximately 6 inches, but longer if used for deep cavity work as in neurosurgery and gynecology. Westcott scissors with either straight or curved blades, and sharp or slightly rounded tips, are useful for fine dissection and trimming of vessel ends. The blunt nature of the tips is essential to dissect around fine structures with safety.

Spring-loaded needleholders, approximately 6 inches long, rest on the web between the index finger and the thumb. The needleholder is held like a pencil and is rolled between the index and middle fingers and the thumb during the motion of inserting sutures. Consequently, needleholders with a rounded surface are preferable. Microsurgery needleholders should have thin jaws with narrow shoulders, capable of grasping and tying sutures as small as 10 microns in diameter. A gentle curve of the jaws is preferred by most microsurgeons. Needleholders should not possess a locking device, because locking and unlocking maneuvers are traumatic to the structures being repaired. A needleholder incorporating these features is shown (Fig. 12–4) (O'Brien and Hayhurst, 1973). With a no. 5 jeweler's forceps held in the nondominant hand and a needleholder in the writing position by the dominant hand, the surgeon is able to complete a vascular anastomosis smoothly without the instruments leaving the hand and without taking his eyes from the microscope.

A 2 or 5 ml syringe with an attached 2 to 3 cm fine-caliber Silastic intracath is useful for irrigation of the microvascular field. A background material of a contrasting color, against which a fine suture is more easily seen, is useful for performing small anasto-

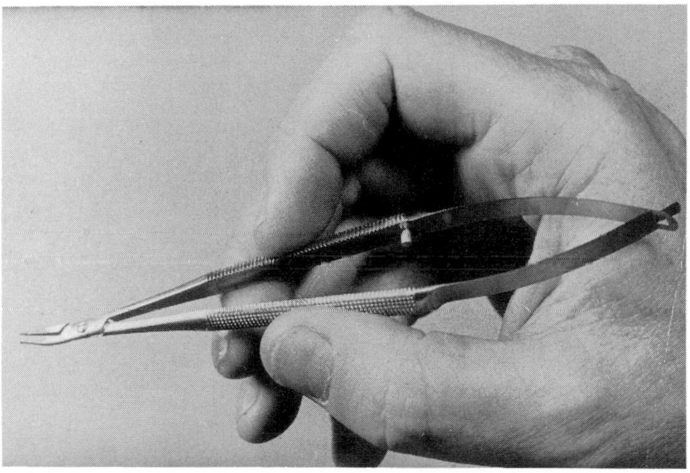

Figure 12–4. The microneedleholder rests in the hand supported by the thenar web.

moses. Any soft plastic sheeting or ordinary toy balloon, preferably yellow or greenish-yellow, may be used as background material. A millimeter ruler may be included in a photograph for easy measurement of vessel size, although use of an ocular micrometer in an eye piece is more accurate.

Clamps

An increasing number of microvascular clamps are now available. Many of the earlier models are obsolete. Small, lightweight atraumatic clamps play a major part in successful microvascular anastomoses. A double microvascular clamp, adjustable by means of a small key and screw mechanism (Fig. 12–5) (Henderson, O'Brien, and Parel, 1970), has been used extensively both experimentally and clinically for a number of years. It is not suitable for vessels smaller than 1.5 mm in diameter. It is applied gently, while the surgeon looks through the microscope in order to minimize damage to the intima of the vessel. Occasionally the clamp is separated into two parts, each of which may be applied to different vessels, the ends of which are then brought together as the two clamps are joined. The clamp causes minimal damage to the vessel wall, but if the pressure is excessive, as has been shown histologically, some damage to the intima can take place. This clamp, however, is not suitable for very small blood vessels or for lymphatics.

A double microvascular clamp has been developed by Acland (Springler & Tritt, West Germany). A small wire rectangle surrounds

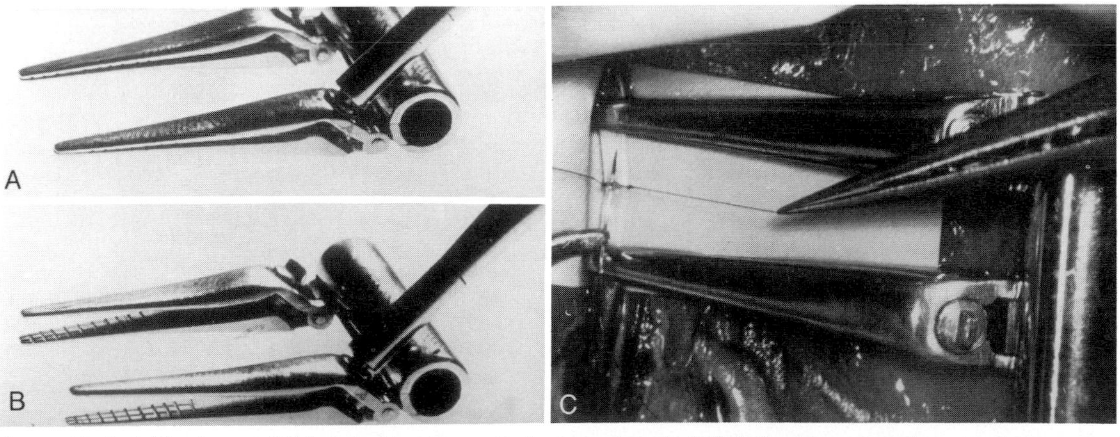

Figure 12–5. *A,* Henderson-O'Brien double clamp with the jaws closed. *B,* With the jaws opened to reveal the serrated surfaces. *C,* Artery 0.8 mm in diameter in the double microvascular clamp being sutured on the anterior wall.

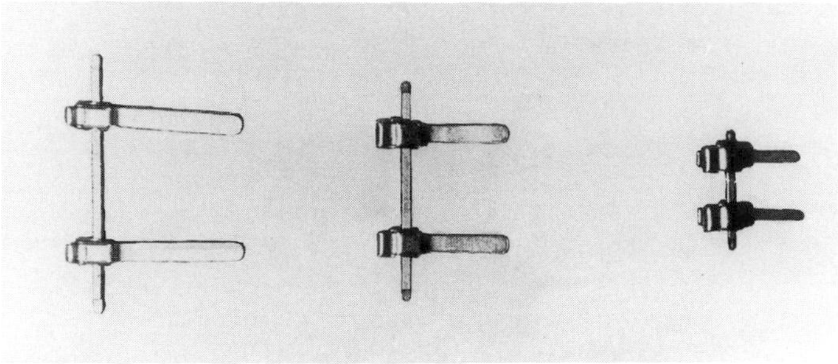

Figure 12–6. A series of adjustable double microvascular clamps of varying sizes (Kleinert-Kutz type).

the jaws of the clamps and incorporates the suture holding device; this feature is helpful to the microsurgeon when working unaided. However, this wire, encircling the jaws of the clamps, necessitates dissection of a longer vessel length. It prevents its insertion into small spaces, as is frequently required in digital replantation and other clinical situations.

Two small microvascular clamps have been incorporated into a sliding bar permitting their approximation (Tamai and associates, 1972). The closing pressure of the clamps is stated to be 80 gm at a point 2 mm from the tips. Subsequently a greatly improved model was produced (Tamai, 1978). A similar clamp (Kleinert-Kutz) was produced with a low pressure of 25 to 30 gm/sq mm. This clamp is also unsuitable for the larger vessels (Fig. 12–6).

A tilted-angle double microvascular clamp has been described by Hendel and Buncke (1980). It is applied to the vessels in such a way that they are anastomosed with the lumina looking at the surgeon. The vessels are angulated upward so that the initial suturing of the posterior wall can be concluded without rotating the vessels. This is a valuable clamp in awkward situations and avoids or lessens the danger of suturing anterior and posterior walls together.

Small, soft, single clamps of different widths have been designed in several centers. These clamps can be applied either with the fingers, with artery forceps, or with special applicators. They have parallel jaws with minimal pressure and are ideal for gently compressing single small vessels, including lymphatics. A series of small clamps of varying sizes, curved and straight, have been produced (Fig. 12–7).

Bipolar Coagulator

A bipolar coagulator is an invaluable aid in coagulating the branches of small vessels during microdissection. It conducts current between the tips of the jeweler's forceps and can safely coagulate small branches near the main vessel. Small increments of current are possible, but the highest levels are excessive and could damage the main vessel. Standard diathermy should not be used under any circumstances for microvascular surgery, as the current extends into the parent vessel and causes rapid destruction. The jeweler's forceps of the bipolar coagulator system are expensive and should be well protected at all times.

Doppler Monitors

Doppler monitors are instruments that detect blood flow in vessels beneath the skin. There are several types equipped with microprobes to detect vessels 1 mm or less in diameter. They are occasionally used to map the course of vessels in proposed microvascular free flaps, and to monitor microvascular

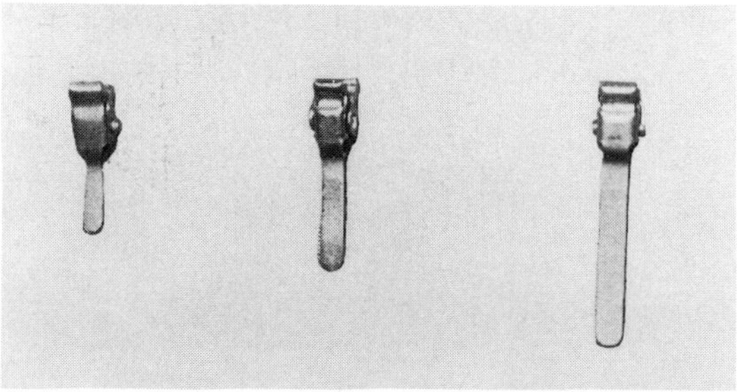

Figure 12–7. A series of single, straight, soft clamps of varying sizes.

free flaps and replanted digits or major extremities. The authors have found their main use to be in the postoperative management of patients with buried microvascular composite tissue transfers, such as muscle or dermolipomatous transfers. However, they should never replace the clinical acumen of the experienced surgeon, but should only aid him in his judgment.

Suction

Small amounts of blood in an operative field may appear negligible, but through the microscope they can totally obscure the field. Their removal is achieved by irrigation and the use of a small Fischer suction tube with an attached fine Zollner tip. Without this additional tip, the suction is usually too powerful and can destroy an anastomosis. The use of suction through small segments of slightly moist hydrocellulose sponge or gauze assists the removal of blood and other fluids from the field. A combined suction irrigation apparatus (Evans, Weightman, and Deane, 1983) has been designed and is useful. On occasions, gauze or the small sponge alone can absorb excess fluid from the field. The Weck-Cell microsponge, which has a tapered, angled joint and is mounted on a plastic spear, affords precise control and immediate absorption.

Van Beek (1983) designed a suction tube that drains fluid through a perforated background plate. A combined suction irrigation device for use in microsurgery was also devised by Evans, Weightman, and Deane (1983) and it incorporates a light, disposable hand piece.

MICROSUTURES

The assessment of sutures that are satisfactory for microvascular repair depends on the size and consistency of the vessel to be anastomosed. The ideal needle for microsutures would be of the same size as the suture material itself. Unfortunately, this has not yet been achieved and the size of the needle remains a critical factor in microsutures.

The successful application of the operating microscope to any branch of surgery requires high quality atraumatic sutures of extremely small caliber (Fig. 12–8). Nylon can be drawn into round, smooth, monofilament fibers of small caliber and high tensile strength, and has proved the most efficient suture material for microvascular surgery. Prolene is also being used in fine microsutures; it is a softer material, possesses less surface tension, and therefore adheres less to itself. It has a light blue color and consequently is poorer in contrast than nylon; it also has the disadvantage that it breaks more easily.

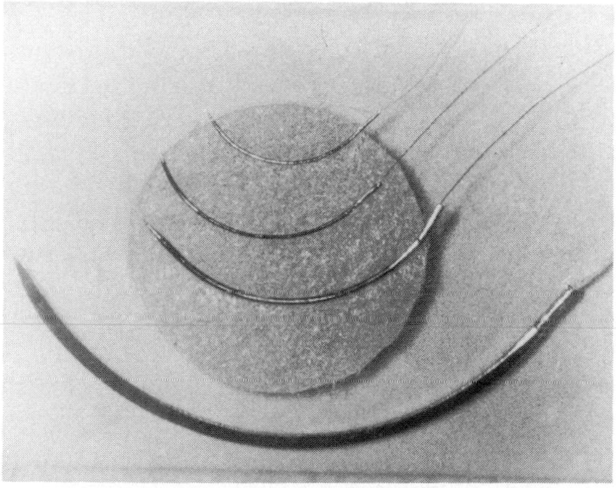

Figure 12–8. A series of microsutures of varying sizes. *From above down:* 11-0 Ethicon, needle diameter, 75 μm, and suture, 18 μm; 10-0 Dermalon (TE-100 Davis & Geck), needle, 100 μm, and suture, 22 μm; 10-0 Ethicon (previously BV-2), needle, 135 μm and suture, 22 μm; 6-0 nylon.

The ratio between the diameter of the suture fiber and the needle for microvascular surgery should be kept to a minimum so that the size of the needle track and fiber are not too disproportionate. For a vessel 0.5 to 1.0 mm in diameter, a needle 60 to 80 μm in diameter with a nylon thread of approximately 20 μm in diameter is essential. Several brands of sutures of this size are available.

All suture labels should bear the diameter of the needle and the suture material in micrometers, the arc length of the needle in millimeters, and the curve of the needle in eighths of a circle. The length of the suture material does not need to exceed 10 cm. Double armed sutures are wasteful and do not appear to have any real place.

The needle and thread should be packaged in a manner that allows the surgeon to lift the needle and its protected point from a soft foam or similar material. When not in use the needle can be placed in the foam in an inclined position ready for easy lifting.

Buncke and McLean (1971) emphasized the advantage of a straight needle (ST nomenclature) but this type of needle, although easy to grasp, can be difficult to maneuver in confined spaces. A slight curve, e.g., 3/8 circle, enables a needle to clear the clamps in cavity-like conditions that may prevail and the posterior wall of the vessels is avoided more easily. Also, after penetrating both vessel edges, a slightly curved needle is more easily picked up by the needleholder. However, in less confined spaces some surgeons prefer the straight needle.

Taper pointed needles are preferred for microneurovascular surgery. Flattening of the needle in its middle segment allows it to be grasped more readily for suture insertion (Acland, 1978). Small, colored background strips (e.g., yellow and blue) included in the package facilitate the microsurgical repair.

The anatomy of a suture needle is illustrated in Figure 12–9. For vessels 0.5 to 1 mm in diameter, usually encountered in children and lymphatics, nylon sutures Ethicon BV 75–3 and BV 100–4 (BV 3/8 circle, needle diameter in micrometers, chord length in millimeters), Davis and Geck TE 70 and 100, Xomed 10–0 70 and 10–0 100, and Springler and Tritt (ST) 7V43 and 10V43 (needle diameter × 10 μm, vessel, chord length in millimeters, 3/8 circle) are suitable. It should be mentioned that the finer the suture material, the less satisfactory is the pigmentation of the nylon fiber, often making it visually unacceptable. Sutures less than 20 μm in diameter have little practical use at the moment.

For vessels 1 to 3 mm in diameter, a 100 to 140 μm needle is easy to handle and is not too large for a microvascular repair. These requirements are satisfied by the Ethicon BV 130–5, Davis and Geck TE 143, Xomed 10–0 140 μm, and Springler and Tritt 14V33.

For vessels greater than 3 mm in diameter, the taper needle diameter of 130 to 150 μm is adequate. For tubes such as the fallopian tube and vas deferens, a cutting edge needle is preferable (e.g., Davis and Geck CE30 8–0 nylon).

Microsutures for nerve repairs follow the same pattern as for vessels.

END TO END ANASTOMOSIS

Position and Preparation

A stainless steel table, approximately 60 cm wide and 75 cm high, with four strong, rubber-covered legs, is suitable for hand surgery and experimental microsurgery. The height of the table allows the surgeon to sit comfortably while observing through the microscope. Hands, forearms, and elbows rest

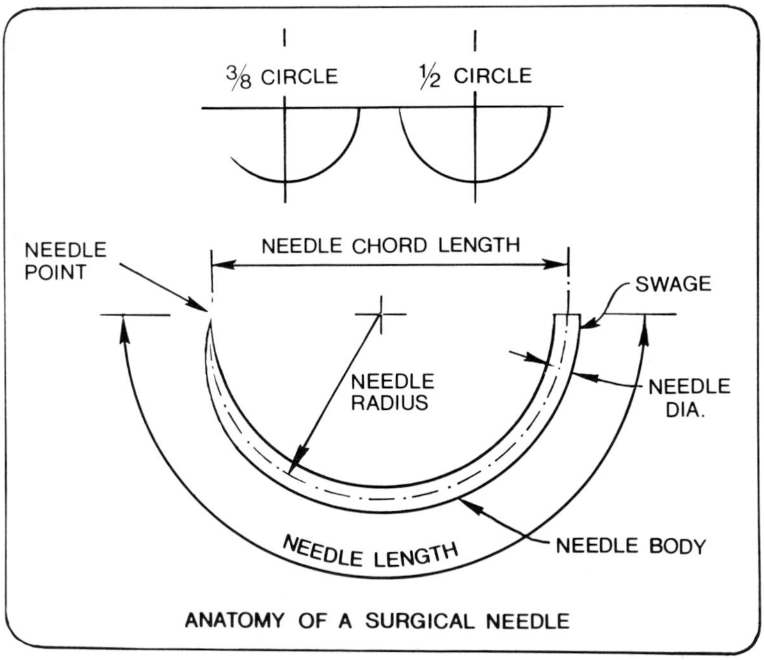

Figure 12–9.

on the table at right angles to the vessels to be anastomosed. The forearm should, as far as possible, be at the same level as the microvascular anastomosis. Folded drapes can be used to provide further support for forearms and hands.

It is much easier to concentrate on the anastomosis if the height of the surgeon's chair allows him to observe through the microscope without undue strain. This height needs to be adjusted during the operation, and chairs that are readily adjustable by the surgeon are preferable.

Exposure

Time spent in obtaining adequate exposure is never wasted. When the surgeon is struggling with a microvascular anastomosis, it is usually due to poor exposure. From a comfortable position, the surgeon should have an unobstructed view of the vessels to be repaired. The incision is occasionally extended to obtain exposure of an adequate length of vessel. The perivascular sheath must be divided, keeping the scissors parallel to or curved away from the vessels.

Technique

Proficiency with microvascular anastomoses should be acquired in the laboratory and maintained either in the operating room or in the laboratory. Microvascular surgeons are fortunate in that they can become proficient in performing microvascular repairs before doing their first clinical case. The microvascular surgeon should be able to achieve patency rates greater than 90 per cent on experimental repairs of 1 mm vessels before undertaking clinical anastomoses. A considerable amount of physical skill is required. After this skill is attained, it is easily maintained with regular clinical work. The ability to achieve dexterity in microvascular repairs is not in itself sufficient to enable a person to become a microvascular surgeon, but it is the basis on which a surgeon can build to acquire experience and judgment and eventually become a competent clinical microvascular surgeon. Clinical microvascular cases are not just vascular problems: they are total reconstructive challenges demanding skills in the broader sense and a strong background in reconstructive surgery. A well-trained assistant and a specialized nurse are essential personnel for a smooth microvascular operation, although sometimes a larger team is necessary.

The following are basic principles of microvascular technique:

1. Repair normal vessels (evaluated through the microscope), providing gentle handling of tissues and adequate debridement.
2. Repair vessels of similar diameter.
3. Repair with normal vessel tension without kinking or twisting.
4. Perform end to end or end to side anastomoses with correct suture tension and spacing.

Repair of Normal Vessels

The need to repair normal vessels is the most important principle in all microvascular surgery. Failure to work with normal vessels leads almost inevitably to impaired flow and a high risk of thrombosis. Vessel normality must be evaluated through the microscope and must be associated with normal flow.

GENTLE HANDLING OF TISSUES

In microvascular surgery the necessity for gentle handling of tissue must be carried to the extreme. Every effort is made to avoid grasping the ends of the vessels to be anastomosed. They should be handled only by grasping a small quantity of loose periadventitia on the external surface (Fig. 12–10). Small veins can readily tolerate a considerable amount of manipulation, including stretching and pinching, but they do not readily withstand the crush of a firm grasp of forceps or clamp (Acland, 1972).

ADEQUATE DEBRIDEMENT

Recipient vessels are frequently in or near the area of trauma, and occasionally the donor vessel may be subjected to trauma, as in digital or major extremity replantation. The extent of the vascular trauma is often far greater than suspected. All vessels are inspected carefully, using the high power of the microscope, for signs of damage that indicate the need for further debridement. Any vessel that contains clots should be resected, as

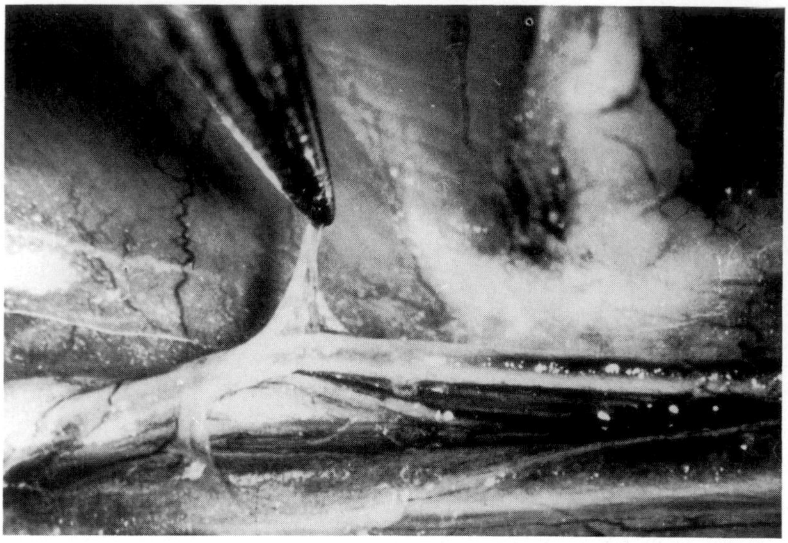

Figure 12–10. The vessels are grasped only by their periadventitial tissues.

these are usually abnormal. The interior of the vessel is irrigated with heparinized saline (without cannulation) and inspected for signs of retained fibrin deposits on the intimal wall. Such fibrin deposits serve as a nidus for platelet thrombus formation and their presence is an indication for further debridement of the vessel; otherwise, further thrombosis is inevitable.

The interior of a vessel is also observed for signs of intimal tears or intimal irregularity such as separation from the media, findings commonly seen proximal and distal to the site of avulsion injuries. These signs call for more aggressive debridement until no vessel damage can be seen through the microscope. Many centimeters of vessel length may require resection. The poorer results obtained in the replantation of avulsed digits and extremities and some composite tissue transfers can usually be attributed to inadequate debridement of vessels proximal and/or distal to the site of injury. Not infrequently the proximal vessel ends are in spasm, and the careful insertion of a no. 2 jeweler's forceps, opened gently in two directions at right angles, relieves the spasm.

After adequate debridement there should be a strong pulsatile flow of blood from the recipient artery. The need for the passage of a catheter to obtain a flow may indicate proximal vascular damage, and further resection of the artery may be necessary until free flow is achieved. These catheters have been shown to strip endothelium, thus exposing thrombogenic subendothelium (Sawyer and associates, 1973).

RELIEF OF SPASM

Spasm may have a number of general causes such as low temperature of the operating theater, suboptimal perfusion, and inadequate levels of anesthesia. Local factors include traumatic handling of the vessels, cold, dryness of the tissues, blood in contact with the vessels, and vascular disease.

Spasm may occur in a peripheral vessel as a result of vasoconstriction of a normal vessel, or it may be associated with a pathologic condition of the vessel. If the vessel is normal, it should be dilated gently with a jeweler's forceps followed by topical application of lidocaine 2 per cent or verapamil, coverage with a moist gauze, and a waiting period. Dependency of the part if possible or alteration of the level of the operating table may be helpful. If the vessel is abnormal and is in a state of spasm, the vessel should be aggressively resected until normal vessel is reached. If the spasm still persists, the same plan as described earlier should be repeated, while the patient is observed. As a last resort, passage of a fine intracath dilatory with heparinized saline or even verapamil can achieve the desired result.

Similar Diameter of Vessels

Vessels with dissimilar diameters, up to 100 per cent or more, can usually be anastomosed satisfactorily; the small vessel is dilated and divided obliquely to give adequate symmetry. Significant difference in the thickness of the vessel walls should not deter the surgeon from an end to end anastomosis. Occasionally an interposing vein graft, each end of which approximates the size of the vessel ends, can resolve the problem.

Normal or Near-Normal Vessel Tension

There should be normal or near-normal tension at the vessel ends. An adjustable approximating clamp aims to bring the vessel ends together for convenient suturing, but it should never be applied with excess tension.

Any kinking or twisting of the vessel distal to the repair predisposes to occlusion of the anastomosis. Such situations are best avoided by adjusting the donor and recipient vessels with normal or near-normal tension and without an excess of vessel, which could cause twisting or kinking. Care should be taken in replacing vessels beneath skin closures or other tissues to avoid kinking or twisting.

Vascular configurations that contribute to turbulent conditions distal to the anastomosis predispose to occlusion. Turbulence initiates platelet reaction and stimulation of blood procoagulants (Leonard, 1972; Jorgensen, Hacrem, and Moe, 1973).

Technique

Descriptions of and modifications to the technical aspects of microvascular repair have been made by many authors including Jacobson and Suarez, 1960; Kleinert and Kasdan, 1965; Cobbett, 1967; Buncke and Schulz, 1967; O'Brien and associates, 1970; Hayhurst and O'Brien, 1975; Urbaniak and associates, 1977; Acland, 1980; and Morrison and O'Brien, 1980.

RESECTION TO NORMAL VESSELS

Any history of avulsion injury, crush, atherosclerosis, or irradiation to the recipient vessel should arouse the suspicion of vascular injury. The vessel must be resected proximal to the level of injury, or alternatively another recipient vessel should be chosen. Microscopic signs of vessel damage include bruising in the wall, medial and intimal prolapse into the lumen, friable walls that readily tear when handled or sutured, and the presence of an intraluminal fixed clot (Fig. 12–11). The vessel should be resected proximal to such areas with fine, straight, sharp scissors and one deft blow (Fig. 12–12).

Forward flow should now be tested (Fig. 12–13). If it does not begin immediately after release of a clamp or if it is weak, an abnormal vessel should be suspected. Spasm may account for some initial delay, and such vessels should be left undisturbed for a few minutes. Antispasmodics may be applied.

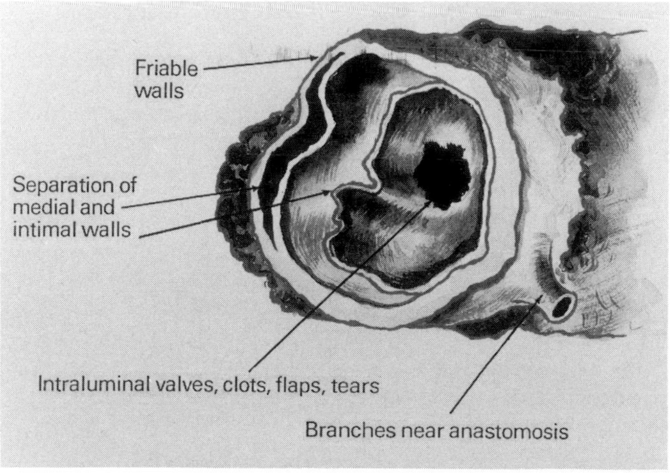

Figure 12–11. Inspection of the damaged vessel end.

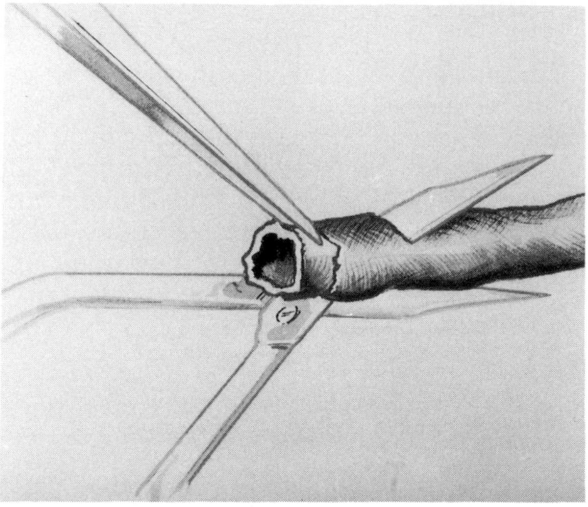

Figure 12–12. Resection of the damaged vessel end with sharp, straight scissors.

CLAMPING OF VESSELS

The two vessel ends to be anastomosed are placed into a double approximating clamp viewed through the microscope. This may be either the screw or spring type. The screw type is particularly valuable for the repair of larger vessels in the clinical situation because of its weight, its stability, and the ability to adjust the jaw pressure to counter any minor distracting forces on the vessels.

A generous length of the vessel end should be included within the clamp for ease of working, and the tips of the jaws should project just beyond the vessel for maximal grip (Fig. 12–14). The assistant pulls the vessel longitudinally while the operator steadies the clamp with his left hand and gently screws the nut with the key, using the other hand. The clamp jaws are approximated so that the vessel ends loosely touch each other.

POSITIONING

Suturing in deep cavities in a vertical plane (Fig. 12–15) or in an oblique horizontal plane (Fig. 12–16), especially from left to right for the right-handed surgeon, are variables that make visualization of the lumina almost impossible and set the stage for failure.

In these unfavorable situations the common denominator is the inability to visualize adequately both lumina, which leads to inaccurate suturing. A gauze swab placed underneath the vessels or a clamp may elevate the vessels into a more favorable position. The position of the surgeon's microscope may be altered so that the right-handed surgeon is able to operate obliquely toward himself from right to left. The use of the heavier clamp offers the advantage of an ability to influence the axis of the vessels (Fig. 12–17).

PREPARATION OF VESSEL ENDS

The periadventitial layer is resected either by scissor dissection or by pulling the adventitial sleeve beyond the end of the vessel and resecting it flush with the underlying vessel end (Fig. 12–18). The periadventitia retracts a sufficient distance to expose the vessel wall for suturing. Sufficient periadventitia should be resected to allow suturing. Excessive stripping of periadventitial and adventitial tissues can diminish the circulation of the wall of the vessel ends.

Urbaniak and associates (1977) reported that stripping of the adventitia caused increased necrosis of the vessel wall at the anastomotic site. If it is technically possible, the adventitia with its vasa vasorum and neural supply should be preserved. Minimal stripping is necessary to visualize the lumen adequately. Eisenhardt and associates (1980)

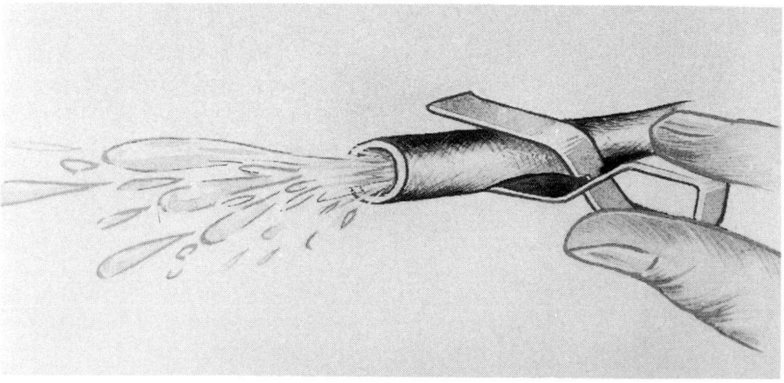

Figure 12–13. Demonstration of forward pulsatile flow from the now normal artery prior to clamping.

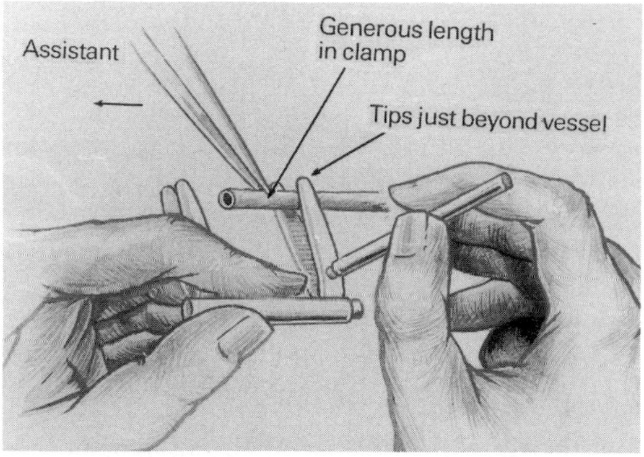

Figure 12–14. Application of the double microvascular clamp. The assistant is pulling the proximal vessel end between the open jaws.

showed that adventitial stripping resulted in an increased rate of false aneurysms.

If the lumen is small or in spasm, it may be dilated gently by inserting the approximated tips of a no. 2 jeweler's forceps and allowing them to separate slowly (Fig. 12–19). The lumen is now irrigated with a solution of heparinized saline (1000 units per 100 ml) (Fig. 12–20).

Slight size discrepancies can often be corrected by taking wider bites on the larger lumen, by cutting the smaller vessel end obliquely, or by dilating the smaller lumen

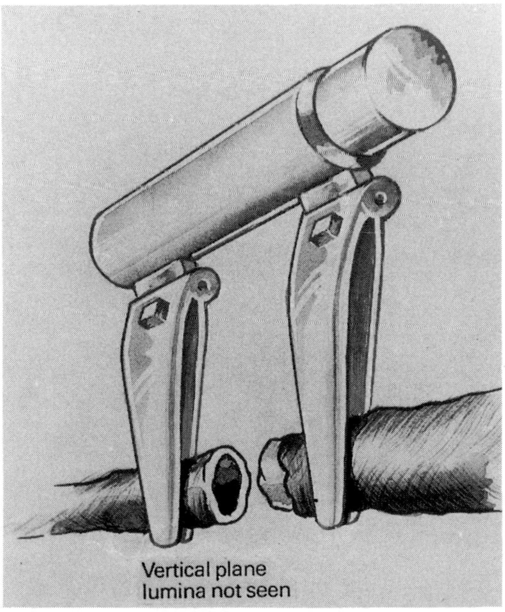

Figure 12–15. Incorrect vertical application of the double clamp.

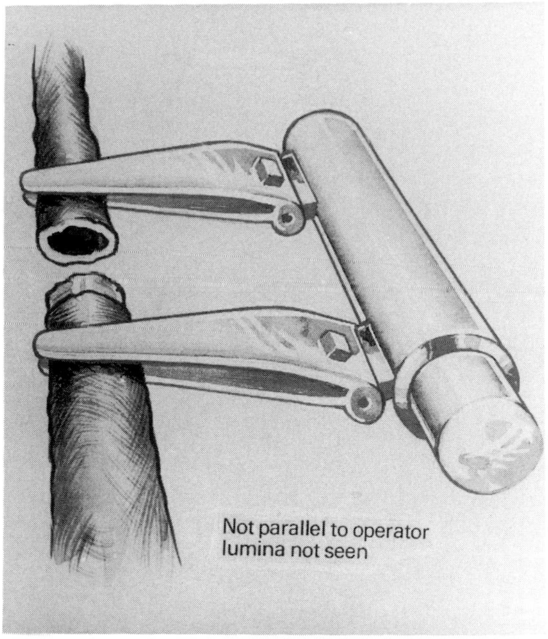

Figure 12–16. Incorrect horizontal application of the double clamp.

(Fig. 12–21). If the discrepancy is greater, the size of a donor flap artery may be enlarged by including a cuff of the parent artery, which is closed with interrupted or continuous suture. The groin flap lends itself to this technique by incorporating a cuff of the femoral artery. The cuff allows an almost symmetric end to end anastomosis (Popov and Trichkova, 1977).

Hamilton (1981) demonstrated that the most favorable arrangement of size-discrepant vessels to achieve high patency is seen when the larger vessel is sutured to the side of the smaller vessel.

SUTURING

End to end anastomosis is the most commonly performed method and this technique is usually possible with vessels of similar diameter (Fig. 12–22). End to side anastomoses are preferable, as spasm is less and there may be only one vital vessel available, especially in lower extremity injuries.

The fewer sutures used the better, and therefore for large vessels such as the radial artery a 9–0 nylon suture should be used. A 10–0 nylon suture is the most versatile for digital replantation and free flap surgery, while 11–0 nylon is reserved for smaller vessels in children and microlymphatic surgery.

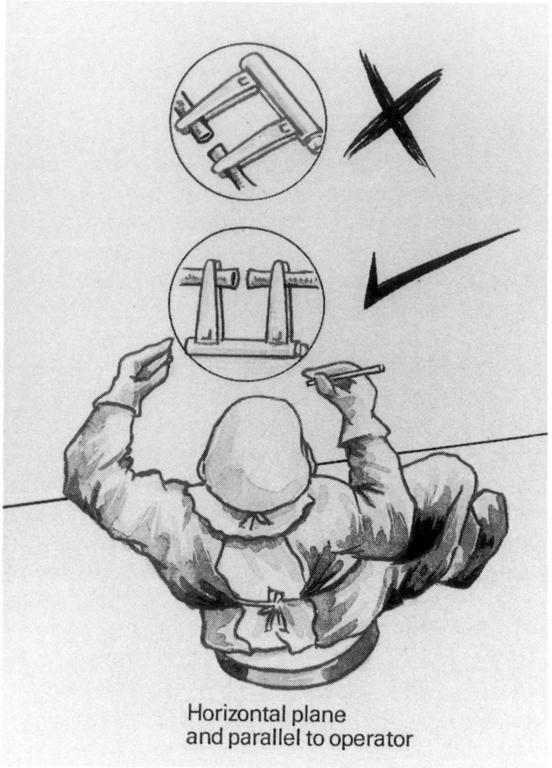

Figure 12–17. Correct horizontal application of the double clamp with the vessel parallel to the operator.

Full-thickness wall sutures are normally used. Wray and O'Brien (1979) in an experimental study showed that extraintimal suturing compared favorably with full-thickness suturing in the diameter range 0.5 to 1.2 mm. However, the method is tedious and for this reason is not recommended.

Either the 180 degree halving or the 120 degree triangulating technique may be used to site the key sutures (Fig. 12–23). For thick-walled arteries in which the walls rarely collapse against each other, the 180 degree method is simpler and quicker. For large-diameter collapsible walled veins the halving method is also easier to judge than triangulation, which must be extremely accurate to avoid vessel discrepancy and dog ears. In thin-walled vessels, however, the method of triangulation has the advantage that the posterior wall drops away when the guy sutures are put under tension, and thereby minimizes the risk of including the posterior wall with an anterior wall suture.

The needleholder is held in the writing position with the thumb and index finger resting on the middle finger. The needle is placed in the operating field and is picked up by the needleholder at its middle with the needletip pointing in the intended direction. If the direction is incorrect, the needle should be steadied with the left hand forceps and regrasped with the needleholder in the correct position. The most natural position of the needleholder, however, is with its curved tips pointing away from the needle point. The most natural range of use is within 30 degrees to the right of the writing position for a right-handed surgeon. The trailing suture is placed on the right so that it can be pulled through the vessel anastomosis in a straight line.

The first suture is inserted at approximately the 150 degree position, since it is technically difficult to begin at the 180 degree position for the halving technique. The second suture is placed directly opposite at approximately −30 degrees. For triangulation they are easiest sited at about 150 and +30 degrees.

The first suture is the most difficult because of lack of stability of the vessel ends. The vessel edge should not be grasped by forceps; either the adventitial layer can be held or, if this is unstable, the forceps tip can be gently inserted into the lumen to act as counterpressure to the needle point (Fig. 12–24).

The needle is passed at right angles to the wall at a distance from the margin slightly

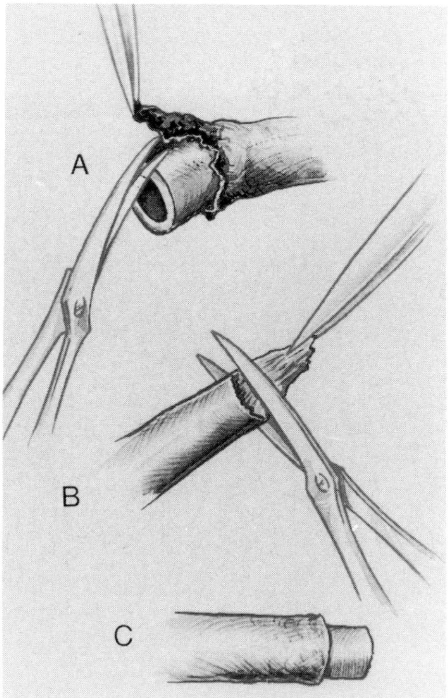

Figure 12–18. *A,* Resection with scissors of adventitial tissue at the vessel end. *B,* Section with scissors of an adventitial sleeve pulled down. *C,* Retraction of the adventitia following resection.

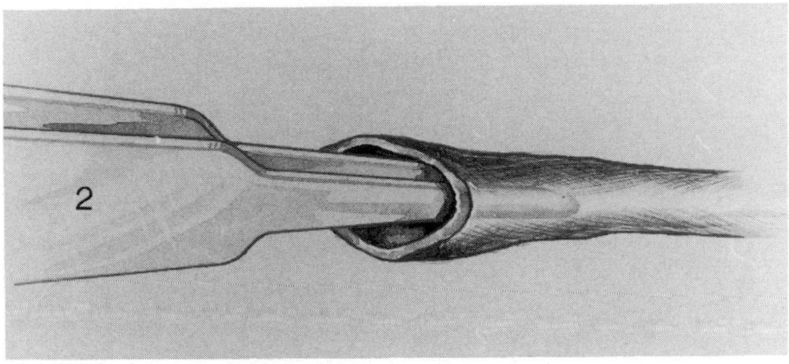

Figure 12–19. Dilatation of the vessel with no. 2 jeweler's forceps.

greater than the thickness of the vessel wall. It is retrieved again by the needleholder pulling it through the wall in the gentle curved arc of the needle (Fig. 12–25).

After a small but sufficient slack of suture is obtained, the needle is inserted into the lumen of the opposite vessel, using the jeweler's forceps in the left hand to steady it. At the corresponding site the needle is passed at right angles through the wall, and counterpressure on the outside of the vessel with the jeweler's forceps in the left hand aids its penetration (Fig. 12–26).

Having penetrated the opposite vessel wall, the needleholder again grasps the needle and the thread is pulled through with a continuous movement, using the jeweler's forceps as a pulley, to prevent sharp angulation of the thread at the vessel edge and tearing of the vessel wall. A change from smooth gliding to irregular shaking of the suture gives a clue that the end is approaching into the microscopic field. Once the end of the suture appears in the periphery of the righthand field, the jeweler's forceps in the left hand grasp the thread at the left hand peripheral of the field, and the needle is blindly dropped from the needleholders outside the field in front of the operator. In a continuous motion the jewelers forceps continue the advancement of the thread through the vessel walls until sufficient length remains for convenient tying (approximately level with the righthand jaw of the clamp). As the jeweler's forceps are advancing the thread to the final desired position, the needleholders are reintroduced into the field to participate in the tying of the knot. This method involves continuous motion and avoids repetition of movement.

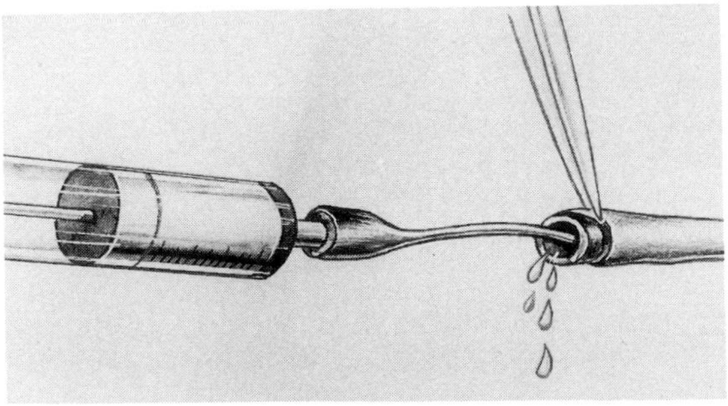

Figure 12–20. Irrigation of the lumen with heparinized saline.

TYING OF KNOT

During knot tying one should ideally use a constant power of magnification, high enough for accurate siting of the needle into the wall and yet with a sufficiently broad visual field to tie the knot. However, for vessels smaller

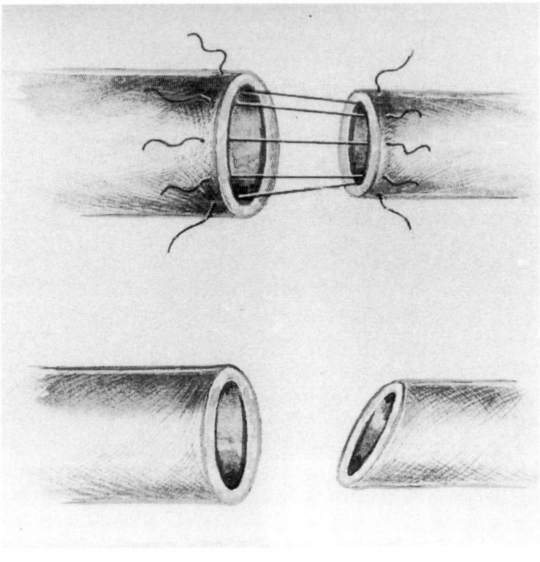

Figure 12–21. *Above,* Correction of slight size discrepancy by larger bites on the bigger vessel. *Below,* Correction of small size discrepancy by oblique cutting of the smaller vessel.

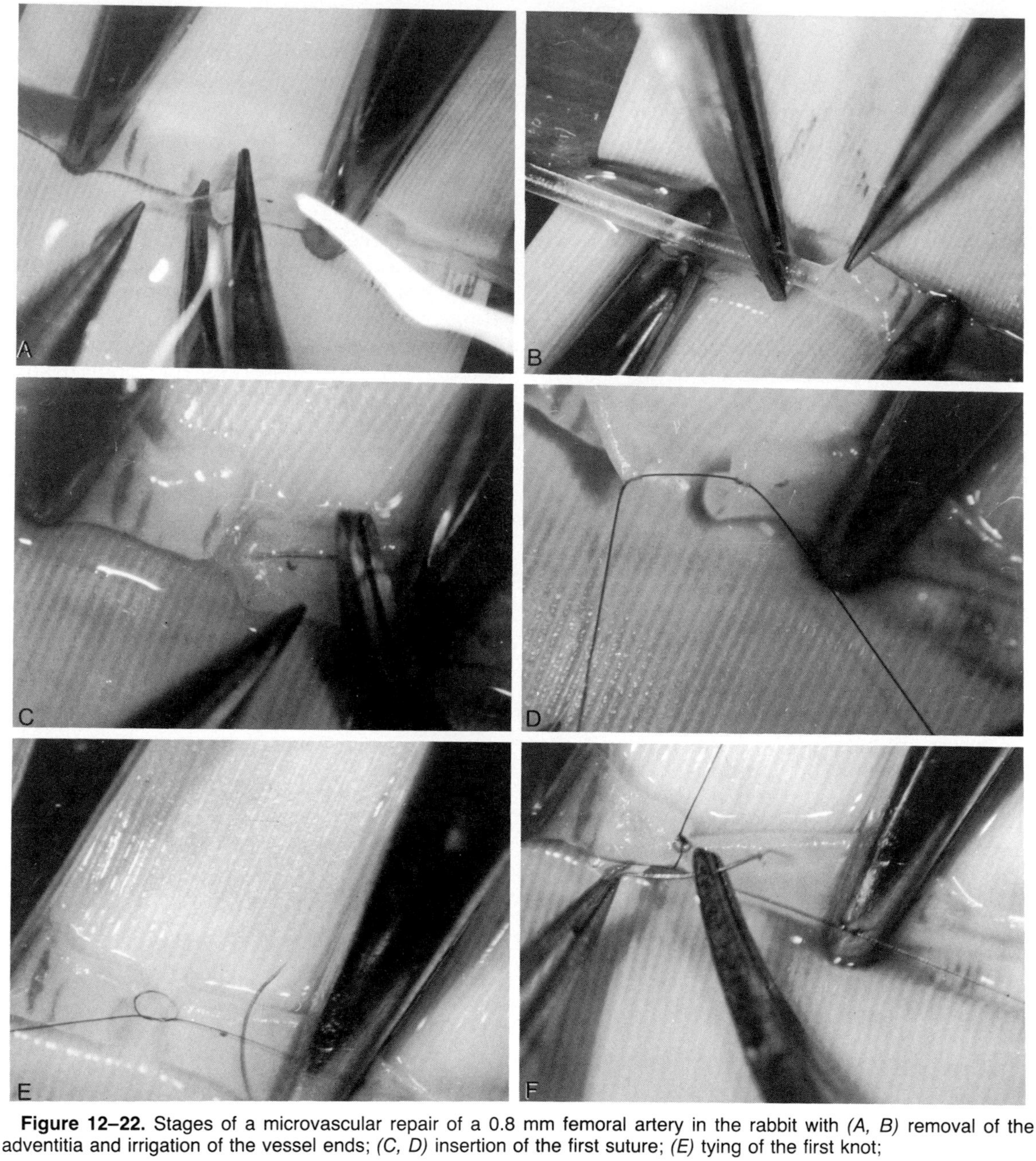

Figure 12–22. Stages of a microvascular repair of a 0.8 mm femoral artery in the rabbit with *(A, B)* removal of the adventitia and irrigation of the vessel ends; *(C, D)* insertion of the first suture; *(E)* tying of the first knot;

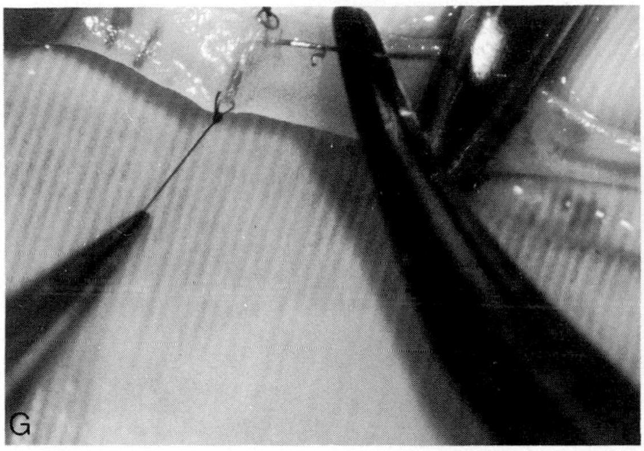

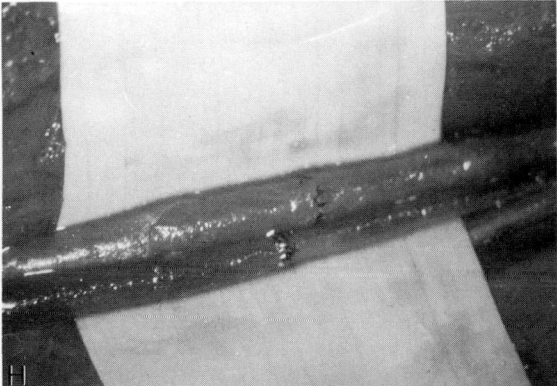

Figure 12–22 *Continued (F, G)* insertion and completion of the second suture and commencement of suturing of the anterior wall; and *(H)* completion of the repair of the artery and adjacent vein with obvious patency.

than 1 mm, higher magnification is needed to insert the sutures and a lower one for knot tying.

In the continuous motion of tying, the jeweler's forceps must grasp the thread sufficiently far from the vessel anastomotic site to allow the thread to be doubly looped around the needleholder jaws (Fig. 12–27). It is a common mistake to grasp this too close to the vessel and pull the distal thread out of the vessel walls during the process of tying. A double throw around the tips of the needleholder for the first knot prevents slipping during tying of the second and third single knots.

The needleholder picks up the short distal thread and draws it to the left side of the field while the long thread simultaneously crosses to the righthand side, thus creating a flat knot (Fig. 12–28). The tension is assessed by sight and not by feel and should just approximate the two vessels' edges rather than strangulate them.

Proper suture tension is extremely important, particularly for microarterial repairs. Sutures tied too tightly cause small mural tears and exposure of the subendothelium, cell walls, and cell contents. All of the latter cause platelet reaction, aggregation, and disintegration, leading to thrombosis formation (MacMillan and Sim, 1970; Spaet and Gaynor, 1970). Sutures that are tied too tightly also cause damage to the media of the arterial wall. If at least one-third of the media does not survive, reendothelization does not occur and occlusion of the anastomotic site invariably follows (Baxter and associates, 1972; Spaet, Gaynor, and Stemerman, 1974).

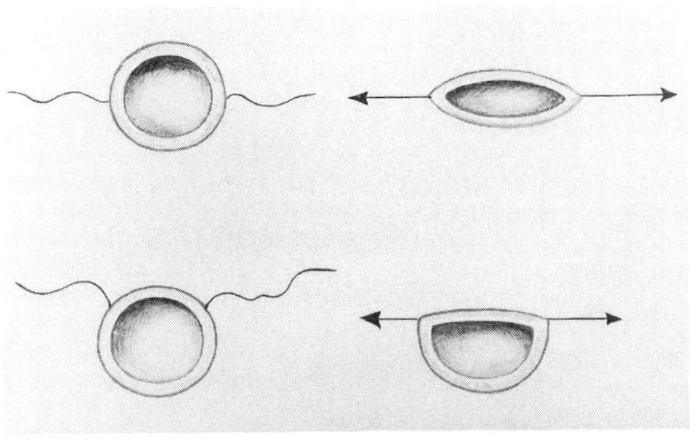

Figure 12–23. *Above,* Insertion of the first two sutures at the 180 degree position gives flattening and traction with approximation of the anterior and posterior wall. *Below,* Insertion of the first two sutures at the 120 degree position allows the posterior wall to fall away on application of traction.

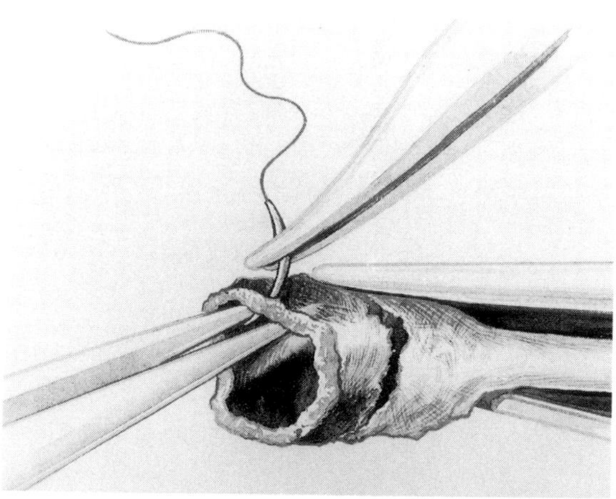

Figure 12–24. Insertion of the first suture with intraluminal counterpressure from jeweler's forceps.

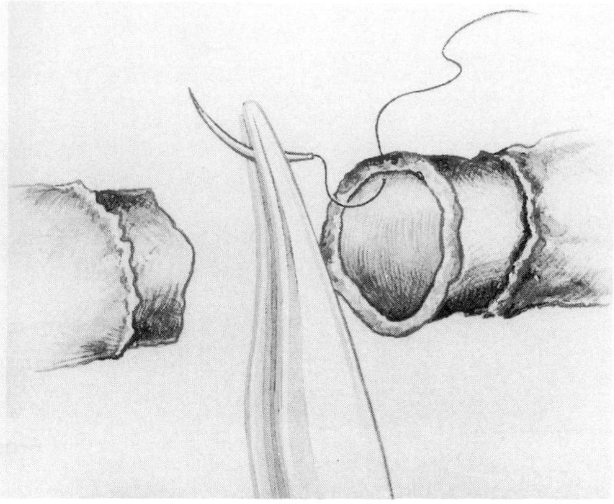

Figure 12–25. Completion of half of the first suture.

The short end in the needleholder is released and the longer lefthand thread wrapped once around the needleholder (Fig. 12–29). The short end is regrasped and pulled tight in a reef knot (Fig. 12–30).

Care should be taken when releasing the short end that it does not fall onto the vessel wall, which makes the thread difficult to pick up because of the filmy surface tension of the adventitia. The assistant is often in a better position to grasp this thread. A final single third tie is now made in a similar fashion. The suture ends should continue to be kept in a horizontal plane as much as possible.

One end is cut short and the other end left long, so that it can be used for intermittent retraction by the assistant. The next suture is inserted at either the 180 degree or 120 degree position as previously described (Fig. 12–31).

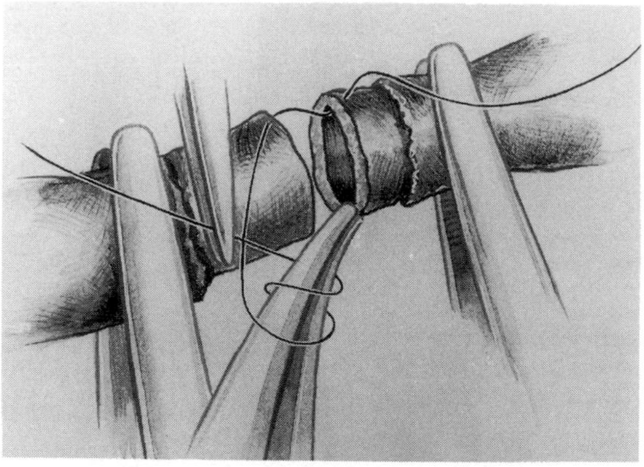

Figure 12–27. Initial double throw of the first suture.

ANTERIOR WALL

When the sutures are inserted it is essential to visualize the lumen so that the full thickness of the wall is included in the suture and the posterior wall is not accidentally caught. The points of the lefthand jeweler's forceps may be carefully inserted into the lumen to aid this maneuver while the assistant retracts on the guy suture (Fig. 12–32). The third suture may be inserted halfway between the two anterior sutures, and additional sutures inserted as required.

The position of the intermediate sutures in the anterior wall is determined by the diameter of the vessel (Fig. 12–33). For large vessels it is safer in continuous fashion to halve the gap until an adequate number of sutures is inserted. For vessels less than 1 mm in diameter, in which only two or three additional sutures are required for the anterior wall, these are estimated directly. If doubt exists at any time that the posterior wall may be caught in a suture, the nearest

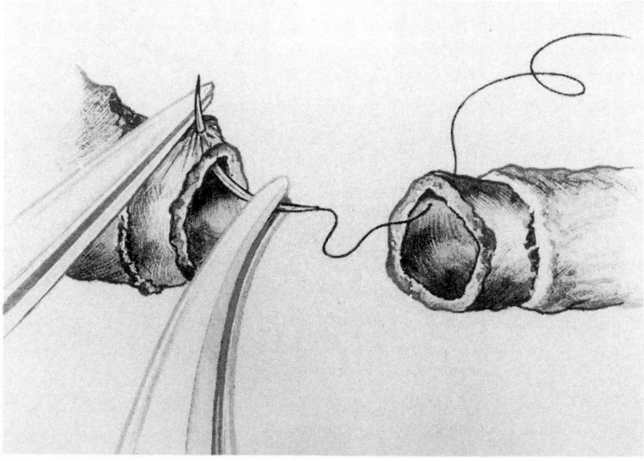

Figure 12–26. Insertion of the needle through the wall of the opposite vessel end.

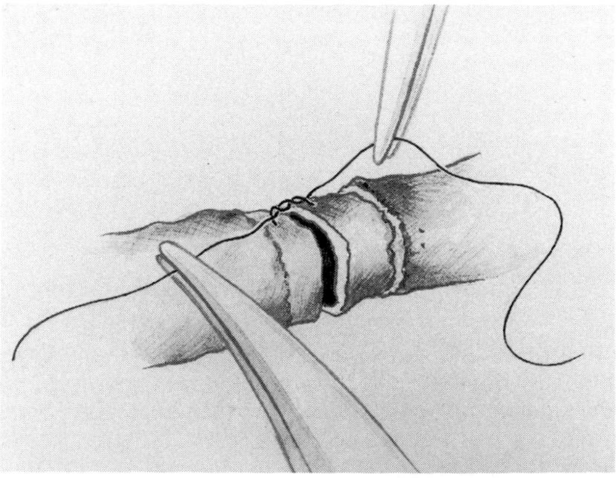

Figure 12–28. Tying of the double throw.

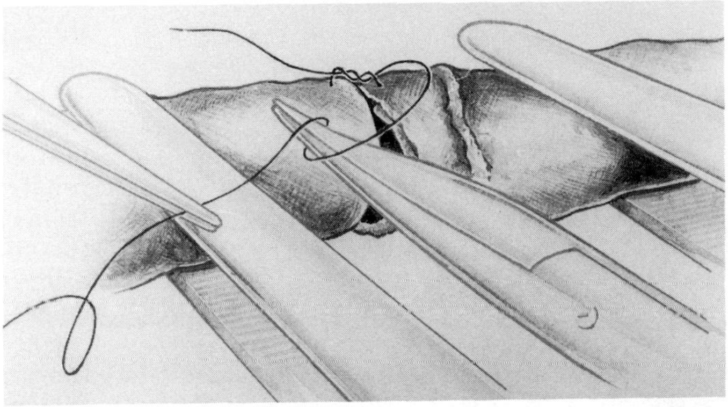

Figure 12–29. Continuation of the tie with a single throw.

lateral guy suture can be elevated and the posterior wall of the vessel pulled away from the anterior wall, thus disclosing any tethering.

POSTERIOR WALL

The clamp is turned over with the jeweler's forceps, while the surgeon observes continuously through the microscope. The guy sutures are rotated in order to bring the posterior wall into full view (Fig. 12–34).

Irrigation aids visualization to check that the posterior wall has not been included in the anterior wall sutures. The same technique for suture insertion, spacing and, tying is used for the posterior wall closure, the assistant again providing traction (Fig. 12–35). With the larger vessels, leaving one end of the completed suture long allows more effective traction for the insertion of the next suture, rather than relying solely on the two main lateral guy threads. Experience is required to estimate the required number of sutures, but the minimal number to prevent leak should be the goal. In an artery 1 mm in diameter, six to eight sutures are usually necessary.

An alternative technique ties the last two sutures of an anastomosis at the same time. The first of these sutures is passed and, without tying, the needle is passed for the last suture. This maneuver enables the anterior and posterior walls to be more freely visualized. The loop between the two sutures is divided and both sutures are tied.

Harashina (1977) inserts sutures at the 180 degree position, completes the anterior wall closure, turns over the clamp, inserts the central posterior suture and leaves it untied, and inserts the rest of the posterior wall sutures so that the central posterior suture is tied last.

The relationship between the number of sutures and the strength of the microvascular anastomosis was studied by Colen, Gonzales, and Buncke (1979). Rats were used and the anastomosis was carried out with the leg amputated except for the vessel. The force required to rupture was determined on a

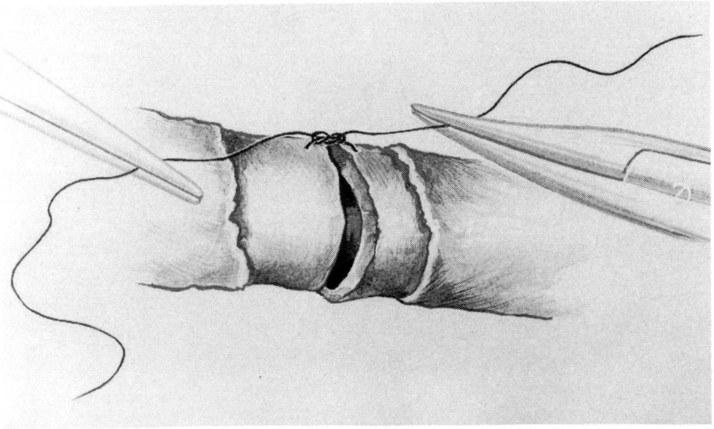

Figure 12–30. Completion of the tie to form a reef knot.

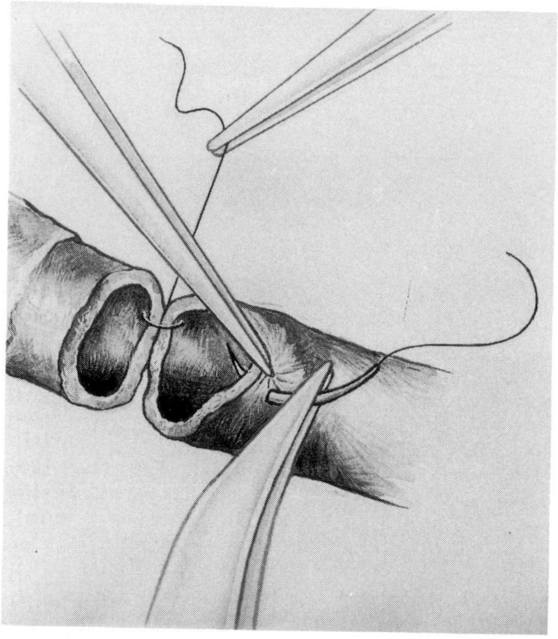

Figure 12–31. Insertion of the second suture at the 120 degree position.

spring scale attached to the foot. The relative strength of microvascular anastomoses in the rat femoral arteries was measured comparing controls (no anastomosis) with those with four, six, eight, ten, 12, and 14 sutures. The ones in which eight sutures were used most closely paralleled the control state, whereas those with only four or six sutures were inferior. For the greater number of sutures the vessels behave as a "shorter" vessel, with the anastomosis becoming the weakest part of the vessel.

Occasionally the vessels must be repaired in a very restrictive cavity, which does not permit satisfactory turning of the clamp to repair the posterior wall. In these circumstances it is advisable to commence the suturing of the posterior wall first by inserting a central posterior suture. Sutures are placed on each side of this and gradually the surgeon works around the circumference, ensuring at the same time that there is proper suture spacing (O'Brien, 1977; Harris, Finseth, and Buncke, 1981).

RELEASE OF CLAMPS

The distal clamp is released first and backflow across the anastomosis is the first indication of patency. Any major leaks at this stage should be dealt with by reapplying the clamp, irrigating, and inserting additional sutures.

Both clamps are now released. Usually a small amount of blood leaks from the anastomosis but stops after a few minutes with the application of sponges. It is unsafe to attempt to insert sutures into a bleeding anastomosis unless it is clamped proximally and distally, because of the high probability of catching the posterior wall with a blind suture. Harashina (1976) stated from experimental work on the femoral vessels in rats that if it is necessary to reapply an arterial clamp, it may be placed either proximal or

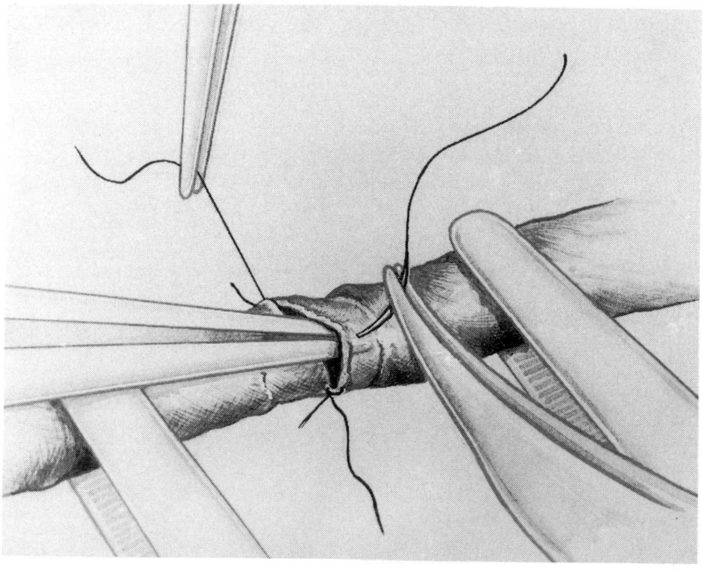

Figure 12–32. Insertion of another suture with delicate counterpressure from the intraluminal jeweler's forceps.

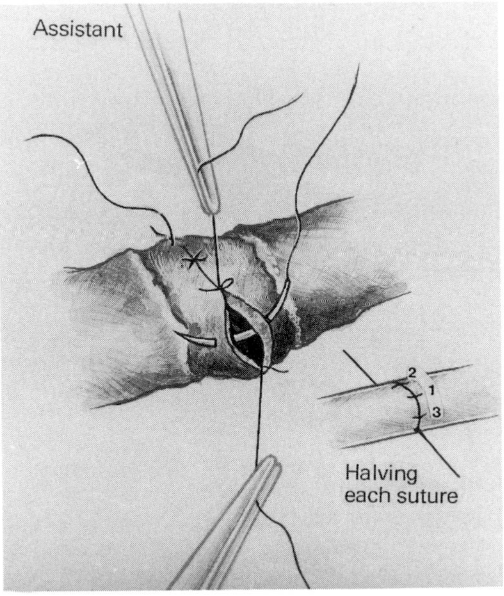

Figure 12–33. The needle penetrates the opposite vessel wall.

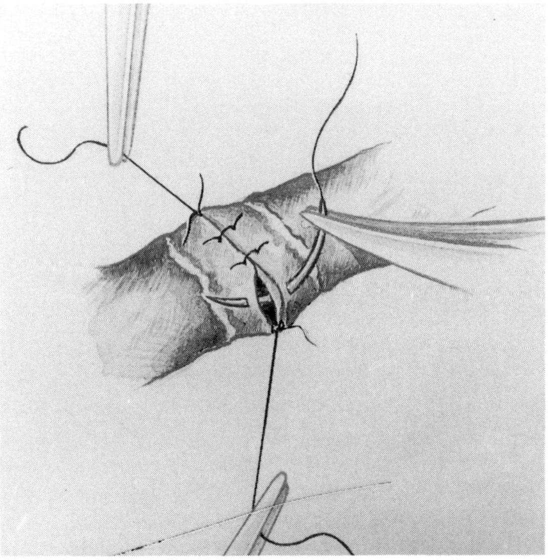

Figure 12–35. Repair of the posterior wall with interrupted sutures.

distal to the anastomosis with almost the same patency resulting.

PATENCY

A number of authors have studied patency rates (Acland, 1972; Hayhurst and O'Brien, 1975; Curtis, Loftis, and Wissinger, 1977).

If there is obviously satisfactory circulation of the part and back-bleeding from the distal wound edges, it can be assumed that all anastomoses are patent. If the circulation appears inadequate, however, the clinical signs of the replanted part indicate whether this is primarily a venous or an arterial problem. Vessels should be checked to ensure that no kinking or spasm exists. Manipulation of the vessels should be avoided, and several minutes or longer are allowed to elapse before the vessel is reinspected. If there still is continued spasm, measures to overcome this should be instituted, as previously described. If at the end of these conservative measures the circulation is still not established, the anastomosis is reinspected. A patency test is carried out distal to the anastomosis of the vein initially. A no. 2 jeweler's forceps is used to grasp the vessel immediately distal to the anastomosis with just sufficient force to occlude the flow of blood. A second no. 2 jeweler's forceps is used to empty the downstream side of the vessel. With the forceps more distal from the anastomosis still occluding the vessel, the forceps nearest the anastomotic site is released (Figs. 12–36, 12–37). If the anastomosis is patent, blood rushes through the anastomosis to fill the empty segment of vessel. This test is used only when there is persistent doubt regarding the patency. If the clinical signs of venous congestion are present, the venous anastomosis should be tested for patency. If the venous anastomosis is not patent, the arterial anastomosis should be checked for patency to exclude secondary arterial obstruction. If pa-

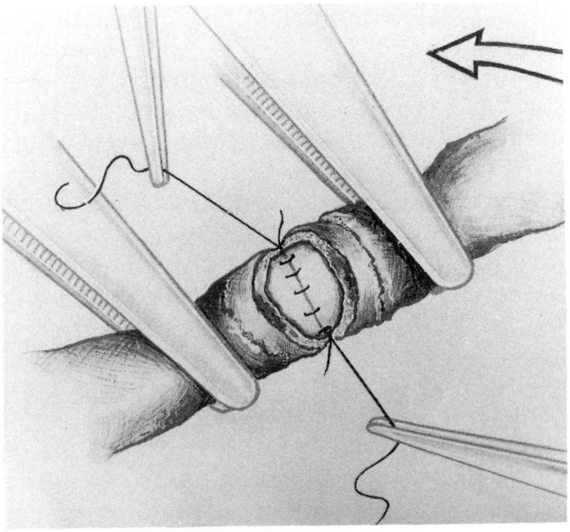

Figure 12–34. The anterior wall completed and the clamp rotated to reveal the posterior wall and lumen.

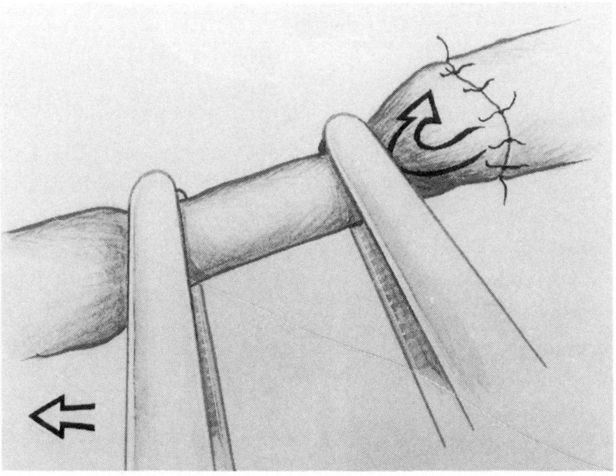

Figure 12–36. Demonstration of patency test by application of two no. 2 jeweler's forceps and emptying a small segment of vessel.

tency is not demonstrated in a repair, it is almost certainly due to a faulty microarterial repair. It is inadequate to dislodge an occluding plug in the hope that the anastomosis will remain open. This treatment of a thrombosis is frequently followed by reocclusion of the vessel at a less opportune time. Any faulty repair must be resected and a better anastomosis performed. The surgeon's assessment of the microvascular anastomosis is the most important measure in the likelihood of success, the degree of vascular spasm and the amount of blood in contact with the external surface of the vessel being less important.

Partial compression distal to the anastomosis may allow flow when seen through the microscope. An expansile pulsation indicates patency but a longitudinal pulsation is not seen in patent vessels—it is a transmitted pulsation.

The uplift test is a more gentle method of evaluating patency. An instrument is placed under the vessel distal to the anastomosis

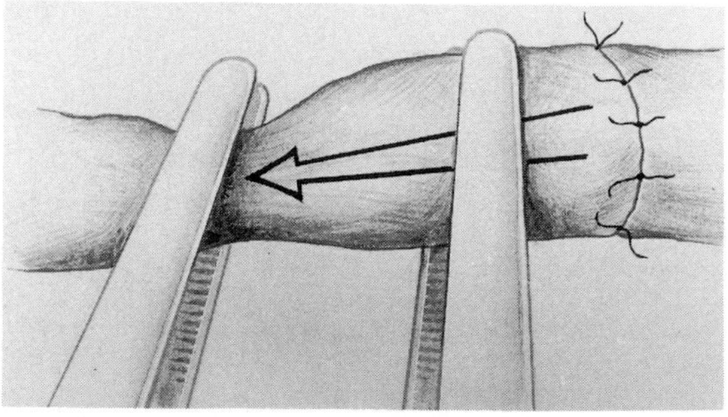

Figure 12–37. Proximal clamp released to fill the segment if the anastomosis is patent.

and lifted upward to put the vessel gently on the stretch and partially occlude the lumen. At the point where the vessel crosses the instrument, an alternating filling and collapsing is seen with each pulse beat if the vessel is patent.

Chow, Huang, and Chan (1982) tested the patency of a microarterial anastomosis in both antegrade and retrograde directions. Experimental and clinical observations have shown that, when patency was achieved in both directions, the subsequent result was much better than in those in which patency was demonstrated only in the antegrade and not in the retrograde direction.

Venous Anastomosis

Excessive suture tension can result in necrosis of the wall and should be avoided. Experimental evidence suggests that this is more critical for arteries than for veins, because large areas of vein wall necrosis sometimes are seen at or near the venous anastomotic site without causing occlusion. Reendothelization of veins also occurs relatively late, sometimes as long as three or four weeks postoperatively (Baxter and associates, 1972). Small veins are sometimes more difficult to repair than arteries, particularly in experimental situations. Under experimental conditions the collapsed vein can be inflated by irrigating with heparinized saline, and the adventitia can then be grasped gently with a no. 5 jeweler's forceps. Human veins are thicker and easier to handle. The anastomosis is completed with a technique similar to that for arteries and the clamp on the downstream side of the anastomosis is always removed first. A 1 mm vessel requires six to eight simple, interrupted sutures for a satisfactory anastomosis.

Fossati, Harashina, and Fujino (1982) demonstrated experimentally that reapplication of clamps proximal or proximal and distal to the venous anastomosis for up to 30 minutes did not impair patency.

Continuous Suturing

Hamilton and O'Brien (1979) reexamined continuous suturing and carried out experiments in the femoral vessels of rabbits (1 mm diameter). The continuous suture technique gave acceptable patency rates (92 per cent arteries and 84 per cent veins), comparable to those with interrupted sutures. While it has the advantage of saving time, the problems associated with entrapment of the suture material in the clamp and breakage of the suture make it a less favorable method.

Lee and associates (1982) compared continuous and interrupted suturing in the saphenous artery of the dog, using high frequency pulse ultrasonography to monitor blood velocity. No statistical differences in the blood velocity profile were found between the two techniques. The pulsatility of the vessels after anastomoses was similar for both techniques. At follow-up examination, the mean being 13 weeks, the patency rate of 100 per cent was demonstrated arteriographically for both the continuous and the interrupted techniques.

Sleeve Anastomosis

Microanastomosis of vessels in the 1 mm external diameter range can be accomplished by means of an invaginating technique with fewer sutures than the end to end method of suture. Lauritzen (1978) presented results that show high patency rates with a two-suture technique in rat femoral vessels (21 out of 21 arteries and 19 out of 21 veins). Functional recovery of the endothelium took place within one week. Meyer and associates (1978) also reported excellent experimental results using a similar "telescoping" method in rat femoral arteries.

If a seemingly easier and more reliable technique of microvascular repair is to be advocated, it must have certain advantages:

1. Speed of completion of anastomosis.
2. Less intraluminal suture exposure.
3. Less vessel trauma owing to fewer sutures and less manipulation of the vessel ends.
4. Prevention of intimal separation.
5. Convenient matching of different sizes of donor and recipient vessels.

Sully and associates (1982) assessed the patency rate of the technique of sleeve anastomosis in a series of femoral arterial repairs in the rabbit, and found that the patency rate was significantly less than that achieved by the conventional end to end anastomosis. The technique of sleeve anastomosis is illustrated in Figures 12–38 and 12–39. The minor advantage of speed of execution of the repair

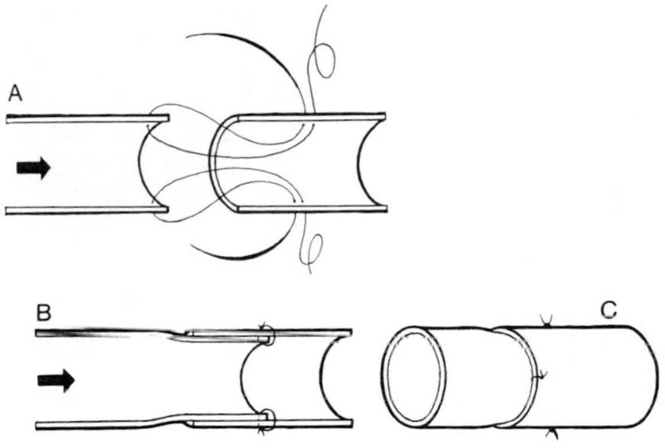

Figure 12–38. Sleeve anastomosis. *A*, Invaginating sutures in place. *B*, The sleeve completed with invaginated sutures tied. *C*, Tacking sutures inserted laterally.

and the supposed advantage of less luminal surface disruption and intraluminal suture exposure did not outweigh the overall lower patency rate as ascertained by direct exploration at varying times. These findings suggest that sleeve anastomosis may not be superior in clinical situations.

Size Discrepancy

If size discrepancies of vessel ends greater than a 3 to 1 ratio are noted, a dilemma arises as to which type of repair achieves the highest patency rate. Using the rabbit's external jugular vein as a graft interposed into resected defects in the femoral artery, Hamilton (1981) showed that the highest patency rates occurred when the larger vessel (jugular vein) was sutured into the side of a smaller one (femoral artery). He evaluated three different types of anastomosis. The end to end repairs confirmed unacceptable failure rates. The tapered vein graft with end to end repair resulted in an improved success rate. The smaller artery sutured into the side of the ligated vein end also had limited patency. However, the best results were obtained by an end to side repair of the vein graft into the artery.

END TO SIDE ANASTOMOSIS

Recipient vessels of 1 to 2 mm diameter are usually prepared for a free flap using end to end anastomoses, and if such large end vessels are present, no problem exists. Occa-

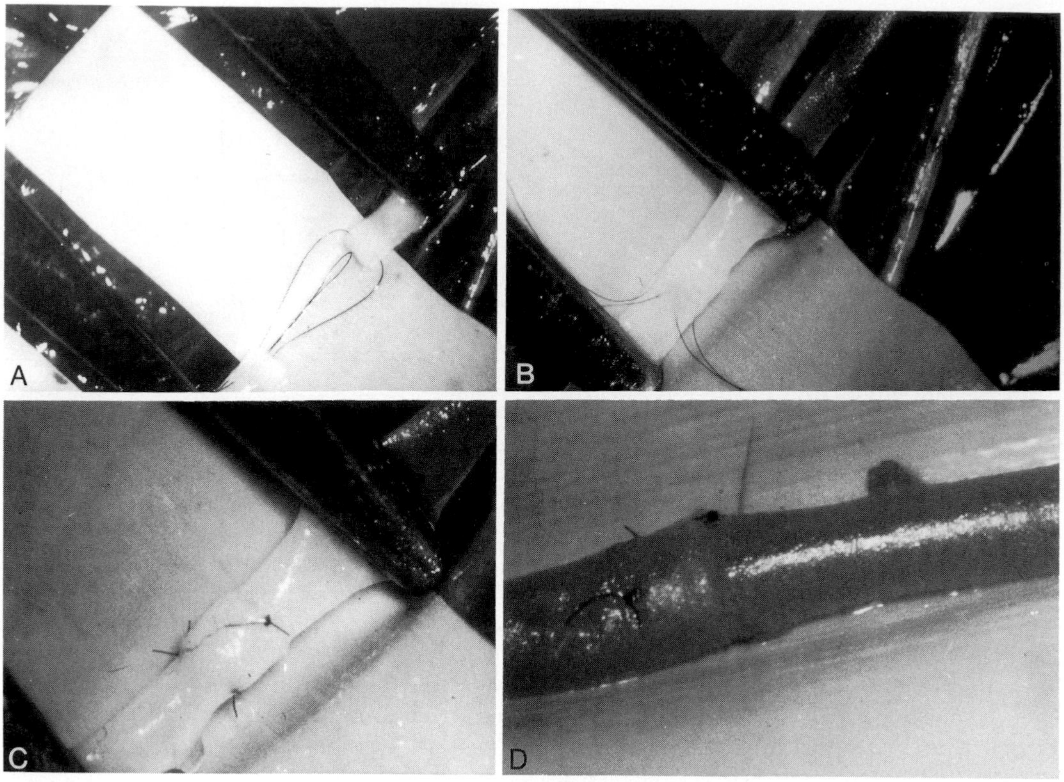

Figure 12–39. *A,* 1 mm femoral artery of the rabbit clamped and divided. The two invaginating sutures are in place. *B,* The proximal end of the same vessel has been drawn into the distal end, but the sutures are not yet tied. *C,* Invaginating sutures tied and tacking sutures inserted. *D,* Clamps released with patency of the vessel.

sionally a larger vessel, principally an artery, has to be divided and used for the anastomosis, the distal end being ligated. This is of little moment in well-vascularized areas such as the face, but in a lower limb, especially in elderly patients, the sacrifice of a major vessel can have a serious effect on distal blood flow. In such circumstances, end to side anastomoses can be used to preserve the patency of the recipient vessels and their normal area of distribution. This type of anastomosis may be necessary even if the recipient vessel is deeply situated.

Ikuta and associates (1975) reported five cases of free groin flaps based on end to side arterial anastomosis. Three of these survived completely and in the others there was only minor necrosis. These authors suggested that the main advantages of this technique are that the search for recipient arteries is simplified and the number of possible sites to which free flaps can be transferred is greatly increased.

Serafin, Georgiade, and Smith (1977) reported 17 free groin flaps to traumatic defects in the lower leg. Ten flaps were totally successful, including the last six, and three flaps were partially successful. In these latter cases a reversed segment of vein graft was used between the recipient artery and the artery to the groin flap. The anastomosis between the recipient artery and the reversed segment of vein graft was carried out by the end to side technique. These authors attributed the increase in success rate to these refinements of technique, although increased familiarity with the procedure could not be excluded.

In the event of no "end artery" being available, it seems logical that an end to side anastomosis be considered. This technique preserves the patency of the recipient artery, and the dependent tissues are not deprived of their blood supply. The search for a recipient artery is also made much easier. The flexibility of the technique can be increased by utilizing larger vascular pedicles or reversed segments of vein grafts.

On the venous side of the circulation a satisfactory patency rate has also been demonstrated. The technique has less application because of the ease in finding a small vein for end to end anastomosis and because there is no interference with the nutrition of the dependent tissues. However, the technique can be used in veins to make use of larger vessels for the anastomosis. A short segment of long saphenous vein may be taken in continuity with the vein draining a groin flap. This gives a vein of more than 5 mm for anastomosis, and by the end to side technique this may be joined to a major vein and the continuity of the latter structure preserved.

The technique has been described by a number of authors (Popov and Trichkova, 1977; Brennen and O'Brien, 1979; Morrison and O'Brien, 1980; Acland, 1980).

End to side anastomosis is difficult to perform in deep areas. The "T" junction tethers the system and prevents adequate rotation of the double clamp. Clear vision of the posterior wall is then impossible. A single clamp is also required to control the incoming vessel, and leaking clamps in areas of difficult access make luminal vision difficult.

Creating a hole into the side of the recipient parent vessel is not easy and requires high quality small scissors (Fig. 12–40). Acland (1980) described a simple technique in small vessels, inserting a 10–0 nylon suture through the wall of the vessel, elevating the wall in a tenting fashion, and cutting a small, ellipic segment out of the vessel wall.

It is preferable to remove an ellipse rather than to make a slit. In thick-walled, small-diameter arteries it is often difficult to visualize the intimal layer clearly because the thick media collapses upon it. In thin-walled veins a filmy adventitia frequently obliterates the hole, and repeated resection of this layer rapidly weakens the vessel wall, thus predisposing to tears and leaks.

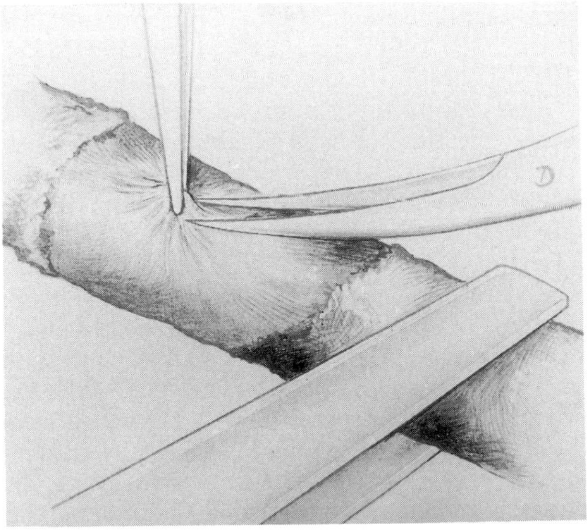

Figure 12–40. Technique of end to side anastomosis, creating a hole in the side wall of the recipient vessel.

The angle of entry of the donor vessel does not appear to alter significantly the blood flow.

The posterior wall is sutured first, beginning at the lefthand corner (Fig. 12–41) and progressing along it to the opposite corner. Spacing of the sutures must be carefully judged. If both corner sutures are inserted first, access to the posterior wall becomes extremely difficult if it is not possible to transfer the entrant vessel forward to expose the posterior wall. If, however, easy access can be gained to the posterior surface, the technique of repair is simplified by inserting the two corner sutures first and then repairing the posterior wall. After the posterior wall is completed, the anterior wall is relatively easy to close (Fig. 12–42).

Occasionally a wider end to side anastomosis can be achieved when a cuff of the major vessel is carried with the donor artery. Other variations are practiced by some surgeons. One apical suture can be inserted, followed by half of the anterior and posterior walls suture by suture. The posterior wall is finished, followed by the anterior wall.

MICROVASCULAR GRAFTS

In clinical microvascular surgery, vessel deficiencies sometimes arise. They occur particularly in replantation surgery of the digits and occasionally in microvascular free flap and toe to hand transfers. The vessel deficiency may involve varying lengths of either arteries or veins. Although there have been numerous reports of arterial and venous grafting of vessels greater than 1 mm in diameter, only a limited number of reports of experimental grafting at the 1 mm vessel level have been published (Yasargil, 1967; Overton and Owen, 1970; Buncke and Murray, 1971; Fujikawa and O'Brien, 1975; Hayhurst and O'Brien, 1975; O'Brien and Hayhurst, 1977; De La Pava and associates, 1979; O'Brien, Browning, and Rosen, 1979; O'Brien, Kubo, and Threlfall, 1979; Das and associates, 1980). The rapid improvement in technique and experience now enables a patency approximating 100 per cent to be achieved.

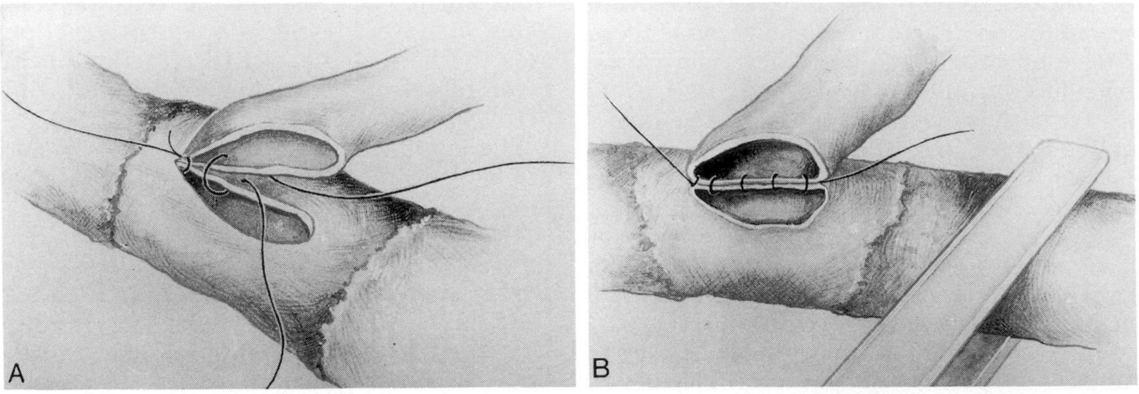

Figure 12–41. *A,* The posterior wall being repaired with a continuous suture. *B,* Completion of the posterior wall with a continuous suture.

The most common clinical method of correcting an arterial deficiency is to use a vein graft, because veins are accessible and dispensable (Biemer, 1977; Buncke, Alpert, and Shah, 1978). Sometimes a small segment of dispensable artery serves as the donor for reconstruction of a vein, but preferably, for venous deficiencies, a vein graft should be obtained. The handling of a small segment of artery is technically easier than that of a similar-sized vein. If the surgeon is confident of the function of a microvascular graft, it greatly extends the range of the clinical applications of microvascular techniques. Factors such as the type of graft, its length, and the value of antispasmodics require consideration.

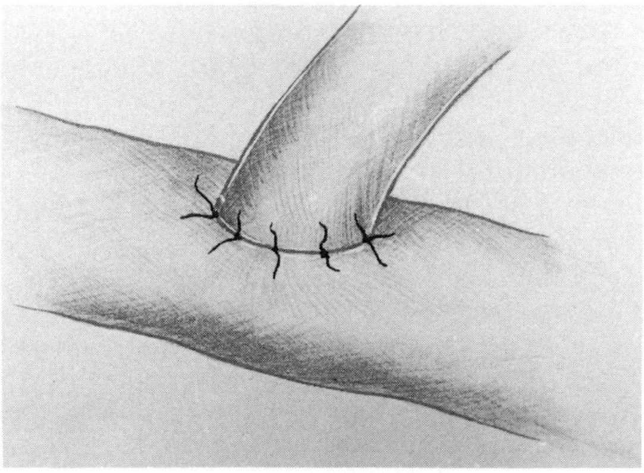

Figure 12–42. Completion of the anterior wall with interrupted sutures.

Microvenous Grafts to Small Arteries

The most common use of microvascular grafts is in bridging defects between small arteries. The exact arterial defect cannot be determined until the vessel ends are resected, appear normal under the microscope, and demonstrate normal flow.

The ideal donor site for digital vessels is the volar aspect of the wrist and lower forearm. Vein grafts can be found of varying sizes with or without branches. Larger and thicker vessels can be obtained from the dorsum of the foot. Arterial grafts taken from nonreplantable digits or from the opposite side of the digit in bilateral damage may give better long-term patency (Melka, Charbonneau, and Bosse, 1979; O'Brien, Browning, and Rosen, 1979; O'Brien, Kubo, and Threlfall, 1979).

The technique of microvascular grafting is based on that of microvascular repairs outlined previously, but varies according to personal choice. Detailed descriptions have been given by Acland (1980) and Morrison and O'Brien (1980).

To harvest the graft a longitudinal incision is made overlying the vein, which can be seen through the skin, and a suitable length of graft selected. The graft is dissected with fine blunt scissors and scalpel. All branches must be ligated. For low flow, low pressure sites in small vessels, such as for replantation, the side branches of grafts are satisfactorily controlled by bipolar coagulation. For higher pressure vessels, particularly with major re-

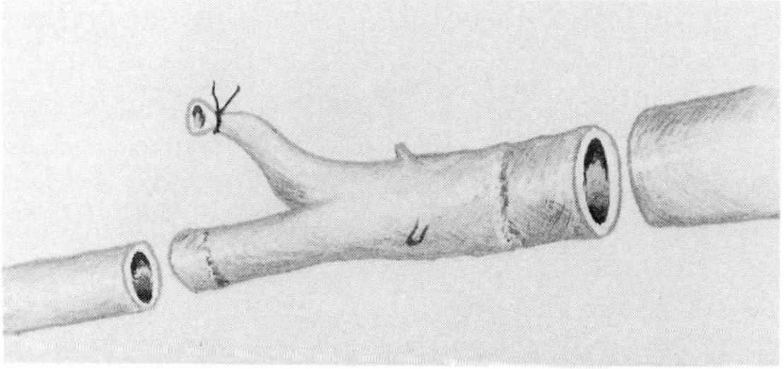

Figure 12–43. Use of one limb of a Y-shaped vein graft to achieve diameter symmetry.

plantation or larger composite tissue transfers, all branches must be meticulously ligated to prevent postoperative reopening. With the branches ligated and the proximal end of the graft occluded, a heparinized saline-filled catheter is inserted into the lumen of the open end and held in place by pinching it between the index finger and thumb. Hydrodistention is then applied to dilate the graft, to unravel kinks, and to demonstrate remaining leaks. This maneuver is extremely important in preventing subsequent graft spasm and the inherent difficulty in interpreting patency.

Grafts should be reversed or occasionally may be used in their original direction, provided that the valves are excluded by catheter irrigation. Small-sized discrepancies can be corrected by taking wider bites on the larger vessel, by cutting the smaller vessel end obliquely, or by dilating the smaller vessel only. A Y-shaped graft can be used for anastomosis to two distal vessels, or only one limb

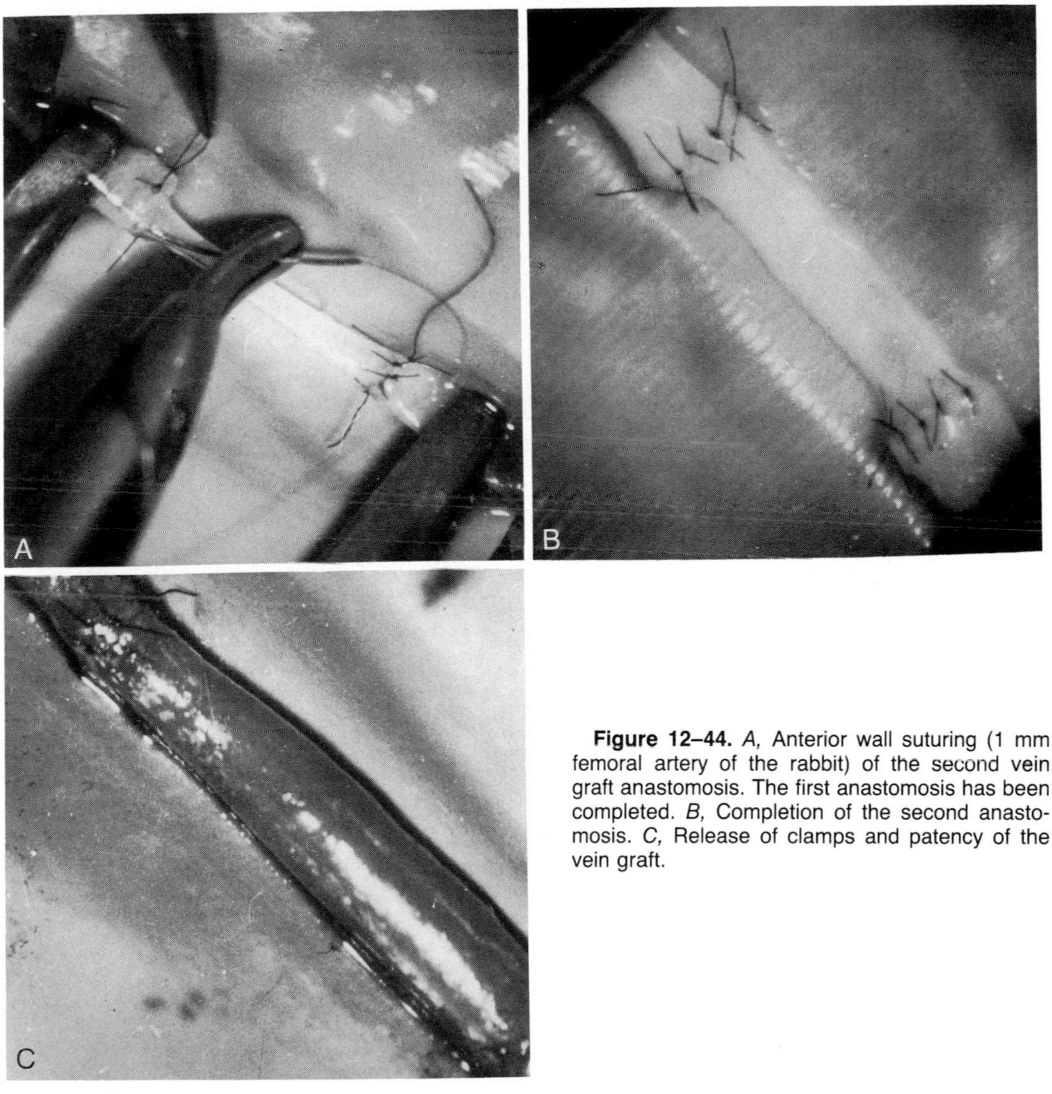

Figure 12–44. *A,* Anterior wall suturing (1 mm femoral artery of the rabbit) of the second vein graft anastomosis. The first anastomosis has been completed. *B,* Completion of the second anastomosis. *C,* Release of clamps and patency of the vein graft.

may be used to accommodate a size discrepancy, the other limb being ligated (Fig. 12–43).

Great care must be taken not to twist or kink the graft. The precise graft length takes some experience to judge, especially when long lengths are involved. They must be inserted under some tension because after release of the clamps the graft elongates. If it is too long, it kinks, twists, or rolls down vertical surfaces, as with grafts spanning the knee or elbow joints.

The vein graft is inserted into the vessel defect, and clamps must be applied to the proximal vessel and to the distal vessel if backflow is present. For short length vein grafts it may be possible to incorporate the whole segment of the graft between the double clamp and allow an anastomosis of each end without the need to change the clamp arrangement (Fig. 12–44). However, in most circumstances separate occlusion clamps are required at the proximal and distal ends of the recipient vessel, as well as a double clamp applied separately at each site of anastomosis. The distal anastomosis should always be performed first and at no time should the graft be permitted to fill with stagnant blood.

In conditions of difficult exposure in which a double clamp cannot be applied and access to the posterior wall cannot be gained by turning the double clamp over, the anterior wall of the first anastomosis can be performed with a single clamp only. The graft is turned upside down to expose the posterior wall for suturing (Fig. 12–45).

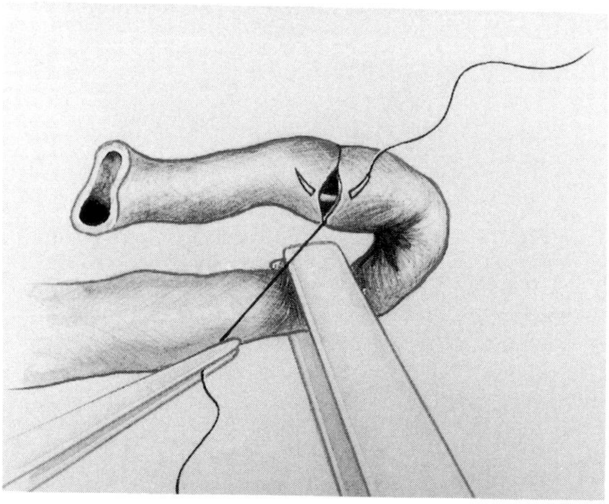

Figure 12–45. Use of a single clamp in conditions of difficult exposure. The anterior wall of the vein graft has been completed at one end and the vein graft is turned over to commence suturing on the posterior wall.

Pribaz and associates (1983) in experimental studies have shown that there is considerable adaptability of vein grafts. They can stretch by 22 per cent of their original length and contract by 30 per cent. Tension leads to thrombosis, but within limits redundancy disappears and is associated with high patency rates (Fig. 12–46). The ideal interposition graft length measured in its donor position before division should be 33 per cent longer than the arterial defect measured in its relaxed state. When such a vein graft is harvested it should measure approximately 30 per cent less than the arterial gap. A vein graft taken to bridge a venous defect, on the other hand, should be the same length as the defect in its relaxed state.

Microvenous Grafts to Small Vein Defects

A similar technique to that used for grafting arterial defects is employed for microvenous grafting to veins, but the venous graft is not reversed as it is in arteries. Patency rates are equivalent to those of vein grafts into arteries, approximately 100 per cent (O'Brien, Browning, and Rosen, 1979; O'Brien, Kubo, and Threlfall, 1979).

Microarterial Grafts to Arteries

The technique used for inserting microarterial grafts into small arteries is similar to that for other previous microvascular grafts. More symmetry of diameter and thickness of wall is possible. The donor artery length needs to be slightly shorter than that of the defect. De La Pava and associates (1979) studied patency rates in Y-shaped arterial grafts from the femoral artery in rabbits and compared these with end to end arterial anastomoses immediately proximal to the bifurcation. No deleterious effects of turbulence were demonstrated and there was no statistical difference in the patency rates (100 per cent and 93 per cent, respectively) in the two groups.

The use of an unrepaired artery as graft material for the repair of a dorsal vein has been encountered infrequently in digital replantation. It reduces the need to search elsewhere for graft material, and the procedure is expedited by the easy handling of the small

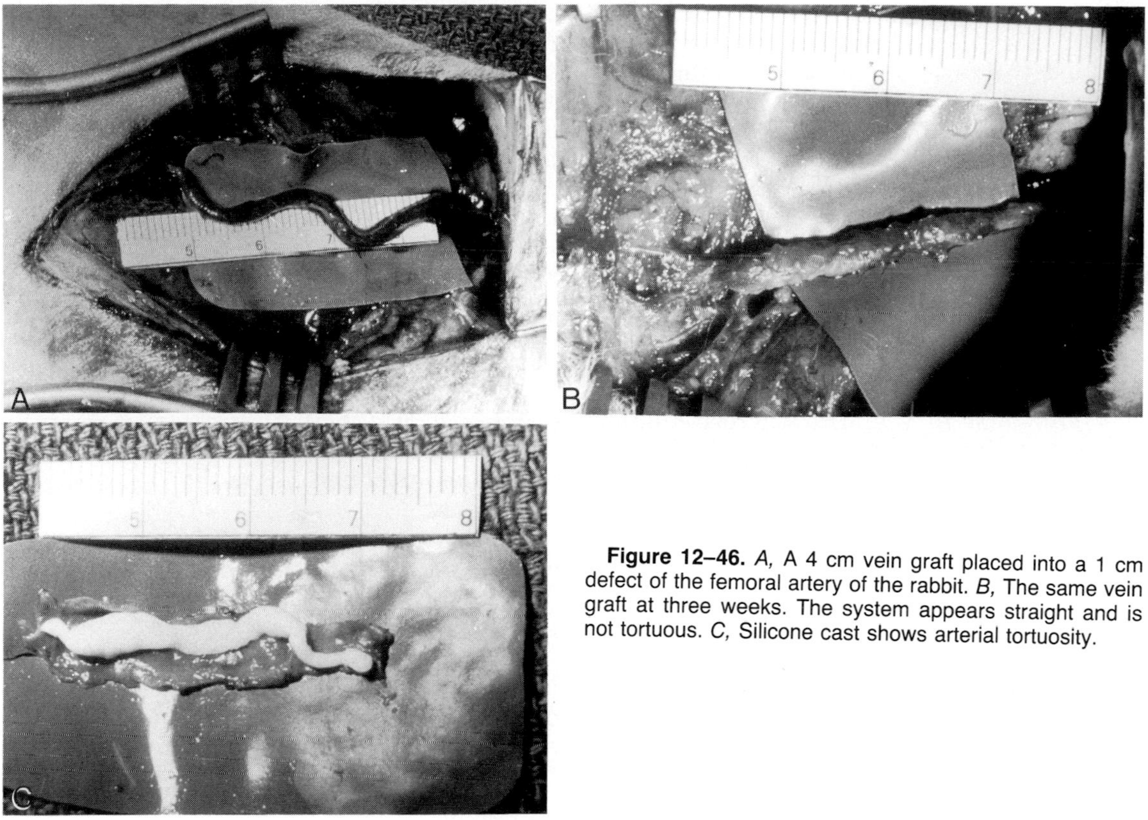

Figure 12–46. *A,* A 4 cm vein graft placed into a 1 cm defect of the femoral artery of the rabbit. *B,* The same vein graft at three weeks. The system appears straight and is not tortuous. *C,* Silicone cast shows arterial tortuosity.

piece of artery. It is preferable to repair both digital arteries in a replanted finger, and hence donor sources are rather limited. In most cases of digital replantation, the bone requires shortening. However, the use of microvascular grafts at times may modify the need for bone shortening. This is particularly applicable in children, in disarticulation replantation, and in digital transposition, when joint surfaces are being preserved.

Preserved Microvascular Grafts

Although autogenous microvascular grafts have achieved a high degree of success, active research is progressing for substitutes, preserved and prosthetic. Harashina (1978) collected common carotid arteries from outbred rabbits and rats. These arteries were preferred because of the unbranched length that could be obtained. The lumen of each was washed with heparinized saline solution and the graft stored in 70 per cent ethyl alcohol for at least three weeks. The longest storage period was six months. The stored arterial grafts were inserted into a 1.2 to 1.5 cm defect in the femoral arteries of rats. The success rate of xenografts was much lower than that of allografts owing to the higher antigenicity, and there was no formation of aneurysms.

Prosthetic Grafts

Parsa and Spira (1979) evaluated patency rates in the laboratory, employing autogenous veins and alloplastic substitute conduit 1 mm internal diameter polytetrafluoroethylene (PTFE) as short length grafts to restore continuity in both arterial and venous defects in rat femoral vessels. The effectiveness of vein grafts was again demonstrated. Recanalization or restoration of blood flow did not occur following thrombosis during the six week period of observation. There was a consistent failure of alloplastic graft to remain patent. Histologic studies revealed an arterialization of the vein grafts when these were used to bridge an arterial defect.

It is apparent from current research that preserved and prosthetic grafts have not yet attained the level of success of autogenous grafts.

NORMAL BLOOD FLOW

An understanding of certain physical properties of blood flow is useful. Full discussion of fluid mechanics in the central areas of the circulation is not pertinent to this discussion. However, factors that apply to blood flow in vessels within the microsurgical range (0.3 to 3 mm) and in the true microcirculation warrant study.

Flow Patterns and Resistance

Flow Patterns. Blood flow (Q) through a segment of vessel is determined primarily by two factors:

1. The *pressure difference* (P) across the length of the vessel.
2. The *resistance to flow* (R) offered by the vessel.

Fluid flowing steadily in a smooth vessel does so in a laminar fashion, as if in concentric layers or laminae, with velocities increasing as the central lamina is approached (Fig. 12–47). There are no sharp boundaries between laminae, but rather a gradual change in flow rate from peripheral to central. Fluid in the faster flowing central lamina tends to remain there and similarly in the other layers.

Laminar flow can be experimentally demonstrated by viewing the interface between two immiscible fluids of different colors in a clear tube (Fig. 12–48). With the fluids stationary, there is a straight interface.

After flow is commenced, the interface assumes a parabolic shape. The marginal fluid molecules tend to adhere to the vessel wall and move forward slowly. The more centrally placed molecules have to slide past the adherent marginal molecules. This type of impedance slows their progress and, in turn, they offer resistance to the next more central molecules, although less so than the marginal molecules.

The least affected molecules are the most centrally located in the vessel where flow is fastest (Fig. 12–49). A smooth parabolic flow pattern is typical of laminar flow.

Factors such as obstruction, vessel angulation, branching, or vessel wall irregularity disturb the orderly flow by deflecting molecules across the stream. In such situations there is fluid flow both across the vessel and along it, breaking up the laminar flow and increasing resistance; this is called *turbulence* (Fig. 12–50).

In a nonpulsatile system the tendency to turbulent flow is proportional to the velocity of flow and vessel diameter, and inversely proportional to the viscosity divided by the

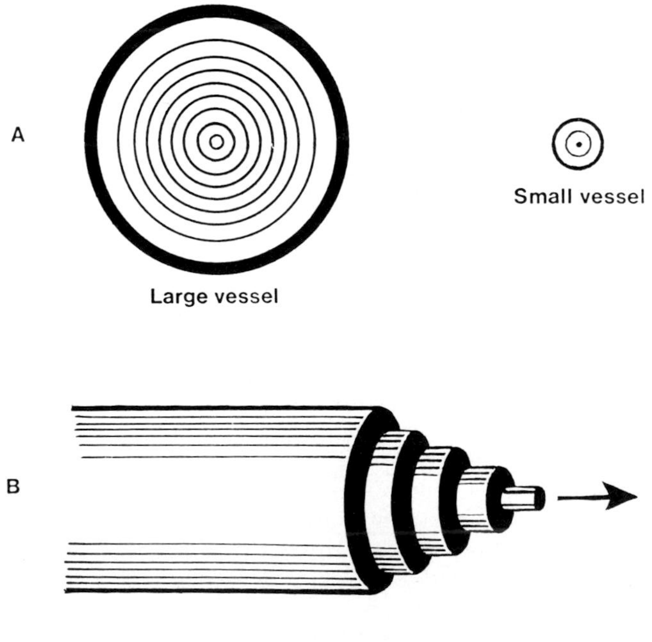

Figure 12–47. *A, B,* Blood flows through straight smooth vessels as if in concentric laminae, the fastest flowing at the center. The smaller the vessel, the closer is the central lamina to the wall.

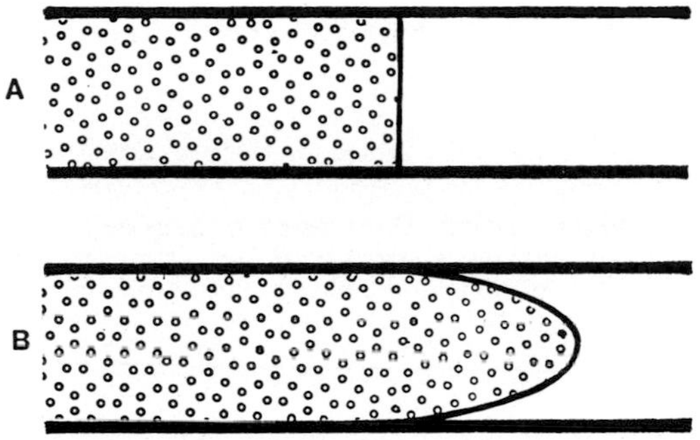

Figure 12–48. *A,* Two stationary immiscible liquids of different color in a clear tube. *B,* With flow, a paraboloid wave front becomes evident.

density. The measure of the tendency for turbulence to occur is called Reynold's number.

In vivo the major arteries are most susceptible to turbulence. This tendency is increased by their pulsatile flow and by sudden changes in vessel diameter. In small vessels under normal circumstances, Reynold's number almost never rises high enough to cause turbulence.

Resistance. Under conditions of laminar flow the resistance of a vessel is produced by the adherence of marginal molecules to the vessel wall. As the diameter of a vessel decreases, the fastest flowing central molecules become progressively closer to the vessel wall and are therefore more affected by the slow-moving marginal molecules, producing a rise in resistance to flow (see Fig. 12–50). The vessel diameter thus is a major factor determining vessel resistance.

It is estimated that under *resting* conditions approximately two-thirds of the systemic peripheral resistance is provided by the arterioles, and the remainder by other vessels, notably the capillaries.

With maximal arteriolar dilatation, the site of maximal resistance moves out to the small vessels.

Elastic Properties

The elastic properties of a blood vessel can be described by Young's modulus (E) (stress). Because arteries are subject to oscillatory stress (pulsatile pressure), the static modulus is less appropriate than the *Dynamic Modulus (EDyn),* in which the frequency of oscillation is defined.

The dynamic modulus is also a determinant of pulse wave velocity, which varies in proportion to EDyn.

Dynamic Impedance

The dynamic impedance rises with:

1. Increase in E(Dyn).
2. Reduction in lumen diameter.
3. Arterial branching.

Arterial branching or obstruction disturbs the paraboloid wave form, causing a rise in impedance. Thus, even in normal vessels turbulence is possible and is increased by:

1. Increased flow.
2. Decreased viscosity.
3. Areas of stenosis or irregularity.
4. Pathologic dilatation.

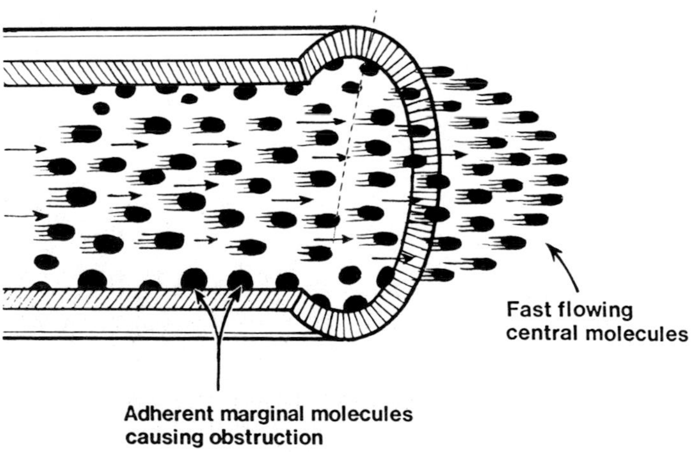

Figure 12–49. The molecules flowing at the center of a vessel are least affected by molecular adherence to the vessel wall.

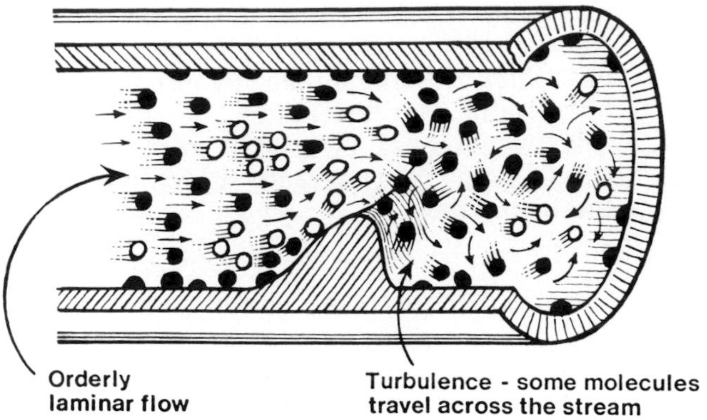

Figure 12–50. Disturbance in laminar flow is called turbulence. Fluid flows across the stream, as well as along it, greatly increasing resistance.

Flow Through Bifurcations

A change in the flow pattern occurs at bifurcations (Fig. 12–51). The laminar flow is disturbed downstream of a branch, and the reflected waves from the bifurcation can produce turbulence and even standing waves within the vessel. Converging venous flow produces different but complex flow patterns.

It must be remembered that blood contains cellular elements that behave differently at branches from the way a homogeneous fluid behaves. The most important parameters governing red cell distribution at the bifurcation of small vessels are the diameter ratio of the cells and vessels, the shape and deformation of the cells, the hematocrit in the main feeder vessel, and the ratio of the flow velocities in the two downstream vessels.

In the microcirculation in which two downstream vessels are of equal diameter, the ratio of the hematocrits in the two downstream vessels is a linear function of the ratio of the two blood velocities, up to a critical velocity ratio, above which essentially all the cells are swept into the vessel with the higher velocity.

Vessel Wall Tension

For expanding vessels, such as aneurysms, vessel wall tension is important since it rises at the same time as the wall itself is thinning, thus predisposing to rupture.

For small vessels this has importance, since as the pressure in a vessel decreases so does the diameter. Since tension is proportional to

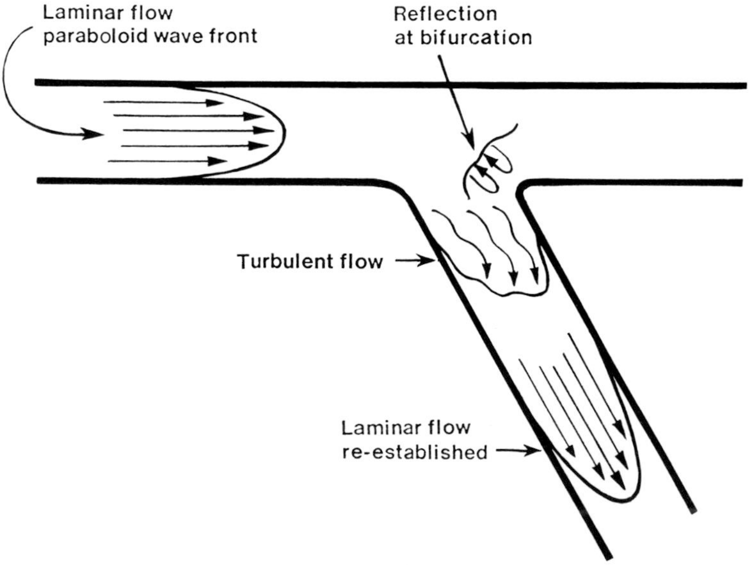

Figure 12–51. Laminar flow is disturbed at vessel bifurcations. Wave reflections may produce turbulence.

diameter times pressure, the tension tending to keep the vessel open against the vasomotor tone and external tissue pressure also drops. A point is reached at which the elastic tension in the vessel wall exceeds the stretching force produced by the pressure and the vessel no longer remains open. This point is the *critical closing pressure*.

Control Mechanisms

Other than adjustments in heart rate and cardiac stroke volume, circulatory adjustments are mediated by alterations in the peripheral resistance vessels—either in a change in total peripheral resistance or in the distribution of blood flow between tissue beds.

Under resting conditions approximately two-thirds of the systemic peripheral resistance is provided by arterioles, and the remainder by other vessels, notably the capillaries. If the arterioles become fully dilated, the site of maximal resistance moves distally to the small venules.

The arterioles also act as a distribution control, varying the distribution of flow between organs and tissues. At any time some of the peripheral resistance vessels are in a state of partial contraction or tone. Superimposed on this there are dual control mechanisms—central via the nervous system and local via conditions in the immediate vicinity of the vessel.

The mechanisms that control the contractile state of the smooth muscle in vessels providing resistance have been diagramatically summarized by Folklow and Neil (1971) (Fig. 12–52). The resistance vessels of some tissues have an intrinsic basal tone, while others require neural input to produce tone.

Removing all external innervation (brain, cardiac, and skeletal muscle) alters the resistance little. This "fail safe" mechanism helps to ensure blood flow to these vital structures. Other tissues, e.g., skin, rely almost entirely on autonomic activity to produce basal vascular tone.

Local control of resistance vessels is called autoregulation. Tissues with this property, when their metabolic demands are stable, can maintain a constant blood flow in the face of varied perfusion pressures and can increase blood flow when metabolic demands increase.

One of the factors responsible for autoregulation is the "myogenic response" described by Bayliss in 1902. Vascular smooth muscle responds to stretch by *active* contraction and to release of stretch by relaxation.

Another local autoregulatory factor is the vascular response to local metabolic demand. The "metabolic hypothesis" holds that with increased metabolic activity certain vasoactive substances accumulate, producing vasodilatation and thereby increased flow, and that, conversely, when metabolic activity declines, the same substances are cleared by the circulation, thus restoring resting vessel tone.

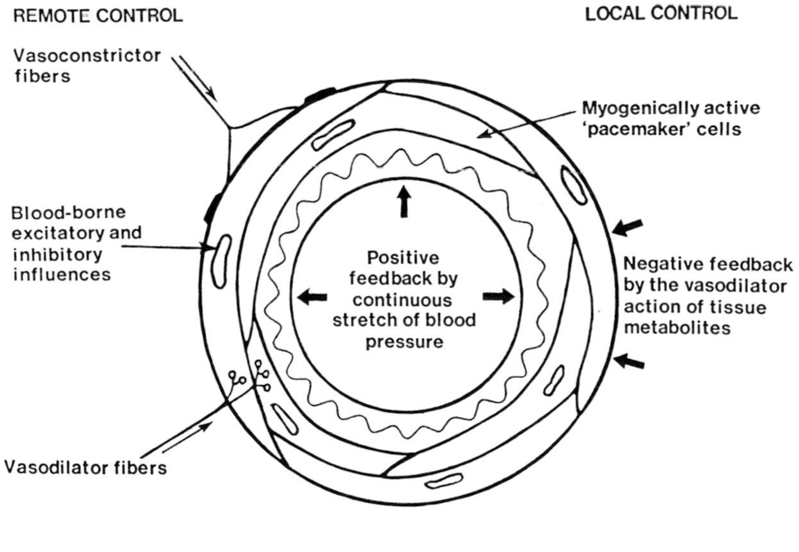

Figure 12–52. The external (remote) and intrinsic (local) mechanisms that control the contractile state of the smooth muscle in the wall of an arteriole. (After Folklow, B., and Neil, E.: Circulation. Oxford, Oxford University Press, 1971.)

Those tissues with the greatest propensity for autoregulation have the least dense sympathetic constrictor innervation. In strongly autoregulated vascular beds, blood flow closely matches metabolic demand. The vascular beds with dense innervation may have a purpose in addition to metabolic needs.

Skin has little capacity for autoregulation but is very sensitive to neural changes. Skin circulation, as well as subserving the metabolic needs of the integument, has an important thermoregulatory role that would not be possible if the circulation was autoregulated. The skin has in fact a unique mechanism for dealing with necessarily reduced flow: its temperature drops and the metabolic demands decrease.

NEURAL CONTROL

Nearly all sections of the vascular tree that contain smooth muscle have an autonomic effector innervation. Probable exceptions are umbilical and placental vessels, the ductus arteriosus, much of the cerebral vasculature, and the precapillary sphincters. It is of note that autonomic nerve endings usually do not occur closer to the vessel lumen than the outer layer of the media. The inner smooth muscle layers are only under the influence of circulating vasoactive substances. This phenomenon is supported by the segregation of adrenergic receptors: the alpha receptors are only in the outer layers of the vessel wall and the beta receptors are only in the inner layers. Figure 12–53 illustrates the distribution of sympathetic nerves to blood vessels.

Sympathetic Innervation. Sympathetic vasoconstrictor action arises in the vasomotor center in the medulla oblongata. A physiologic center rather than a defined anatomic collection of cells, the center is tonically active. Stimulation causes norepinephrine release at the effector site, eliciting the alpha-adrenergic response of vasoconstriction. Inhibition reduces the tonic activity, resulting in vasodilatation. The sympathetic vasoconstrictor fibers supply the arterioles, the veins, and perhaps the precapillary sphincters. Although arteries and larger veins also receive

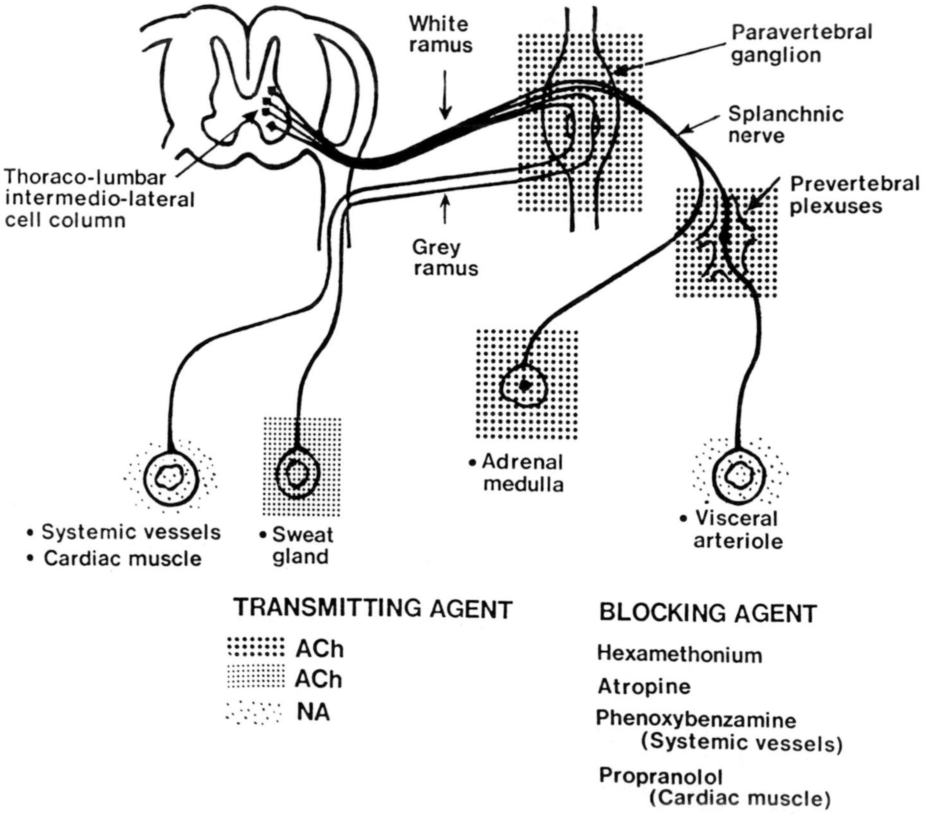

Figure 12–53. The distribution of the sympathetic nerves to blood vessels and endocrine glands relevant to the vasculature. (Reproduced by permission from the Royal Australasian College of Surgeons.)

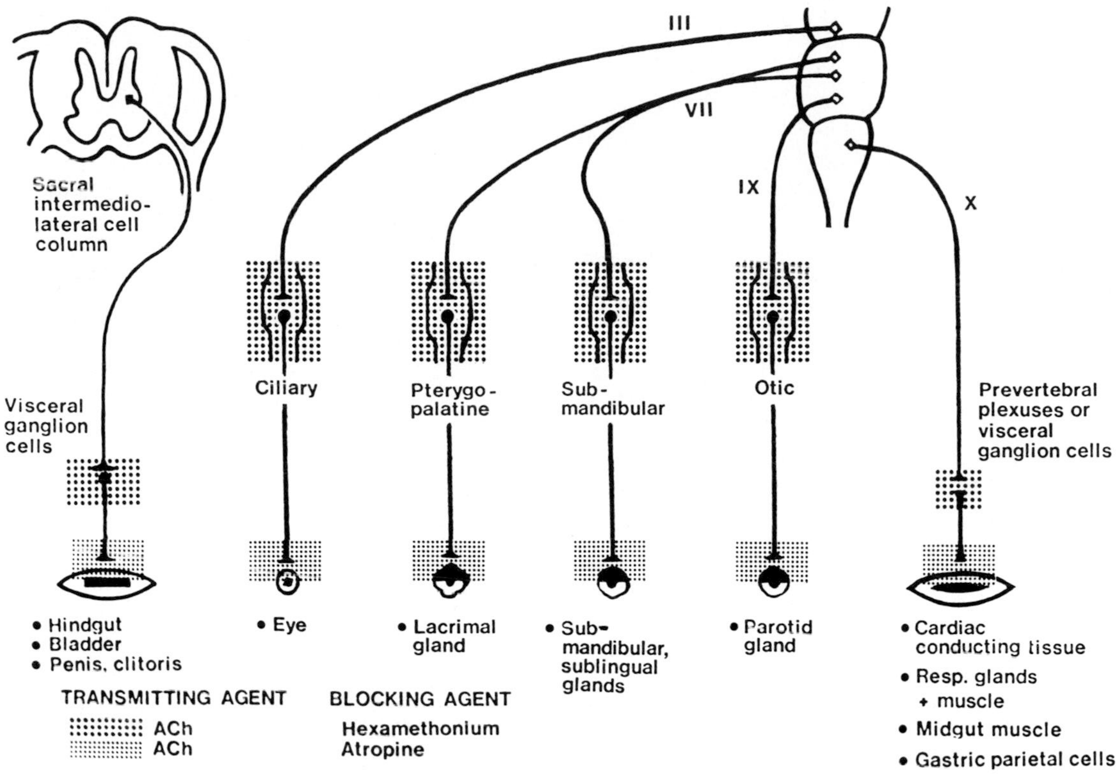

Figure 12–54. The distribution of the parasympathetic nerves to blood vessels, exocrine glands and the gastrointestinal and genitourinary tracts. (Reproduced by permission from the Royal Australasian College of Surgeons.)

some sympathetic innervation, this is a less important function than the action on the microcirculation.

There are, in addition, sympathetic cholinergic vasodilator fibers innervating resistance vessels in skeletal muscle and skin. There is no evidence of any tonic activity in this system. Activation produces a relatively large transient initial increase in blood flow, followed by a smaller sustained increase during continued nerve stimulation. The action may be to cause an anticipatory increase in muscle blood flow at times of impending stress.

Parasympathetic Innervation. The parasympathetic autonomic system is also active in the control of blood flow. Figure 12–54 illustrates the distribution of parasympathetic nerves to blood vessels. Efferent cranial fibers supply head and visceral blood vessels, and sacral parasympathetics supply vessels of the genitalia, bladder, and large bowel. Skeletal muscle and skin do not receive parasympathetic supply. The vasodilator effect of the cholinergic fibers on total peripheral resistance is only small.

HUMORAL CONTROL

Of the vasoactive humoral substances, the adrenomedullary hormones are the most important. However, this group of substances is known to include antidiuretic hormone, angiotensin, serotonin, kinins, histamine, and prostaglandin (most important, prostacyclin).

From the standpoint of overall circulatory control, neural and humoral stimuli combine to exert similar or dissimilar effects on different segments of the vasculature, altering blood flow, tissue blood volume, or extravascular volume to meet physiologic requirements.

Blood

The laws of hemodynamics are derived from the study of the steady flow of conventional fluids in straight, uniform bore tubes. Poiseuille's law, for instance, does not apply fully to the flow of blood, which exhibits non-newtonian properties. In fact, the faster blood flows, the lower is its viscosity. This can be

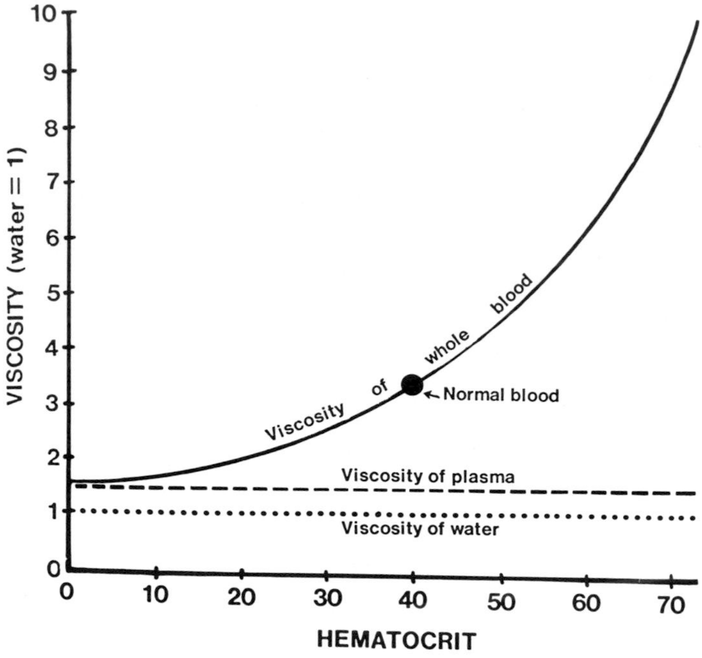

Figure 12–55. The effect of hematocrit on blood viscosity. (After Guyton, A. C.: Textbook of Medical Physiology. 7th Ed. Philadelphia, W. B. Saunders Company, 1986.)

demonstrated in vitro and is chiefly determined by the red cell concentration and plasma concentrations of fibrinogen and globulin.

The higher the hematocrit of blood, the greater is the friction between successive layers of blood, and therefore viscosity rises. Figure 12–55 illustrates the relationship between hematocrit and viscosity.

The size and shape of the conduit greatly influences blood flow properties. The Fahraeus-Lindqvist phenomenon (Fig. 12–56) be-

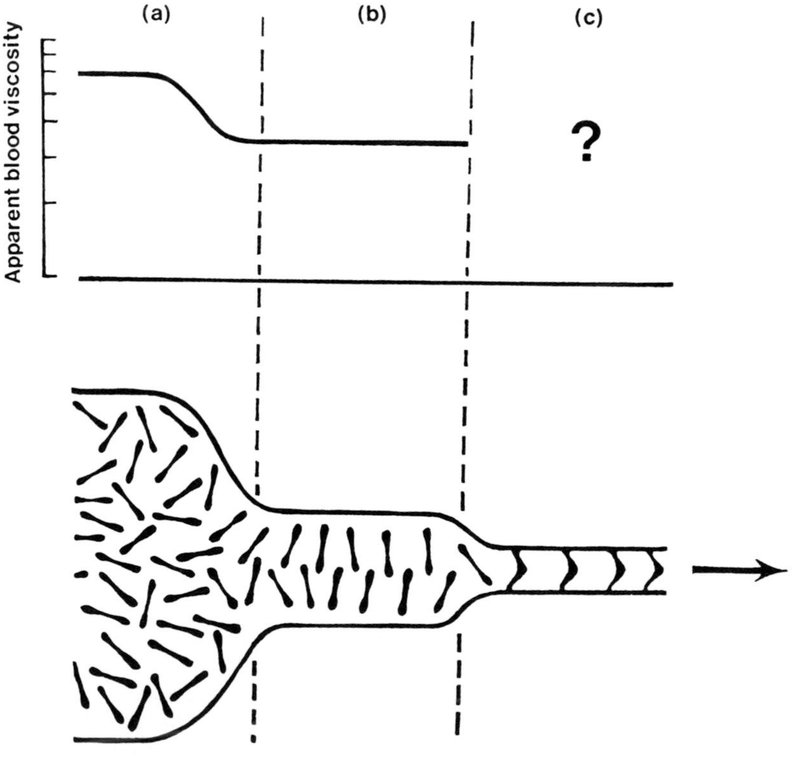

Figure 12–56. Red cell behavior and blood viscosity in the microcirculation. (*a*), 100 m arteriole with random orientation of red cells. (*b*), 15 m metarteriole, with more regular orientation of red cells, a relatively large, red cell–free boundary zone, and a fall in apparent blood viscosity (Fahreus-Lindqvist effect); (*c*), Capillary, with single file movement of red cells as paraboloids rather than biconcave discs. The effective viscosity of blood in a capillary is unknown. (Reproduced by permission from Ludbrook, J., and Walsh, J. A.: *In* Birnsting, M. (Ed.): Peripheral Vascular Surgery. London, Heinemann, 1973.)

gins to appear when vessel diameter falls below approximately 1.5 mm. Below this vessel size, blood flow is far less viscous than in larger vessels. In fact, in vessels as small as capillaries the effect is so prominent that the viscosity of whole blood is as little as one-half that in large vessels. The effect is probably due to red cells aligning themselves in the smaller vessels rather than moving independently, thus reducing the viscous resistance within the blood itself. Sutera and Hochmuth (1968) found that, in models, rigid particles produce 30 to 40 per cent less drop in pressure when flowing in groups than when traveling separately.

Visual observation of blood flowing in small tubes has also given rise to the axial streaming model of blood flow, with the cells appearing to congregate at the center of the stream and leaving an apparently cell-poor marginal layer, thus significantly lowering resistance. Bloch (1962), however, found that the appearance is one of a cell-free layer adjacent to a vessel because of two factors: (1) there are occasional plasma gaps in the vicinity of the wall; and (2) since no red cells can have their center at the wall, the hematocrit in the wall region is reduced (Fig. 12–57).

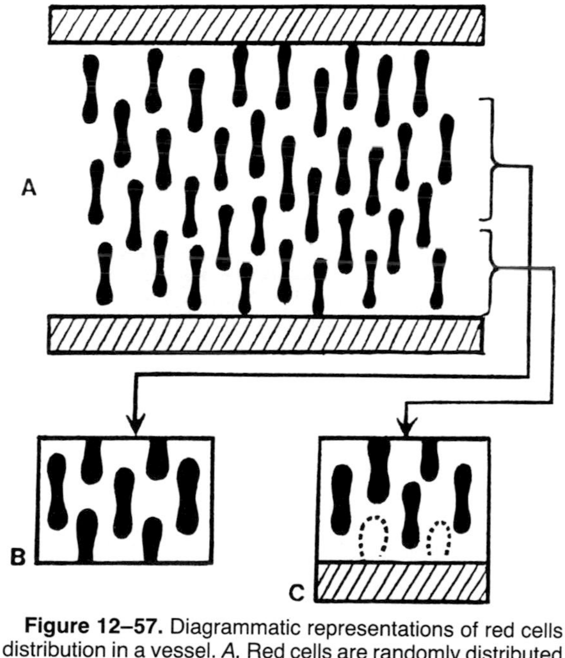

Figure 12–57. Diagrammatic representations of red cells distribution in a vessel. *A*, Red cells are randomly distributed in a vessel. *B*, Red cell distribution in the center of the vessel. *C*, At the vessel wall, no red cell can have its center. Red cell concentration is correspondingly less.

Other experimental studies have demonstrated that, if a truly cell-free marginal layer exists, it is very small. In fact, Wiederhielm and Billig (1968) showed that red cells are distributed throughout the flow stream.

The Microcirculation

Knowledge of the anatomy and function of the microcirculation is desirable. The components of the microcirculation are illustrated in Figures 12–58 to 12–60.

The arterioles are the major site of peripheral resistance under resting conditions. Precapillary sphincters determine the flow or no-flow status of the capillaries they serve. Their activity is thought to be controlled by local metabolic demand, and as such they control the distribution of blood between capillaries.

The precapillary sphincter is only one smooth muscle cell thick, its efficacy being dependent on the small vessel diameter and flow pressure. Metarterioles and arterioles also have smooth muscle activity, serving to redistribute blood flow between larger areas of tissue.

Capillaries have no smooth muscle but are elastic, their diameter varying with transmural pressure. It is across the walls of the true capillaries and venous capillaries that the metabolic exchange between tissues and blood takes place.

ABNORMAL BLOOD FLOW

Virchow's triad has long formed the basis for the classification of factors producing vascular thrombosis, the triad being abnormalities of the (1) vessel wall, (2) flow of blood, and (3) constituents of the blood. This triad also forms a convenient basis for discussion of the abnormalities of blood flow pertinent to microvascular surgery.

Abnormal Vessels

TRAUMA

Microvascular repair is a reliable procedure when both proximal and distal vessels are normal. Reendothelization of the repair occurs in two to four weeks (Harashina, 1976; Nightingale, Fogdestam, and O'Brien, 1980). Minor degrees of intimal damage, such as

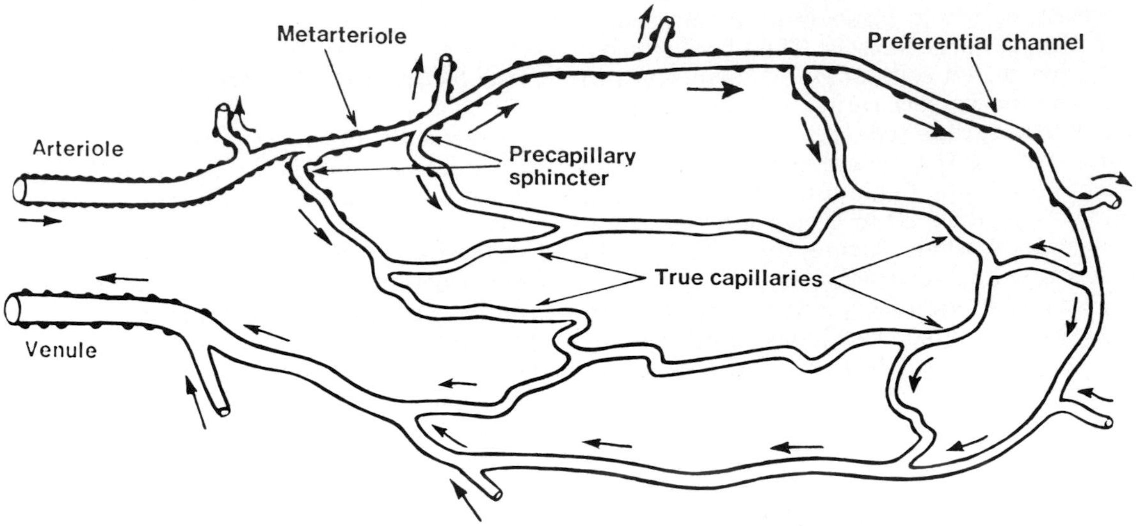

Figure 12–58. Overall structure of the capillary bed. (After Zweifach: Factors regulating blood pressure. Josiah Macy, Jr. Foundation, 1950.)

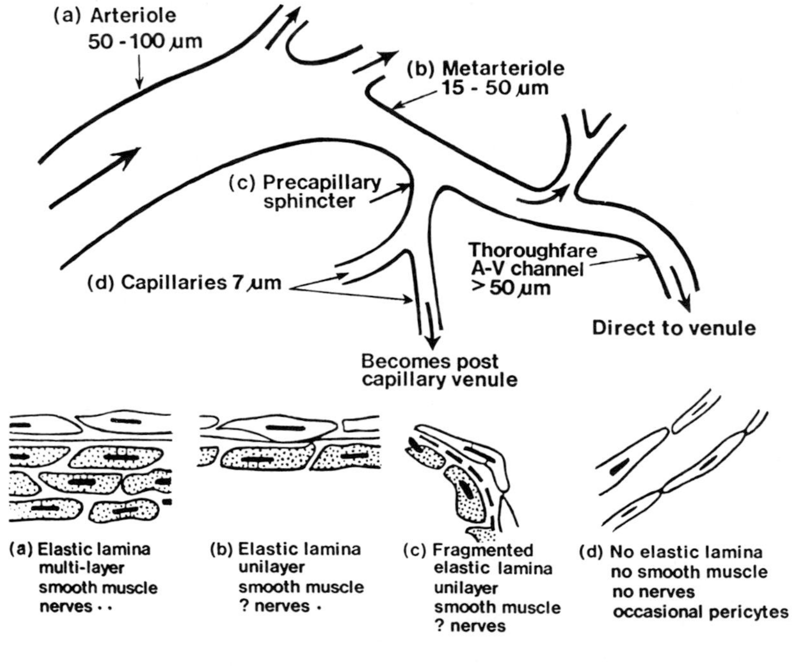

Figure 12–59. The microstructure of the arterioles and capillaries. (After Rhodin, J. A.: J. Ultrastruct. Res., *18*:181, 1967.)

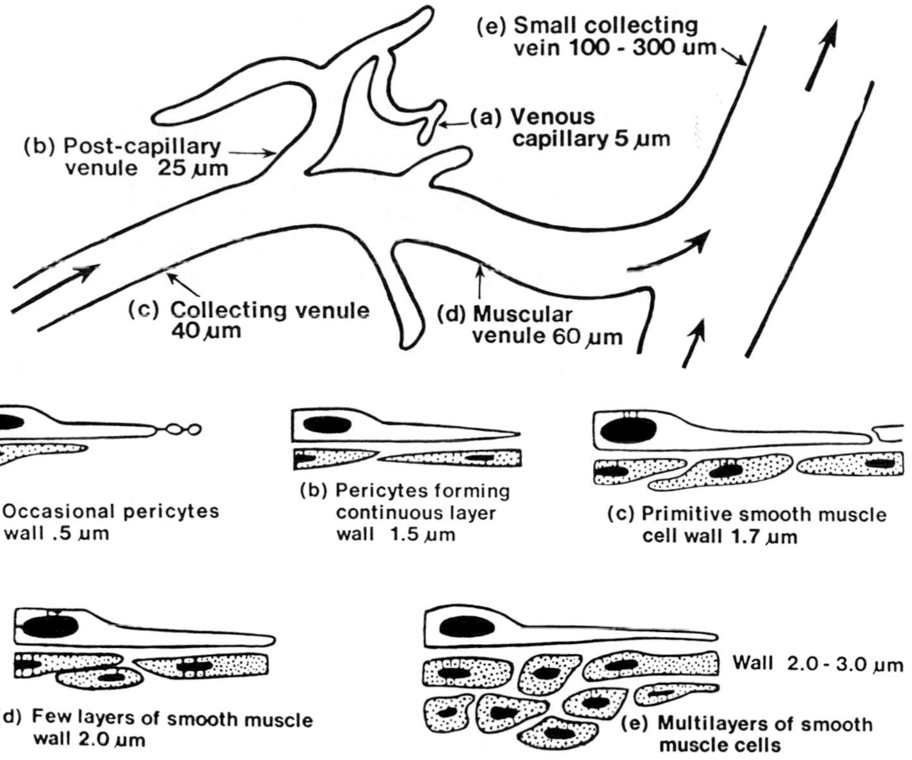

Figure 12–60. The microstructure of the venous capillaries and venules. (After Rhodin, J. A.: J. Ultrastruct. Res., *25*:452, 1967.)

that caused by mechanical vessel dilatation or vessel clamping, do not necessarily impair vessel healing or lead to thrombosis. However, as grades of vessel damage increase, the likelihood of anastomotic failure also increases.

The degree and extent of trauma varies with the type of vessel injury.

Type of Lesion

1. *Sharp* injuries cause damage to a small length of vessel. The amount of necessary resection is correspondingly small, and end to end anastomosis is usually possible.

2. *Crush* injuries have a wider zone of injury and often require a vein graft to bridge the defect caused by resection of the damaged vessel. Inadequate resection or failure to perform a vein graft when necessary results in thrombosis. Forward flow should be demonstrated before anastomosis.

3. *Avulsion* injuries are more complex, and the survival rate of the replanted part is lower with this type of surgery.

Mitchell and associates (1985) demonstrated that, particularly in avulsed arteries, significant intimal damage is found up to 4 cm from the site of vessel rupture. Since veins rupture more readily than arteries, the extent of avulsion damage to veins is much less than that seen in the arteries. These findings correlate with the clinical experience that repaired avulsed arteries occlude more frequently than repaired avulsed veins (Morrison, O'Brien, and MacLeod, 1977).

In practice, vessel resection is continued until microscopically normal vessel is seen and a satisfactory forward flow demonstrated. One predictable site of avulsion injury is at the first significant proximal arterial branch. Inspection at this point may reveal a lesion that will obstruct flow.

ANASTOMOSIS TECHNIQUE

The value of various techniques has been described earlier.

VESSEL WALL DRYING

Prolonged procedures where all concentration is directed to only a portion of the wound or wounds leaves exposed structures vulnerable to the risk of drying.

INFLUENCE OF HEALING ON MICROVASCULAR ANASTOMOSES

Wound healing favorably influences the normalization of postmicroarteriorrhaphy hemodynamics. Blair and associates (1985) studied the influence of wound healing on microvascular anastomoses, using a rat model and Doppler flowmetry.

Their findings confirmed that hemodynamic variables do not return to normal immediately after microarteriorrhaphy but do so three weeks after wound healing. There was also no difference in the return of blood flow to normal between repairs with either interrupted or continuous suture.

LOCAL VESSEL ABNORMALITIES

Variations in vascular anatomy, by altering flow direction and pressure, have implications for microvascular surgery. Any pathologic condition in a vessel wall raises the risk of anastomotic failure or has an adverse effect on flow.

Local Artery Thrombosis and Aneurysms

While collateral circulation usually provides satisfactory circulation following ligation or obstruction of a single forearm artery, thrombosis of certain hand vessels produces abnormalities that go beyond the mere interruption of blood flow in those vessels.

Although other arteries in the hand may be affected, the most frequent site of such pathology is the ulnar artery in Guyon's canal. Etiologic factors associated with thrombosis of the ulnar artery are closely related to those of ulnar artery aneurysm. Repetitive trauma to the hypothenar eminence may produce either pathologic condition. Most patients are men of working age whose jobs subject their hands to repetitive blunt trauma, although cases in women have been reported. Temporal arteritis may be a far less common cause.

Ulnar artery thrombosis may cause a tender and painful mass, ischemic symptoms in the digits, sensory damage in the fingers, or a combination of these. Sensory abnormalities may be related either to the etiologic trauma or to compression by the thrombosed vessel, which may be dilated.

Vascular changes are more complex and not explained purely on the basis of interruption of flow, since excision of the damaged vessel frequently effects a cure.

Leriche, Fontaine, and Dupertuis (1937) proposed that the vascular effects are due to alterations in the sympathetic plexus surrounding the diseased vessel. Numerous reports support this contention and, in fact, simple resection is curative.

Most upper extremity aneurysms are caused by trauma, producing vessel wall weakness and a fusiform dilatation. Penetrating trauma may cause a pseudoaneurysm. Symptoms may be due to Raynaud's phenomenon. Pain and pallor of the digits can result from embolic showers, or local nerve compression. The region of the aneurysm may be locally tender and erythematous, mimicking an abscess or bone tumor.

Treatment involves resection with or without reconstruction, depending on local vascular factors, distal perfusion, and ease of anastomosis.

Arteriovenous Fistulas

Arteriovenous fistulas are of interest to microsurgeons in several areas:

1. They may be used to salvage a digital replant in which no distal veins are available by anastomosing the nondominant distal artery to a proximal vein. Smith, Sonneveld, and van der Meulen (1983) described three successful cases. No patient developed the usual features of an AV fistula or claudication. It was presumed that angiogenesis followed, with restoration of a more normal venous outflow.

Nichter, Haines, and Edgerton (1985) investigated this concept, using a rabbit ear model with inadequate venous outflow. They speculated that metabolic exchange occurred proximal to the capillaries, encouraged by the high tissue CO_2 that shifts the oxygen dissociation curve to the right by the Bohr effect.

2. Erol and Spira (1980) described using an arteriovenous fistula constructed with a vein graft from artery to vein and laid in a tissue bed. New vessels from the fistula provided sufficient vascularity to the skin and subcutaneous tissue, allowing elevation as a flap.

3. Arteriovenous fistulas are frequently constructed in patients with renal insufficiency to facilitate dialysis. Significant vascular congestion of the thumb may be seen after arteriovenous shunt. A painful, en-

gorged thumb results. Reversion to normal follows ligation of the shunt.

4. Congenital or traumatic arteriovenous fistulas may attract the attention of the microsurgeon for ablative and reconstructive reasons.

Generalized Vascular Pathology

There are many generalized conditions that adversely alter vessels: (1) atherosclerosis, (2) diabetes, (3) Buerger's disease, and (4) other inflammatory vascular disorders.

Abnormalities of Blood Flow

Although excessive blood flow is rarely, if ever, a problem, except in arteriovenous shunts, loss of perfusion pressure, increased peripheral resistance, or turbulence adversely affect circulation. Normal blood flow is smooth and laminar, blood flow being determined by the pressure difference along a vessel and the resistance of that vessel, a factor related to the fourth power of the vessel radius.

General factors of cardiovascular function alter blood flow, but only abnormalities of blood flow pertinent to microvascular surgery are discussed below.

EXTERNAL COMPRESSION

Tight wound closure exacerbated by swelling, a wound hematoma, vessel angulation over bony fractures, or fixation are the most common external causes of abnormal blood flow (Fig. 12–61). Swelling or hematoma, when combined with tight wound closure and bandaging, produces vascular compression. The lower pressure venous system is most susceptible to compression, which results in venous congestion. A rise in the venous pressure may overcome the external compression force and maintain blood flow, but if the compression totally prevents venous flow, the venous pressure rises until arterial input becomes obstructed. This leads to vascular stasis, progressive cellular damage, thrombosis, and eventual tissue death.

Hydrodistention of vein grafts is useful for three reasons. This maneuver abolishes spasm, displays leaks, and helps to maintain orientation. When the proximal end of a vein graft is clamped and heparinized saline is injected into the distal lumen, the vessel distends and any rotation is seen to unwind. By clamping the vessel distally the distention is maintained, enabling a long vein graft to be passed through a subcutaneous tunnel without loss of orientation.

A gentle rotation of an arterial repair becomes a tight choking of the vessel on clamp release. The forward flow forces the twist along the vessel up to the first distal branch, at which point forward progression stops. The twist tightens and obstructs flow (Fig. 12–62).

Other external factors may obstruct flow such as a repaired nerve under tension running across a vessel, a metal internal fixation device, or angulation over a bone prominence.

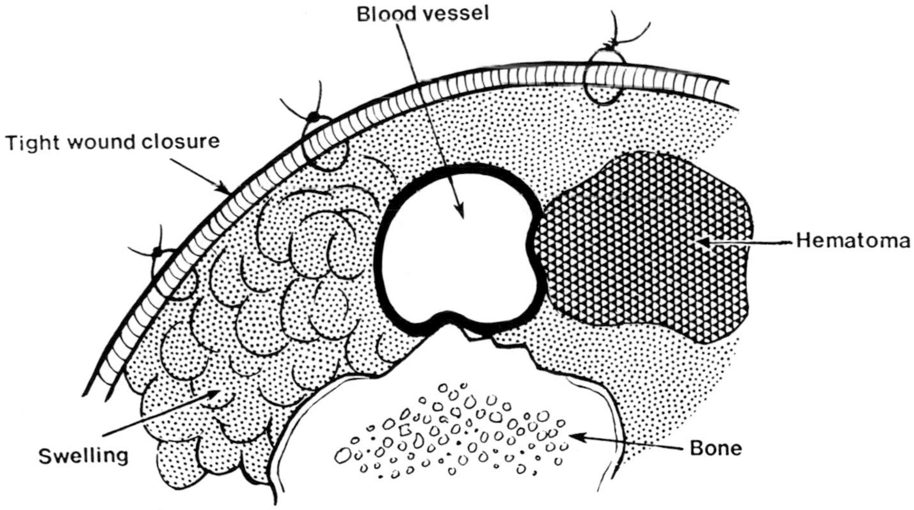

Figure 12–61. Causes of external compression of blood flow.

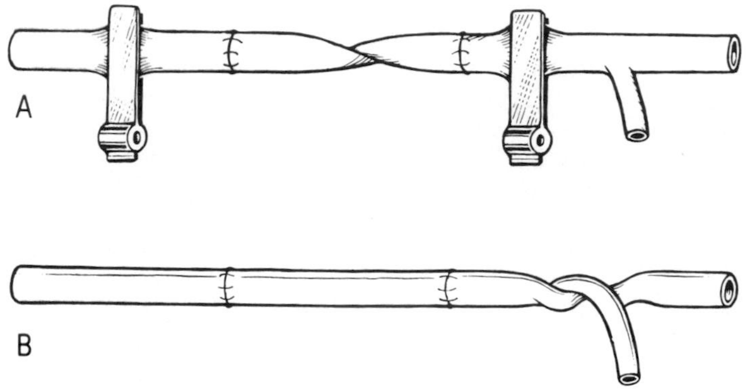

Figure 12–62. External compression of blood flow. *A,* Rotation of arterial repair. *B,* Flow forces the vessel to twist forward to the first distal branch.

Vigilance is required to avoid these external factors. Wounds over anastomoses should be closed without tension after adequate hemostasis is obtained. Some surgeons use small Z-plasties, even in replanted digits, to prevent annular wound constriction. If midaxial incisions have been used for exposure, the longitudinal portion of the wound on the side opposite the arterial repair may need to be left open or skin grafted when only one artery has been repaired. Careful design of skin flaps, away from the course of the vessels, allows the flaps to cover repaired vessel even if the wound cannot be closed completely.

INFECTION

Luk and Chow (1985) have studied the effect of infection on the patency of microvascular anastomoses in the rat femoral artery. The presence of infection did *not* significantly lower the patency rate in this experimental study. Infection in the clinical setting has long been considered detrimental to the patency of repaired small vessels (Hayhurst and O'Brien, 1975).

VASOSPASM

Vasospasm may be pathologic, as in Raynaud's disease. It also occurs in connective tissue disorders, such as scleroderma, and in cryoglobulinemia.

Cryoglobulinemia is one of a group of disorders labeled dysproteinemia in which abnormal proteins are found circulating in the plasma. Cryoproteins precipitate on cooling and redissolve on warming. Their presence often does not cause symptoms, but they may cause peripheral vascular insufficiency and even gangrene. Cryoglobulins are often associated with multiple myeloma or macroglobulinemia, and occasionally with systemic lupus erythematosus or other connective tissue diseases.

Posttraumatic

The choice of a recipient artery in a traumatized field sometimes creates a dilemma. Although distal pulsation may be palpable preoperatively, the vessel, once dissected, may not flow. Lidman and Daniel (1981) have shown internal skip lesions at a distance from original vessel transection in 12 clinical cases, despite normal arterial biopsy at the original surgery.

Arteriograms may not demonstrate the abnormality. These lesions, in combination with vessel spasm, impair blood flow.

While veins within a scarred, traumatized bed may demonstrate significant spasm, some appear not to contract, which tempts the surgeon to use them as recipients. These, in fact, appear open when divided owing to dense circumferential scarring that allows them to neither contract nor expand. Flow through these channels is often poor and there is no capacity to tolerate the increased flow from a flap. These vessels should be avoided and more proximal vessels sought outside the zone of injury. Irrigation of a vein with heparinized saline from distal to proximal end helps to confirm adequate flow capability and vessel expansion.

Physiologic Vasospasm

Vasospasm is a normal protective mechanism that minimizes blood loss from traumatized vessels. Spasm can be induced in the normal vessel by a number of means including cold, vessel dissection, adventitial handling, and the application of vasoconstrictive drugs. Although several vasoconstrictive agents are important in the causation of spasm, experimental work has demonstrated that norepinephrine is most likely to be the main agent responsible.

In the nontraumatized vessel when conditions are restored to normal, vasospasm gradually decreases and flow is reestablished. Despite the low volume or even cessation of flow, coagulation does not occur within the normal vessel since the intact endothelium is not thrombogenic.

To the microsurgeon, even such "normal" spasm is of great importance. Dissection to expose recipient vessels commonly produces spasm. This is most marked in the lower limb in which both the arteries and veins are thicker walled and demonstrate degenerative vascular changes at an earlier age than in the upper limb.

The surgeon must be assured of a forward flow in a donor artery before relying on the vessel to feed a free tissue transfer. This is extremely difficult when intense refractory spasm is present, and much delay may occur while spasm resolution is awaited. Venous spasm, similarly, makes vein dissection and anastomosis more difficult. In vessels traumatized by dissection, clamping, vascular repair, or injury, the diminished flow may allow thrombus formation.

In our laboratory, Papadopoulos and associates (unpublished data) have shown that spasm of the feeding artery lasting longer than one hour in the dog saphenous artery free flap does not prejudice survival. Nevertheless a point is reached at which spasm is present for sufficient time to create ischemic changes in the flap tissue.

Pharmacologic Spasm

Vasospasm is seen following the accidental intra-arterial administration of drugs. Some drugs, in addition to causing vasospasm, damage the endothelium and cause irreparable vessel occlusion.

Nicotine is a vasoconstrictor commonly used in the community, and it warrants more detailed consideration. Cigarette smoking is often cited as the single most preventable cause of death, and the long-term deleterious effects to health are well known. Nicotine is the principal active component of tobacco smoke and it is known that each cigarette yields 0.4 to 1.6 mg of nicotine. A colorless alkaloid, it is known to stimulate central and peripheral nervous systems with release of catecholamines, causing vasoconstriction, a rise in blood pressure, and tachycardia (Goodman, Gilman, and Gilman, 1980). Smoking one cigarette produces a decrease in distal blood flow velocity of 42 per cent (Sarin, Austin, and Nickel, 1974). Hladovec (1978) demonstrated that nicotine caused endothelial injury in rats, and Booyse, Osikowiez, and Quanfoot (1981) showed endothelial disorders in rat aortas after nicotine administration. Brinson and Chakrabarti (1974) concluded that nicotine inhibited platelet aggregation in rabbit blood in vitro.

Rao, Morrison, and O'Brien (1983) studied the effect of nicotine on microvascular anastomoses. A single large dose of nicotine injected into the repaired dog saphenous artery produced marked vasoconstriction in a dose-dependent fashion, which then underwent natural decay over ten minutes. A second study investigated the long-term effect on arterial anastomoses. The rabbit femoral artery was used as a model, being an approximation in size to the vessels commonly repaired in microsurgery. Twice daily intraperitoneal injections of nicotine, the equivalent of smoking six cigarette packs per day, were continued over three weeks in preoperative, perioperative, and postoperative combinations. There was no marked increase in the incidence of thrombosis even with the high nicotine doses used. Perhaps the suggested inhibition of platelet aggregation combined to balance the vasoconstriction effects on these clean surgical repairs.

In the context of trauma or more extensive surgery, in which vessel spasm can be a significant problem even without nicotine, the known vasoconstrictor effect of nicotine should justify its prohibition, particularly during the first two weeks after surgery during which time the vascular repair site is being reendothelized (Nightingale, Fogdestam, and O'Brien, 1980).

Management of Vasospasm

Mechanical Dilatation. Mechanical dilatation of vessel ends before repair relieves local spasm. Although jeweler's forceps are frequently used, special dilating forceps are preferable. These are rounded in cross section at their tips and polished to remove any sharp edges. The squared shape of regular jeweler's forceps may be responsible for the internal damage seen on scanning electron microscopy after vessel dilatation, although this amount of damage does not seem to cause vessel occlusion.

Hydrodistention. Hydrodistention of vein grafts is an effective way of abolishing the spasm produced by dissection and preventing later spasm when flow is reestablished. In addition, the heparin adheres to the endothelium, and distention helps to prevent vessel twisting.

Controlled limb dependency is efficacious and is suitable for intraoperative use. When spasm threatens the circulation to foot or hand tissue, lowering that part over the operating table increases the hydrostatic pressure within the limb and tends to expand the contracted vessel. This maneuver is continued only for a few minutes and frequently is effective even when the usual pharmacologic methods of relieving spasm fail.

Pharmacologic Measures. External application of 2 per cent lidocaine or other local anesthetic agents is the most common method of relieving vessel spasm. There are some circumstances, however, when 2 per cent lidocaine is ineffective. Increasing the concentration of lidocaine increases its effectiveness; in practice, 10 per cent lidocaine, available as an infusion concentrate used in cardiac surgery, is satisfactory.

For more refractory spasm, verapamil (Isoptin) applied undiluted in small amounts provides the most assured vasodilatation. Clinical experience to date shows an absence of cardiovascular side effects from this calcium antagonist.

Intra-arterial injection or infusion of vasodilators is sometimes required. Phentolamine mesylate (Regitine), papaverine, procaine and lidocaine have been used for this purpose.

Sympathetic Blockade. Useful as an adjunct to the management of vasospasm, sympathetic block is commonly already in effect, at least in upper limb surgery performed under brachial plexus anesthesia.

Sympathectomy has long been established as a reliable and lasting procedure for lower limb peripheral vascular disorders. Upper limb sympathectomy, however, has proved unreliable. Certainly, transient vasomotor improvement occurs, but the long-term results are disappointing. Gifford, Hines, and Craig (1958) reported that only 54 per cent of women with Raynaud's disease had a satisfactory long-term result from proximal sympathectomy, despite encouraging initial results.

Anatomic features lie behind the failure of proximal sympathectomy. The brachial plexus receives its sympathetic fibers not only from the cervicosympathetic trunk, but also from the sinuvertebral nerve, from the carotid plexus, and from the nerve of Kunz. Intermediate sympathetic ganglia, lying in the nerve root canals, bypass the sympathetic trunk (Pick, 1970). Cervical sympathectomy frequently fails to clear these accessory pathways.

The upper limb arterial sympathetic supply is not fully established in the proximal limb. Sympathetic axons travel with the peripheral nerves and send frequent branches to arteries throughout their course (Morgan, Reisman, and Wilgis, 1983), even to the level of the digital arteries. The sympathetic axons apparently are then distributed only within the adventitia of the arteries.

Flatt (1980) proposed that, if the aim of sympathectomy is to relieve finger symptoms, it seems logical that it be carried out as far distally as possible. He described stripping as much adventitia as possible from a 3 to 4 mm length of proper digital artery under microscope control. This maneuver removes as reliably as possible the sympathetic innervation of the digital vessels. Flatt has performed this procedure in eight patients followed over 20 years with pulse volume recordings and skin temperature monitoring. In this group with mixed etiology (frostbite, post-traumatic vascular spasm, and scleroderma), all had a permanent rise in finger skin temperature and variable, but rewarding, symptomatic improvement.

Wilgis (1981) reported his results with digital sympathectomy in 18 digits of ten patients. Nine of the ten gained verifiable improvement in digital blood flow. Pain was reduced in all patients with digital ulcers, and cold intolerance was relieved in all but one. Wilgis stressed that only those who have a positive response to local anesthetic digital block should have this surgery and that all connections between the adjacent nerve and vessel be severed. In addition, there should be circumferential removal of all the loose adventitia over a distance of 2 cm. It is important that the vessel be not damaged; in particular, the media and intima must be left untouched to prevent thrombosis.

Pharmacologic sympathetic blockade produces vasodilatation, and can be a useful adjunctive measure when peripheral vascular spasm threatens a replantation or free tissue transfer to an extremity. Although a catheter can be positioned near the stellate ganglion for continuous sympathetic block, brachial plexus anesthesia is the most straightforward method of providing sympathetic block.

In the long-term management of vasospastic conditions, intravenous regional perfusion with guanethidine, a drug that decreases the norepinephrine stores in the peripheral adrenergic synapses (a chemical sympathectomy), may be of value. Its use, although still experimental, can produce gratifying circulatory improvement. The effect of guanethidine lasts a variable period, but it may be of use when digital infarcts are occurring in the patient with scleroderma.

Sympathetic block, however, should not be used as the first line of intervention with a failing flap or replant, since mechanical factors of wound tension, external compression by hematoma, or technical anastomosis failure are more likely causes. Immediate wound exploration and correction of these factors are indicated.

BLOOD VOLUME

The success of free tissue transfers or replantation depends on adequate flow across repaired vessels and perfusion of tissue fed by these vessels, thus allowing oxygen transfer and clearance of metabolic products. Low perfusion pressure, hyperviscosity states, or low oxygen-carrying capacity therefore adversely affect the outcome.

Microvascular procedures and free tissue transfer are often extended procedures involving blood loss and changes in intravascular volume. Appropriate fluid management is important. Basic fluid balance theory teaches that:

1. Dextrose solution, after the glucose is metabolized, is distributed rapidly among all tissue compartments.

2. Saline and other electrolyte solutions distribute to the extracellular fluid space.

3. Colloid solutions remain intravascular, at least until they are metabolized.

Any of the fluids can be used, but only colloids continue to support blood volume for any significant period. Volume should be replaced predominantly with colloid, and the question is, which colloid should be selected? Relevant considerations are:

1. Blood viscosity should not be increased and a decrease is desirable.

2. Oxygen transport should not be impaired. Since it is known that the rheologic properties of blood are enhanced by a measure of anemia, some centers aim to allow the hemoglobin to fall. Usually a hemoglobin of 10 (or hematocrit of 30) is the accepted level. Others feel that there is little to be gained from lowered hemoglobin levels except lowered oxygen-carrying capacity, and they aim to maintain normal hemoglobin levels.

In practice, depending on the length of time banked blood has been stored, maintenance of laboratory values with blood transfusion does not fully correct the oxygen-carrying capacity of blood, since many of the red cells are affected and unable to perform normally.

Since satisfactory results are experienced from both therapeutic approaches, the difference is not critical. However, the important factors are adequate volume replacement with colloid solution, and maintenance of oxygen-carrying capacity by keeping the hemoglobin level above 10.

Blood Constituents

The tendency to vascular thrombosis, all other factors being equal, increases with abnormalities that increase coagulability or reduce blood flow by increasing blood viscosity.

Conditions in which platelet numbers are elevated may be associated with intravascular thrombosis, even in normal vessels. Platelet numbers are transiently raised following parturition, trauma, and severe hemorrhage. Splenectomy may be followed by a protracted thrombocytosis, a state that is also persistent in polycythemia vera. Platelet adhesiveness is increased in patients with brain tumors, multiple sclerosis, or hyperlipidemia and probably after trauma.

Clotting time is shortened after severe hemorrhage, somewhat after trauma and infection, and following the administration of corticosteroids and estrogens. Hyperlipidemia shortens clotting time and inhibits fibrinolysis.

Blood viscosity changes that affect blood

flow in the clinical situation are usually secondary to dehydration. Inflammation can produce a local rise in viscosity, and systemic conditions such as polycythemia also increase viscosity.

Dintenfass (1982) has outlined the following blood viscosity factors:

1. Viscosity of whole blood.
2. Plasma viscosity.
3. Aggregation of red cells.
4. Rigidity (deformability) of red cells.
5. Tendency for formation of red and white thrombi or white thrombi.

A hyperviscosity syndrome can be present when at least one viscosity factor is elevated.

ANTICOAGULATION

A worldwide survey of anticoagulation practice in microvascular surgery (Davies, 1982) revealed that the use of anticoagulants was by no means standardized and was not even universally practiced.

The aim of anticoagulation must be to protect either the patency of microvascular repair or blood flow through damaged vessels and tissue beds by the prevention of intravascular coagulation or by lysis of thrombi. To this end the agents used may

1. Decrease platelet aggregation or adhesiveness.
2. Interfere with the coagulation cascade.
3. Use the complex effect of dextran.
4. Act to break down thrombus.

Agents That Affect Platelet Function

Acetylsalicylic Acid (ASA). The ability of ASA to inhibit platelet adherence to collagen and subendothelium has been shown experimentally (Cazenave and associates, 1978). Its influence on platelets manifests itself as ASA-induced prolongation of the bleeding time by influencing primary hemostasis. Its action is thought to be due to inhibition of prostaglandin synthesis via an irreversible effect on an enzyme that remains throughout the life of the platelet, thus producing a long duration of action.

This effect occurs at *low* doses of ASA, while, owing to a combination of enzyme effects, high ASA doses can in fact have a thrombogenic effect (Kelton and associates, 1978).

When ASA is used in microvascular surgery it seems wise to consider a low dose, a bonus in producing less side effects, with dosage continued at least until vascular repairs and areas of trauma have reendothelized.

Dipyridamole (Persantin). Originally used as a vasodilator, this substance inhibits platelet aggregation but does not affect platelet adhesiveness.

Other Agents. These include sulfinpyrazone, hydroxychloroquine, and flurbiprofen.

Anticoagulants

Heparin is used for intravenous anticoagulation. It acts principally by inactivating thrombin, which prevents it from acting on fibrinogen. It also acts earlier in the clotting pathway by accelerating the combination of antithrombin with factors Xa, IXa, and XIa. Factor Xa is inactivated by a much lower concentration of heparin than is required to inactivate thrombin. This explains why low dose heparin, although without influence on the clotting time, can reduce postoperative venous thrombosis.

All coagulation tests are altered by heparin; however, the usual monitor of heparin function is the partial thromboplastin time. Heparin clearance is via the liver. An average dose has a half-life of approximately two hours and is cleared from the blood, excreted in the urine, by six hours.

Heparin is commonly indicated in the management of questionable anastomoses, injured vessels, or distal flow impairment due to trauma, ischemia, or coagulation. It may be administered intravenously as a continuous monitored infusion or by intermittent injections. Complications include hemorrhage, thrombocytopenia, and (occasionally) allergy and osteoporosis.

Dextran

Dextran is a polysaccharide unit of approximately 450 glucose molecules, about the same molecular weight as albumin. While it was being investigated as a plasma substituting agent, it was found to induce hemorrhage and have a thromboprophylactic property.

Dextran has an effect on a number of physiologic systems:

1. It has a colloid osmotic effect. Dextran binds more water per gram than does albumin. The water is not available in the

circulatory system and is absorbed from the extracellular fluid, and in this way expands the plasma volume.

2. Blood flow improvement is attributed to
   a. An effect on red cell aggregation.
   b. Hemodilution.
   c. Passive capillary dilatation as a result of the colloid osmotic pressure.

Dextran infusion does not alter the number of platelets, but platelet adhesiveness to foreign surfaces decreases. Dextran adheres to the platelet surface and the negative charge of the platelets increases. Both properties are believed capable of reducing platelet adhesiveness.

Factor VIII is the only coagulation factor affected by dextran, its level falling considerably more than can be explained by hemodilution. Other effects of dextran on the fibrin system and plasminogen system are controversial.

Possible complications of the use of dextran are cardiac overload, hemorrhage, anaphylactoid reactions, and renal damage.

Fibrinolytic Substances

As yet, no clinical series have been published on the use of fibrinolytic substances such as streptokinase and urokinase in microvascular surgery. These substances convert plasminogen to plasmin, which leads to clot lysis.

Jelalian and associates (1985) reported the use of continuous, low dose, intraarterial streptokinase in the treatment of six patients with ischemia of the hand secondary to distal arterial occlusion. Following an initial bolus of 100,000 units of streptokinase, 5000 units per hour were infused and titrated against the patient's coagulation profile. Perfusion continued for 16 to 96 hours and was successful in achieving recanalization in four of the six patients.

The disadvantages of fibrinolytic agents relate to their efficacy in lysis of the clot. Internal or external hemorrhage can result if there are any vessel wounds sealed by thrombus. In the clinical situation in which a failing flap can be locally perfused through its feeding artery and the venous drainage discarded, the use of such agents is justified and has been effective.

Activation of the fibrinolytic system may be impaired after prolonged ischemia, a factor that may contribute to the no-reflow phenomenon (May and associates, 1978). Puckett, Misholy, and Reinisch (1983) studied the effect of streptokinase on the survival of ischemic rat island flaps, and found a moderate but statistically significant improvement.

Topical Heparin

Sinclair (1980) drew attention to the topical use of heparin. In a rat model he found that free flaps based on small vessels (superficial epigastric) consistently failed when saline only was used to irrigate the open ends of the repaired vessels, whereas 80 per cent of identical flaps survived when heparinized saline was instilled.

Heparin binds to the endothelium, probably at the intercellular cement lines, and has a half-life on the cell of perhaps five hours (Glimelius, Busch, and Hook, 1978). Heparin concentrations on the endothelium rise well above that in the circulating blood, and this may prevent platelet adherence and the initiation of thrombosis.

Topical heparin should be used and, when possible, applied immediately after the vessels are divided. It should be continued frequently throughout microvascular procedures, since endothelial saturation with heparin requires more than two hours.

GENERAL ASPECTS OF FREE FLAP TRANSFERS

A microvascular free flap is defined as the transfer in a single operation of a composite segment of skin and subcutaneous tissue to a distant site, using microvascular surgery. This one-stage transfer is made possible by the anastomosis of usually a single artery and vein in the flap to an artery and vein at the recipient site. In appropriate circumstances other tissues such as bone, nerve, muscle, or tendon can be included to form a compound flap.

The first experimental flaps transferred to a distant site by microvascular anastomoses were in dogs and were reported by Goldwyn, Lamb, and White (1963). Three of their five flaps survived, and these for 48 hours only, but they pointed to the feasibility of the survival of flaps based on an anastomosed artery and vein. The first long-term successful experimental free flaps were transferred from the groin in dogs and made use of small vascular cuffs from the femoral vessels without the need for microvascular anastomoses (Krizek and associates, 1965). Strauch and Murray (1967), using microvascular anastomoses for vessels approximately 1 mm in diameter, transferred skin flaps in rats from the groin to the neck. They achieved an overall survival rate of 61 per cent in a transfer of 33 groin flaps. Fujino, Harashina, and Mikata (1972) obtained a 59 per cent survival in transferring 12 groin flaps in dogs, using a microvascular stapler for the vascular anastomoses. O'Brien and Shanmugan (1973) reported 100 per cent survival of 27 groin flaps in rabbits, using microvascular anastomoses on femoral vessels approximately 1 mm in diameter. Pigs have also been used for the transfer of microvascular flaps and an 80 per cent survival of 15 groin flaps, somewhat larger vessels being used, was reported (Daniel and Williams, 1973).

Concurrent with the developments in microsurgical experimental technique and instrumentation was the new clinical emphasis on cutaneous vascularization. At the same time there was the development of the concept of axial pattern flaps. The deltopectoral flap (Bakamjiam, 1965) and the groin flap (McGregor and Jackson, 1972; Smith and associates, 1972) particularly paved the way for the one-stage transfer by microvascular anastomosis of skin flaps.

Antia and Buch (1971) reported the transfer, done several years previously, of a free vascularized buried dermolipomatous graft to the face for a contour defect. The abdominal skin and fat were vascularized on the superficial epigastric system and a cuff of femoral artery and saphenous vein were included; 7.0 silk was used for the repair and "brisk bleeding was noted from the cut edges of the flap following release of the clamps." Edema persisted for several weeks followed by oily discharge, but the wound healed by six weeks although there had been considerable resorption of volume.

Kaplan, Buncke, and Murray (1973) reported a microvascular free groin flap based on the superficial circumflex iliac artery transferred to the floor of the mouth. It was raised as an island initially and delayed for 72 hours before transfer. The flap was vascularized and remained viable until the patient's discharge from the hospital. Three weeks postoperatively the flap became necrotic. The area had been irradiated and healing was insecure.

In 1971 Harii and Ohmori (1973) raised a tube pedicle on the left lower abdomen incorporating the superficial epigastric artery in its lower end. After ten days the tube was divided at its lower end and the artery of the tube pedicle anastomosed microsurgically to the gastroepiploic vessels, which had been transposed extra-abdominally. Ten days later the tube pedicle was disconnected from its other abdominal attachment and spread over the right chest wall after excision of an irradiated section of chest wall.

McLean and Buncke (1972) transferred the omentum by microvascular techniques to resurface a scalp in 1970.

The first completely successful microvascular skin flap reported was by Daniel and Taylor (1973), who used a groin flap based on the superficial epigastric vessels and transferred to the ankle. Harii, Ohmori, and Ohmori (1974a) had in fact transplanted free scalp flaps as early as 1972. Other single case reports followed (O'Brien and associates, 1973; Don-Yoa, 1973). Soon several centers reported a series of free flap transfers (Harii, Ohmori, and Ohmori, 1974b; O'Brien and associates, 1974; Ikuta and associates, 1975; Baudet, Guimberteau, and Nascimento, 1976).

May and associates (1978) studied the no-reflow phenomenon following reconstitution of blood flow in free epigastric flaps in the rabbit. Microscopic, histologic, angiographic, and hematologic studies demonstrated the progressive nature of the obstruction to the peripheral blood flow after increasing periods of ischemia. The obstruction reached the point of irreversibility after 12 hours of ischemia. The study suggested that the no-reflow phenomenon was caused by cellular swelling, intravascular aggregation, and the leakage of intravascular fluid into the interstitial space. Chait and associates (1978) studied the effects of perfusion of several fluids on the free epigastric flap of the rabbit after normothermic ischemic periods of eight or 12 hours. The perfusions were carried out either after or before the ischemic periods. Although the three perfusion fluids studied were shown to penetrate to all levels of a flap after such ischemic periods, none of them had a beneficial effect on skin survival. However, the solution containing mannitol did have a protective effect on fat survival.

To date, the exact mechanism of the no-reflow phenomenon remains unclear. Work in several centers has implicated reperfusion injury due to the production of oxygen-free radicals (Parks, Bulkley, and Granger, 1983; Korthuis and associates, 1985) as one potential mechanism. These highly reactive molecules are produced in large amounts after significant ischemic periods and lead to subsequent damage to the microvascular system. Manson and associates (1986) showed increased survival of free skin transfers in rats after ischemic periods by perfusion with free radical scavengers before reestablishment of flow.

Black and associates (1978) developed a microvascular free flap in pigs and ligated the supplying vessels at varying intervals after transfer in order to study the effect of revascularization from the recipient bed. At eight days or later following transfer, survival routinely occurred. Earlier than eight days, although necrosis was not inevitable, the results were unpredictable.

Donski and associates (1980) studied cooling in the epigastric flap in the rabbit and reported that cooling to 6° to 7°C significantly increases ischemic tissue survival to 48 hours and probably 72 hours. Inflammatory changes developed in direct proportion to the duration of the cold ischemia time, while vessels within the flap appeared to be minimally affected by cold ischemia. However, fat and muscle demonstrated significant areas of necrosis.

Gould and associates (1985) perfused Ross solution into inferior epigastric free flaps in rabbits before cold storage for periods ranging from three to five days, and found that the perfusion was deleterious. It is significant that more flap necrosis occurred than in a control group of cooled flaps in which no perfusion was used. Late perfusion of similar flaps performed after the period of cooling was not deleterious to flap survival when compared with cold storage alone. These findings suggested that perfusion would not be indicated either before or after the cooling phase in free flap transfers.

Das and O'Brien (1982, 1983) investigated the survival of microvascular skin flap allografts in rabbits. With the administration of steroid perfusion of the flap and parenteral steroid to the recipient, flap survival could be prolonged for as long as 100 days, compared with the control survival of approximately 11 days.

Knight and associates (1985) studied the pharmacologic modification of blood flow in the rabbit microvasculature with prostacyclin and related drugs. They used the rabbit inferior epigastric free flap and concluded that the vasodilatory properties of prostacyclin and carbacyclin, together with their known platelet antiaggregatory properties, caused an increase in blood flow, with a maximal twofold increase. The use of thromboxane synthetase inhibitors had no demonstrable effect on normal flap blood flow.

Indications

The simplest procedure that provides adequate esthetic coverage of a defect is the wisest approach. Skin grafts or local flaps that are simpler and require less time with less risk to the patient should always take precedence. Only if these are not possible should the surgeon consider flaps from a distance. Each surgeon develops his own indications for the use of microvascular free flaps and these indications are influenced by training and unit organization. In some circumstances the microvascular flap is the only method of treatment, but in others conventional methods ultimately achieve a similar result. However, as a surgeon gains facility with the use of the microvascular flaps, his application of them is likely to increase. Increased technical sophistication and the multiplicity of donor flaps currently available allow transfer of specific tissue qualities to achieve a functional and esthetic result as well as the most favorable secondary defect. In many circumstances, therefore, free tissue transfer is the preferred method of treatment, even though conventional local or distant flaps are available.

Advantages

The free transfer of a full-thickness flap of skin and subcutaneous tissue to cover a defect has great advantages.

One-Stage Procedure. In contrast, cross-leg, abdominal flaps, and distant pedicle flaps require two, three, or more procedures, more hospitalization, and greater expense. It must be remembered that distant flaps have an established morbidity rate. Difficult bone, tendon, or nerve surgery may be performed primarily under a free flap in which the defect is closed at the same operation. Large traumatic defects resulting in exposure of bone, tendon, or joints can also be closed primarily by free flap transfer, permitting salvage of the underlying tissues.

Failure of a free flap may not be disastrous. In a significant percentage of such cases healing can be achieved by split-thickness skin grafts, since the deepest layers of the flap can survive to receive such a graft (Khoo and Bailey, 1982).

Variety of Donor Tissues. With the myriad of free tissue transfers now available, it is possible to be highly selective in terms of flap size, texture, thickness, color, innervation, finger-printed or hair-bearing skin, or compound tissue transfers involving skin and bone, tendon, or muscle.

Size. Many conventional flaps, either local or distant, are limited in size of available tissue. Free transfers allow massive amounts of tissue to be transferred in one stage.

Cosmetically Acceptable Donor Defects. Microvascular free flaps can often be taken from inconspicuous areas, such as the groin, where primary closure is possible on nearly all occasions. Such a site is easily concealed and is more acceptable to the patient than the multiple scars caused by distant pedicle flaps or even by some local flaps. Some free flap donor sites such as the forehead, deltopectoral, and saphenous areas leave grafted sites that may be embarrassingly noticeable and are therefore rarely indicated.

Early Mobilization. Distant pedicle flaps often require immobilization of one or more extremities in a flexed position for a considerable time. These positions may be particularly disadvantageous or even impossible in older patients, or in patients with stiff joints or with concomitant fractures of the pelvis or lower extremities. Microvascular free flaps require only mild elevation if in the extremities and little, if any, immobilization.

Improved Vascularity of Flap. The microvascular free flap with its unique vasculature has a circulation that is more than adequate for its own needs and provides additional blood supply to the recipient area. The recipient vessels have often been peripherally divided or destroyed by trauma, burns, or irradiation. The anastomosis of their normal proximal segments to the vessels of the flap establishes satisfactory circulation to the flap and to the surrounding area. Wound healing is enhanced by the superior circulation. On the other hand, distant pedicle flaps provide a vascular input to the recipient area only so long as they remain attached to their donor site. After the pedicle is detached from its origin, the vascularity of the flap is dependent on vessels that grow through the surrounding circumferential scar.

Disadvantages

Lengthy Operations. Most microvascular free flaps require approximately three to eight hours of operating time. However, compared with the time required for the series of operations necessary for a distant pedicle flap, the difference in total operating time may be minimal. With experience and with simultaneous dissection of donor and recipient sites, operating time is reduced significantly. Thin flaps can be elevated and transferred, inset, and anastomosed with greater speed than thick flaps from obese individuals. Generally, flaps to the head and neck, and to a lesser extent the upper limb, can be performed more quickly than flaps to the lower limb because of the greater number, greater accessibility, and lack of spasm of the recipient vessels.

Lack of Availability of Recipient Vessel. The distal areas of the extremities are sites that frequently require flap coverage. Fortunately the dual arterial supply to the hand and foot is such that the loss of a major artery is easily tolerated. On occasion, no recipient vessel is available owing to the nature of the original injuries, and this may preclude the use of microvascular free flaps. The only major vessel in the area may be vital to the supply of the hand or the foot. A reasonably sized branch may be available for anastomosis, otherwise a conventional flap is preferable. End to side anastomosis to the remaining artery is a possibility, but such a step introduces a major risk that would not be acceptable unless there was no alternative. In such circumstances, conventional transfers may be streamlined by temporary microvascular attachment of the free flap to a carrier such as the wrist or opposite leg. In this way the flap can be immediately inset into the defect, thus eliminating one stage of the conventional pedicle transfer (Morrison and Pribaz, 1980). Advanced age is a contraindication only if the recipient or donor site vessels are involved with degenerative disease. The state of both recipient and donor vessels can often be assessed only during dissection. Atheroma in limb vessels is a sinister finding at an anastomotic site, but the patchy nature of the degeneration may allow the anastomosis to be sited in a normal segment. In head and neck surgery, however, it appears to have little influence on patency.

In the head and neck the blood supply is such that the sacrifice of almost any recipient microvessel (1 to 3 mm in diameter) is entirely safe. The trunk is likewise supplied generously with multiple small vessels in such a way that the loss of any single microvessel is well tolerated.

Vascular Thrombosis. Even with maximal expertise, care, and preoperative planning, a certain risk factor remains with microvascular transfers. Most vascular complications are directly related to inadequate planning or technique and are reduced by the use of the largest vessels possible. The nature of the recipient vessels is the area of greatest concern. Despite all precautions, however, a certain caprice remains as to vascular patency and a definite risk factor must be accepted with free tissue transfers.

Preoperative Evaluation

When the merits of a microvascular free flap coverage for a particular defect are being evaluated, consideration is given to both the recipient site and the donor area.

Recipient Site. When presented with an acute wound that requires a distant flap, the reconstructive surgeon should not overlook the possibility of primary free flap coverage. Although it would be injudicious to attempt a primary microvascular coverage in most wounds, it would be equally unfortunate to miss an opportunity for an appropriate one-stage primary repair, particularly for compound losses with exposed joints or tendons. A primary free flap taken from a nonreplantable amputated segment of tissue may offer a once only opportunity to resurface the residual defect with uniquely suitable tissue. This is particularly applicable in lower limb amputations where the dorsal foot or sole can be used to cover below knee stumps and possibly avoid above knee amputation. The condition of some wounds is optimal at the first operation, and primary coverage with a well-vascularized flap may offer the best chance of maximal salvage and preservation of function.

A more conservative approach, and usually the correct one, is to prepare the wound for delayed primary or secondary coverage. Every effort should be made first to eliminate as much necrotic and infected tissue as possible. Temporary coverage with split-thickness skin graft may be necessary. A well-vascularized microvascular free flap is relatively resistant to infection and can perform a considerable amount of biologic debridement. This conservative approach usually provides the optimal conditions for a free flap transfer.

Recipient vessels of an appropriate size must be available close to the margins of the defect. Large defects, particularly on the extremities, often interrupt the course of an appropriate vessel, the free end of which can be found in or near the edge of the defect. Use can often be made of a long vascular pedicle either on the microvascular flap itself or from nearby recipient vessels, or from a combination of both. Otherwise, the gap between recipient and donor vessels must be bridged by a vein graft so that the vascular repairs are sited well away from the zone of injury. Normal skin surrounding the recipient defect may occasionally need to be excised or elevated in order to approximate the recipient and donor vessels. In these circumstances the defect must be made to fit the flap. The placement of arterial and venous repairs on opposite sides of the flap may sometimes be helpful. If the original injury has interrupted the course of a significant vessel, it may be possible to reconstitute the vessel by use of the flap artery. If a flap is nourished from side branches of a vessel, e.g., the dorsalis pedis artery flap or the fibula bone on the peroneal vessels, the proximal and distal ends of the flap vessel can be anastomosed to each end of the limb vessel. Alternatively, a branch of the vessel to a flap can be used as the outflow path to join to the distal vessel of the limb. By restoration of the runoff, the vascular anastomosis is theoretically protected from thrombosis because of increased flow across it.

Insetting a flap upside down frequently facilitates the vascular repair by improving access and siting the anastomoses away from the zone of injury.

Spasm in the lower limb vessels is the rule after dissection and can frequently be intense. It is impossible to assess the normality of a vessel because of the absence of forward flow predisposing to anastomotic thrombosis or to mistaken use of damaged vessels. Prolonged flap ischemia risks the no-reflow phenomenon.

The aim in free tissue transfer is to use as large a vessel as possible both at the recipient and donor sites. The vascular repair must be in a site situated well away from injury zones and should avoid atheromatous vessels.

The recipient vessels (arteries and veins) must always be resected back to normal tissue. In the coverage of areas of irradiation damage, a long vascular pedicle helps to avoid the use of irradiated vessels. A precise chart of an irradiated area must be obtained from the radiotherapist before surgery; two flaps in the authors' series have been lost because of inaccurate information. Irradiated vessels are not suitable for microvascular surgery (Tan, O'Brien, and Brennen, 1978).

Arteriography of donor or recipient vessels is rarely required. In most cases not only is it unreliable and unnecessary, but there is considerable debate as to whether contrast dye damages microvascular endothelium (Branemark, Jacobsson, and Sorensen, 1969; Franklin and associates, 1979; May, Athanasoulis, and Donelan, 1979; Yaremchuk and associates, 1981; Sheppard and Dell, 1983). Recipient vessels, with normal arteriography, were found to be abnormal on exploration (Sharzer and associates, 1975) and vice versa. Frequently, insufficient definition of peripheral vessels is obtained by routine angiography and a femoral puncture may render the groin area, for example, unsuitable as a donor site. An angiogram demonstrating a patent vessel does not indicate whether it is *microsurgically normal.* Clinical examination, with palpation of the respective pulses for forward and reverse flow, combined with a knowledge of the original pathology and the nature of the wound, usually provides an accurate preoperative assessment of the circulation. Doppler flow probing may help, but only surgery finally reveals the precise state of the recipient vessels. Venography may be more relevant than arteriography, particularly in the lower limb following trauma, where clinical assessment of the venous state may be impossible. It should be emphasized that a sclerosed vein unsuitable for microsurgical repair may appear patent on the venogram.

Digital subtraction angiography offers a noninvasive alternative that shows the promise of being simple, practical, and reliable and is nonpainful and noninjurious to vessels.

Clinical evaluation of the pulses and a detailed knowledge of the anatomy of the area remain the key factors in evaluating and locating suitable recipient vessels.

In the head and neck region, the trunk, and the proximal portion of the limbs, sufficient recipient vessels are usually available to allow end to end vascular repair immediately adjacent to the site of the flap.

For tissue transfers to the hand and digits, the radial artery and cephalic vein in the anatomic snuffbox region are the favored recipient vessels. Flaps to the hand are frequently from the foot, from which a long dorsalis pedis artery pedicle can be obtained to run directly to the snuffbox when end to side arterial anastomosis is preferred.

In the lower limb considerable difficulty can arise in locating adequate recipient vessels situated away from the site of previous trauma. In the upper and middle thirds of the lower leg, the major arteries are inaccessible from the anterior aspect and may themselves be damaged. Vein grafts anastomosed end to side to the femoral artery above the knee can overcome the difficulty; however, they prolong the procedure and introduce the added intrinsic problems of vein grafts. The flap pedicle may be passed through the interosseous membrane for anastomosis to recipient vessels in the popliteal fossa, but this maneuver necessitates turning the patient. Alternatively, a first-stage fistula can be created by anastomosing a long saphenous vein graft proximally to the side of the femoral artery above the knee and running the graft distally to the proximal limit of the defect, where it is passed back and anastomosed end to end to the long saphenous vein. At the time of flap transfer approximately one week later, the fistula is divided at the apex of the loop, thereby making available a large diameter artery and vein directly at the proximal site of the recipient defect (Threlfall, Little, and Cummine, 1982).

In the middle to lower thirds of the lower limb the flap may be joined to the anterior tibial vessels if these are not traumatized, or it may be reversed in order that the anastomosis is situated distal in the leg. In this situation the artery of the flap may be anastomosed end to side to the posterior tibial or end to end to the anterior tibial or dorsalis pedis artery, which is divided distal to the flap and passed backward. The flap may even be vascularized by retrograde flow from the divided dorsalis pedis artery. When the flap is reversed in such a manner, however, the vein must also be anastomosed distally in the leg, and patent recipient veins at this level must be confirmed before anastomosis. Generally the deep venous system is more reliably patent than the superficial system in the traumatized leg.

Flaps to the heel area can usually be vascularized via an end to side anastomosis to the posterior tibial artery and end to end to the venae comitantes system at the medial malleolar level, while flaps to the dorsum of the foot allow easy access to the terminal portion of the anterior tibial artery and its venae comitantes or to the long saphenous vein.

The size of the recipient defect should equal the exact size of the donor flap. Allowance should be made for flaps passing around convex surfaces. The donor flap should not be detached from its vascular pedicle until the recipient site dissection is completed and the recipient vessel ends have been prepared and are ready for immediate anastomosis.

Donor Site. An ideal donor flap should be of adequate size (with dependable constant axial vessels of good length and diameter), should create a mild secondary defect, and should possess esthetic and functional qualities appropriate to the defect it is replacing. If an area has contact with other axial pattern systems, extensive enlargement of the free flap is possible.

A vast array of donor flaps, both cutaneous and compound, have now been developed. From the head and neck region, scalp, forehead, nasolabial, postauricular, cervical, and facial flaps are available. From the trunk the deltopectoral, lateral thoracic (both cutaneous and myocutaneous), intercostal, scapular and parascapular, epigastric (on both superficial and deep vessels), and groin flaps can be raised. The upper limb provides the deltoid flap, the medial upper arm flap on the ulnar collateral artery, the lateral upper arm flap on the radial collateral artery, the cubital flap, the radial and ulnar artery forearm flaps, and segmental transfers of digital skin. In the lower limb, the buttock flaps on the superior and inferior gluteal vessels; the gracilis and tensor fascia lata myocutaneous flaps; the anterior, medial, lateral, and posterior thigh flaps; the saphenous and dorsal foot flaps; and the first web space flaps and toe pulps, as well as the midsole fasciocutaneous flaps, can be transferred.

Compound skin and bone can be obtained from the groin with the underlying iliac crest, from the dorsal foot with its second metatarsal bone, from the forearm with the radius and ulna, from the lateral arm skin with the humerus, and from the fibula or rib with overlying skin. Skin and tendon can be obtained from the dorsal foot with the extensor hallucis brevis or longus, or from the forearm radial or ulnar artery flaps with the palmaris longus or extensor carpi ulnaris.

Despite the large number of flaps available, the groin flap and the myocutaneous lateral thoracic flap remain the most popular. Both have a reliable anatomic pattern. The lateral thoracic flap is simpler to dissect and has long pedicle vessels of larger diameter. Its disadvantages are that it is bulky and the secondary defect may be difficult to camouflage. The groin flap has smaller vessels of shorter length and variable anatomy and the dissection is more difficult, although the secondary defect is by far the most acceptable of all flaps described.

In deciding which donor flap to use, consideration should also be given to the required positioning of the patient so that simultaneous recipient and donor dissections can be performed to streamline the operation. There is no flap ideal for all circumstances and the surgeon should choose the most appropriate of the many flaps available for the particular patient.

Technique

Donor Site Dissection. Details of donor site anatomy, dissection, and the specific advantages and disadvantages are discussed elsewhere (see Chaps. 9, 10, 11, 18, 76, 79, 82).

Recipient Site Dissection. The recipient site is prepared simultaneously with the donor flap dissection by a second surgical team. The recipient dissection should not be an exploratory procedure but should be conducted strictly according to preoperative planning decisions, particularly with regard to the choice and location of the recipient vessels.

Atraumatic technique is vital, especially when the vessels of the lower limb are dissected, because of their marked propensity for spasm. This problem is aggravated by hypovolemia and anxiety. In microvascular transfers in which simultaneous dissection is performed in two separate areas, considerable blood loss and exposure results and every precaution must be made to replace blood volume. The operating room should be warmed or electric blankets should be applied to the patient, and adequate long-acting regional anesthetic blocks, which allay anxiety and produce sympathetic blockade, should be performed.

Vascular Repair. The venous repair should be made first to minimize blood loss and avoid engorgement of the flap. After the arterial repair has been performed, it is undesirable to clamp the arterial side because of the risk of thrombosis. Therefore, if the artery is anastomosed first, one has to accept bleeding from the edge of the flap during the venous repair. End to end repairs are preferred to end to side. However, once the technical expertise of end to side anastomosis is mastered, it is a safe form of repair and should be frequently considered for arterial anastomoses in the periphery of the limbs where limited vessels are available. The desirability of using as large a vessel as possible, both in the donor flap and the recipient site, has already been mentioned. This conversion of microvascular surgery to macrovascular surgery has greatly increased the reliability of free flap transfer. Flaps with long vascular pedicles, such as the latissimus dorsi myocutaneous flap, facilitate transfer and increase their reliability. Vein grafts should be used when necessary, but the intrinsic problems of two anastomoses, kinking, twisting, and the need to judge the correct length increase the risk of vascular problems. The problems of diameter discrepancy in anastomoses are discussed elsewhere.

Postoperative Management

Flaps should be exposed to allow maximal observation, and circumferential bandaging must be avoided because of the risk of postoperative swelling or hematoma causing compression of the vascular pedicle. Most microvascular free flaps exhibit some edema, owing to the ischemic period and to lymphatic obstruction, but mild elevation, if practical, helps to minimize this. No anticoagulant therapy is given, since the vessels are usually greater than 1.5 mm in diameter and troublesome bleeding, particularly from the donor site, may be induced.

Hourly observations of the flap for color, warmth, and capillary return are essential; this routine is followed for the first 24 hours, after which observations made every two or four hours are adequate. Most vascular complications occur within the first 24 hours, the great majority in fact immediately after the anastomosis, but it may be many hours before the problem becomes clinically recognizable. Arterial thrombosis has been observed as late as the tenth postoperative day.

Following revascularization, most free flaps are initially pinker than normal and have a more brisk capillary return. This usually subsides over the first 12 to 24 hours. However, transferred flaps are occasionally pale and difficult to interpret. This is particularly true of the groin flap. If the flap should develop arterial insufficiency, pallor, or sluggish capillary return, a drop in temperature and an empty feeling develop. The most reliable sign of adequate arterial supply is bright red bleeding from the flap edge. If this cannot be elicited by rubbing with dry gauze or by stabbing the flap with a needle, arterial insufficiency is certain. If venous obstruction occurs, cyanosis, rapid capillary return, and a full tense feeling in the flap are noticed. Following venous obstruction there may initially be excessive bleeding of a dark color from the flap margins, but this eventually ceases. As most vascular problems stem directly from an intraoperative fault, it is good policy to observe the patient for a considerable period in the recovery room before he is allowed to return to the ward. It is usually during this period that the earliest signs of vascular insufficiency occur.

Machine Monitoring. Monitoring of flaps by Doppler recordings over the vascular pedicle can be particularly valuable in doubtful cases or in patients with buried flaps.

Temperature probes are probably the simplest objective method of monitoring flaps and are particularly valuable for inexperienced nursing staff.

Results

Shaw (1984) collated the results of 2233 flaps pooled from multiple microsurgery centers around the world. The overall success rate was 93 per cent; 10 per cent required reexploration and 40 per cent of these were salvaged. No correlation was made between success and type of donor flap or recipient site. The wide variance of numbers and variety of donor flaps and recipient sites reflect the type of surgery done at each center as much as individual preferences.

At St. Vincent's Hospital, Melbourne, from 1973 until December 1983, 295 flaps were transferred. The great majority (102) were from the groin. The latter has remained the flap of choice when simple skin cover is required to achieve esthetic reconstruction with minimal donor morbidity. The latissimus dorsi flap has increased in popularity, having the special attraction of a long, large-diameter vascular pedicle; it is rapid and simple to raise and safe to transfer. However, it is considerably more bulky than the groin and the secondary defect is less acceptable. The donor flaps used, and their frequency of survival, are listed in Table 12–1. One hundred and eight of these flaps were composite transfers (Table 12–2).

Recipient sites for these free flaps have been in all areas of the body. The predominant site has been in the upper limb, reflecting the bias of the authors' unit to upper limb and hand surgery.

Survival overall in this series has been 89 per cent (Table 12–3). Various factors suggest that survival is related more to the recipient site than to the donor flap chosen (Table 12–4), although the groin flap, because of its small vessels, must be considered less safe than larger vessel flaps.

The time taken for free flap transfer has varied considerably, depending on the type of transfer and the associated surgery required. With two teams operating, transfer times have ranged from three hours to longer than 12 hours. For simple cutaneous flaps, particularly to the head and neck, the average operating time would be expected to be four hours or less. Ischemia times for the flaps have ranged considerably, but should be less than one hour if the operation proceeds according to plan and the recipient site is fully prepared, including the vessels, before the donor flap is detached.

The survival rate in patients over 50 years of age has been distinctly lower than in younger patients.

Secondary flap revision has often been required after free tissue transfer. This usually involves thinning of the subcutaneous tissues and revision of the scar margins with Z-plasties. Although free flap transfers are frequently purported to enable multistaged procedures to be avoided, the absence of a thin donor flap from a cosmetically acceptable site usually means that a second-stage thinning procedure is required. The latissimus dorsi

Table 12–1. Breakdown of Free Flap Transfers at St Vincent's Hospital, Melbourne

Donor Sites	No.	Total and Partial Survival	%
Groin	102	85	84
Forehead	2	2	100
Deltopectoral	1	1	100
Dorsum of foot	30	28	93
Toes and first web	40	37	92
Latissimus dorsi	25	23	92
Tensor fascia lata	6	5	83
Myocutaneous gracilis	11	11	100
Scapular	5	5	100
Parascapular	4	4	100
Sole foot	3	3	100
Instep flap	5	5	100
Scalp	7	6	100
Deltoid	1	1	100
Radial artery	9	8	88
Osteocutaneous fibula	5	3	60
Ulnar artery	5	5	100
Lateral arm	7	7	100
Rectus abdominis	19	19	100
Free foot flaps	8	7	87
TOTAL	295	265	89

Table 12–2. Breakdown of Free Flap Composite Transfers at St Vincent's Hospital, Melbourne

Composite Free Flaps	
Groin and iliac bone	21
Dorsum of foot and second metatarsal	10
Dorsum of foot and extensor tendon	4
Myocutaneous latissimus dorsi	17
Myocutaneous tensor fascia lata	6
Myocutaneous gracilis	6
Myocutaneous rectus abdominis	10
Neurovascular (foot to hand)	30
Osteocutaneous fibula	2
Osteocutaneous radial artery	2
TOTAL	108

Table 12–3. Results of Free Flap Transfers at St Vincent's Hospital, Melbourne, March, 1973

Cases	283
Flaps	295
Flap survival	265 (89%)
Flap necrosis	30 (11%)

Table 12–4. Free Flap Failures at St Vincent's Hospital, Melbourne

Recipient Site		Donor Site
Head and neck	5:1	groin
	2	dorsalis pedis (foot)
	1	scalp
	1	radial artery
Trunk	4:	groin
Upper limb	8:4	groin
	2	wrap-around
	1	first web foot
	1	osteocutaneous fibula
Lower limb	13:9	groin
	2	latissimus dorsi
	1	tensor fascia lata
	1	osteocutaneous fibula
TOTAL	30	

flap particularly requires secondary thinning despite some degree of spontaneous muscle atrophy.

Complications

Complications of free flap surgery may be general or local.

General complications are those of prolonged surgery: anesthesia, positional problems such as neuropraxia, deep venous thrombosis, and postoperative respiratory difficulties. Three cases of pulmonary emboli have been encountered in the authors' series and this complication resulted in one death, seven days postoperatively, in an elderly patient with inoperable carcinoma. Another death occurred following groin flap transfer to a mutilated limb after a gunshot wound. The patient developed pulmonary edema on the third postoperative day for a reason that remained obscure, even at postmortem examination. The incidence of complications that could be related to prolonged anesthesia in this series, as well as over 400 cases of replantation involving similar anesthetic times, has been remarkably low. Local nerve blocks are used when possible to minimize the extent of general anesthesia, and a urinary catheter is inserted preoperatively to avoid patient restlessness.

Local complications of the flap transfer relate mainly to vascular problems. Infection is rare. Most problems with vascular patency stem from the failure to join normal vessel to normal vessel.

As discussed under Preoperative Evaluation, vascular anastomoses should be situated away from the zone of injury, irradiation, and atheromatous damage. Technical problems of anastomosis are always a factor influencing patency, and meticulous microvascular technique is essential. Size discrepancy and the intrinsic problems of vein grafts are discussed elsewhere. In this series, arterial thrombosis has been by far the most common complication. Vascular complications in general have been more frequent in the lower limb. Compression from tight skin closure, compressive bandaging, hematoma formation, or vessels kinking across adjacent anatomic structures may lead to vascular compromise. In the St. Vincent's Hospital series, 62 flaps developed vascular complications of which 41 (66 per cent) were arterial thrombosis and 14 (23 per cent) were venous in location. Combined arterial and venous thrombosis occurred in seven flaps (11 per cent). Analysis of the causes of the vascular complications is outlined in Table 12–5. Fifteen per cent of cases developed nonthrombotic complications and these included arterial spasm, hematoma, infection, flap tension, and no-reflow. At the first sign of vascular compromise, the flap should be checked for the possibility of

Table 12–5. Microvascular Free Flap: Complications at St Vincent's Hospital, Melbourne

Arterial Thrombosis			41
Recipient artery disease		20	
Trauma	10		
Atherosclerosis	8		
Irradiation	2		
Compression or kinking of artery		4	
Inadequate artery to flap		4	
Technical error		5	
Anesthetic		2	
Donor artery disease (spasm)		6	
Venous Thrombosis			14
Kinking		6	
Technical error		1	
Abnormal vein		5	
2° to arterial thrombosis		2	
Arterial and Venous Thrombosis			7
Trauma		2	
Pharmacologic		2	
Technical		2	
Irradiation		1	
TOTAL			62

compression from bandages, tight sutures, or hematoma, and the limb should be elevated or made dependent, according to whether the diagnosis is venous or arterial obstruction, respectively. Surgical reexploration is mandatory as soon as possible and anastomotic revision, which may necessitate grafting, is always worthwhile. Partial flap necrosis may occur as a result of a prolonged period of ischemia. Despite flap necrosis, sufficient deep tissue may survive to allow closure of the original defect by a more simple method, such as skin grafting (Khoo and Bailey, 1982). If a portion of the flap fails to vascularize immediately following arterial anastomosis, one may suspect that the flap has been raised over an area not supplied by the donor vessels. This may represent an error in technique or a vascular anomaly. The authors have encountered two cases of groin flap dissection in which the superficial circumflex iliac artery failed to vascularize the standard groin flap distribution.

Secondary Defects

By and large the secondary defects resulting from free flap transfer do not constitute a significant long term problem (Colen, Shaw, and McCarthy, 1986). The groin flap leaves by far the most satisfactory secondary defect from the point of view of cosmetic appearance. No matter what the size of the flap, almost all groin defects can be closed in a linear fashion by flexion of the hip. The scar, however, may stretch significantly and extend above the bikini line. Dissection of the groin flap involves considerable interference with the major lymphatic channels in the groin, and two cases of mild lymphedema following groin flap elevation have been observed in the authors' series. The dissection of the groin flap on the deep vessels, including the iliac crest, requires meticulous closure of the muscle layers to avoid hernia formation, and the authors have encountered a significant hernia in one case. Paresthesia in the distribution of the lateral cutaneous nerve of the thigh is particularly debilitating and there is little excuse for this to occur, since both the superficial and deep vessels routinely pass superficially to the nerve.

The dorsalis pedis flap potentially has a high donor site complication rate because of poor skin graft take and the possibility of exposure of the extensor tendons. Healing may be delayed as a result, but despite this long-term morbidity is unusual. If the flap is elevated distally in the foot, just proximal to the web space, a hyperkeratotic lymphedematous-type thickening frequently occurs distal to the graft. The more proximal the flap is elevated from the foot, the better is the secondary defect. Web space and toe pulp defects can result in contractures and may require secondary release with skin grafting or Z-plasty. Latissimus dorsi flaps leave surprisingly little functional disability, but the scar commonly stretches and often causes an indentation as a result of the inability to reconstitute the underlying muscle layer.

Rectus abdominis myocutaneous flaps create a very long scar and risk hernia formation, while radial artery flaps leave a significant cosmetic deformity and sacrifice a major vessel.

Whatever the donor site, meticulous attention to detail needs to be devoted to closure lest the whole raison d'être of the transfer, which is to improve the overall esthetics of the patient, is forgotten in the pursuit of the surgery on the recipient site.

Acknowledgement: The illustrations in this chapter have been reproduced from the authors' chapters in Barron, J. N., and Saad, M. N. (Eds.): Operative Reconstructive Plastic Surgery, 1980, and O'Brien, B. M., and Morrison, W. A.: Reconstructive Microsurgery, 1987, by permission of Churchill Livingstone, Edinburgh.

REFERENCES

Acland, R. D.: Signs of patency in small vessel anastomosis. Surgery, *72*:744, 1972.

Acland, R. D.: Photomicrography through the operating microscope. Plast. Reconstr. Surg., *60*:730, 1977.

Acland, R. D.: A flat-bodied needle for microvascular surgery. Plast. Reconstr. Surg., *61*:793, 1978.

Acland, R. D.: Microsurgery. A Practice Manual. St. Louis, C. V. Mosby Company, 1980.

Antia, N. H., and Buch, V. I.: Transfer of abdominal dermo-fat graft by direct anastomosis of blood vessels. Br. J. Plast. Surg., *24*:15, 1971.

Bakamjiam, V. Y.: A two stage method for pharyngoesophageal reconstruction with a primary pectoral skin flap. Plast. Reconstr. Surg., *36*:173, 1965.

Baudet, J., Guimberteau, J. C., and Nascimento, E.: Successful clinical transfer of two free thoracodorsal axillary flaps. Plast. Reconstr. Surg., *58*:680, 1976.

Baxter, T. J., O'Brien, B. M., Henderson, P. N., and Bennett, R. C.: The histopathology of small vessels following microvascular repair. Br. J. Surg., *59*:617, 1972.

Biemer, E.: Vein grafts in microvascular surgery. Br. J. Plast. Surg., *30*:197, 1977.

Black, M. J., Chait, L., O'Brien, B. M., Sykes, P. J., and Sharzer, L. A.: How soon may the axial vessels of a surviving free flap be safely ligated: a study in pigs. Br. J. Plast. Surg., *31*:295, 1978.

Blair, W. E., Pedersen, D. R., Joos, K., Green, E. R., and Bondi, D.: Microarteriorrhaphy: blood flow after wound healing. Microsurgery, *6*:116, 1985.

Bloch, E. H.: A quantitative study of the hemodynamics in the living microvascular system. Am. J. Anat., *110*:125, 1962.

Booyse, F. M., Osikowiez, G., and Quanfoot, A. J.: Effects of chronic oral consumption of nicotine on the rabbit aortic endothelium. Am. J. Pathol., *102*:229, 1981.

Branemark, P. I., Jacobsson, B., and Sorensen, S. E.: Microvascular effects of topically applied contrast media. Acta Radiol. [Diagn.], *8*:547, 1969.

Brennen, M. D., and O'Brien, B. M.: Patency rates in end to side anastomoses in the rabbit. Br. J. Plast. Surg., *32*:24, 1979.

Brinson, K., and Chakrabarti, B. K.: Effect of nicotine on rabbit blood platelet aggregation. Atherosclerosis, *20*:527, 1974.

Buncke, H. J., Jr., Alpert, B., and Shah, K. G.: Microvascular grafting. Clin. Plast. Surg., *5*:185, 1978.

Buncke, H. J., Jr., and McLean, D. H.: The advantage of a straight needle in microsurgery. Plast. Reconstr. Surg., *47*:602, 1971.

Buncke, H. J., Jr., and Murray, D. E.: Autogenous arterial interposition of grafts less than 1 mm in external diameter in rats. Transactions of the Sixth International Congress of Plastic and Reconstructive Surgery. London, Butterworths, 1971, p. 572.

Buncke, H. J., Jr., and Schulz, W. P.: Experimental digital amputation and reimplantation. Plast. Reconstr. Surg., *36*:62, 1965.

Buncke, H. J., Jr., and Schulz, W. P.: The suture repair of 1 mm vessels. *In* Donaghy, R. M. P., and Vasargil, M. G. (Eds.): Microvascular Surgery. St. Louis, C. V. Mosby Company, 1967, p. 24.

Cazenave, J. P., Kinlough-Rathbone, R., Packham, M. A., and Mustard, J. F.: The effect of acetylsalicylic acid and indomethacin on rabbit platelet adherence to collagen and the subendothelium in the presence of a low or high hematocrit. Thromb. Res., *13*:971, 1978.

Chait, L. A., May, J. W., Jr., O'Brien, B. M., and Hurley, J. V.: The effects of the perfusion of various solutions on the no-reflow phenomenon in experimental free flaps. Plast. Reconstr. Surg., *61*:421, 1978.

Chow, S. P., Huang, C. D., and Chan, C. W.: Microvascular anastomosis of arteries under tension. Br. J. Plast. Surg., *35*:82, 1982.

Cobbett, J.: Small vessel anastomosis. A comparison of suture techniques. Br. J. Plast. Surg., *20*:16, 1967.

Colen, L. B., Gonzales, F. P., and Buncke, H. J.: The relationship between the number of sutures and the strength of microvascular anastomoses. Plast. Reconstr. Surg., *64*:325, 1979.

Colen, S. R., Shaw, W. W., and McCarthy, J. G.: Review of the morbidity of 300 free-flap donor sites. Plast. Reconstr. Surg., *77*:948, 1986.

Curtis, L. M., Loftis, J. W., and Wissinger, H. A.: Objective signs of patency following microvascular arterial anastomoses: a controlled study. J. Hand Surg., *2*:22, 1977.

Daniel, R. K., and Taylor, G. I.: Distant transfer of an island flap by microvascular anastomoses. A clinical technique. Plast. Reconstr. Surg., *52*:111, 1973.

Daniel, R. K., and Williams, H. B.: The free transfer of skin flaps by microvascular anastomoses. An experimental study and a reappraisal. Plast. Reconstr. Surg., *52*:16, 1973.

Das, S. K., and O'Brien, B. M.: Fate of microvascular skin flap allograft in the rabbit. Am. Coll. Surg. Forum, *33*:567, 1982.

Das, S. K., and O'Brien, B. M.: Microvascular skin flap allografts in rabbits. *In* Williams, H. B. (Ed.): Transactions of the Eighth International Congress of Plastic and Reconstructive Surgery. Montreal, Canada, Eighth Int'l. Congress of Plastic Surgery, 1983, pp. 30–31.

Das, S. K., O'Brien, B. M., Browning, F. S., Nicholls, B. W., and Nightingale, G. M.: Segmental microvenous graft to artery. Br. J. Plast. Surg., *33*:365, 1980.

Davies, D. M.: A world survey of anticoagulation practice in clinical microvascular surgery. Br. J. Plast. Surg., *35*:96, 1982.

De La Pava, D., Nightingale, G. M., Shafiroff, B. B., and O'Brien, B. M.: Patency of anastomoses adjacent to the bifurcation of the rabbit femoral artery and a comparison with Y-shaped microarterial grafts. Br. J. Plast. Surg., *32*:158, 1979.

Dintenfass, L.: Blood viscosity factors and hyperviscosity: a noninvasive method for determination of tissue perfusion and cardiovascular status. J. Microsurg., *3*:185, 1982.

Don-Yoa, Y.: Editorial addendum. Plast. Reconstr. Surg., *52*:116, 1973.

Donaghy, R. M. P., and Yasargil, M. G.: Microvascular Surgery. St. Louis, C. V. Mosby Company, 1967.

Donski, P. K., Franklin, J. D., Hurley, J. V., and O'Brien, B. M.: The effects of cooling on experimental free flap survival. Br. J. Plast. Surg., *33*:353, 1980.

Eisenhardt, H. J., Hennecken, H., Klein, P. J., and Pichlmaier, H.: Experiences with different techniques of microvascular anastomosis. J. Microsurg., *1*:341, 1980.

Erol, O. O., and Spira, M.: New capillary bed formation with a surgically constructed arteriovenous fistula. Plast. Reconstr. Surg., *66*:109, 1980.

Evans, D. M., Weightman, B., and Deane, G.: A new suction-irrigation device: uses in microsurgery and plastic surgery. Br. J. Plast. Surg., *36*:273, 1983.

Fisher, B. S.: Microvascular surgical techniques in research with special reference to renal transplantation in the rat. Surgery, *58*:904, 1965.

Flatt, A. E.: Digital artery sympathectomy. J. Hand Surg., *5*:550, 1980.

Folklow, B., and Neil, E.: Circulation. Oxford, Oxford University Press, 1971.

Fossati, E., Harashina, T., and Fujino, T.: Reapplication of microvascular clamps after venous anastomosis: an experimental study. J. Microsurg., *3*:239, 1982.

Franklin, J. D., Withers, E. H., Madden, J. J., Jr., and Lynch, J. B.: Use of free dorsalis pedis flap in head and neck repairs. Plast. Reconstr. Surg., *63*:195, 1979.

Fujikawa, S., and O'Brien, B. M.: An experimental evaluation of microvenous grafts. Br. J. Plast. Surg., *28*:244, 1975.

Fujino, T., Harashina, T., and Mikata, A.: Autogenous en bloc transplantation of the mammary gland in dogs, using microsurgical technique. Plast. Reconstr. Surg., *50*:376, 1972.

Gifford, R. W., Jr., Hines, E. A., Jr., and Craig, W. M.: Sympathectomy for Raynaud's phenomenon. Follow up study of 70 women with Raynaud's phenomenon. Circulation, *17*:5, 1958.

Glimelius, B., Busch, C., and Hook, M.: Binding of

heparin on the surface of cultured human endothelial cells. Thromb. Res., *12*:773, 1978.

Goldwyn, R. M., Lamb, D. L., and White, W. L.: An experimental study of large island flaps in dogs. Plast. Reconstr. Surg., *31*:528, 1963.

Goodman, L. S., Gilman, A. G., and Gilman, A.: The Pharmacological Basis of Therapeutics. 6th Ed. New York, MacMillan, 1980.

Gould, J. S., Sully, L., O'Brien, B. M., Das, S. K., Knight, K. R., and Hurley, J. V.: The effects of combined cooling and perfusion on experimental free-flap survival in rabbits. Plast. Reconstr. Surg., *76*:104, 1985.

Guyton, A. C.: Textbook of Medical Physiology. 7th Ed. Philadelphia, W. B. Saunders Company, 1986.

Hamilton, R. B., and O'Brien, B. M.: An experimental study of microvascular patency using a continuous suture technique. Br. J. Plast. Surg., *32*:153, 1979.

Hamilton, S.: Presented at Sixth International Society of Reconstructive Microsurgery. Melbourne, February, 1981.

Harashina, T.: Site of reapplication of microvascular clamps. Plast. Reconstr. Surg., *58*:719, 1976.

Harashina, T.: Use of the untied suture in microvascular anastomoses. Plast. Reconstr. Surg., *59*:134, 1977.

Harashina, T.: Arterial allografts and heterografts in microvascular surgery. Br. J. Plast. Surg., *31*:6, 1978.

Harashina, T., Fujino, T., and Watanabe, S.: The intimal healing of microvascular anastomoses. Plast. Reconstr. Surg., *58*:608, 1976.

Harii, K., and Ohmori, S.: Use of the gastroepiploic vessels as recipient or donor vessels in the free transfer of composite flaps by microvascular anastomoses. Plast. Reconstr. Surg., *52*:541, 1973.

Harii, K., Ohmori, K., and Ohmori, S.: Hair transplantation with free scalp flaps. Plast. Reconstr. Surg., *53*:410, 1974a.

Harii, K., Ohmori, K., and Ohmori, S.: Free deltopectoral skin flaps. Br. J. Plast. Surg., *27*:231, 1974b.

Harris, G. D., Finseth, F., and Buncke, H. J.: Posterior-wall—first microvascular anastomotic technique. Br. J. Plast. Surg., *34*:47, 1981.

Hayhurst, J. W., and O'Brien, B. M.: An experimental study of microvascular technique, patency rates and related factors. Br. J. Plast. Surg., *28*:128, 1975.

Hendel, P. M., and Buncke, H. J.: Use of a tilted double clamp in microvascular anastomosis. J. Microsurg., *1*:470, 1980.

Henderson, P. N., O'Brien, B. M., and Parel, J. M.: An adjustable double microvascular clamp. Med. J. Aust., *1*:715, 1970.

Hladovec, J.: Endothelial injury by nicotine and its prevention. Experientia, *34*:1585, 1978.

Hoerenz, P.: The operating microscope. I. Optical principles, illumination systems, and support systems. J. Microsurg., *1*:364, 1980.

Hoerenz, P.: The operating microscope. V. Maintenance and cleaning. J. Microsurg., *2*:179, 1981.

Ikuta, Y., Watari, S., Kawamura, K., Shima, R., and Matsuishi, Y.: Free flap transfer by end-to-side arterial anastomosis. Br. J. Plast. Surg., *28*:1, 1975.

Jacobson, J. H., and Suarez, E. L.: Microsurgery in anastomosis of small vessels. Surg. Forum, *11*:243, 1960.

Jelalian, C., Mehrhof, A., Cohen, I. K., Richardson, J., and Merritt, W. H.: Streptokinase in the treatment of acute arterial occlusion of the hand. J. Hand Surg., *10*:534, 1985.

Johnson, P. C.: Hemodynamics. Annu. Rev. Physiol., *31*:331, 1969.

Jorgensen, L., Haerem, J. W., and Moe, N.: Platelet thrombosis and non-traumatic intimal injury in mouse aorta. Thromb. Diath. Haemorr., *29*:470, 1973.

Kaplan, E., Buncke, H. J., and Murray, D. E.: Distant transfer of cutaneous island flaps in humans by microvascular anastomoses. Plast. Reconstr. Surg., *52*:301, 1973.

Kelton, J. G., Hirsch, J., Carter, C. J., and Buchanan, M. R.: Thrombogenic effect of high-dose aspirin in rabbits. J. Clin. Invest., *62*:892, 1978.

Khoo, C. T., and Bailey, B. N.: The behaviour of free muscle and musculocutaneous flaps after early loss of axial blood supply. Br. J. Plast. Surg., *35*:43, 1982.

Kleinert, H. E., and Kasdan, M. L.: Anastomosis of digital vessels. J. Kentucky Med. Assoc., *63*:106, 1965.

Knight, K. R., Crabb, D. J., Niall, M., Martin, T. J., O'Brien, B. M., and Angus, J. A.: Pharmacological modification of blood flow in the rabbit microvasculature with prostacyclin and related drugs. Plast. Reconstr. Surg., *75*:692, 1985.

Korthuis, R. J., Granger, D. N., Townsley, M. I., and Taylor, A. E.: The role of oxygen-derived free radicals in ischemia-induced increases in canine skeletal muscle vascular permeability. Circ. Res., *57*:599, 1985.

Krizek, T. J., Tasaburo, T., Desprez, J. D., and Kiehn, C. L.: Experimental transplantation of composite grafts by microsurgical vascular anastomoses. Plast. Reconstr. Surg., *36*:538, 1965.

Kurze, T.: Micro technique in microneurological surgery. Clin. Neurosurg., *11*:128, 1964.

Lauritzen, C.: A new and easier way to anastomose microvessels. An experimental study in rats. Scand. J. Plast. Reconstr. Surg., *12*:291, 1978.

Lee, B. Y., Thoden, W. R., Brancato, R. F., Kavner, D., Shaw, W., and Madden, J. L.: Comparison of continuous and interrupted suture techniques in microvascular anastomoses. Surg. Gynecol. Obstet., *155*:353, 1982.

Lendvay, P. G.: Replacement of the amputated digit. Br. J. Plast. Surg., *26*:398, 1973.

Leonard, E. F.: The role of flow in thrombogenesis. Bull. N.Y. Acad. Med., *48*:273, 1972.

Leriche, R., Fontaine, R., and Dupertuis, S. M.: Arterectomy with follow up studies on 78 operations. Surg. Gynecol. Obstet., *64*:149, 1937.

Lidman, D., and Daniel, R. K.: Evaluation of clinical microvascular anastomoses—reasons for failure. Ann. Plast. Surg., *6*:215, 1981.

Luk, K. D., and Chow, S. P.: An experimental study of the effect of infection on microvascular anastomosis. Microsurgery, *6*:113, 1985.

MacMillan, D. C., and Sim, A. K.: Thromboembolism: a manifestation of the response of blood to injury. Circulation, *42*:1, 1970.

Manson, P. N., Narayan, K. K., Im, M. J., Bulkley, G. B., and Hoopes, J. E.: Improved survival in free skin flap transfers in rats. Surgery, *99*:211, 1986.

May, J. W., Jr., Athanasoulis, C. A., and Donelan, M. B.: Preoperative magnification angiography of donor and recipient sites for clinical free transfer of flaps or digits. Plast. Reconstr. Surg., *64*:483, 1979.

May, J. W., Jr., Chait, L. A., O'Brien, B. M., and Hurley, J. V.: The no-reflow phenomenon in experimental free flaps. Plast. Reconstr. Surg., *61*:256, 1978.

McGregor, I. A., and Jackson, I. T.: The groin flap. Br. J. Plast. Surg., *25*:3, 1972.

McLean, B. H., and Buncke, H. J., Jr.: Autotransplant of omentum to a large scalp defect, with microsurgical revascularization. Plast. Reconstr. Surg., *49*:268, 1972.

Melka, J., Charbonneau, R., and Bosse, J.-P.: Experimental evaluation of microarterial grafts in rats and rabbits: long-term histological studies. Plast. Reconstr. Surg., *63*:245, 1979.

Meyer, V. E., Donski, P., Smahel, J., Scholzel, E., and Baratti, C.: Fifth Symposium of the International Society of Reconstructive Microsurgery, Brazil, 1978.

Michon, J., and Masse, P.: Le moment optimum de la suture nerveuse dans les plaies du membre supérieur. Rev. Chir. Orthoped., *50*:205, 1964.

Mitchell, G. M., Morrison, W. A., Papadopoulos, A., and O'Brien, B. M.: A study of the extent and pathology of experimental avulsion injury in rabbit arteries and veins. Br. J. Plast. Surg., *38*:278, 1985.

Morgan, R. F., Reisman, N. R., and Wilgis, E. F.: Anatomic localization of sympathetic nerves in the hand. J. Hand Surg., *8*:283, 1983.

Morrison, W. A., and O'Brien, B. M.: Microsurgical techniques. *In* Barron, J. N., and Saad, M. N. (Eds.): Operative Plastic and Reconstructive Surgery. Vol. 1. New York, Churchill Livingstone, 1980, pp. 57–72.

Morrison, W. A., O'Brien, B. M., and MacLeod, A. M.: A long-term review of digital replantation. Aust. N.Z. J. Surg., *47*:767, 1977.

Morrison, W. A., and Pribaz, J. J.: Vascularized tube pedicle: a case report. Br. J. Plast. Surg., *33*:25, 1980.

Nichter, L. S., Haines, P. C., and Edgerton, M. T.: Successful replantation in the face of absent venous drainage: an experimental study. Plast. Reconstr. Surg., *75*:686, 1985.

Nightingale, G., Fogdestam, I., and O'Brien, B. M.: Scanning electron microscope study of experimental microvascular anastomoses in the rabbit. Br. J. Plast. Surg., *33*:283, 1980.

Nylen, C-O.: The microscope in aural surgery, its first use and later development. Acta Otolaryngol. Suppl., *116*:226, 1954.

Nylen, C-O.: The otomicroscope and microsurgery 1921–1971. Acta Otolaryngol., *73*:453, 1972.

O'Brien, B. M.: Microvascular Reconstructive Surgery. New York, Churchill Livingstone, 1977.

O'Brien, B. M., Browning, F. S., and Rosen, P.: Experimental micro-arterial grafts to small arteries. Br. J. Plast. Surg., *32*:155, 1979.

O'Brien, B. M., and Hayhurst, J. W.: Metallized microsutures and a new micro needle holder. Plast. Reconstr. Surg., *52*:673, 1973.

O'Brien, B. M., and Hayhurst, J. W.: Principles and techniques of microvascular surgery. *In* Converse, J. M. (Ed.): Reconstructive Plastic Surgery. 2nd Ed. Philadelphia, W. B. Saunders Company, 1977, pp. 340–391.

O'Brien, B. M., Henderson, P., Bennett, R. C., and Crock, G. W.: Microvascular surgical technique. Med. J. Aust., *1*:722, 1970.

O'Brien, B. M., Kubo, T., and Threlfall, G. N.: Autogenous micro-arterial grafts to the femoral vein in rabbits. Br. J. Plast. Surg., *32*:167, 1979.

O'Brien, B. M., MacLeod, A. M., Hayhurst, J. W., and Morrison, W. A.: Successful transfer of a large island flap from the groin to the foot by microvascular anastomoses. Plast. Reconstr. Surg., *52*:271, 1973.

O'Brien, B. M., Morrison, W. A., Ishida, H., MacLeod, A. M., and Gilbert, A.: Free flap transfer with microvascular anastomoses. Br. J. Plast. Surg., *27*:220, 1974.

O'Brien, B. M., and Shanmugan, N.: Experimental transfer of composite free flaps with microvascular anastomoses. Aust. N.Z. J. Surg., *43*:285, 1973.

Overton, J. H., and Owen, E. R.: The successful replacement of minute arteries. Surgery, *68*:713, 1970.

Papadopoulos, O., MacLeod, A., O'Brien, B. M., Roberts, A., and Mitchell, G.: The role of arterial spasm in the survival of experimental free flaps. Unpublished data.

Parks, D. A., Bulkley, G. B., and Granger, D. N.: Role of oxygen free radicals in shock, ischemia and organ preservation. Surgery, *94*:428, 1983.

Parsa, F. D., and Spira, M.: Experimental evaluation of autogenous and prosthetic vein grafts in microsurgery. Intl. J. Microsurg., *1*:36, 1979.

Perritt, R. A.: Recent advances in corneal surgery. *In* American Academy of Ophthalmology and Otolaryngology Course No. 280, 1950.

Pick, J.: The Autonomic Nervous System: Morphological, Comparative, Clinical and Surgical Aspects. Philadelphia, J. B. Lippincott Company, 1970.

Popov, D. G., and Trichkova, P. I.: A new technique for end-to-side anastomoses in microvascular surgery. Plast. Reconstr. Surg., *59*:444, 1977.

Pribaz, J. J., Schneider, P., Asaadi, M., Russell, R., and Zook, E.: An experimental study of microvenous grafting. Presented at the Royal Australasian College of Surgeons, Melbourne, 1983.

Puckett, C. L., Misholy, H., and Reinisch, J. F.: The effects of streptokinase on ischemic flaps. J. Hand Surg., *8*:101, 1983.

Rao, V. K., Morrison, W. A., and O'Brien, B. M.: Effect of nicotine on blood flow and patency of experimental microvascular anastomosis. Ann. Plast. Surg., *11*:206, 1983.

Sarin, C. L., Austin, J. C., and Nickel, W. O.: Effects of smoking on digital blood-flow velocity. J.A.M.A., *229*:1327, 1974.

Sawyer, P. N., Stanczewski, B., Pomerance, A., Lucas, T., Stoner, G., and Srinivasan, S.: Utility of anticoagulant drugs in vascular thrombosis: electron microscopic and biophysical study. Surgery, *74*:263, 1973.

Serafin, D., Georgiade, N. G., and Smith, D. H.: Comparison of free flaps with pedicle flaps for coverage of defects of the leg or foot. Plast. Reconstr. Surg., *59*:492, 1977.

Sharzer, L. A., O'Brien, B. M., Horton, C. E., Adamson, J. E., Mladick, R. A., et al.: Clinical applications of free flap transfer in the burn patient. J. Trauma, *15*:766, 1975.

Shaw, W.: Microvascular free flaps: survey. *In* Buncke, H., and Furnas, D. (Eds.): Symposium on Clinical Frontiers in Reconstructive Microsurgery. St. Louis, C. V. Mosby Company, 1984, pp. 3–10.

Sheppard, J. E., and Dell, P. C.: The effect of preoperative arteriography on vascular endothelium and replant survival in rabbit ears. J. Hand Surg., *8*:145, 1983.

Sinclair, S.: The importance of topical heparin in microvascular anastomoses: a study in the rat. Br. J. Plast. Surg., *33*:422, 1980.

Smith, A. R., Sonneveld, G. J., and van der Meulen, J. C.: AV anastomosis as a solution for absent venous drainage in replantation surgery. Plast. Reconstr. Surg., *71*:525, 1983.

Smith, J. W.: Microsurgery of peripheral nerves. Plast. Reconstr. Surg., *33*:317, 1964.

Smith, P. J., Foley, B., McGregor, I. A., and Jackson, I. T.: The anatomical basis of the groin flap. Plast. Reconstr. Surg., *49*:41, 1972.

Spaet, T. H., and Gaynor, E.: Vascular endothelial damage and thrombosis. Adv. Cardiol., *4*:47, 1970.

Spaet, T. H., Gaynor, E., and Stemerman, M. B.: Thrombosis, atherosclerosis, and endothelium. Am. Heart J., *87*:661, 1974.

Strauch, B., and Murray, D. E.: Transfer of composite graft with immediate suture anastomosis of its vascular pedicle measuring less than 1 mm. in external diameter using microsurgical techniques. Plast. Reconstr. Surg., *40*:325, 1967.

Sully, L., Nightingale, G. M., O'Brien, B. M., and Hurley, J. V.: An experimental study of the sleeve technique in microarterial anastomoses. Plast. Reconstr. Surg., *70*:186, 1982.

Sutera, S. P., and Hochmuth, R. M.: Large scale modelling of blood flow in the capillaries. Biorheology, *5*:45, 1968.

Tamai, S.: Digital replantation. Clin. Plast. Surg., *5*:195, 1978.

Tamai, S., Sarauchi, N., Hori, Y., Tatsumi, Y., and Okuda, H.: Microvascular surgery in orthopaedics and traumatology. J. Bone Joint Surg., *54B*:637, 1972.

Tan, E., O'Brien, B. M., and Brennen, M.: Free flap transfer in rabbits using irradiated recipient vessels. Br. J. Plast. Surg., *31*:121, 1978.

Threlfall, G. N., Little, J. M., and Cummine, J.: Free flap transfer—preliminary establishment of an arteriovenous fistula: a case report. Aust. N.Z. J. Surg., *52*:182, 1982.

Urbaniak, J. R., Soucacos, P. N., Adelaar, R. S., Bright, D. S., and Whitehurst, L. A.: Experimental evaluation of microsurgical techniques and small artery anastomoses. Orthop. Clin. North Am., *8*:249, 1977.

Van Beek, A. L.: Presented at Seventh Symposium of International Society of Reconstructive Microsurgery Meeting, New York, 1983.

Wiederhielm, C. A., and Billig, L.: Effects of erythrocyte orientation on light transmission through blood flowing through microscopic blood vessels. *In* Copey, A. L. (Ed.): Proceeding of 1st International Conference of Hemorheology. New York, Pergamon, 1968.

Wilgis, E. F.: Evaluation and treatment of chronic digital ischemia. Ann. Surg., *193*:693, 1981.

Wray, R. C., and O'Brien, B. M.: The effects of suturing technique and vessel size on patency after microarterial repair. Ann. Plast. Surg., *2*:223, 1979.

Yaremchuk, M. J., Bartlett, S. P., Sedacca, T., and May, J. W., Jr.: The effect of preoperative angiography on experimental free-flap survival. Plast. Reconstr. Surg., *68*:201, 1981.

Yasargil, M. G.: Experimental small vessel surgery in the dog including patching and grafting of cerebral vessels in the formation of functional extracranial shunts. *In* Donaghy, R. P., and Yasargil, M. G. (Eds.): Microvascular Surgery. St. Louis, C. V. Mosby Company, 1967, p. 87.

13

Louis C. Argenta
Eric D. Austad

Principles and Techniques of Tissue Expansion

In his discussion of Radovan's landmark paper in 1982, Grabb wrote, "Although many innovations are advanced, only a few have had the impact of microsurgery techniques and of muscle flaps. I predict that over the next five years the technique of tissue expansion will be of equal importance" (Radovan, 1982). Since 1982, tissue expansion has added new dimensions to reconstructive surgery (Radovan, 1984; Argenta, Marks, and Pasyk, 1985). As with microsurgery and free flap techniques, tissue expansion has permitted the achievement of surgical goals that were previously impossible by conventional means.

Tissue expansion is based on the observation that all living tissues respond in a dynamic fashion to the mechanical stresses placed upon them. The growth of the "skin envelope" from fetal life through maturity illustrates the ability of soft tissue to accommodate to skeletal growth. The normal skin and subcutaneous tissue developed over the gravid abdomen further illustrate physiologic tissue expansion. Normal skin, mucosa, or scalp over large benign tumors demonstrates the focal ability of these structures to respond to stimuli that are clearly nongenetic. Surgically induced tissue expansion allows the reconstructive surgeon an entirely new approach: donor tissue generated in situ and used for reconstruction without compromise of innervation, vascularity, or external physical appearance. Attractive in its simplicity and encouraging in its clinical applications to date, tissue expansion may be viewed as a judicious manipulation of normal physiologic processes: a biologic dividend (Austad, Thomas, and Pasyk, 1986).

HISTORY

As early as 1905, attempts at distraction techniques for bone lengthening resulted in concomitant, but unrecognized, expansion of soft tissue (Codivilla, 1905; Matev, 1970). Neumann (1957) described the use of a subcutaneously placed implant in an attempt to reconstruct an external ear deformity. Although strikingly similar to current tissue expanders, the prosthesis was externally filled and made of rubber (Fig. 13–1). The surgical result was acceptable but Neumann's work was treated as anecdotal and generally forgotten.

Working independently in 1975, Radovan and Austad developed the concept of tissue expansion with a silicone implant. Radovan's first implant was delivered to him in January

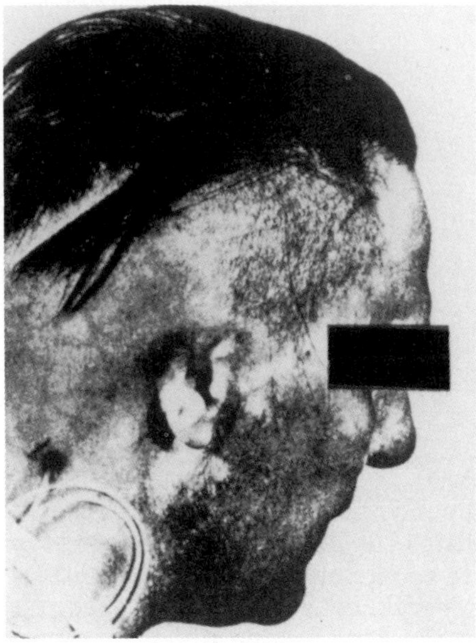

Figure 13–1. First clinical application of tissue expansion—Neumann's attempt at partial (right) ear reconstruction. A polyethylene tube leading from the balloon is shown. (From Neumann, C. G.: The expansion of an area of skin by progressive distention of a subcutaneous balloon. Plast. Reconstr. Surg., *19*:124, 1957.)

1976, and his first tissue expansion procedure was performed on January 26, 1976. At the same time, Austad was developing a self-inflating silicone prosthesis. Radovan proceeded immediately to clinical trials, presenting his initial experience at the American Society of Plastic and Reconstructive Surgeons in 1976 and 1977. This work was met with skepticism. Austad continued studying the histologic changes of tissue expansion in the laboratory and presented them in 1978. In the period between 1976 and 1978, considerable laboratory and clinical experience with tissue expansion was gained. In 1979, Austad and Rose received first prize in the Clinical Research Competition of the American Society of Plastic and Reconstructive Surgeons for their evaluation of the clinical and histologic aspects of tissue expansion. Subsequent presentations at national meetings by Radovan, Argenta, Austad, and other surgeons have resulted in wide clinical acceptance of tissue expansion as a new technique with an established basis of safety and efficacy.

TYPES OF IMPLANTS

Many cultures throughout the world have induced expansion in various anatomic regions by applying spacers of progressively increasing size (Rees, 1980). The common feature of these primitive "expanders" is their ability to apply controlled tension to adjacent soft tissue. To provide this stimulus in a clinically useful way, a variety of implants have evolved.

Radovan's initial expander consisted of a silicone prosthesis with two valves, each connected to the main reservoir with a segment of silicone tubing. One valve was used for injection of saline, while the other served as a means for withdrawal if overinflation occurred. A single, self-sealing port was soon developed. In the latter form, the Radovan expander continues to be available in different sizes and shapes.

The incorporation of the filling reservoir into the dome of the main reservoir was developed by Lapin and associates (1980). This prosthesis circumvents localization or placement of a remote port. It does have the disadvantage, however, of being a difficult port to palpate when placed beneath muscle or scar tissue. Theoretical objection to this prosthesis is that inflation of the implant thrusts the semirigid valve into the dome of the flap, the point of maximal stress (Cohen, 1985).

The Austad prosthesis is a self-inflating device consisting of a sealed, collapsed silicone balloon (Austad and Rose, 1982). It contains an osmotic substance that causes migration of extracellular water through the silicone, and results in continuous inflation at a constant rate. The inflation rate is controlled by varying the thickness of the implant shell or by modifying the amount or type of osmotic material within the implant. This device has been used experimentally, but currently awaits U.S. Food and Drug Administration approval.

"Permanent" expanders have also been developed (Becker, Cohen, and Scheflan, 1982; Becker, 1984). They are both gel-containing and double-lumen implants, which may be enlarged by percutaneous injection of saline. Both have remote ports that can later be removed after appropriate implant size has been attained. These devices are primarily for breast reconstruction, but long-term studies are still unavailable. The possibility of eliminating the second stage of a breast reconstruction remains an attractive goal.

Prostheses that expand asymmetrically or differentially have been used on a limited basis. Through modifications in the thickness of the implant or in the actual design, these prostheses expand to a specific shape rather than the usual round shape. They may have potential in both scalp and breast reconstruction. "Low-profile" implants have been devised by Austad and van Beek (1987), designed to eliminate fold flaw erosion by minimizing tension on the overlying skin early in the course of inflation. A wide variety of other implants will undoubtedly be developed for specific purposes. Many surgeons with extensive experience in tissue expansion feel that the technical ability and ingenuity of the surgeon are probably more important than the specific type of implant used.

BIOLOGY OF TISSUE EXPANSION

Histologic Studies

Most of the information regarding the biology of tissue expansion has been derived from animal experiments, since human tissue is difficult to obtain. Pasyk has recently published preliminary studies on expanded human tissue (Pasyk, Argenta, and Austad, 1987). In general, the results parallel the changes seen in animal studies. Extensive well-controlled studies in tissue expansion in the guinea pig and pig model have been reported (Fig. 13–2) (Austad and associates, 1982; Pasyk, Austad, and Cherry, 1984; Pasyk, Argenta, and Austad, 1987).

Epidermis

Statistical analysis of multiple sites over the implant and at its periphery revealed no significant variation in epidermal thickness during tissue expansion. One week after placement of the prosthesis, significant thickening may occur. Since this is also seen in sham-operated controls, the thickness probably represents postoperative edema. By four weeks after placement of the prosthesis, epidermal thickness decreases to its normal baseline and essentially remains unchanged throughout the process of expansion. Accessory skin structures, such as hair follicles, show some element of compression but no evidence of degeneration. An increase in melanocytic activity has been noted during expansion, but this returns to near normal several months after completion of the reconstruction. It has been hypothesized that this phenomenon may contribute to the hyperpigmentation observed in expanding tissues, which disappears spontaneously after reconstruction.

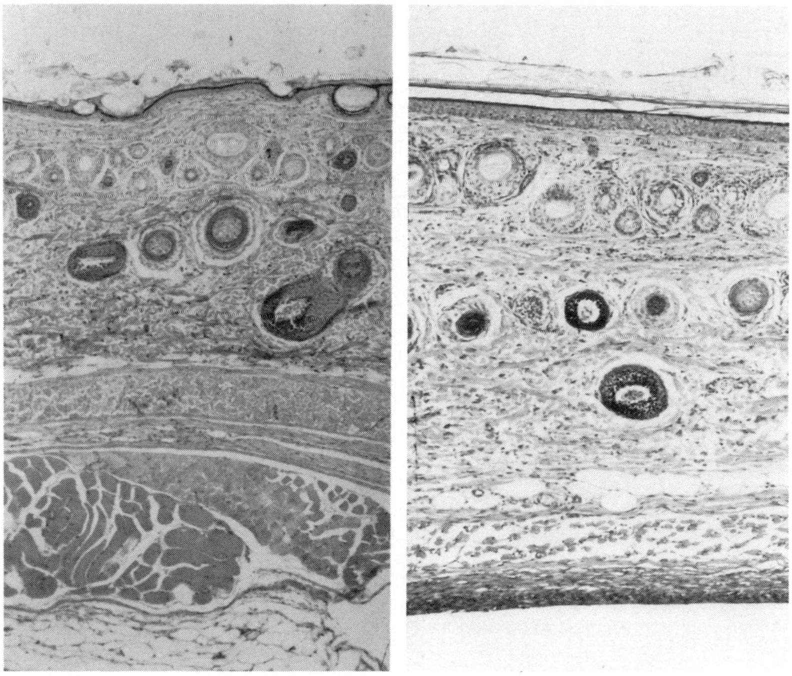

Figure 13–2. *Left,* low power view of tissue over an implant at four weeks demonstrating (1) intact, normal-appearing stratified squamous epithelium, (2) slight compression of the hair follicles, (3) moderate atrophy of the panniculus carnosus muscle, and (4) a well-formed fibrous connective tissue capsule. *Right,* Normal nonexpanded tissue. Note the thickness of the panniculus carnosus muscle, compared with that of the treated animal on the left (200×).

Dermis

In contrast to the epidermis, there is a rapid decrease in dermal thickness over the entire implant during expansion. This finding is most pronounced in the first weeks after implant placement and persists throughout the entire period of implant expansion. A dense, fibrous capsule is formed around the implant. An inflammatory cell response has not been observed around the implant unless extrusion or infection occur. With passage of time, the capsule becomes less cellular and progressively more collagenized. Dystrophic calcification or ossification have not been observed. No evidence of dysplastic changes or loss of normal cell maturation has been observed in either the epidermis or dermis.

Muscle

Significant atrophy of muscle (Fig. 13–3) occurs during the process of expansion, whether the expander is placed above or below the specific muscle. Muscle function, however, remains active. After removal of the expander, muscle mass is diminished, but it probably resumes its normal state over time.

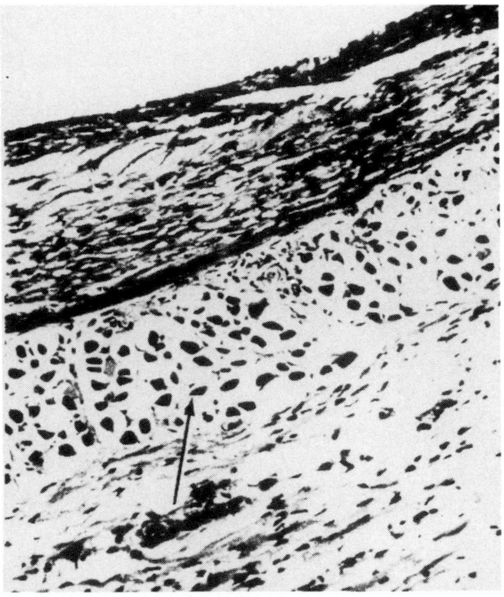

Figure 13–3. High power view of the atrophic panniculus carnosus muscle (*arrow*) and the adjacent edematous connective tissue in animals implanted for two weeks (400×).

Ultrastructural Studies

Electron microscopy studies of expanded tissue have confirmed the relatively innocuous nature of tissue expansion, as has been observed at the light microscope level (Pasyk and associates, 1982). The epidermis displays a reduction of intercellular distance, and a significant increase in undulation of the basal lamina is seen in expanded specimens. The dermis displays large, compact bundles of collagen fibers, oriented in an orderly, parallel fashion over the implant surface. Active fibroblasts are identified in the expanded dermis, and intracellular collagen has been identified within these cells. Myofibroblasts are also identified in the deep dermis, near the capsule. The subcutaneous tissue displays a paucity of adipose tissue, but no changes in the vessels of the subcutaneous space have been noticed. Skeletal muscle demonstrates changes suggestive of pressure atrophy, with numerous mitochondria and abnormally arranged sarcomeres. The small blood vessels within the skeletal muscles, however, appear normal.

Vascularity of Expanded Tissue

The clinical observation that expanded tissue is extremely well vascularized was made long before laboratory studies verified this phenomenon. It has been histologically demonstrated that a large number of new vessels are formed in the area adjacent to the capsule. The mechanism of formation of these vessels, and information as to how long they persist after expansion, remain unknown.

Cherry and associates (1983) demonstrated that a dramatic increase in vascularity occurs during tissue expansion (Fig. 13–4). Comparing expanded flaps to delayed flaps and acutely raised flaps, they were able to show that flaps elevated in expanded tissue had the greatest increase in survival length, averaging 117 per cent over control flaps (Fig. 13–5). Similar experiments with labeled microspheres have demonstrated increase of flap length survival, as well as increased blood flow to the expanded tissue (Sasaki and Pang, 1984). Thus, rather than resulting in vascular compromise, tissue expansion appears to elicit additional tissue with vascular characteristics similar to those of delayed flaps.

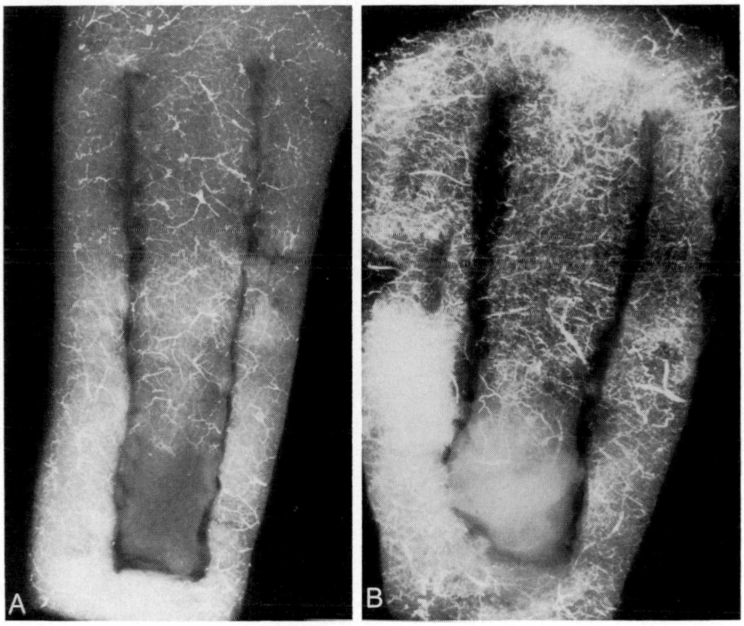

Figure 13–4. A barium injection roentgenogram of the vessels in (*A*) a random pattern skin flap in a pig and (*B*) an expanded flap in the same animal model. A dramatic increase in the vascularity of the expanded flap is evident.

TISSUE EXPANSION: DIVIDEND OR LOAN?

In the clinical setting and in laboratory tissue, expansion results in a readily apparent and measurable increase in tissue surface area. The source of this tissue has been the subject of many investigations. The increase in tissue seems to arise from two sources. There is a significant recruitment from tissue of adjacent areas (Brobmann and Huber, 1985). Increasing surface area of the expansion prostheses carries with it some of the loose skin of adjacent areas.

Austad, Thomas, and Pasyk (1986), using audioradiographic techniques, demonstrated increased mitotic activity in the epidermis

MEAN SURVIVING LENGTH OF RANDOM PATTERN SKIN FLAPS RAISED IN EXPANDED TISSUE

Control Flaps (Acutely Raised)	Flaps Raised In Nonexpanded Skin With Radovan Expander	Delay Flaps	Flaps Expanded With Radovan Expander
*6.6 ± 1.4 (5)	9.7 ± 2.4 (5)	11.4 ± 1.7(5)	14.3 ± 0.9 (5)
	Percentage Increase Over Control		
	+47%	+73%	+117%

*Mean ± S.D. (N)

Figure 13–5. Survival of expanded skin flaps. Expanded flaps survived 117 per cent more than the control flaps. (From Cherry, G. W., Austad, E. D., Pasyk, K. A., et al.: Increased survival and vascularity of random-pattern skin flaps elevated in controlled, expanded skin. Plast. Reconstr. Surg., *72*:680, 1983.)

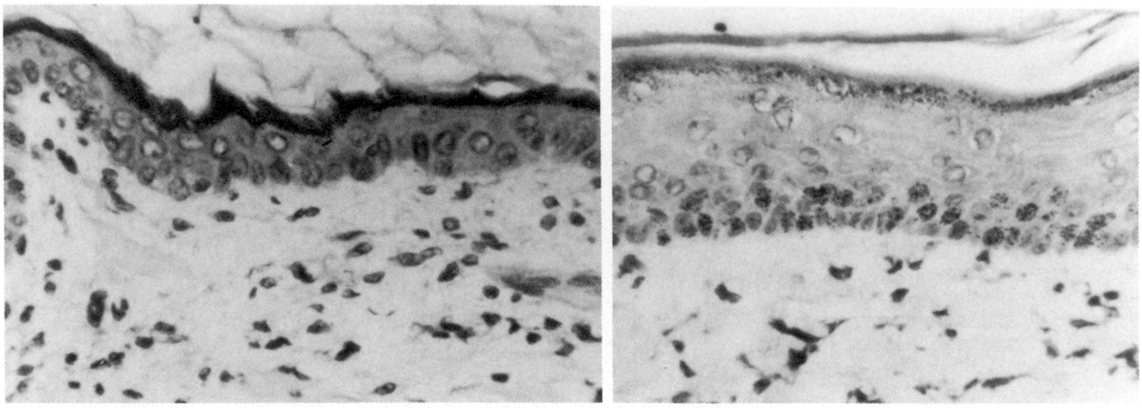

Figure 13–6. Tritiated thymidine labeling of unexpanded (*left*) and expanded (*right*) epidermis (H&E, ×400). Note the dramatic increase in the uptake of thymidine, indicating an increased rate of mitosis in the expanded epidermis.

overlying the expansion prostheses during the process of expansion (Figs. 13–6, 13–7). They noted a significant increase in mitotic rate following each inflation of the prosthesis. With deflation of the implant, a significant decline in the rate of epidermal mitosis below normal baseline was seen. It is clear that the epidermis is exquisitely sensitive to these physical stimuli, but no mechanism of action has been clarified.

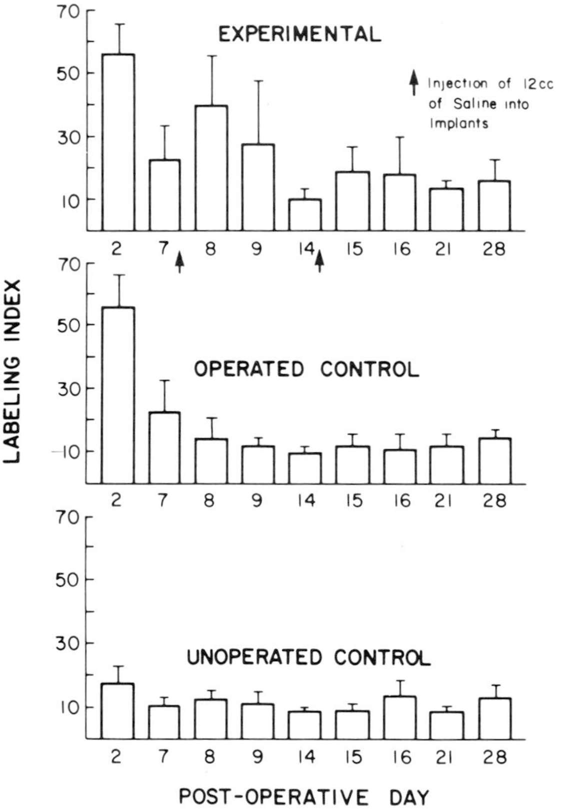

Figure 13–7. Epidermal thymidine labeling during tissue expansion. *T* indicates 2 standard deviations. An increased rate of thymidine uptake indicates that an increased rate of mitosis occurred after each inflation (arrow) of the prosthesis.

BASIC PRINCIPLES

Patient Selection

Tissue expansion has a potential role in the treatment of any soft tissue defect that cannot be closed primarily, or in which closure under tension is contraindicated. Informed consent, as with any other procedure, is important since temporary, but significant, cosmetic deformity occurs. In general, the process of tissue expansion is well tolerated by emotionally stable patients of all ages, although the presence of the implant may interfere with social and other activities. Noncompliant and mentally impaired patients are obviously poor candidates.

The presumptive donor sites in each patient must be individualized. Areas that have undergone significant radiation are not categorically excluded but should be approached with caution. Irradiated tissue can be expanded with a higher risk of complications over a longer period than normal tissue. After mastectomy, radiation therapy has been performed concomitant with tissue expansion, again with a greater complication rate. Tissue expansion can be commenced during chemotherapy but should be carried out at a tempered rate.

In general, tissue expansion is best performed as a secondary reconstructive procedure, rather than an acute, post-trauma reconstruction. Expansion of the scalp, however, has been carried out acutely (Leonard and Small, 1986), as has been expansion of the soft tissue of the upper and lower extremity.

Implant Choice and Placement

The implant selected is approximately the size and shape of the donor area. The potential donor site should be measured, and an implant of equal or slightly smaller base diameter selected. The nominal volume of the specific implant is relatively unimportant, since implants may be hyperinflated to many times their specified volumes and still maintain their integrity. After the size of the implant has been established, it is likely that a standard implant is available from the vast assortment of sizes and shapes currently supplied by manufacturers. Occasionally an unusually shaped donor site or complicated case may require the services of a manufacturer to fabricate a custom shape and size of prosthesis. Most standard expanders incorporate a remotely placed filling port, which decreases the risk of inadvertent implant puncture during inflation. This factor becomes more important when the prostheses are placed in the submuscular position, as in breast reconstruction, or when seroma occurs around the prosthesis.

Expanders are generally placed under the skin and subcutaneous tissue. In areas where the subcutaneous tissue is thin, or risk of possible extrusion is significant, the prosthesis may also be placed under the muscle. Careful planning is necessary to select an incision for placement of the prosthesis in order that possible alternative flaps are not compromised. Optimally the incisions should be incorporated into the projected incision ultimately left by implant removal and flap rotation or advancement. Some surgeons prefer a radial incision adjacent to the area undergoing expansion to minimize tension on the suture line. However, this is often difficult to accomplish without creating new scars. The key to successful expansion is careful preoperative planning and consideration of the alternatives before any incision is made.

Prostheses have been placed in almost every area of the body. Transient neuropraxia from adjacent nerves has been reported. However, prostheses have been placed directly over the facial nerve and major nerves in the forearm and leg without causing significant complications. Likewise, prostheses may be expanded over a major vessel or the trachea without significant risk. A severely debilitated patient or a patient with atherosclerosis may suffer complications from compression of previously compromised vessels.

The remote filling port should be located in an area where it is easy to palpate and easily removed. Bony prominences should be avoided. The connector tube joining the implant and filling port should not traverse a joint since both ends of the prosthesis become rapidly fixed in scar. Sudden movement of the joint may result in rupture of the implant. Occasionally, it is possible to position a filling port in a relatively anesthetic area, which minimizes discomfort during inflation.

Implant Inflation

If wound tension is minimal at the time of tissue expander placement, a moderate volume of saline may be introduced without delay. This lubricates the interior of the implant and may reduce the likelihood of fold flaw erosion. The immediate introduction of saline may also place enough tension on the margins of the wound to lessen seroma and hematoma formation. Only sufficient saline should be placed at the time of implant placement to fill the dissection space without placing any undue tension on the suture line.

Inflations are generally begun one to two weeks after implant placement, although inflation schedules must be individualized to the nature and anatomic location of the deformity. For practical reasons, most prostheses are inflated at weekly intervals, but highly accelerated inflation schedules have been successfully carried out (Marks and associates, 1985, 1986). Each inflation proceeds to a point of patient discomfort or blanching of the skin overlying the implant. In anesthetic regions, such as in the treatment of pressure sores, objective changes in flap vascularity should be evaluated with particular care. Although a variety of pressure transducers, oxygen tension monitors, and other types of perfusion monitoring devices are available as adjuncts to inflation of tissue expanders, objective inspection and patient response are usually reliable indicators of appropriate implant inflation. In each subsequent inflation, saline is placed into the implant through a 23 gauge, or smaller, needle. The use of the butterfly needle with the small connecting piece of tubing is especially useful and allows some patient motion without dislocation of the syringe. Implant expansion should proceed until adequate additional soft tissue has been generated to accomplish the specific surgical goal.

In the case of breast reconstruction in which a permanent implant is anticipated, overinflation of the expander by 20 to 25 per cent is frequently carried out. The expanded breast is maintained at that volume for three to four months before placement of a permanent implant in an effort to reduce the likelihood of capsular contracture.

BREAST RECONSTRUCTION

A wide variety of techniques are available for reconstruction of the female breast. Simple implant placement suffices for a large number of women who have undergone modified radical mastectomy. Small-breasted women are ideal for this technique, especially when healthy skin has been preserved at mastectomy. Patients who have undergone extensive modified radical mastectomy or radical mastectomy, or have an extremely large ptotic breast on the opposite side, are best reconstructed with transfer of tissue from other areas. The small number of patients who have a distinct inability to tolerate silicone implants should likewise be reconstructed with autogenous tissue. The transverse rectus abdominis musculocutaneous flap and the latissimus dorsi myocutaneous flap have stood the test of time for such reconstructions and are dependable (see Chap. 79).

Tissue expansion is applicable to those patients who have qualitatively good tissue remaining on the chest wall but who have quantitatively insufficient skin to cover a silicone prosthesis that will give them symmetry with the opposite side. Most of these patients have an intact pectoralis muscle, usually with some atrophy of the lower half and varying amounts of soft tissue and skin. Patients who require an implant greater than 300 ml may also require expansion to accommodate a prosthesis in the subpectoral plane.

Advantages

Placement of an expansion prosthesis for breast reconstruction is a simple, straightforward procedure that can be carried out under general or local anesthesia, usually in less than one hour. Since extensive dissection is not necessary, rehabilitation is rapid. This procedure is ideally suited to debilitated individuals, the elderly, and those whose life style precludes prolonged recovery time. A second procedure in which the prosthesis is removed and replaced with a permanent implant is likewise a minor procedure that depends on reconstruction of the inframammary fold and contouring of the opposite breast.

Tissue expansion allows for ideal color and texture match of the reconstructed breast with the remaining chest wall, since the breast is generated from existing chest wall skin. With transfer of flaps from distant areas, the color, texture, and hair-bearing characteristics of the donor site remain on the neobreast. Breast reconstruction by tissue expansion usually can be performed through the original mastectomy site without the addition of new scars. At the second operation, an incision in the new inframammary fold may be necessary if accentuation or modification of this area is necessary. The range of breast sizes that can be created with expansion is considerable. Hyperinflation of prostheses up to 1500 ml has been carried out routinely. Large silicone prostheses can be placed within the expanded space to allow for reconstruction of even the largest breast. The incidence of fibrous contracture after tissue expansion seems to be less than in breasts reconstructed with a simple implant. The mechanism for this is poorly understood but may be related to the prolonged resistance afforded by progressive expansion.

Disadvantages

Two operations are required to reconstruct the breast successfully by tissue expansion: one in which the expander is placed and a second in which a permanent prosthesis is placed. The development of a permanent expansion prosthesis has obviated the need for a second procedure in some cases. However, proper positioning of the neobreast as well as reconstruction of an acceptable inframammary fold frequently necessitates a second procedure. Reconstruction of the nipple may be performed during the second procedure but ideally is delayed in most cases, since some redistribution of the breast skin does occur. Multiple visits to the office are required for inflation of the expander. Usually, four to six inflations at weekly or biweekly intervals are needed. If hyperinflation is to be performed to create a large breast or an accentuated inframammary fold, more visits may be required. Capsular contractures can develop in such reconstructed breasts.

Surgical Technique

Correct preoperative positioning of the expander reduces secondary reconstructive procedures. Before the procedure the inframammary fold and the extent of undermining are marked in permanent ink with the patient in a standing position.

Radovan's initial technique (Radovan, 1982) involved placing the expander in the subcutaneous space above the pectoralis muscle. As with all reconstructions in this plane, the frequent result was a firm, round breast with less than an ideal cosmetic appearance.

Most surgeons currently place expanders and prostheses beneath the pectoralis muscle (Argenta, Marks, and Grabb, 1983; Argenta, 1984a,b; Seckel and Hyland, 1985). If an intact serratus anterior muscle is found, the prosthesis may be placed behind it also. If the serratus is atrophic, the inferior one-third to one-half of the expander is left in the subcutaneous space.

General anesthesia is preferred, although local anesthesia with sedation can be tolerated by some patients. The hands are positioned on the iliac crest, thus removing tension from the pectoralis muscle and facilitating dissection beneath it. The lateralmost aspect of the patient's original mastectomy scar is used for placement of the expander. Dissection is carried down to the pectoralis muscle, which is split in the direction of its fibers several centimeters from the lateral border. Splitting of the muscle allows for better closure than can usually be achieved by dissecting laterally to the lateral margin of the muscle. Dissection beneath the pectoralis is done bluntly down to the level of the serratus, where dense adhesions occur and require sharp dissection. Electrocautery is usually employed at this point. A round inflatable prosthesis of 700 ml or more is usually placed. The base of the prosthesis should be slightly larger than the base of the opposite breast. The base size of the prosthesis is more important than its actual volume, since the prosthesis may be overinflated. If prostheses with distant reservoirs are used, the inflation reservoir is ideally placed in the subcutaneous space in the axilla or beneath what will be the patient's brassiere line. The muscle is closed with absorbable sutures, and isotonic saline is infused into the implant until mild tension of the overlying musculature is observed. Subcuticular monofilament sutures are used for skin closure and left in place for at least one month.

Inflation follows the general plan for expansion as previously described. The patient returns at weekly or biweekly intervals for serial percutaneous inflation with a 23 gauge butterfly needle. During this period the overlying skin frequently becomes hyperemic. The erythema usually resolves after inflation has been terminated or the prosthesis has been removed. After volumetric symmetry with the opposite side is achieved, hyperinflation of at least 250 to 400 ml should be carried out (Versaci, 1987). If a large amount of ptosis is to be developed or extensive repositioning of the breast is necessary, additional hyperinflation may be required. The fully expanded prosthesis should be left in place for at least three to four months in order that natural ptosis of the breast will develop and symmetry with the mature breast on the opposite side will evolve. Prostheses may be left in place for many months or even years before being exchanged for permanent implants.

At a second procedure the permanent silicone implant is placed. Sufficient saline is removed from the expansion prosthesis immediately before surgery to achieve symmetry with the opposite side. The remaining saline can then be measured to determine the size of the prosthesis, which is inserted. If ptosis is minimal, the expander can be placed through the original mastectomy scar. If repositioning of the inframammary fold or definition of the fold is required, an incision should be made at the projected inframammary fold. This allows creation of ptosis by infolding and uplifting the expanded tissue and advancing of the lower abdominal flap (Pennisi, 1979; Ryan, 1982). The expander is deflated to volume symmetry with the opposite side, and the expanded tissue is moved up or down so that the apices of the breasts are on an equal level (Fig. 13–8). The capsule is left intact unless the prosthesis needs to be repositioned. Stable reconstruction of the inframammary fold can be achieved by tacking the anterior capsule to the posterior chest wall capsule. Thus, the new breast is at the same level as the opposite side. Permanent

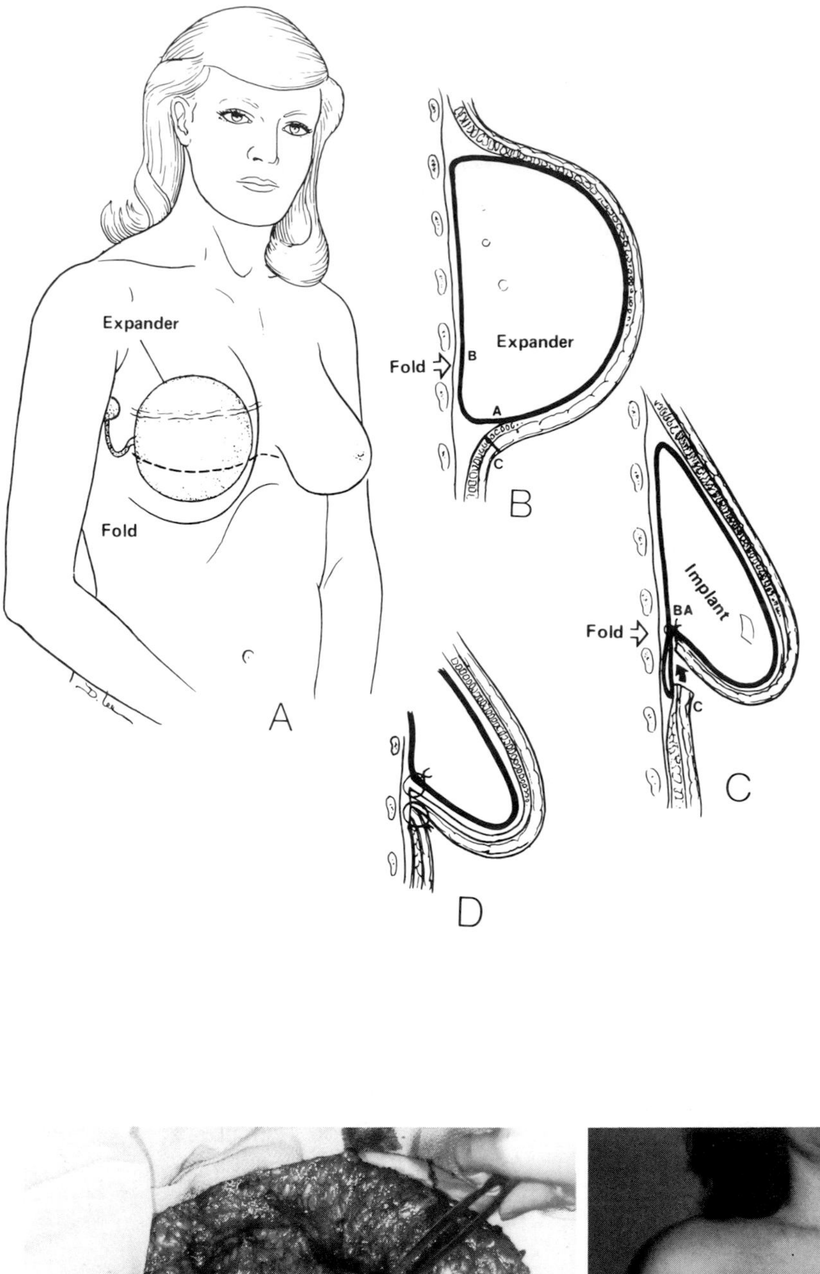

Figure 13–8. Technique of creating a ptotic breast by moving the inframammary fold. *A,* The prosthesis is overexpanded to create excess tissue. *B,* The position of the desired fold (*point B*) is determined on the thoracic wall. *C, D,* Through an inframammary incision (*point C*) the expander is removed and the skin and capsule are moved cephalad and sutured to point B. The abdominal wall is undermined above the fascia and advanced into the inframammary defect.

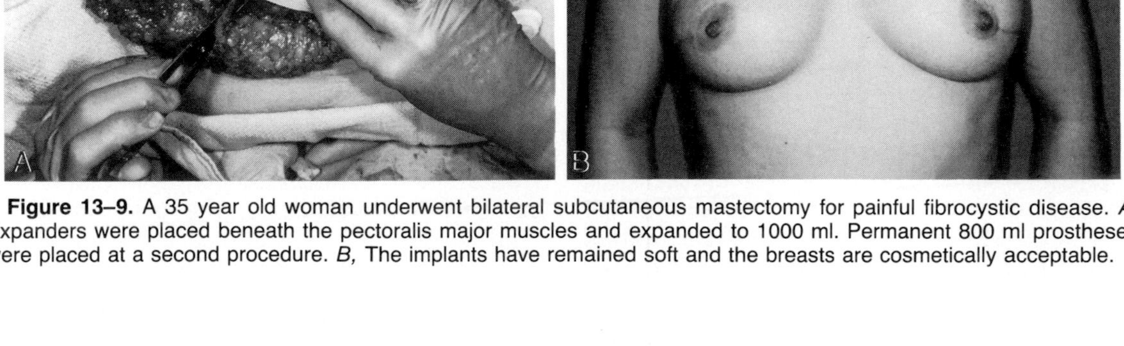

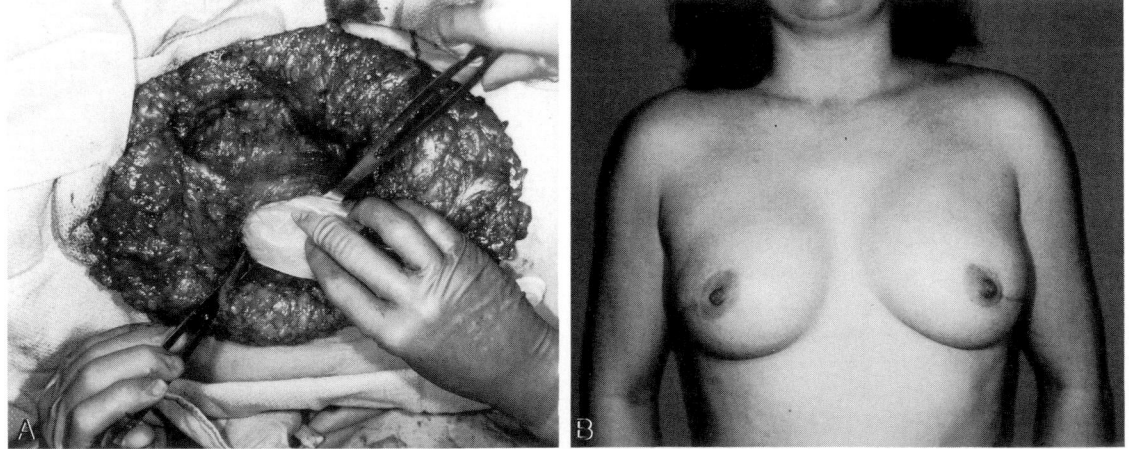

Figure 13–9. A 35 year old woman underwent bilateral subcutaneous mastectomy for painful fibrocystic disease. *A,* Expanders were placed beneath the pectoralis major muscles and expanded to 1000 ml. Permanent 800 ml prostheses were placed at a second procedure. *B,* The implants have remained soft and the breasts are cosmetically acceptable.

large sutures are usually required for stability. The abdominal skin is undermined above the fascia and is advanced superiorly into the inframammary cleavage to close the posterior wall defect. The breast is taped into an appropriate position. A second piece of foam tape is placed across the superior aspect of the breast to prevent the implant from being displaced in a cephalad direction. The tape is removed and vigorous massaging begun five days after the procedure (Fig. 13–9).

Bilateral Breast Reconstruction

Bilateral reconstruction of the breast can be performed by tissue expansion, following the same techniques previously outlined. Since there is usually a paucity of tissue, expansion may take slightly longer, making very large breasts more difficult to reconstruct. In practice, bilateral reconstruction is frequently simpler than unilateral reconstruction since symmetry can be more easily achieved (Fig. 13–10).

Immediate Breast Reconstruction

With mammography and periodic breast examination, breast neoplasms are being discovered earlier in the course of the disease. In consultation with general surgeons, patients with a low risk of metastatic disease can be identified, and reconstruction can be carried out at the time of modified radical mastectomy (Albo, Gruber, and Kahn, 1980; Georgiade and associates, 1982). Expansion techniques allow reconstruction of almost any breast without compromise of the ablative surgery.

Correct positioning for breast reconstruction must be done with the patient in the erect position before the induction of anesthesia. As with delayed reconstruction, the inframammary fold is marked from the sternum laterally beyond the surgical site. Ptosis or a large opposite breast frequently requires the inframammary fold of the new breast to be displaced caudally (Fig. 13–11).

After the general surgeon has completed his procedure, a 700 ml round expansion prosthesis is placed beneath the pectoralis muscle and, if possible, the upper portion of the serratus anterior. Displacement of the prosthesis into the axillary dissection is prevented by tacking the lateral margins of the pectoralis muscle to the chest wall with absorbable sutures. Occasionally the skin flaps may be tacked to the chest wall as well. Absence of the fascia over the pectoralis muscle following radical mastectomy makes closure of the submuscular space more tenuous than in a delayed reconstruction. Closure is meticulously done with absorbable sutures.

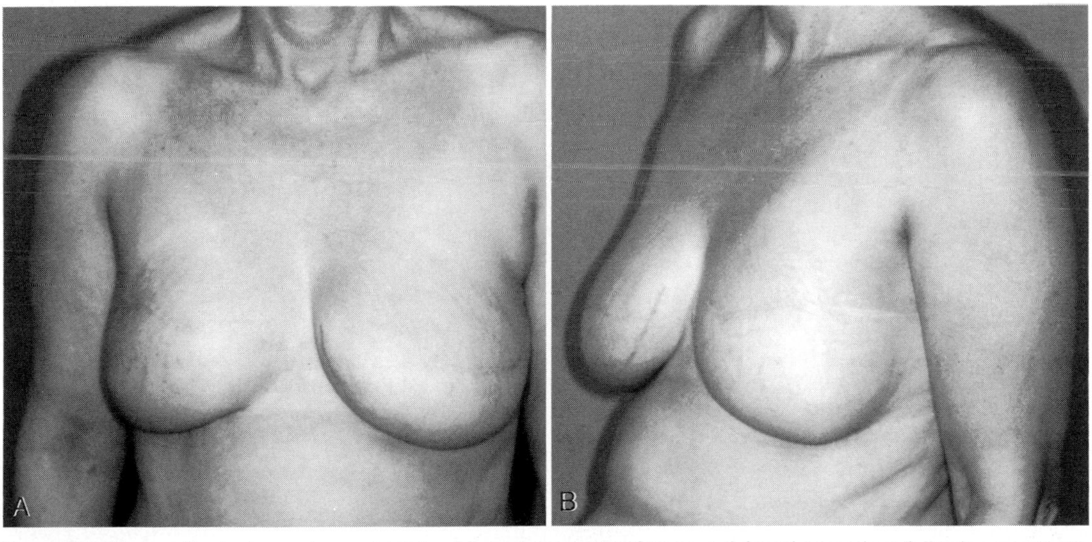

Figure 13–10. A patient who underwent bilateral breast reconstruction as a delayed procedure following mastectomy. 700 ml prostheses were expanded over eight weeks and left in place for four months. Using the technique illustrated in Figure 13–8, ptotic and cosmetically acceptable breasts were reconstructed using 480 ml permanent implants. *A,* Frontal view. *B,* Oblique view.

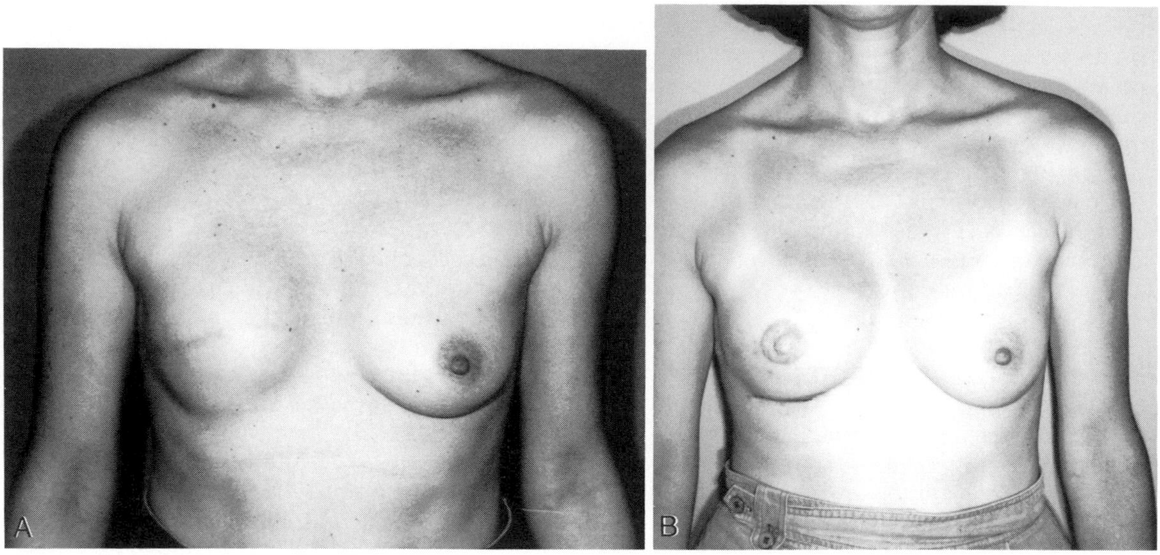

Figure 13–11. Immediate breast reconstruction was achieved by placing a tissue expander at the time of mastectomy. *A,* The prosthesis was expanded over two months. *B,* The patient five years after permanent implant placement and nipple reconstruction.

The inflation reservoir is situated in the subcutaneous tissue below the inframammary fold. Because lymphatic and serous collection often occurs in the axilla, the inframammary position is preferable in order to avoid migration of the filling reservoir; this fluid collects around the prosthesis and may serve as a nidus for infection. Antibiotics are given perioperatively and continued for at least one week postoperatively.

Two to three weeks after healing of the modified radical mastectomy, inflation can begin. Since a fresh wound is present, inflation should be carried out more cautiously than with delayed reconstruction. At biweekly intervals the prostheses are expanded until appropriate size and symmetry are achieved. The process is then identical to that outlined for delayed reconstruction.

Despite the most careful preoperative diagnostic efforts, metastatic disease may be found after mastectomy and placement of the expansion prostheses. Adjuvant chemotherapy is usually prescribed and need not be delayed. Inflation is carried out more slowly in these patients than in those not undergoing chemotherapy. A permanent implant is not placed until chemotherapy is completed. Radiation therapy may also be given with an expander in place if deemed necessary.

Permanent Expansion Prostheses

Several new prostheses designed to avoid a second procedure have been developed (Becker, 1984). The expanders are intended to remain in place as a permanent breast prosthesis after expansion has been accomplished. Initial experience with these devices has been favorable (Fig. 13–12). The prosthesis is placed in an identical position as in secondary or immediate breast reconstruction. The reservoir is usually located either below the brassiere line or in the axilla. The expander is inflated and hyperinflated by at least 200 ml for three months. The excess fluid is removed to create a more naturally ptotic breast.

In approximately 50 per cent of patients a second procedure to reposition the prosthesis or to redefine the inframammary fold is thus avoided. The expansion device is especially useful in women who have a minimally or mildly ptotic breast and whose inframammary fold is not well defined. The inflation reservoir and tubing may be removed in a brief office procedure under local anesthesia. It may not be necessary to consider removing the inflation reservoir if it is placed in the

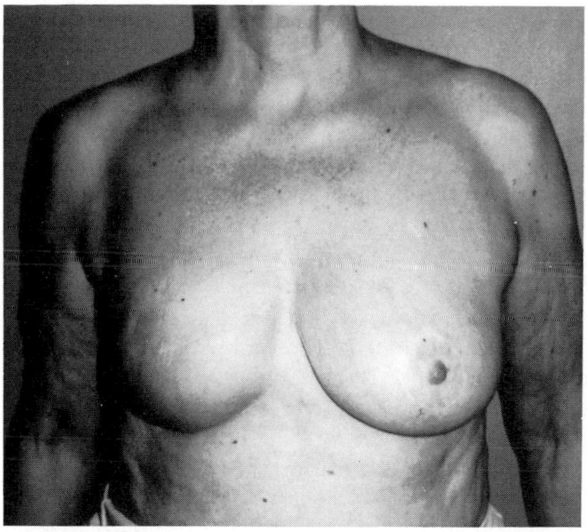

Figure 13–12. A 52 year old woman who underwent a right mastectomy with simultaneous placement of a Becker permanent expander. The prosthesis was expanded over one month and no other procedures have been performed.

axilla of a woman with sufficient subcutaneous tissue.

The long-term stability of these implants is unknown. In view of previous problems with spontaneous deflation of inflatable implants, the authors caution against describing them to patients as "permanent."

Reconstruction in Conjunction with Distant Flaps

Patients with inadequate or insufficient tissue of the chest wall may require a transfer of full-thickness tissue from elsewhere in the body (Fig. 13–13). The latissimus dorsi myocutaneous flap and the transverse rectus abdominis flap have become standard procedures for this type of reconstruction (see Chapter 79). Following removal of large areas of skin grafts or large areas of abnormal skin,

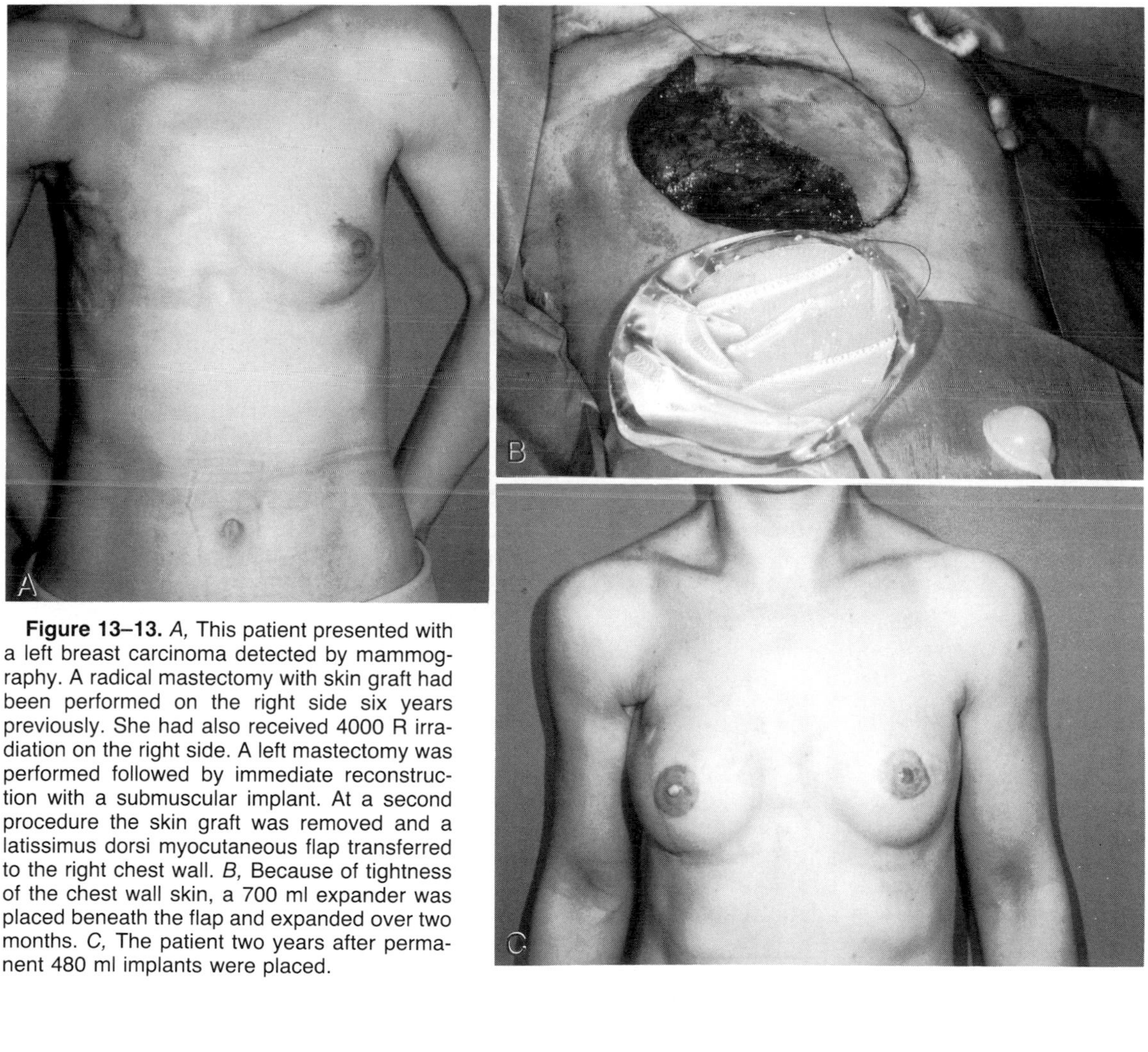

Figure 13–13. *A,* This patient presented with a left breast carcinoma detected by mammography. A radical mastectomy with skin graft had been performed on the right side six years previously. She had also received 4000 R irradiation on the right side. A left mastectomy was performed followed by immediate reconstruction with a submuscular implant. At a second procedure the skin graft was removed and a latissimus dorsi myocutaneous flap transferred to the right chest wall. *B,* Because of tightness of the chest wall skin, a 700 ml expander was placed beneath the flap and expanded over two months. *C,* The patient two years after permanent 480 ml implants were placed.

the amount of skin transferred in a flap may be insufficient to achieve symmetry with the opposite side. Expansion prostheses have been placed beneath the latissimus dorsi as well as the transverse rectus abdominis flaps when additional volume is necessary.

Congenital Breast Abnormalities

Maldevelopment of the breast may have numerous causes. Bilateral hyperplasia and bilateral hypoplasia are often related to systemic factors. Diagnosis of their etiology requires appropriate consultation with pediatricians, endocrinologists, or gynecologists. Unilateral hypoplasia may likewise be due to multiple factors, including injury to the breast from radiation or surgical misadventure, trauma, or Poland's syndrome. The cause of most cases of unilateral hypoplasia, however, remains unknown. The severity may vary from extreme hypoplasticity of the breast and adjacent structures, as occurs in Poland's syndrome, to a slightly hypoplastic breast that does not require treatment.

These patients have a small nipple-areola complex that remains in a cephalad position. Tissue expanders have allowed reconstruction for such patients by mimicking normal development of the breast (Argenta, Marks, and Pasyk, 1985).

TREATMENT OF THE MATURE BREAST

In the normal female, full breast development has usually been achieved by 18 to 19 years of age. Hormonal changes, weight gain, or pregnancy may result in later changes in volume or shape of the breast. If the asymmetry is minor and the nipple-areola complex is in a normal position, augmentation of the affected side in combination with a ptosis correction or reduction of the normal side often allows symmetry. In moderate to severe cases, however, expansion of the hypoplastic side allows not only the achievement of volumetric symmetry but also the development of a more normally positioned nipple-areola complex.

In severe cases, a tissue expander can be placed through either an inframammary or an axillary incision into the submuscular space. The prosthesis is gradually expanded until volumetric symmetry is achieved. During this process the nipple-areola complex not only is increased in diameter, but over time is moved inferiorly to assume a more normal (mature) position. Overinflation allows development of additional ptosis. The expander should be left in place for at least three to four months after overinflation has been achieved. The weight of the saline prosthesis permits development of a more pendulous breast to achieve symmetry with the opposite side (Fig. 13–14).

At a second procedure the permanent implant is placed. An incision can be made either in the inframammary fold or through the axilla. The expander is removed and the capsule of the expander incised if repositioning of the prosthesis is necessary. An appropriate permanent prosthesis is placed.

TREATMENT OF THE IMMATURE BREAST

Many young females with significant breast asymmetry present in early adolescence. Social pressures placed upon an adolescent female, in combination with the awareness of a developing physique, can cause severe psychologic conflict. She may refuse to participate in athletics and may avoid summer clothing. Placement of an expansion prosthesis beneath the hypoplastic breast has allowed correction of many of these deformities early in adolescence.

A small axillary incision is used to develop a plane behind the pectoralis muscle. A 700 ml round prosthesis is placed beneath the muscle and positioned beneath the hypoplastic breast, with the inflation reservoir placed high in the axilla on the thoracic wall. At three to six month intervals the prosthesis is inflated to maintain symmetry with the growth of the normal breast. The nipple-areola complex gradually enlarges and is displaced caudally to a more normal position. No activity restraints are placed on the patient during this period.

When the patient reaches approximately 19 years of age, the expander is removed and a permanent prosthesis is placed. The procedure performed is similar to that previously described for correction of the mature breast.

CORRECTION OF POLAND'S SYNDROME

Poland's syndrome involves maldevelopment not only of the breast but also of other

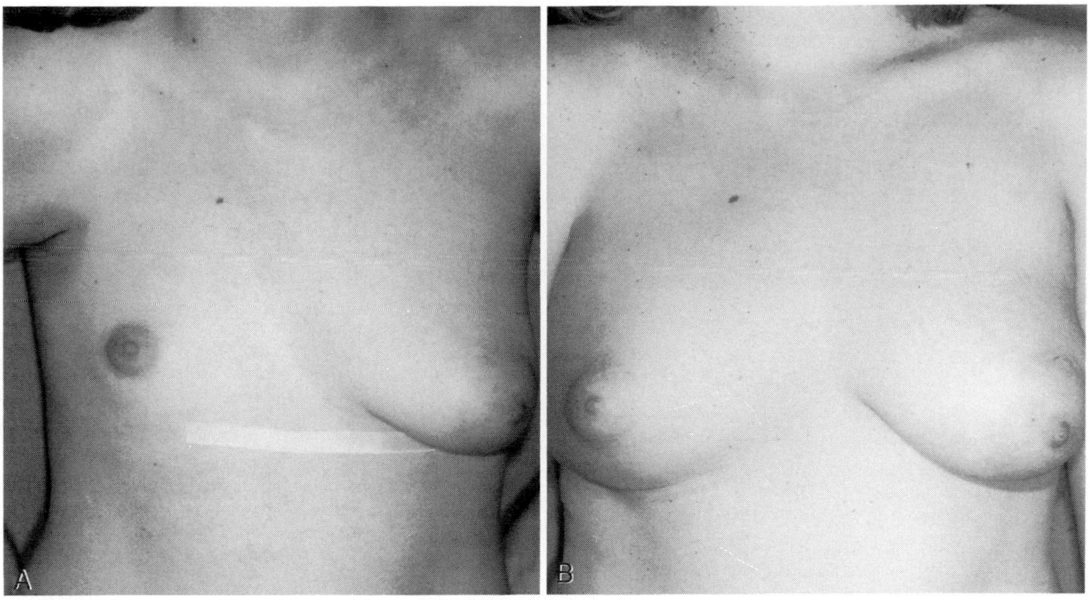

Figure 13–14. *A,* A 19 year old woman with Poland's syndrome had completed growth of the normal breast. To correct the deformity an expander was placed through the axilla and expanded to 500 ml. Six months later the implant was removed and the latissimus muscle transferred over a 300 ml permanent prosthesis. *B,* The breast has remained soft and symmetric. The nipple has moved to a more mature position and is of normal size. (From Argenta, L., Vanderkolk, C., Friedman, R., and Marks, M.: Refinements in reconstruction of congenital breast deformities. Plast. Reconstr. Surg., *76*:76, 1985.)

anatomic structures. The pectoralis muscle may be absent along with other muscles of the thorax. Subcutaneous tissue on the affected side is frequently hypoplastic, and bony chest wall deformities may occur secondary to the abnormal stresses placed upon the thorax by the asymmetric musculature.

In the *mature* female, expansion allows for translocation of the nipple caudally and development of an adequate skin envelope to achieve symmetry with the opposite side (see Fig. 13–14). Overinflation is useful to develop ptosis. At the time at which the permanent implant is placed, transfer of the latissimus dorsi muscle to cover the prosthesis and create an anterior axillary fold is possible. A small incision on the anterior border of the latissimus dorsi is adequate both to expose and transpose the muscle and to place the permanent implant. At the same operation and through the same incision, contouring of ribs can be performed to achieve better symmetry. The costochondral junctions are frequently flared, and to achieve adequate projection of the breast, removal of some of the cartilage is helpful. In severe chest wall deformities, additional implants or transfer of a transverse rectus abdominis myocutaneous flap may be required to correct the underlying abnormality (see also Chap. 79).

In the *immature* female with Poland's syndrome, the expanders are placed through a small incision in the axilla and inflated gradually until the patient is approximately 19 years of age. The technique followed is the same as that used for the immature breast, previously described. After the patient has achieved maturity, the latissimus dorsi muscle is transferred and a permanent implant is placed (Fig. 13–15). Some authors feel that early transfer of the latissimus dorsi muscle may be beneficial in minimizing subsequent development of a chest wall deformity. However, there have been only a few cases in which the latissimus dorsi has been transferred early in life, and this technique is not yet recommended.

THE TUBEROUS BREAST

Unilateral or bilateral tuberous breast deformity may result in asymmetric, hypoplastic, and irregularly shaped breasts. When the abnormality becomes apparent, it is useful to place an expander beneath the abnormal breast, making an incision in the inframam-

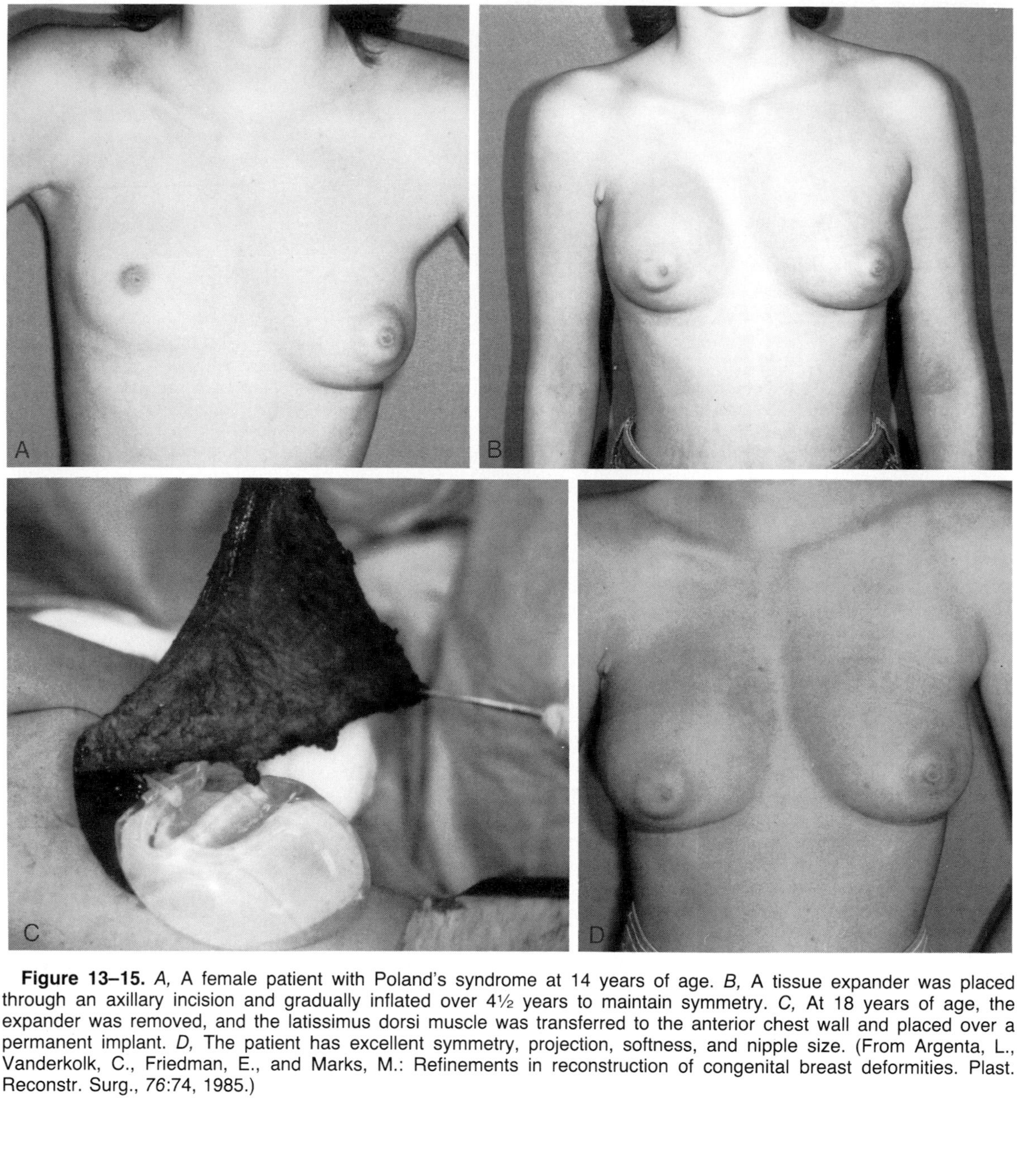

Figure 13–15. *A,* A female patient with Poland's syndrome at 14 years of age. *B,* A tissue expander was placed through an axillary incision and gradually inflated over 4½ years to maintain symmetry. *C,* At 18 years of age, the expander was removed, and the latissimus dorsi muscle was transferred to the anterior chest wall and placed over a permanent implant. *D,* The patient has excellent symmetry, projection, softness, and nipple size. (From Argenta, L., Vanderkolk, C., Friedman, E., and Marks, M.: Refinements in reconstruction of congenital breast deformities. Plast. Reconstr. Surg., *76*:74, 1985.)

mary area or the axilla. Since the nipple-areola complex in these patients is often abnormally large, it is best to avoid incisions in the areola at this time. No attempt to reduce the size of the nipple complex should be made before or during expansion. After an adequate skin envelope has been developed and a permanent implant placed, the nipple-areola complex can be reduced to an appropriate size.

SCALP RECONSTRUCTION

Tissue expansion has become the method of choice for reconstruction of major scalp defects (Manders and associates, 1985; Anderson and Argenta, 1987). It is the only procedure that allows the development of relatively normal hair-bearing tissue to cover areas of alopecia. Tissue expansion allows closure of large defects in a shorter time than previously required with multiple procedures and many serial excisions.

Correction of Post-traumatic Alopecia

Areas of alopecia may result from traumatic, thermal, radiation, neoplastic, or infective processes (see also Chap. 31). Tissue expanders have been useful in correcting these defects. The process of tissue expansion results in a redistribution of the remaining hair follicles. New follicles are *not* created in the process. Individual hair follicles may be separated by a factor of 2 without producing a noticeable thinning. Blondes and redheads may undergo even more expansion without creating visible thinness of the hair.

To achieve homogenous distribution of hair follicles, as much of the remaining normal scalp as possible should be expanded. Consideration must be given to the normal areas of the scalp that remain, as well as to previous scars and incisions. Careful planning for the creation of advancement or transposition flaps is essential to achieve optimal results. Multiple expanders around the defect are helpful in creating maximal scalp expansion in the shortest time (Fig. 13–16).

The prostheses are best placed through small incisions at the margins of the defect and normal scalp. The dissection is extended to the subgaleal plane and wide undermining is performed bluntly. The dissected pocket should be sufficiently large to accommodate the prosthesis so that its edge does not abut the suture line. Proper placement of the inflation reservoir is important in order that there is no inordinate pressure when the patient is sleeping. Complications may be expected when attempts are made to place the reservoir beneath existing skin grafts.

The scalp extends from the brows to the occiput and on each side to the ear. Expansion of the forehead and manipulation of the junction of the forehead and scalp can be useful, especially in the reconstruction of large defects. The forehead surface area can be increased or decreased 10 to 15 per cent without its being significantly visible if coverage of the scalp becomes difficult.

Initial inflation usually produces transient discomfort. Small amounts of saline can be placed in the first several injections. Following this, a significant loosening of the galea occurs and large amounts of saline can be infused without difficulty. Inflation to over 1000 ml has been carried out in both adults and children. Most scalp expansion can be accomplished in six to eight weeks (Figs. 13–17, 13–18).

After adequate expansion the prostheses are removed through the original incisions at the junction of the defect and the normal scalp. As much of the scalp as possible is undermined so that rotation and manipulation of the remaining scalp can be achieved for a homogeneous distribution of hair follicles. Any type of advancement, transposition, or rotation flap can be employed after expansion. The increased blood flow after expansion allows the design of much larger flaps. Wounds are closed with permanent monofilament sutures, which are left in place for at least three weeks to minimize scalp retraction. Some scalp retraction can be expected to occur, especially when extensive expansion has been performed.

Serial expansion of the scalp may be necessary in young patients or when large areas of the scalp have been lost. In these patients, expansion is carried out until the overlying tissue becomes excessively thinned. Flaps are then advanced as far as possible to remove some of the area of alopecia, which is excised only after the surgeon is certain that that flap can cover that area. The expander can be left in place, and after a period of several months the scalp can be reexpanded (Fig. 13–

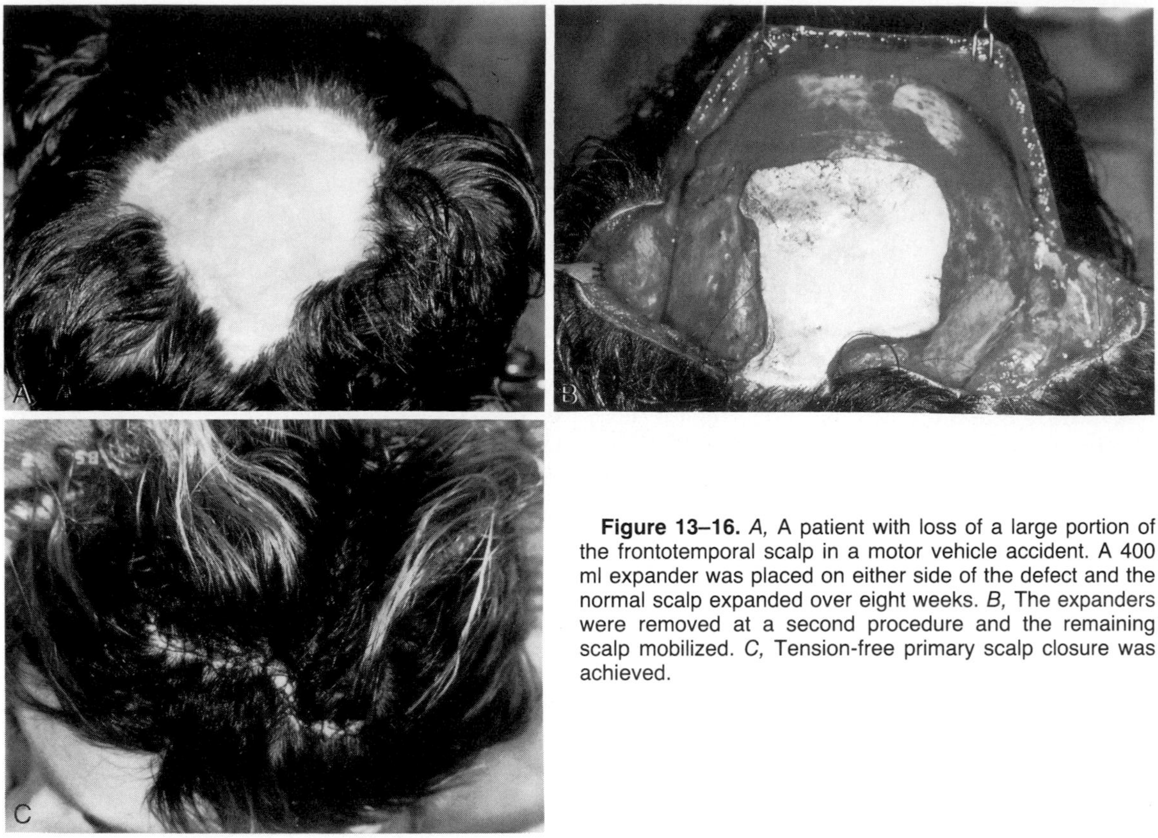

Figure 13–16. *A,* A patient with loss of a large portion of the frontotemporal scalp in a motor vehicle accident. A 400 ml expander was placed on either side of the defect and the normal scalp expanded over eight weeks. *B,* The expanders were removed at a second procedure and the remaining scalp mobilized. *C,* Tension-free primary scalp closure was achieved.

19). In young children the scalp becomes thin during extended expansion and it may be necessary to wait six to eight months for a second expansion. Serial expansion of the same tissue can be carried out several times without difficulty.

Long-term results have been most satisfactory. There is widening of the scar over time, particularly in children. Occasionally the scalp that has been vigorously expanded loses the hair follicles for several months. At least four to six months should be allowed to pass before removal of any area of scalp in which it appears that hair follicles have failed to grow.

Treatment of Male Pattern Baldness

Tissue expansion has become an important adjunctive procedure in the treatment of male pattern baldness (Adson, Anderson, and Argenta, 1987; Anderson, 1987). Previous techniques such as scalp reduction and rotation of hair-bearing flaps can be used in conjunction with tissue expansion to achieve optimal and often dramatic results (see also Chap. 31).

In patients with vertex baldness, in whom scalp reduction may be conventional treatment, tissue expansion significantly expedites reconstruction. Expansion of the remaining temporal and occipital hair can achieve in two months what may previously have required multiple scalp reduction procedures. Expanders are placed through incisions that would be used for scalp reduction. As with all types of scalp expansion, some deformity and discomfort occur. Full expansion requires six to eight weeks. The cosmetic deformity is minimal during the first three weeks, but may become significant at the fourth week or later.

Serial expansion for scalp reduction may be indicated in some patients who are unable to accept the deformity that becomes apparent with one-stage expansion. In such pa-

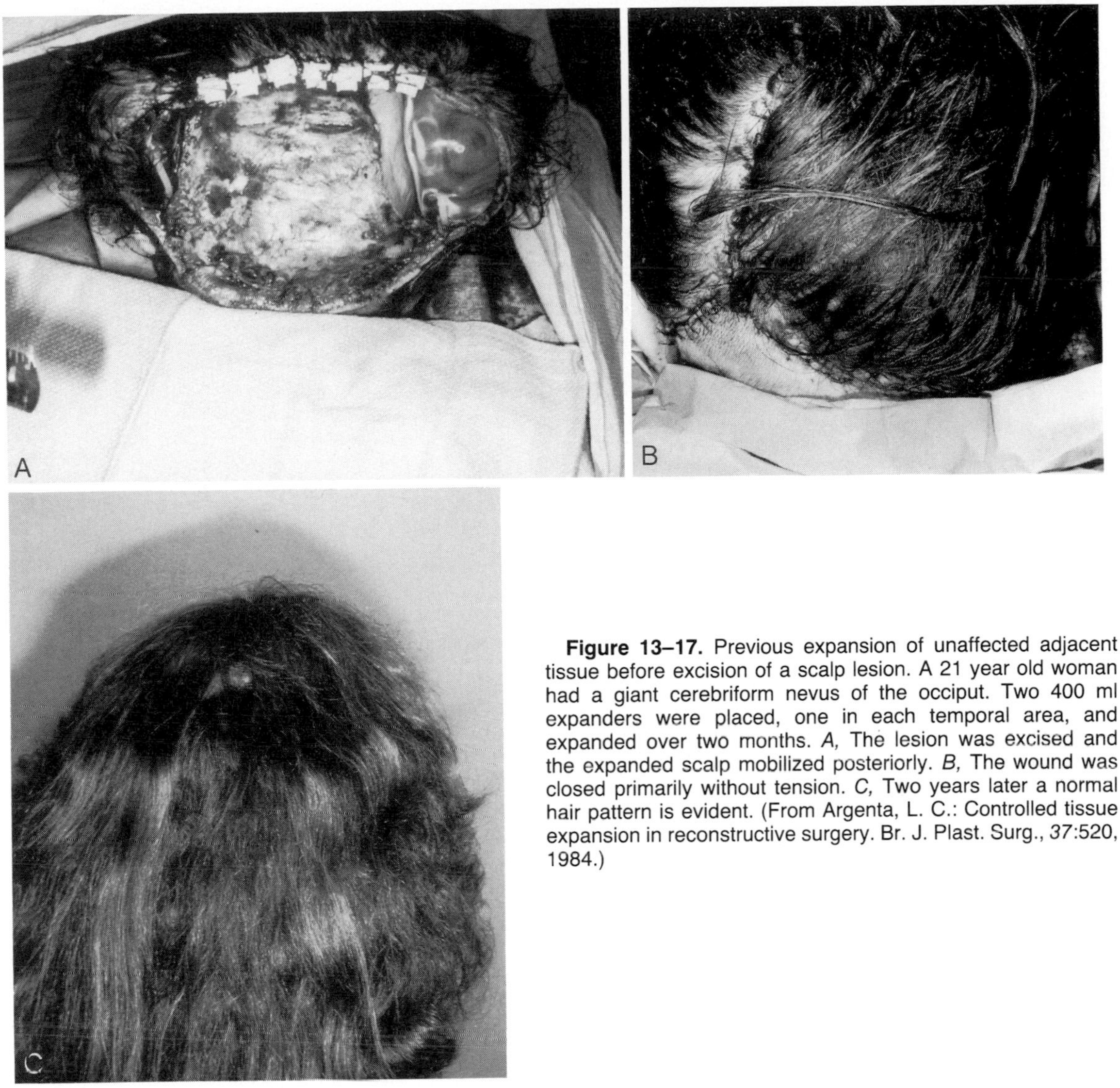

Figure 13–17. Previous expansion of unaffected adjacent tissue before excision of a scalp lesion. A 21 year old woman had a giant cerebriform nevus of the occiput. Two 400 ml expanders were placed, one in each temporal area, and expanded over two months. *A,* The lesion was excised and the expanded scalp mobilized posteriorly. *B,* The wound was closed primarily without tension. *C,* Two years later a normal hair pattern is evident. (From Argenta, L. C.: Controlled tissue expansion in reconstructive surgery. Br. J. Plast. Surg., *37*:520, 1984.)

tients the prostheses are inflated until deformity becomes visible. The expanders are deflated and the hair-bearing flaps advanced as far in a cephalad direction as possible. The prostheses are left in place, and a second or even third expansion is carried out until the entire bald area is removed.

Patients with anterior baldness present a special problem. Expansion and simple advancement of the remaining temporal scalp results in a straight, unnatural hairline. Transposition flaps to create an anterior hairline are helpful in developing a more pleasing result. Standard Juri temporoparietal flaps are limited in size and require multiple delays (Juri and Juri, 1982). Expanders may be used to expand the temporal area and a very large Juri flap may be developed. These flaps are transposed to create an anterior hairline. Bilateral flaps may be placed one behind the other to cover a larger area.

Detailed planning of such flaps is critical to their success. Flaps are outlined on the hair-bearing scalp and an incision is made along the most cephalad margin of the flap. The prostheses are placed beneath the galea. When full expansion has been achieved, the prostheses are removed through the original incision, which becomes one of the edges of the flap. Very wide flaps can be created by

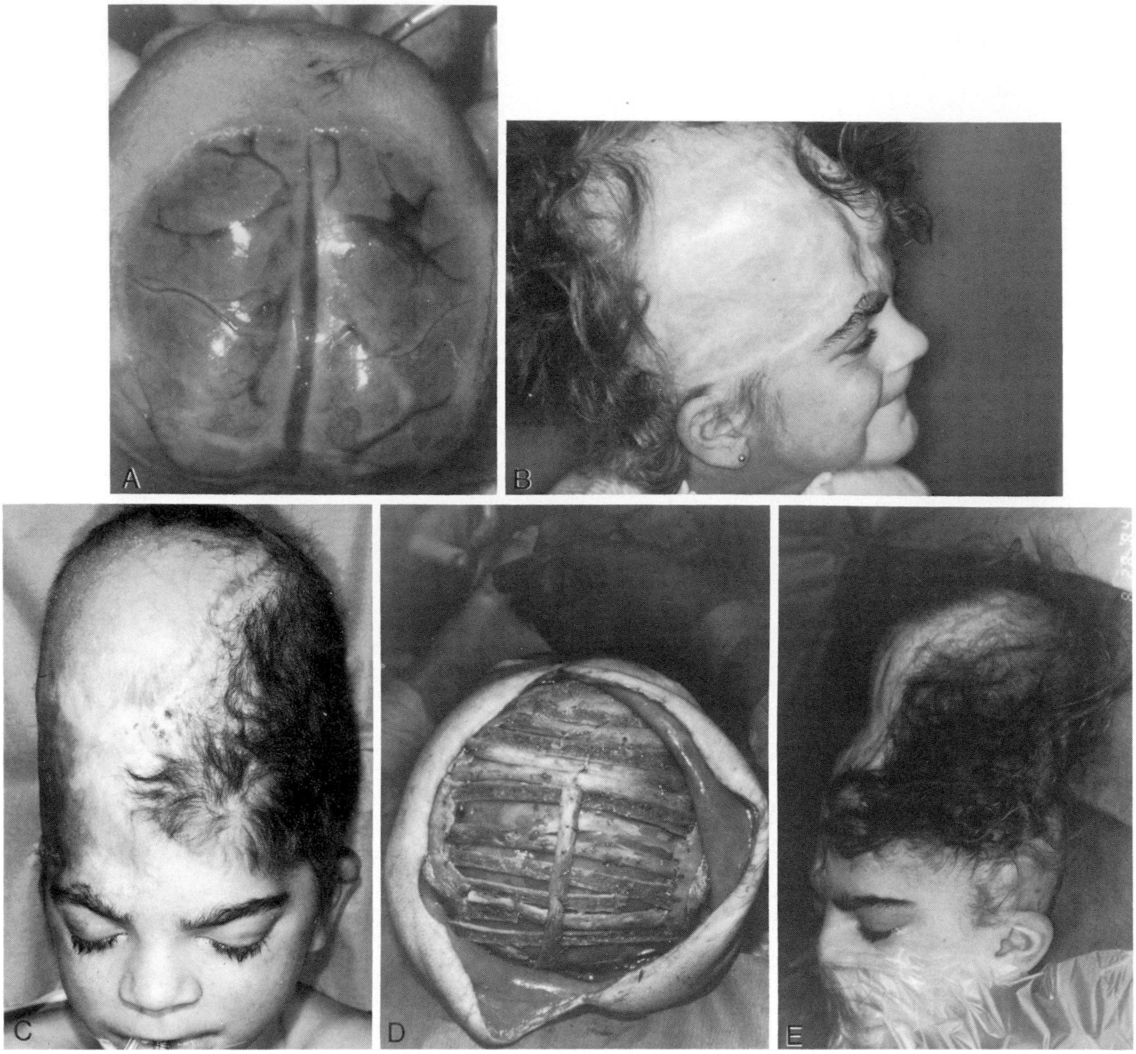

Figure 13–18. *A,* An infant with severe aplasia cutis congenita involving the scalp, skull, and dura. *B,* The brain was covered at birth by two large scalp-forehead advancement flaps. Absence of the cranium prevented the patient from attending school. *C,* The flaps were separated from the underlying brain; a reinforced polyethylene sheet was secured across the cranial defect; and an expander was placed over the sheet. The scalp was expanded over three months. *D,* The cranium was reconstructed with multiple split rib grafts within the expanded capsule. *E,* One year later the scalp was reexpanded to over 1000 ml to remove the skin grafts and reconstruct the forehead and scalp.

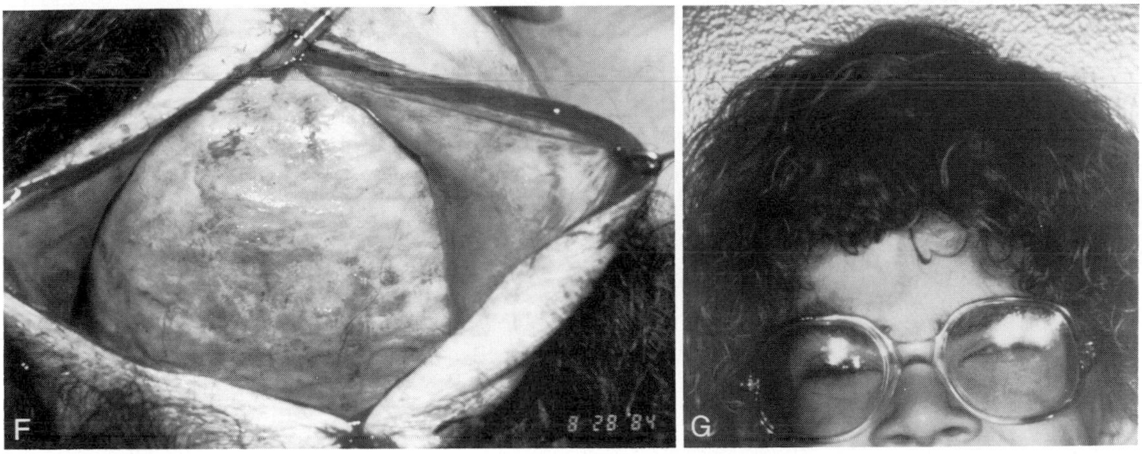

Figure 13–18 *Continued F,* The reconstructed skull suffered no ill effects during reexpansion. *G,* One year postoperatively the patient has an intact skull with normal scalp and forehead coverage.

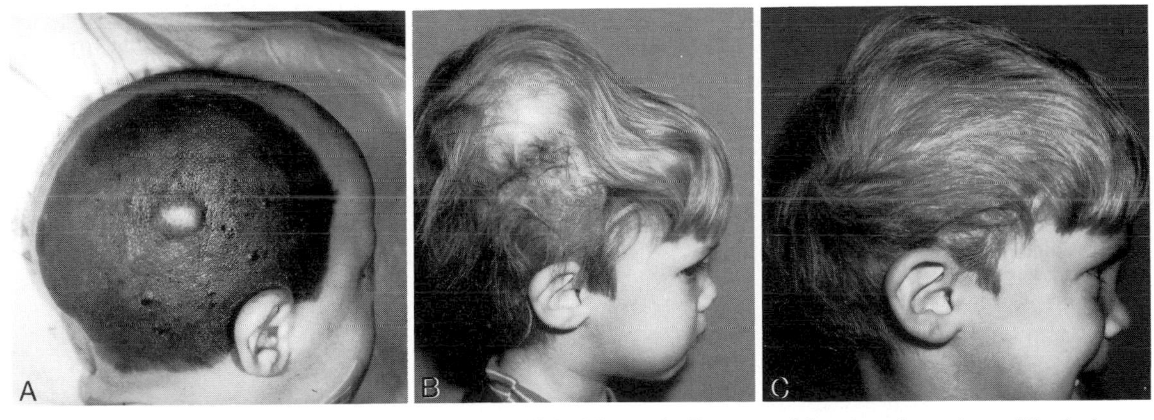

Figure 13–19. *A,* A child born with a nevus of one-third of the scalp. Because of the changing nature of the lesion on biopsy, excision was undertaken. At two years the normal scalp was expanded, allowing removal of one-half of the lesion. The expander was left in place and four months later reexpanded. *B,* The patient is shown after 400 ml of saline had been instilled. *C,* Advancement of the scalp after the second expansion allowed removal of almost all the lesion.

means of this technique, with primary closure of the donor site. The remaining expanded scalp is advanced in a cephalad direction to replace other areas of alopecia.

FACE RECONSTRUCTION

Many different types of skin exist on the face. Esthetic reconstruction is best achieved by mobilization of local tissue rather than by the transfer of distant tissue that does not match in color, texture, or hair-bearing capability. Tissue expansion allows excellent reconstruction by use of a specifically matched donor area to reconstruct a defect (Argenta, Watanabe, and Grabb, 1983; Argenta, 1984a,b).

The skin of the face can be divided into three specific areas. The *forehead and nose* are covered by thick skin that contains a large number of sebaceous glands and little hair. The *neck, upper lip, and cheek area* has fewer sebaceous glands; the skin is thinner; and the hair pattern is significantly different in quality and quantity from that on the remainder of the body. The *skin of the periorbital areas* is extremely thin and pliable, and contains a minimal number of sebaceous glands.

There is a limited amount of tissue on the human face, so it is essential that any procedure be performed correctly the first time. Consideration should be given to the area of the defect, the quality of the remaining tissue, existing scars, and possible future reconstructive needs. Possible secondary alternatives should also be planned before the placement of the prosthesis is undertaken.

Expansion prostheses in the face and neck are placed in the subcutaneous space. Because of the relative thinness of the overlying tissue, meticulous careful dissection for placement of the expansion prosthesis should always be accomplished under direct vision. Placing the prosthesis beneath the platysma muscle in the neck is useful to provide an extra layer of coverage (Fig. 13–20).

Reconstruction that requires the mobilization of expanded tissue to the area of the *eyelids and mouth* is particularly difficult. Since some degree of contraction does occur with expanded flaps, it is most important that the flaps be fixed to stable underlying tissue. Fixation to the infraorbital rim or the pyriform margin with permanent sutures is helpful (Fig. 13–21). To minimize the amount of flap retraction, the implant may be overexpanded and left in place for several weeks after expansion is completed (Fig. 13–22).

The *forehead* area is anatomically a portion of the scalp. Because of its lack of hair and vulnerability to injury, this region presents a particular problem. In conjunction with the adjacent scalp, however, it can be expanded with relative ease. Prostheses are placed beneath the frontalis muscle, since this plane is more easily dissected than a plane anterior to the muscle. Expansion may at first be difficult and uncomfortable. Like the scalp, however, a point is reached at which expansion proceeds rapidly. Flaps may be developed in any direction and are usually simple advancement flaps. In areas where tissue has been lost, the remaining forehead should be expanded to correct the defect (Fig. 13–23). If an inadequate amount of forehead remains, expansion of the adjoining scalp may be useful. A reduction of 15 to 20 per cent in the surface area of the forehead is not readily visible with appropriate hair styling (Fig. 13–24).

Vertical discrepancies of the forehead may also be corrected by tissue expansion in cases where an inadequate amount of non–hair-bearing tissue exists. This problem frequently occurs with various congenital abnormalities characterized by an abnormally low hairline. In these cases, the forehead is expanded and moved into a cephalad direction. The intervening hair-bearing scalp is excised. Fixation of the forehead to the underlying skull with several small wire sutures helps to reduce the amount of flap retraction.

Expansion of the frontalis muscle in conjunction with the scalp allows preservation of frontalis function. Cases have been described in which frontalis slings have been approximated to expanded tissue to correct ptosis (Fig. 13–25).

Total *nose* reconstruction may be facilitated by expansion of the forehead skin. Expansion allows development of large flaps and achieves primary closure of the forehead donor site without skin grafts. Since the color and texture match of the forehead are ideally suited to the nose, this procedure makes reconstruction of almost any nasal defect possible. Any of the standard forehead flaps may be employed in conjunction with the expander. If lining is also necessary, expansion of a Converse scalping flap (see Chap. 37) is

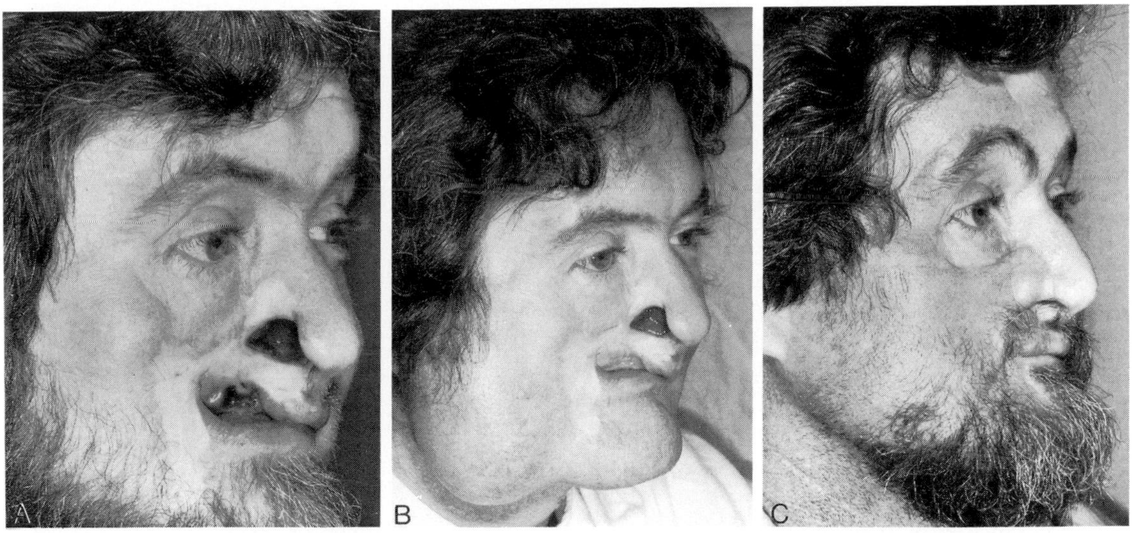

Figure 13–20. *A,* A male patient who underwent excision of a soft tissue sarcoma of the face and had no recurrence after five years. *B,* A 250 ml expander was placed in the right face and expanded over 12 weeks. The defect was reconstructed in one stage with a forehead flap to the nose, an Abbé flap from the lower to the upper lip, and advancement of the expanded cheek flap. *C,* Two years after reconstruction there is normal hair distribution over the face with a beard and mustache. (From Argenta, L. C., Watanabe, M. J., and Grabb, W. C.: The use of tissue expansion in head and neck reconstruction. Ann. Plast. Surg., *11*:31, 1983.)

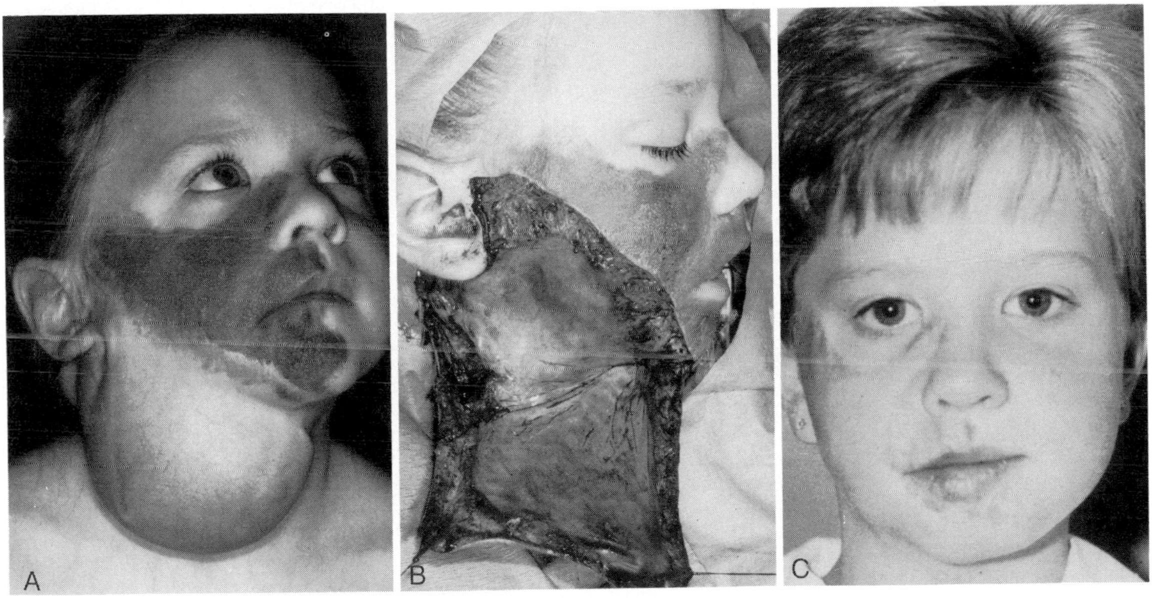

Figure 13–21. *A,* A 5 year old child with a giant hairy nevus of the face. The neck was expanded to 700 ml over two months (prosthesis placed below the platysma muscle). *B,* A large cheek rotation flap was mobilized using the expanded skin. The flap was sutured to the orbital rim after the nevus was removed, and the upper lip was reconstructed with a full-thickness skin graft. *C,* The patient five years after completion of expansion. There is no evidence of ectropion or retraction of the flap. (From Argenta, L. C.: Controlled tissue expansion in reconstructive surgery. Br. J. Plast. Surg., *37*:520, 1984.)

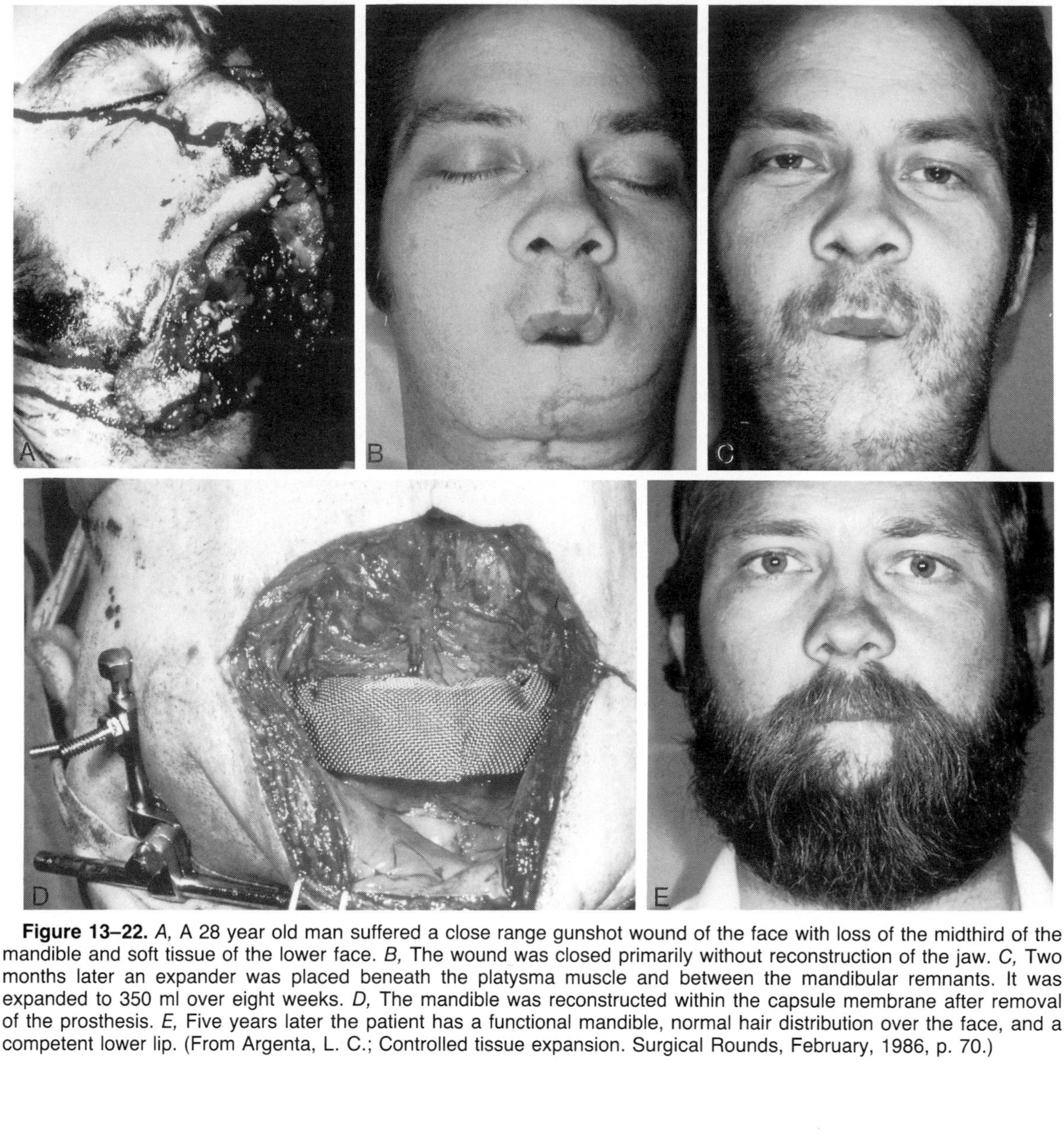

Figure 13–22. *A,* A 28 year old man suffered a close range gunshot wound of the face with loss of the midthird of the mandible and soft tissue of the lower face. *B,* The wound was closed primarily without reconstruction of the jaw. *C,* Two months later an expander was placed beneath the platysma muscle and between the mandibular remnants. It was expanded to 350 ml over eight weeks. *D,* The mandible was reconstructed within the capsule membrane after removal of the prosthesis. *E,* Five years later the patient has a functional mandible, normal hair distribution over the face, and a competent lower lip. (From Argenta, L. C.; Controlled tissue expansion. Surgical Rounds, February, 1986, p. 70.)

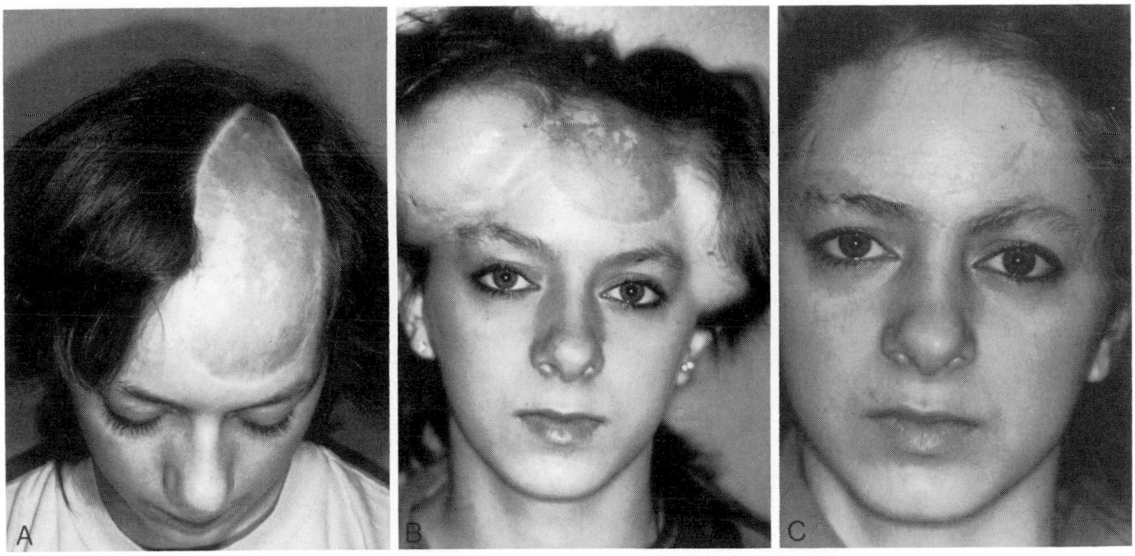

Figure 13–23. *A,* A 15 year old girl suffered an avulsion injury of the forehead and scalp as a child. An unstable skin graft covered the skull and forehead. *B,* Expanders were placed on either side of the defect to expand the scalp and the forehead. 450 ml of saline were instilled over two months. *C,* Advancement flaps of the expanded skin allowed closure with an excellent cosmetic result. (From Argenta, L. C.: Controlled tissue expansion. Surgical Rounds, February, 1986, p. 69.)

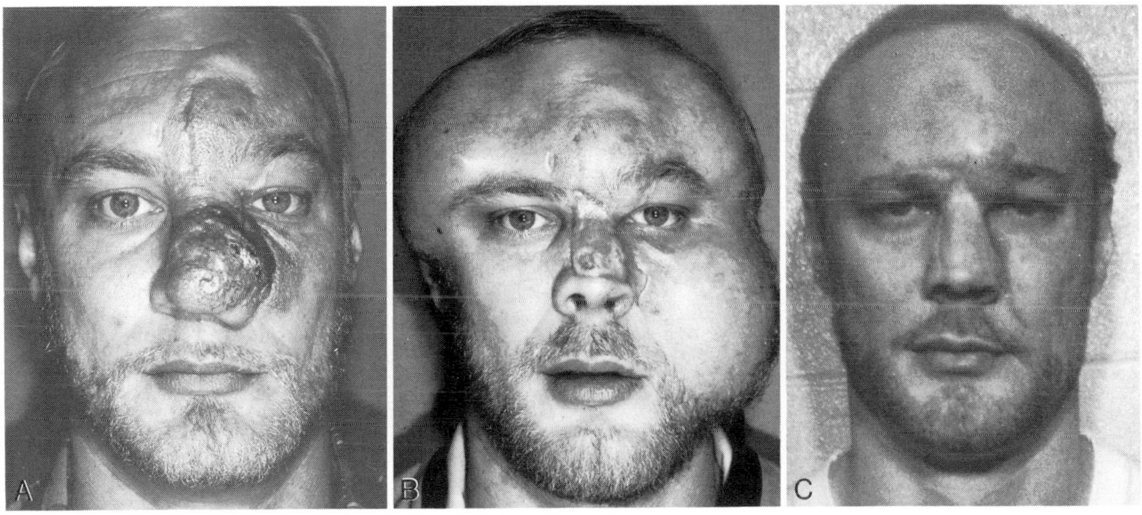

Figure 13–24. *A,* An ulcerating hemangioma of the central third of the face. The lesion of the nose was excised and skin grafted over a transferred pericranial flap. *B,* Three expanders were placed, two in the forehead and one in the cheek, and expanded over ten weeks. The lesion was totally excised and the expanded flaps advanced. *C,* Result two years postoperatively shows no distortion of the face or eyelids. (Reproduced by permission from Argenta, L. C., Watanabe, M. J., and Grabb, W. C.: The use of tissue expansion in head and neck reconstruction. Ann. Plast. Surg., *11*:31, 1983.)

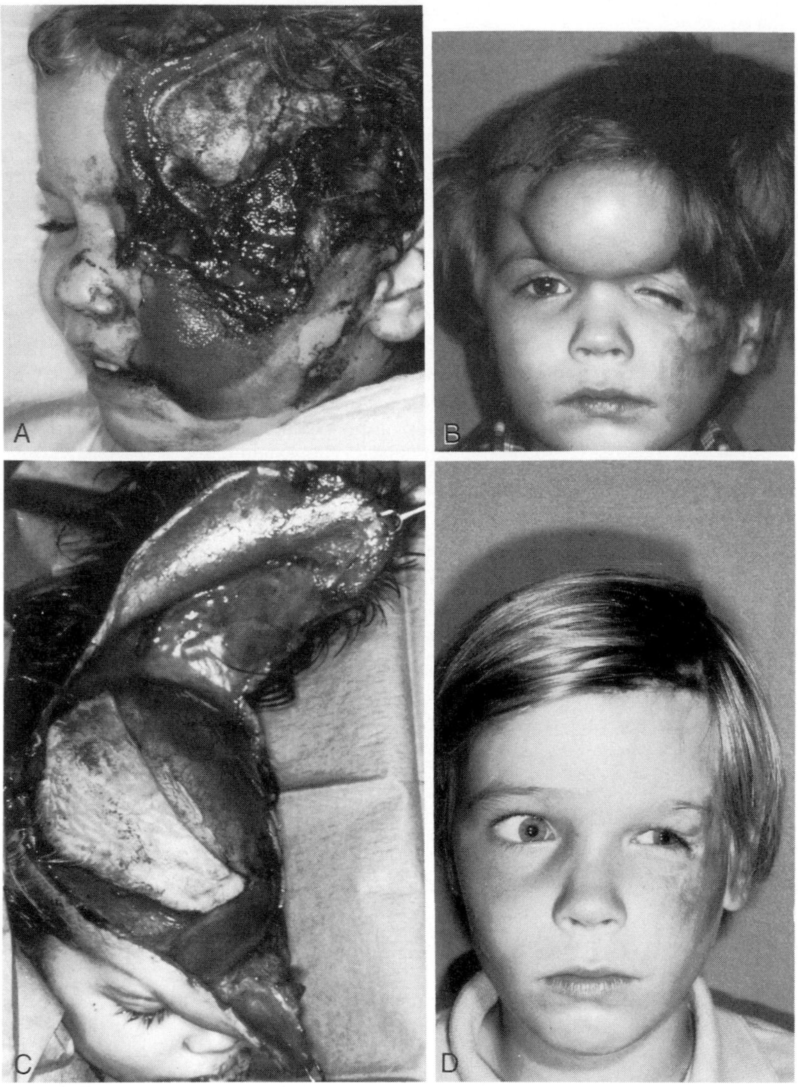

Figure 13–25. *A,* A child who suffered extensive soft tissue loss of the forehead, scalp, and lateral eyelid. An occipitally based scalp flap was used to close the defect primarily. *B,* Three months after the injury three expanders were placed under the remaining forehead and scalp. *C,* After expansion over two months, the prostheses were removed and the expanded scalp and forehead used to resurface the defect. *D,* Appearance six months after surgery. The patient is able to overcome a post-traumatic ptosis with a sling of the expanded and advanced frontalis muscle attached to the left upper lid.

particularly useful, since thinning of the resulting tissue allows folding of the expanded tissue upon itself. Prostheses are usually placed through a transcoronal incision beneath the frontalis muscle and galea, and expanded over four to six weeks until adequate tissue is developed. The forehead flap is based on a supraorbital or supratrochlear vessel. If large amounts of lining are necessary, the flap can be carried into the hairline and the hair follicles excised when the flap is thinned. The flap is transposed into position and the donor site closed primarily. Occasionally the scalp or remaining forehead must be undermined to achieve a tension-free reconstruction (Fig. 13–26).

Contraction of the expanded tissue occurs after the forehead flap has been transferred. It is important that there be an adequate underlying structure to maintain the projection and contour of the nose. Cartilage grafts (concha) are useful in reconstructing a nasal tip. The projection and size of the nose are maintained by incorporating a bone graft into the forehead flap at the time of flap rotation. Cranial bone grafts are thin and ideally suited for this purpose. They are securely wired to the remaining nasal bone. The flap is divided two weeks following rotation. Since swelling and retraction of tissue occur, secondary touch-up procedures are best deferred for at least several months. Nasal reconstruction is discussed in more detail in Chapter 37.

EAR RECONSTRUCTION

Most cases of microtia or post-traumatic ear deformity result in an inadequate amount of skin. As with all reconstructions of the ear, it is best to wait until the child is 4 to 5 years of age before beginning reconstruction. Custom tissue expanders are placed beneath the remaining non–hair-bearing tissue adjacent to the ear remnant. The expanders are gradually filled until an adequate amount of soft tissue is developed for placement of a custom-carved cartilage framework or silicone implant.

The expansion prosthesis is best placed through an incision in the posterior hair-bearing tissue. This allows preservation of the temporoparietal tissue for possible later reconstruction. A plane is developed around the remaining ear remnant. Particular care is taken to avoid the auditory canal. Expansion in this area usually takes eight to ten weeks, but in most cases sufficient soft tissue coverage can be developed for almost any reconstruction.

At a second procedure, the implant is removed and the framework of the ear reconstructed with carved costal cartilage or a

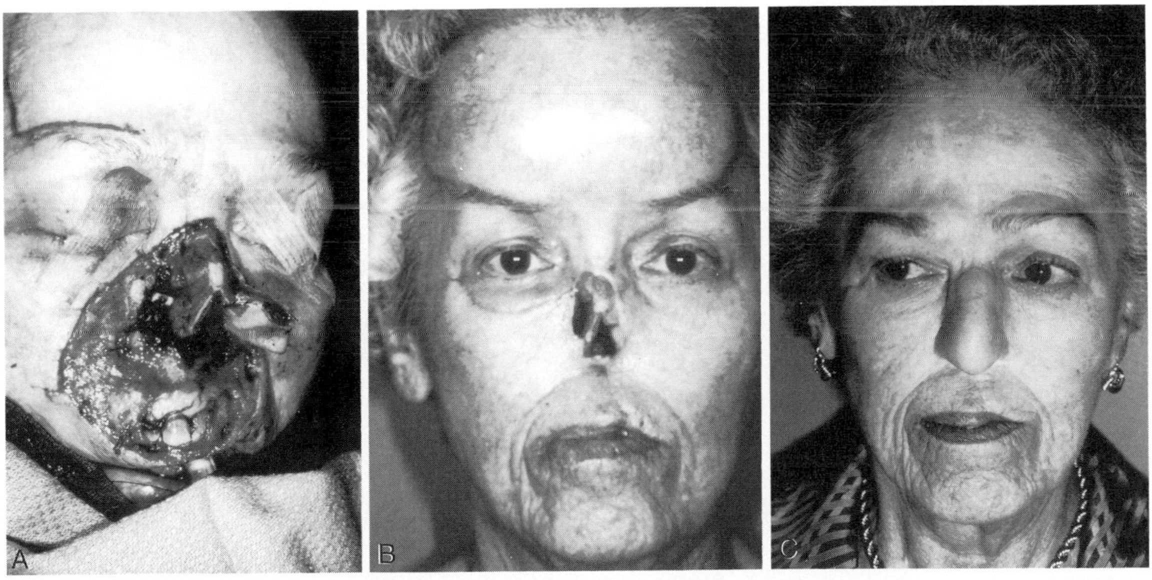

Figure 13–26. *A,* A patient who underwent resection of the nose, upper lip, medial cheek, and frontoethmoidal sinuses for a large microcystic adnexal carcinoma. The upper lip and face were reconstructed with cheek advancement flaps. *B,* A 400 ml expander was placed in the forehead and expanded over six weeks. *C,* An expanded forehead flap allowed reconstruction of the skin and lining of the nose over a cantilevered bone graft.

silicone prosthesis. When cartilage is used, the bulk of the infrastructure should be exaggerated to overcome some distortion, which may occur when the expanded tissue retracts. Overinflating the prosthesis and leaving the expander prosthesis in place for at least two months may help to overcome some of the problems with later retraction and distortion. In cases in which exposure or excessive thinness of the expanded skin occurs, a temporoparietal flap can be turned down over the cartilage graft to provide coverage. Silicone prostheses (ear framework) obviously should not be used when contamination of the expansion device has occurred. Ear reconstruction is discussed in more detail in Chapter 40.

EXPANSION TECHNIQUES OF THE TRUNK

The thorax and abdomen lend themselves to tissue expansion in individuals of all ages. The prostheses are usually placed through incisions in the margin of the defect above the fascia. Because of the large adjoining surface area from which tissue can be recruited, large prostheses can be placed and large flaps quickly expanded. Expansion can be performed over the abdominal wall without fear of compromise of internal structures. If contour defects are present, expansion can be carried out and the excess expanded tissue imbricated into the wound to correct a contour deformity.

Multiple expanders placed around a specific defect minimize distortion during expansion and more rapidly develop adequate amounts of tissue for completion of the procedure (Argenta, Marks, and Pasyk, 1985). Expansion of the trunk may produce sufficient deformity to affect the patient's day to day activities. Expansion of the back and buttock areas is particularly difficult for the patient because it interferes with sitting and sleeping. Fortunately, the expansion process can be rapidly expedited in these areas by inflating prostheses weekly or even twice a week (Fig. 13–27).

Particularly large deformities such as burns, giant hairy nevi, or other congenital abnormalities, may require multiple serial expansions to be carried out because of the area to be covered. In such cases, expanders are inflated maximally and the flap is advanced. Prostheses can be left in place and reexpansion carried out several weeks later. Multiple sequential expansions have been successfully performed without difficulty.

The chest and abdomen are particularly well suited for the development of myocutaneous flaps. Placement of expanders beneath the standard myocutaneous flap develops an extremely large flap in a short time. The increased vasculature associated with expansion allows a large adjacent random area to be carried with the original flap (Forte, Middleton, and Briant, 1985). Experimental studies have demonstrated that the vascular leash of such a flap remains intact and may in fact be elongated (Hong, Stark, and Futrell, 1987). Standard myocutaneous flaps such as the pectoralis and latissimus dorsi can be considerably increased to allow coverage of almost any defect of the hemithorax (Thornton and associates, 1987). Expanders of 1000 ml volume have been placed beneath the latissimus dorsi muscle and expanded to over 2000 ml without difficulty. The immense flaps generated can be transferred either as pedicle flaps or as free flaps. Such flaps have been used for reconstruction of extensive areas of osteoradionecrosis and recurrent chest wall tumors.

The latissimus dorsi myocutaneous flap can

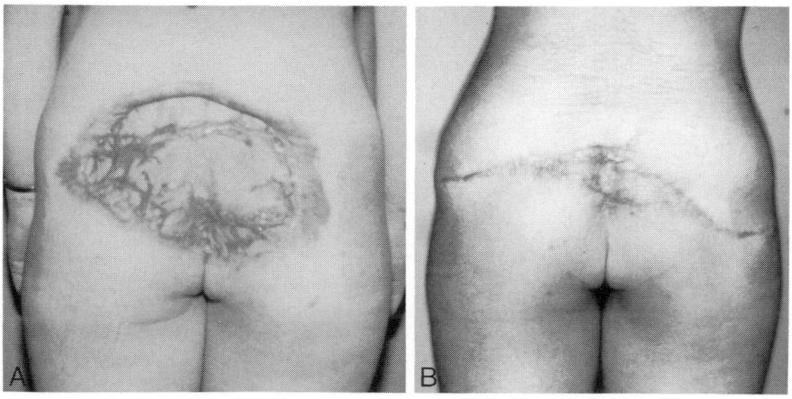

Figure 13–27. *A,* A woman who suffered a deep thermal burn to the buttocks area. The wound had been resurfaced with a skin graft. Two years after injury four large expanders were placed around the defect. *B,* The patient one year after removal of the expanders and advancement of sensate tissue.

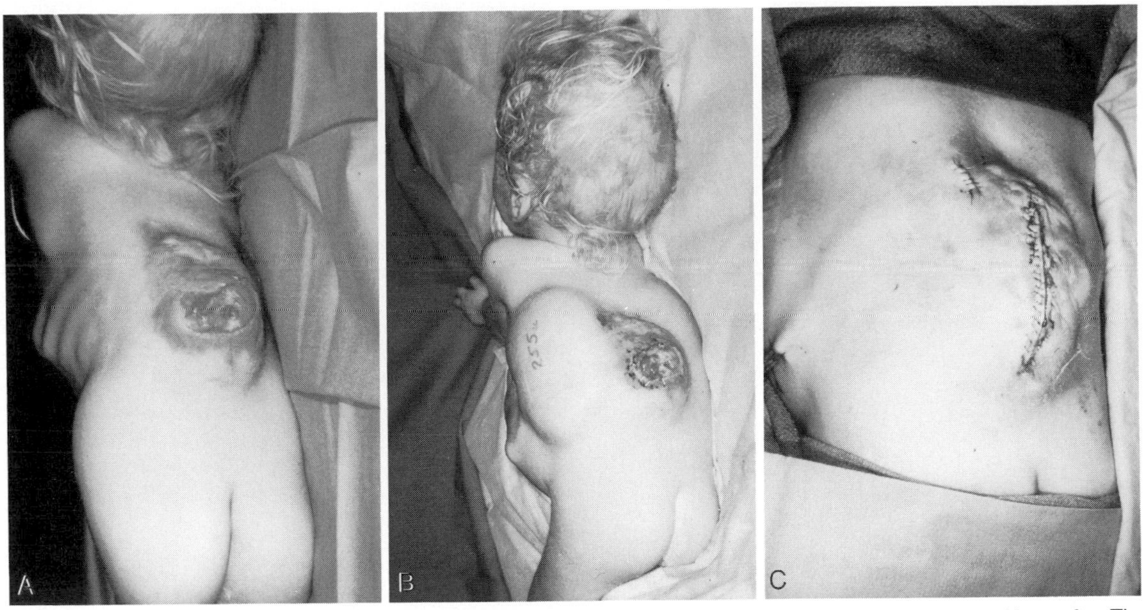

Figure 13–28. *A,* A child born with a large myelomeningocele that was covered with split-thickness skin grafts. The latter had broken down and the patient was referred for reconstruction. *B,* Expanders were placed beneath the latissimus dorsi muscle on each side. With daily inflations in the hospital expansion to 250 and 300 ml respectively was accomplished on either side without difficulty. *C,* At a second procedure the flaps were transposed primarily over the defect. The function of the latissimus dorsi muscle has been maintained.

be rapidly expanded bilaterally in children to cover large meningoceles (Fig. 13–28). The prostheses are placed beneath the latissimus dorsi muscle through incisions in the lateral margins of the muscle. After inflation, standard myocutaneous flaps are elevated on each side and transposed over the midline. Such flaps not only provide coverage without a donor defect but also preserve function of the muscle. Permanent sutures are used to fix the latissimus muscle and capsule to the vertebra to ensure a normal excursion of the muscle.

The deltopectoral and pectoralis major flap can be expanded rapidly to over 1000 ml volume. Such flaps allow coverage of the large areas of the chest wall or face in cases of tumor reconstruction. The thinness of the flap after expansion enhances the esthetic value of this flap. Expansion also allows primary closure of the chest wall donor defect, thus minimizing breast distortion and obviating the need for skin grafts.

EXPANSION TECHNIQUES OF THE EXTREMITIES

The skin and soft tissue of the extremities adapt well to tissue expansion (Gruss and MacKinnon, 1985). Tissue defects resulting from trauma, tumor, congenital abnormalities, tattoos, and irradiation injuries can be corrected. The capsule that develops adjacent to the expander provides a smooth gliding surface that can be transposed over joints and tendons to decrease tethering.

Defects of the extremity are best corrected by the placement of multiple expanders in a position axial to the defect (Fig. 13–29). Although expanders may be placed longitudinally on the arm or the leg, clinical experience has shown that a greater amount of expansion is necessary to achieve reconstruction. The use of multiple expanders has the advantages of rapid generation of tissue, less distortion of the extremities, and more comfort by distribution of the expansion forces.

Significant anatomic distortion of the underlying musculature in the arm and leg frequently occur during expansion, but function and strength are maintained. Patients are able to walk and use their upper extremities without difficulty during the process of expansion. Several cases of neuropraxia have been encountered in the lower extremity, particularly in the distribution of the sural nerve. Neuropraxia has been uncommon in the upper extremity even when expansion is carried out over major nerve branches. When

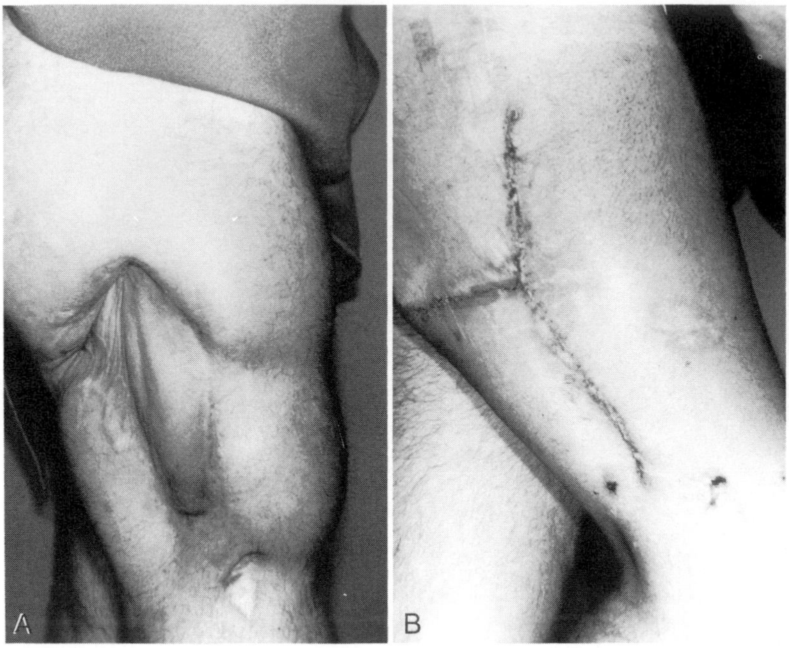

Figure 13–29. *A,* A young man who suffered a 10 by 19 cm avulsion injury of the lower extremity. Three expanders were placed around the defect and expanded over two months. *B,* After the expanders were removed, the flaps were advanced to cover the defect and achieve primary closure. Excess expanded tissue was deepithelized and buried to correct the contour defect. (From Argenta, L. C.: Controlled tissue expansion in reconstructive surgery. Br. J. Plast. Surg., *37*:528, 1984.)

neuropraxia occurs, it is best to deflate the prosthesis and reinflate at a slower rate. Custom expanders may be necessary in the upper extremity, particularly in the hand and finger areas. The dorsum of the hand lends itself well to expansion, whereas the volar surface is particularly painful and resistant to expansion.

Expanders have been used to correct single and multiple digit syndactyly. Successful expansion has been carried out in a significant number of patients and skin grafting avoided. In such cases, custom prostheses have been fabricated for the dorsal surface of finger syndactyly. A small incision is made on the dorsum of the hand and a tunnel created between the digits. Standard interdigitating Z-plasties are performed on the expanded tissue, as well as on the volar surface. In the cases of glove syndactyly, individual expanders between each digit are recommended. Staged division of the lateral most digits is recommended, the central digits being delayed until the vascularity to these digits has been ensured.

While the upper leg can be easily expanded, a significant number of complications have been encountered during inflation of tissue expanders below the knee. Isolated defects resulting from avulsion injuries or excision of tumors may be treated by expansion of adjacent tissue in a position axial to the defect. Multiple expanders are preferable to a single large device. When significant avulsion injury with compromise of adjacent lymphatics and vasculature has occurred, the risk of complications from tissue expansion rises significantly. Cellulitis and tissue compromise frequently occur during expansion in this area and are thought to be secondary to obstruction of the remaining lymphatic and blood flow in an already compromised lower extremity. *Myocutaneous and microvascular free flaps are recommended for reconstruction in this particularly difficult area.* The dorsum of the foot can be expanded with some difficulty. Care must be taken to avoid areas that have been excessively traumatized, and whose lymphatics and vascularity have been impaired. Lower extremity reconstruction is discussed in more detail in Chapter 82.

COMPLICATIONS

Initial attempts at tissue expansion are associated with a uniformly high complication rate. However, this decreases dramatically as more experience is gained by the individual surgeon (Manders and associates, 1984). Most complications of tissue expansion are relatively minor and usually do not interfere with successful completion of the procedure.

Implant Failure

Successive refinements in prosthesis design by manufacturers have markedly decreased the rate of mechanical failure. Implants marketed in the 1970's occasionally failed because of manufacturing defects. Implant failure is now rare and most prostheses are able to tolerate inflation up to three to five times their intended volume. Puncture of the prosthesis occurs most frequently with devices in which the inflation reservoir is incorporated into the main reservoir. Leakage from the inflation reservoir is uncommon if small gauge needles (23 gauge or smaller) are used. All prostheses should be tested before being placed into the patient.

Deflation is treated by replacement of the prosthesis. There is a significant decrease in the rate of mitosis of the overlying tissue after deflation (Austad, Thomas, and Pasyk, 1986). Replacement of the prosthesis is not an emergency and may be delayed several days without loss of significant amounts of the tissue that has been previously developed. If significant expansion has taken place before rupture, the generated tissue should be advanced with resurfacing of as much of the defect as possible. A new expander is then placed and serial expansion carried out.

Infection

Infection may occur, as with the placement of all kinds of prostheses in the human body. Perioperative introduction of infection is the most common cause and may be avoided by attention to sterile technique. Meticulous hemostasis, avoidance of drains when possible, and perioperative antibiotic therapy are all employed. The collection of body fluids around the implant, especially following excision of hemangiomas and lymphangiomas or in immediate breast reconstruction, exposes the patient to a higher risk of infection. Long-term antibiotic therapy is given if any collection of fluids around the prosthesis is anticipated. Late infection is the result of hematogenous contamination or invasion from adjacent contaminated wounds, or is iatrogenically caused. Inflation of the expansion prosthesis should be performed under sterile conditions in the office. Iodine solutions are used to sterilize the injection site.

The diagnosis of infection may be difficult since erythema does occur over the prosthesis following inflation. Persistent pain and warmth of the expansion site are indications that infection may be present. Since fluid around the infected prosthesis is in continuity with the inflation reservoir, cultures may be taken by aspirating around the inflation port.

If infection occurs in the perioperative period or early in the course of expansion, the prosthesis should be removed, the wound irrigated, and the procedure aborted. A second attempt may be made three to four months after healing has occurred. If infection occurs late in the course of expansion, the prosthesis can be removed and the expanded tissue advanced after copious irrigation of the infected cavity. Multiple flaps have been successfully rotated even though clinical infection of the prosthesis was apparent. Bone grafts and synthetic prostheses should never be placed after removal of an infected implant.

Implant Exposure

Exposure or extrusion of an expansion prosthesis is most often related to surgical error. Inadequate dissection or an excessively large prosthesis that abuts on the wound closure is the most frequent cause of early exposure. The prosthesis should be of such size that several centimeters of relatively normal tissue are not violated adjacent to the suture line. Substitution of a smaller prosthesis usually is not a problem if a larger prosthesis cannot be easily accommodated. Overinflation of a smaller prosthesis accomplishes the same result. Excessively rapid and overzealous inflation is the second most common cause of implant exposure. There are few situations in which rapid expansion is indicated. Since most expansion is carried out in situations in which there is an adequate amount of local tissue for an optimal reconstruction, it behooves the surgeon to proceed at a judicious rate. A third reason for implant extrusion is improper positioning of the implant. The best available adjacent tissue should be expanded for coverage of the defect. If local tissues are compromised but must be expanded, a higher risk of exposure can be anticipated. This is particularly true in cases of irradiated and burned tissues (Marks, Argenta, and Thornton, 1987). Implants placed on the lower extremity, back, and buttock area are particularly prone to trauma during normal daily activities. Exposure of the implant is frequent in these areas.

Treatment of the exposed implant depends on the degree to which exposure occurs and the amount of expansion that has been accomplished. If the implant becomes exposed early after placement, it is best to remove it and repeat the procedure three to four months later. If minimal or late exposure occurs, the procedure need not be aborted. A topical antibiotic cream is applied to the exposed implant and the area washed frequently. Expansion is continued as long as overt signs of infection do not occur. More frequent and smaller inflations may be helpful in overcoming tissue resistance. Temperature and white blood count levels are monitored; if these become elevated, the prosthesis is removed.

Compromise of Adjacent Structure

Expansion has been carried out in virtually all areas of the body. Impairment of adjacent nerve function is unusual except in the area of the sural nerve. Successful expansion has been carried out over the facial nerve, as well as the major nerves of the extremities, without difficulty. If neuropraxia becomes apparent, the prosthesis should be deflated and more gradual expansion accomplished later. If neuropraxia recurs, the prosthesis should be removed. Erosion of adjacent major blood vessels has not been encountered, although expansion has been carried out over the major vessels of the neck, upper extremity, and lower extremity. Aggressive expansion in a compromised host with underlying vascular disease should be avoided.

Flap Necrosis

Tissue expansion exerts changes in living tissue similar to the phenomenon of flap delay. Both expansion and delay result in an increase of blood vessels to the tissue, and there is accumulating evidence that these two types of flaps are similar in their sensitivity to epinephrine (Milton, 1969; Reinisch and Myers, 1974). Several cases of expanded flap death have been reported (Austad, 1987), all associated with the use of epinephrine solution injected during the insetting of previously expanded flaps. Since this phenomenon is poorly understood, epinephrine should be avoided in all expanded tissues, which are potentially marginal.

REFERENCES

Adson, M. H., Anderson, R. D., and Argenta, L. C.: Scalp expansion in the treatment of male pattern baldness, Plast. Reconstr. Surg., *79*:906, 1987.

Albo, R. J., Gruber, R., and Kahn, R.: Immediate breast reconstruction after modified mastectomy for carcinoma of the breast. Am. J. Surg., *140*:131, 1980.

Anderson, R.: Expansion-assisted treatment of male pattern baldness. Clin. Plast. Surg., *14*:477, 1987.

Anderson, R. D., and Argenta, L. C.: Tissue expansion for the treatment of alopecia. *In* Unger, W. P. (Ed.): Hair Transplantation. 2nd Ed. New York, Marcel Dekker, 1987.

Argenta, L. C.: Reconstruction of the breast by tissue expansion. Clin. Plast. Surg., *11*:257, 1984a.

Argenta, L. C.: Controlled tissue expansion in reconstructive surgery. Br. J. Plast. Surg., *37*:520, 1984b.

Argenta, L. C., Marks, M. W., and Grabb, W. C.: Selective use of serial expansion in breast reconstruction. Ann. Plast. Surg., *11*:188, 1983.

Argenta, L. C., Marks, M. W., and Pasyk, K. A.: Advances in tissue expansion. Clin. Plast. Surg., *12*:159, 1985.

Argenta, L. C., VanderKolk, C., Friedman, R. J., and Marks, M.: Refinements in reconstruction of congenital breast deformities. Plast. Reconstr. Surg., 76:73, 1985.

Argenta, L. C., Watanabe, M. J., and Grabb, W. C.: The use of tissue expansion in head and neck reconstruction. Ann. Plast. Surg., *11*:31, 1983.

Austad, E. D.: Complications in tissue expansion. Clin. Plast. Surg., *14*:549, 1987.

Austad, E. D., Pasyk, K. A., McClatchey, K. D., and Cherry, G. W.: Histomorphologic evaluation of guinea pig skin and soft tissue after controlled tissue expansion. Plast. Reconstr. Surg., *70*:704, 1982.

Austad, E. D., and Rose, G. L.: A self-inflating tissue expander. Plast. Reconstr. Surg., *70*:588, 1982.

Austad, E. D., Thomas, S. B., and Pasyk, K.: Tissue expansion: dividend or loan? Plast. Reconstr. Surg., *78*:63, 1986.

Austad, E. D., and van Beek, A. L.: Personal communication, 1987.

Becker, H.: Breast reconstruction using an inflatable breast implant with detachable reservoir. Plast. Reconstr. Surg., *73*:678, 1984.

Becker, H., Cohen, I. K., and Scheflan, M.: Breast reconstruction after modified radical mastectomy. South. Med. J., *75*:1335, 1982.

Brobmann, G. F., and Huber, J.: Effects of different-shaped tissue expanders on transluminal pressure, oxygen tension, histopathologic changes, and skin expansion in pigs. Plast. Reconstr. Surg., *76*:731, 1985.

Cherry, G. W., Austad, E. D., Pasyk, K. A., McClatchey, K. D., and Rohrich, R. J.: Increased survival and vascularity of random-pattern skin flaps elevated in controlled, expanded skin. Plast. Reconstr. Surg., *72*:680, 1983.

Codivilla, A.: On the means of lengthening in the lower limbs, the muscle and tissues which are shortened through deformity. Am. J. Orthop. Surg., *2*:353, 1905.

Cohen, I.: Silicone expander with self-contained valve. Plast. Reconstr. Surg., *75*:279, 1985.
Forte, V., Middleton, W. G., and Briant, T. D.: Expansion of myocutaneous flaps. Arch. Otolaryngol., *111*:371, 1985.
Georgiade, G., Georgiade, N., McCarty, K. S., Jr., and Seigler, H. F.: Rationale for immediate reconstruction of the breast following modified radical mastectomy. Ann. Plast. Surg., *8*:20, 1982.
Gruss, J. S., and MacKinnon, S. E.: Soft tissue expanders in upper limb surgery. J. Hand. Surg., *10A*:749, 1985.
Hong, C., Stark, G. B., and Futrell, J. W.: Elongation of axial blood vessels with a tissue expander. Clin. Plast. Surg., *14*:465, 1987.
Juri, J.: Use of parieto-occipital flaps in the surgical treatment of baldness. Plast. Reconstr. Surg., *55*:456, 1975.
Juri, J., and Juri, C.: Temporo-parieto-occipital flap for the treatment of baldness. Clin. Plast. Surg., *9*:255, 1982.
Lapin, R., Daniel, D., Hutchins, H., et al.: Primary breast reconstruction following mastectomy using a skin expander prosthesis. Breast, *6*:97, 1980.
Leonard, A. G., and Small, J. O.: Tissue expansion in the treatment of alopecia. Br. J. Plast. Surg., *39*:42, 1986.
Manders, E. K., Schenden, M. J., Furrey, J. A., Hetzler, P. T., Davis, T. S., and Graham, W. P., III: Soft-tissue expansion: concepts and complications. Plast. Reconstr. Surg., *74*:493, 1984.
Manders, E. K., Graham, W. P., III, Schenden, M. J., and Davis, T. S.: Skin expansion to eliminate large scalp defects. Ann. Plast. Surg., *12*:305, 1985.
Marks, M. W., Argenta, L. C., and Thornton, J.: Burn management: the role of tissue expansion. Clin. Plast. Surg., *14*:543, 1987.
Marks, M. W., Burney, R. E., Mackenzie, J. R., and Knight, P. R.: Enhanced capillary blood flow in rapidly expanded random pattern flaps. J. Trauma, *26*:913, 1986.
Marks, M. W., Mackenzie, J. R., Burney, R. E., Knight, P. R., and Anderson, S. H.: Response of random skin flaps to rapid expansion. J. Trauma, *25*:947, 1985.
Matev, I.: Thumb reconstruction after amputation at the metacarpophalangeal joint. J. Bone Joint Surg., *52*:957, 1970.
Milton, S.: The effects of "delay" on the survival of experimental pedicled skin flaps. Br. J. Plast. Surg., *22*:244, 1969.
Neumann, C. G.: The expansion of an area of skin by progressive distention of a subcutaneous balloon. Plast. Reconstr. Surg., *19*:124, 1957.
Pasyk, K. A., Argenta, L. C., and Austad, E.: Histopathology of human expanded tissue. Clin. Plast. Surg., *14*:435, 1987.
Pasyk, K. A., Austad, E. D., McClatchey, K. D., and Cherry, G. W.: Electron microscopic evaluation of guinea pig skin and soft tissues expanded with a self-inflating silicone implant. Plast. Reconstr. Surg., *70*:37, 1982.
Pasyk, K. A., Austad, E. D., and Cherry, G. W.: Intracellular collagen fibers in the capsule around self-inflating silicone expanders in guinea pigs. J. Surg. Res., *36*:125, 1984.
Pennisi, V. R.: Making a definite inframammary fold under a reconstructed breast. Plast. Reconstr. Surg., *60*:523, 1979.
Radovan, C.: Breast reconstruction after mastectomy using the temporary expander. Plast. Reconstr. Surg., *69*:195, 1982.
Radovan, C.: Tissue expansion in soft-tissue reconstruction. Plast. Reconstr. Surg., *74*:482, 1984.
Rees, T.: Aesthetic Plastic Surgery. Vol. 1. Philadelphia, W. B. Saunders Company, 1980, p. 10.
Reinisch, J., and Myers, B.: The effect of local anesthesia with epinephrine on skin flap survival. Plast. Reconstr. Surg., *54*:324, 1974.
Ryan, J. J.: A lower thoracic advancement flap in breast reconstruction after mastectomy. Plast. Reconstr. Surg., *70*:153, 1982.
Sasaki, G. H., and Pang, C. Y.: Pathophysiology of skin flaps raised on expanded skin. Plast. Reconstr. Surg., *74*:59, 1984.
Seckel, B. R., and Hyland, W. T.: Soft tissue expander for delayed and immediate breast reconstruction. Surg. Clin. North Am., *65*:383, 1985.
Thornton, J., Marks, M., Izenberg, P., and Argenta, L. C.: Expanded myocutaneous flaps: their clinical use. Clin. Plast. Surg., *14*:529, 1987.
Versaci, A.: Reconstruction of a pendulous breast utilizing a tissue expander. Clin. Plast. Surg., *14*:499, 1987.

14

David T. W. Chiu
Bradford W. Edgerton

Repair and Grafting of Dermis, Fat, and Fascia

The autogenous transplantation of dermis, fat, and fascia has been established as a useful modality for soft tissue augmentation, coverage of vital structures, elimination of dead space, or reconstruction of ligamentous or fascial structures. Until the mechanism of foreign material recognition and rejection has been fully understood and harnessed, autogenous tissues remain the most reliable and applicable materials available for reconstructive surgeons.

DERMIS TRANSPLANTATION

Dermis transplantation is defined as transferring dermis as a free graft (all layers of the skin remaining after removal of the epidermis as a thin split-thickness graft). The dermis graft, therefore, contains the deep layer of the papillary dermis and the entire reticular layer of the dermis along with a minimal amount of adherent subcutaneous fat and the indigenous subepidermal extensions of the epithelial appendages, i.e., the hair follicles, sebaceous glands, and sweat glands (Fig. 14–1).

History

Successful clinical application of an autogenous dermal graft was first reported in 1913 by Loewe, who abraded the epidermis from a graft of full-thickness skin with a knife, and used the dermal graft as a substitute for fascia in hernia repair and as a tendon substitute in the repair of severed tendons.

In 1914 Rehn reported a similar application of the dermal graft in which the surface epidermis was removed as a split-thickness skin graft with a razor or a graft knife. In the same year, the application of a buried dermal graft for the augmentation of a soft tissue depression in the reconstruction of facial contour was reported by Lexer, who used the dermal graft in the nasal tip and in the helix of the ear. Eitner (1920) reported the use of a dermal graft for correction of sunken cheeks, and found the results more permanent than those obtained by using fat or fascia.

In 1929, there appeared a follow-up report by Loewe on his experience with the application of the dermal graft in more than 100 cases, including the repair of hernias and dura mater; the internal fixation of fractured long bones; arthroplasty of the knee, hip, and elbow; and recurrent dislocation of the shoulder. In 1932, Straatsma first reported the

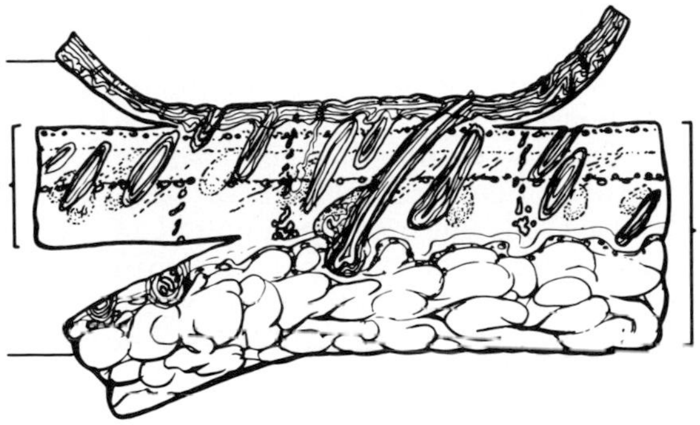

Figure 14–1. *A, B,* Dermis graft contains the deeper layer of the papillary dermis and the entire reticular layer of the dermis, along with a minimal amount of adherent subcutaneous fat and indigenous subepidermal extensions of the epithelial appendages.

successful application of the dermal graft for the correction of a minor saddle nose deformity. A review by Uihlein (1939) of 104 cases of the application of a dermal graft in Rehn's clinic between 1929 and 1939 stimulated widespread interest in dermal grafting far beyond the borders of Germany. In Rehn's clinic, dermal grafting was used mainly for hernia repair; however, the application also extended to the reinforcement of extra-articular ligaments in the knee joint, temporomandibular joint, fingers, and elbows. Dermal grafts were also used to repair ruptured and lacerated tendons.

In the United States, Cannaday (1943, 1945) adopted the technique of dermal grafting and expanded its application to the treatment of ankylosis of the mandible by interposing a dermal graft into the line of a high osteotomy. Gebauer (1950) reported the application of the dermal graft to repair stenotic bronchial tubes. The application of the dermal graft was also extended to the repair of major diaphragmatic defects, as reported by Metheny, Lundmark, and Morcom (1952). For the treatment of unstable adherent scars of the lower extremity, Hynes (1954) described the application of a dermal graft in an upside-down manner in which the deepithelized superficial papillary surface of the dermis was applied directly over the wound while the adipose tissue–laden reticular dermis was exposed to the surface. A thin layer of split-thickness skin graft was often used as a temporary coverage of the reticular surface of the dermal graft. Stallings, Huffman, and Bernstein (1969) experimentally demonstrated the superior revascularization of the reversed dermal graft as compared with the conventional full-thickness and split-thickness skin grafts. The use of the dermal graft to protect the carotid artery was also reported by Corso and Gerold (1961, 1963). In addition, the dermal graft has been used for cosmetic augmentation of the soft tissue mound of the thenar muscles in patients with leprosy (Johnson, 1961), for replacement of the articular disc after meniscectomy of the temporomandibular joint (Georgiade, 1962), and for repair of a dura mater defect (Guiot, Rougerie, and Tessier, 1967).

Fate of Dermal Grafts

Experimental Studies. Routine survival of a full-thickness skin graft depends on the viability of the dermis layer. Several experimental studies were performed to investigate the fate of the epithelial elements in dermal grafts in animals. In dogs, dermal grafts show no surviving epithelial cells after 15 weeks in the subcutaneous pocket (Swenson, 1950), and only slightly longer survival in the intraperitoneal cavity (Horton and associates, 1953; Armistead, 1956), intrathoracic cavity (Horton and associates, 1955), and intracranial cavity (Crawford, 1957). In pigs, sebaceous glands were observed to disappear in two weeks and hair follicles in eight weeks. However, sweat glands survived the observation period of eight weeks, while the dermal collagen and elastic tissue showed no evidence of abnormality (Sawhney, Banerjee, and Chakravarti, 1969). However, as pointed out by Thompson in 1960, the fate of epithelial elements in dermal implants in animals bears little significance to human grafts in view of the absence of sweat glands in all the animals studied and the relatively hairless condition of man.

Nonetheless, information gathered from experimental studies on animals has led to speculation about the possibility of mesodermal metaplasia in response to functional stimulation of dermal grafts. Rehn (1914) described a successful experiment in which he used plaited strips of dermis to replace the

Achilles tendon in dogs. It was noted that the epithelial elements disappeared and the dermis was replaced by connective tissue microscopically identical with that of tendon in approximately ten weeks; the observation was confirmed by Schwartz in 1922. In 1962, Georgiade observed that a dermis implant in the mandibular joints of monkeys developed the histologic appearance of an articular disc within six months. It was rationalized that mesodermal metaplasia occurs as a response to the functional stimulus, mainly *tension* in the transformation into a tendon-like structure and *pressure* in the transformation into a cartilage-like structure.

Histologic Data in Human Study. Observations of the histologic changes of the dermal graft in humans were made by Peer and Paddock (1937), Uihlein (1939), Peer (1955), and Thompson (1960). These findings suggest that removal of surface epidermis ensures early vascularization of the graft. Both the inosculation process (see Chap. 8) and the ingrowth of host vessels are evident by the fourth day (Peer, 1959). The sebaceous glands usually disappear within two weeks (Peer and Paddock, 1937; Thompson, 1960). Hair follicles generally disappear within two months, but most of the sweat glands survive permanently and continue to function. The excretory sweat ducts end blindly at the surface of the graft. The sweat gland secretion is internally absorbed into adjacent capillaries. In addition, the remaining blind-ended sweat glands are functionally active, as demonstrated by the histochemical evidence of succinic dehydrogenase content and the depletions of glycogen after secretory stimulation as in normal glands (Thompson, 1960). Microscopic epidermoid cyst formation derived mainly from the hair follicles, and less so from the sebaceous glands, is common after the second week. The accumulating keratinous epithelial debris within the lumen of the cyst causes the epithelial wall to stretch and eventually become necrotic. Direct contact of the retained epithelial product with the surrounding mesodermal stroma led to an intense foreign body, giant cell, and granulomatous reaction and eventually to complete replacement fibrosis, as originally observed by Stewart in 1912 (Fig. 14–2).

Surgical Technique

The basic prerequisites for successful dermal grafting are the following:

1. An inconspicuous donor site.
2. A favorable recipient bed, free of infection and scar tissue.
3. Meticulous hemostasis.
4. Adequate immobilization.

The scheme for correction of a saddle nose with a dermal graft is illustrated in Figure 14–3. Through an intracartilaginous incision, a suitable subcutaneous pocket is prepared over the nasal bridge. The pocket is developed with blunt and sharp dissection following a previously planned outline representing the exact area where the dermal graft is to be inserted (Fig. 14–3*A*). Hemostasis is achieved by a saline pack. The dermal graft is harvested from one of the following donor sites:

1. Groin.
2. Gluteal fold.
3. Lateral gluteal region.
4. Submammary region in females.
5. Lower abdomen.

In excising the graft, a 25 per cent excess of surface area should be removed to allow for contraction. The graft is harvested as an ellipse, hemostasis is obtained, and the donor site is closed in a linear fashion. The graft is deepithelized with a Reese dermatome. The excessive fat adherent to the reticular dermis is removed. The graft is tailored to the size and shape of the defect. For an area of deep depression, a double layer of dermal graft should be planned (Fig. 14–3*B*). At the circumference of the graft, the edge of the dermal graft should be beveled to minimize the step-off appearance after the graft is inserted. The grafts are layered and fixed with nylon sutures. The needles are then discarded. Both free ends of each of the two sutures are passed through the eye of an autopsy needle, and are then exteriorized through the skin individually. The free ends of each suture are tied over a dental roll or a rolled-up piece of Xeroform gauze (Fig. 14–3*C*). This maneuver ensures maximal contact between the graft and the undersurface of the skin of the nasal dorsum. After the graft is inserted, the intracartilaginous incision is closed with interrupted absorbable sutures.

Complications

The most common complications after dermal grafting are hematoma and wound infections, the incidence of which was reported as 5 per cent and 14 per cent, respectively, by Uihlein (1939). Subsequent reports demonstrated declining rates of hematoma and

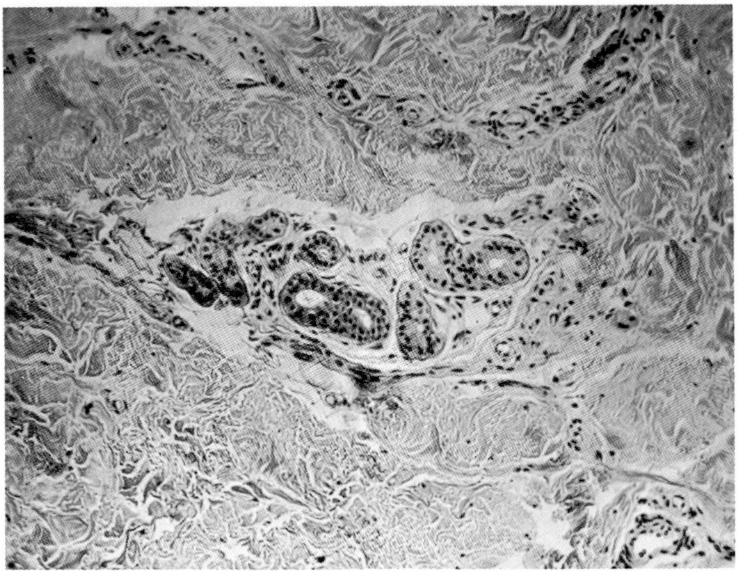

A

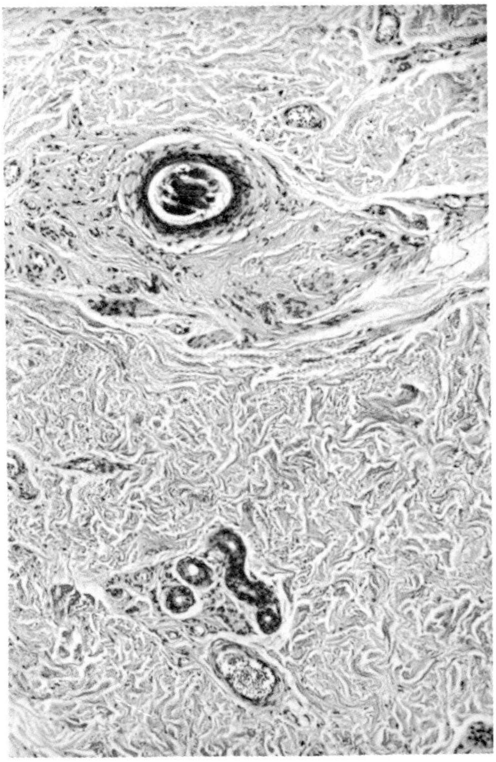

B

Figure 14–2. *A,* Human autogenous dermal graft buried subcutaneously for four years. The essentially normal secretory coil of a sweat gland is shown. H & E, × 120. *B,* From the same section as *A.* The greatly dilated excretory duct containing a secretion cast in its lumen *(above)* is shown with its associated sweat gland (*below*). H & E, × 75.

Illustration continued on following page

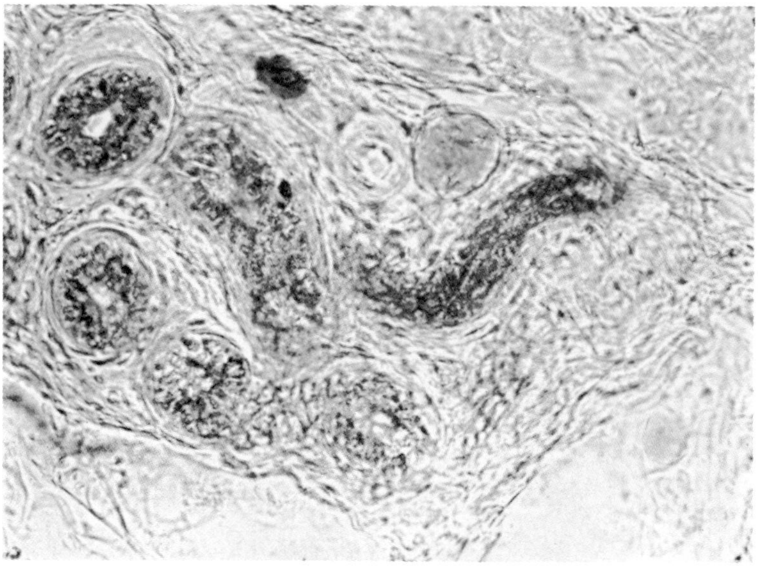

C

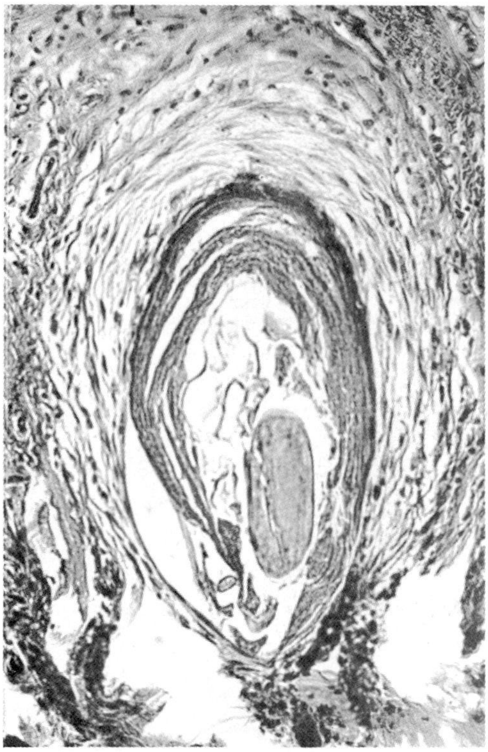

D

Figure 14–2 *Continued C,* Human autogenous dermal graft buried subcutaneously for four years. The dark granules represent sites of succinic dehydrogenase activity inside the cells of a surviving sweat gland. Succinic dehydrogenase, an enzyme in the Krebs citric acid cycle, is essential for the vital processes of mammalian cells. Neo-tetrazolium method, × 300. *D,* Human autogenous dermal graft buried subcutaneously for five months. An epidermoid cyst derived from a hair follicle is shown at an intermediate stage of disintegration. The epithelial lining is becoming thinned after the accumulation of keratohyaline debris inside the cyst. There is considerable surrounding reactive fibrosis. H & E, × 210.

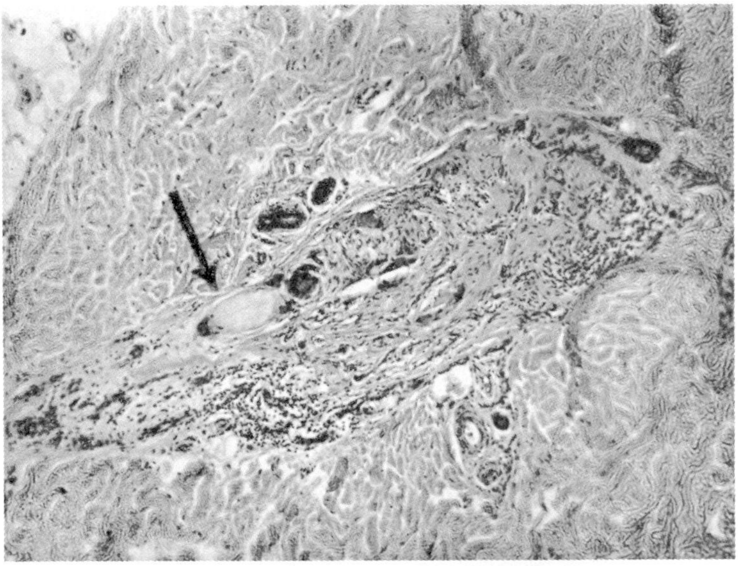

E

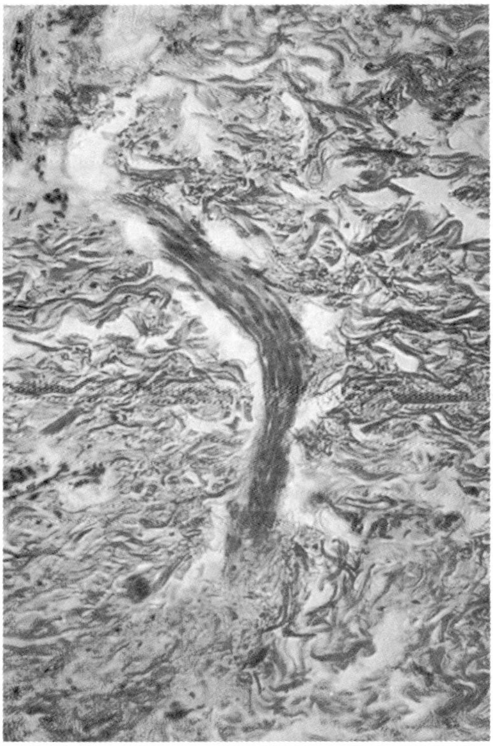

F

Figure 14–2 *Continued E,* Human autogenous graft buried subcutaneously for 15 months. An epidermoid cyst originating from a hair follicle is shown at a late stage of disintegration. All epithelial elements have disappeared, but a hair shaft fragment *(arrow)* persists. The cyst has become replaced by organizing granulation tissue with many foreign body giant cells and appreciable lymphocytic infiltration. H & E, × 60. *F,* Human autogenous dermal graft buried subcutaneously for five years. Surviving arrector pili muscle in the graft dermis. H & E, × 120.

Illustration continued on following page

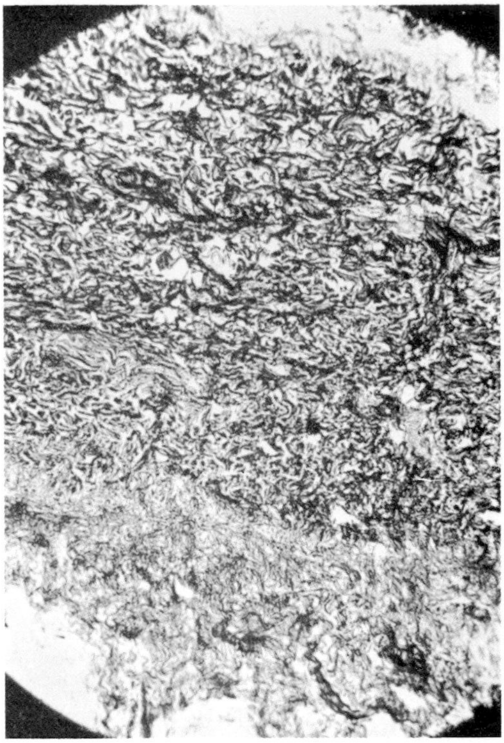

G

Figure 14–2 *Continued G,* Human autogenous dermal graft buried subcutaneously for five years. Elastic tissue showing a pattern of distribution resembling that found in normal skin. Orcein, × 50.

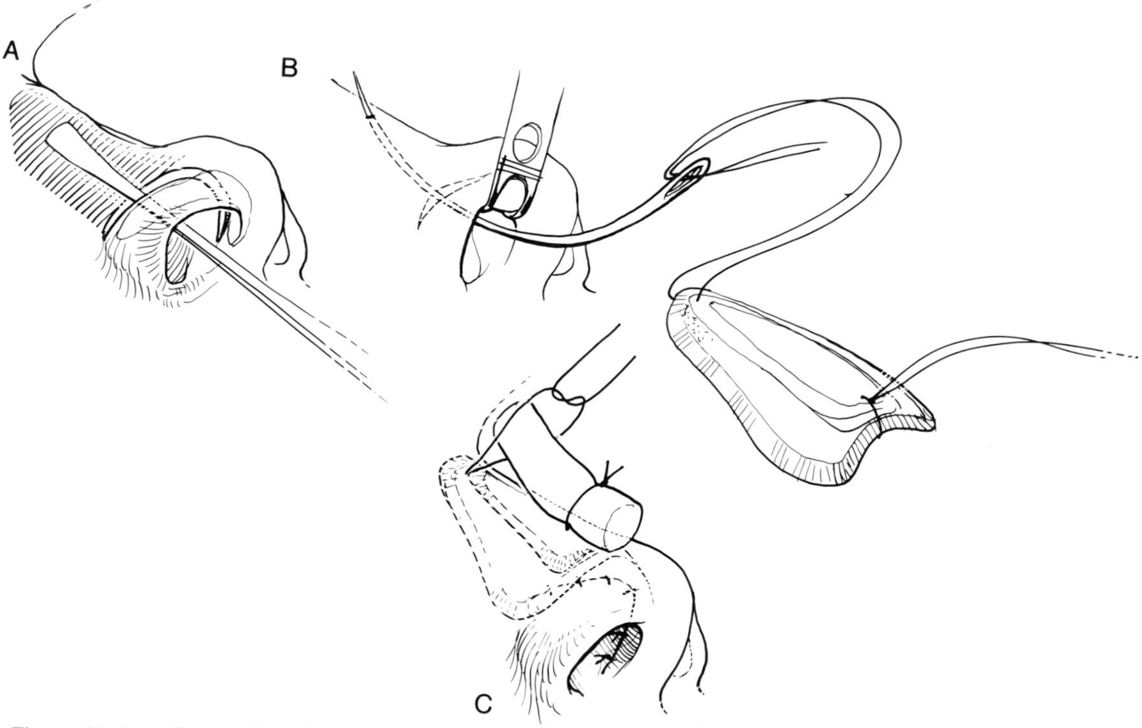

Figure 14–3. *A,* Preparation of the recipient site for a dermal graft to the nasal dorsum. *B,* Suture stabilization of the dermal graft (double layered) and introduction of the graft into the pocket. *C,* Fixation of the dermal graft unit with a tie-over dressing.

wound infection. Cannaday (1945) reported the rate of hematoma formation and wound infection as 3.5 per cent and 5.4 per cent, respectively, and Schuessler and Steffanoff (1949) reported 1.25 per cent for each. According to the latter study, the rate of clinical cyst formation and necrosis was 2.5 per cent. In Thompson's 1960 series of 43 subcutaneous dermal grafts, he reported 90 per cent satisfactory graft survival and no evidence of clinical epidermoid cyst formation, the usual cause of failure being necrosis followed by complete resorption of the graft. In the application of a dermal graft for carotid artery coverage, epithelization of the dermal graft may occur during the period of wound dehiscence or drainage.

An epithelized dermal graft over an exposed carotid artery is desirable as it provides a viable biologic coverage of the vessel. However, the reepithelized dermal graft may also result in persistent draining sinuses. In fact, removal of the full-thickness dermal graft during the time of definitive flap coverage of the carotid artery is recommended to obviate the possibility of having to set in a flap over an epithelized recipient bed (Dedo and associates, 1975).

The Future

With a better understanding of the induction effect of dermal elements on epidermal growth and differentiation, dermal grafting may assume a more prominent role in reconstructive surgery.

On the horizon is the application of frozen dermal allografts to support the engraftment and expansion of autologous epidermis. Heck, Bergstresser and Baxter (1985) reported success from the resurfacing of full-thickness skin burn wounds with previously frozen allograft skin followed by the application of trypsin-disaggregated syngeneic epidermal cells five days after original grafting. At that juncture, the epidermis on the allograft skin is rejected and removed, exposing the denuded dermal surface on which the epidermal autograft is transplanted. Successful engraftment with complete epidermal coverage has been observed within seven to ten days. This technique was also applied clinically in eight patients by the same investigators. The necrotic epidermis is removed surgically in four days and a vacuum-blister–prepared sheet of autologous epidermal graft is used to resurface the denuded dermal surfaces. The patient was followed for up to four months with no demonstration of graft loss or significant wound contracture.

Griffiths and Shakespeare (1982) reported a three year study of the histologic sequence of formalin-treated human fibrous dermal collagen as an allograft. There was no immune or inflammatory response and no fibrous encapsulization around the graft. The implants were reportedly colonized by host fibroblasts and blood vessels with no signs of collagen resorption. This preparation offers the advantages of being cell free and causing no donor site scarring, and it may serve as an alternative to autogenous dermal grafts.

The importance of the dermal papilla, a discrete population of specialized fibroblasts, in the growth of hair has been recognized. Papillae can induce hair growth when implanted in the follicles and can interact with skin epidermis to develop new hair follicles (Oliver, 1967, 1970).

Jahoda, Horne, and Oliver (1984) reported that serial cultured adult papillar cells can induce the growth of hair when implanted into follicles that otherwise would not grow hair, thus substantiating the induction effect of dermal cells in the reformation of organized epidermal stuctures (Worst, MacKenzie, and Fusenig, 1982). This observation may pave the way for a new technique in the treatment of baldness (see Chap. 31).

FAT TRANSPLANTATION

Autogenous fat transplantation is defined as the heterotopic transfer of fat cells along with their stromal tissues by one of the following means:

1. Free adipose tissue transplantation.
2. Transplantation of adipose tissue with dermal tissue as a carrier in the form of dermis-fat graft.
3. Transplantation of adipose tissue with microvascular free tissue transfer technique.

History

The abundance of adipose tissue throughout the body invites imagination on its application for replacement of soft tissue defects, for obliteration of dead space, and for creation of a favorable tissue interface. Neuber (1893) pioneered the application of fat transplantation and made the first attempt in humans. Lexer (1910, 1919, 1925) employed adipose tissue transplantation extensively and reported success in establishing normal contour in hemifacial atrophy and in enlargement of small breasts. Adipose tissue autograft has been used to fill the orbit at the time of enucleation as early as the beginning of the nineteenth century (Barraquer, 1901; López, 1902–1903; Lauber, 1910; Marx, 1910; Key, 1919).

Excellent results have been reported following the application of autogenous fat implants to fill the dead space left behind by stripping of the frontal sinuses (Montgomery and Pierce, 1963; Schenck, 1974, 1975). To establish a favorable barrier limiting the growth of cicatrix into the spinal canal, autogenous fat transplants are also used to resurface denuded dura mater during lumbar spine operations. With the advent of microsurgery, the application of fat transplantation has been greatly expanded. Omental free flap transfers have been applied for resurfacing of scalp defects, for the restoration of facial contour, and for the carrying of skin flaps.

Fate of Transplanted Fat Cells

There are two schools of thought about the fate of fat cells after transplantation in man. The first group is of the opinion that in free fat transfers, the fat cells do not survive and that the host histiocytes phagocytize the lipid released from the decomposed fat cells and become new adipose cells. This is known as the "host cell replacement theory" (Peer, 1977).

The other school maintains that some adipose tissue indeed survives and that the cells collectively represent the fatty tissue ultimately remaining in the transplant. This is known as the "cell survival theory" (Peer, 1955, 1959) (Fig. 14–4).

Peer's observation by serial histologic study suggested that in human fat transplantation, circulation is established in the graft approximately four days after transplantation, in a manner similar to that observed in skin grafts (Fig. 14–5). The host histiocytes invade all fat grafts and appear to serve only as scavengers in removing fat from broken-down fat cells (Fig. 14–6). Peer also noted that traumatized fat cells lose much more weight in volume than do gently handled transplants. This observation favors the "cell survival theory" (Peer and Paddock, 1937; Peer, 1939, 1950).

Clinical Applications

Transplantation of adipose tissue as a *free graft* has been used experimentally and clinically. In the experimental situation, adipose tissue has been utilized for obliteration of the denuded frontal sinus. According to the study by Bright, Thacker, and Brunner (1983), circulation of the free nonvascularized fat graft was reestablished by means of blood vessel to vessel reanastomosis, also known as inosculation. These authors observed that, if the graft failed to become revascularized, it was often replaced by fibrous tissue and bone ingrowth caused by osteoneogenesis.

In the clinical setting, autogenous fat transplants have been applied to resurface denuded dura mater during lumbar spine operations. Bryant, Bremer, and Nguyen (1983) demonstrated the viability of the fat transplant with computed tomographic (CT) scans in their series of 44 consecutive surgical procedures performed primarily for discogenic or spondylytic disease from 1979 to 1982. Autogenic fat transplants were found to be well accepted by all recipients during a one to 32 month follow-up. There was no incidence of wound infection. Fat grafts greater than 1 cm in thickness were identified on subsequent CT scans and were considered as signs of viability of fat grafts. It was believed that fat grafts have a surface barrier limiting the growth of cicatrix into the spinal canal.

The second technique in the application of fat grafts is the *dermis-fat graft,* which was used extensively in the early nineteenth century to obliterate the dead space after enucleation of the orbit. The feasibility of dermis-fat grafts for operative implantation was confirmed by the experience of Smith and associates (1983). In addition, dermis-fat grafts were widely used to correct soft tissue deficits, such as retromandibular depression, secondary to either postradical parotid resection or congenital facial asymmetry (Fig. 14–7).

The basic technique in dermis-fat grafting involves:

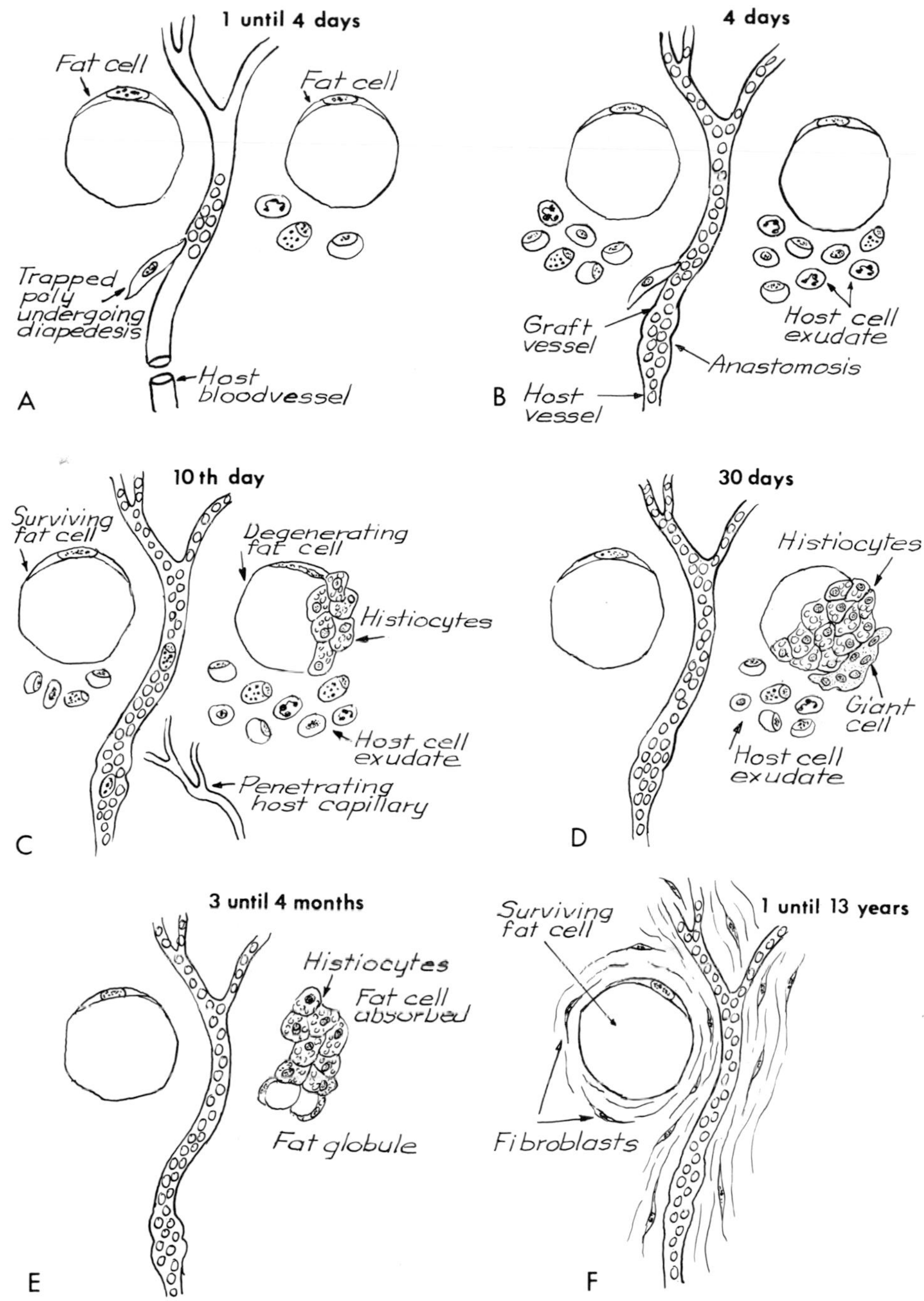

Figure 14–4. *A* to *F,* The contrasting fate of two adipose cells in an autogenous human fat transplant. The fat cell on the right fails to survive transplantation, and its fatty content is removed by host histiocytes and other host cells. The fat cell on the left survives transplantation and constitutes part of the apparently normal adipose cells seen in the grafted area one year or more after transplantation. The drawings are based on a series of autogenous human fat grafts removed and examined histologically (Peer).

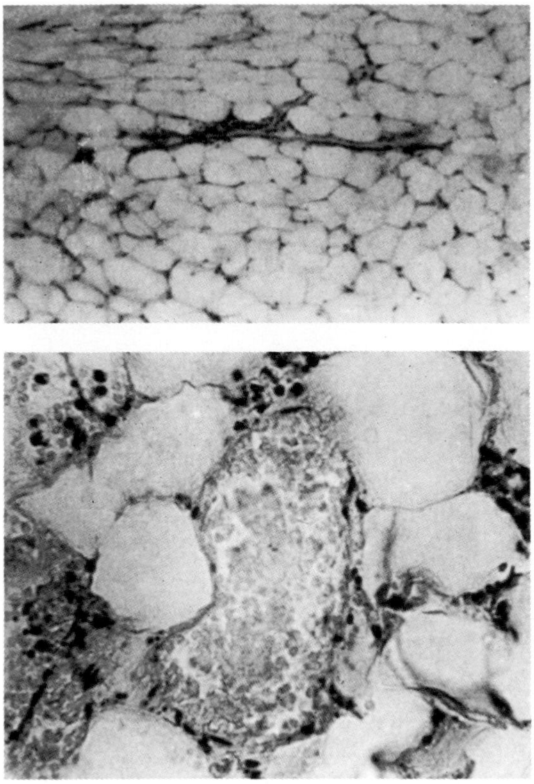

A

B

Figure 14–5. *A,* Autogenous human dermis-fat graft buried four days on pull-out sutures. Note the absence of cell infiltration, the unruptured fat cells, and the empty graft blood vessel. × 100. *B,* The same graft showing an area with two blood vessels engorged with red blood cells and the adjacent adipose cells. × 400. (Peer.)

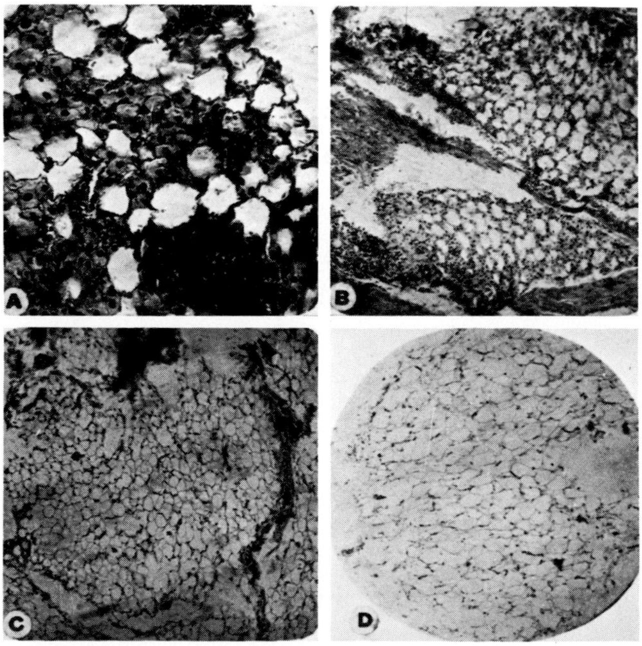

Figure 14–6. *A,* Autogenous human fat graft buried in muscle for 21 days. Note the surviving fat cells and large histiocytes. The histiocytes are resorbing fat cells that have failed to survive. *B,* Autogenous human fat graft buried in muscle for 40 days. Note that there are surviving fat cells and that large histiocytes are removing broken-down fat. *C,* Autogenous human fat graft buried in muscle for 14 months. Note the normal-appearing fatty tissue. Graft loss was approximately 50 per cent of its volume. *D,* Autogenous human fat graft buried in muscle for 13 years. Its appearance is that of normal fatty tissue. Graft loss was approximately 50 per cent of its volume.

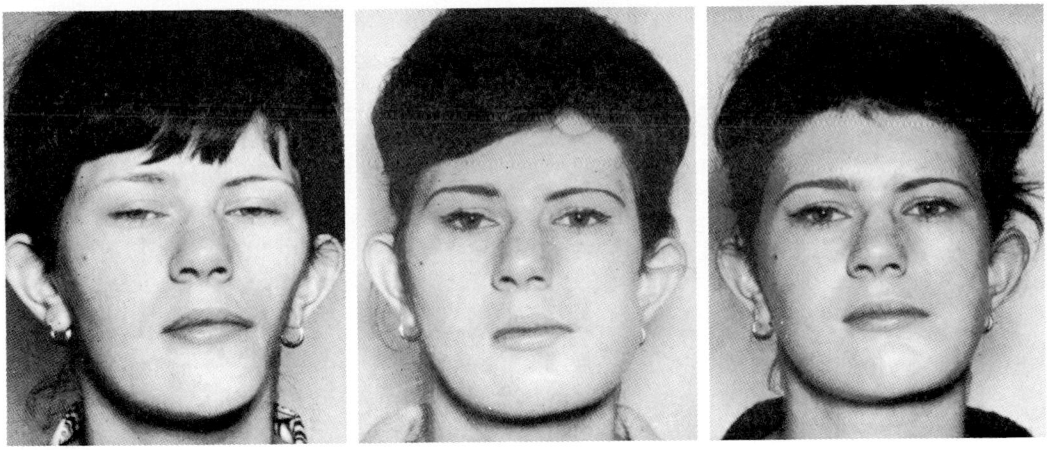

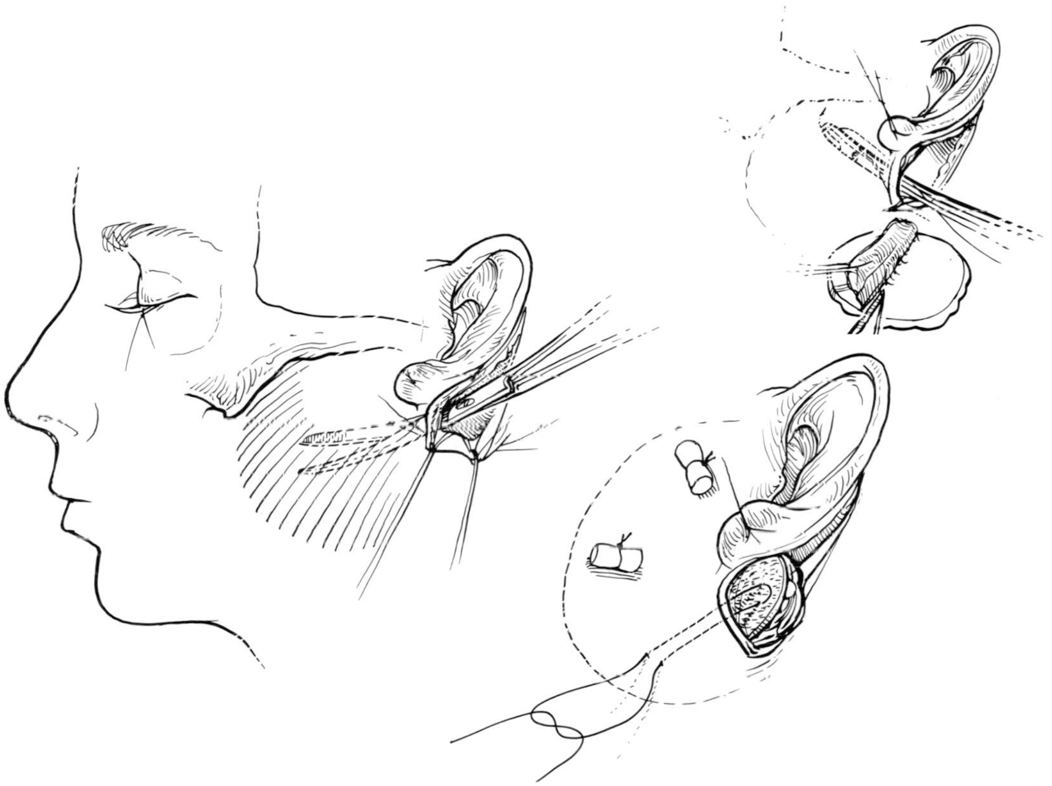

Figure 14–7. *Above,* A 21 year old female with congenital facial asymmetry. *Left,* Preoperative appearance. *Center,* Early postoperative appearance 17 days after the insertion of a dermis-fat graft, taken from the lower abdomen, into the left cheek through a preauricular incision, with limited overcorrection of the defect. *Right,* Appearance six months after transplantation. *Below,* Dermis-fat graft inserted in a parotid defect. Details of the technique.

1. Selection of a concealed donor site.
2. Preparation of the graft, including deepithelization.
3. Gentle handling of the graft.
4. Secure placement of the graft into the recipient site.
5. Meticulous hemostasis.
6. Absence of infection.
7. Moderate overcorrection.

The groin, lateral gluteal area, and gluteal fold are ideal donor sites as they yield an adequate amount of adipose tissue and spareable skin, and leave relatively inconspicuous scars that are easily concealed by clothing (Fig. 14–8). Deepithelization is most readily achieved by the application of a Reese dermatome set at 14/1000ths of an inch. The grafts should be handled with utmost gentleness. As Peer (1977) demonstrated, the surgical incision alone may lead to fat cell death and destruction and subsequent volume loss. Therefore, the grafts should be tailored to the size and shape of the defect and transferred as one piece of tissue rather than as multiple small pieces (Peer, 1977). The grafts should be secured to the recipient site by anchoring sutures to ensure contact and subsequent revascularization. Hematomas are catastrophic for dermis-fat grafts and should be avoided at all costs. Meticulous cauterization and the application of pressure and Avitene will enhance clotting of the bleeding vessels. The avoidance of rubbing of the tissue surface and the application of a gentle stream of Ringer's lactate as an irrigant will prevent the rebleeding of quiescent small vessels. A catastrophe for the dermis-fat graft is wound infection.

Peer's report (1950) indicated that approximately 50 per cent of the weight and volume is lost one year after transplantation. This observation may serve as a guideline, but actual 50 per cent overcorrection is rarely justified. In most cases, correction of soft tissue depression on the face is for esthetic enhancement. A patient is rarely happy to carry 50 per cent overcorrection for as long as a year to wait for the natural, gradual self-correction to materialize. The authors have found that a 20 per cent overcorrection is well tolerated by the patient and is adequate to compensate for the volume reduction. More-

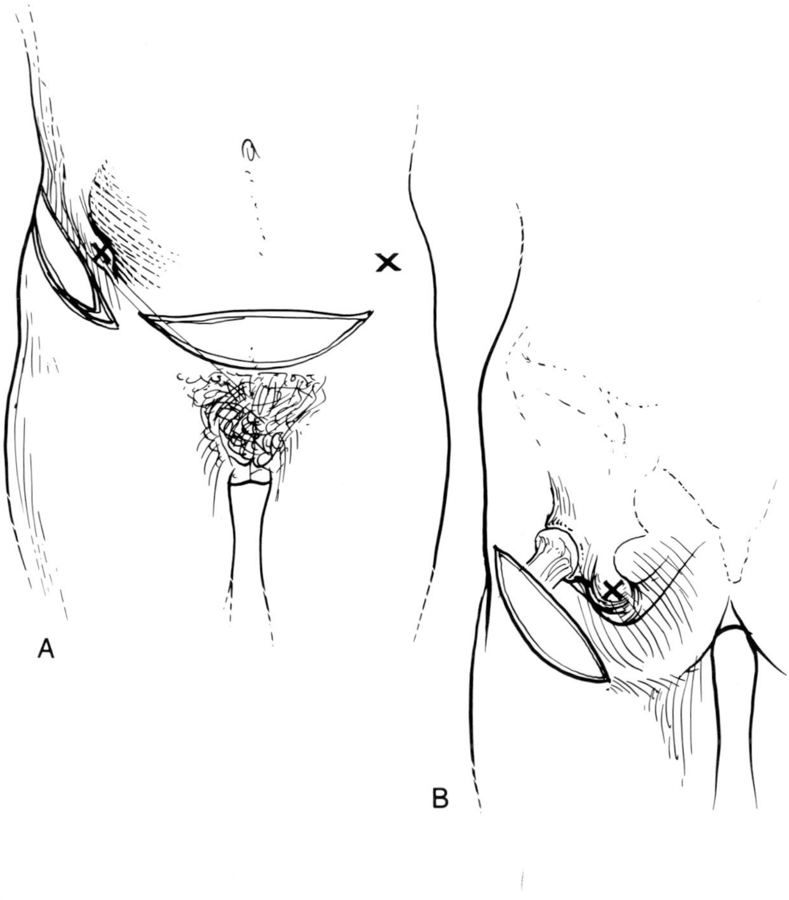

Figure 14–8. Common dermis-fat graft donor sites. *A,* Suprapubic and subiliac sites. *X* designates the iliac spines. *B,* Gluteal crease site. *X* designates the ischial tuberosity.

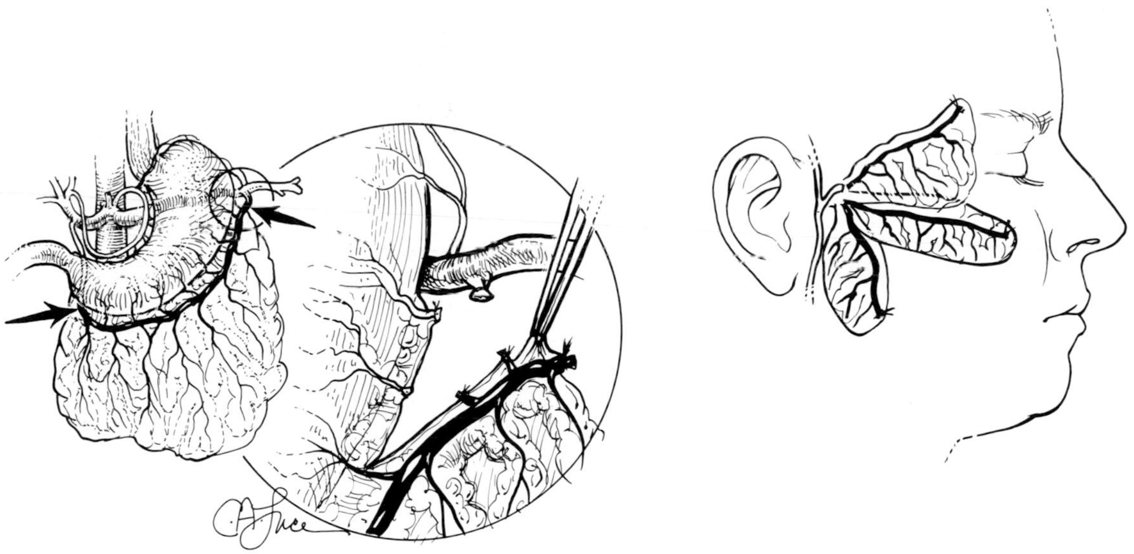

Figure 14–9. Omental transfer as a free flap based on the gastroepiploic pedicle. Note that the flap can be tailored to the defect.

over, if the volume reduction is indeed excessive, one can always resort to an additional augmentation in the future.

The uncertainty in terms of the volume reduction after free fat tissue transfers has rendered *vascularized omental transfers* an attractive alternative. With the development of microsurgical technique (see Chap. 12), the transfer of vascularized autologous fat tissue becomes readily feasible and, in fact, desirable.

Vascularized autologous omental transfers have the advantage of being predictable in terms of ultimate volume retention, and often serve to decrease the number of procedures required for the reconstruction. Omental free flaps also enjoy the distinct advantage of their malleability. Since their introduction by McClean and Bunke in 1972, omental free flaps have been widely used for facial soft tissue reconstruction, particularly for reconstruction of hemifacial atrophy (see Chap. 63) and craniofacial microsomia (see Chap. 62) (Fig. 14–9) (Upton and associates, 1980).

An omental free flap can also be used to tailor a skin flap. The principle for creating a transferable skin flap based on the greater omentum cutaneous axial flap was reported by Shen and associates (1981). The basic principle of this technique is to revascularize random skin flaps with the axial vessels of the omentum and to transfer this skin flap based on the axial vessels of the greater omentum.

An innovative application of dermis-fat transfers for soft tissue augmentation is the deepithelized flap with microvascular transfer. This technique ensures blood supply and in all likelihood brings some predictable results (Fujino, Rytinzaburo, and Sugimoto, 1975; Wells and Edgerton, 1977).

The Future

Autogenous fat transplantation may continue to serve a useful function when used as a small graft, such as for denuded sinuses. When a moderate amount of tissue replacement is required, the dermis-fat graft is still a useful technique, such as for retromandibular tissue augmentation for defects secondary to parotidectomy. However, graft resorption is unpredictable. Large volume replacement, such as breast augmentation and facial reconstruction for craniofacial microsomia, is best treated by vascularized tissue transfer.

Recently the widespread application of suction assisted lipectomy (SAL) has been followed by a surge of interest in the fat injection technique to correct soft tissue depressions and prominent nasolabial folds or wrinkles (see Chap. 81). However, the key questions remain: (1) will the fat cells, after the trauma caused by suctioning and injecting, survive as grafts?; and (2) if so, how much atrophy may be expected? A seemingly logical answer to this question is that, if "proper" injection pressure and needles of appropriate diameter are used, a certain percentage of the transferred fat cells may survive. However, until the "proper" values of these "variables" are determined, fat injection as a method of fat grafting will only be an experimental technique courted with unpredictable results. The answers await critical and quantitative longitudinal studies.

FASCIA TRANSPLANTATION

Fascia transplantation is defined as the free transfer of fascial tissues with or without a vascular supply.

History

McArthur (1901, 1904) was credited as the first to utilize the strips of aponeurosis of the external oblique muscle as biologic sutures to repair inguinal hernias.

Transplantation of fascia to reconstruct other structures soon followed. Kirshner (1909) and Busch (1913) used slings of autogenous fascia lata to correct facial nerve palsy, a technique subsequently refined and popularized by Blair (1926) and which continues to be employed today. Fascia lata is also used to form a loop to stabilize the tongue for the treatment of the Robin sequence described by Lewis, Lynch, and Blocker (1968). Fascia may be used as an interposition material between bony edges after resection osteotomy to correct ankylosis of the temporomandibular joint.

Physical Property

Crawford (1968, 1969) reported the specific gravity of fascia lata to be 1.31 and its average tensile strength to be approximately 7000 lb per square inch. Fresh fascia lata has an average strength of 10.73 lb when meshed in ¼ inch strips. The tensile strength of fascia decreases with advancing age.

Harvesting of Fascia Lata Grafts

Fascia lata is the most common donor site for a fascial graft. A strip 10 to 15 mm wide may be harvested from the lateral aspect of the thigh with no significant morbidity. If a wider strip of fascia is removed, muscle may herniate through the fascial defect. For harvesting of a small strip of fascia lata graft, a fascia stripper is recommended.

A refined version of a fascia stripper was popularized by Wilson and Castroviejo (Fig. 14–10). It has a guillotine that permits resection of the fascia lata through a short incision over the iliotibial tract above the knee joint. The incision is made transversely, exposing the fascia. Two small incisions made parallel to the fibers of the fascia lata, joining at right angles with the transverse incision, permit the fascia to be raised as a small flap. The fascial flap is passed through the distal end of the stripper and is secured by a clamp. While downward traction on the fascia is maintained with the clamp, the fascia lata is stripped by upward movement of the stripper, tension being maintained constantly downward upon the fascia so that the stripper severs the fascia as it moves upward parallel to the fibers. The fascia stripper is advanced proximally by a steady upward movement until it reaches the muscle belly of the tensor fascia lata. The guillotine mechanism is activated to sever the upper end of the graft. The cutaneous wound is sutured and a compressive dressing is applied. A longitudinal incision can be made parallel to the direction of the fibers, allowing subdivision of the graft into smaller strips. Handling of the fascial grafts should be gentle, and drying of the graft should be avoided.

Clinical uses of fascial grafts include the correction of facial palsy, the repair of urethral fistulas, the closure of nasal septal defects, and the coverage of exposed implants.

Vascularized Fascial Transfers

The advent of microsurgical techniques has inspired a better understanding of vascular anatomy, and fascia on various parts of the body has been transferred as free flaps. Among them is the temporoparietal fascia free flap (Crawford, 1968, 1969; Abul-Hassan, von Drasek Ascher, and Acland, 1986), which is advantageous because it is ultra-thin and leaves a minimal donor site defect. Excellent results have been reported from its application for external ear reconstruction, avulsed scalp resurfacing, reconstitution of soft tissues, and replacement of soft tissue deficits of the hand (Fig. 14–11) (Brent and associates, 1985; Upton and associates, 1986).

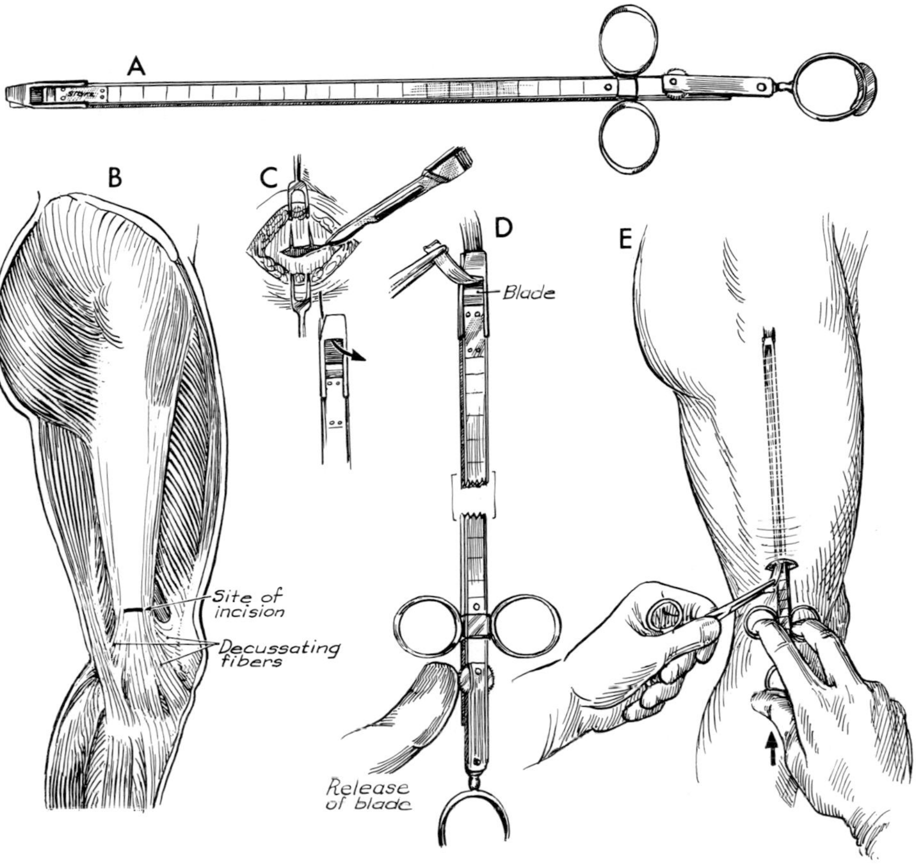

Figure 14–10. Method of obtaining a strip of fascia lata. *A,* Fascia stripper. *B,* Anatomy of the fascia lata and the incision site. Note the decussation of the fascial fibers. *C,* A flap of fascia is raised parallel to the direction of the fibers. *D,* The flap of fascia is introduced into the stripper and held by a heavy clamp. *E,* The stripper is advanced while downward traction is maintained on the clamp. The knee should be flexed, thus maintaining the fascia lata under tension. When a fascial strip of sufficient length is obtained, the upper end of the strip is severed by means of the guillotine.

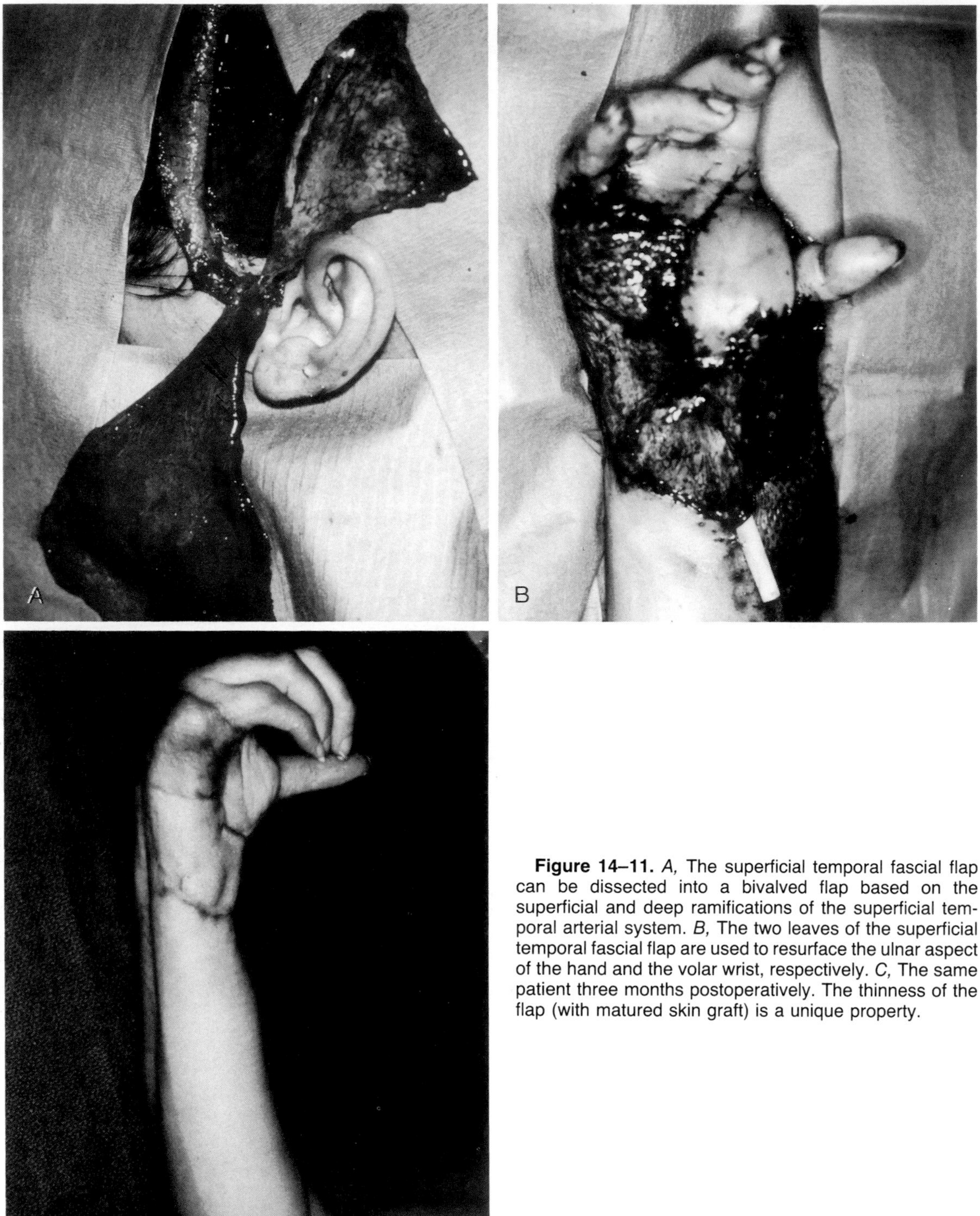

Figure 14–11. *A,* The superficial temporal fascial flap can be dissected into a bivalved flap based on the superficial and deep ramifications of the superficial temporal arterial system. *B,* The two leaves of the superficial temporal fascial flap are used to resurface the ulnar aspect of the hand and the volar wrist, respectively. *C,* The same patient three months postoperatively. The thinness of the flap (with matured skin graft) is a unique property.

REFERENCES

Abul-Hassan, H. S., von Drasek Ascher, G., and Acland, R. D.: Surgical anatomy and blood supply of the fascial layers of the temporal region. Plast. Reconstr. Surg., *77*:17, 1986.

Armistead, W. W.: The experimental use of skin autografts intraperitoneally. Plast. Reconstr. Surg., *18*:9, 1956.

Barraquer, J.: Enucleacion con injerto de tejido adiposo en copsula de Tenon. Arch. Oftal. Hispano-Am., Madrid, *1*:82, 1901.

Blair, V. P.: Notes on the operative corrections of facial palsy. South Med. J., *19*:116, 1926.

Brent, B., Upton, J., Acland, R. D., Shaw, W. W., Finseth, F. J., et al.: Experience with the temporoparietal fascial free flap. Plast. Reconstr. Surg., *76*:177, 1985.

Bright, R. M., Thacker, H. L., and Brunner, R. D.: Fate of autogenous fat implants in the frontal sinuses of cats. Am. J. Vet. Res., *44*:22, 1983.

Bryant, M. S., Bremer, A. M., and Nguyen, T. Q.: Autogeneic fat transplants in the epidural space in routine lumbar spine surgery. Neurosurgery, *13*:367, 1983.

Busch, H., von: Kosmetische Besserung der durch Fazialislähmung bedingten Enstellung. Z. Ohrenheilkd., *68*:175, 1913.

Cannaday, J. E.: Some of the uses of the cutis graft in surgery. Am. J. Surg., *59*:409, 1943.

Cannaday, J. E.: An additional report on some of the uses of cutis graft material in reparative surgery. Am. J. Surg., *67*:238, 1945.

Corso, P. F., and Gerold, F.: Use of autogeneous dermis for protection of the carotid artery and pharyngeal suture line in radical head and neck surgery. Surg. Forum, *12*:483, 1961.

Corso, P. F., and Gerold, F. P.: Use of autogenous dermis for protection of the carotid artery and pharyngeal suture lines in radical head and neck surgery. Surg. Gynecol. Obstet., *117*:37, 1963.

Crawford, H.: Dura replacement. An experimental study of derma autografts and preserved dura homografts. Plast Reconstr. Surg., *19*:299, 1957.

Crawford, J. S.: Fascia lata: its nature and fate after implantation and its use in ophthalmic surgery. Trans. Am. Ophthalmol. Soc., *66*:673, 1968.

Crawford, J. S.: Nature of fascia lata and its fate after implantation. Am. J. Ophthalmol., *67*:900, 1969.

Dedo, D. D., Sessions, D. G., Alonso, W. A., and Ogura, J. H., Complications of dermal graft protection of carotid artery. Arch. Otolaryngol., *101*:649, 1975.

Eitner, E.: Über Unterpolsterung der Gesichtshaut. Med. Klin., *16*:93, 1920.

Fujino, T., Rytinzaburo, T., and Sugimoto, C.: Microvascular transfer of free deltopectoral dermal-fat flap. Plast. Reconstr. Surg., *55*:428, 1975.

Gebauer, P. W.: Plastic reconstruction of tuberculous bronchostenosis with dermal grafts. J. Thorac. Surg., *19*:604, 1950.

Georgiade, N. G.: The surgical correction of temporomandibular joint dysfunction by means of autogenous dermal grafts. Plast. Reconstr. Surg., *30*:68, 1962.

Griffiths, R. W., and Shakespeare, P. G.: Human dermal collagen allografts: a three year histological study. Br. J. Plast. Surg., *35*:519, 1982.

Guiot, G., Rougerie, J., and Tessier, P.: La greffe dermique. Procédé de protection cérébro-méningée et de blindage duremerien. Ann. Chir. Plast., *12*:93, 1967.

Heck, E. L., Bergstresser, P. R., and Baxter, C. R.: Composite skin graft: frozen dermal allografts support the engraftment and expansion of autologous epidermis. J. Trauma, *25*:106, 1985.

Horton, C., Campbell, F., Connar, R., McWhirt, J., and Pickrell, K.: Behavior of split-thickness, dermal, and full-thickness skin grafts in the thoracic cavity; experimental study. A.M.A. Arch. Surg., *70*:221, 1955.

Horton, C., Georgiade, N., Campbell, F., Masters, F., and Pickrell, K.: The behavior of split thickness and dermal skin grafts in the peritoneal cavity. An experimental study. Plast. Reconstr. Surg., *12*:269, 1953.

Hynes, W.: The skin-dermis graft as an alternative to the direct or tubed flap. Br. J. Plast. Surg., *7*:97, 1954.

Jahoda, C. A., Horne, K. A., and Oliver, R. F.: Induction of hair growth by implantation of cultural dermal papilla cells. Nature, *311*:560, 1984.

Johnson, H. A.: Dermis graft for post-leprosy muscular wasting in the hand. Plast. Reconstr. Surg., *27*:624, 1961.

Key, B. W.: Fat implantations. Arch. Ophthalmol., *48*:292, 1919.

Kirschner, M.: Ueber freie Shenen-und Faszientransplantation. Beitr. Klin. Chir., *65*:472, 1909.

Lauber, H.: Ueber Enukleation mit Fettimplantation. Ztschr. Augenheilkd, *23*:426, 1910.

Lewis, S. R., Lynch, J. B., and Blocker, T. G., Jr.: Fascial slings for tongue stabilization in the Pierre Robin syndrome. Plast. Reconstr. Surg., *42*:237, 1968.

Lexer, E.: Freie Fettgewebstransplantation. Dtsch. Med. Wochenschr., *36*:640, 1910.

Lexer, E.: Free transplantation. Ann. Surg., *60*:166, 1914.

Lexer, E.: Fettgewebstransplantation, in die freien Transplantationen. Part I. Neue Deutsche Chir., *25*:272, 1919.

Lexer, E.: Zwanzig Jahre Transplantationsforschung in der Chirurgie. Arch. Klin. Chir., *138*:294, 1925.

Loewe, O.: Ueber Haut Implantation on Stelle der freien faszien Plastik. München. Med. Wochenschr., *60*:1320, 1913.

Loewe, O.: München. Med. Wochenschr., *76*:2125, 1929. Cited by Cannaday (1942).

López, F.: Valor comparativo de las diversas operaciones propuestas para reemplazar à la enucleación del ojo y especialmente de las implantaciones de grasa. An. Oftal., Mexico, *5*:335, 1902–1903.

Marx, G.: Ueber Fetttransplantation nach Evisearatio und Enucleatio bulbi. Arch. Augenheikd., *66*:15, 1910.

Metheny, D., Lundmark, V. O., and Morcom, T.: Use of dermal graft to supply defect in the diaphragm. West. J. Surg., *60*:156, 1952.

McArthur, L. L.: Autoplastic sutures in hernia and other diseases. Preliminary report. J.A.M.A., *37*:1162, 1901.

McArthur, L. L.: Autoplastic sutures in hernia and other diseases. J.A.M.A., *43*:1039, 1904.

Montgomery, W. W., and Pierce, D. L.: Anterior osteoplastic fat obliteration for frontal sinus: clinical experience and animal studies. Trans. Am. Acad. Ophthalmol. Otolaryngol., *69*:46, 1963.

Neuber, G. A.: Fetttransplantation. Verh. Dtsch. Ges. Chir. Kong. Verh., *22*:66, 1893.

Oliver, R. F.: The experimental induction of whisker growth in the hooded rat by implantation of dermal papillae. J. Embryol. Exp. Morphol., *18*:43, 1967.

Oliver, R. F.: The induction of follicle formation in the adult hooded rat by vibrissa dermal papillae. J. Embryol. Exp. Morphol., *23*:219, 1970.

Peer, L. A.: Fate of buried skin grafts in man. Arch. Surg., *39*:131, 1939.

Peer, L. A.: Loss of weight and volume in human fat grafts. Plast. Reconstr. Surg., *5*:217, 1950.

Peer, L. A.: Transplantation of Tissues. Vol. 1. Baltimore, Williams & Wilkins Company, 1955, pp. 396, 397, 404, 406.

Peer, L. A.: Transplantation of Tissues. Vol. 2. Baltimore, Williams & Wilkins Company, 1959, pp. 25, 26, 229, 230.

Peer, L. A.: Transplantation of fat. *In* Converse, J. M. (Ed.): Reconstructive Plastic Surgery. 2nd Ed. Philadelphia, W. B. Saunders, 1977, p. 251.

Peer, L. A., and Paddock, R.: Histologic studies on the fate of deeply implanted dermal grafts; observations on sections of implants buried from one week to one year. Arch. Surg., *34*:268, 1937.

Rehn, E.: Das kutane und subkutane Bindegewebe als plastisches Material. München. Med. Wochenschr., *61*:118, 1914.

Sawhney, C. P., Banerjee, T. N., and Chakravarti, R. N.: Behaviour of dermal fat transplants. Br. J. Plast. Surg., *22*:169, 1969.

Schenck, N. L.: Frontal sinus disease. I. An historical perspective on research. Laryngoscope, *84*:1031, 1974.

Schenck, N. L.: Frontal sinus disease. III. Experimental and clinical factors in failure of the frontal osteoplastic operation. Laryngoscope, *85*:76, 1975.

Schuessler, W. W., and Steffanoff, D. N.: Dermal grafts for correction of facial defects (series of 80 cases). Plast. Reconstr. Surg., *4*:341, 1949.

Schwartz, E.: Ueber die anatomischen Vorgange bei der Sehnenregeneration und dem plastischen Ersatz von Sehnendefekten durch Sehne, Fascie und Bindegewebe; eine experimentelle Studie. Dtsch. Ztschr. Chir., *173*:301, 1922.

Shen, Z. Y., Wang, S. H., Cheng, X. X., Lu, J. Z., Yin, D. Q., et al.: Greater omentum-cutaneous axial flap: a method to create transferable skin flap. Chin. Med. J., *944*:718, 1981.

Smith, B., Bosniak, S., Nesi, F., and Lisman, R.: Dermis-fat orbital implantation: 118 cases. Ophthalmic Surg., *14*:941, 1983.

Stallings, J. O., Huffman, W. C., and Bernstein, L.: Skin graft on bare bone. Plast. Reconstr. Surg., *43*:152, 1969.

Stewart, M. J.: On the occurrence of irritation giant cells in dermoid and epidermoid cysts. J. Pathol. Bacteriol., *17*:502, 1912.

Straatsma, C. R.: Use of the dermal graft in the repair of small saddle defects of the nose. Arch. Otolaryngol., *16*:506, 1932.

Swenson, S. A., Jr.: Cutis grafts; clinical and experimental observations. Arch. Surg., *61*:881, 1950.

Thompson, N.: Tubular resorption of secretion in human eccrine sweat glands. Based on a histochemical study of buried autogenous dermis grafts in man. Clin. Sci., *19*:95, 1960.

Uihlein, A., Jr.: Use of the cutis graft in plastic operations. Arch. Surg., *38*:118, 1939.

Upton, J., Mulliken, J. B., Hicks, P. D., and Murray, J. E.: Restoration of facial contour using free vascularized omental transfer. Plast. Reconstr. Surg., *66*:560, 1980.

Upton, J., Rogers, C., Durham-Smith, G., and Swartz, W. M.: Clinical applications of free temporoparietal flaps in hand reconstruction. J. Hand Surg., *11A*:475, 1986.

Vélez, D.: Valor comparativo de las diversas operaciones propuestas para reemplazar à la enucleación y especielmente de las implantaciones de grasa. An. Oftal., Mexico, *5*:303, 1902–1903.

Wells, J. H., and Edgerton, M. T.: Correction of severe hemifacial atrophy with a free dermis-fat flap from the lower abdomen. Plast. Reconstr. Surg., *59*:223, 1977.

Worst, P. K., MacKenzie, I. C., and Fusenig, N. E.: Reformation of organized epidermal structure by transplantation of suspensions and cultures of epidermal and dermal cells. Cell Tissue Res., *225*:65, 1982.

15

David T. W. Chiu
Bradford W. Edgerton

Repair and Grafting of Tendon

The property of tendon to be successfully transferred after transection of its vascular supply has been clinically exploited for many years. Recent advances in the understanding of the anatomy and biology of tendon transplantation have given surgeons the ability to proceed with their clinical work with a greater understanding of the underlying basic science.

ANATOMY

Tendons. A tendon is a white fibrous cord that connects a muscle to a bone or other structure. It may unite with a muscle at its extremity or it may accompany the muscle for a distance, receiving muscular fibers along its lateral border. It may lie in a loose areolar tissue called a *paratenon,* or it may pass through a tube of condensed fibrous tissue called a *tendon sheath.*

Paratenon. The word "paratenon" was proposed by Mayer (1916) to describe the connective tissue surrounding a tendon that is traversing a straight course and is not subject to pressure. It is a loose elastic tissue, organized as a multilayered structure, which connects the tendon to the surrounding tissues (Fig. 15–1) (Nisbet, 1960; Colville, Callison, and White, 1969; Winckler, 1970).

These layers enclose a semifluid, filmy, homogenous material and drape over a mesotenon that contains the blood supply to the tendon in this region. Paratenon contains mucopolysaccharide components that allow motion (Peacock, 1971) and fine collagen fibers that are loosely arranged (Fig. 15–2) (Potenza, 1964).

Palmar Bursae. As tendons proceed in their course from the musculofascial planes in the forearm to the fingers, they are enclosed in distinct palmar bursae. These provide no structural support, but enclose the tendons and define pathways for the spread of infections that have long been known to hand surgeons (Kanavel, 1939). These are open to the thumb and the little finger flexor tendon sheaths, but do not communicate with the digital tendon sheaths of the middle three digits (Fig. 15–3). They incorporate mesotenon blood vessels in the carpal and metacarpal regions.

Tendon Sheath. From an area overlying the metacarpal heads proximally to the midportion of the distal phalanges, fully devel-

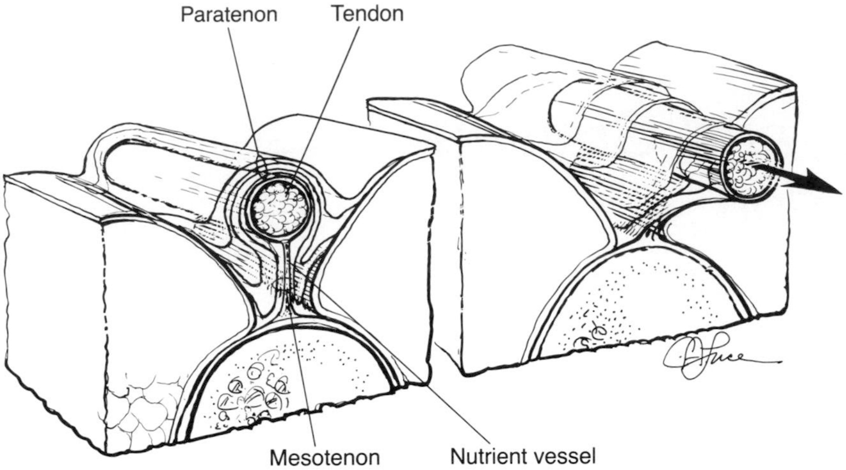

Figure 15–1. The multilayered paratenon forms a barrier between the tendon and the surrounding structure and serves as a source of nutrition via the vincular vessels. The mesotenon is the part of the paratenon draped over the nutrient vessels functioning as an umbilicus. Its pliability and length allow the tendon to glide and yet maintain continuous perfusion.

oped fibrous sheaths are attached to the underlying bone and palmar plates at the metacarpophalangeal, proximal interphalangeal, and distal interphalangeal joints and enclose the flexor tendons. These sheaths have been designed both to prevent "bowstringing" of the flexor tendons by holding the tendons close to the bones at certain locations and to allow acute flexion at the interphalangeal joints. There are broad, dense condensations of fibrous tissue at several locations overlying the proximal and middle phalanges, and thinner annular bands directly overlying the interphalangeal joints. Between these lie collapsible segments of tendon sheath that contain two cruciate ligaments proximal to each interphalangeal joint through which the vincular vessels penetrate (Fig. 15–4) (Strauch and deMoura, 1985).

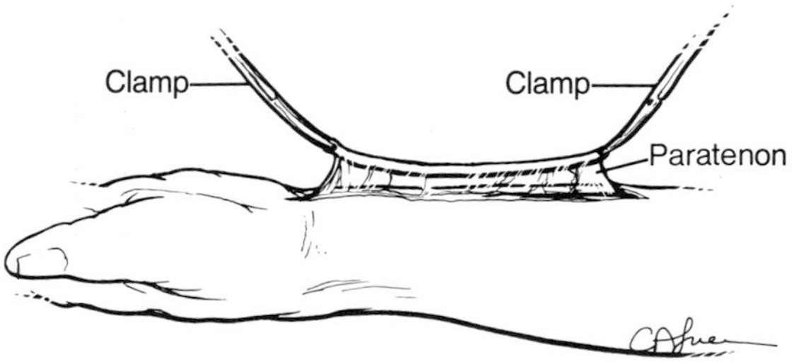

Figure 15–2. The paratenon at the forearm is a filmy homogenous material containing mucopolysaccharide components that facilitate the gliding motion. The paratenon is composed of fine collagen fibers arranged as a loosely laced network that contributes to its pliability.

The sheath is lined by a parietal layer similar to the synovial lining of a joint (Winckler, 1970). In addition to the mechanical aid to flexion provided by the flexor

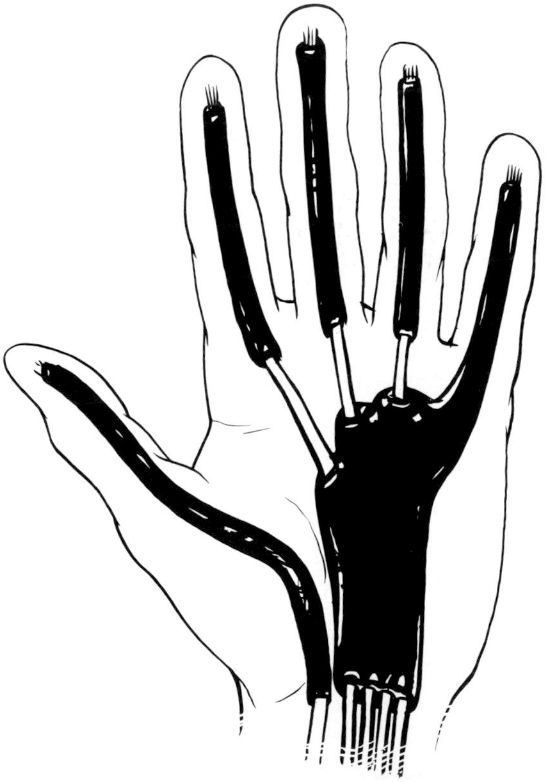

Figure 15–3. The palmar fascia can be divided into the radial palmar bursa, which communicates with the thumb, and the ulnar palmar fascia, which communicates directly only with the flexor tendon sheath of the little finger.

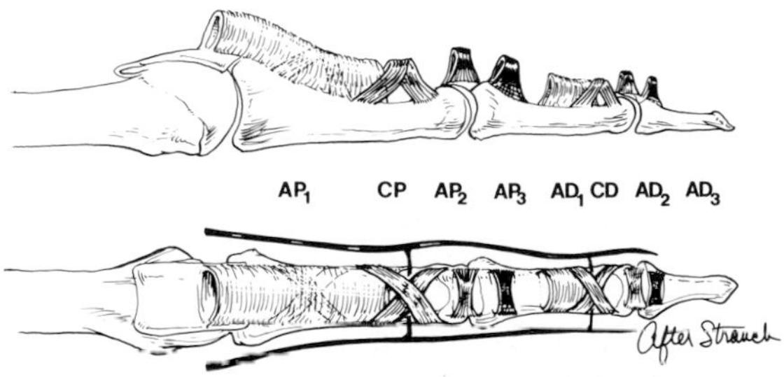

Figure 15–4. The digital flexor tendon sheath is characterized by the presence of annular condensation of fibrous tissue overlying segments of the proximal and middle phalanges (AP_1, AD_1) (annular proximal 1 and annular distal 1) and thinner annular bands directly overlying the interphalangeal joints (AP_2, AD_2, AP_3, AD_3). In between lie the collapsible segments of tendon sheath with two cruciate ligaments proximal to each interphalangeal joint (CP, CD) (cruciate proximal and cruciate distal).

tendon sheath, this layer allows for smooth gliding of the tendinous structures and provides an enclosed bursal environment for synovial fluid nutrition. Diffusion of nutrients through the fluid in this closed space is considered an important contribution to tendon nutrition after transplantation.

Blood Supply. Mayer (1916) provided the first accurate description of the blood supply of tendons. A mesotenon in the forearm and proximal palm provides the blood supply to tendons on their deep surface in a segmental fashion (see Fig. 15–1). The mesentery is condensed into two specific vincula in the digits that provide distinct vessels entering on the deep side of the flexor tendons proximal to each interphalangeal joint. Subsequent studies (Edwards, 1946; Brockis, 1953; Nisbet, 1960; Smith, 1965; Schatzker and Branemark, 1969) further detailed this delicate anatomy. Within the substance of the tendon exists a longitudinal, intrafascicular vascular pattern paralleling the collagen fibers. Chaplin (1973) noted that these vessels were concentrated on the dorsal aspect of the tendons. Lundborg, Myrhage, and Rydevik (1977) noted areas of consistent avascularity in flexor tendons. Ochiai and associates (1979) performed further studies that identify specific patterns of vincular blood flow and suggest patterns of variation in some patients, with the absence of vincular vessels in some specimens. Armenta and Lehrman (1980) suggested classification of four types of vincula. Zbrodowski, Gajisin, and Grodecki (1981) described the mesotenons of the flexor tendons in detail in the palmar bursae. Azar, Culver, and Fleegler (1983) detailed the blood supply of the flexor pollicis longus tendon. Strauch and deMoura (1985) noted a constant penetrating vessel at each interphalangeal joint. As the understanding of the precise anatomic details of the vascular supply of the flexor tendons is enhanced, the debate continues over the relative nutritional importance of the blood supply versus the synovial fluid. One clinical series (Amadio and associates, 1985) showed inferior functional results in tendon repairs in which the vincular supply had been disrupted.

HISTOLOGY AND BIOCHEMISTRY

Tendon is composed of collagen, ground substance, elastin, tenocytes, and associated blood vessels, nerves, and lymphatics. Collagen is in a higher concentration in tendons than in any other tissue of the body, being approximately 70 per cent dry weight (Harkness, 1968). Collagen is a complex protein and the basic unit is the fibril. A fibril is composed of tropocollagen macromolecules, which in tendons (Type I collagen) consist of two identical and one dissimilar polypeptide chains, each containing approximately 1000 amino acid residues. The fibrils are combined in a triple helix in tendons (Klein, 1976). Glycine is the most common amino acid residue (30 per cent), and hydroxyproline and proline (28 per cent combined) are also common. Crosslinking of the macromolecules provides the tensile strength inherent in tendons.

The collection of tendon fibrils lying parallel are called tendon fibers, which are approximately 300 μ in diameter (Elliot, 1965). The primary tendon fibers are grouped into "fasciculi." A third level of aggregation into tendon bundles then occurs (Fig. 15–5).

The tension from the muscle is transmitted from a myofibril into a tendon fibril. At the osseous junction, the primary tendon bundles attach to fibrocartilage, mineralized fibrocartilage, and bone itself (Cooper and Misol, 1970).

Ground substance in tendon is present in small amounts and is composed of glycosaminoglycans, glycoproteins, and noncollagenous protein (Jackson and Bentley, 1968). Glycosaminoglycans are large molecular weight carbohydrates composed of amino acids and uronic acids. They are involved in the matu-

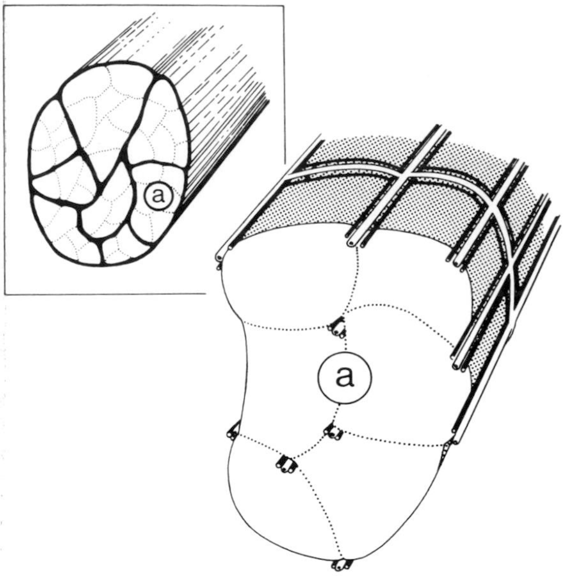

Figure 15–5. Cross section of a tendon showing the arrangement of the fasciculi and vascular bundles. (Modified from Braithwaite, F., and Brockis, J. G.: The vascularization of a tendon graft. Br. J. Plast. Surg., *4*:130, 1951. Reproduced by permission of E & S Livingstone.)

ration, aggregation, and cementing of collagen fibrils and fibers (Jackson, 1953; Edwards and Dunphy, 1958). They also facilitate the lubrication of fibrils and fibers during deformation.

Cellular Histology of Tendons. Much confusion reigns about the exact function of the various cells in and around tendons. Three distinct populations have been identified: (1) *epitenon* cells, a thin cellular layer on the outer margin of the tendon; (2) *endotenon* cells, the continuation of the epitenon projection into tendon bundles—the intratendinous vasculature is located in the interfascicular area; and (3) *tenocytes,* sparsely distributed cells within the tendon bundles. It has not been clearly defined whether the cells in the epitenon and endotenon and within the tendon bundles (the tenocytes) have differing characteristics and functions (Manske, Gelberman, and Lesker, 1985).

PHYSIOLOGY OF TENDON NUTRITION

The current thinking is that both perfusion (vascular supply) and diffusion (through synovial fluid) contribute to the nutrition of tendons. The well-defined vascular pathways contribute to the transport of nutrients in the intact tendon, but the ability of lengthy devascularized segments of tendon to survive and undergo healing signifies that diffusion is also an important source of nutrition for a tendon graft.

In a series of studies (Manske, Bridwell, and Lesker, 1978; Manske, Lesker, and Bridwell, 1979; Manske and Lesker, 1982, 1983), radioactive tracer materials were used in several animals and showed that diffusion is more efficient than perfusion in the delivery of the tracer to tendons. In the absence of all vascular connections, diffusion alone provided adequate nutrition for tendon healing. A scientific debate has been raging as to the relative importance of the two phenomena.

Of interest is the study by Winckler (1970), who observed that the small vascular conglomerates in human tendons did not penetrate tendon fascicles. He concluded that tendon nutrition is dependent on diffusion of fluid through the vessel walls, and suggested that nutrients emerged from the vascular channels and diffused into the tendon. McDowell and Snyder (1977) observed vascular loops and canaliculi in tendons and suggested that synovial fluid could adequately nourish all segments of a tendon. Weber (1979) noted conduits and channels on scanning electron microscopy and suggested that synovial fluid was delivered through these channels. Lundborg, Holm, and Myrhage (1980), using sulfur 35 and methyl-3H-glucose, and Hooper, Davies, and Tothill (1984) using radioactive microspheres, also noted more predominant roles of diffusion in dog models.

PHYSIOLOGY OF TENDON GRAFT HEALING

For a transplanted tendon to function, it must form connections to the distal structure (bone or tendon) and the proximal tendon. Revascularization of the entire transplanted tendon must also occur to ensure long-term viability. The tendon graft must also glide freely through the intervening tissues to have any functional benefit.

Healing of Tendon Ends. To explain how tendons heal to bone and other tendons, a brief description of the three phases of wound healing follows (Weiner and Peacock, 1971).

Cellular Phase. After tendon transplantation the space between the tendon ends and between tendon and bone is first filled with blood clot. Fibrinous material and a mesh of granulation tissue containing erythrocytes, macrophages, and inflammatory cells invade the space. Epitenon cells (from the surface of the tendon) proliferate and invade the repair site, and change their appearance to that of fibroblasts (Fig. 15–6) (Gelberman and associates, 1985).

Collagen Synthesis Phase. Collagen synthesis may be detected by the sixth day and proceeds for several weeks. The number of fibroblasts reaches a peak at two weeks and then declines. Revascularization of the tendon begins during this period. Continued strengthening of the wound occurs as the collagen fibers reorient (Potenza, 1962).

Remodeling Phase. The functioning of a tendon transplant is most dependent on the third phase of healing in which the tendon union gains strength and the peritendinous adhesions lose strength. This development allows mobility of the tendon graft. By eight weeks in favorable conditions the adhesions between the graft and the peritendinous tissues are filmy and loose. However, it is nine months before the collagen fibers in the healing ends resemble normal tendon bundles.

Intrinsic versus Extrinsic Healing

Although there is reasonable agreement about the general course of events in tendon healing, a controversy exists in the scientific community over the source of the active healing cells. This revolves around whether cells within the tendon (tenocytes, endotenon), cells on the surface of the tendon (epitenon), or cells in the surrounding tissue (fibroblasts)

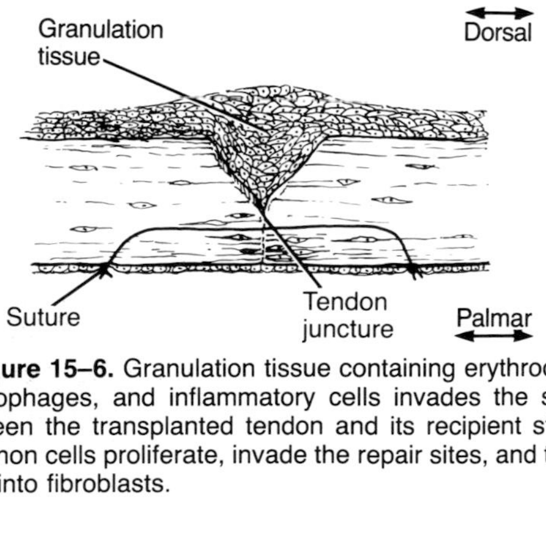

Figure 15–6. Granulation tissue containing erythrocytes, macrophages, and inflammatory cells invades the space between the transplanted tendon and its recipient stump. Epitenon cells proliferate, invade the repair sites, and transform into fibroblasts.

are the agents for healing and the production of new collagen. Classical teaching on how to resect large areas of tendon sheath to permit the ingrowth of adhesions (Potenza, 1969; Verdan, 1975) has been challenged by a series of experiments indicating that the tendon does have an "intrinsic" ability to heal from epitenon surface cells, endotenon cells, tenocytes, or all three. The evidence for intrinsic healing is as follows. Furlow (1976) observed healing human tendon anastomoses without the evidence of adhesions from the surrounding tissues. Richards (1977) and Matthews (1979) noted that lacerated flexor tendons that had retracted into the flexor tendon sheath "rounded off" and healed their ends without evidence of adhesion attachment. A series of experiments in chicken tendons (Lindsay and Thomson, 1959; Lindsay, Thomson, and Walker, 1960; Lindsay and McDougall, 1961) indicated that healing is initiated by epitenon cells and augmented by endotenon cells after a delay of several days. Tenocytes also participated in the repair after two or three weeks. Adhesions were not essential to the healing process. However, Lindsay and Birch (1964) also found, in studying rat tendons, that repair was primarily due to extrinsic fibroblasts migrating from the tendon sheath. Fibroblasts within the tendons were not capable of proliferation and collagen production in the rat model.

Another series of experiments (Matthews and Richards, 1974, 1975, 1976; Eiken, Lundborg, and Rank, 1975) produced tendon lacerations in rabbit tendons while maintaining the integrity of the flexor synovial sheath environment. These authors observed healing of the tendon lacerations in the absence of peripheral adhesions. The resting tenocytes were transformed to active tenoblasts that proliferated and produced new collagen. Central necrosis was noted in the tendons, but the superficial layers were characterized by fibroplasia and the synthesis of new collagen fibers without adhesion formation. McDowell and Snyder (1977) confirmed these findings in dog flexor tendons.

Lundborg, in a series of experiments (Lundborg, 1976; Lundborg and Rank, 1978, 1980; Lundborg and associates 1980), investigated the healing of rabbit and human flexor tendons within the rabbit knee joint. The tendons demonstrated cellular fibroplasia in the superficial layers and bridging of the suture gap in the absence of peripheral adhesions.

The central layer of the tendon was characterized by no cellular activity. Lundborg and Rank (1980), Lundborg and associates (1980), Katsumi and associates (1980), and Katsumi and Tajima (1981) studied rabbit flexor tendon healing in pouches with a dialyzing membrane and noted complete healing in six weeks. These experiments all support the concept that tendon healing is performed by *intrinsic* cells.

These in vivo experiments were supported by several in vitro studies by Manske and Lesker (1984) and Gelberman and associates (1984), which demonstrated that the tendons of monkeys, chickens, dogs, and rabbits exhibited a healing potential for up to 12 weeks in tissue culture media. Epitenon cells migrated into the wound and initiated the repair process with phagocytosis. Collagen synthesis was a function of the endotenon cells. The tendons remained viable for 12 weeks with no evidence of central necrosis.

In contradistinction, Landi and associates (1980) repeated Lundborg's "in situ tissue culture" experiment with rabbit knee joints and found the tendon segments completely covered by adhesions. Potenza and Herte (1982) and Chow, Hooper, and Chan (1983) demonstrated in the dog and rabbit that nonviable, freeze-dried acellular tendons were recellularized and healed by seeding of cells from the synovial lining cells. Thus, these experiments showed a role for *extrinsic* healing in certain in vivo models. It is not clear in human situations whether *intrinsic* or *extrinsic* healing is more significant.

Revascularization of Graft

Tendon transplants consist of initially avascular grafts. It is not known whether autograft tendons survive completely or become reorganized. Peacock (1959a) and Potenza (1963) showed that a tendon deprived of its blood supply undergoes cellular necrosis (within an impervious sheath) by nine days. By the third week there is a loss of cohesiveness between the collagen bundles (Peacock, 1957). To survive, the autograft must be revascularized either "primarily" by direct anastomoses with vessels in the bed, or "secondarily" by the ingrowth of capillaries and the establishment of a new vascular network. Although there have been several reports of direct evidence of "primary" revascularization in tendon grafts in nonsheath areas (Peer, 1955; Bergljung, 1968; Chaplin 1973), there has been no direct evidence for this type of "primary" revascularization in tendon grafts enclosed by sheaths.

A study by Eiken and Lundborg (1983) in chickens provided strong evidence of "secondary" revascularization in tendon grafts. In their experiment the longitudinal microvascular system of the tendon was established by eight weeks, but vessels were evenly distributed on the dorsal and volar surfaces. (A normal anatomic relationship has no vessels on the volar aspect of flexor tendons within a sheath.) By 16 weeks, tendon grafts within a sheath had restored a normal pattern of only dorsal vascular distribution. Tendon grafts not enclosed by a sheath showed continued volar and dorsal intratendinous vessels at both eight and 16 weeks. These authors found that revascularization in sheathed tendon grafts occurred in the absence of significant adhesions. "Secondary" revascularization most likely ensures the survival of tendon grafts with sheaths. The initial survival, however, must depend on synovial fluid nutrition.

Tendon Gliding

To be successful, a tendon transplant must slide through the surrounding tissues. When a tendon graft covered with paratenon is utilized within a sheath, the paratenon may become the source of proliferation of fibroblasts and scar tissue (Weiner and Peacock, 1971). If the paratenon is removed by scraping, the epitenon will presumably be violated and increased adhesions will ensue (Skoog and Persson, 1954). Thus, extreme care must be exercised in removing the paratenon atraumatically in order not to violate the epitenon.

CLINICAL TRANSPLANTATION

In the 1960's and 1970's several authors demonstrated superior results in repairing tendon lacerations acutely (Kleinert and associates, 1969; Lister and associates, 1977), and the indications for tendon grafting have narrowed. Tendon transplantation is now reserved for situations in which there is a delay in management, when a delayed primary repair is not feasible, or when the circumstances of the injury or condition of the bed require preparations before tendon reconstruction. It is presently advocated that the tendon sheath needs to be reconstructed in tendon grafting to achieve a satisfactory result. "In any circumstance in which primary flexor tendon repair or secondary tendon graft is being undertaken, the flexor tendon sheath should be restored" (Lister, 1985).

Technique

Incisions. Incisions in the hand should be designed to allow complete exposure but avoid subsequent scar contracture of an adjacent joint. Midaxial or volar zigzag incisions (Fig. 15–7) accomplish these aims in the digit. The proximal juncture may be performed in the palm (Fig. 15–8) if unscarred, but care should be taken to have the proximal juncture beneath a skin flap. Junctures may also be performed in the wrist, and the incision should course in an ulnar direction to avoid the palmar cutaneous branch of the median nerve.

Graft Bed Preparation. If the tendon sheath needs to be opened, it should be at a membranous portion, preserving the annular pulleys. When dissecting near a joint, it is essential to remain volar to the palmar plate to prevent joint stiffness. If a vincular vessel is divided, it should be cauterized to prevent bleeding. A 1 cm stump of distal profundus tendon is preserved and split. The stump of superficialis tendon, if present over the proximal interphalangeal joint, should be left in

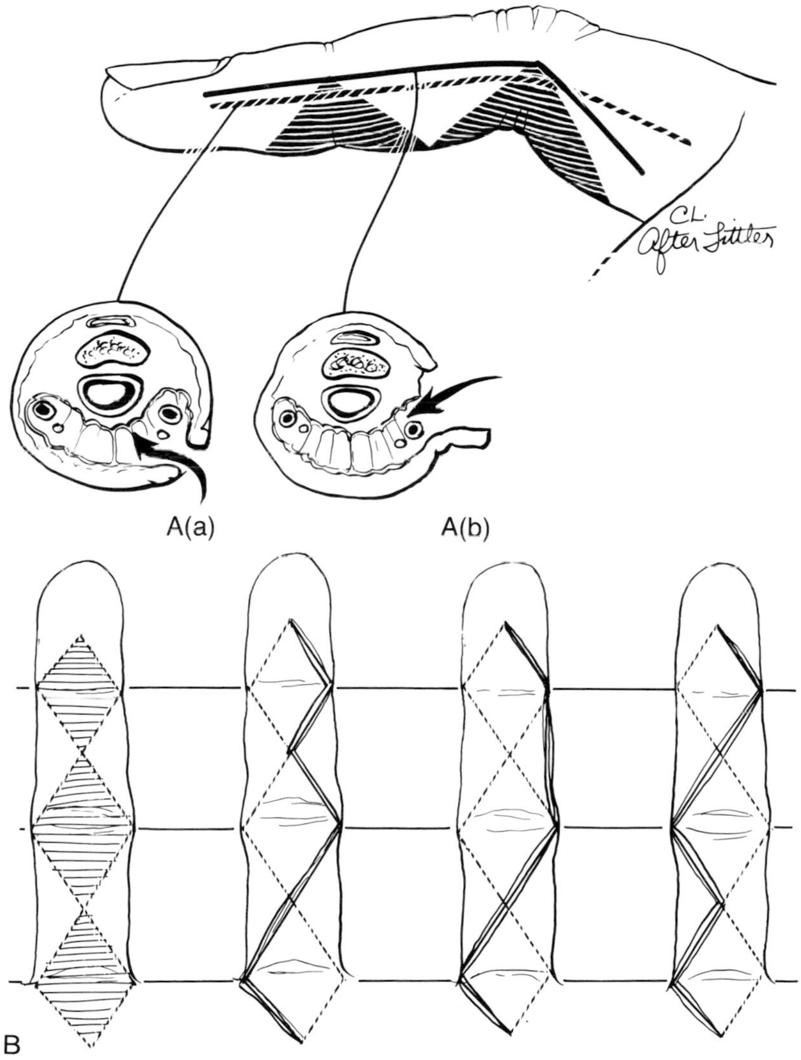

Figure 15–7. The basic principles to follow when performing a skin incision in a digit in order to obtain full exposure of the digit and to avoid transgressing the flexion surfaces of the joints. A midaxial incision *(A)* or a volar zigzag incision *(B)* accomplishes this purpose. If a midaxial incision is utilized, it is preferable to elevate the neurovascular bundle with the volar flap (as in *A(b)*).

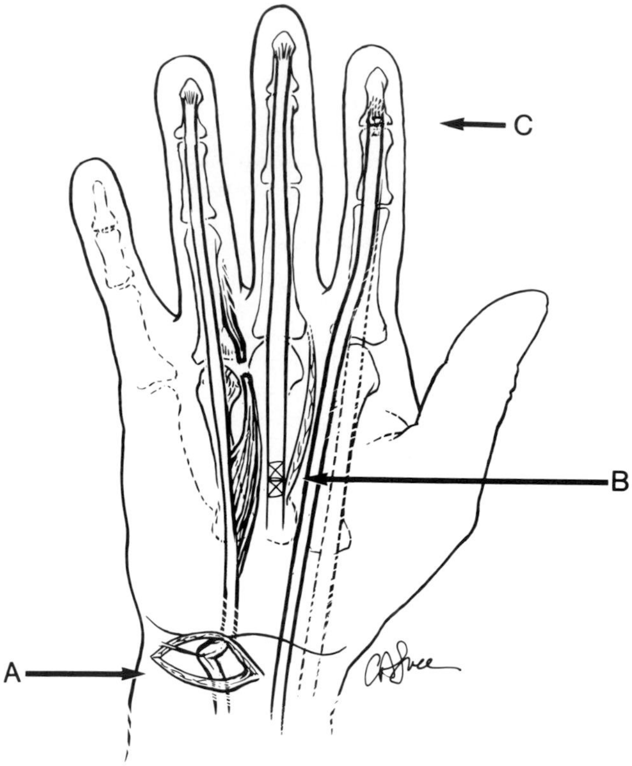

Figure 15–8. The proximal junction of the tendon graft can either be at the midpalmar level *(B)* or at the wrist level *(A)*. However, if the tenorrhaphy is performed at the wrist level, the distal lumbrical insertion should be disrupted to avoid a "lumbrical-plus" hand. The Silastic rod is sutured distally to a stump of approximately 4 mm of flexor digitorum profundus *(C)*. The proximal end of the Silastic rod should be free and is usually placed to the ulnar side of the prospective donor site.

place to allow a smooth bed and provide a tenodesis effect. If that joint is hyperextensible, a formal proximal interphalangeal tenodesis should be performed. In the palm, any scarred palmar fascia should be excised. The lumbrical muscle is dissected from any adhesions to the retracted profundus stump to prevent a "lumbrical-plus" finger (Fig. 15–9) (Parkes, 1971). A judgment on which motor to use must then be made. A motor that has not undergone myostatic contracture (Weeks and Wray, 1978) must be selected. The ulnar three profundus tendons have a common muscle belly, so if only one tendon is divided it will not retract. A 35 mm tendon excursion is necessary for a satisfactory arc of motion; this can be checked by assessing the passive stretch on a muscle unit. The fibro-osseous tendon sheath needs to be assessed and gently stretched to allow placement of the graft. If the pulleys have to be reconstructed, two-stage tendon reconstruction is indicated and a silicone rod should be placed (see below). The proximal juncture is performed by means of a Pulvertaft "fishmouth weave" (Fig. 15–10), using 4.0 braided polyester suture. The distal juncture is made by passing the tendon just volar to the pulp, securing it to the stump of the profundus, and suturing the end to the nail plate (Fig. 15–11). It should be set at slightly more tension than that of the adjacent digits, as stretching of the transplant will occur postoperatively.

Donor Sites

The ideal donor tendon has the following characteristics: (1) it is always present; (2) it is consistent in all its dimensions; (3) it is of sufficient length to bridge completely the defect at the recipient site; (4) it is superficially located for ease of access; (5) its loss does not affect the function of the donor area; (6) it is thin enough for adequate revascularization; and (7) it is sufficiently strong for its new task.

Commonly used tendons include the palmaris longus; the plantaris; the extensor digitorum longus tendons to the second, third, and fourth toes; a flexor digitorum superficialis tendon; or an undamaged tendon in an amputated digit. None of these has all the ideal attributes of the perfect donor tendon, but each has some of them.

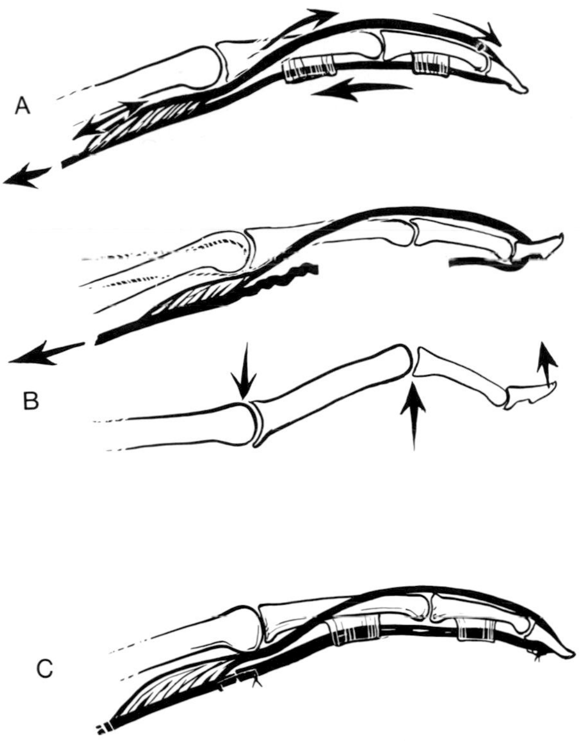

Figure 15–9. *A,* Excessive tension on the lumbrical muscle caused by contraction of the unrepaired profundus muscle leads to excessive tension on the intrinsic system via the lumbrical tendon. *B,* Inappropriate extension of the distal interphalangeal joint during attempted flexion of the digit is known as a "lumbrical-plus" finger. *C,* The appropriate tendon graft restores the physical continuity of the profundus tendon and restores the balance between the extensor and flexor systems.

PALMARIS LONGUS

Anatomy. Showing the features of phylogenetic degeneration, this vestigial muscle (Last, 1966), like the plantaris, has a long tendon and a short muscle belly. It lies immediately deep to the deep fascia of the forearm between the flexor carpi radialis and flexor carpi ulnaris, and is one of the superficial flexor group of forearm muscles; its nerve supply is from the median nerve (C6, C7) (Gray's 1973). The tendon, usually 10 to 12 cm long, 3 to 5 mm wide, and 1 to 2 mm thick, emerges from the muscle belly at the mid-forearm level and passes distally to be inserted partly into the volar aspect of the flexor retinaculum and partly into the central part of the palmar aponeurosis. In the distal forearm the tendon is enclosed in the antebrachial fascia (Hollingshead, 1982). In addition to these commonly described attachments, slender fibers may diverge from the

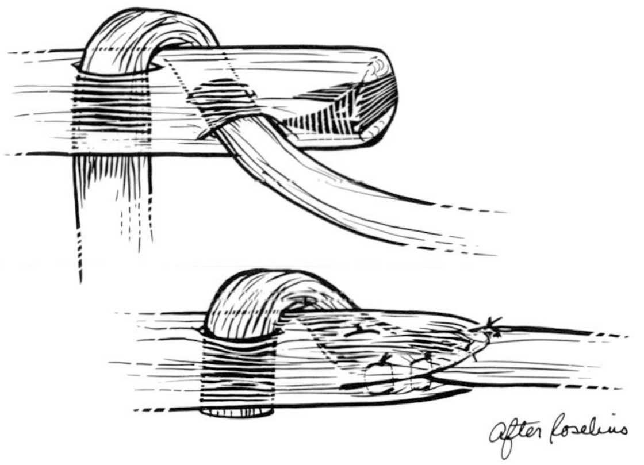

Figure 15–10. Pulvertaft "fishmouth" weaving technique allows for a strong union of two tendons with significantly different diameters, and is appropriate for the proximal junction of the tendon graft.

distal part of the tendon to gain attachment to the deep fascia of the forearm.

Just proximal to the wrist the palmaris longus tendon lies superficial to the median nerve, covering its ulnar side. The tendon of the flexor carpi radialis, a thicker structure, lies on the radial side of the tendon. Both of these structures have been mistaken for the palmaris longus tendon.

The palmaris longus tendon may be demonstrated by forcible opposition of the tips of the thumb and little finger, with the wrist in slight flexion. If present in a slim wrist, the tendon projects clear of the deeper structures, raising a ridge on the overlying skin and the median line of the wrist region; if the arm is

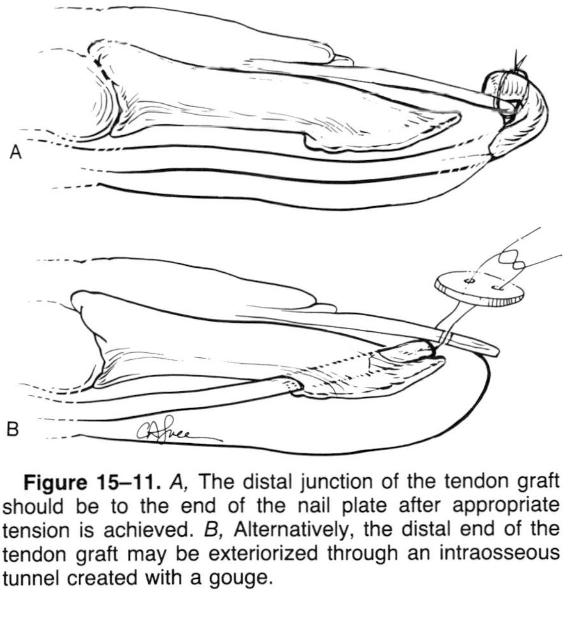

Figure 15–11. *A,* The distal junction of the tendon graft should be to the end of the nail plate after appropriate tension is achieved. *B,* Alternatively, the distal end of the tendon graft may be exteriorized through an intraosseous tunnel created with a gouge.

fat, the presence of the tendon may be confirmed by palpation.

Technique of Removal. After exsanguination and the application of a tourniquet, a transverse incision 1 to 2 cm long in the wrist crease is made overlying the palmaris tendon. After the skin is incised, a combination of blunt and sharp dissection reveals the tendon lying below the deep fascia. Dissection is extended distally to deliver all available tendon in this direction. If necessary, and when positive identification of the tendon is assured, it is divided just distal to a hemostat. Traction on this instrument then allows palpation of the remaining tendon. A second small transverse incision then allows exposure of the proximal palmaris longus tendon. The tendon can be divided at the musculotendinous junction under direct vision.

Possible Anomalies. The palmaris longus is one of the most variable muscles in the human body. A recent survey of 658 cadavers (1316 limbs) showed agenesis in 20.9 per cent of limbs. It was not demonstrable in right arms alone in 8.1 per cent and in left arms alone in 8.8 per cent. It was bilaterally absent in 12.5 per cent of cadavers. Absence of the palmaris did not predispose to absence of the plantaris (Harvey, Chu, and Harvey, 1983).

Advantages. The presence of the palmaris longus may be confirmed by observation and palpation. It is often considered the ideal donor for replacement of the long flexors of the fingers by the "short graft" method (in which the proximal anastomosis is performed in the palm), and for replacement of the flexor pollicis longus tendon. It is also ideal for use as a simple static support in the treatment of facial paralysis, one end being split to enclose the affected half of the oral sphincter.

Access is excellent and removal causes no permanent functional sequelae. Indeed, if the recipient site is the same hand or forearm as the donor forearm, all immediate postoperative symptomatology is localized to the same area of the body. It is not too thick to prevent adequate revascularization, yet is rarely too thin or weak to act as a flexor tendon replacement graft.

Disadvantages. Absence can be detected preoperatively, but any anomalous malformation rendering the tendon unsuitable as a graft is usually discovered only at operation. The palmaris longus is too short for use as a "long" (digit to wrist) flexor tendon replacement graft, except for the little finger and for the thumb.

PLANTARIS

Anatomy. The plantaris is also a vestigial muscle showing the characteristics of phylogenetic degeneration—a short muscle belly and a long tendon (Last, 1966). It forms, with the gastrocnemius and soleus, the superficial group of the posterior crural muscles (Fig. 15–12). The small fusiform muscle belly of the plantaris, usually 7 to 10 cm long (Gray, 1973), arises from the lower part of the lateral supracondylar line and the oblique popliteal ligament (Fig. 15–13). The long slender tendon passes distally between the gastrocnemius and soleus to lie on the medial side of the Achilles tendon, gaining insertion with it into the calcaneus. It is innervated by the tibial nerve (S1, S2) (Gray, 1973). Owing to the arrangement of its collagenous fasciculi, this tendon has the unusual property that it can be expanded into a wide ribbon.

Technique of Removal. A longitudinal incision of approximately 2 to 3 cm is made anterior to the Achilles tendon on the medial aspect of the ankle region, about 1 to 2

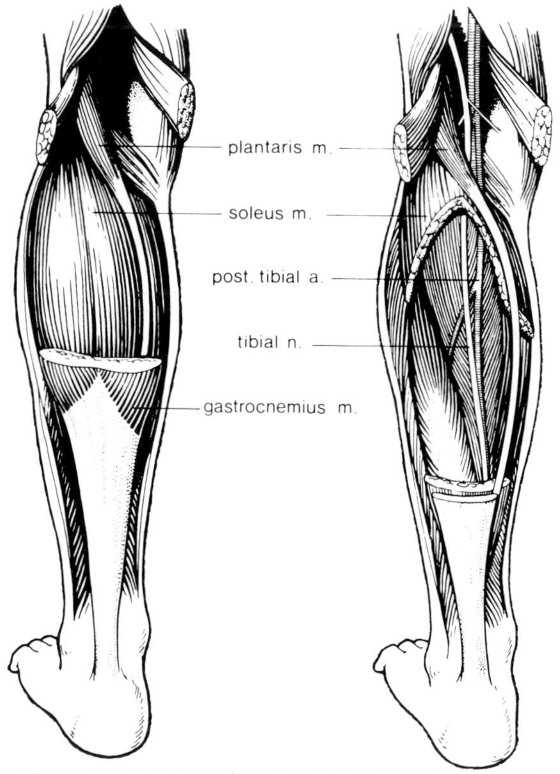

Figure 15–12. The anatomic relationships of the plantaris tendon. (Modified from White, W. L.: Tendon grafts: a consideration of their source, procurement and suitability. Surg. Clin. North Am., *40*:403, 1960.)

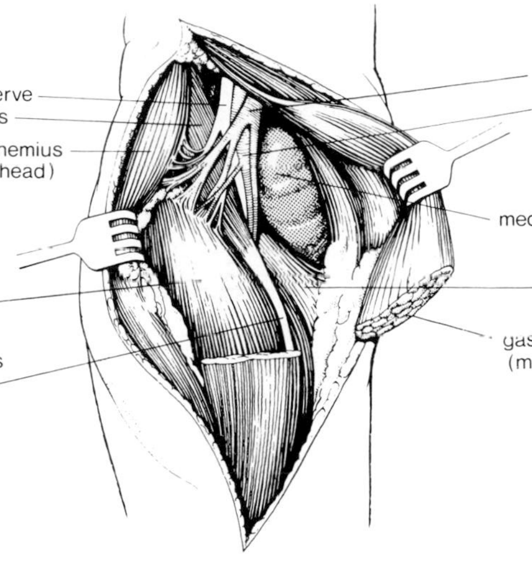

Figure 15–13. The anatomic relationships of the plantaris muscle and tendon in the popliteal fossa, illustrated to emphasize the importance of ensuring impaction of the stripper into the plantaris muscle belly to avoid injury to the adjacent vessels and nerves. (Modified from White, W. L.: Tendon grafts: a consideration of their source, procurement and suitability. Surg. Clin. North Am., *40*:403, 1960.)

fingerbreadths proximal to the most proximal part of the calcaneus (Fig. 15–14).

Deep to the skin, blunt dissection easily penetrates the loosely knit subcutaneous fat to reveal the Achilles tendon, with the plantaris tendon usually lying closely applied to its medial aspect. This should be differentiated from an accessory slip of the Achilles tendon, which will show tendon fibers devoid of paratenon on dissection, and movement of the Achilles tendon with traction (White, 1960b). Following isolation by blunt dissection, a hemostat is applied close to its insertion, and the tendon is divided.

Using the hemostat as a retractor, one can isolate the tendon from the surrounding tissue until proximally an "edge" of the deep fascia is reached. A Brand tendon stripper, designed for this purpose (Brand, 1961), is slipped over the free end of the tendon, which is again gripped by a hemostat. In order to ensure security of this grip, the tendon should be wound over the end of the hemostat and gripped again by another hemostat (Fig. 15–14).

As tension is maintained on the tendon by traction on the hemostats, the stripper is advanced, gently at first, until it has passed deep to the inferior "edge" of the superior extensor retinaculum. With the knee in extension, the stripper is advanced further along the tendon until resistance is felt at approximately 20 to 25 cm; resistance indicates impaction of the cutting edge into the muscle belly. This impaction, with the maintenance of full knee extension, prevents damage to deep structures of the tendon.

Firmer movement of the stripper cuts through the muscle and allows the tendon to be withdrawn through the ankle incision; it is immediately trimmed and transplanted.

Before transplantation the tendon is stretched horizontally between two hemostats so that the surplus paratenon may be trimmed, extreme care being taken to preserve the surface of the tendon intact from damage and desiccation.

The skin wound is closed, a dressing is applied, and the leg, from popliteal fossa to toes, is firmly bandaged with a pressure dressing and an elastic bandage before the tourniquet is released. To decrease the chance of thromboembolism, ambulation is encouraged on the first or second postoperative day.

Possible Anomalies. The tendon is absent in approximately 18.2 per cent of extremities. It was absent from the right alone in 6.1 per cent and absent from the left alone in 4.9 per cent. If the tendon is absent on one side, the chance of finding it on the other is one in three. No relationship is found between presence and absence of the palmaris and plantaris tendons (Harvey, Chu, and Harvey, 1983). When present, 60 per cent of the tendons are inserted with the Achilles tendon, while about 32 per cent gain their insertion directly to the calcaneus at a position 0.5 to 2.5 cm anterior to the Achilles tendon. Of the remaining anomalous insertions, the most common is that inserted into the distal end of the Achilles tendon itself (Daseler and Anson, 1943). It is possible to palpate the tendon only if its course is separate from that of the Achilles tendon (Pilcher, 1939).

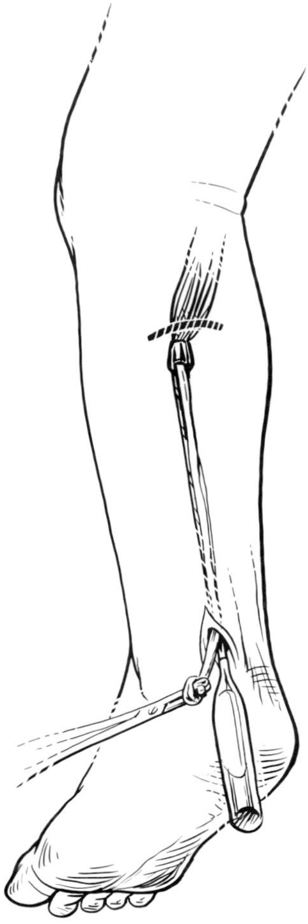

Figure 15–14. Securing the distal stump of the plantaris tendon with a hemostat avoids the embarrassment of losing the tendon graft when advancing the tendon stripper. The maneuver also allows fine adjustments of tension when advancing the tendon stripper.

Advantages. The plantaris is frequently present. It is long enough for use as a "long" flexor tendon replacement graft (wrist to digit) or as two "short" grafts. Its loss does not affect function of the limb. Its strength is usually adequate for flexor tendon replacement grafting, and it is not too thick for revascularization. The tendon can be stretched laterally. Owing to the parallel arrangement of the fibers, the tendon may be split into two or more slips or tails if necessary.

Disadvantages. It is usually not possible to determine the presence of the plantaris before surgery. It is uncommon for the prospective recipient site to be on the same extremity; thus, there are two operative sites. It may be anomalous. Splitting or lateral stretching interferes with the integrity of the intact tendon surface, thus encouraging collagenous adhesions. The latter is a factor if the graft is used in a dynamic situation requiring a long excursion.

EXTENSOR DIGITORUM LONGUS

Anatomy. The extensor digitorum longus arises in the proximal part of the anterior compartment of the leg, where it is innervated by the deep peroneal (anterior tibial) nerve (L5, S1) (Gray, 1973). The tendon forms over the lower part of the tibia deep to the superior extensor retinaculum. The tendon divides into four slips that pass distally in a compartment of the inferior extensor retinaculum, emerging to spread over the dorsum of the foot, immediately deep to the deep fascia. As they reach the dorsal aspects of the metatarsophalangeal joints, the tendons to the second, third, and fourth toes are joined on their lateral sides by the tendons of the extensor digitorum brevis before passing distally to their insertions.

As both muscles are extensors of the toes, loss of the extensor digitorum longus to the second, third, and fourth toes produces no disability. If the long extensor tendon to the fifth toe is required, its distal stump should be anastomosed to the tendon of the extensor digitorum brevis supplying the fourth toe.

Technique of Removal. Serial transverse incisions are made over the course of the tendon, but if more than one is required a curved oblique incision is preferred (Figs. 15–15, 15–16). Care should be taken to avoid damage to the branches of the superficial

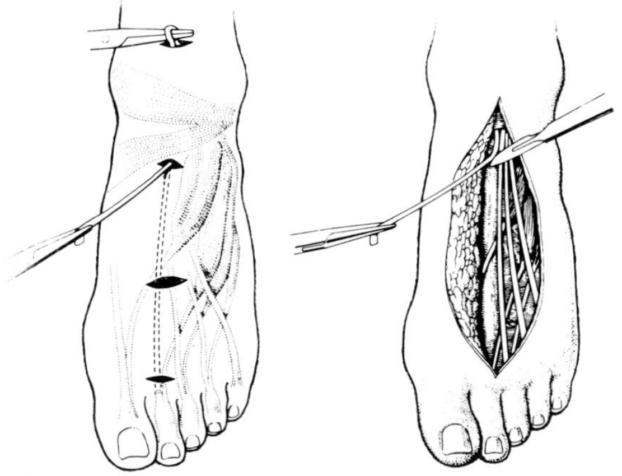

Figure 15–15. The anatomic relationship between the long and short toe extensors and the "closed" and "open" methods of tendon removal. (Modified from White, W. L.: Tendon grafts: a consideration of their source, procurement and suitability. Surg. Clin. North Am., *40*:403, 1960.)

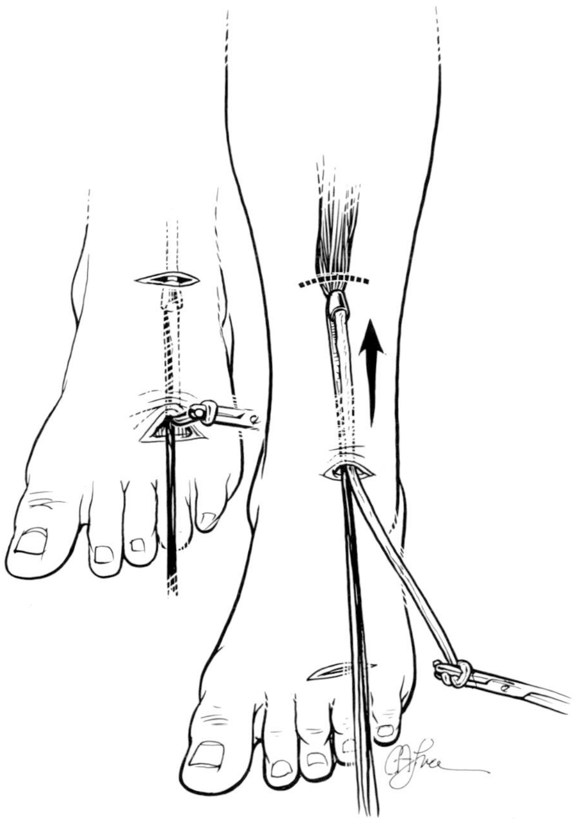

Figure 15–16. To obtain a single, long toe extensor, serial transverse incisions are made over the course of the tendon. The authors recommend using a fine small tendon stripper, which may obviate the need to incise the extensor retinaculum.

peroneal (musculocutaneous) nerve lying in the subcutaneous fat. The deep peroneal nerve and anterior vascular bundle lie on a plane slightly deep to the tendons in the ankle region, and on the dorsum of the foot the tendons diverge laterally. The skin is closed in one layer; a pressure and elastic bandage is applied before the tourniquet is released.

Possible Anomalies. The arrangement of the tendons on the dorsum of the foot varies in that they may be duplicated, or extra slips may pass to the corresponding metatarsal bones (Quain's, 1923).

Advantages. The extensor digitorum longus is always present and easily demonstrable preoperatively. A graft containing up to three tendon slips arising from a common tendon can be provided. The average length of the graft is 12 to 15 cm. Access is excellent. The slips are slender enough for full revascularization, and yet are sufficiently strong for all purposes.

Disadvantages. The division of the frequently present accessory slips leaves the tendon surface devoid of epitenon, thus encouraging adhesions. Although the demands of reconstruction may require that this risk be taken, the common tendon stump, if two or three slips are used, may be too thick for satisfactory revascularization. When the foot is used as a donor site, two separate operative fields are necessary.

FLEXOR DIGITORUM SUPERFICIALIS

Anatomy. The flexor digitorum superficialis muscle is one of the two extrinsic flexor muscles of the fingers. Its belly lies in the proximal two-thirds of the forearm superficial to the other extrinsic flexor of the fingers, the flexor digitorum profundus. The median nerve is applied to its deep surface and innervates it (C7, C8) (Gray, 1973). In the distal forearm the muscle belly divides into four slips, which in turn give rise to the four tendons passing beneath the flexor retinaculum to enter the palm, where they spread out toward their respective fingers. In the region of the proximal digital compartment, each tendon decussates around the appropriate tendon of the flexor digitorum profundus to gain insertion by the radial and ulnar slips into the middle phalanx of each finger. They are the primary flexors of the proximal interphalangeal joints.

Technique of Removal. The tendon may be removed by means of two incisions. The first is placed proximal to the base of the selected digit, and the other is made in the distal forearm, the tendon being withdrawn through either. North and Littler (1980) described in detail the technique for safe removal of the flexor digitorum superficialis to prevent a flexion or hyperextension deformity at the proximal interphalangeal joint. The incision should be placed distal to the palmar crease, the tendon retracted and the finger flexed.

Advantages. The tendon is always available, is within the same operative field, is sturdy, and is reasonably accessible.

Disadvantages. Removal of a superficialis tendon from a finger may lead to a recurvatum deformity. Its removal from a normal finger may also reduce the efficiency of digital flexion (White, 1960a). Power grasp is diminished. The tendons have occasional tendinous or muscular connections with the flexor digitorum profundus tendons (Quain's, 1923).

When used as a graft, the thickness of the tendon renders it likely to undergo central avascular necrosis (Bunnell, 1970). This tendon is seldom taken from a normal finger for a tendon transplant, as there are better alternatives. It is sometimes used when transfer of a musculotendinous unit is needed to restore flexion to the thumb or as an intrinsic transfer. Its major utility in tendon transplantation is when the tendon is present in a lacerated condition, is not to be repaired, and can be used as a short graft to replace the profundus.

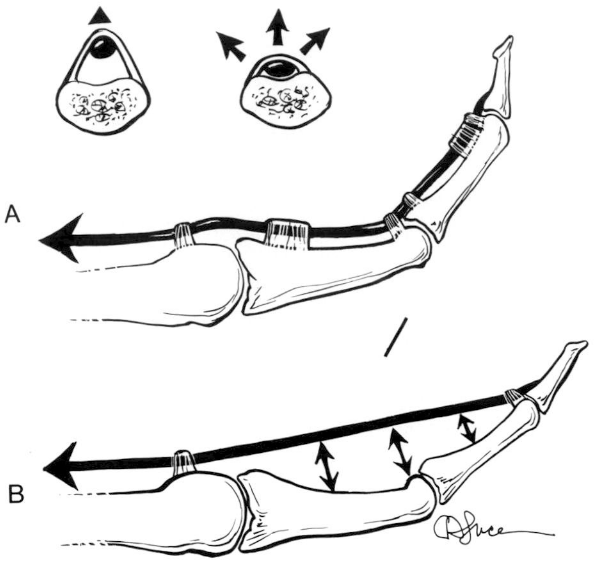

Figure 15–17. The retinacular pulley system prevents bowstringing of the flexor tendon. *A,* A five-pulley system is optimal, with pulleys bridging each side of the metacarpophalangeal and proximal interphalangeal joints and lying proximal to the distal interphalangeal joint. *B,* Disruption of the key pulleys allows bowstringing.

Tendon Sheath Reconstruction

In more recent years the importance of the tendon sheath has been recognized and its anatomy detailed (Doyle and Blythe, 1975; Ochiai and associates, 1979; Hunter and Cook, 1982; Strauch and deMoura, 1985). To prevent bowstringing, multiple pulleys need to be reconstructed. A five-pulley system is optimal with pulleys bridging each side of the metacarpophalangeal and proximal interphalangeal joints and lying proximal to the distal interphalangeal joint. If the pulleys are absent, the tendon pulls away from the bone and increased adhesions dorsal to the tendon graft occur (Fig. 15–17) (Hunter and Cook, 1982).

A second functional requirement of tendon sheath reconstruction is to restore the synovial environment so that adequate nutrition of the avascular graft may occur. Eiken and Rank (1977) performed experimental and clinical studies (Eiken and associates, 1980; Eiken, Hagberg, and Lundborg, 1981) showing improved functional results when tendon sheaths were completely reconstructed with autologous grafts of extensor retinaculum or tendon sheath from the foot. Several authors (Benjamin and associates, 1955; Anzel, Lipscomb, and Grindlay, 1961; Biro, 1980) used autologous veins to reconstruct tendon sheaths experimentally and clinically (Forgon and Biro, 1980) over silicone rods. Strauch and associates (1985) showed that vein patches over tendon repairs in chickens improved the functional and histologic results.

These efforts have been stimulated by a desire to improve the results after two-stage tendon grafting. First proposed by Bassett and Carroll (1963) and Hunter (1965), the technique of implantation of a silicone rod and reconstruction of strategic pulleys followed by tendon grafting three months later has been an excellent salvage procedure in many digits (Weeks and Wray, 1976; Chuinard, Dabezies, and Mathews, 1980; Wilson and associates, 1980; LaSalle and Strickland, 1983; Schneider, 1985). Key to the issue of whether autologous tissue grafts are preferable to the smooth scar tissue that forms around a silicone implant are the biologic observations of the nature of the fluid. Does it function as synovial fluid or merely as foreign body reaction fluid that is of no nutritional benefit to the tendon (Eiken, Hagberg, and Lundborg, 1981)? Hunter and associates (1983) described the pseudosynovial sheath in a primate model and noted three layers: an intima, a media, and an adventitia. It showed no propensity for longitudinal contracture in their study. There is one case report of a progressive flexion contracture of a finger after implantation of a silicone tendon prosthesis (Chamay and Gabbiani, 1978). Many myofibroblasts were seen and presumably were the initiators of the contracture. However, another electron microscopic study of pseudosheaths showed no myofibroblasts (Eskeland and associates, 1977).

Two-Stage Tendon Grafting

The technique of two-stage tendon grafting was first described by Bassett and Carroll (1963) and Hunter (1965) and is necessary when there is an unsuitable bed for tendon grafting. These are salvage cases in which excellent results often are not achieved, but the technique is useful in carefully selected patients. In the first stage, if necessary joint contractures are released, skin cover is provided, the nerves are repaired, the tendon ends and scar tissue are debrided, and the retinacular pulleys are reconstructed. Many techniques for pulley reconstruction utilizing remnants of tendons or extensor retinaculum have been described (Kleinert and Bennett, 1978; Lister, 1979; Manske and Lesker, 1977; Hunter and Cook, 1982). It is optimal to reconstruct pulleys on each side of each joint (five in all). Other techniques of autologous tissue transplantation of extensor or flexor retinaculum or vein patch may improve the results (see the above discussion of tendon sheath reconstruction.) A flat silicone implant with a Dacron tip (Swanson-Hunter design) is preferred in order to prevent tearing of the implant by the distal fixation suture to the profundus stump (see Fig. 15–8*C*). A snug fit, usually over a 4 mm implant in an adult, is necessary. The proximal end is placed in the ulnar side of the distal forearm and is not fixed. After the scars are soft and supple (which takes three months or longer), incisions are made distally over the fingertip and proximally over the distal forearm. A tendon graft is sutured to the silicone rod, the rod is withdrawn as the tendon graft is implanted, the tension is established, and the junctures are performed as in one-stage tendon grafting.

Vascularized Tendon Transfers

Recent reports on vascularized tendon transfer with microvascular surgical technique indeed open a new dimension in tendon grafting. A potential donor tendon is the extensor hallucis brevis based on the dorsalis pedis pedicle. Such a transfer fits well to a scarred recipient bed that is not conducive to conventional tendon grafts. However, formidable technical hurdles remain. The tightness of the flexor tendon sheath does not allow adequate space for safe replacement of both the tendon and the vascular pedicle. Enlargement of the pulley systems becomes a necessary adjunctive measure that may compromise the overall functional result. Thus, vascularized tendon transfer remains an *experimental* pursuit (Leitner, Gordon, and Buncke, 1985; Hing, 1987).

EXPERIMENTAL TRANSPLANTATION

Allografts

A considerable body of literature exists relating to experimental allograft tendon transplantation in many animal models. Most of the studies indicate an unacceptable amount of host reaction and adhesions, the results being inferior to those of autografts (Crockford, 1977). Nevertheless, there is some promise in this field of transplantation.

Tendon is a structure with a low level of antigenicity, presumably because it is relatively hypocellular and collagen is species specific (Adelmann, Glynn, and Kirrane, 1968; Michaeli, Martin, and Benjamini, 1970). The antigenicity of a tissue lies principally in its cells and ground substance (Peacock, 1959a). Many methods have been used to reduce the antigenicity: trypsin, Cialit (an organic mercurial with strong antibacterial properties) (Seiffert, 1971), freezing, prolonged storage, irradiation, and lyophilization. Cialit has received the most attention. However, it may be unnecessary to reduce the antigenicity of the transplant, since the "dose" of cells and ground substance transferred is much smaller than in whole organ transplants, and although transient lymphadenopathy may occur, rejection does not appear to be a clinical problem (Peacock, 1981).

Human experiments have provided some support for the use of allografts in tendon transplantation. Liu (1983) reported the use of allografts simply refrigerated at 20°C after harvest (no chemical treatments) and used as second-stage tendon grafts (after silicone rod insertion). The results were satisfactory in some patients but not as good as those from autograft use in similar patients.

Peacock and Madden (1967) reported the allograft transplantation of the complete flexor apparatus, including both flexor tendons, the periosteum and palmar plates, and the complete tendon sheath in ten humans. These had been stored for a few days at 4°C. In seven of the ten patients satisfactory function resulted. Other work has been performed in composite allografts (Peacock, 1959b; Hueston, Hubble, and Rigg, 1967; Furlow, 1969; Cameron, Conrad, and Latham, 1970; Cameron and co-workers, 1971; Liu, 1975). As transplantation biology is better understood, there may be a larger role for these transplants in the future.

Xenografts

Xenografts suffer the disadvantage that collagen transplanted across species induces an antigenic response. Klein and Lewis (1972) found that rat tendons lost mass and morphologic integrity rapidly when transplanted into guinea pigs, a finding in contrast to allografts transplanted into other rats.

The success of porcine valve glutaraldehyde-treated xenograft implantation in cardiac surgery has stimulated research on a xenograft bioprosthesis. To be useful, a xenograft must satisfy several criteria (McMaster and associates, 1976): (1) it should not be antigenic, (2) it should not be carcinogenic, (3) it should be easily stored and implanted, (4) it should be incorporated by the host, and (5) its function must simulate that of the original part.

Smith and associates (1986) utilized mammalian xenografts, treated with glutaraldehyde, in chickens. They observed satisfactory healing and tissue incorporation of the bioprosthesis ends, and noted a lack of significant adhesions within the tendon sheath when it was intact. This research is promising and may lead to a reliable method of one-stage tendon reconstruction.

REFERENCES

Adelmann, B. C., Glynn, L. E., and Kirrane, J.: Delayed-type hypersensitivity reactions of native and denatured rat and calf skin-collagen in sensitized guinea pigs. Fed. Proc., *27*:263, 1968.

Amadio, P. C., Hunter, J. M., Jaeger, S. H., Wehbe, M. A., and Schneider, L. H.: The effect of vincular injury on the results of flexor tendon surgery in zone 2. J. Hand Surg., *10A*:626, 1985.

Anzel, S. H., Lipscomb, P. R., and Grindlay, J. H.: Construction of artificial tendon sheaths in dogs. Am. J. Surg., *101*:355, 1961.

Armenta, E., and Lehrman, A.: The vincula to the flexor tendons of the hand. J. Hand Surg., *5*:127, 1980.

Azar, C. A., Culver, J. E., and Fleegler, E. J.: Blood supply of the flexor pollicis longus tendon. J. Hand Surg., *8*:471, 1983.

Bassett, C. A. L., and Carroll, R. E.: Formation of tendon sheath by silicone rod implants. J. Bone Joint Surg., *45A*:884, 1963.

Benjamin, H. B., Wagner, M., Zett, W., and Ausman, R. K.: The use of an endothelial cuff in tendon repair. Med. Times, *83*:697, 1955.

Bergljung, L.: Vascular reactions after tendon suture and tendon transplantation. A stereo-microangiographic study on the calcaneal tendon of the rabbit. Scand. J. Plast. Reconstr. Surg. (Suppl.), *4*:7, 1968.

Biro, V.: Experimental formation of tendon sheaths from a vein. Handchir. Mikrochir. Plast. Chir., *12*:193, 1980.

Brand, P. W.: Tendon grafting. Illustrated by a new operation for intrinsic paralysis of the fingers. J. Bone Joint Surg., *43B*:444, 1961.

Brockis, J. G.: The blood supply of the flexor and extensor tendons of the fingers in man. J. Bone Joint Surg., *35B*:131, 1953.

Bunnell, S.: *In* Boyes, J. H. (Ed.): Surgery of the Hand. 5th Ed. Philadelphia, J. B. Lippincott Company, 1970.

Cameron, R. R., Conrad, R. N., and Latham, W. D.: Preserved composite tendon allografts: a comparative study of changes in length, elasticity and anastomotic and lineal tensile strength. Surg. Forum, *21*:506, 1970.

Cameron, R. R., Conrad, R. N., Sell, K. W., and Latham, W. D.: Freeze-dried composite tendon allografts: an experimental study. Plast. Reconstr. Surg., *47*:39, 1971.

Chamay, A., and Gabbiani, G.: Digital contracture deformity after implantation of a silicone prosthesis: light and electron microscopic study. J. Hand Surg., *3*:266, 1978.

Chaplin, D. M.: The vascular anatomy within normal tendons, divided tendons, free tendon grafts and pedicle tendon grafts in rabbits. J. Bone Joint Surg., *55B*:269, 1973.

Chow, S. P., Hooper, G., and Chan, C. W.: The healing of freeze-dried rabbit flexor tendon in a synovial fluid environment. Hand, *15*:136, 1983.

Chuinard, R. G., Dabezies, E. J., and Mathews, R. E.: Two-stage superficialis tendon reconstruction in severely damaged fingers. J. Hand Surg., *5*:135, 1980.

Colville, J., Callison, J. R., and White, W. L.: Role of mesotendon in tendon blood supply. Plast. Reconstr. Surg., *43*:53, 1969.

Cooper, R. R., and Misol, S.: Tendon and ligament insertion. A light and electron microscopic study. J. Bone Joint Surg., *52A*:1, 1970.

Crockford, D. A.: Transplantation of tendon. *In* Converse, J. M. (Ed.): Reconstructive Plastic Surgery. 2nd Ed. Philadelphia, W. B. Saunders Company, 1977, pp. 266–292.

Daseler, E. H., and Anson, B. J.: The plantaris muscle. An anatomical study of 750 specimens. J. Bone Joint Surg., *25*:822, 1943.

Doyle, J. R., and Blythe, W.: The finger flexor tendon sheath and pulleys: anatomy and reconstruction. *In* Am. Acad. Orthop. Surgeons Symposium on Tendon Surgery in the Hand, Philadelphia, 1974. St. Louis, C. V. Mosby Company, 1975, p. 81.

Edwards, D. A. W.: The blood supply and lymphatic drainage of tendons. J. Anat., *80*:147, 1946.

Edwards, L. C., and Dunphy, J. E.: Wound healing. An injury and normal repair. N. Engl. J. Med., *259*:224, 1958.

Eiken, O., Hagberg, L., and Lundborg, G.: Evolving

biologic concepts as applied to tendon surgery. Clin. Plast. Surg., *8*:1, 1981.

Eiken, O., Holmberg, J., Ekerot, L., and Sälgeback, S.: Restoration of the digital tendon sheath. A new concept of tendon grafting. Scand. J. Plast. Reconstr. Surg., *14*:89, 1980.

Eiken, O., and Lundborg, G.: Experimental tendon grafting within intact tendon sheath. Scand. J. Plast. Reconstr. Surg., *17*:127, 1983.

Eiken, O., Lundborg, G., and Rank, F.: The role of the digital synovial sheath in tendon grafting. Scand. J. Plast. Reconstr. Surg., *9*:182, 1975.

Eiken, O., and Rank, F.: Experimental restoration of the digital synovial sheath. Scand. J. Plast. Reconstr. Surg., *11*:213, 1977.

Elliot, D. H.: The structure and function of mammalian tendon. Biol. Rev., *40*:392, 1965.

Eskeland, G., Eskeland, T., Hovig, T., and Teigland, J.: The ultrastructure of normal digital flexor tendon sheath and of the tissue formed around silicone and polyethylene implants in man. J. Bone Joint Surg., *59B*:206, 1977.

Forgon, M., and Biro, V.: Reconstruction of tendon sheaths from veins in "no-man's land" of the hand. Handchirurgie, *12*:189, 1980.

Furlow, L. T., Jr.: Homologous flexor mechanism replacement in four fingers of one hand. Case report. Plast. Reconstr. Surg., *43*:531, 1969.

Furlow, L. T., Jr.: The role of tendon tissues in tendon healing. Plast. Reconstr. Surg., *57*:39, 1976.

Gelberman, R. H., Manske, P. R., Vande Berg, J. S., et al.: Flexor tendon repair in vitro: comparative histologic study of rabbit, chicken, dog and monkey. J. Orthop. Res., *2*:39, 1984.

Gelberman, R. H., Vande Berg, J. S., Manske, P. R., and Akeson, W. H.: The early stages of flexor tendon healing: a morphologic study of the first fourteen days. J. Hand Surg., *10A*:776, 1985.

Gray's Anatomy. 35th Ed. Warwick R., and Williams, P. L. (Eds.). London, Longmans, 1973.

Harkness, R. D.: Mechanical properties of collagenous tissues. *In* Gould, B. S., and Ramchandran, G. S. (Eds.): Treatise on Collagen. Vol. 2A. New York, Academic Press, 1968, p. 254.

Harvey, F. J., Chu, G., and Harvey, P. M.: Surgical availability of the plantaris tendon. J. Hand Surg., *8*:243, 1983.

Hing, D. N.: Extensor digitorum brevis. *In* Buncke, H. J. (Ed.): Clinical Atlas of Reconstructive Microsurgery and Replantation. Philadelphia, Lea & Febiger (in press).

Hollingshead, W. H.: Anatomy for Surgeons: The Back and Limbs. 3rd Ed. Philadelphia, Harper & Row, 1982.

Hooper, G., Davies, R., and Tothill, P.: Blood flow and clearance in tendons. J. Bone Joint Surg., *66B*:441, 1984.

Hueston, J. T., Hubble, B., and Rigg, B. R.: Homografts of the digital flexor tendon system. Aust. N.Z. J. Surg., *36*:269, 1967.

Hunter, J.: Artificial tendons. Early development and application. Am. J. Surg., *109*:325, 1965.

Hunter, J. M., and Cook, J. F., Jr.: The pulley system: rationale for reconstruction. *In* Strickland, J. W., and Steichen, J. B. (Eds.): Difficult Problems in Hand Surgery. St. Louis, C. V. Mosby Company, 1982, p. 94.

Hunter, J. M., Jaeger, S. H., Matsui, T., and Miyaji, N.: The pseudosynovial sheath—its characteristics in a primate model. J. Hand Surg., *8*:461, 1983.

Jackson, D. S.: Chondroitin sulphuric acid as a factor in the stability of tendon. Biochem. J., *54*:638, 1953.

Jackson, D. S., and Bentley, J. P.: Collagen glycosaminoglycan interactions. *In* Gould, B. S., and Ramchandran, G. S. (Eds.): Treatise on Collagen. Vol. 2A. New York, Academic Press, 1968.

Kanavel, A. B.: Infections of the Hand. A Guide to the Surgical Treatment of Acute and Chronic Suppurative Processes in the Fingers, Hand and Forearm. 7th Ed. Philadelphia, Lea & Febiger, 1939.

Katsumi, M., Kameda, I., Tachikawa, K., et al.: Experimental investigation of healing process of tendons with or without synovial coverage in or outside of synovial cavity. Seikei Geki, *31*:1394, 1980.

Katsumi, M., and Tajima, T.: Experimental investigation of healing process of tendons with or without synovial coverage in or outside of the synovial cavity. J. Niigata Med. Assoc., *95*:532, 1981.

Klein, L.: Collagen structure and metabolism. *In* Krizek, T. J., and Hoopes, J. E. (Eds.): Symposium on Basic Science in Plastic Surgery. St. Louis, C. V. Mosby Company, 1976, p. 80.

Klein, L., and Lewis, J.: Simultaneous quantification of ^{3}H-collagen loss and ^{1}H-collagen replacement during healing of rat tendon grafts. J. Bone Joint Surg., *54A*:137, 1972.

Kleinert, H. E., and Bennett, J. B.: Digital pulley reconstruction employing the always present rim of the previous pulley. J. Hand Surg., *3*:297, 1978.

Kleinert, H. E., Kutz, J. E., Ashbell, T. S., and Martinez, E.: Primary repair of lacerated flexor tendons in "no man's land." J. Bone Joint Surg., *49A*:577, 1969.

Landi, A. P., Altman, F. P., Pringle, J., et al.: Oxidative enzyme metabolism in rabbit intrasynovial flexor tendons. II. Studies of nutritional pathways. J. Surg. Res., *29*:281, 1980.

LaSalle, W. B., and Strickland, J.: An evaluation of the two-stage flexor tendon reconstruction technique. J. Hand Surg., *8*:263, 1983.

Last, R. J.: Anatomy, Regional and Applied. 4th Ed. London, J. & A. Churchill, 1966.

Leitner, D. W., Gordon, L., and Buncke, H. J.: Case report. The extensor digitorum brevis as a muscle island flap. Plast. Reconstr. Surg., *76*:777, 1985.

Lindsay, W. K., and Birch, J. R.: The fibroblast in flexor tendon healing. Plast. Reconstr. Surg., *34*:223, 1964.

Lindsay, W. K., and McDougall, E. P.: Digital flexor tendons: an experimental study. Part III. The fate of autogenous digital flexor tendon grafts. Br. J. Plast. Surg., *13*:293, 1961.

Lindsay, W. K., and Thomson, H. G.: Digital flexor tendons: an experimental study. Part I. The significance of each compartment of the flexor mechanism in tendon healing. Br. J. Plast. Surg., *12*:289, 1959.

Lindsay, W. K., Thomson, H. G., and Walker, F. G.: Digital flexor tendons: an experimental study. Part II. The significance of a gap occurring at the line of suture. Br. J. Plast. Surg., *13*:1, 1960.

Lister, G. D.: Reconstruction of pulleys employing extensor retinaculum. J. Hand Surg., *4*:461, 1979.

Lister, G. D.: Indications and techniques for repair of the flexor tendon sheath. Hand Clin., *1*:85, 1985.

Lister, G. D., Kleinert, H. E., Kutz, J. E., et al.: Primary flexor tendon repair followed by immediate controlled mobilization. J. Hand Surg., *2*:441, 1977.

Liu, T. K.: Transplantation of preserved composite tendon allografts. An experimental study. J. Bone Joint Surg., *57A*:65, 1975.

Liu, T. K.: Clinical use of refrigerated flexor tendon allografts to replace a silicone rubber rod. J. Hand Surg., *8*:881, 1983.

Lundborg, G.: Experimental flexor tendon healing without adhesion formation—a new concept of tendon nutrition and intrinsic healing mechanisms. A preliminary report. Hand, *8*:235, 1976.

Lundborg, G., Hansson, H. A., Rank, F., et al.: Superficial repair of severed flexor tendons in synovial environment. An experimental, ultrastructural study on cellular mechanisms. J. Hand Surg., *5*:451, 1980.

Lundborg, G., Holm, S., and Myrhage, R.: The role of the synovial fluid and tendon sheath for flexor tendon nutrition. Scand. J. Plast. Reconstr. Surg., *14*:99, 1980.

Lundborg, G., Myrhage, R., and Rydevik, B.: The vascularization of human flexor tendons within the digital synovial sheath region—structural and functional aspects. J. Hand Surg., *2*:417, 1977.

Lundborg, G., and Rank, F.: Experimental intrinsic healing of flexor tendons based upon synovial fluid nutrition. J. Hand Surg., *3*:21, 1978.

Lundborg, G., and Rank, F.: Experimental studies on cellular mechanisms involved in healing of animal and human flexor tendons in synovial environment. Hand, *12*:3, 1980.

Manske, P. R., Bridwell, K., and Lesker, P. A.: Nutrient pathways to flexor tendons of chickens using tritiated proline. J. Hand Surg., *3*:352, 1978.

Manske, P. R., Gelberman, R. H., and Lesker, P. A.: Flexor tendon healing. Hand Clin., *1*:25, 1985.

Manske, P. R., and Lesker, P. A.: Strength of human pulleys. Hand, *9*:147, 1977.

Manske, P. R., and Lesker, P. A.: Nutrient pathways of flexor tendons in primates. J. Hand Surg., *7*:436, 1982.

Manske, P. R., and Lesker, P. A.: Comparative nutrient pathways to the flexor profundus tendons in Zone II of various experimental animals. J. Surg. Res., *34*:83, 1983.

Manske, P. R., and Lesker, P. A.: Biochemical evidence of flexor tendon participation in the repair process. An in vitro study. J. Hand Surg., *9B*:117, 1984.

Manske, P. R., Lesker, P. A., and Bridwell, K.: Experimental studies in chickens on the initial nutrition of tendon grafts. J. Hand Surg., *4*:565, 1979.

Matthews, P.: The pathology of flexor tendon repair. Hand, *11*:233, 1979.

Matthews, P., and Richards, H.: The repair potential of digital flexor tendons. J. Bone Joint Surg., *56B*:618, 1974.

Matthews, P., and Richards, H.: The repair reaction of flexor tendon within the digital sheath. Hand, *7*:27, 1975.

Matthews, P., and Richards, H.: Factors in the adherence of flexor tendons after repair: an experimental study in the rabbit. J. Bone Joint Surg., *58B*:230, 1976.

Mayer, L.: The physiological method of tendon transplantation. I. Historical: anatomy and physiology of tendons. II. Operative technique. III. Experimental and clinical experiences. Surg. Gynecol. Obstet., *22*:182, 298, 472, 1916.

McDowell, C. L., and Snyder, D. M.: Tendon healing: an experimental model in the dog. J. Hand Surg., *2*:122, 1977.

McMaster, W. C., Kouzelos, J., Liddle, S., et al.: Tendon grafting with glutaraldehyde-fixed material. J. Biomed. Mater. Res., *10*:259, 1976.

Michaeli, D., Martin, G. R., and Benjamini, E.: Localization of the antigenic determinants of collagen. *In* Balazs, E. A. (Ed.): Chemistry and Molecular Biology of the Intercellular Matrix. Vol. I. New York, Academic Press, 1970.

Nisbet, N. W.: Anatomy of the calcaneal tendon of the rabbit. J. Bone Joint Surg., *42B*:360, 1960.

North, E. R., and Littler, J. W.: Transferring the flexor superficialis tendon. Technical considerations in the prevention of proximal interphalangeal joint disability. J. Hand Surg., *5*:498, 1980.

Ochiai, N., Matsui, T., Miyaji, N., Merklin, R. J., and Hunter, J. M.: Vascular anatomy of flexor tendons. I. Vincular system and blood supply of the profundus tendon in the digital sheath. J. Hand Surg., *4*:321, 1979.

Parkes, A.: The "lumbrical plus" finger. J. Bone Joint Surg., *53B*:236, 1971.

Peacock, E. E.: Vascular basis of tendon repair. Surg. Forum, *8*:65, 1957.

Peacock, E. E.: A study of the circulation in normal tendons and healing grafts. Ann. Surg., *149*:415, 1959a.

Peacock, E. E.: Some problems in flexor tendon healing. Surgery, *45*:415, 1959b.

Peacock, E. E.: The influence of modern connective tissue biology upon surgery of the hand. *In* Cooper, P., and Nyhus, L. M. (Eds.): Surgery Annual. Vol. 3. London, Butterworths, 1971.

Peacock, E. E.: Research in tendon healing. *In* Tubiana, R.: The Hand. Philadelphia, W. B. Saunders Company, 1981, pp. 511–540.

Peacock, E. E., and Madden, J. W.: Human composite flexor tendon allografts. Ann. Surg., *166*:624, 1967.

Peer, L. A.: Transplantation of Tissues. Vol. 1. Cartilage, Bone, Fascia, Tendon and Muscle. Baltimore, Williams & Wilkins Company, 1955.

Pilcher, R.: Repair of hernia with plantaris tendon graft. A.M.A. Arch. Surg., *38*:16, 1939.

Potenza, A. D.: Tendon healing within the flexor digital sheath in the dog. An experimental study. J. Bone Joint Surg., *44A*:49, 1962.

Potenza, A. D.: Critical evaluation of flexor-tendon healing and adhesion formation within artificial digital sheaths. An experimental study. J. Bone Joint Surg., *45A*:1217, 1963.

Potenza, A. D.: The healing of autogenous tendon grafts within the flexor digital sheath in dogs. J. Bone Joint Surg., *46A*:1462, 1964.

Potenza, A. D.: Mechanisms of healing of digital flexor tendons. Hand, *1*:40, 1969.

Potenza, A. D., and Herte, M. C.: The synovial cavity as a "tissue culture in situ"—science or nonsense? J. Hand Surg., *7*:196, 1982.

Quain's Elements of Anatomy. Vol. IV. 11th Ed. Part II. Myology. Bryce, T. H. (Ed.). New York, Longmans, Green & Company, 1923.

Richards, H. J.: Digital flexor tendon repair and return of function. Ann. R. Coll. Surg. Engl., *59*:25, 1977.

Schatzker, J., and Branemark, P. I.: Intravital observations on the microvascular anatomy and microcirculation of the tendon. Acta. Orthop. Scand. (Suppl.), *126*:1, 1969.

Schneider, L. H.: Staged tendon reconstruction. Hand Clin., *1*:109, 1985.

Seiffert, K. E.: Preserved grafts in reconstructive surgery. Trans. Internatl. Soc. Plast. Surgeons, Fifth Congress, 1971. Australia, Butterworths, 1971.

Skoog, T., and Persson, B. H.: An experimental study of the early healing of tendons. Plast. Reconstr. Surg., *13*:384, 1954.

Smith, D. J., Jr., Jones, C. S., Hull, M., and Kleinert, H. E.: Evaluation of glutaraldehyde-treated tendon xenograft. J. Hand Surg., *11A*:97, 1986.

Smith, J. W.: The blood supply of tendons. Am. J. Surg., *109*:272, 1965.

Strauch, B., and deMoura, W.: Digital flexor tendon sheath: an anatomic study. J. Hand Surg., *10A*:785, 1985.

Strauch, B., deMoura, W., Ferder, M., et al.: The fate of tendon healing after restoration of the integrity of the tendon sheath with autogenous vein grafts. J. Hand Surg., *10A*:790, 1985.

Verdan, C. E.: Primary and secondary repair of flexor and extensor tendon injuries. *In* Flynn, J. E.: Hand Surgery. 2nd Ed. Baltimore, Williams & Wilkins Company, 1975, p. 160.

Weber, E. R.: Synovial fluid nutrition of flexor tendons. Orthop. Res. Soc., *4*:227, 1979.

Weeks, P. M., and Wray, R. C.: Rate and extent of functional recovery after flexor tendon grafting with and without silicone rod preparation. J. Hand Surg., *1*:174, 1976.

Weeks, P. M., and Wray, R. C.: Management of Acute Hand Injuries. A Biological Approach. 2nd Ed. St. Louis, C. V. Mosby Company, 1978, p. 331.

Weiner, L. J., and Peacock, E. E.: Biologic principles affecting repair of flexor tendons. *In* Welch, C. E., and Handy, J. W. (Eds.): Advances in Surgery. Vol. 5. Chicago, Year Book Medical Publishers, 1971.

White, W. L.: Tendon grafts: a consideration of their source, procurement and suitability. Surg. Clin. North Am., *40*:403, 1960a.

White, W. L.: The unique, accessible and useful plantaris tendon. Plast. Reconstr. Surg., *25*:133, 1960b.

Wilson, R. L., Carter, M. S., Holdeman, V. A., and Lovett, W. L.: Flexor profundus injuries treated with delayed two-staged tendon grafting. J. Hand Surg., *5*:74, 1980.

Winckler, G.: Caractères des vaisseaux para—et pertendineux des flechisseurs des doigts. C.R. Assoc. Anat., *148*:581, 1970.

Zbrodowski, A., Gajisin, S., and Grodecki, J.: Mesotendons of digital flexor muscles and their vasculature. Hand, *13*:231, 1981.

16

Timothy A. Miller

Repair and Grafting of Skeletal Muscle

In reconstructive surgery it is routine to transfer all varieties of tissue from one anatomic location to another with a high expectation of success. Grafts of skin, bone, tendon, cartilage, and nerve are common; the notable exception has been skeletal muscle. Until recently it was generally agreed that this metabolically demanding tissue could not be grafted (Peer and Walker, 1951). However, the successful transfer of contractile muscle into a functionless area must be considered a goal of the highest priority in reconstructive surgery.

In order to graft other tissue such as skin or cartilage, for example, it is only necessary to acquire a new blood supply to be successful. Muscle grafting is much more complex, involving other variables such as the balance of physiologic tension between points of origin and insertion, innervation, and blood supply. Altering any of these factors even in situ results in compromise of muscle function or death.

Striated muscle makes up 30 to 40 per cent of body weight and is the organ system responsible for all movement. The design of different muscles is quite variable: some are made up of fibers oriented parallel to their origin and insertion; others consist of shorter fibers that course obliquely to the long axis, taking their origin from fascial envelopes and planes within the muscle (e.g., the bipennate muscle, whose fibers resemble a feather).

Each individual muscle fiber is a syncytium containing multiple nuclei oriented just beneath the sarcolemmal (cell) membrane. Each fiber receives a single twig of nerve that provides innervation at the motor end plate (neuromuscular junction) by the secretion of acetylcholine. A motor unit designates a group of fibers innervated by a single alpha motor neuron. It is the neural innervation that determines the metabolic activity, enzyme content, and histochemical pattern of the muscle. Each fiber contains thousands of filaments of myosin and actin whose alignment results in the characteristic striation pattern. The fibrillar elements lie within sarcoplasm, the intracellular fluid that contains large quantities of potassium, magnesium, phosphate, and protein enzymes. Large numbers of mitochondria lie between the myofibrils, supplying the adenosine triphosphate (ATP) necessary for contraction.

The function of muscle is to *contract,* to shorten resting length, thus moving its tendon of insertion and the anatomic structure to which it attaches proximally. This process is accomplished by a sliding mechanism that takes place on a molecular level, pulling the actin filaments inward between the myosin chains, thus shortening length. Although there is variability, most muscles shorten by approximately 40 per cent of their length during full contraction.

In general there is a linear relationship between the force of contraction of a muscle and its weight. The cross sectional area is directly proportional to muscle weight and inversely related to individual fiber length (Wickiewicz and associates, 1983). Tension production is greater for muscles with shorter fibers, whereas muscles made up of long fibers do not generate as much force but contract with much greater velocity.

Although individual muscle fibers appear similar when examined in cross section by conventional microscopic techniques, there are significant differences in enzymatic and chemical structure. These differences can be detected by special histochemical staining techniques, the most useful of which detects variations in the content of myosin ATPase and its isoforms. Using specific histoenzymatic methods, two basic fiber systems can be identified: Type I fibers are rich in myoglobin ("red"), metabolize ketones and fatty acids aerobically, and contain abundant mitochondria; Type II fibers are rich in phosphorylase but low in oxidative enzymes, mitochondria, and myoglobin (therefore "white"). The latter are "fast" contracting, relying on the metabolism of glycogen as their primary energy source. In man, most muscles contain a mixture of fibers oriented on cross section in a mosaic fashion, one type usually predominating, depending on the function (Fig. 16–1). The soleus muscle in the cat and man, for example, contains almost entirely Type I fibers.

INNERVATION

It is known that following motor nerve severance muscle atrophies and is eventually replaced by fibrous tissue. Detailed investigations into the denervation process have been summarized by Gutmann (1962).

Innervation provides continuing synthesis of acetylcholinesterase at the motor end plate (Filogamo and Gabella, 1966). The neural influence on muscle is responsible for the type of enzymatic composition of fibers, and thus the histochemical profile. If the nerve to a predominantly fast (anaerobic) muscle is transferred to a slow (aerobic) muscle and vice versa, the contractile and histochemical staining characteristics of the two muscles are reversed (Close, 1965; Romanul and Van der Meulen, 1967). The fact that the enzyme content of muscle fibers (and therefore the histochemical staining pattern) is neural dependent has been used by Karpati and Engel (1968) to document reinnervation. The appearance of clusters of muscle fibers of the same histochemical type ("type grouping") replacing the usual mosaic pattern is indicative of axonal regeneration and reestablishment of neural innervation (Fig. 16–2).

Denervated muscle or a muscle graft can

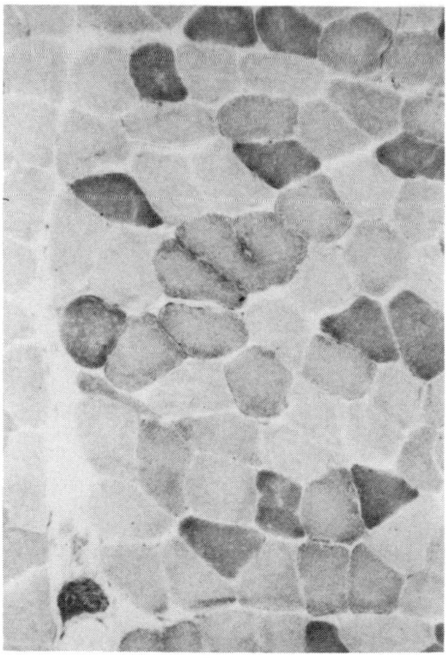

Figure 16–1. Myosin ATPase histochemical stain at pH 9.4. Note the checkerboard pattern with dark Type II fibers and light Type I fibers randomly distributed.

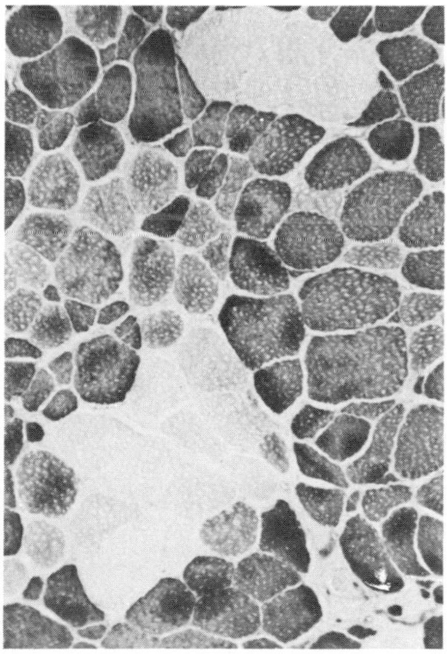

Figure 16–2. Denervation atrophy (similar ATPase reaction as in Figure 16–1) with reinnervation indicated by histochemical fiber type grouping.

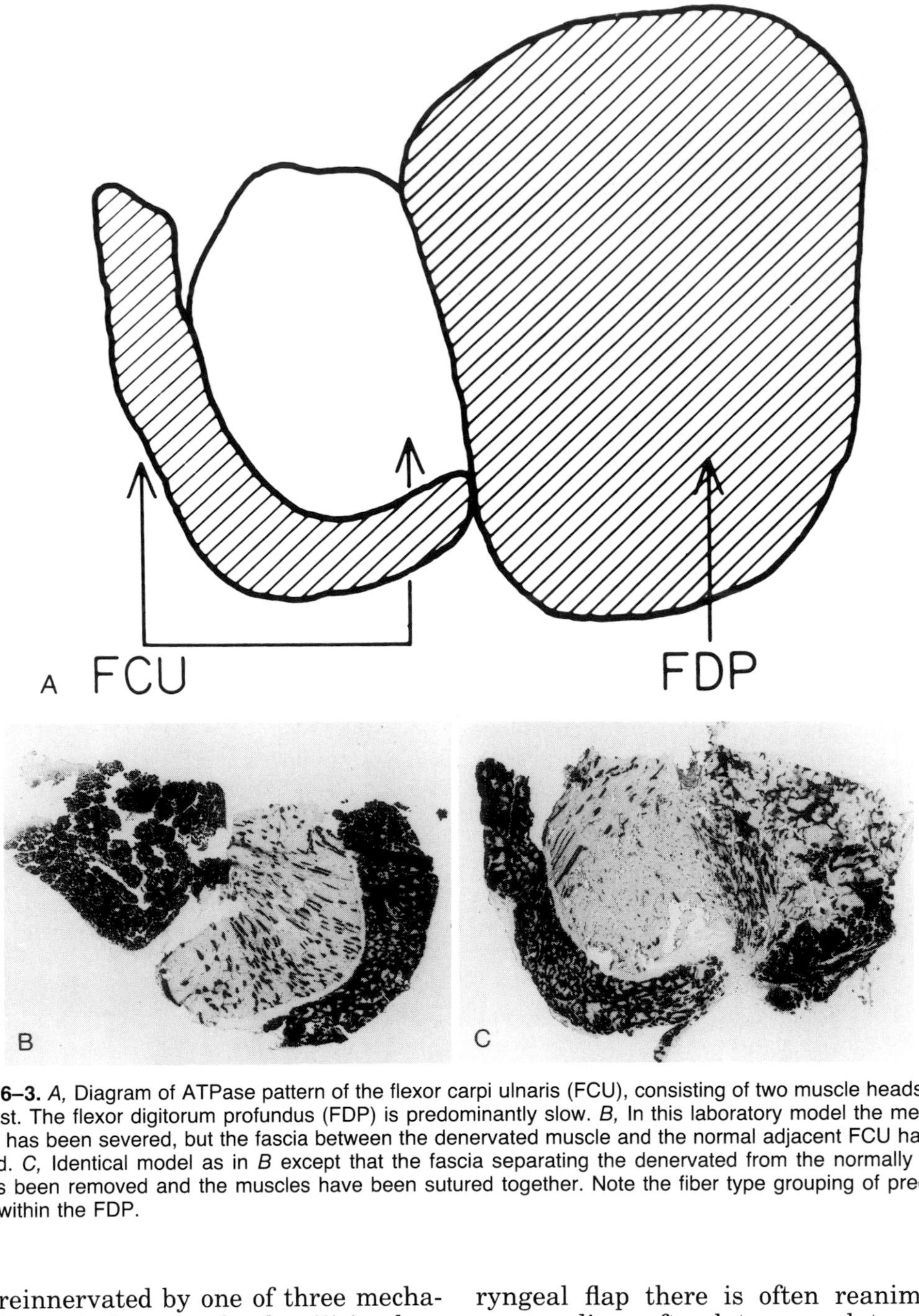

Figure 16–3. *A,* Diagram of ATPase pattern of the flexor carpi ulnaris (FCU), consisting of two muscle heads, one slow and one fast. The flexor digitorum profundus (FDP) is predominantly slow. *B,* In this laboratory model the median nerve to the FDP has been severed, but the fascia between the denervated muscle and the normal adjacent FCU has been left undisturbed. *C,* Identical model as in *B* except that the fascia separating the denervated from the normally innervated muscle has been removed and the muscles have been sutured together. Note the fiber type grouping of predominantly fast fibers within the FDP.

become reinnervated by one of three mechanisms: (1) surgical neurorrhaphy; (2) implantation of nerve directly into the muscle; and (3) sprouting of nerves from adjacent normal muscle, i.e., muscular neurotization. In clinical situations in which a nerve is not available, the latter mechanism is predominant. The phenomenon of one muscle reinnervating another has been observed clinically (Erlacher, 1915; Owens, 1951). Harii, Ohmori, and Torii (1976) noted that following a pharyngeal flap there is often reanimation of surrounding soft palate musculature.

Muscular neurotization has also been documented in the laboratory using histochemical and electromyographic methods (Miller and associates, 1978). However, in the experimental denervated muscle, in which the other variables of tension and blood supply are left undisturbed, considerable muscle atrophy occurs despite evidence of reinnervation (Fig. 16–3). Since this type of reinnervation process takes place over the entire surface of the muscle, it is difficult to test the functional recovery of the muscle because it is intimately adherent to surrounding muscles. However, it is generally agreed that this process is not as efficient as nerve-nerve repair or nerve-muscle implantation (Gutmann, 1969; Kugelberg, Edstrom, and Abbruzzese, 1970; Hakelius, 1974; Miller and associates, 1978; Faulkner and associates, 1981; Frey and associates, 1982).

It is likely that fascia is a barrier to reinnervation between muscles. Most reports of successful free muscle grafts in humans have occurred in the reconstruction of facial and anal muscles, neither of which have fascial coverings.

Reinnervation is probably the single most important aspect of the repair process of muscle as well as the most time-consuming, even when surgical neurorrhaphy is performed. Schenck (1977) has reported that after successful microneurovascular transfer no muscle contraction was identified for five months.

It is not known how long a muscle can exist before irreversible atrophy and fibrosis makes attempts to introduce neural innervation unsuccessful. It is likely that different muscles undergo atrophy at different rates. It has been observed that intrinsic muscles of the hand atrophy within months after denervation, yet successful reinnervation of facial muscles has been reported one year after facial nerve injury (Sunderland, 1968; Tolhurst, 1980). There seems little question, however, that the longer the period of denervation, the more unsuccessful is the reinnervation process (Gutmann and Young, 1944).

It is also difficult to evaluate precisely the extent of muscle reinnervation. Following denervation, motor end plates degenerate and they are reformed by axonal growth. Choline acetyltransferase levels correlate closely with the level of reinnervation in the experimental model (Carlson, Hansen-Smith, and Magon, 1979). In clinical situations, however, where biopsy is not possible, one must rely on the more imprecise methods of clinical examination (grip manometers) and electromyography.

Electromyography. Like the brain and heart, there is electric potential within skeletal muscle. This is discharged upon voluntary activity. At rest, normal muscle is electrically silent. Other than the slight irritability seen upon insertion of the monopolar electrode, no activity is seen.

Denervated muscle (whether due to nerve severance or neuropraxia) consistently demonstrates a fibrillation pattern and positive sharp waves. Evidence of reinnervation is seen as the appearance of large polyphasic units (Fig. 16–4).

TENOTOMY

Alterations in the normal physiologic length of muscle adversely influence function. It is well known from clinical experience that after an unrecognized tendon laceration, reduction of the resting length of the muscle results in atrophy, fibrosis, and loss of normal elasticity within a few weeks of injury. If insufficient resting tension exists, the muscle fibers decrease in cross sectional area and shorten in length, thus limiting motor function and strength (Wickiewicz and associates, 1983). It is also true that increasing the length of a muscle and applying excessive stretch results in fibrosis and loss of contractile force (Zierler, 1974).

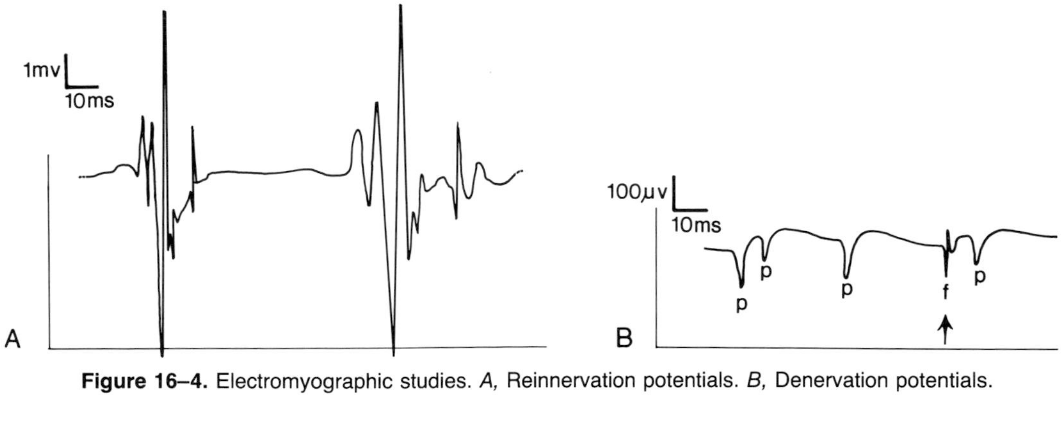

Figure 16–4. Electromyographic studies. *A,* Reinnervation potentials. *B,* Denervation potentials.

The fact that resting tension affects muscle is illustrated by the laboratory studies of Terzis and associates (1978), which investigated the functional capacity of muscle transplants. It was found that tenotomy (division of the origin and insertion) was more damaging than severance of the nerve and blood supply, followed by immediate microscopic repair.

It is reasonable to assume that in clinical situations in which microvascular muscle transfers are required, the variations in physiologic length imposed by the special demands of the recipient area have substantial and detrimental effects on the eventual functional result. Manktelow and McKee (1978) selected the gracilis and pectoralis muscles in the reconstruction of forearm defects. The muscle fibers run parallel to the line of contraction, allowing the muscle to shorten approximately 40 per cent of its length and thus providing excursions of 12 and 10 cm, respectively—adequate distance to replace finger flexion (6 to 8 cm excursion). The difference in excursion is probably equalized as the transplanted muscles undergo an inevitable degree of fibrosis secondary to the neurovascular transfer and alteration in resting tension.

Frey and associates (1983) advocated a technique of placing a silk suture along the long axis of the donor muscle prior to harvest. During resuturing in a heterotopic position, the suture should ideally be stretched, thus reestablishing normal resting tension.

BLOOD SUPPLY

Because of its high metabolic demands, muscle is extraordinarily sensitive to anoxia. In clinical situations of extremity replantation following trauma, muscle is undoubtedly the time-limiting tissue. Periods of normothermic ischemia that exceed one hour result in muscle damage (Tamai and associates, 1970).

The metabolic effects of ischemia on muscle have been studied after tourniquet application (Dahlbäck, 1970; Wilgis, 1974). All investigators confirmed that following deflation (after two hours at 300 mm Hg) there was increased capillary permeability to protein and fluid. This resulted in edema formation due to depressed levels of pO_2 (Kennedy and associates, 1981; Wilgis, 1974) and there was still increased blood flow with significant arteriovenous shunting (Kennedy and associates, 1981). The fluid collection within the muscle caused increases in pressure sufficient to result in focal areas of necrosis.

During oxygen deprivation, muscle metabolism relies solely on glycolysis to produce ATP. This is associated with accumulation of lactic acid, which is converted to glycogen aerobically when blood flow is reestablished. Muscle metabolites and tissue gas tensions return to normal 1.5 hours after tourniquet deflation (Miller and associates, 1978).

Much of the information regarding the effects of anoxia on muscle have been gathered from early clinical experience with neurovascular transplantation. Following an ischemic period of one hour, Tamai and associates (1970) observed an inflammatory cell infiltration at three days and proliferation of interstitial connective tissue and myonuclei at one week. At two weeks, irregularity in muscle fiber shape and vacuolization within the intermyofibrillar spaces were observed. By two months the cross striation pattern, which had been lost, had returned to normal. Electron microscopic changes were more prominent: one week postoperatively there was atrophy of mitochondria and destruction of sarcoplasmic reticulum. Evidence of repair appeared in the fourth and fifth weeks: increased glycogen granules and mitochondria and decreased fibrous tissue were seen, although focal areas of fiber degeneration were still evident throughout the muscle.

The repair process that follows ischemia takes a long time. Five months postoperatively, biopsies of transplanted human muscle have demonstrated continuing restoration of the microscopic anatomy and the presence of atrophy (Harii, Ohmori, and Torii, 1976). Manktelow and McKee (1978) noted continuing improvement with the observation that there was less evidence of fiber atrophy and fibrosis in muscle biopsies taken during the seventh and 14th months after the ischemic episode.

The *maximal* time for which muscle can endure temporary periods of anoxia is not precisely known. It is likely, however, that after approximately six hours of normothermic ischemia (and eight hours if cooled) successful replantation is unlikely, owing to irreversible muscle necrosis (Bunche, 1985).

MUSCLE INJURY

It has been recognized that skeletal muscle has the potential for repair following injury or disease (Forbus, 1926; Le Gros Clark and Blomfield, 1945). Sporadic reports have suggested that muscle has the regenerative capability of healing after crush injury, small lacerations (Millar, 1934; Le Gros Clark, 1946; Allbrook, Baker, and Kirkaldy-Willis, 1966), and infection such as typhus (Forbus, 1926; Volkmann, 1926).

Although lacerations of muscle are common in clinical practice, little attention has been focused on the study of functional recovery. In a laboratory study, Garrett and colleagues (1984) found that completely lacerated (transected) muscles recovered approximately 50 per cent of their ability to produce tension and were able to contract (against a minimal weight) at a level 80 per cent of normal. After partial lacerations of the muscle, 60 per cent of tension production and normal shortening were observed. The muscle laceration was noted to heal by scar formation, but it should be pointed out that the extremities of the animals used in this study were not immobilized following injury. The portion of the muscle distal to the transection showed microscopic evidence of denervation atrophy: small, irregular-shaped muscle cells with central positioning of the nuclei, and an increased amount of fibrous tissue. The denervated segment did not stretch during contraction, probably because of the increased content of fibrous tissue.

The importance of innervation to the repair or regeneration process within muscle is profound. Following injury, regenerative activity takes place but does not continue unless a nerve supply is present (Denny-Brown, 1951; Walton and Adams, 1956). Palmaris longus muscles have been grafted in the rhesus monkey with and without surgical repair of the median nerve. No vascular repair was performed. Muscle fibers regenerated in all grafts in which neural repair was done, but in only three of eight autografts without nerve repair (Maxwell and associates, 1979).

MUSCLE GRAFTS

A muscle graft is a muscle completely removed from its origin, insertion, and nerve and blood supply and replaced into the original bed (orthotopic) or another anatomic location (heterotopic).

From the earliest investigations of muscle grafting without neurovascular anastomosis, disagreements have arisen. Zielonko (1874) was the first to make an unsuccessful attempt. Shortly thereafter, however, Gluck (1881) claimed success, and the controversy began. To summarize the work of the next 80 years, until 1960 it was generally agreed that muscle could not be successfully grafted (Peer, 1955). In retrospect, however, the literature reveals that several investigators observed that muscle possessed regenerative capabilities (Forbus, 1926; Millar, 1934). Studies of muscle regeneration in mammals have been comprehensively summarized by Carlson (1973).

Some of the earliest and most extensive laboratory work on free muscle grafting was done by Studitsky in Russia. In 1960 Studitsky and Bosova performed what may be the first successful muscle graft, transferring the middle third of the gastrocnemius of the rat. Subsequently the regenerative capacity of muscle was confirmed when "minced" muscle (cut into 1 mm cubes) was found to reform the rat gastrocnemius muscle provided that the tendon of insertion and the nerve were left in place (Studitsky, 1963, 1964). Studitsky believed that mincing stimulated myoblasts into "mitotic division." At this time the concept of preoperative denervation was also introduced, a maneuver thought to induce a "plastic state" of regenerative activity within the muscle: "enlargement and division of nuclei, amitotic division of nuclei, the growth of sarcoplasm masses. . . , the formation of myofibrils." (Studitsky, 1964).

In 1971, Thompson was the first to report successful free muscle grafts in humans, principally in the surgical efforts to reanimate the face following seventh nerve palsy in which he used predenervated palmaris longus grafts (Fig. 16–5). He also presented experimental evidence of free muscle graft survival in dogs to substantiate his clinical studies (Thompson, 1971). Predenervation, performed three weeks before grafting to alter the muscle's metabolism, was felt to be essential, as was the transplantation of the entire muscle length so that muscle fibers were undamaged. Success, however, was attributed to the *survival* of muscle fibers within the

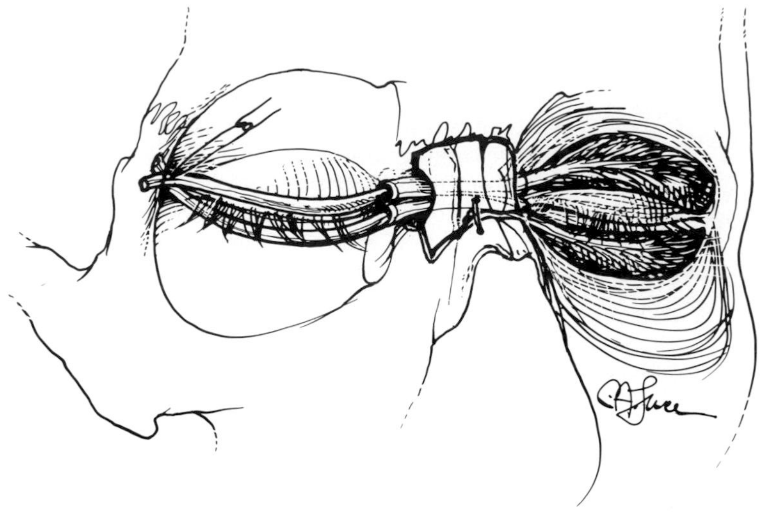

Figure 16–5. Muscle graft of the extensor digitorum brevis muscle (longitudinally split into two muscle and tendon halves) applied to contralateral obicularis oculi to restore eyelid closure in a patient with facial paralysis. (After Thompson, N.: Autogenous muscle grafts in the reconstruction of the paralyzed face. *In* Converse, J. M. (Ed.): Reconstructive Plastic Surgery. 2nd Ed. Philadelphia, W. B. Saunders Company, 1977, p. 1841.)

graft rather than to the result of any regenerative process.

Other investigators did not experience clinical success with free muscle grafts. Before 1971 the vast majority of surgeons were unaware of the pioneering research in Russia and were influenced by the pessimistic viewpoint of Peer and Walker (1951) as well as by the more recent unsuccessful attempts to graft muscle in dogs (Roy, 1966). Following Thompson's clinical and laboratory success, free muscle grafts were again attempted (Lavine and Cochran, 1976; Watson and Muir, 1976). One study (Watson and Muir, 1976) included the concepts of preoperative denervation, transplantation of the entire muscle belly length, restoration of physiologic tension, and removal of all fascia. The graft was positioned at right angles to the recipient muscle for later identification. Histologic, histochemical and contraction studies were employed to evaluate the results. No viable muscle was identified. It was suggested that the observed failure could be attributed to the excessive size of the muscle graft (Watson and Muir, 1976).

The effective use of free muscle grafts for patients with facial palsy, and in the reconstruction of the anal sphincter in cases of incontinence, has been reported (Thompson, 1974; Hakelius, 1974, 1975, 1981; Hakelius and Stalberg, 1974; Freilinger, 1975). In most of these clinical reports the technique relied on the placement of the muscle graft over normal muscle, in the expectation that neural innervation would be provided through muscular neurotization (Fig. 16–5). The palmaris longus muscle was used most commonly as the graft, and it was denervated three weeks preoperatively. To reconstruct the oral sphincter the muscle belly of the graft was divided and sutured over both the paralyzed and the normal orbicularis oris muscles. Support and elevation of the oral commissure was obtained by fixing the tendon to the zygomatic arch.

The documentation of muscle graft function can be difficult. The electromyographic studies of Hakelius and Stalberg (1974) are convincing, employing single fiber techniques. It is not unreasonable to state that positive documentation such as this is the exception rather than the rule in clinical reports. There seems to be little question that the technique of muscle grafting was often beneficial in reconstructing eyelid and oral sphincter function. It was not clear, however, whether the observed motion was due to actual contraction of the muscle graft itself. A failed graft could function effectively as a static or passive sling by tightening as the normal (adjacent) muscle contracted (Miller and associates, 1978).

The clinical experience with free muscle grafting has not been uniformly encouraging and failures have been encountered (Miller and associates, 1978; Nicolai, 1981; Tolhurst, 1985). Despite the lack of uniformity of results with this method, it seems apparent that under certain, as yet incompletely defined, circumstances it can be of value. It is questionable, however, whether it can be considered a reliable, consistent reconstructive technique. It may be that the clinical applications are limited. Hakelius (1985b) has effectively used free muscle grafts (extensor brevis; palmaris longus) for restoration of eyelid closure and reconstruction of *partial* facial paralysis (Hakelius, 1985b).

Perhaps one of the principal difficulties in evaluating the conflicting data on free muscle grafts is the fact that many of the basic concepts originally presented are now open to question. The early reported clinical success with free muscle grafts, in spite of so many previously negative experiments by others, was attributed to: (1) transplantation of an entire muscle belly, thereby including only undamaged muscle fibers; and (2) preoperative denervation, to render the transplanted muscle more suitable metabolically for the initial anoxic period associated with grafting (Thompson, 1971). Neither of these concepts, however, is entirely supported by experimental or clinical evidence.

The Abbé lip flap, for example, has been used successfully as a composite graft (nonvascularized) from lower to upper lip (Walker and Sawhney, 1972). When the lip is transferred as a flap, the technique certainly divides the majority, if not all, of the orbicularis oris muscle cells contained within it, yet the technique is effective. The mincing of muscle grafts in successful laboratory experiments also seems a strong argument against the need to transplant the entire muscle length.

Conflicting data also exist regarding the need for preoperative denervation. Muscle metabolism is highly complex. It was originally suggested that denervation altered the metabolic demands of the graft, thus allowing a greater chance of graft *survival* (Thompson, 1971). It is now clear from experimental work that after grafting, most muscle fibers die of ischemia necrosis, and a regenerative process ensues. Denervation provides a stimulus for dormant cells possessing myogenic potential, the satellite cell (Verna, 1979). It also reduces the bulk of muscle and increases capillary circulation (Gutmann, 1962). The beneficial effect of predenervation to improve graft survival has not been substantiated in laboratory conditions (Carlson and Gutmann, 1975; Carlson, 1976). However, predenervation is usually employed when muscle grafts are used clinically.

Histology of Free Muscle Grafts. The microscopic events that follow free muscle grafting have been studied in several animal species and they demonstrate a consistent pattern, particularly in grafts that weigh less than 4 gm. Within hours after grafting, all muscle fibers die of ischemic necrosis with the exception of a thin rim of cells around the periphery of the graft (Fig. 16–6). These fibers (less than 5 per cent of the total) apparently survive by diffusion of fluid from the recipient site. A wave of vascular ingrowth begins to penetrate the graft within two days and brings with it leukocytes and macrophages (Hansen-Smith and Carlson, 1979), which begin to remove the dead sarcoplasm but leave the basal laminae intact. This wave of phagocytosis progresses centripetally ahead of the ingrowing capillary bed. After a few days a cross section of a free muscle graft discloses three distinct circular zones: (1) the peripheral rim of surviving muscle fibers, which is adjacent to (2) a ring of muscle regeneration surrounding (3) a core of necrotic fibers that have not yet been removed by the macrophages.

Regeneration of new muscle is first apparent three days after grafting in the smallest and most extensively studied graft, the extensor digitorum longus of the rat, which weighs 100 mg (Carlson and Gutmann, 1975; Carlson, 1976). The first evidence of regeneration appears at the edge of individual necrotic muscle fibers where small, flat nuclei develop cytoplasm and become round cells (Cedars and associates, 1983). The round cells produce myofilaments, fuse into multinucleated myotubes that mature into muscle fibers, and eventually form a fascicular pattern within the muscle.

It appears that the size of the graft is a critical factor in determining whether or not complete regeneration will occur or whether a residual area of central fibrosis will remain. Complete regeneration occurs throughout the entire muscle in the rat extensor digitorum longus (100 mg) (Carlson and Gutmann, 1975) and the rabbit flexor digitorum sublimis (1.5 gm) (Cedars and associates, 1983). However, a persistent core of necrosis, which is eventually replaced by scar tissue, has been observed in the cat extensor digitorum longus (3.5 gm) and the monkey palmaris longus (4.5 gm) (Maxwell and associates, 1978, 1979). This difference suggests that a critical factor in regeneration is the radius of the graft. This may be due to the time necessary for centripetal vascular penetration to reach the center of the graft and provide nourishment to the residual myogenic cells. The regener-

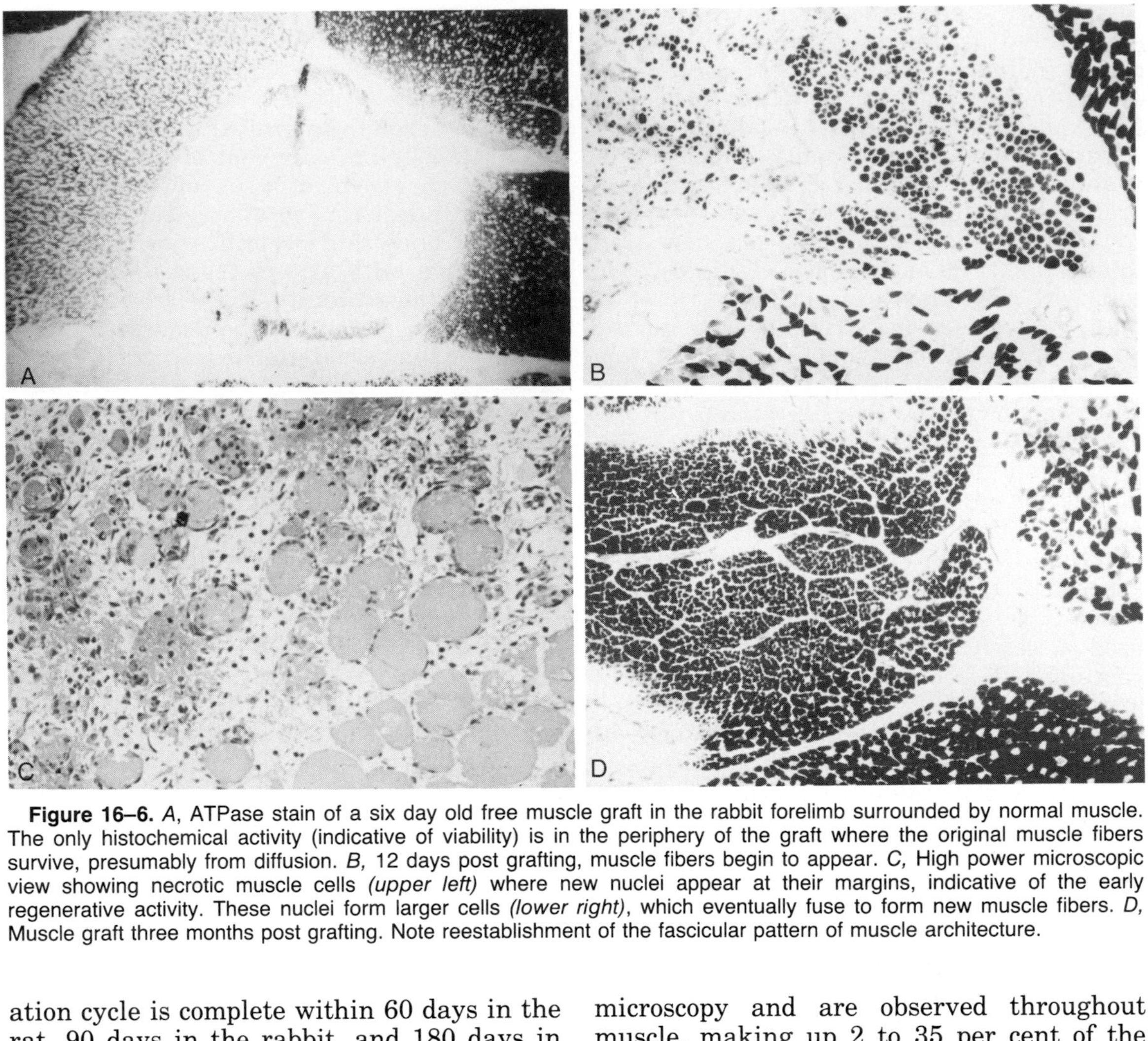

Figure 16–6. *A*, ATPase stain of a six day old free muscle graft in the rabbit forelimb surrounded by normal muscle. The only histochemical activity (indicative of viability) is in the periphery of the graft where the original muscle fibers survive, presumably from diffusion. *B*, 12 days post grafting, muscle fibers begin to appear. *C*, High power microscopic view showing necrotic muscle cells *(upper left)* where new nuclei appear at their margins, indicative of the early regenerative activity. These nuclei form larger cells *(lower right)*, which eventually fuse to form new muscle fibers. *D*, Muscle graft three months post grafting. Note reestablishment of the fascicular pattern of muscle architecture.

ation cycle is complete within 60 days in the rat, 90 days in the rabbit, and 180 days in the cat (Maxwell and associates, 1978; Faulkner and associates, 1981).

No investigation other than that of Thompson (1971) has reported successful grafts using larger muscles. As previously mentioned, attempts by other investigators (Roy, 1966; Watson and Muir, 1976; Lavine and Cochran, 1976) with large (± 50 gm) muscle grafts in dogs have resulted uniformly in failure. This discrepancy remains unexplained.

It is generally believed that the source of the regenerative process is the activation of the dormant stem cell known as the satellite cell identified by Mauro in 1961 (Church, Noronha, and Allbrook, 1966; Moss and Leblond, 1971; Snow, 1978). These cells are located beneath the basement membrane of the muscle fiber, and under conventional light microscopy appear identical to muscle cell nuclei. They can be identified only by electron microscopy and are observed throughout muscle, making up 2 to 35 per cent of the total number of nuclei, depending on the age of the animal (Schmalbruch and Hellhammer, 1976). The number of satellite cells has been shown to increase after denervation (Schultz, 1978; Verna, 1979).

It appears that the satellite cell is capable of surviving periods of ischemia that result in necrosis of mature muscle fibers and initiating the regeneration process when the neovascularization wave moves through the graft. The potential for longer survival by the satellite cell may be attributed to a low metabolic rate due to a very small amount of cytoplasm, thus allowing these cells to survive by plasmic imbibition (Snow, 1977, Mayr, 1981).

The factors that influence the regeneration process are only partially understood. Some factor associated with the grafting of muscle, perhaps the ischemic necrosis that follows, initiates myogenesis. In the same laboratory model in the rabbit forelimb, it appeared that *more* muscle volume was achieved after grafting than was observed after denervation in situ followed by muscular reinnervation (Miller and associates, 1978; Miller and Das, 1981). There seems little question that young age in the recipient is associated with more muscle regeneration. Muscle grafts in young rabbits regenerated entire muscles at a faster rate and with less connective tissue and became more completely reinnervated than those of mature animals (Das and associates, 1982; Cedars and associates, 1983). Muscle grafts from older rats placed into young ones developed better function (generating greater tension on functional testing) compared with those of the reverse graft exchange (Gutmann and Carlson, 1975). This finding suggests superior reinnervation, and perhaps revascularization occurs in the younger animal.

MICRONEUROVASCULAR MUSCLE TRANSFERS

In 1970 Tamai and associates transferred the rectus femoris muscle in dogs and documented the histologic, histochemical, and electromyographic events that followed. These studies firmly established for the first time that entire muscles could be successfully moved to a new anatomic position by immediate microscopic revascularization and neural repair. This method was subsequently used clinically with satisfactory results in the reconstruction of forearm defects (Sixth Peoples Hospital, 1976; Schenck, 1977; Manktelow and McKee, 1978) and in the reanimation of the face following VII nerve injury (Harii, Ohmari, and Torii, 1976; O'Brien, Franklin, and Morrison, 1980; Tolhurst, 1980, 1985).

The principles defined in this pioneering effort (Tamai and associates, 1970) can be summarized as efforts to expedite the technical aspects of the procedure and to maximize reinnervation potential: (1) selection of a donor muscle with a single artery and nerve that can be removed with little residual functional disability; (2) reduction of the length of ischemia time; and (3) proximal neural repair. Subsequently, refinements in donor muscle selection have been made, with emphasis placed on obtaining functional characteristics that closely parallel the specific anatomic deficit (Manktelow and McKee, 1978; Harrison, 1985).

The functional results from these efforts are generally satisfactory but variable. Biopsies and electromyographic studies have been employed to document survival, and several reports indicate that adequate muscle function can be documented after transplantation. Detailed physiologic evaluations have been carried out in controlled laboratory conditions. Terzis and associates (1978) reported that after microneurovascular transfer the weight of the muscle correlated with the force of contraction. Although the transplanted muscles showed evidence of survival, function tests (fatigue rate and tetanic tension) indicated that after complete reinnervation, maximal work capacity was only 25 per cent of normal. Reinnervation required at least eight to nine months and electromyographic wave forms were observed in different locations within the graft. Nerve conduction velocity exceeded 15 m/sec.

This study points out some of the complexities in evaluating muscle function as well as the variable response of muscle to alterations in its normal physiologic state. While one would suspect that disturbance of only one of the three variables that affect muscle function (blood supply, innervation, tension) would be preferable to interruption of two or three, this may not be the case. It was found that muscle function was more adversely altered by tenotomy alone (detaching origin and insertion) than by microneurovascular repair (Terzis and associates, 1978).

Variability in experimental results has also been reported. Frey and associates (1983), using essentially the same experimental model as discussed above (rabbit rectus femoris; weight 10 gm), reported acquisition of muscle function (measured by maximal tetanic tension) of 55 per cent of normal. Aside from possible differences in technique, such as shorter ischemia time, the twofold difference cannot be explained.

There have been reports of successful microneurovascular transplantation by using the gracilis muscle (Harii, Ohmori, and Torii, 1976) and pectoralis minor muscle (Harrison, 1985) to reconstruct facial nerve palsy defects. However, a question has been raised as to whether these donor muscles are too large in volume to reconstruct the muscle responsible for smiling, the zygomaticus major. The latter is approximately 5 cm in length and shortens 1.5 to 2 cm during smiling (Manktelow and Zuker, 1984). To reconstruct this comparatively small muscle, a *portion* of the gracilis muscle, centered on the neurovascular pedicle, has been used (Manktelow and Zuker, 1984). Harii, Ohmori, and Torii (1976) have effectively transferred half of the gracilis muscle, relying on a cross facial nerve graft to provide a new source of reinnervation and synchronous expression (Fig. 16–7).

It is obviously difficult to evaluate accurately the return of muscle function in clinical situations. Early reports suggested that approximately 50 per cent of pretransplant muscle mass could be expected to survive (Harii, Ohmori, and Torii, 1976; Terzis and associates, 1978). However, the position of the muscle transfer as well as individual patient effort are significant considerations. Transplants placed in the forearm are more available to voluntary exercise and subsequent hypertrophy than those placed in the face. Fourteen months after pectoralis major muscle reconstruction of finger flexion, survival of normal muscle volume and the ability to generate 35 lb grip strength have been reported (Manktelow and McKee, 1978).

In all clinical and laboratory reports the investigators have emphasized the prolonged period necessary for the return of muscle function. Schenck (1977, 1978) did not observe muscle function until at least five months postoperatively, and muscle biopsies showed diminishing numbers of atrophic fibers and less evidence of fibrosis 14 months after surgery (Manktelow and McKee, 1978).

Muscle transfers are also discussed in Chapters 42 and 100.

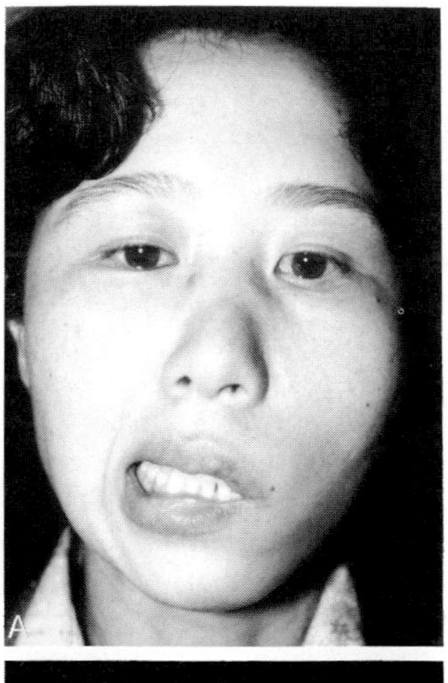

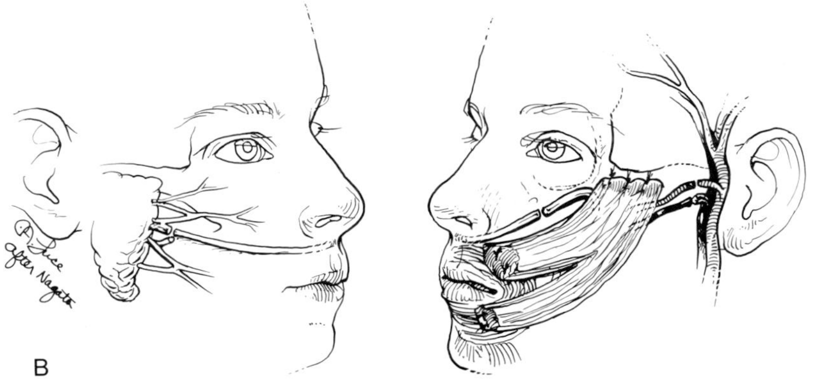

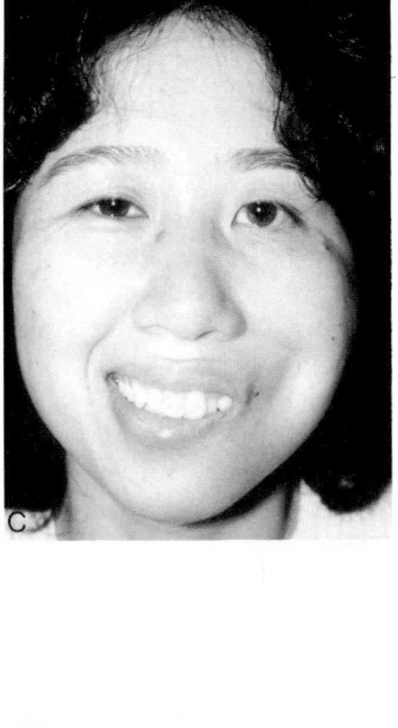

Figure 16–7. *A,* Preoperative animation view of a 35 year old female with chronic left-sided Bell's palsy in whom a cross facial sural nerve graft had been placed on the unaffected side one year earlier. A Tinel's sign has been present at the distal nerve graft stump for two months. (Courtesy of Kiyonori Harii, M.D.) *B,* Less than half of the gracilis muscle is placed into the paralyzed side, suturing the muscle into the zygomatic arch and the lower and upper lips after microneurovascular anastomoses (cross face sural nerve graft) as illustrated. *C,* Animation view one year postoperatively.

REFERENCES

Allbrook, D.: An electron microscopic study of regeneration in skeletal muscle. J. Anat., *96*:137, 1962.

Allbrook, D., Baker, W. de C., and Kirkaldy-Willis, W. H.: Muscle regeneration in experimental animals and in man. J. Bone Joint Surg. (Br.), *48*:153, 1966.

Bunche, U.: Personal communication, 1985.

Carlson, B. M.: The regeneration of skeletal muscle. A review. Am. J. Anat., *137*:119, 1973.

Carlson, B. M.: A quantitative study of muscle fiber survival and regeneration in normal, predenervated, and Marcaine-treated free muscle grafts in the rat. Exp. Neurol., *52*:421, 1976.

Carlson, B. M., and Gutmann, E.: Regeneration in grafts of normal and denervated rat muscles. Pflugers Arch., *353*:215, 1975.

Carlson, B. M., Hansen-Smith, F. M., and Magon, D. K.: The life history of a free muscle graft. *In* Mauro, A. (Ed.): Muscle Regeneration. New York, Raven Press, 1979, p. 493.

Cedars, M. G., Das, S. K., Roth, J. C., and Miller, T. A.: The microscopic morphology of orthotopic free muscle grafts in rabbits. Plast. Reconstr. Surg., *72*:179, 1983.

Church, J. C. T., Noronha, R. F. X., and Allbrook, D. B.: Satellite cells and skeletal muscle regeneration. Br. J. Surg., *53*:638, 1966.

Close, R.: Effects of cross-union of motor nerves to fast and slow skeletal muscles. Nature, *206*:831, 1965.

Dahlbäck, L. O.: Effects of temporary tourniquet ischemia on striated muscle fibers and motor end-plates. Scand. J. Plast. Reconstr. Surg., Suppl. 7, 1970.

Das, S. K., Cragun, J. R., Idler, R., and Miller, T. A.: Autogenous free muscle grafts and regeneration in rabbits: a preliminary study. Plast. Reconstr. Surg., *69*:500, 1982.

Denny-Brown, D.: The influence of tension and innervation in the regeneration of skeletal muscle. J. Neuropathol., *10*:94, 1951.

Erlacher, P.: Direct and muscular neurotization of paralyzed muscles: experimental research. Am. J. Orthop. Surg., *13*:22, 1915.

Faulkner, J. A., Markley, J. M., Jr., and White, T. P.: Skeletal muscle transplantation in cats with and without nerve repair. *In* Freilinger, G., Holle, J., and Carlson, B. M. (Eds.): Muscle Transplantation. New York, Springer-Verlag, 1981, p. 47.

Filogamo, G., and Gabella, G.: Cholinesterase behavior in the denervated and reinnervated muscles. Acta Anat., *63*:199, 1966.

Forbus, W. D.: Pathologic changes in voluntary muscle II. Experimental study of degeneration and regeneration of striated muscle with vital stains. Arch. Pathol., *2*:486, 1926.

Freilinger, G.: A new technique to correct facial paralysis. Plast. Reconstr. Surg., *56*:44, 1975.

Frey, M., Gruber, H., Havel, M., Steiner, E., and Freilinger, G.: Experimental free muscle transplantation with microneurovascular anastomoses. Plast. Reconstr. Surg., *71*:689, 1983.

Frey, M., Gruber, H., Holle, J., and Freilinger, G.: An experimental comparison of the different kinds of muscle reinnervation: nerve suture, nerve implantation, and muscular neurotization. Plast. Reconstr. Surg., *69*:656, 1982.

Garrett, W. E., Jr., Seaber, A. V., Boswick, J., Ubaniak, J. R., and Goldner, J. L.: Recovery of skeletal muscle after laceration and repair. J. Hand Surg., *9*:683, 1984.

Gluck, T.: Ueber Muskel-und Schenplastik. Langenbecks. Arch. Klin. Chir., *26*:61, 1881.

Gutmann, E. (Ed.): The Denervated Muscle. Prague, Publishing House Czechoslovak Academy of Science, 1962.

Gutmann, E.: Physiological control mechanisms: nervous and hormonal mechanisms in the aging process of the neuromuscular system. *In* 8th International Congress of Gerontology. Proceedings-Vol. 1. International Association of Gerontology, Washington, DC, 1969, p. 143.

Gutmann, E., and Carlson, B. M.: Regeneration in grafts of normal and denervated rat muscles. Contractile properties. Pflugers Arch., *353*:215, 1975.

Gutmann, E., and Young, J. Z.: The re-innervation of muscle after various periods of atrophy. J. Anat., *78*:15, 1944.

Hakelius, L.: Transplantation of free autogenous muscle in the treatment of facial paralysis. Scand. J. Plast. Reconstr. Surg., *8*:220, 1974.

Hakelius, L.: Free autogenous muscle transplantation in two cases of total anal incontinence. Acta Chir. Scand., *141*:69, 1975.

Hakelius, L.: Treatment of facial paralysis with free autogenous muscle transplants. *In* Freilinger, G., Holle, J., and Carlson, B. M. (Eds.): Muscle Transplantation. New York, Springer-Verlag, 1981, p. 215.

Hakelius, L.: Personal communication, 1985a.

Hakelius, L.: Long-term results of free muscle grafting without vascular anastomoses in long-standing facial palsy. *In* Portmann, M. (Ed.): Proceedings of the Fifth International Symposium on the Facial Nerve. New York, Masson, 1985b, p. 137.

Hakelius, L., and Stalberg, E.: Electromyographical studies of free autogenous muscle transplants in man. Scand. J. Plast. Reconstr. Surg., *8*:211, 1974.

Hansen-Smith, F. M., and Carlson, B. M.: Cellular response to free grafting of the extensor digitorum longus muscle of the rat. J. Neurol. Sci., *41*:149, 1979.

Harii, K., Ohmori, K., and Torii, S.: Free gracilis muscle transplantation with microneurovascular anastomoses for the treatment of facial paralysis. Plast. Reconstr. Surg., *57*:133, 1976.

Harrison, D. H.: The pectoralis minor vascularized muscle graft for the treatment of unilateral facial paralysis. Plast. Reconstr. Surg., *75*:206, 1985.

Karpati, G., and Engel, W. K.: "Type grouping" in skeletal muscle after experimental reinnervation. Neurology, *18*:447, 1968.

Kennedy, T. J., Miller, S. H., Nellis, S. H., Buck, D., Flaim, S. F., et al.: Effects of transient ischemia on nutrient flow and arteriovenous shunting in canine hindlimb. Ann. Surg., *193*:255, 1981.

Kugelberg, E., Edstrom, L., and Abbruzzese, M.: Mapping of motor units in experimentally reinnervated rat muscle. Interpretation of histochemical and atropic fibre patterns in neurogenic lesions. J. Neurol. Neurosurg. Psychiatry, *33*:319, 1970.

Lavine, D., and Cochran, T.: The failure to survive of autogenous free grafts of whole gracilis muscles in dogs. Plast. Reconstr. Surg., *58*:221, 1976.

Le Gros Clark, W. E.: An experimental study of the regeneration of mammalian striped muscle. J. Anat. (Lond.), *80*:24, 1946.

Le Gros Clark, W. E., and Blomfield, L. B.: The efficiency of intramuscular anastomoses with observation on the regeneration of devascularized muscle. J. Anat., *79*:15, 1945.

Manktelow, R. T., and McKee, N. H.: Free muscle trans-

plantation to provide active finger flexion. J. Hand Surg., *3*:416, 1978.
Manktelow, R. T., and Zuker, R. M.: Muscle transplantation by fascicular territory. Plast. Reconstr. Surg., *73*:751, 1984.
Maxwell, L. C., Faulkner, J. A., Markley, J. M., Jr. and Winborn, D. R.: Neuroanastomosis of orthotopically transplanted palmaris longus muscles. Muscle and Nerve, *2*:44, 1979.
Maxwell, L. C., Faulkner, J. A., Mufti, S. A., and Turowski, A. M.: The free autografting of entire limb muscle in the cat: histochemistry and biochemistry. J. Appl. Physiol., *44*:431, 1978.
Mayr, R.: The muscle satellite cell and its role in muscle transplantation (a short review). *In* Freilinger, G., Holle, J., and Carlson, B. M. (Eds.): Muscle Transplantation. New York, Springer-Verlag, 1981, p. 19.
Millar, W. G.: Regeneration of skeletal muscle in young rabbits. J. Pathol. Bacteriol., *38*:145, 1934.
Miller, T. A., and Das, S. K.: An early report of free muscle grafts in rabbits. *In* Freilinger, G. (Ed.): Proceedings of Vienna Muscle Symposium. St. Louis, C. V. Mosby Company, 1981, p. 83.
Miller, T. A., Korn, H. N., Wheeler, E. S., and Eldridge, L.: Can one muscle reinnervate another? A preliminary study of muscular neurotization in the rabbit. Plast. Reconstr. Surg., *61*:50, 1978.
Moss, F. P., and Leblond, C. P.: Satellite cells as the source of nuclei in muscles growing in rats. Anat. Rec., *170*:421, 1971.
Nicolai, J. P.: Free muscle grafting in facial paralysis. Br. J. Plast. Surg., *34*:91, 1981.
O'Brien, B. M., Franklin, J. D., and Morrison, W. A.: Cross-facial nerve grafts and microneurovascular free muscle transfer for long established facial palsy. Br. J. Plast. Surg., *33*:202, 1980.
Owens, N.: The surgical treatment of facial paralysis, collective review. Plast. Reconstr. Surg., *7*:61, 1951.
Peer, L. A.: Transplantation of Tissues. Baltimore, Williams & Wilkins Company, 1955.
Peer, L. A., and Walker, J. C.: The behavior of autogenous human tissue grafts. II. Plast. Reconstr. Surg., *7*:73, 1951.
Romanul, F. C., and Van der Meulen, J. P.: Slow and fast muscles after cross-innervation. Enzymatic and physiological changes. Arch. Neurol., *17*:387, 1967.
Roy, P. R.: Behavior of a free autogenous muscle graft into the skeletal muscle of dog. J. Exp. Med. Sci., *9*:78, 1966.
Schenck, R. R.: Free muscle and composite skin transplantation by microneurovascular anastomoses. Orthop. Clin. North Am., *8*:367, 1977.
Schenck, R. R.: Rectus femoris muscle and composite skin transplantation by microneurovascular anastomoses for avulsion of forearm muscles: a case report. J. Hand Surg., *3*:60, 1978.
Schmalbruch, H., and Hellhammer, U.: The number of satellite cells in normal human muscle. Anat. Rec., *185*:279, 1976.
Schultz, E.: Changes in the satellite cells of growing muscle following denervation. Anat. Rec., *190*:299, 1978.
Shafiq, S. A., and Gorycki, M. A.: Regeneration in skeletal muscle of mouse: some electron microscope observations. J. Pathol. Bacteriol., *90*:123, 1965.
Sixth Peoples Hospital, Microvascular Service, Shanghai: Free muscle transplantation by microsurgical neurovascular anastomoses. Report of a case. Chinese Med. J., *2*:47, 1976.
Snow, M. H.: Myogenic cell formation in regenerating rat skeletal muscle injured by mincing. I. A fine structural study. Anat. Rec., *188*:181, 1977.
Snow, M. H.: An autoradiographic study of satellite cell differentiation into regenerating myotubes following transplantation of muscles in young rats. Cell. Tissue Res., *186*:535, 1978.
Studitsky, A. N.: Dynamics of the development of myogenic tissue under conditions of explanation and transplantation. *In* Rose, G. G. (Ed.): Cinemicrography in Cell Biology. New York, Academic Press, 1963, p. 171.
Studitsky, A. N.: Free auto- and homographs of muscle tissue experiments on animals. Ann. N.Y. Acad. Sci., *120*:789, 1964.
Studitsky, A. N., and Bosova, N. N.: Development of atrophic muscular tissue transplanted to supply a defect of mechanically injured muscles. Arch. Anatomii, Gistologii i Embryologii, *39*:18, 1960.
Sunderland, S. (Ed.): The capacity of human muscles to function efficiently following reinnervation after prolonged denervation. *In* Nerves and Nerve Injuries. Baltimore, Williams & Wilkins Company, 1968.
Tamai, S., Komatsu, S., Sakamoto, H., Sano, S., Sasauchi, N., et al.: Free muscle transplants in dogs, with microsurgical neurovascular anastomoses. Plast. Reconstr. Surg., *46*:219, 1970.
Terzis, J. K., Sweet, R. C., Dykes, R. W., and Williams, H. B.: Recovery of function in free muscle transplants using microneurovascular anastomoses. J. Hand Surg., *3*:37, 1978.
Thompson, N.: Autogenous free grafts of skeletal muscle. A preliminary experimental and clinical study. Plast. Reconstr. Surg., *48*:11, 1971.
Thompson, N.: A review of autogenous skeletal muscle grafts and their clinical application. Clin. Plast. Surg., *1*:349, 1974.
Tolhurst, D. E.: Free revascularised muscle grafts reinnervated by cross facial nerve grafts. Ann. Acad. Med. Singapore, *9*:361, 1980.
Tolhurst, D. E.: Personal communication, 1985.
Verna, V.: Satellite cell in denervated muscles. Experientia, *35*:40, 1979.
Volkmann, J.: Ueber die Regeneration des quergestreiften Muskelgewebes beim Menschen und Sugetier, 1883; cited in Forbus, W. D.: Pathologic changes in voluntary muscle. Arch. Pathol., *2*:486, 1926.
von Zielonko, J.: Ueber die Entwicklung und Proliferation von Epithelien und Endothelien. Bonn, C. Georgi, 1874.
Walker, J. C., Jr., and Sawhney, O. P.: Free composite lip grafts. Plast. Reconstr. Surg., *50*:142, 1972.
Walton, J. N., and Adams, R. D.: The response of the normal, the denervated and the dystrophic muscle-cell to injury. J. Pathol. Bacteriol., *72*:273, 1956.
Watson, A., and Muir, A.: Failure of free muscle grafts in dogs. Br. J. Plast. Surg., *29*:27, 1976.
Wickiewicz, T. L., Roy, R. R., Powell, P. L., and Edgerton, V. R.: Muscle architecture of the human lower limb. Clin. Orthop., *179*:275, 1983.
Wilgis, E. F. S.: Tourniquet ischemia, muscle anoxia and operative edema. *In* Littler, J. W., Cramer, L. M., and Smith, J. W. (Eds.): Symposium on Reconstructive Hand Surgery. Vol. 9. St. Louis, C. V. Mosby Company, 1974, p. 59.
Zierler, K. L.: Mechanism of muscle contraction and its energetics. *In* Mountcastle, V. B. (Ed.): Medical Physiology. 13th Ed. St. Louis, C. V. Mosby Company, 1974.

17

Burt Brent

Repair and Grafting of Cartilage and Perichondrium

The versatility of autogenous cartilage makes it unique within the surgeon's armamentarium of grafting materials for tissue transfer. One can delicately sculpt cartilage to form an ear, or use it as living "fill" to obliterate depressions. It can be employed to correct contour defects; to provide architectual support; to mimic the finest of details, such as Montgomery glands in a nipple-areola complex; or even to restore function in joint reconstruction.

Cartilage grafts do not bear the risks of extrusion as do alloplastic implants. Unlike bone, autogenous cartilage grafts are indifferent to functional stress for survival. They may be carved to any desired shape and can be expected to retain long-term form and bulk, if the surgeon has provided an adequate vascular pocket and avoided tension, dead space, and hematoma. These unique properties render autogenous cartilage an indispensable graft tissue for the contemporary plastic surgeon.

Although irradiated cartilage and thimerosal- (Merthiolate)-preserved allografts have occasional, isolated clinical applicability, the use of living or preserved cartilage allografts and xenografts has been found to be disappointing. The spark of initial enthusiasm for cartilage allografts has been extinguished by late findings of gradual, progressive absorption (Dupertuis and Musgrave, 1959; Hagerty and associates, 1967; Krutchinskij and Schved, 1984).

In contrast, autogenous cartilage grafts not only have demonstrated long-term success, but have been found to grow in size (Dupertuis, 1941 and 1950; Stoll and Furnas, 1970; Tanzer, 1978; Brent, 1988) or to survive even when grafted as tiny particles of cartilage (Brent, 1979a). The author has employed more than 400 clinical rib cartilage autografts over a period of 15 years without experiencing a single case of resorption, except in unusual situations such as hematoma or infection—an incidence of 2 per cent.

Sheen (1987b) made similar observations in his extensive rhinoplasty practice, in which he performs more than 300 cartilage autografts per year. In his total experience, which includes 4500 septal grafts and 1000 conchal cartilage grafts, he has seen only two cases of cartilage resorption without an underlying cause. Only one of these remains inexplicable, whereas the other was probably related to severe circulatory compromise that existed before graft placement; i.e., the patient's nose had been irradiated and the skin was thin, atrophic, and deficient.

Considering the evidence against cartilage allografts, it is surprising that surgeons still use them (Donald and Col, 1982), except in a few specific instances, which will be discussed later in this chapter.

PHYSIOLOGY AND GROWTH

The cartilage is a unique tissue in that it has a comparatively low metabolic rate, one hundredth to one five hundredth of that for other human tissues (Hagerty and associates, 1960a). The glycolytic activity and oxygen consumption of cartilage approaches anaerobic conditions, properties that are generally attributed both to sparsity of its cell population and to avascularity (Curran and Gibson, 1956). Chondrocytes are nourished by tissue fluid diffusion, and metabolize sulfur to produce chondroitin sulfate, the mucopolysaccharide constituent of the protective cartilage matrix. This function provides a basis for chondrocyte viability tests by labeled sulfate (^{35}S) uptake (Curran and Gibson, 1956). Radioactive sulfur is incorporated into chondroitin sulfate within three minutes of presentation to the cartilage cells; the rate can be increased by stimulation with growth hormone.

In the young animal, cartilage proliferates by the deep perichondrial cells differentiating into chondrocytes (appositional growth), and by the young chondrocytes dividing by mitosis (interstitial growth). The tissue mass enlarges as the cartilage cells surround themselves with the substantial matrix they generate.

The chondrocyte efficiently produces chondromucoprotein, elastin, and collagen to generate continually a surrounding matrix (Fig. 17–1). When one injects papain into baby rabbits, it degrades and removes the cartilaginous ground substance; the ears soften and collapse (Thomas, 1956). Uniquely, the chondrocytes rapidly regenerate their surrounding matrix, and the ears regain their normal convolutions and erect positions within days (Fig. 17–2). Therefore, it is not surprising that the long-term success of a cartilage graft depends on living chondrocytes that service and maintain the graft's bulk, and likewise that dead, preserved cartilage grafts eventually resorb.

Dupertuis (1941) and Stoll and Furnas (1970) demonstrated that young cartilage grafts grow. Brent (1987d) determined the

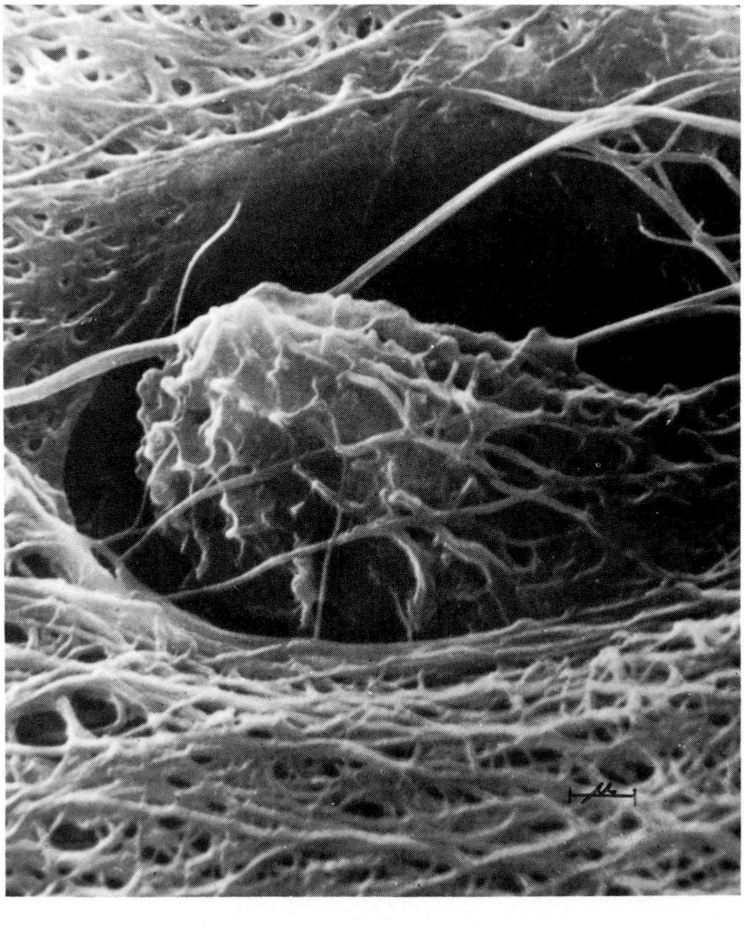

Figure 17–1. The chondrocyte is a versatile cell that produces all structures of the cartilage matrix. Through the scanning electron microscope, it is noted that the chondrocyte is spinning the fine interlaced fibers that surround it. (Courtesy of Dr. J. G. McCall.)

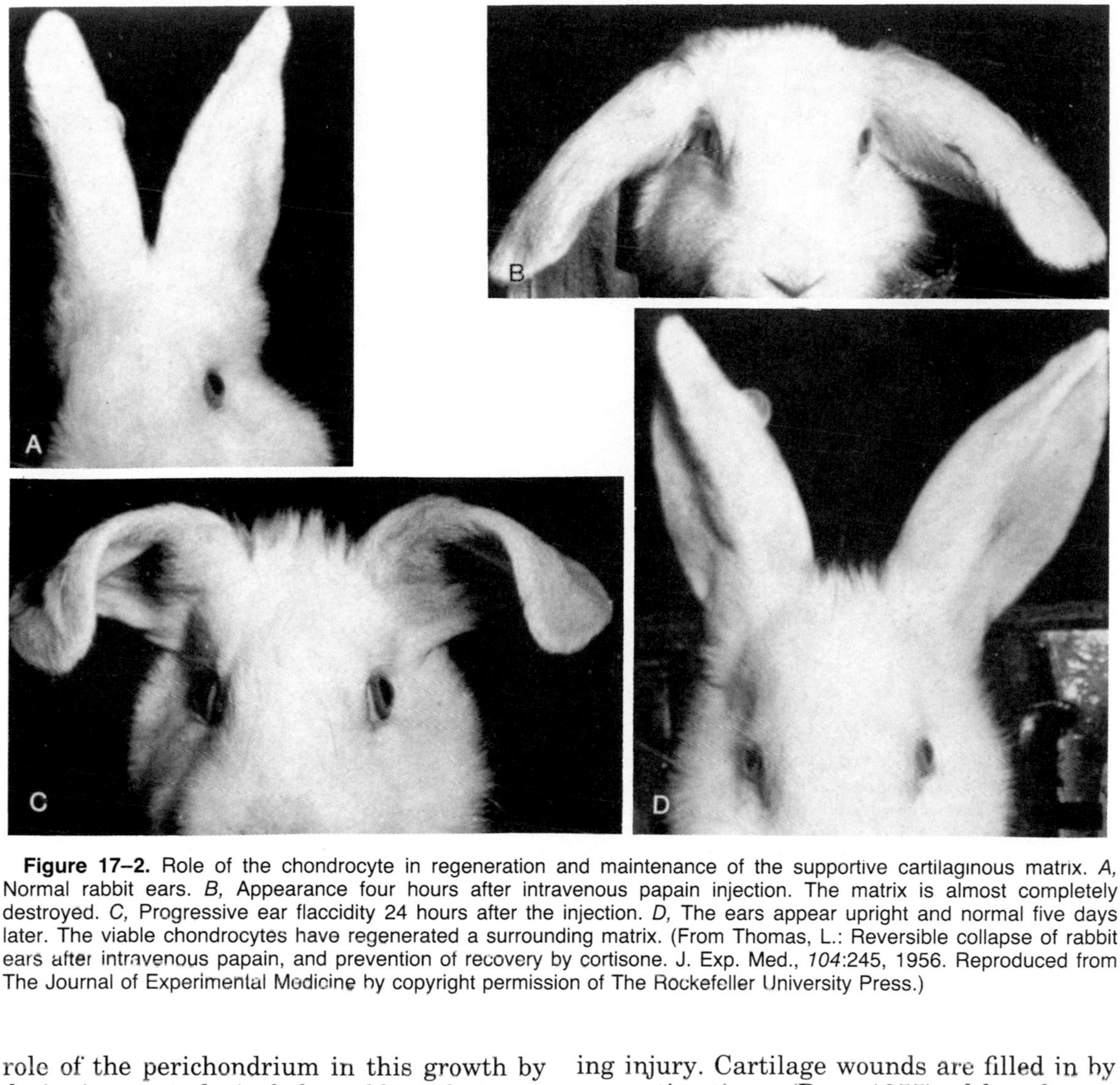

Figure 17–2. Role of the chondrocyte in regeneration and maintenance of the supportive cartilaginous matrix. *A,* Normal rabbit ears. *B,* Appearance four hours after intravenous papain injection. The matrix is almost completely destroyed. *C,* Progressive ear flaccidity 24 hours after the injection. *D,* The ears appear upright and normal five days later. The viable chondrocytes have regenerated a surrounding matrix. (From Thomas, L.: Reversible collapse of rabbit ears after intravenous papain, and prevention of recovery by cortisone. J. Exp. Med., *104*:245, 1956. Reproduced from The Journal of Experimental Medicine by copyright permission of The Rockefeller University Press.)

role of the perichondrium in this growth by designing a study in baby rabbits that contrasted perichondrial-covered cartilage grafts with perichondrial-stripped grafts (Fig. 17–3). He found that the perichondrial-covered grafts grew 77.5 per cent, whereas the stripped grafts grew an average of 42.6 per cent (Fig. 17–3*C*).

It is wise to include perichondrium on *any* cartilage graft to ensure its mechanical strength (Duncan, Thompson and Mancer, 1984) and to enhance its healing to surrounding tissues. Brent's study (1988) further suggested that one should always include perichondrium when grafting cartilage in young patients to ensure the production of new cartilage cells via appositional growth.

In adults, cartilage stops growing, and probably has less regenerative ability following injury. Cartilage wounds are filled in by connective tissue (Peer, 1955), although neochondrogenesis can occur from the undersurface of perichondrium that has been separated from its cartilage (Skoog, 1974a,b; Skoog, Ohlsén, and Sohn, 1972, 1975; Skoog and Johansson, 1976; Brent and Ott, 1978). As the cartilage ages, the proteoglycan content decreases, collagen content increases (Quintarelli, Ippolito and Roden, 1975), and it progressively calcifies (Hass, 1943; Brent, 1979b). Consequently, cartilage sculpting is difficult in an older patient (Fig. 17–4).

PHYSICAL PROPERTIES

Cartilage is composed of cells (chondrocytes), a surrounding chondromucoprotein

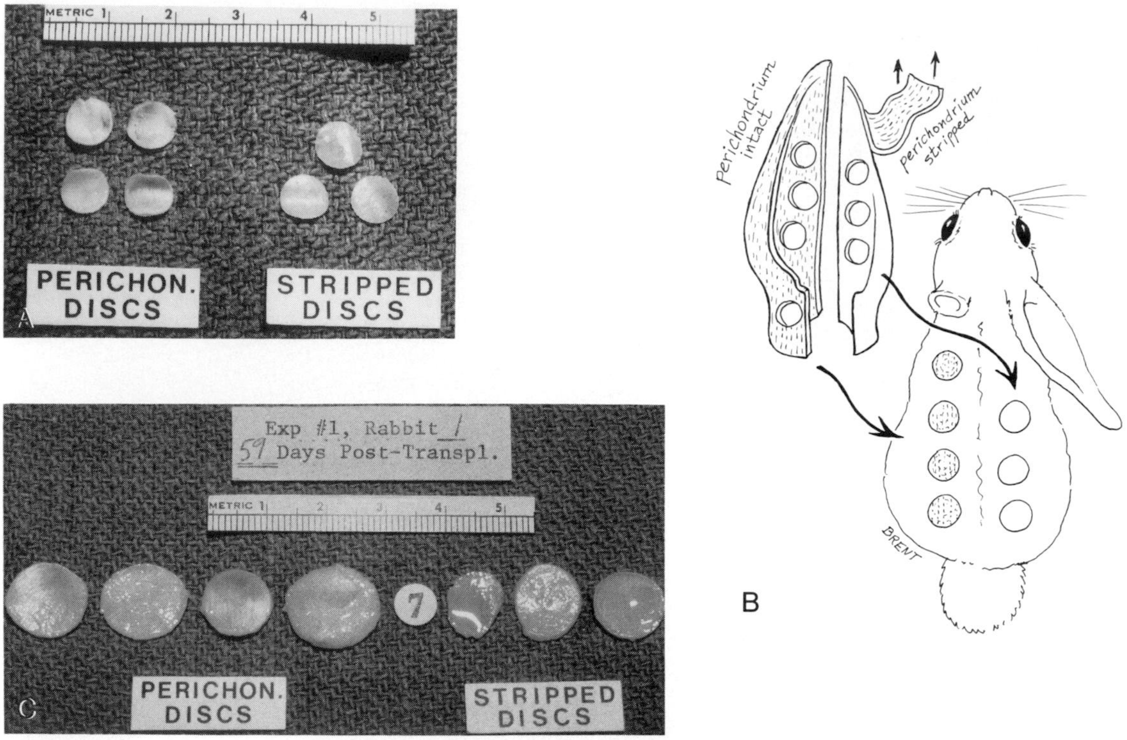

Figure 17–3. Contrasted growth potentials of perichondrial-covered and perichondrial-stripped autogenous cartilage grafts in the 3 week old rabbit. *A,* Preparing cartilage grafts for growth studies by cutting discs with a 7 mm dermal punch. The perichondrium is intact on the left discs, but stripped from those on the right. *B,* The comparative study. In each baby rabbit, an ear was amputated, skinned, and longitudinally divided and the perichondrium was stripped from one-half. Equal cartilage discs were cut with a dermal punch, the perichondrial-covered grafts being placed subcutaneously to the left of the midline, the stripped grafts to the right. When the normal contralateral ear doubled in size, the disc grafts were harvested and studied. *C,* Compared with the 7 mm paper disc, which represents the discs' original size when placed two months previously, the perichondrial-covered grafts had grown considerably larger than the denuded ones. The perichondrial-covered grafts are sturdy tissue buttons that grew an average of 77.5 per cent, whereas the denuded grafts are flimsy and friable and grew an average of 42.6 per cent. This study defines the role of chondrocytes and perichondrocytes in interstitial and appositional growth.

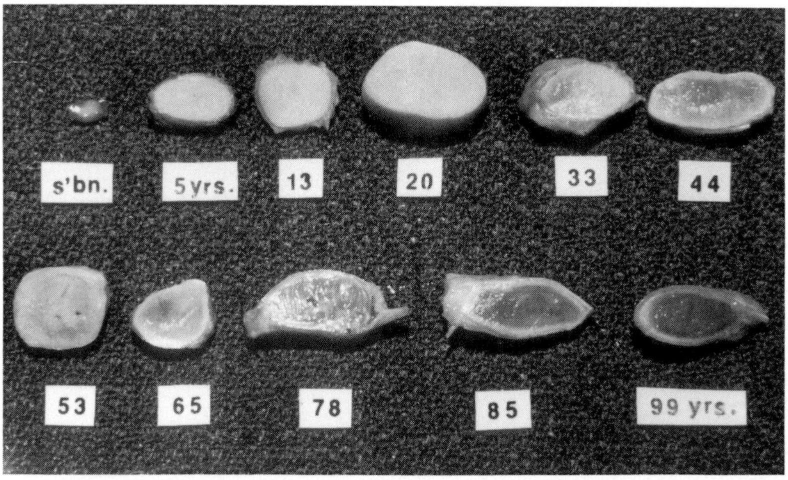

Figure 17–4. Rib cartilage calcification. Progressive ossification of the costal cartilage makes it more difficult to sculpt in the aging patient. The degree of medullary calcification is shown in rib cartilage cross sections obtained from cadavers ranging in age from stillborn infancy to 99 years. (From Brent, B.: The versatile cartilage autograft: current trends in clinical transplantation. Clin. Plast. Surg., *6*:163, 1979.)

ground substance, and a fibrous network (see Fig. 17–1). The type of fiber that weaves through the ground substance to create a supporting tissue determines the actual property of the matrix and the subsequent specific function of the cartilage. Hence, one can roughly categorize cartilage tissue as being either *hyaline, elastic*, or *fibrocartilage*, depending on the character of its matrix.

Hyaline cartilage covers the articular surface of bones; connects bony ribs to the sternum; and forms the skeletal substance of the larynx, trachea, bronchi, and nasal alae and septa. Each of the cartilages within this group has unique, specific functions. The rib cartilages act as springy bars that return the thoracic cage to neutral position between inspiratory and expiratory movements; articular cartilages provide frictionless joint movement; nasal cartilages are sufficiently flexible to control air intake yet provide support and contour; laryngeal cartilages control voice modulations; and tracheal and bronchial cartilages maintain airway patency (Gibson, 1965).

Elastic cartilages occur where flexible support is required, as in the external ear, the epiglottis, and portions of the larynx.

Fibrocartilage exists where firm support or tensile strength is required, as in intervertebral discs and in certain ligaments and tendon attachments to bone. In their unique role, the discs serve as brain- and viscera-protecting shock absorbers as well as spinal movement control mechanisms.

Certain chondrocytes are adapted for extremely specific functions, the most highly specialized being those within growing epiphyseal cartilage. As emphasized by Gibson (1965), not only do these precursors of bone precisely control the relative length of various bones, but they do so in a symmetric and synchronous fashion. One also finds specialized chondrocytes in the hyaline matrices of nasal septal and rib cartilages in which they secrete ground substance under varied pressures to produce a system of locked stresses within the cartilage (Gibson and Davis, 1958).

While a balanced stress system is necessary for the torsion spring function of rib cartilage, it plays havoc with the plastic surgeon who attempts to carve and shape a costal cartilage graft that ultimately twists and warps. Gillies (1920) proposed that the distortion occurred when perichondrium was retained on only one side of a carved strut. However, Gibson and Davis (1958) demonstrated that, in costal cartilage, the taut and compact outer subperichondrial cartilage layer regulates the tendency of the main, loose inner mass to expand and distort (Fig. 17–5). Thus, uneven removal of the peripheral cartilage results in undesirable warping. When carving a straight strut for nasal augmentation, therefore, one must respect the stresses and sculpt cartilage grafts with symmetrically distributed stresses (Figs. 17–6, 17–7).

In contrast, when carving an ear framework one can deliberately cause cartilage to warp by thinning the helical strut on the outer convex surface only (Brent, 1987a,d), thus producing the acute flexion necessary to simulate a helix (see Chap. 40).

In actual clinical practice, unfavorable cartilage warping is most striking in nasal reconstructions, where a carved strut has been placed beneath the relatively loose and mobile dorsal nasal skin. Warping is not a problem in ear reconstructions, perhaps because the sculpted cartilage framework is contained

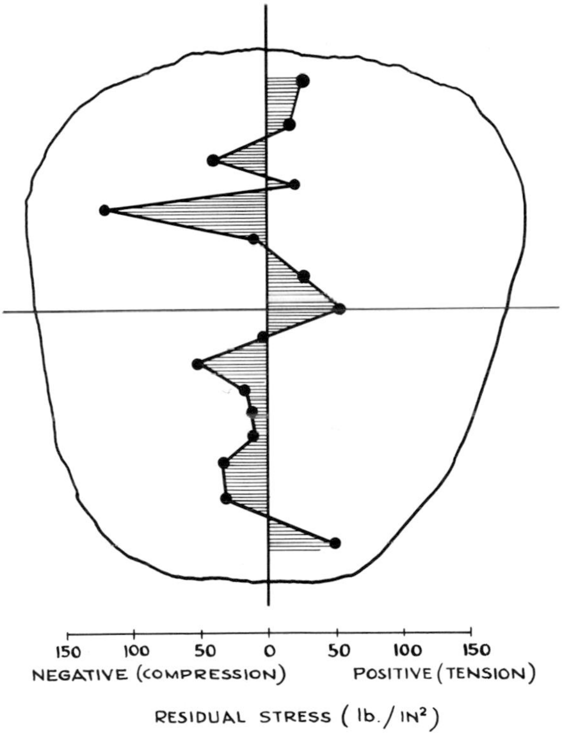

Figure 17–5. Engineering analysis of the alternating compression and tension stresses in a cartilaginous rib from a 50 year old male, shown graphically and superimposed on the cross sectional outline of the rib. (From Gibson, T.: Cartilage grafts. Br. Med. Bull., *21*:153, 1965.)

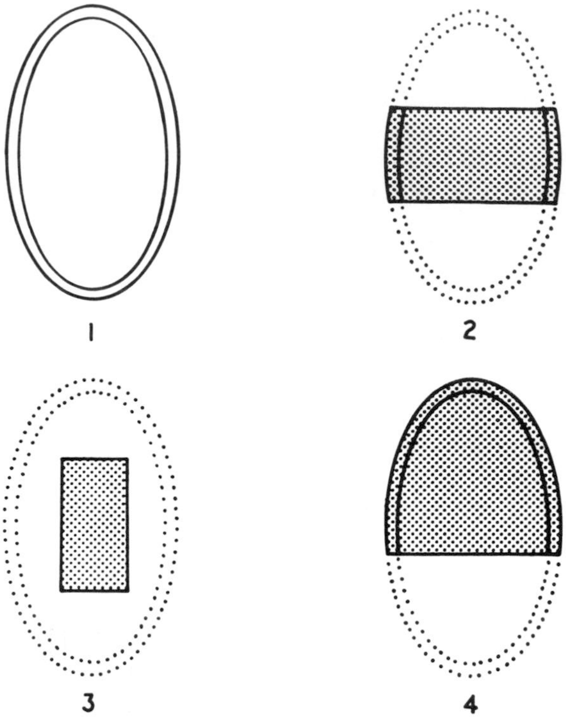

Figure 17–6. Four basic, balanced cross sections of rib cartilage (assuming a symmetric distribution of stresses). While this assumption does not always hold true, adherence to these configurations produces nonbending grafts in a high proportion of cases. (From Gibson, T., and Davis, W. B.: The distortion of autogenous grafts: its cause and prevention. Br. J. Plast. Surg., *10*:257, 1958.)

by a relatively tight and unyielding auricular skin pocket.

Cartilage warping in nasal reconstruction is compounded by the time it takes for maximal distoration to occur; a straight strut placed beneath the nasal skin may produce a pleasing *immediate* postoperative result, but it *later* twists and distorts.

Unaware of the interlocked cartilaginous stresses and carving methods to combat them, early plastic surgeons sought interesting solutions to deal with the time element in cartilage warping. Perhaps the most curious scheme was proposed by Mowlem (1938, 1941), who noted that, if a cartilage graft were going to warp, it would do so within three months after surgery. Frustrated by the development of distorted rib cartilage grafts in the nasal dorsum, Mowlem banked the carved graft in an abdominal pocket for three months, then removed it for examination. If the graft had not warped, he placed it in the nose. If it had warped, he recarved the graft before its insertion.

After Gibson and Davis had described the physiologic mechanism of rib cartilage warping and its prevention (1958), Abrahams and Duggan (1965) noted that carved cartilage fully distorts within 30 minutes. They suggested that one should allow this period of time to elapse before inserting the graft.

Having proposed that similar stresses exist in nasal septal cartilage, Fry (1966, 1967) demonstrated that septal cartilage grafts distort upon being disrupted by uneven, traumatic blows. He corrected septal warping by scoring the opposite, intact side with a scalpel, and concluded that this maneuver equalized the "breaching" of tensile stresses on both sides of the septum, bringing them into balance. Gorney (1987) utilized this principle to its maximal advantage when he straightened the cartilaginous septum (Fig. 17–8).

ANTIGENICITY

Because cartilage is reputed to be an "immunologically privileged" transplant tissue

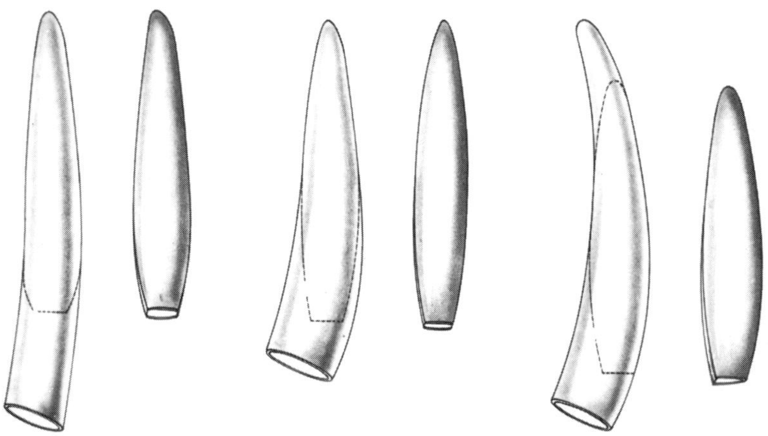

Figure 17–7. The tip of the eighth rib is a useful source of cartilage grafts to support the nasal bridge, since little trimming is usually required. Carving as shown maintains balanced cross sections. (From Gibson, T., and Davis, W. B.: The distortion of autogenous cartilage grafts: its cause and prevention. Br. J. Plast. Surg., *10*:257, 1958.)

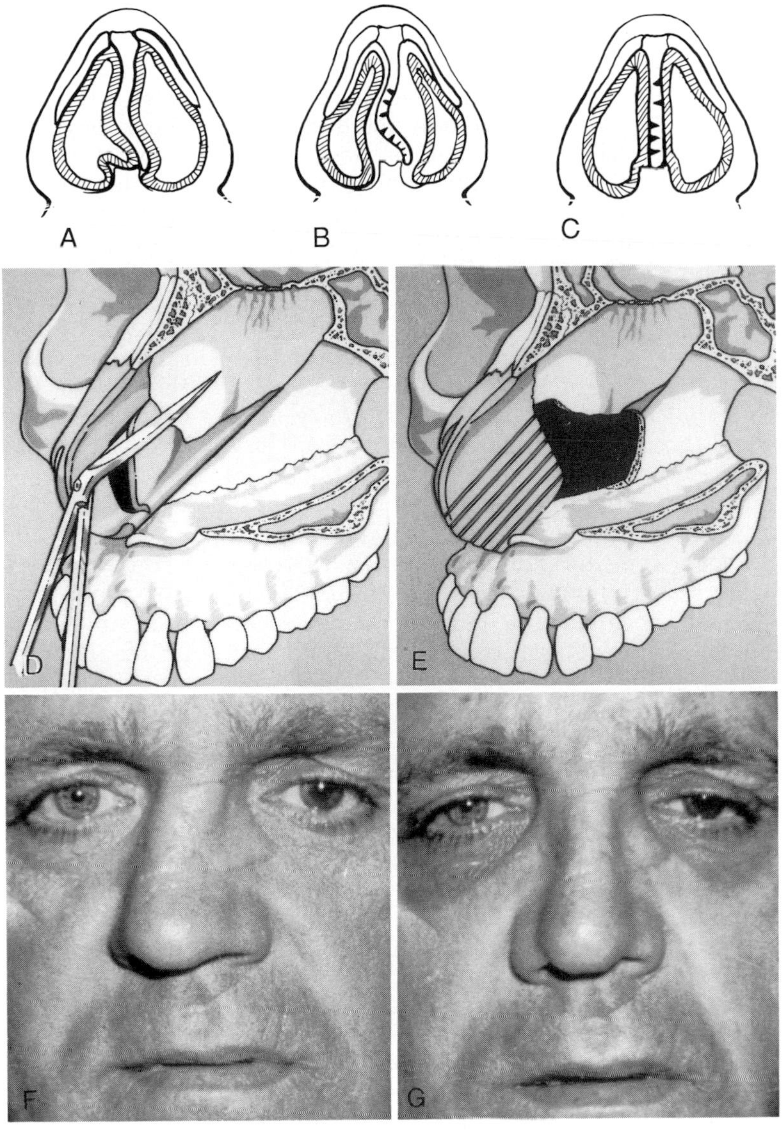

Figure 17–8. Repairing the deviated nasal septum by cartilage scoring to restore the balanced stress system (after Fry). *A,* Septal deviation. *B,* Partial-thickness incisions on the concave side only. *C, D, E,* As the incised regions bend toward opposite intact cartilaginous surfaces (combined with a submucous resection), the nasal deviation is corrected. *F,* A patient with severe post-traumatic nasal deviation. *G,* Correction by the method illustrated. (From Gorney, M.: Correction of the deviated nose. Clin. Plast. Surg., *8*:201, 1981.)

that is weakly (if at all) antigenic, it has been hypothesized that cartilage allografts fare nearly as well as autografts. This simply is not true. A careful study of the literature reveals that allograft enthusiasts have been misled by encouraging *early* results.

It is possible to find *portions* of allograft cartilage still viable at two years (Gibson, Davis, and Curran, 1958), but when proclaimed "successful" cartilage allografts are critically examined over a *long* period, the results are disappointing. Extensively studying a volume of living human rib cartilage, Hagerty and associates (1960a,b, 1967) elucidated the reality of long-term allografting. Before transplantation into recipient hosts, each cartilage allograft exhibited an initial cellular viability of 75 per cent, measured by radioactive sulfur uptake. After two years, the investigators harvested half of the grafts and found that viability had declined to 55 per cent. After six years, the same grafts, being gradually and progressively resorbed and involved in fibroinvasive host reactions, had a viability of only 15 per cent.

Review of the literature discloses additional evidence. In 1920, Gillies began using maternal ear cartilages to repair the ears of microtic children. He performed 37 such transplants during the next two decades. In 1960, Gibson and Davis enthusiastically reported living chondrocytes in *one* of Gillies' microtic patients, although they did not describe the gross condition of the reconstructed ear. However, Converse painted the true picture in 1977 when he evaluated 21 of Gillies' original 37 patients. Converse noted that cartilage persisted in only one patient; in the other 20, the maternal auricular transplants underwent shrinkage and resorption. Converse attributed the one surviving allograft, as well as that noted by Gibson and Davis, to a close tissue-typing match between mother and child.

In 1984, Krutchinskij and Schved reported the completion of 13 similar living allograft maternal ear reconstructions. *Initially*, they found the results satisfactory, but after three to five years they noted the beginning of shrinkage and effacement of ear details. Microscopic examination revealed degenerative changes and the allotransplanted cartilage being replaced with connective tissue.

From these careful documentations of allograft failure, one must conclude that cartilage is not a "privileged" transplant tissue. Instead, the host's immune response is merely retarded by the chondrocytes being protected both by the presence of a thick surrounding matrix, and by the absence of vascular channels that normally provide easy access for attacking host cells. However, as a river bank yields to persistent erosive forces of the river's adjacent current, transplanted allograft cartilage eventually yields to the immune response system of its host.

As to cartilage being "weakly antigenic," this should not be attributed solely to the protective surrounding matrix, but also to the sparse cell population of cartilage, which produces a low dose of antigen. Indeed, there is sufficient laboratory evidence to show that the chondrocytes themselves evoke an immune response. Both Craigmyle (1958a,b, 1960) and Heyner (1973) used chondrocytes removed from their surrounding matrix to sensitize laboratory animals. After a suitable waiting period, they challenged the recipient animals with skin grafts from the cartilage donors to elicit an accelerated reaction similar to that observed in a second set graft rejection phenomenon.

By isolating chondrocytes through enzymatic degradation of the matrix, Moskalewski, Kawiak, and Rymaszewska (1966) designed a unique study of cartilage antigenicity. They injected the "exposed" chondrocytes into the muscles of recipient host animals and compared the ensuing cellular reaction with that evoked by implanting whole cartilage fragments into the same muscles. After 28 days, the isolated allogenic chondrocyte clusters exhibited massive leukocytic cell infiltrates, whereas the intact cartilage fragments demonstrated negligible reactions.

All these studies suggest that grafted cartilage does evoke transplantation antigens, and that the rejection response is merely delayed by the physical barrier that the matrix interposes between the chondrocytes and the cells of the immune surveillance system of the recipient host.

BANKING AND PRESERVATION

Before the discouraging reports of the resorption of living homologous cartilage, many profitable studies resulted from the search for an ideal condition in which to "bank" living cartilage for ready use. These investigations provided much useful information about cartilage.

Chondrocytes are known to survive somatic death for at least 48 hours. Hence, Curran and Gibson (1956) obtained and banked fresh cadaver cartilage under various conditions: they found by ^{35}S uptake studies that storage at 39°C resulted in a short survival, and that freezing resulted in cellular death, but that storage in Tyrode's solution at 4°C maintained cartilage in a living state for as long as six weeks. Their conclusive proof of banked cartilage viability was likewise confirmed by Hagerty and associates (1960b), who further deduced that cartilage survival was more successful when stored in sterile containers and moist air at 3° to 5°C. Gibson (1972) subsequently endorsed moist air as the preferred storage medium. Hagerty and associates found an average cellular viability of approximately 95 per cent in cartilage stored under the above conditions for one week, and a viability of 80 per cent after one month's storage; this declined to less than 20 per cent after six to eight weeks.

In an additional study, Krüger (1964) noted that by supravital staining of the chondrocytes there were no perceptible changes in cartilage grafts stored for two weeks in Ringer's solution or in air at 3°C. During the two weeks, Krüger transplanted a number of the grafts into human recipients; upon removal, each graft demonstrated viability by supravital staining.

The evidence extracted from the above studies strongly suggests that cartilage removed from an individual should exhibit no difference in survival rate whether used immediately as an autogenous graft, or used autogenously after sterile banking in moist air at 3° to 5°C for periods of one or two days. To obtain further support for the above findings, Brent (1974) conducted an investigation using both rabbits and humans, in which equal portions of autogenous cartilage were transplanted both as immediate controls and following periods of refrigeration for 24 hours, 48 hours, 72 hours, and seven days. The results supported the aforementioned supposition.

Because sculpting an ear framework from costal cartilage initially took the author considerable time, he undertook this study to justify dividing the operation into two separate phases. He harvested the rib cartilage, awakened the patient, and sent him to the recovery room. The framework was leisurely carved, banked in the refrigerator overnight, and implanted under local anesthesia the following day. Since the entire operation (rib harvest, framework fabrication, and insertion beneath the periauricular skin) currently takes the author less than four hours, he no longer performs this two-stage procedure.

Before silicone rubber implants, a great deal of interest arose in developing an inert implant by killing and preserving cartilage from human cadavers, cattle, and other mammals. As one would expect, xenograft (bovine) cartilage undergoes progressive resorption (Gibson and Davis, 1953), and preserved allograft cartilage usually fares no better. When examined critically, enthusiastic reports of "success" usually reflect inadequate follow-up, the writer's evaluation often being conceived by "somewhat of a guess" or a "biased opinion clouded by the surgeons' desires for their patients to do well" (Donald and Col, 1982).

The best visual documentation of preserved allograft failure came from Steffensen (1952, 1955), who reconstructed auricles with detailed frameworks carved from preserved rib cartilage. Not content with merely showing his initial good results in 1952, he conscientiously published follow-up photographs of the same patients three years later. All the auricles had begun to shrink and lose detail (Steffensen, 1955).

In 1959, Rasi conducted the longest and largest follow-up study on 59 Merthiolate-preserved allografts that had been carried out almost two decades earlier by Straith and Slaughter (1941). He reported that more than 60 per cent were substantially reduced in bulk, and that the rest were progressively resorbing.

A unique exception to the usual fate of an allograft was reported by Mühlbauer, Schmidt-Tintemann, and Glaser in 1971, when they employed Merthiolate-preserved allograft rib cartilage to correct saddle nose deformities. Unexpectedly, a number of grafts in this series calcified to persist and produce satisfactory long-term results. This phenomenon approximates the normal aging of living cartilage in which the matrix becomes calcified and the chondrocytes die as they are buried in an impermeable mineral tomb.

Similar changes are seen in cartilage that has been irradiated in preparation for implantation (Dingman and Grabb, 1961; Agris, 1976). In the irradiated cell, a considerable quantity of calcium crystal is seen along the cell surface. As radiation is increased to 3 million rep., the free ribosomes gradually disappear and an increased density of calcium deposits is seen along the lacunae that formerly housed the chondrocytes. In some cells, dense bodies and calcium crystals appear in the former region of the nucleus. Eventually all that remains is a lattice framework of mineral matrix totally lacking all cellular structures. Although this creates the seemingly ideal, inert, implantable material, it is brittle, undependable, and still susceptible to resorption.

When the author questioned Grabb and Dingman on separate occasions in the 1970's, both concurred that irradiated cartilage was a "reasonable alternative" for onlay grafts, from which one could expect "varying degrees of resorption." They both felt it was an unpromising medium for repairs requiring fine detail such as ear reconstruction. In this context, irradiated cartilage is perhaps a "reasonable alternative" when one augments the chin or cheeks and wishes to avoid silicone implants, or when patients refuse an additional operation and scar. Such patients should be frankly warned that their correction will suffer a loss of bulk as time passes.

AUTOGENOUS CARTILAGE GRAFTING

Of all buried autogenous grafts, plastic surgeons most commonly use cartilage. Like corneal or epidermal tissue, cartilage has no blood vessels and receives its nourishment via tissue fluid diffusion. This property allows the cartilage autograft to acclimatize itself to almost any tissue environment, since the chondrocytes survive as living cells that continue to service and maintain their surrounding matrix.

Once transferred as a free graft, autogenous cartilage undergoes no metaplastic changes. Hyaline matrix remains hyaline; thus, rib cartilage remains firm upon being fashioned into an ear and transferred to the auricular region. Ear cartilage retains its unique elastic properties upon transfer as a graft to a myriad of heterotopic sites.

Although even the meniscal cartilage of the knee has been used for a cartilage autograft (Mir y Mir, 1952), the rib, nasal septum, and ear represent the customary donor sources.

Auricular Cartilage Grafts

Because of its unique characteristics, the auricular cartilage graft is not only an ideal transfer tissue but perhaps the most versatile of all cartilage grafts. Auricular cartilage can be obtained easily under local anesthesia, and a significant portion of the concha can be removed without donor deformity (Adams, 1955; Gorney, Murphy, and Falces, 1971; Brent, 1979b) (Fig. 17–9).

Furthermore, auricular cartilage can easily be fashioned and contoured into various shapes for a variety of uses (Peer, 1944; Stark and Frileck, 1969; Brent, 1979b) (Fig. 17–10). It is an indispensable aid in secondary rhinoplasty (Falces and Gorney, 1972; Sheen, 1987a), and has been employed as a framework for total ear reconstruction (Davis, 1972; Gorney, 1974). When auricular cartilage is incorporated into a composite graft,

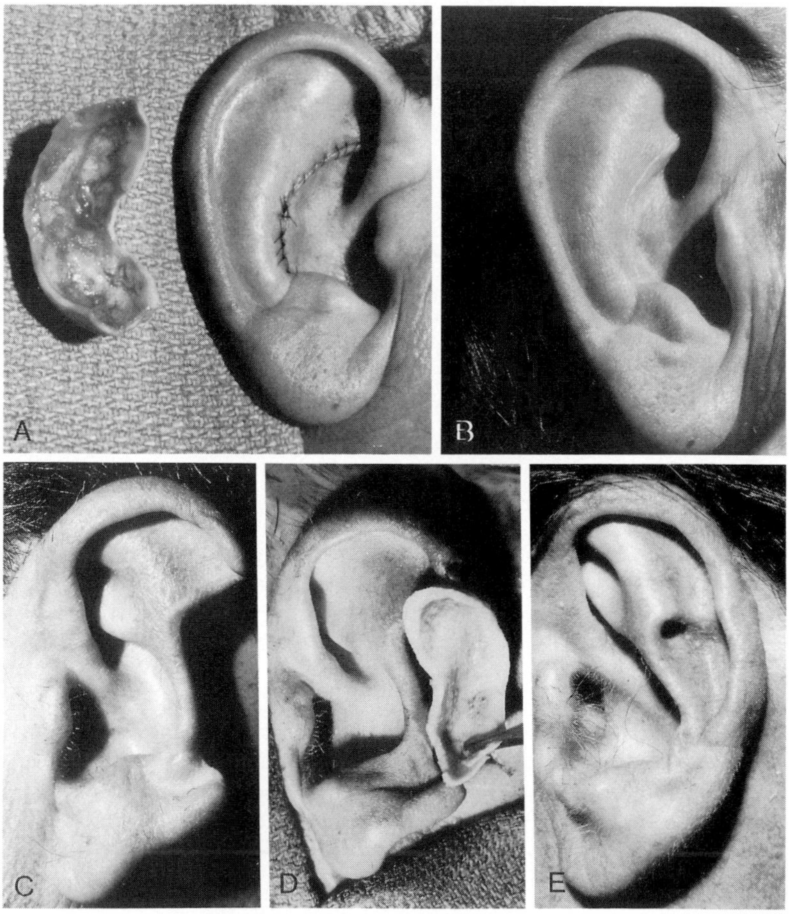

Figure 17–9. Repair of partial ear deformity with autogenous conchal cartilage graft. *A,* Donor conchal cartilage is excised through an "anteromedial approach." *B,* Healed donor ear. Note the almost imperceptible scar. *C,* Middle-third postsurgical auricular defect. *D,* Conchal cartilage graft from the contralateral ear. *E,* Result obtained by the "tunnel procedure" of Converse (see Chap. 40). Secondary procedures will be necessary to release the ear and improve helical contour. (From Brent, B.: The acquired auricular deformity: a systematic approach to its analysis and reconstruction. Plast. Reconstr. Surg., *59*:475, 1977.)

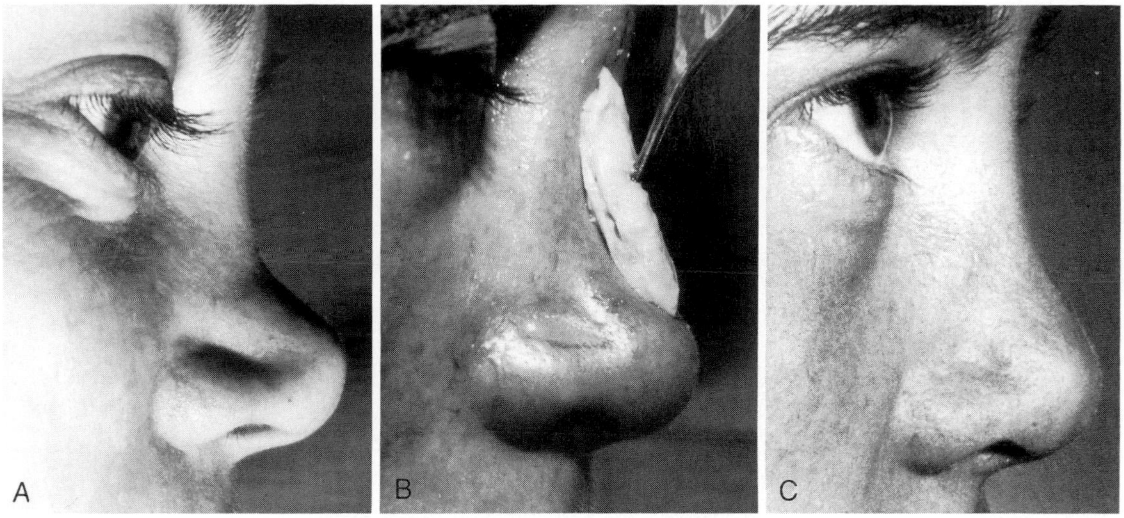

Figure 17–10. Auricular cartilage employed as a laminated contour graft. *A,* Post-traumatic saddle nose deformity. A previous submucous resection eliminated the septum as a possible cartilage graft source. *B,* A laminated auricular cartilage graft was fabricated from a bilateral conchal cartilage excision. *C,* Final result. (From Brent, B.: The versatile cartilage autograft: current trends in clinical transplantation. Clin. Plast. Surg., *6*:163, 1979.)

the author has successfully employed it in patients as old as 82 (Fig. 17–11). Small pieces are useful in middle ear surgery (Duncan, 1962; Brockman, 1965); when shaped into a ring, auricular cartilage can be used to maintain fallopian tube patency (Barsky and Blinick, 1953).

Most significantly, auricular cartilage not only survives as a successful heterotopic autograft in an unlimited variety of transplant conditions, but seems immune to resorption (Gorney, 1974–1987; Sheen, 1978–1987; Brent, 1987b).

The author has employed conchal cartilage as single-layered grafts in auricular, nasal, tarsal, and nipple reconstructions (see Figs. 17–9, 17–12); as laminated grafts to correct such defects as saddle nose deformity (see Fig. 17–10) and inverted nipples (Brent and Bostwick, 1977); and as tiny dices beneath skin grafts to simulate Montgomery glands (Brent, 1979a) (Fig. 17–13). The long-term survival of grafted auricular cartilage in such diversified situations attests to its versatility and dependability as a donor tissue.

Nasal Cartilage Grafts

Although not available in large quantities, nasal cartilage is nonetheless a valuable donor source. This cartilage has been employed as a composite chondromucosal graft to restore support and lining for eyelid reconstruction. While Millard (1962) and Mustardé (1969) obtained tissue for chondromucosal grafts from the nasal septum, Tessier (1976) used upper lateral nasal cartilage for the same purpose. Tessier's chondromucosal graft seemingly provides more appropriate contour incorporated with a more delicate, tarsal-like cartilage, but its removal runs the risk of shortening the nose.

Septal cartilage, readily obtained by submucous resection, is an invaluable repair material for secondary rhinoplasty (Fig. 17–14) (Peer, 1948; Sheen, 1975, 1987a). As in resecting distorted septal cartilage to relieve obstruction during a septorhinoplasty, secondary deformity must be circumvented by careful harvesting of septal cartilage. To avoid nasal collapse, it is essential to preserve an L-shaped septal strut for adequate nasal support (see Fig. 17–8*E*). Sheen has employed over 4000 septal cartilage grafts as individual struts, layered transplants, and crushed "fill" (see Chap. 36). His experience and results have been impressive, and resorption appears to be almost nonexistent (Sheen, 1975, 1987b; Brent, 1987b).

Rib Cartilage Grafts

Costal cartilage grafts serve best when a large quantity of living, grafted tissue is

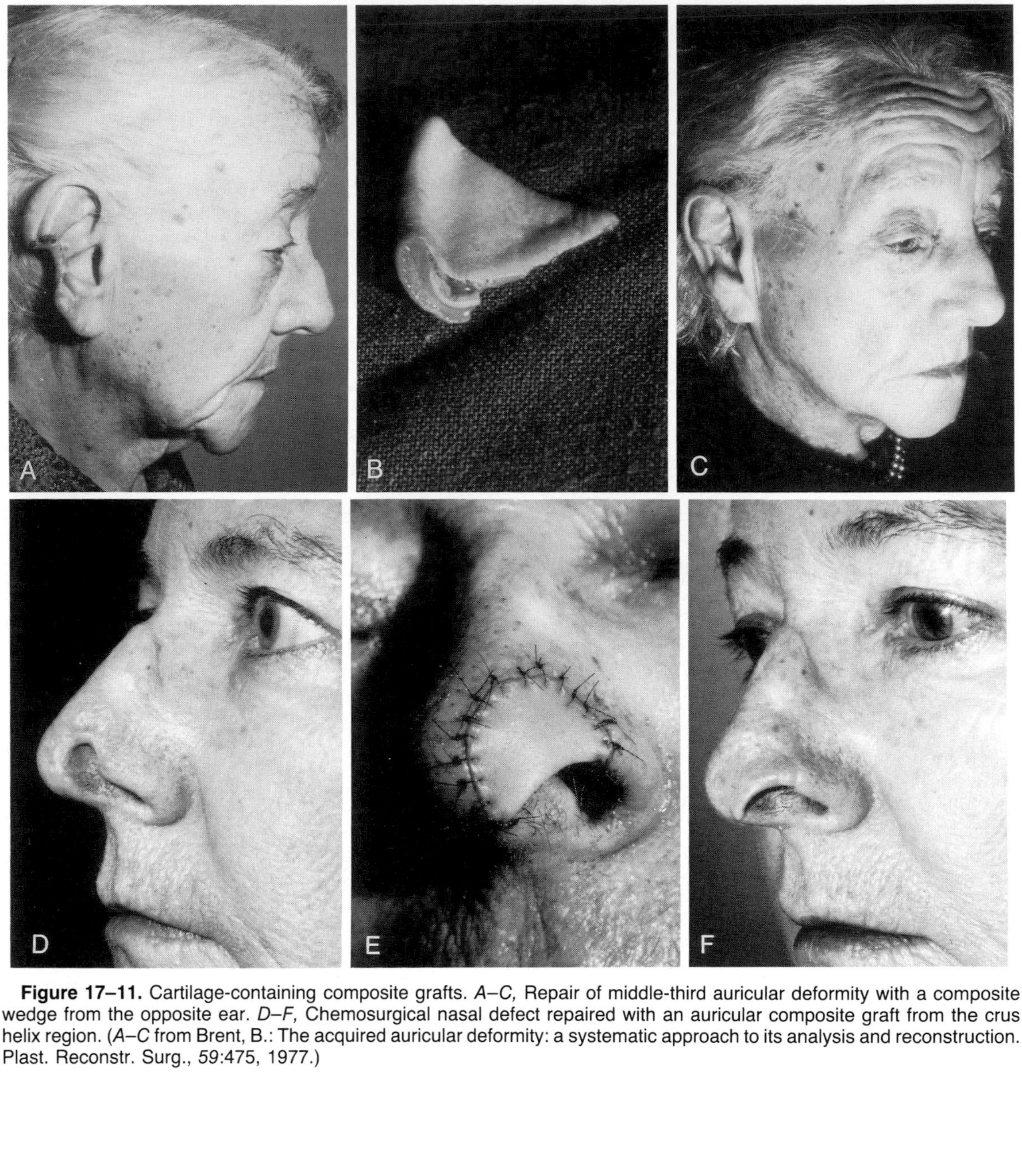

Figure 17–11. Cartilage-containing composite grafts. *A–C,* Repair of middle-third auricular deformity with a composite wedge from the opposite ear. *D–F,* Chemosurgical nasal defect repaired with an auricular composite graft from the crus helix region. (*A–C* from Brent, B.: The acquired auricular deformity: a systematic approach to its analysis and reconstruction. Plast. Reconstr. Surg., *59*:475, 1977.)

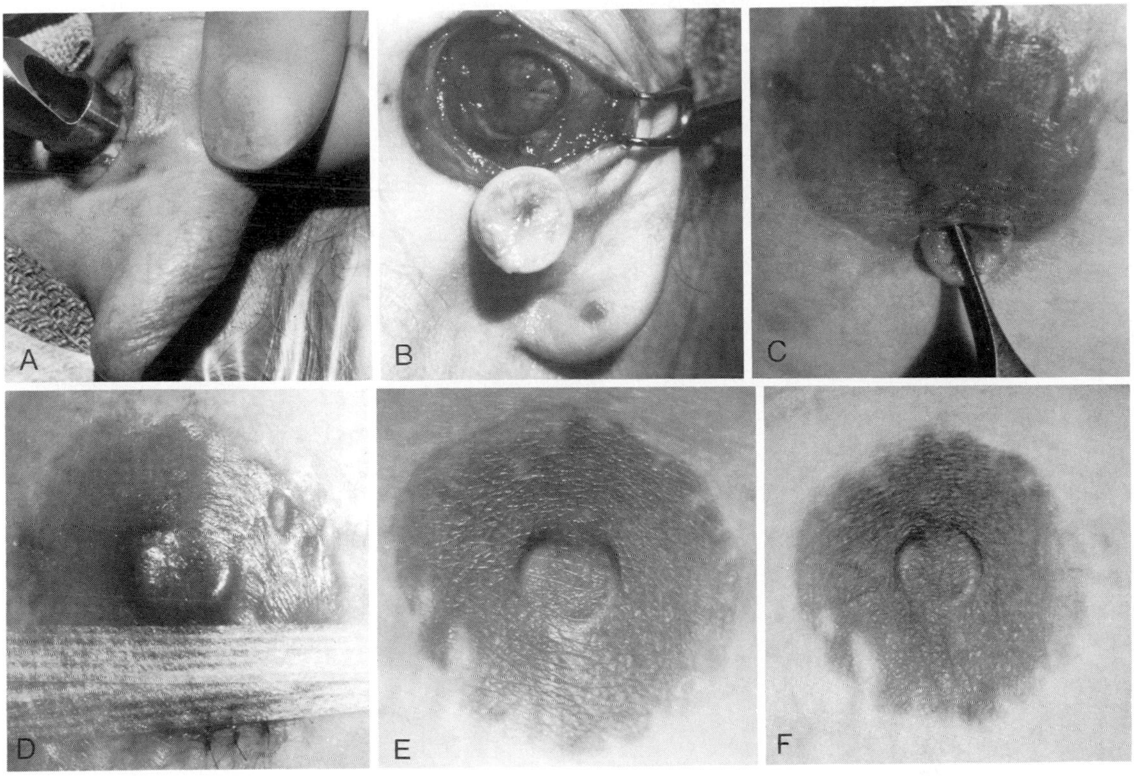

Figure 17–12. Nipple reconstruction with an auricular cartilage disc. *A, B,* Removal of a 10 mm disc from the concha with a dermal punch. *C, D,* Insertion of the disc beneath the previous areolar graft. *E,* Result at nine months. *F,* Unchanged appearance at five years. Although the author does not use the technique today, the long-term result demonstrates the unequaled reliability of autogenous cartilage grafts. (From Brent, B., and Bostwick, J., III: Nipple-areola reconstruction with auricular tissues. Plast. Reconstr. Surg., *60*:353, 1977.)

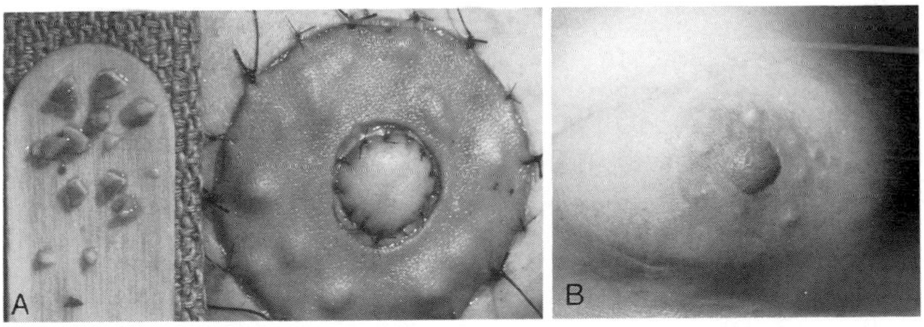

Figure 17–13. Simulating Montgomery glands with diced autogenous auricular cartilage. *A,* Diced ear cartilage inserted randomly under an areolar skin graft. *B,* Appearance of the reconstructed breast and nipple-areola complex four years postoperatively. The long-term survival of grafted autogenous cartilage under such adverse conditions attests to its versatility and dependability. (From Brent, B.: Nipple-areola reconstruction following mastectomy: mimicry with assorted tissue grafts and tattoo pigments. *In* Brent, B. (Ed.): The Artistry of Reconstructive Surgery. St. Louis, C. V. Mosby Company, 1987, pp. 933–946.)

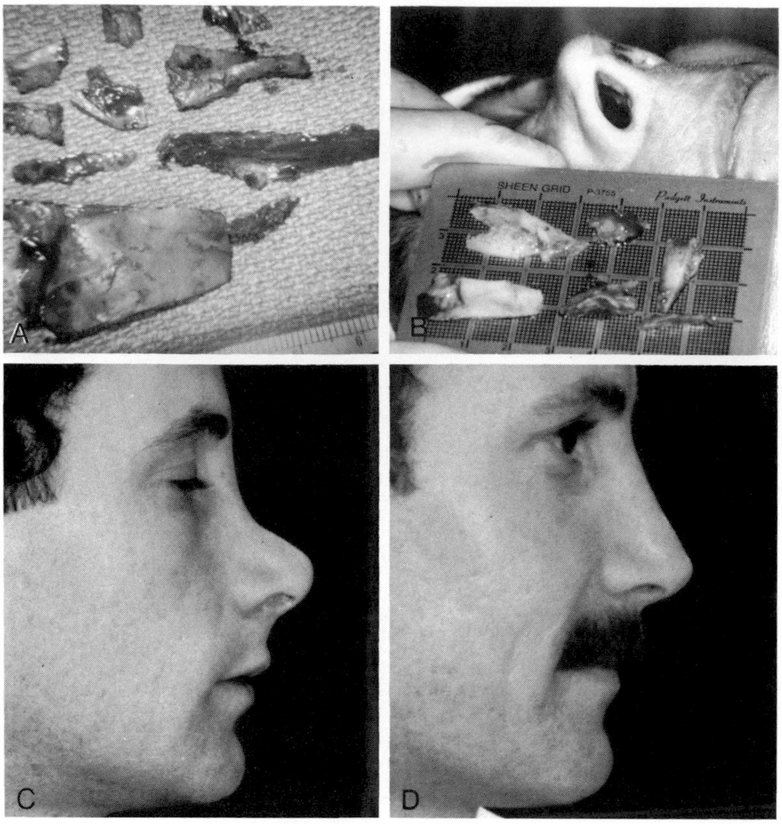

Figure 17–14. Autogenous septal cartilage grafts in nasal repair. *A,* Note the large quantity and sizes of grafts available from the nasal septum. *B,* The harvested cartilage fashioned into grafts. *C,* Postsurgical saddle nose depression. *D,* Repair achieved with autogenous septal cartilage grafts (eight years postoperatively). (Courtesy of Dr. Jack H. Sheen.)

required. Indifferent to functional stress for its survival, autogenous rib cartilage can be contoured into any desired shape and it retains form and bulk if basic surgical principles are followed.

Although a sizable operation is required to harvest this tissue (Fig. 17–15), and progressive calcification renders it difficult to sculpt in the older patient (see Fig. 17–4), a variety of applications make rib cartilage an invaluable medium for the plastic surgeon.

Costal cartilage can be included on the terminus of an osseous rib graft to reconstruct the mandibular ramus and temporomandibular joint (Gillies and Millard, 1957; Bromberg, Song, and Craig, 1972), or it can be used in bulk form to obliterate major contour deformities (see Fig. 17–18) (Young, 1944; Peer, 1955). It has long been employed as an onlay graft to provide malar or mandibular contour (Dupertuis, 1950) in cases in which bone grafts predictably would suffer resorption. Rib cartilage grafts have long been used to provide nasal support and to correct major saddle nose deformities. The grafts must be fashioned to comply with Gibson's principles of balanced cross sectional carving. Like septal cartilage (Fry, 1966, 1967), built-in stresses within rib cartilage necessitate a careful sculpting technique so that the sur-

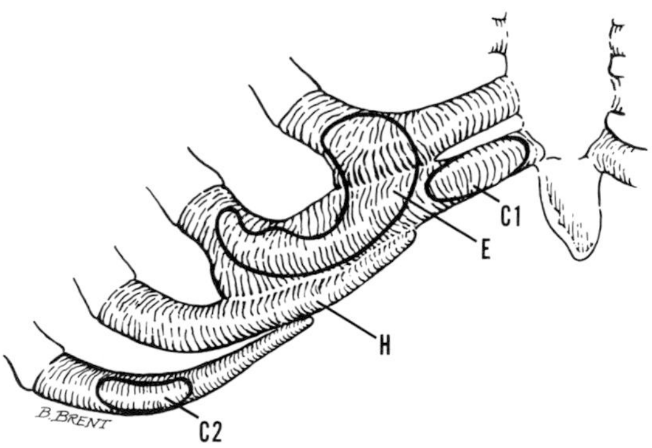

Figure 17–15. Donor site for costal cartilage grafts in auricular framework and chin graft construction. E = ear base block; H = helix; C1 = chin graft, first layer; C2 = chin graft, second layer. (From Brent, B.: Chin contouring with a laminated cartilage graft. *In* Brent, B. (Ed.): The Artistry of Reconstructive Surgery. St. Louis, C. V. Mosby Company, 1987, p. 597.)

geon is not confronted with undesirable warping (Mowlem, 1938; Gibson and Davis, 1958).

Total reconstruction of the ear (see Chap. 40) has been most consistently successful when accomplished with a framework of autogenous rib cartilage (Tanzer, 1959, 1971; Fukuda and Yamada, 1978; Brent, 1974, 1980, 1987a) (Fig. 17–16). Autogenous cartilage grafts are also helpful in contour restorations (Figs. 17–17, 17–18).

AUTOGENOUS PERICHONDRIAL GRAFTING

A unique aspect of cartilage grafting is the transfer of free perichondrial tissue to generate *new* cartilage at the recipient site. In 1959, Lester first documented the production of neocartilage by perichondrium separated from its underlying cartilage, although it seems that its clinical potential went unrecognized at that time. In a series of surgical corrections of pectus excavatum, Lester noted recurrence of the deformity in two patients who had undergone subperichondrial resections of costal cartilage. Repeat surgery in these patients revealed cartilaginous regeneration. Histologic examination demonstrated distinct demarcation at the resection site, a finding that implied that the cartilage probably regenerated from the perichondrium.

More than a decade later, Skoog and associates (Skoog, Ohlsén, and Sohn, 1972, 1975; Skoog, 1974a,b) investigated the pathogenesis of "cauliflower ear" and demonstrated that the source of cartilage overproduction was the undersurface of the displaced perichondrium. Formation of a "cauliflower ear" begins when the perichondrium is traumatically elevated by a hematoma. Skoog, Ohlsén, and Sohn (1972, 1975) demonstrated that neocartilage from the displaced perichondrium invaded the hematomatous substrate, and deduced that chondrogenesis resulted from the perichondrium's loss of "contact inhibition" with the underlying cartilage (Ohlsén, Skoog, and Sohn, 1975). These findings stimulated the authors to investigate intensely the chondrogenic potential of the perichondrium as a free graft, specifically for trachea (Sohn and Ohlsén, 1974) and joint reconstruction (Engkvist and associates, 1975; Skoog and Johansson, 1976).

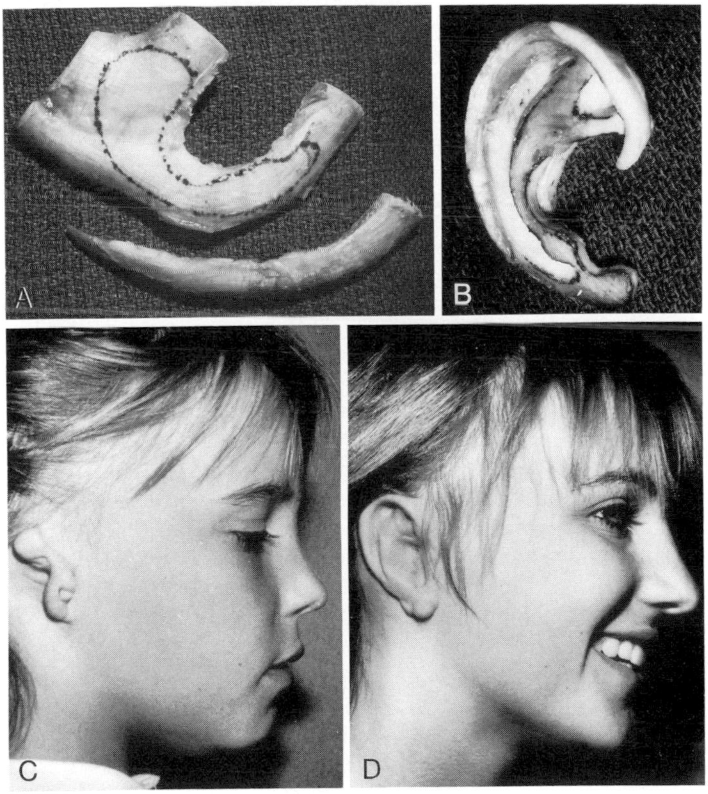

Figure 17–16. Total ear reconstruction with a sculpted graft of autogenous rib cartilage. *A,* Excised costal cartilage grafts serve as a sculpting medium. *B,* Completed framework. *C,* A child with a variation of microtia. *D,* Result achieved with autogenous rib cartilage graft (six years postoperatively).

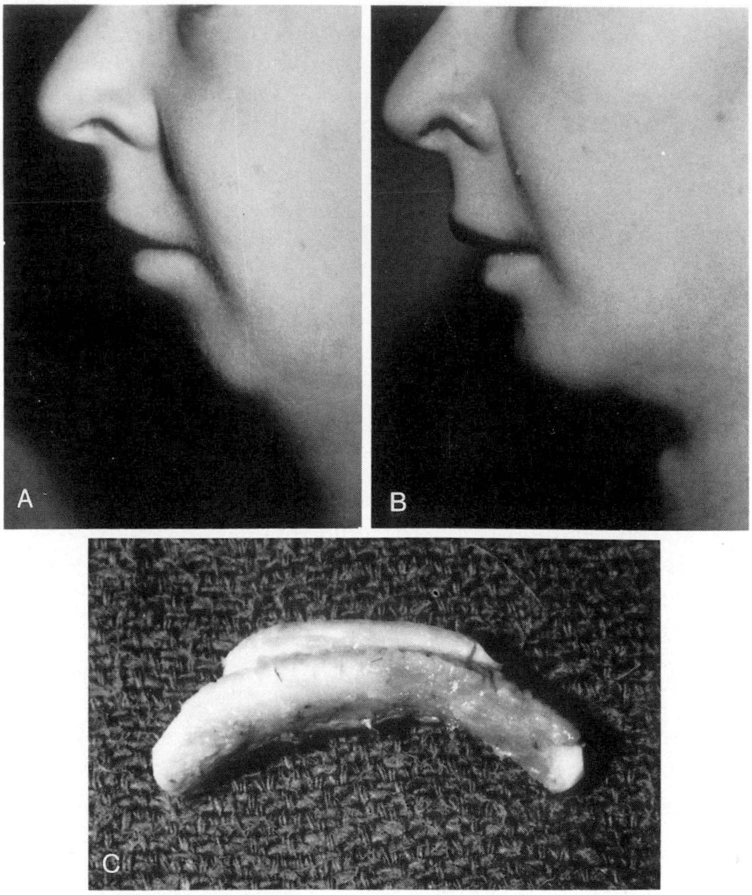

Figure 17–17. A chin augmentation with autogenous rib cartilage graft. *A,* A Treacher Collins patient with microgenia. *B,* Result achieved with laminated costal cartilage. *C,* The two-layered graft fashioned from the patient's rib cartilage (see Fig. 17–15). The intact perichondrium on the graft's concave surface facilitates its adherence to the bony chin surface and provides the graft with growth potential. (From Brent, B.: Chin contouring with a laminated cartilage graft. *In* Brent, B. (Ed.): The Artistry of Reconstructive Surgery. St. Louis, C. V. Mosby Company, 1987, p. 597.)

Perichondrial Grafts for Joint Repair

Although perichondrial grafts occasionally have been used for support in ear reconstruction (Brent, 1977; Ohlsén, 1978), they have been most useful in repairing damaged joint surfaces. Neochondrogenic activity apparently exists over a wide age spectrum, but the cartilage yield from any type of perichondrial graft seems likely to be influenced by age. Skoog and Johansson (1976) reported an excellent result in repairing the traumatically ankylosed metacarpophalangeal joint in a young individual, although they experienced somewhat disappointing results in several older patients. It would seem that this is related to the well-known physiologic changes that occur in aging rib cartilage (Hass, 1943; Brent, 1979b), or to a decreased neochondrogenic potential in the older individual. Both the laboratory findings and the clinical experience of the author coincide with those of other investigators in suggesting that perichondrial arthroplasty be restricted to the young patient free from degenerative disease (Brent and Ott, 1978; Engkvist and Johansson, 1980; Upton, Sohn, and Glowacki, 1981).

When surgeons first used perichondrium in joint reconstruction, they restricted the donor site to ribs. Although Skoog (1974a) employed auricular perichondrial flaps in an otoplastic technique to form the antihelix, he avoided

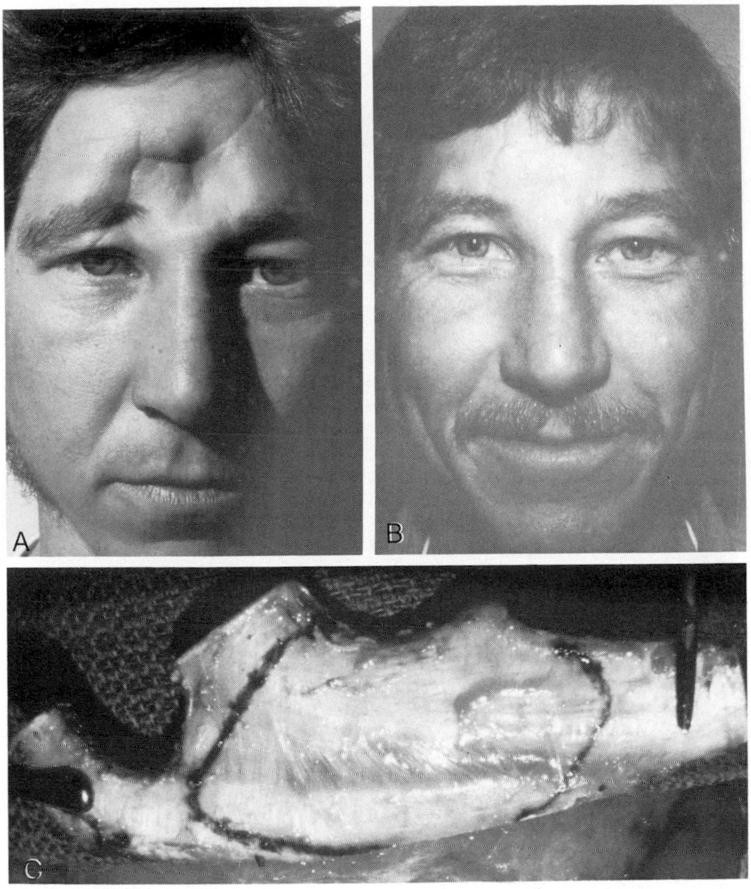

Figure 17–18. Contour restoration with an autogenous rib cartilage graft. *A*, Post-traumatic forehead deformity. *B*, Result achieved with autogenous rib cartilage graft. *C*, The rib graft. A block of cartilage was used to fill the defect, and a "floating" rib cartilage was employed to restore the right supraorbital rim. (From Brent, B.: The versatile cartilage autograft: current trends in clinical transplantation. Clin. Plast. Surg., *6*:163, 1979.)

using this tissue as a free graft for his phalangeal joint reconstructions. For this purpose, he consistently used rib perichondrium (Skoog and Johansson, 1976). Likewise, Tajima, Aoyagi, and Maruyama (1978) employed perichondrial grafts harvested from rib cartilage for the correction of temporomandibular joint ankylosis. Using an auricular perichondrial graft to correct an ankylosed temporomandibular joint in a young patient (Fig. 17–19), Brent (1979b, 1987c) found that substantial perichondrial grafts can be obtained with great care from the posteromedial auricular surface. Thus, a large operation associated with significant patient discomfort can be avoided. If necessary, one can use both ears as donor sites to obtain sufficient perichondrial grafts to line both joint surfaces.

In both laboratory and clinical situations, most investigators have routinely placed perichondrial grafts with their chondrogenic "active surface" facing toward the joint space (Engkvist and Johansson, 1980; Tajima, Aoyagi, and Maruyama, 1978; Upton, Sohn, and Glowacki, 1981). Although the most advantageous position to place the grafts within a joint has not been established conclusively, a pilot study by Kulick, Brent, and Ross (1984) suggested that the histologic appearance or thickness of the generated neocartilage is uninfluenced by graft orientation. This controversial point is provocative, for even though one finds the optimal manner of restoring the cartilage of a defective joint surface to be perichondrial grafting, the unique articular surface of a *normal* joint contains no perichondrium!

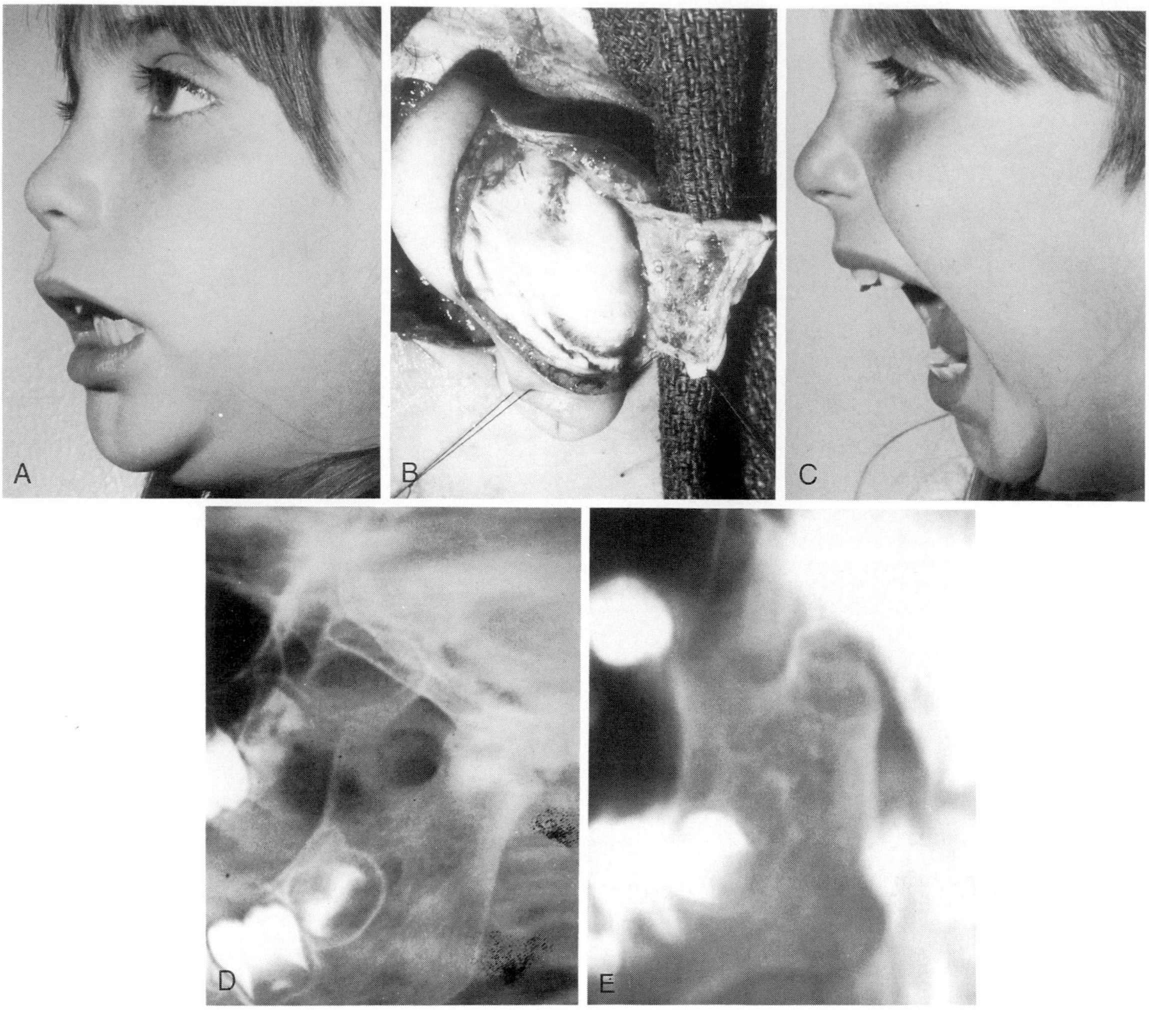

Figure 17–19. Reconstruction of an ankylosed temporomandibular joint with a graft of auricular perichondrium. *A,* This 7 year old patient had right-sided temporomandibular joint ankylosis; the range of motion was 2 mm. *B,* Elevation of the perichondrial graft from the posteromedial auricular surface. *C,* Following reconstruction of the temporomandibular joint with perichondrial grafts. Note the range of motion at nine months. *D,* Preoperative radiographic appearance of the affected temporomandibular joint. *E,* Radiographic appearance after reconstruction with an auricular perichondrial graft. Note the smooth contour of the new "condyle." (From Brent, B.: The versatile cartilage autograft: current trends in clinical transplantation. Clin. Plast. Surg., *6*:163, 1979.)

Perichondrocutaneous Graft

An interesting variation of cartilage-generating grafts incorporates auricular perichondrium and skin as a composite unit to create a perichondrocutaneous graft (Brent and Ott, 1978) (Fig. 17–20). This unique graft differs from classical cartilage-containing composite grafts in that it is apparently limited neither by the size that can be expected to "take," nor by the inherent contours dictated by usual donor sources. Furthermore, it is sufficiently pliable to fit any shaped recipient defect, and it has the potential to produce its own underlying support, which ultimately conforms to the recipient bed upon which the graft is maturing. Hence, the perichondrium-lined skin graft has clinical potential in facial reconstruction of a defect that requires both coverage and support.

The perichondrocutaneous graft can be used to resurface external nasal defects in which the lining is preserved (Fig. 17–21), and to restore the nasal lining itself. Likewise, it can be utilized to provide cover and support in repairing partial auricular defects,

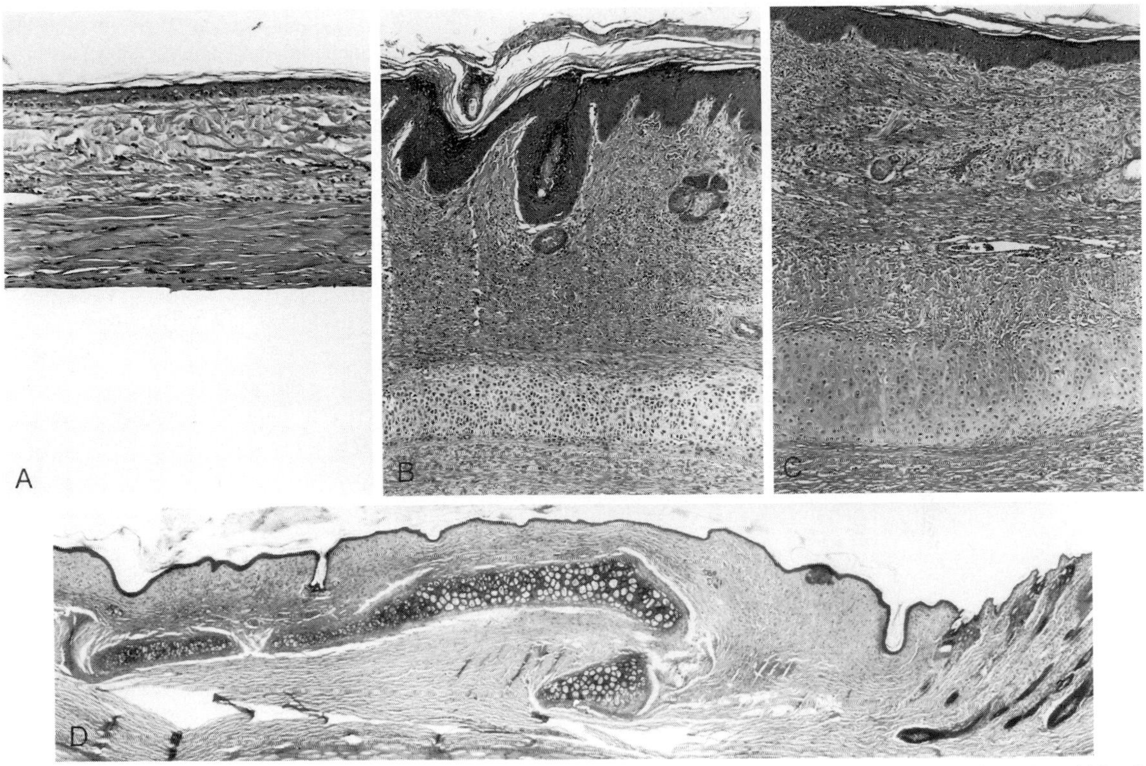

Figure 17–20. Maturation of neocartilage generated from a perichondrocutaneous graft in a 21 day old rabbit. *A,* Histologic appearance of a perichondrocutaneous graft from the anterior auricular surface, before transplantation. Note the intimate relationship of the two components and the minimal interposition of the subcutaneous tissue. *B,* At seven days, a distinct sheet of closely packed mesenchymal cells is apparent. These rounded cells, the precursors of cartilage, arise from the graft's perichondrial component. *C,* At 14 days, the cells have become noticeably separated by increasing amounts of intracellular substance, a result of chondroblastic activity. Note that a distinct layer of perichondrium surrounds the cartilaginous growth, and that differentiation of the chondrocytes has also begun. (H & E stain, × 75.) *D,* Perichondrocutaneous graft at six weeks. Note the plate of normal-appearing, mature cartilage, and the junction of the graft with the follicular skin of the rabbit's back. (H & E stain, × 10.) (From Brent, B., and Ott, R.: Perichondro-cutaneous graft. Plast. Reconstr. Surg., *62*:1, 1978.)

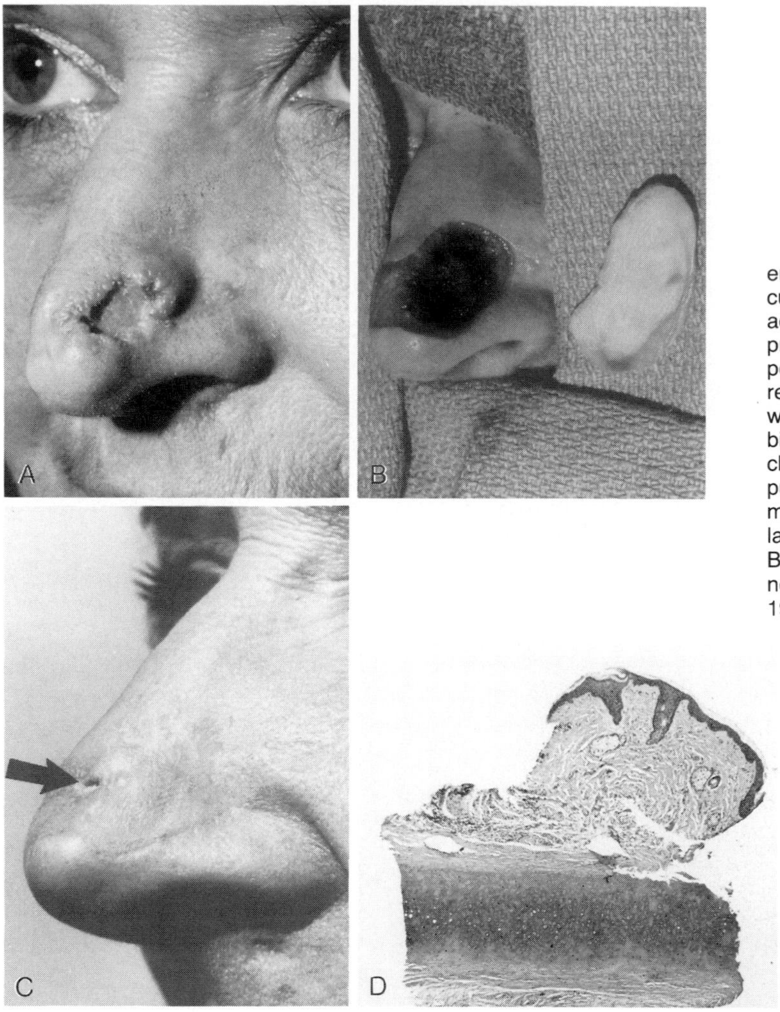

Figure 17–21. Provision of nasal coverage and support with a perichondrocutaneous graft. *A,* Recurrent keratoacanthoma. *B,* Excision of the lesion with preservation of nasal lining; note the perichondrocutaneous graft obtained for repair. *C,* Appearance of the graft at six weeks. The arrow points to the healing biopsy site. *D,* A specimen of the perichondrocutaneous graft was obtained by punch biopsy. The full-thickness specimen strikingly resembles normal auricular tissue (H & E stain, × 30.) (From Brent, B., and Ott, R.: Perichondrocutaneous graft. Plast. Reconstr. Surg., *62*:1, 1978.)

or to reconstruct the external auditory canal. This unique graft also seems applicable to specific cases of eyelid reconstruction and severe ectropion.

The donor source for a perichondrocutaneous graft is restricted to the anterolateral auricular surface, as the abundant subcutaneous tissue that loosely separates the posterior auricular skin from its underlying perichondrium would be likely to prevent "take" of a large posteromedial graft. The donor source should be restricted to the concha in order to prevent deformity (Fig. 17–22). Therefore, the available size of a perichondrocutaneous graft corresponds to individual conchal variance (Fig. 17–23). A somewhat larger graft can be obtained by including the triangular fossa, which permits a graft as large as 2.5 × 4.0 cm.

This small but unique graft has shown promise in the variety of clinical applications described above. Like any perichondrial graft, cartilage production from a perichondrocutaneous graft is not completely predictable. However, it seems fair to state that "take" of this composite unit, even if not accompanied by subsequent chondrogenesis, produces a graft that is more substantial and supportive than a full-thickness skin graft (see Fig. 17–21).

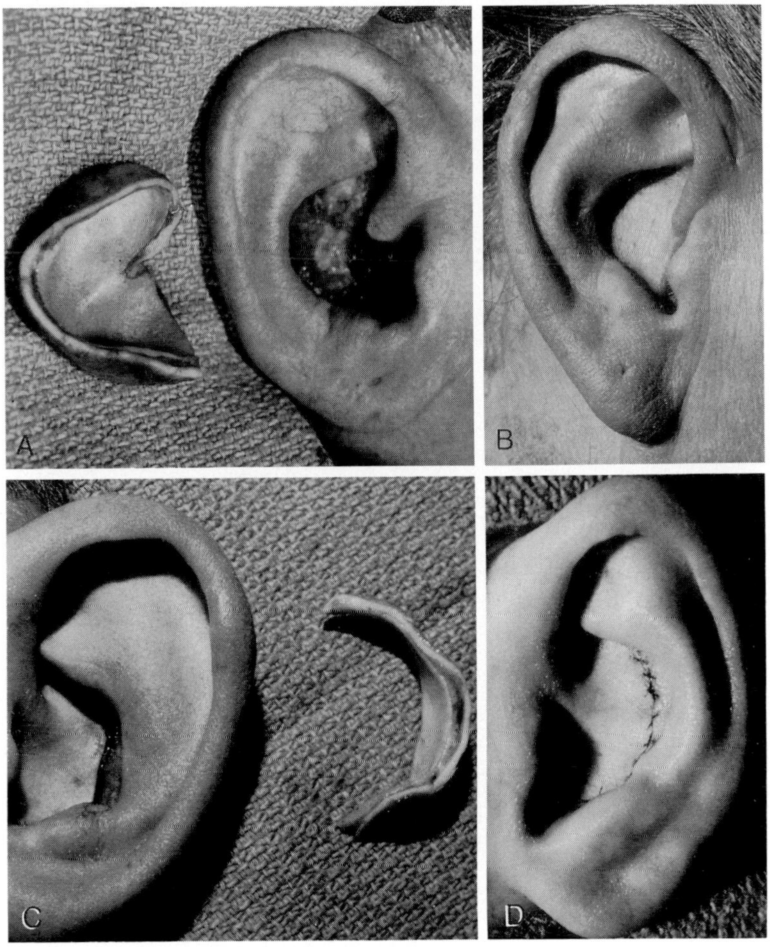

Figure 17–22. Donor site of a perichondrocutaneous graft. *A,* Excision of a full-thickness concha before the perichondrocutaneous graft is stripped (see Fig. 17–23). The maximal size is obtained by a carefully placed incision extended through the skin, perichondrium, and cartilage. The conchal excision is begun deep in the cymba, the inferior crus being split along its margin. The incision continues 3 to 4 mm within the antihelical crest, hides within the inner edge of the antitragus, sweeps upward several millimeters behind the meatus, and curves around the helical root to converge with the initial incision. The entire concha is extracted easily from its bed by scissor dissection. *B,* Healed donor ear at six months. The conchal bed has been resurfaced with full-thickness abdominal skin. *C,* Excision of a narrow conchal wedge before the perichondrocutaneous graft is stripped for restoration of the nasal lining. *D,* Primary closure of the donor site. (From Brent, B., and Ott, R.: Perichondrocutaneous graft. Plast. Reconstr. Surg., *62*:1, 1978.)

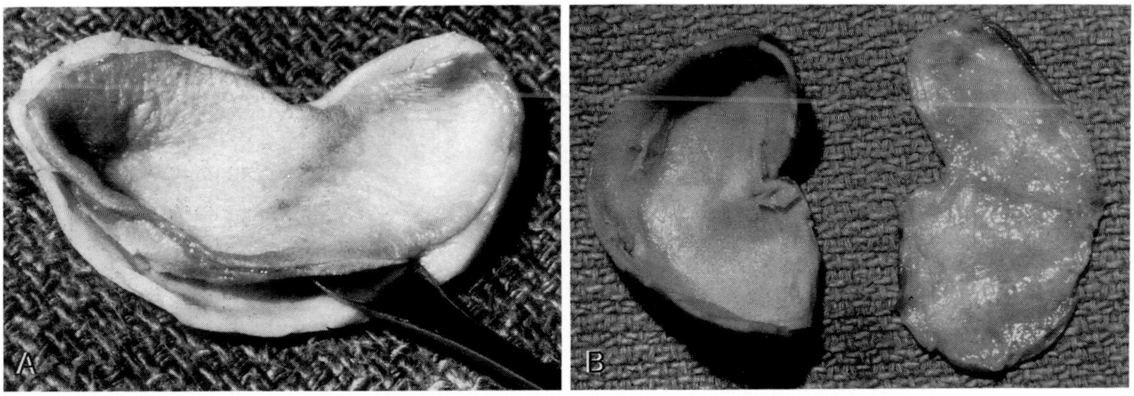

Figure 17–23. Stripping a perichondrocutaneous graft from the excised concha. *A,* The graft is stripped with the sharp end of a Freer elevator. Note the two adherent components of the graft, allowing easy stripping as a single unit. *B,* The stripped perichondrocutaneous graft. Note the glistening surface of the perichondrial component. The stripped conchal cartilage can be "banked" as desired. (From Brent, B.: The versatile cartilage autograft: current trends in clinical transplantation. Clin. Plast. Surg., *6*:163, 1979).

REFERENCES

Abrahams, M., and Duggan, T. C.: The mechanical characteristics of costal cartilage. *In* Kenedi, R. M. (Ed.): Biomechanics and Related Bio-engineering Topics. Proceedings of Symposium held in Glasgow. London, Pergamon Press, 1965, p. 285.

Adams, W. M.: Construction of upper half of auricle utilizing composite conchal cartilage graft with perichondrium attached on both sides. Plast. Reconstr. Surg., *16*:88, 1955.

Agris, J.: Irradiated homograft cartilage. Presented at the Annual Meeting of the American Society of Plastic and Reconstructive Surgeons Boston, MA, September 30, 1976.

Barsky, A., and Blinick, G.: The use of cartilage grafts to maintain patency of the fallopian tubes. Plast. Reconstr. Surg., *11*:87, 1953.

Brent, B.: Ear reconstruction with an expansile framework of autogenous rib cartilage. (Includes laboratory investigations and clinical application of overnight cartilage refrigeration.) Plast. Reconstr. Surg., *53*:619, 1974.

Brent, B.: The acquired auricular deformity. A systematic approach to its analysis and reconstruction. Plast. Reconstr. Surg., *59*:475, 1977.

Brent, B.: Nipple-areola reconstruction following mastectomy: an alternative to the use of labial and contralateral nipple-areolar tissues. Clin. Plast. Surg., *6*:85, 1979a.

Brent, B.: The versatile cartilage autograft: current trends in clinical transplantation. Clin. Plast. Surg., *6*:163, 1979b.

Brent, B.: The correction of microtia with autogenous cartilage grafts: I. The classic deformity. Plast. Reconstr. Surg., *66*:1, 1980.

Brent, B.: The correction of microtia with autogenous cartilage grafts: II. Atypical and complex deformities. Plast. Reconstr. Surg., *66*:13, 1980.

Brent, B.: Total auricular construction with sculpted costal cartilage. *In* Brent, B. (Ed.): The Artistry of Reconstructive Surgery. St. Louis, C. V. Mosby Company, 1987a, pp. 113–127.

Brent, B.: Auricular repair with a conchal cartilage graft. *In* Brent, B. (Ed.): The Artistry of Reconstructive Surgery. St. Louis, C. V. Mosby Company, 1987b, p. 110.

Brent, B.: Temporomandibular joint repair with an auricular perichondrial graft. *In* Brent, B. (Ed.): The Artistry of Reconstructive Surgery. St. Louis, C. V. Mosby Company, 1987c, p. 539.

Brent, B.: A comparative study in growth potential of perichondrial-covered autogenous cartilage grafts versus perichondrial-stripped grafts. Perspect. Plast. Surg. (in press).

Brent, B., and Bostwick, J., III: Nipple-areola reconstruction with auricular tissues. Plast. Reconstr. Surg., *60*:353, 1977.

Brent, B., and Ott, R.: Perichondro-cutaneous graft. Plast. Reconstr. Surg., *62*:1, 1978.

Brockman, S. J.: Cartilage graft tympanoplasty type III. Laryngoscope, *75*:1452, 1965.

Bromberg, B., Song., I. C., and Craig, G. T.: Split-rib mandibular reconstruction. Plast. Reconstr. Surg., *50*:357, 1972.

Converse, J. M.: The absorption and shrinkage of maternal ear cartilage used as living homografts: follow-up report of 21 of Gillies' patients. *In* Converse, J. M. (Ed.): Reconstructive Plastic Surgery. 2nd Ed. Philadelphia, W. B. Saunders Company, 1977, p. 308.

Craigmyle, M. B. L.: Antigenicity and survival of cartilage homografts. Nature (Lond.), *182*:1248, 1958a.

Craigmyle, M. B. L.: Regional lymph node changes induced by cartilage homo- and heterografts in the rabbit. J. Anat., *92*:467, 1958b.

Craigmyle, M. B. L.: A study of cartilage homografts in rabbits sensitized by a skin homograft from the cartilage donor. Plast. Reconstr. Surg., *26*:150, 1960.

Curran, R. C., and Gibson, T.: The uptake of labelled sulfate by human cartilage cells and its use as a test for viability. Proc. R. Soc. (Biol)., *155*:572, 1956.

Davis, J. E.: On auricular reconstruction. Internatl. Microform J. Aesth. Plast. Surg., Otoplasty, 1972–C.

Dingman, R. O., and Grabb, W. C.: Costal cartilage homografts preserved by irradiation. Plast. Reconstr. Surg., *28*:562, 1961.

Donald, P. J., and Col, A.: Cartilage implantation in head and neck surgery: report of a national survey. Otolaryngol. Head Neck Surg., *90*:85, 1982.

Duncan, M. J., Thompson, H. G., and Mancer, J. F.: Free cartilage grafts: the role of perichondrium. Plast. Reconstr. Surg., *73*:916, 1984.

Duncan, R. B.: Cartilage grafting in stapes surgery: report of two cases. N.Z. Med. J., *61*:278. 1962.

Dupertuis, S. M.: Actual growth of young cartilage transplants in rabbits. Arch. Surg., *43*:32, 1941.

Dupertuis, S. M.: Growth of young human autogenous cartilage grafts. Plast. Reconstr. Surg., *5*:486, 1950.

Dupertuis, S. M., and Musgrave, R. H.: Experiences with reconstruction of the congenitally deformed ear. Plast. Reconstr. Surg., *23*:361, 1959.

Engkvist, O., Johansson, S. H., Ohlsén, L., and Skoog., T.: Reconstruction of the articular cartilage using autologous perichondrial grafts: a preliminary report. Scand. J. Plast. Reconstr. Surg., *9*:203, 1975.

Engkvist, O., and Johansson, S. H.: Perichondrial arthroplasty: a clinical study in twenty-six patients. Scand. J. Plast. Reconstr. Surg., *14*:71, 1980.

Falces, E., and Gorney, M.: Use of ear cartilage grafts for nasal tip reconstruction. Plast. Reconstr. Surg., *50*:147, 1972.

Fry, H.: Cartilage and cartilage grafts: the basic properties of the tissue and the components responsible for them. Plast. Reconstr. Surg., *40*:426, 1967.

Fry, H. J. H.: Interlocked stresses in human nasal septal cartilage. Br. J. Plast. Surg., *19*:276, 1966.

Fukuda, O., and Yamada, A.: Reconstruction of the microtic ear with autogenous cartilage. Clin. Plast. Surg., *5*:351, 1978.

Gibson, T.: Cartilage grafts. Br. Med. Bull., *21*:153, 1965.

Gibson, T.: Personal communication with B. Brent, October 18, 1972.

Gibson, T., and Davis, W. B.: The fate of preserved bovine cartilage grafts in man. Br. J. Plast. Surg., *6*:4, 1953.

Gibson, T., and Davis, W. B.: The distortion of autogenous cartilage grafts: its cause and prevention. Br. J. Plast. Surg., *10*:257, 1958.

Gibson, T., and Davis, W. B.: A bank of living homograft cartilage: a preliminary report. Trans Int. Soc. of Plastic Surgeons, 2nd Congress, London, Edinburgh, E. & S. Livingstone, 1960, p. 452.

Gibson, T., Davis, W. B., and Curran, R. C.: The long-term survival of cartilage homografts in man. Br. J. Plast. Surg., *11*:177, 1958.

Gillies, H. D.: Plastic Surgery of the Face. London, Oxford University Press, 1920.

Gillies, H. D.: Reconstruction of external ear with special

reference to use of maternal ear cartilage as supporting structure. Rev. Chir. Structive, *7*:169, 1937.

Gillies, H. D., and Millard, D. R., Jr.: The osteo-chondral graft. *In* Gillies, H. D., and Millard, D. R., Jr. (Eds.): The Principles and Art of Plastic Surgery. Boston, Little, Brown & Company, 1957, p. 527.

Gorney, M.: The ear as a donor site: anatomic and technical guidelines. *In* Tanzer, R. C., and Edgerton, M. T. (Eds.): Symposium on Reconstruction of the Auricle. St. Louis, C. V. Mosby Company, 1974, p. 106.

Gorney, M.: Personal communications, 1974–1987.

Gorney, M.: Correction of the deviated nose. *In* Brent, B. (Ed.): The Artistry of Reconstructive Surgery. St. Louis, C. V. Mosby Company, 1987, p. 43.

Gorney, M., Murphy, S., and Falces, E.: Spliced autogenous conchal cartilage in secondary ear reconstruction. Plast. Reconstr. Surg., *47*:432, 1971.

Hage, J.: Collapsed ala strengthened by conchal cartilage (the butterfly cartilage graft). Br. J. Plast. Surg., *18*:92, 1965.

Hagerty, R. F., Braid, H. L., Bonner, W. M., Jr., Hennigar, G. R., and Lee, W. H., Jr.: Viable and nonviable human cartilage homografts. Surg. Gynecol. Obstet., *125*:485, 1967.

Hagerty, R. F., Calhoon, T. B., Lee, W. H., and Cuttino, J. T.: Characteristics of fresh human cartilage. Surg. Gynecol. Obstet., *110*:3, 1960a.

Hagerty, R. F., Calhoon, T. B., Lee, W. H., and Cuttino, J. T.: Human cartilage grafts stored in air. Surg. Gynecol. Obstet., *110*:433, 1960b.

Hass, G. M.: Studies of cartilage. Part IV. A morphologic and chemical analysis of aging human costal cartilage. Arch. Pathol., *35*:275, 1943.

Heyner, S.: The antigenicity of cartilage grafts. Surg. Gynecol. Obstet., *136*:298, 1973.

Krüger, E.: Absorption of human rib cartilage grafts transplanted to rabbits after preservation by different methods. Br. J. Plast. Surg., *17*:254, 1964.

Krutchinskij, G. V., and Schved, I. A.: Attempt to reconstruct the auricle using the ear cartilage from a living donor. Acta Chir. Plast., (Prague) *26*:100, 1984.

Kulick, M. I., Brent, B., and Ross, J.: Free perichondrial graft from the ear to the knee in rabbits (a study to determine most favorable orientation of grafts in perichondrial arthroplasty). J. Hand Surg., *9A*:213, 1984.

Lester, C. W.: Tissue replacement after subperichondrial resection of costal cartilage: two case reports. Plast. Reconstr. Surg., *23*:49, 1959.

Millard, D. R., Jr.: Eyelid repairs with a chondromucosal graft. Plast. Reconstr. Surg., *30*:367, 1962.

Mir y Mir, L.: Role of the meniscus of the knee in plastic surgery. Plast. Reconstr. Surg., *10*:431, 1952.

Moskalewski, S., Kawiak, J., and Rymaszewska, T.: Local cellular response evoked by cartilage formed after auto- and allogeneic transplantation of isolated chondrocytes. Transplantation, *4*:572, 1966.

Mowlem, R.: Use and behavior of iliac bone grafts in restoration of nasal contour; clinical and radiographic observations. Rev. Chir. Structive, *8*:23, 1938.

Mowlem, R.: Bone (iliac) and cartilage transplants to ear and nose; their use and behaviour. Br. J. Plast. Surg., *29*:182, 1941.

Mühlbauer, W. D., Schmidt-Tintemann, U., and Glaser, M.: Long-term behaviour of preserved homologous rib cartilage in the correction of saddle nose deformity. Br. J. Plast. Surg., *24*:325, 1971.

Mustardé, J. C.: Repair and Reconstruction in the Orbital Region. Edinburgh, E & S Livingstone, 1969, p. 192.

Ohlsén, L.: Cartilage formation from free perichondrial grafts: an experimental study in rabbits. Br. J. Plast. Surg., *29*:262, 1976.

Ohlsén, L.: Cartilage regeneration from perichondrium: experimental studies and clinical applications. Plast. Reconstr. Surg., *62*:507, 1978.

Ohlsén, L., Skoog, T., and Sohn, S. A.: The pathogenesis of cauliflower ear. Scand. J. Plast. Reconstr. Surg., *9*:34, 1975.

Peer, L. A.: Cartilage grafting. Surg. Clin. North Am., *24*:404, 1944.

Peer, L. A.: The neglected septal cartilage graft. Arch. Otolaryngol., *42*:384, 1948.

Peer, L. A.: Cartilage grafting. Br. J. Plast. Surg., *7*:250, 1955.

Quintarelli, G., Ippolito, E., and Rodén, L.: Age-dependent changes on the state of aggregation of cartilage matrix. Lab Invest., *32*:111, 1975.

Rasi, H. B.: The fate of preserved human cartilage. Plast. Reconstr. Surg., *24*:24, 1959.

Schuller, D. E., Bardach, J., and Krause, C. J.: Irradiated homologous costal cartilage for facial contour restoration. Arch. Otolaryngol., *103*:12, 1977.

Sheen, J. H.: Secondary rhinoplasty. Plast. Reconstr. Surg., *56*:137, 1975.

Sheen, J. H.: Personal communications, 1978–1987.

Sheen, J. H.: Aesthetic Rhinoplasty. 2nd Ed. St. Louis, C. V. Mosby Company, 1987a.

Sheen, J. H.: Personal communication, 1987b.

Skoog, T.: Reconstructing the antihelix by perichondrioplasty. In Plastic Surgery. Philadelphia, W. B. Saunders Company, 1974a, pp. 264–283.

Skoog, T.: Cartilage regeneration. In Plastic Surgery. Philadelphia, W. B. Saunders Company, 1974b, p. 287.

Skoog, T., and Johansson, S. H.: The formation of articular cartilage from free perichondrial grafts. Plast. Reconstr. Surg., *57*:1, 1976.

Skoog, T., Ohlsén, L., and Sohn, S. A.: Perichondrial potential for cartilaginous regeneration. Scand. J. Plast. Reconstr. Surg., *6*:123, 1972.

Skoog, T., Ohlsén, L., and Sohn, S. A.: The chondrogenic potential of the perichondrium. Chir. Plast., *3*:84, 1975.

Sohn, S. A., and Ohlsén, L.: Growth of cartilage from a free perichondrial graft placed across a defect in a rabbit's trachea. Plast. Reconstr. Surg., *53*:55, 1974.

Stark, R. B., and Frileck, S. P.: Conchal cartilage grafts in augmentation rhinoplasty and orbital floor fracture. Plast. Reconstr. Surg., *43*:591, 1969.

Steffensen, W. H.: Comments on total reconstruction of the ear. Plast. Reconstr. Surg., *10*:186, 1952.

Steffensen, W. H.: Comments on reconstruction of the external ear. Plast. Reconstr. Surg., *16*:194, 1955.

Stoll, D. A., and Furnas, D. W.: The growth of cartilage transplants in baby rabbits. Plast. Reconstr. Surg., *45*:356, 1970.

Straith, C. L., and Slaughter, W. B.: Grafts of preserved cartilage in restoration of facial contour. J.A.M.A., *116*:2008, 1941.

Tajima, S., Aoyagi, F., and Maruyama, Y.: Free perichondrial grafting in the treatment of temporomandibular joint ankylosis. Preliminary report. Plast. Reconstr. Surg., *61*:876, 1978.

Tanzer, R. C.: Total reconstruction of the external ear. Plast. Reconstr. Surg., *23*:1, 1959.

Tanzer, R. C.: Total reconstruction of the auricle. The evolution of a plan of treatment. Plast. Reconstr. Surg., *47*:523, 1971.

Tanzer, R. C.: Microtia—a long-term follow-up of 44

reconstructed auricles. Plast. Reconstr. Surg., *61*:161, 1978.

Tessier, P.: Secondary treatment of the injured and mutilated eyelid. *In* Tessier, P., Callahan, A., Mustardé, J. C., and Salyer, K. E. (Eds.): Symposium on Plastic Surgery in the Orbital Region. St. Louis, C. V. Mosby Company, 1976, p. 57.

Thomas, L.: Reversible collapse of rabbit ears after intravenous papain and prevention of recovery by cortisone. J. Exp. Med., *104*:245, 1956.

Upton, J., Sohn, S. A., and Glowacki, J.: Neocartilage derived from transplanted perichondrium: what is it? Plast. Reconstr. Surg., *68*:166, 1981.

Young, F.: Cast and precast cartilage grafts. Surgery, *15*:735, 1944.

18

Court B. Cutting
Joseph G. McCarthy
David M. Knize

Repair and Grafting of Bone

"Bone is fluid."
J. G. M.

MICROANATOMY AND HISTOCHEMISTRY

Bone is a dynamic living substance that shows marked structural alterations in response to injury, changes of stress, and vascular, endocrine, genetic, and nutritional influences. It is one of the few human organs that can undergo regeneration rather than repair with formation of scar tissue. Bone is a specialized form of connective tissue that provides support and protection for the vital and delicate organs of the body and also allows for locomotion. It is characterized by the presence of bone cells *(osteocytes)* that occupy cavities *(lacunae)*. Long, branching processes from these cells lie in fine canals *(canaliculi)*, which course through a hard, dense matrix consisting of collagenous fibers embedded in an amorphous ground substance *(cement)* impregnated with calcium phosphate complexes. The primary structural unit of bone is the *osteon* (Fig. 18–1), laid down in laminated layers around central blood vessels in the haversian canal (Fig. 18–2).

According to its origin, bone may be divided into *chondral* and *mesenchymal* forms. Growth of any long bone, a chondral bone, is occasioned by cartilaginous growth of the epiphysis, which is gradually replaced by new bone from the diaphysis. Membranous bone is formed by the replacement of a membrane of preexisting condensed mesenchyme. The regenerative powers of bone are limited except in the very young.

Every bone contains two types of tissue: The outer layer is *compact cortical bone,* the surface of which is penetrated by canals (Volkmann's canals), which carry blood vessels that anastomose with those of the haversian canals (Fig. 18–3). Blood from the haversian canals supplies the osteocytes through the canaliculi. The osteons of the long bones are oriented in the general direction of the longitudinal axis (see Fig. 18–2). Cortical bone is covered with periosteum,

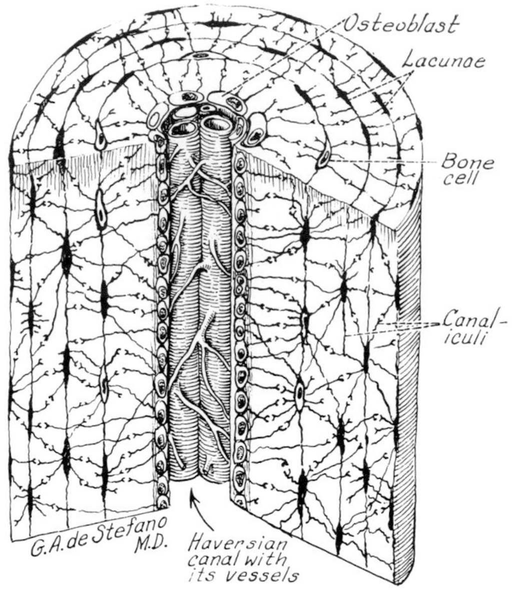

Figure 18–1. A single osteon of the haversian system.

which has two layers of cells. The cells of the outer layer resemble fibrocytes, while those of the deeper (cambium) layer resting on the cortical bone surface are plump and round. The latter layer contains the blood vessels, and its cells differentiate into osteoblasts, which add new bone to the cortical surface (Fig. 18–3*A*).

The inner layer is *coarse cancellous bone* (Fig. 18–3*B*), open and trabeculated but similar in structure to compact bone. It differs in that complete osteons are present only in the thickened trabeculae, which branch out to form the framework surrounding the marrow-filled spaces. The surfaces of the trabeculae are covered with resting osteoblasts.

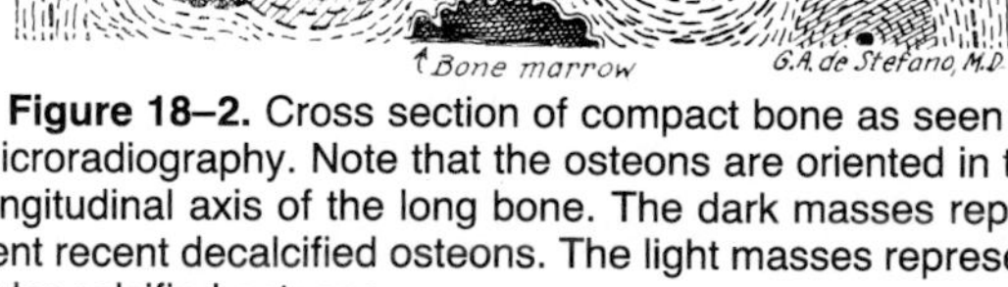

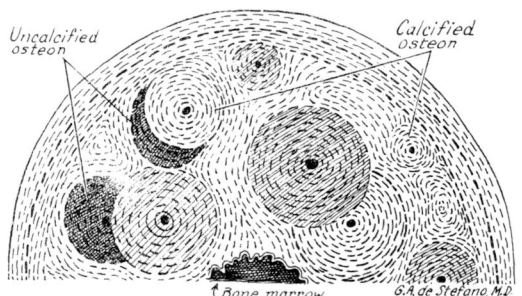

Figure 18–2. Cross section of compact bone as seen by microradiography. Note that the osteons are oriented in the longitudinal axis of the long bone. The dark masses represent recent decalcified osteons. The light masses represent older calcified osteons.

Bone is a highly specialized form of connective tissue. The principal element that differentiates it from other connective tissue is that it is hard. This characteristic is the result of mineral deposition within a soft organic matrix. The mineral component is a complex of calcium, phosphate, carbonate, and citrate. The interstitial substance is made up of fibers common to other types of connective tissue in a mucopolysaccharide, proteoglycan, and glycoprotein ground substance (McLean and Urist, 1961; Triffitt, 1980). The fibers are principally collagen with some reticular fibers as well.

With the exception of its tendency to calcify, bone is closely related to cartilage. Most of the embryonic skeleton is laid down first as hyaline cartilage. The cells hypertrophy and change their chemical characteristics immediately before their replacement by bone. After fracture of this type of bone, cartilage and fibrocartilage appear in the first stage of bone healing, which is callus formation (Ham, 1930; Leriche and Policard, 1928). The membranous bones of the skull and face are exceptions to this pattern and are not first formed as cartilage.

Although the nonliving components of bone provide the structural strength essential to bone function, it must be kept in mind that bone is living tissue. The cellular components of bone control the distribution of the nonliving elements. The quotation that opens this chapter is a reflection of this fact. All too often a skeletal reconstruction is undertaken in the spirit of carpentry. The nonliving elements of bone are positioned in a pleasing configuration initially. The surgeon is often horrified with the long-term result because of his failure to consider the cellular elements of bone. *Bone is fluid!* Although it may not flow immediately at the time of operation, it will certainly flow thereafter with the passage of years. This fluid nature is due to the cellular responses of living bone.

The traditional cell types unique to bone are *osteoblasts, osteocytes,* and *osteoclasts* (Mathews, 1980). It is useful, however, to consider only two cell lines in bone: osteoblasts and osteoclasts. Osteoblasts are derived from an osteoprogenitor cell line, while osteoclasts develop from a hematopoietic stem cell. Osteoblasts are seen on the surface of growing and remodeling bone. These cuboidal cells are basophilic owing to the large number of ribosomes within the cytoplasm reflecting

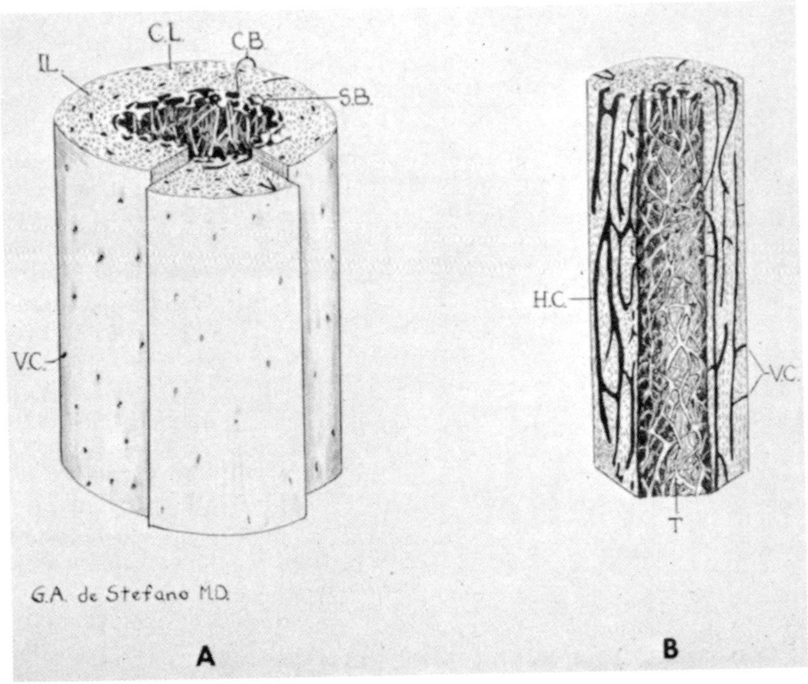

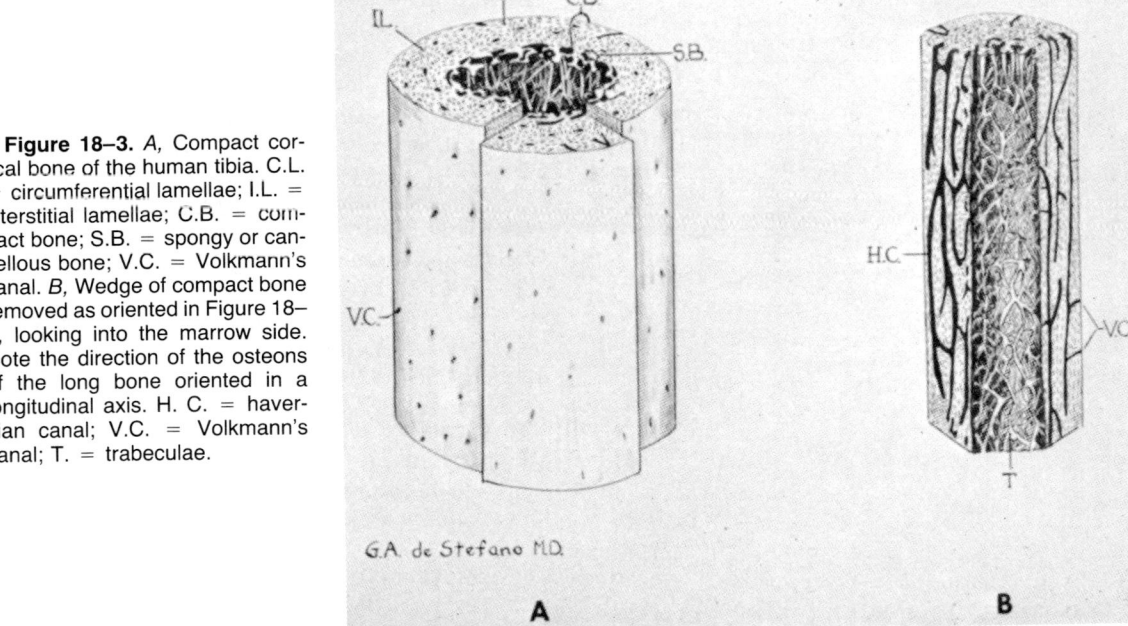

Figure 18–3. *A,* Compact cortical bone of the human tibia. C.L. = circumferential lamellae; I.L. = interstitial lamellae; C.B. = compact bone; S.B. = spongy or cancellous bone; V.C. = Volkmann's canal. *B,* Wedge of compact bone removed as oriented in Figure 18–1, looking into the marrow side. Note the direction of the osteons of the long bone oriented in a longitudinal axis. H. C. = haversian canal; V.C. = Volkmann's canal; T. = trabeculae.

active protein synthesis. The cells are actively producing the organic bone matrix.

Osteocytes are osteoblasts that have become totally entrapped by the matrix they produce. With the subsequent mineralization of the matrix, osteoblasts become trapped in their lacunar space and soon take on the characteristic appearance of osteocytes. They have cytoplasmic processes that extend out of this space through canaliculi in the bone. Under circumstances of resorption of the surrounding matrix, osteocytes are capable of again taking on the character of osteoblasts and resuming bone production (Young, 1967).

Osteoclasts are multinucleated giant cells that are responsible for bone resorption and are found on bone surfaces in areas of resorption. They arise from a different cell line from that of the osteocyte, most likely a blood-borne monocyte. The evidence for this comes from the study of osteopetrotic mutant mice who lack osteoclasts. These animals can be provided with normal-appearing osteoclasts by transplanting spleen cells from normal mice into the mutants. A few human cases of osteopetrosis have been successfully treated by immunosuppression and thymic tissue transplantation. Other studies also confirm that lymphoid tissue provides the osteoclast stem cell (Walker, 1975; Milhaud and associates, 1978; Ballet and Griscelli, 1978; Marks, 1984; Yabe and Hanaoka, 1985). Osteoclasts have been observed to envelop the tip of bone spicules that are undergoing resorption in the spongy bone of rapidly growing animals. Osteoclasts are covered with a surface membrane of microvilli that greatly increases the resorptive surface area of the cell.

Bone is covered on the outer surface with periosteum and on the inner with endosteum. The largely collagenous periosteal connective tissue carries blood vessels, nerves, and lymphatics to the outer surface of the bone, as well as serving as the site of bone attachment for muscles and tendons. The endosteum is a thin layer of reticular cells that lines the walls of bone marrow cavities and the haversian canal system of compact bone. Endosteum has both hematopoetic and osteogenic potential. Both endosteum and periosteum are active in the healing of fractures.

Bone marrow contains many of the cellular elements of loose connective tissue that are absent from compact bone. Although bone marrow is usually thought of in terms of its hematopoietic function, it is also active in osteogenesis. The reticular cells of marrow stroma readily transform into cells of bone. Marrow is richly supplied with blood vessels, nerves, and lymphatics, which may also be seen to extend somewhat into the haversian canal system of compact bone along with the blood vessels.

During the period of skeletal growth the formation of new bone outweighs resorption. In the healthy adult both processes are in balance. In the aged, regenerative apposition lags behind resorption, leading to senile osteoporosis. The presence of resting or reversal lines in a section of bone permits the reconstruction of a history of that area in much the same manner as a geologist reconstructs the past from studying the rock strata of a region. The biophysical investigations of bone by Engström, Amprino, and Finean (1946, 1953, 1955, 1960) and Holmstrand (1957) make it possible to study the differentiation of the newly laid-down bone from the old, the degree of calcification, and the orientation of the inorganic hydroxyapatite crystals along with the orientation of collagen fibrils embedded in or resting on the bone. The collagen fibrils in a lamella are arranged in bundles that encircle the canal in continuous spirals, resulting in a trellis-like arrangement. This arrangement imparts maximal structural strength to the tissue; it gives a characteristic appearance when viewed in polarized light. The inorganic crystals of hydroxyapatite are deposited in this highly ordered matrix of collagen and ground substances. The crystals are aligned with their long axes parallel to the longitudinal axis of the fibril. The distribution of the crystals can be studied by microradiography and their direction determined by microdiffraction.

In order to resist mechanical strain in the most efficient manner, the trabeculae of the cancellous bone are oriented along the lines of maximal stress. It is thought that the size and orientation of the trabeculae can change in response to altered mechanical demands. This concept of the functional adaptation of bone was first advocated by Wolff (1892). The work of Holmstrand (1957) has challenged Wolff's law by showing that the direction of the vessels growing into a compact bone graft in rabbits accounts for the orientation of the bone crystallites in the new osteons of the graft, and that mechanical forces, in spite of previous assertions, do not influence the ultrastructural organization of the substituting bone. In 1960 Holmstrand, Longacre, and deStefano were able to confirm this finding further in the study of a series of split rib autografts and allografts used to reconstruct skull defects in seventeen *Macaca* rhesus monkeys. The "healing-in" time of the grafts varied from two weeks to two years. Microdiffraction studies again showed that the structure of the original split rib graft and its placement either sagittally or transversely in the skull defect are the deciding factors in the ultrastructure of the new substituting bone in the graft. The following is a summary of the findings of these experiments:

1. Vascularization of the graft is brought about by vessels originating from the host skull bone, entering the graft primarily at its ends, and extending along the old haversian systems of the graft. This has been observed by microangiography as early as two weeks after implantation (Fig. 18–4).

2. Demineralization of the graft is the main activity during the first six months. This is followed by replacement of the old haversian systems by new osteons that are only slightly mineralized. These follow the original pattern of the original osteons of the graft.

3. During the first six months postoperatively, the vascularization and demineralization in autografts take place sooner than in fresh allografts (Fig. 18–5), but after an interval of two years there is little discernible difference.

4. Studies by microradiography and in polarized light disclose the fate of the graft after a "healing-in" period of 16 months. Both autografts and allografts retain their original orientation and their morphologic characteristics.

5. The osseous union between adjacent rib grafts and between rib grafts and skull results in a structure that in many respects resembles the normal calvarium after the final formation of an inner and outer table. The direction of the osteons in the newly laid-down bone corresponds to the direction of the osteons of the donor site.

6. The fibrous union between adjacent rib grafts and between rib grafts and skull has the morphologic characteristics of a normal cranial suture.

7. Microdiffraction studies prove that the ultrastructural organization of the inorganic hydroxyapatite crystals depends on the direction of the osteons of the original graft (Fig. 18–6).

CELLULAR MECHANISMS OF BONE TURNOVER

For the purposes of bone reconstruction, what is the source of bone-forming cells? Bone

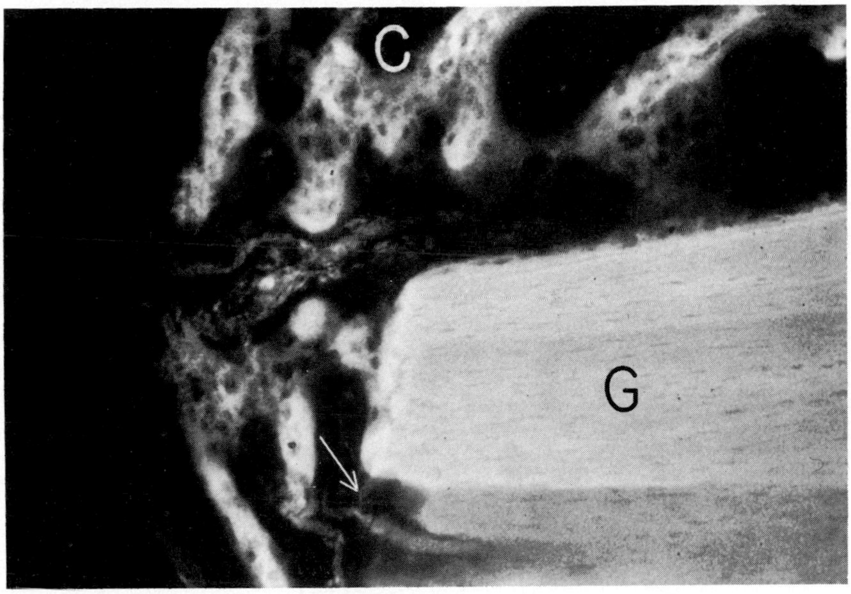

Figure 18–4. Microradiogram of an 80 micron thick sagittal section of a split rib graft (the rib is sectioned lengthwise) two weeks after surgery. Callus structures are seen at C. Note the large lacunae of the osteocytes in the callus in comparison with the finer lacunae seen in the graft at G. The arrow points to a contrast-filled vessel that enters an old haversian system in the graft. Note the demineralization occurring around this vessel. Recorded with Cu K alpha radiation at 27 kv. Primary magnification × 80.

is one of the few human tissues that undergo regeneration rather than repair with the formation of scar tissue. Reticular cells of bone marrow appear to have the capacity to differentiate into all types of blood and bone-forming cells. Mature bone cells appear to be capable of de-differentiating into reticular cells. They may then differentiate into osteoblasts and begin the process of bone formation. It is well established that if living bone cells of any type are transferred from one site to another, osteoblasts are capable of being formed in the transferred tissue.

What is less clear is the extent to which nonosseous connective tissue is capable of dedifferentiation and modulation into an osteoprogenitor cell (Young, 1967). All connective tissue cells derive from embryonic mesenchyme, some of which persist undifferentiated in the adult organism. These cells are certainly capable of differentiating into osteoblasts or any other type of connective tissue cell. What is uncertain is how many of the cells persist and what constitutes a proper stimulus to induce their transformation into osteocytes. The cells most likely exist as undifferentiated, perivascular, spindle-shaped cells that may be seen throughout the body. Whether nonosseous fibroblasts and other differentiated connective tissue cells are capable of back-differentiating into mesenchymal cells is still an area of active debate. This subject is discussed later in the chapter.

Mineral Equilibrium in Bone

The organic fraction of compact bone makes up 35 per cent of its dry weight; the remainder is inorganic bone matrix. The mineral crystals of bone matrix are rods approximately 200 angstroms long and 50 angstroms in diameter. These crystals are interwoven into the collagen fibers of compact bone along with the mucopolysaccharide chondroitin sulfate. The basic bone salt is hydroxyapatite with the chemical composition:

$$Ca_{10}(PO_4)_6(OH)_2$$

This salt is in a *metastable* equilibrium in the normal ion concentrations of extracellular fluid. They are below the concentration necessary for spontaneous precipitation of hydroxyapatite, but are well above the concentration needed for spontaneous crystal growth once a nidus has been formed (Neuman, 1980). Hydroxyapatite can be made in the laboratory and is now being used as a bone substitute in reconstructive surgery (Holmes, 1979; Hoogendoorn and associates, 1984) (see Chap. 20). Bone can be shown to grow into pores on the outer surface of the implant,

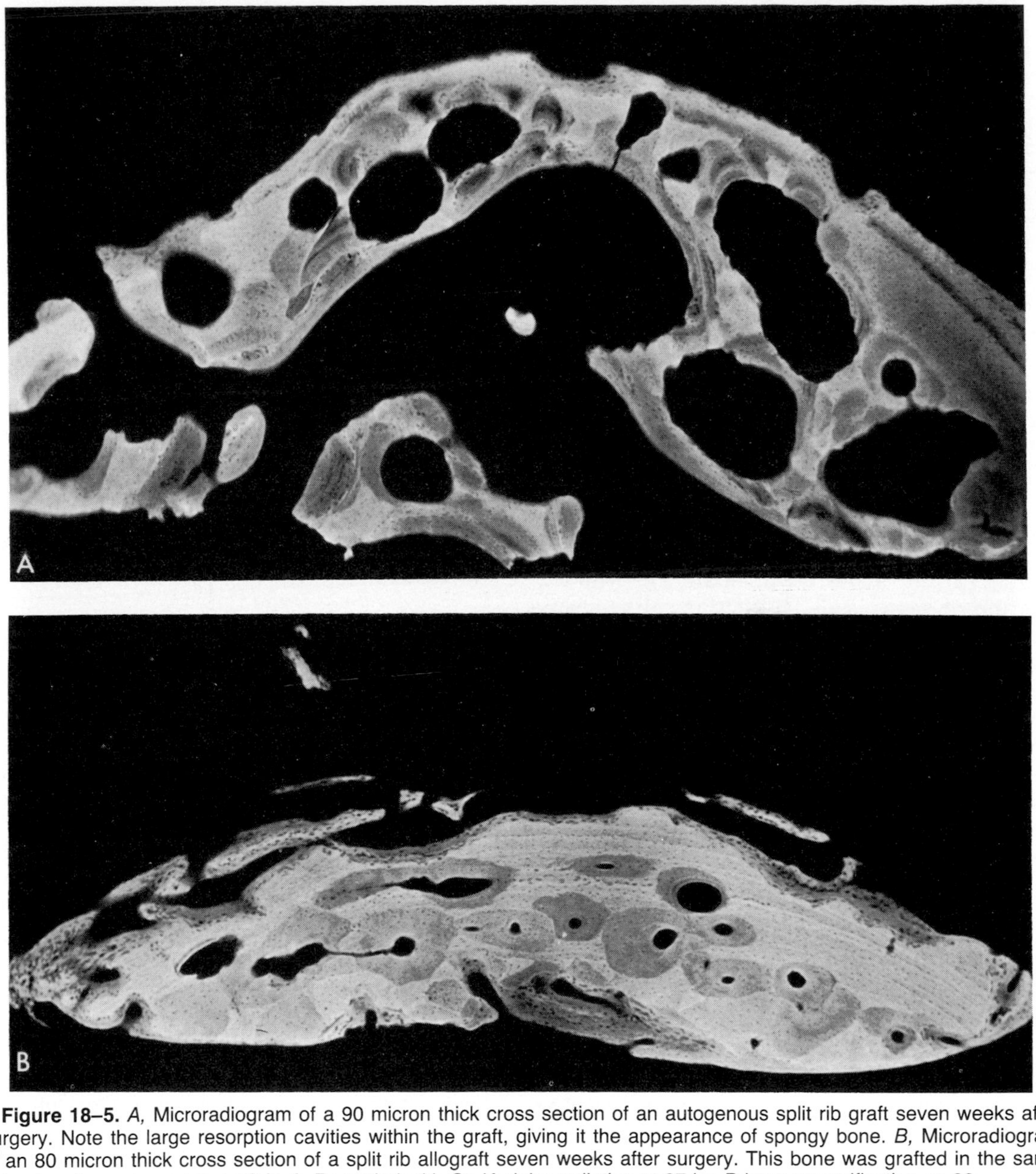

Figure 18–5. *A,* Microradiogram of a 90 micron thick cross section of an autogenous split rib graft seven weeks after surgery. Note the large resorption cavities within the graft, giving it the appearance of spongy bone. *B,* Microradiogram of an 80 micron thick cross section of a split rib allograft seven weeks after surgery. This bone was grafted in the same animal as the autogenous graft in *A.* Recorded with Cu K alpha radiation at 27 kv. Primary magnification × 20.

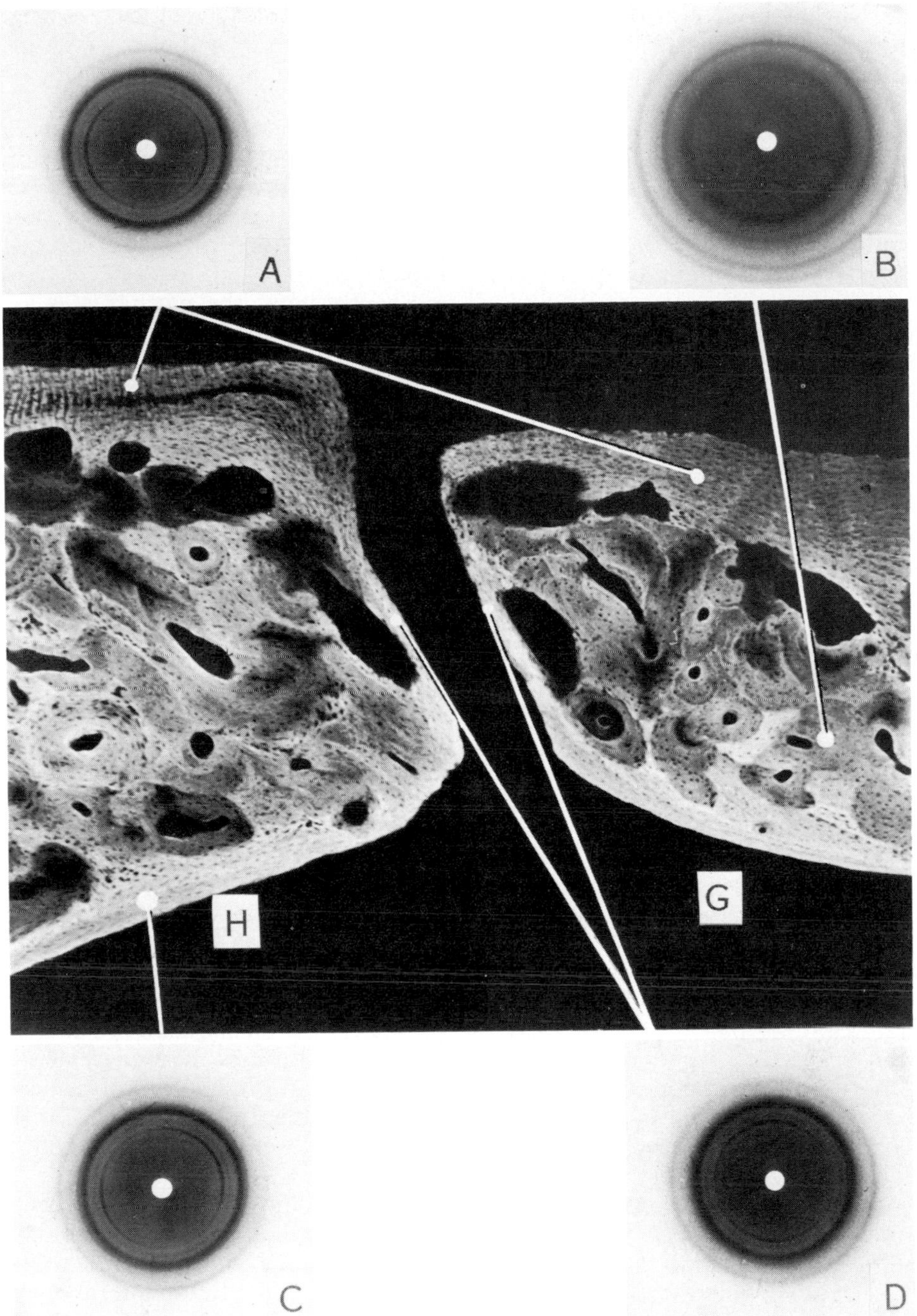

Figure 18–6. Microradiogram of an 85 micron thick cross section of an allograft 16 months after surgery. Letters H and G refer to the host bone and the rib graft, respectively. Diffractogram *D* was recorded from the osseous union between the graft and host bone, and shows that the orientation of the bone crystallites is perpendicular to the skull roof and parallel to the plane of the picture; therefore, it is the same as the orientation of the collagen fibers in a fibrous union between a graft and skull bone. Microradiogram and diffractograms recorded with Cu K alpha radiation at 27 kv. Primary magnification × 20.

depending on pore size. The material does not appear to resorb significantly. It should be remembered that pores in a foreign substance may also harbor bacteria. The long-term usefulness of hydroxyapatite as a bone substitute will be evaluated as clinical experience with the material accumulates.

A bone scan is a test frequently misinterpreted by the clinician. A radionucleotide (e.g., strontium, fluoride, gallium, technetium pyrophosphate) is injected into the patient, followed some time later by the imaging of skeletal structures by a gamma camera. It is important that the mechanism of uptake of the radionucleotide by the bone be understood. It occurs by *inorganic ion exchange*. If the radionucleotide is in contact with bone minerals, diffusion will allow the ions to exchange. *This should not be mistaken for blood flow!* It is true that blood flow will bring the circulating radiolabel in contact with bone mineral and result in the bone lighting up on bone scan. On the other hand, dead bone in contact with well-vascularized soft tissue also results in ion uptake by the bone. For this reason a bone that lights up on bone scan may not be assumed to be well vascularized. While it is true that well-vascularized bone lights up faster than nonvascularized bone, quantitative evaluation of blood flow using this method is discouraged (Stein and Shapiro, 1971; Horowitz, 1971). Microspheres and washout methods are preferred (Shim, 1968). Bone cell viability is even more difficult to assess with certainty. Tetracyclines are taken up by living osteocytes and are incorporated into the bone matrix they produce. Ultraviolet microscopy reveals fluorescent rings around active osteocytes in response to pulses of tetracycline (Milch, Rall, and Tobie, 1957). This technique provides a method of demonstrating bone cell viability. Tetracycline labeling can give false-negative results. If the osteocyte is alive, but not actively producing matrix, tetracycline labeling does not correctly identify a live cell. Autoradiography following uptake of radiolabeled cytidine is currently the most accurate experimental method to assess cell viability.

As a salt in solution, hydroxyapatite must be in equilibrium with the ions that make it up. Through a complex set of enzymatic and inorganic interactions, parathyroid hormone regulates serum calcium concentration. Robison (1932) proposed a dual mechanism for the calcification of hypertrophic cartilage:

1. Alkaline phosphatase produced by bone cells breaks down phosphoric acid esters which increase the local concentration of phosphate. This type of local supersaturation favors calcium salt deposition in bone.
2. Local factors also serve as a nidus for calcification in a supersaturated solution. Collagen can be shown to provide such a nidus. Its interactions with chondroitin sulfate have also been felt to be responsible for selective crystal deposition in bone. Differences in pH also alter the solubility of hydroxyapatite.

Exactly what the mechanisms are that determine the deposition of calcium salts in bone is a matter of continuing research.

Under certain conditions calcium salts may be deposited in other tissues of the body. Myositis ossificans is the best example. If a rabbit muscle is injected with alcohol, intramuscular calcium salt deposition and true bone formation result (Heinen, 1949). Ectopic calcification may also be found in the aorta and in other connective tissue sites (Huggins, 1931). It is important that calcification be distinguished from living bone.

The cellular mechanisms of bone resorption are debated. Osteoclasts play the major role in bone resorption, although osteocytic osteolysis has also been well described. Electron micrographs of osteoclasts reveal a brush border at the cell surface that greatly increases the surface area in contact with bone. Koelliker in 1873 (Urist, 1980) concluded that the osteoclast eroded bone by chemical means, although this mechanism was not specified. It has been discovered that chelating agents such as EDTA are capable of decalcifying bones in neutral or even strongly alkaline solutions. It was hypothesized that the osteoclast produces a substance at the cell surface with a greater affinity for the calcium ion than hydroxyapatite, and that this is the mechanism by which it produces local decalcification. The collagenase enzyme is also produced and is responsible for dissolving the organic element of bone matrix. Many efforts are being made to understand the cellular control mechanisms of osteolysis. It is hoped that as understanding of the mechanisms increases, it may be possible to delay or prevent bone graft resorption.

HEALING OF FRACTURES

The mechanisms of bone healing after fracture have been extensively studied (Gordon and Ham, 1950; Koekenberg, 1963; Trueta, 1968; Rhinelander, 1968, 1974; Brookes, 1971; Burchardt and Enneking, 1978; Heppenstall, 1980). At the site of a fracture, healing begins with the clotting of extravasated blood. The fibrin trellis that connects the two sides of the fracture serves as the pathway for ingrowth of cells into the gap. The torn ends of the periosteum, endosteum, and bone marrow proliferate and differentiate into fibrous connective tissue, fibrocartilage, and hyaline cartilage. The blood-borne cells of inflammation are also present and aid in the clearing of the necrotic material in the bone gap. The deposition of a cartilaginous precursor into the callus is most prominent in large bone gaps in the long bones. For small gaps and in membranous bones, osteoblasts grow out from the injured bone ends and fill the gap directly. In many cases, in particular widely separated fractures in membranous bones, osseous union does not develop and only a fibrous union persists (Pritchard, 1946; Mulholland and Pritchard, 1959). This is the reason why upper facial–calvarial fractures that are several years old often appear on radiographic study as if they were new. In long bone fractures the cartilaginous callus is replaced with bone as osteoblasts from the bone ends enter and replace it. New bone formation appears within 48 hours of injury on the inner and outer surfaces of the bone. The periosteum and endosteum contribute to the new bone formation.

In a widely separated fracture, healing may be viewed as a race between *fibrosis* produced by connective tissue that surrounds the bone gap and *osteogenesis* from the cells at the bone ends (Mulholland and Pritchard, 1959). If the gap is too wide, fibrosis prevails and the bone ends are sealed off in a fibrous union. If osteogenesis wins, a bony union results. Experiments have been performed in which a plastic tube has been used to bridge the bone gap in a widely separated fracture where fibrous union would normally occur. The tube prevents fibrous tissue ingrowth from the surrounding connective tissue. New vessel proliferation and ingrowth of osteogenic cells from the bone ends are noted within the tube, and an osseous union develops within. This mechanism is analogous to the events at nerve trunk anastomosis. Axonal growth from one side to the other must occur before connective tissue from the surroundings seals off the nerve endings.

For this reason, fracture healing is best promoted by minimizing the gap between the bone ends and by applying compression between the two fragments. In this way, little osteogenesis is required to unite the two bone ends. This is the conceptual framework for the AO and Luhr plate methods of fracture treatment in which compression plates are used (Fig. 18–7). The disadvantage of this method is that the periosteum must be widely stripped to allow application of the plate. For this reason, AO fracture healing is primarily endosteal in character. Intramedullary pin fixation such as the Küntscher type of nailing obliterate the marrow space, allowing only periosteal healing. Interosseous twisted wiring methods may also produce compression, although stabilization of fragment position is not as precise. Kirschner wire, Steinmann's

A

B

C

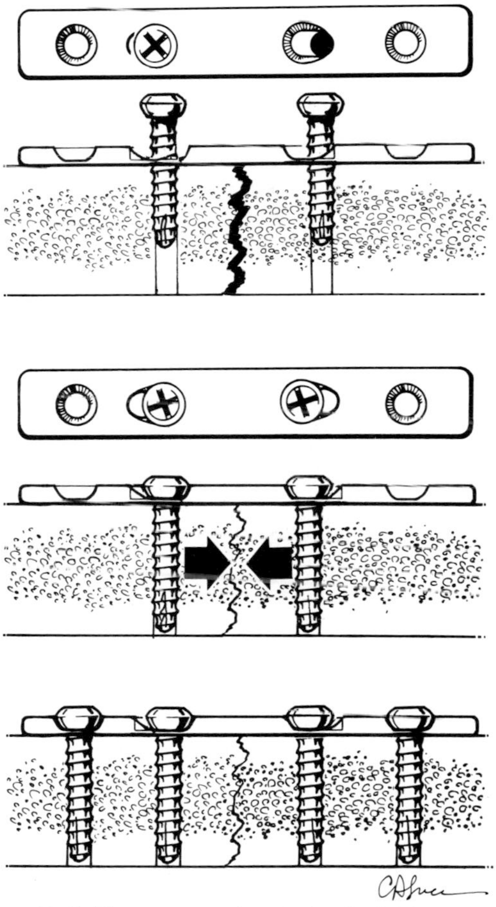

Figure 18–7. The compression mode of miniplate fixation. *A*, A four-hole plate. Note that the inner holes are eccentrically shaped so that, as the screws are tightened, the heads fall into the wider portion and compress the bony margins (*B*). *C*, Completed view of the skeletal fixation.

pin, or similar rigid pin methods produce excellent stabilization of fragment position, but compression is often lacking. External fixation devices such as the Hoffmann apparatus or the Morris biphase appliance produce satisfactory stabilization without periosteal stripping at the fracture site. Some element of compression is also possible with the latter devices. The principal disadvantages of external fixation are that it is usually clumsy and uncomfortable during the healing period and requires a separate procedure for removal. Treatment methods must be individualized to the situation; often a combination of methods is best.

The importance of adequate bone blood supply for fracture healing is well established (Koekenberg, 1963; Trueta, 1963; Rhinelander, 1968, 1974). Vascular outgrowth from bone ends accompanied by rapid proliferation of well-nourished osteogenic cells is essential for satisfactory fracture healing (Fig. 18–8). Intramedullary nails that obliterate the marrow space have been criticized for poor fracture healing due to the interruption of the nutrient artery supply of the long bones (Huggins and Wiege, 1939; Trueta and Cavadius, 1964). The blood supply to bone is further discussed later in the chapter.

After a period of immobilization that allows new-woven bone to join the fractured segments, reapplication of the normal biologic stresses to the bone causes the bone at the fracture site to remodel and mature. Much of the remodeling of fracture callus is currently thought to be mediated by the electrical potentials that result from stressing the fractured bone ends. Electrical potentials produced by artificial means can result in healing of fracture non-unions (Becker, Bassett, and Bachman, 1964; Friedenberg and Kohanim, 1968; Bassett, 1982; Brighton, 1984; Pollack, 1984; Black, 1984).

The mechanisms for bone remodeling are discussed later. Bone morphogenetic protein (BMP) (Urist and McLean, 1952) may also be released from fractured bone ends and may induce the production of osteoblasts.

TRANSPLANTATION OF BONE-PRODUCING TISSUE

For the past two centuries surgeons have investigated the possibility of producing bone where it had not existed previously. The earliest work involved identifying the tissue most responsible for bone production in postfetal life. Duhamel (1742) placed silver wires subperiosteally and found later that they were covered by bone. This led him to conclude that the new bone had been produced as a result of the osteogenic properties of the periosteum. Heine (1836) completely resected

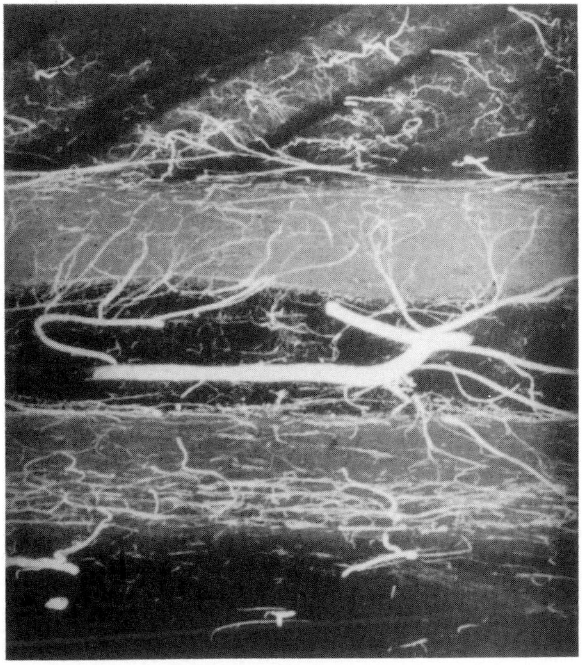

Figure 18–8. Microangiogram showing the development of anastomoses between the nutrient artery and the diaphyseal periosteal vessels in response to fracture. (From Rhinelander, F. W.: The normal microcirculation of diaphyseal cortex and its response to fracture. J. Bone Joint Surg., *50A*:784, 1968.)

ribs and found that they regenerated. In 1867 Ollier reported his series of exhaustive scientific studies on periosteum. He concluded that periosteum was osteogenic and its transplantation was capable of producing bone at the recipient site (Bonome, 1886; Lexer, 1929; Cestero and Salyer, 1975). Axhausen (1907) confirmed the osteogenic capacity of periosteum and further discovered that the effect was marked in autografts, less noted in allografts, and virtually absent in xenografts.

Macewen (1912) performed a series of ingenious studies disputing the notion that the periosteum was the source of all osteogenesis. He discovered that multiple strippings of the periosteum from the diaphysis of a long bone in a living animal resulted in large increases in the diameter of the bone. Removing the periosteum, drilling a hole in the cortex, and inserting a long glass tube into the hole in a living animal also produced unique findings. Bone was found to grow out of the tube in the absence of periosteum. These and a number of other studies led Macewen to conclude that the periosteum was merely a limiting membrane that prevented further outgrowth from living bone. He considered that the bone itself was the source of osteogenesis.

In the years that followed a large number of studies were directed toward the production of bone after the transplantation of periosteum alone. In some of these studies the periosteum was transplanted as a free graft, and in others as a vascularized flap. In some studies new bone was produced, and in others no bone was formed. This controversy was reviewed extensively by Ritsila, Alhopuro, and Rintala (1972). Their conceptual resolution of the dilemma is appealing. They believed that the site of osteogenesis occurs at the interface between bone and periosteum, and that the differences in experimental results are accounted for by the methods used to strip the periosteum. If, in the harvesting of the periosteum, the bone surface is scraped aggressively, osteoblasts at the interface stay on the periosteal surface. If, on the other hand, the periosteum is peeled away, particularly in older animals, the osteogenic cells may not strip with the periosteum and no new bone will form. The interface layer is called the cambium layer of the periosteum. The experiments of Ollier (1867) and Macewen (1912) cannot be disputed. It is evident that under some circumstances periosteum forms new bone (Skoog, 1967). It is also clear that living vascularized bone is capable of generating new bone. These concepts should not be viewed as mutually exclusive.

HISTORY OF AUTOGENOUS BONE GRAFTING

In 1682 Van Meekren transplanted canine skull bone to a calvarial defect with reported success (Rogers, 1930; Chase and Herndon, 1955; Prolo and Rodrigo, 1985). The surgeon was forced to remove the graft, however, or face excommunication from the Church. As time passed, bone grafting became more widely practiced on the basis of the empiric success of the procedure. Ollier (1867) reported the transfer of periosteum and bone and concluded that both must be alive to account for the osteogenesis he observed. Barth (1893) was the first to challenge this doctrine. His studies revealed that several days after bone graft transfer, the graft was entirely dead. Barth felt that bone grafting worked via gradual resorption and replacement of the dead bone by *creeping substitution* of the dead graft by live bone growing into it from the living bone in contact with it. Creeping substitution is now widely referred to as *osteoconduction*.

Axhausen (1907) performed a series of experiments demonstrating that periosteally covered bone grafts exhibited osteogenesis from the surface cells surviving at the periosteum. Phemister (1914) published an extensive series of studies demonstrating conclusively that some of the osteogenic cells on the surface of a bone graft survive by diffusion of oxygen and nutrients from the recipient bed (Ham and Gordon, 1952; Hancock, 1963). Phemister agreed with Barth (1893) that the vast majority of the bone in the center of a large graft was dead, since empty lacunae were observed ten days after transfer. On the other hand, he emphasized the importance of cell survival at the surface of the graft. Bone-forming cells on the surface of the graft were important for the resorption and replacement of the central necrotic portions of the graft with new bone. Boiling the bone killed the cells, producing a deleterious effect on graft survival. Phemister also discovered that a hematoma was detrimental to bone graft survival, as it formed a diffusion block between the recipient bed and the bone graft, a situation analogous to skin grafting. The skin graft is dependent on diffusion from the recipient bed for its survival until vascular microanastomoses can develop (Hancox, 1947; Ray, 1972; Goldberg and Lance, 1972; Albrektsson, 1980). The same is true for an autogenous bone graft. Phemister (1914) performed his studies using cortical bone grafts. Gallie and Robertson (1918) agreed that survival of cells on the surface of a bone graft was important. They also noted that survival and osteogenesis were much better with the use of cancellous bone than with cortical bone. It is now known that cancellous bone is a much richer source of osteoprogenitor cells than is cortical bone. The diffusion necessary for early cell survival occurs much more readily through the interstices of cancellous bone than through the dense, calcified matrix of cortical bone. More recent studies (Ham and Gordon, 1952; Heslop, Zeiss, and Nesbit, 1960; Zeiss, Nesbit, and Heslop, 1960) showed that bone cells survive for a distance of only 200 to 300 microns from the surface of cortical bone.

Mowlem (1944, 1963) popularized the use of cancellous bone grafts and demonstrated their superiority to cortical bone grafts in a wide variety of clinical situations. According to Mowlem, "The method should be directed to the creation of circumstances under which the maximum cellular survival is insured under conditions which will make the subsequent activity of the cells most effective. No longer is a bone graft that inorganic bridge which is to be completely resorbed and slowly replaced. Instead it is only the scaffold to carry these cells which can rapidly envelop it with new bone and incorporate it in the new repair."

It is the survival of the surface cells in autogenous bone grafts that results in their superiority to freeze dried autogenous grafts, allografts, bone implants, and inorganic bone substitutes (Oklund and associates, 1985). If an autogenous graft is interposed into a large bone gap, not only will creeping substitution occur from contact with the recipient bone ends, but resorption and replacement of the dead bone in the center of the graft will be contributed to by live bone cells from the surface. The surgeon should be aware of this fact when handling an autogenous bone graft in the operating room. High speed drills and saws generate heat that has been shown to kill bone cells. Adequate irrigation should always be used to cool the bone when these devices are employed. If a bone graft is dropped on the floor during a procedure, autoclaving it before use will kill every living cell within the graft.

Osteoinduction is the last major factor that contributes to the success of a bone grafting procedure. Undifferentiated mesenchymal cells are induced to differentiate into bone-forming cells in response to an inducing substance in the implant. The inducing substance, *bone morphogenetic protein* (BMP), is released by the graft. Autogenous bone grafts share this mechanism with other types of bone implants. Although banked bone is capable of resorption while hydroxyapatite implants are not, it does contain BMP, which stimulates new bone formation. Isolating BMP and combining it with autogenous bone has been shown to produce results superior to autogenous bone grafting alone (Sato and Urist, 1985; Prolo and Rodrigo, 1985; Oklund and associates, 1985). This is an exciting area for further research. Osteoinduction is discussed in greater detail below.

Kazanjian (1952) articulated four clinical rules for bone grafting in the mandible that are guidelines for all bone grafting situations:

1. The recipient site must have adequate blood supply, which is essential to ensure the survival of any live cells of the surface of the graft.

2. Bone to bone contact must be established between the graft and the host bone. This obviously facilitates "creeping substitution."

3. Rigid fixation of the fragments must be maintained during the healing period. In this way, as bone ingrowth occurs by osteoconduction, the connection is not broken with motion at the fracture site.

4. The bone graft should be placed only into healthy tissue. A bacterially contaminated tissue bed precludes successful grafting.

We might also add to these rules that an autogenous bone graft should be treated with respect for the preservation of the living cells within it.

OSTEOINDUCTION

A bone transplant transfers viable bone cells, whereas a bone implant does not transfer living cells. Living bone grafts revascularize by the development of microanastomoses with host vessels, while implants vascularize by the invasion of capillary sprouts from the host bed during the process of resorption of the old matrix. In the bone transplant, living osteogenic precursor cells on the surface of the graft survive by diffusion of oxygen and nutrients from the host bed. These cells actively contribute to the repopulation of the bone transplant with living bone-forming cells. This process does not occur in the bone implant. The bone implant is replaced by living bone via osteoconduction or "creeping substitution" of the implant by the living bone that abuts the implant and by osteoinduction.

Urist and McLean (1952) and Urist (1980) described osteoinduction as the last major factor that contributes to the success of a bone grafting procedure. They transplanted various substances devoid of living bone-forming cells to the anterior chamber of the eye in rats and observed the formation of new bone. These authors postulated that undifferentiated mesenchymal cells were induced to differentiate into bone-forming cells in response to an inducing substance in the implant. This work spawned a major research effort by Urist and his group to characterize and manipulate this phenomenon. The evidence for osteoinduction is now well established. Autogenous bone grafts share this mechanism with other types of bone implants. The Urist group discovered a diffusible bone morphogenetic protein (BMP) that incites this differentiation. It has been shown that if a piece of demineralized bone matrix is placed in a diffusion chamber and implanted into rat muscle without bone contact, bone cells develop (Urist and associates, 1970; Harakas, 1984). The protein is capable of evoking a cross-species bone morphogenetic response. For this reason, xenograft bone implants retain a potential for bone formation.

Heterotopic bone formation has also been shown when muscle is placed in contact with cells of the urinary bladder, HeLa cells, placenta, and vaccinia transformed fibroblasts (Huggins and Wiege, 1939; Wlodarski, Hancox, and Brooks, 1973; Oikarinen and Korhonen, 1979). Presumably a chemical stimulus is also responsible for these demonstrations of the bone induction phenomenon.

IMMUNE RESPONSE TO BONE ALLOGRAFTS AND XENOGRAFTS

For some years after World War II there was a certain amount of enthusiasm for the use of preserved bovine bone implants (xenografts). Several years of careful follow-up revealed such a high percentage of failures and resorption that the technique fell into disfavor. A second wave of enthusiasm for the use of lyophilized calf bone implants has developed in the United States. Carefully controlled experimental work by Stringa (1957) showed that the fresh living autograft was quickly vascularized, whereas there was delayed vascularization and a high rate of complications when allografts were used. However, in a xenograft there was an immediate walling off of the foreign body by the tissues of the host. The xenograft was never incorporated or vascularized, and eventually the chances of extrusion were comparable with those for other foreign bodies.

Studies of the antigen-antibody reaction demonstrate that in the case of the bone allograft the main antigens are associated with the nucleated marrow cells, while in the xenograft the matrix and the serum proteins are antigenic.

According to Enneking (1962), bone tissue antigens are not different from other tissues. They stimulate cellular antibodies and hemoagglutinins, which in turn destroy the proliferating transplanted cells and remaining matrix. However, bone is antigenic for only a limited time, and the intensity and effectiveness of the immune response vary considerably. These factors in combination may lead to temporary immunoparalysis.

The success of a graft depends on its early vascularization. Holmstrand (1957) demonstrated that new blood vessels from the bed enter the haversian systems of the bone graft as early as the second week (see Fig. 18–4).

Burwell (1962) showed that primary fresh allografts are less well vascularized than autogenous bone, and that substances were carried directly to the lymph nodes draining the area, producing a proliferative response of the lymphocytes within three days. However, when "second set grafts" were introduced into the host, the reaction was much more rapid and violent, with marked lymphoid hyperplasia and enlargement of the regional nodes. The large and medium lymphoid cells quickly destroyed all exposed cells of the graft, and there was no new bone formation.

In an attempt to reduce the immune response to the xenograft, cobalt irradiation has been used to sterilize the bone. Short-term observations of these implants showed that there was less reaction on the part of the host. Long-term studies, however, revealed that 95 per cent of the implant remained after 20 months and that there was no "creeping substitution," as noted in fresh allografts. Bassett, Hurley, and Stinchfield (1962) concluded that further clinical use was not indicated.

Although the work by Burwell (1968) confirmed the existence of intrinsic osteogenic inductors, it is increasingly apparent that cells of the graft (particularly those on its surface) may survive and form bone shortly after transplantation. For this reason, fresh, autogenous, cancellous bone continues to be the best material to aid osteogenesis in the recipient region.

The state of cell viability is involved not only in the function of a bone graft but also in the semantics of bone grafting. Viable bone transplants should be considered as grafts, while nonviable ones (allografts and xenografts) must be classified as implants, since their behavior is similar to that of metallic or alloplastic implants. A graft must be defined as anything inserted that becomes an integral part of the host. Finally, it is not sufficient to have merely a stimulus for bone formation. It is necessary to have a satisfactory vascular bed, since in the absence of a proper nutritional and physical milieu, the osteocytes may not synthesize the organic precursors of an osseous matrix.

Using the accelerated rejection of a skin allograft as a test to demonstrate the immune response to a previously implanted fresh bone allograft, according to the technique of Chalmers (1959), Brooks and associates (1963) investigated the immune response to various types of bone implants. These included fresh allografts; frozen allografts; frozen, irradiated allografts; freeze dried allografts; frozen, dried, and irradiated allografts; deproteinized, frozen allografts; and decalcified allografts. In a first stage, the various transplants were placed into the lateral thigh muscles of the anesthetized C57 mouse. The bone allografts were removed from C3H donors. After a three week delay, to allow the C57 mouse recipient to become sensitized to the C3H bone allografts, a full-thickness graft from another C3H donor was transplanted to the C57 recipient of the allografts. Both C57 and C3H mice were isogenic strains. The accelerated rejection of the skin allograft was used as a test to demonstrate that the recipient had undergone an immune response to the implanted bone. As judged from the accelerated rejection of the skin allograft, fresh bone allografts have antigens in common with skin. Freezing and freeze drying the bone allograft seemed to inactivate the antigens. Decalcification, deproteinization, and freezing of the bone allografts appeared to leave intact a sufficient quantity of common antigens with skin to produce an acceleration of the skin allograft rejection.

It should be noted that in this experimental series, virtually all the calcium had been removed, but the organic matrix that remained seemed to retain antigenic properties. It was also obvious that freezing and drying from the frozen state altered the antigens and provoked a lesser response to the challenge by the skin allografts.

Much of the difficulties with allogeneic bone implants center around the rejection phenomenon (Burwell, Friedlaender, and Mankin, 1985). Foreign antigens in the bone implant initiate cell mediated immunity, as is common in other transplantation situations. With a chronic rejection reaction the allogeneic bone implant is sequestered by the body in a covering of fibrous tissue. Much of the work on banking of allogeneic bone involves analysis of the method of treating the bone in terms of the host immune response. One common method of allogeneic bone preparation involves freeze drying the implant. Unfortunately, freeze drying does not reduce the antigenicity of allogeneic bone (Burchardt and Enneking, 1978). The BMP from the implant is blocked from bone induction by the surrounding immune reaction.

The best allogeneic implant preparations attempt to eliminate bone antigenicity (Urist, 1980). The more cellular the bone, the greater is the antigenicity. For this reason, cancellous allografts are seldom used. Cortical bone is preferred because of its large proportion of collagen, which has low antigenic activity. BMP appears to be denatured by autoclaving and high dose radiation. For this reason, only low dose radiation should be used to kill bone cells if this is part of the preparative technique. Since irradiation has minimal influence on decreasing antigenicity, it is not frequently used. Xenograft bone is seldom used owing to the wide disparity between the antigenic make-up of the donor and that of the recipient.

Antigen-extracted, autolyzed, allogeneic (AAA) bone is the most conceptually well founded of the allogeneic implants (Urist, 1980). The aim of this preparation method is to sterilize cortical bone without loss of BMP activity, while lowering the antigenicity of the implant. The osteocytes are removed by autolytic digestion and the antigens are extracted using chloroform and methanol. The BMP content of the resultant matrix does not appear to be destroyed by this process. The antigenicity of the bone is also lowered significantly. Although it is capable of osteoinduction, it should be used whenever possible in such a manner that osteoconduction from adjacent living bone is also possible. While none of the bone implants is as satisfactory as living autogenous bone, there are circumstances in which the use of bone implants is desirable. Implants offer the potential of an unlimited supply of bone graft, the absence of donor site morbidity, and decreased operative time. It is hoped that future research into bone implants and the isolation and characterization of BMP may some day revolutionize skeletal surgery, but that day is not yet at hand. Most of the efforts to use the induction principle alone for bone reconstruction yield bone, but it is not of high quality. Reports of the application of this principle to cranioplasty have been somewhat encouraging (Mulliken and Glowacki, 1980). At present, autogenous living bone remains the skeletal reconstructive material of choice.

BONE REMODELING

The growth pattern of enchondral and membranous bone differs significantly. In the long bones (i.e., enchondral bones), bone is deposited in a preformed cartilage precursor. With further growth, a cartilaginous growth plate between the bony epiphysis and diaphysis serves as a center for bone deposition as the length of the bone increases. The mechanism by which compression at the epiphysis stimulates bone formation will be discussed. In membranous bones (e.g., the calvarial bones), new bone deposition is a more passive process. The primary ossification centers of the bones of the calvaria gradually increase in radius until they come into contact with one another at the sutures. The lack of bone fusion at the sutures allows the growth of the brain to increase according to the size of the gap at the sutures. Bone growth continues as the edges of the bone fill the gap. When brain growth is complete, the sutures fuse. The mechanism and control processes that mediate suture fusion are discussed in Chapter 61, dealing with the pathophysiology of premature suture fusion in the craniosynostoses.

In 1870 and 1892 Wolff described the relationship between bone structure and function on the basis of his own work and the earlier observations of von Meyer (1867) (see also Roux, 1893; Koch, 1917). It was observed that bone cortex and trabeculae were oriented in such a way that the bone could best withstand the muscular and gravitational stresses to which it was subjected. Wolff's law of bone remodeling continues to stand the test of time. Teleologic reasoning was often put forth in describing this biomechanical phenomenon.

In 1957 Fukada and Yasuda made a critical observation that paved the way to an understanding of bone remodeling as theorized by Wolff. They discovered that if a bone was subjected to mechanical stress, an electric charge was generated. As news of the discovery spread, it became evident that bone deposition occurred in areas of electronegativity, while bone resorption was associated with electropositivity (Becker, Bassett, and Bachman, 1964; Friedenberg and Kohanim, 1968; Brighton, 1984; Black, 1984; Bassett, 1982). Fukada and Yasuda (1957) attributed the separation of charge to the piezoelectric effect. There is evidence that electrokinetic mechanisms may also be active (Pollack, 1984). Figure 18–9 illustrates how mechanical stress that generates an electric charge results in bone remodeling. Following improper reduction of a tibial fracture, the bone may initially heal with an angle at the fracture line rather than being straight. As compression forces are applied to the ends of the bone, the mechanical stresses at the fracture site differ, depending on whether one views the concave or the convex cortical surface. On the concave side there is compression of the cortex. On the convex side the cortex

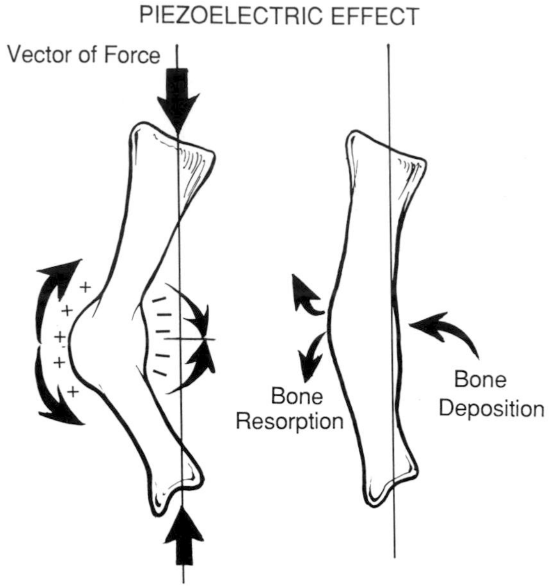

Figure 18–9. A long bone that has been allowed to heal with an angulation at the fracture site will remodel to become straighter through a bioelectric mechanism. Weight bearing causes compression on the concave side of the bone, producing electronegativity, which in turn results in bone deposition. On the convex side of the callus the bone is actually being stretched, producing electropositivity. Bone resorption occurs on the convex side. This mechanism results in a gradual straightening of the angulated long bone.

is actually under stretch. This induces an electric charge that is negative on the concave side and positive on the convex side. The charge causes bone deposition on the concave side and resorption on the convex side. As the remodeling process continues, the bone once again become straight. Bassett (1982) and others used artificially induced electric current to stimulate bone growth in malunions and other pathologic states.

Enlow (1963) viewed craniofacial skeletal structure as being defined by the muscular forces applied to it. Figure 18–10 is modified from his concept of the development of the mandibular angle. In the newborn there is little evidence of a mandibular angle, with the ramus and body lying in nearly a straight line. The pull of the masseter muscle causes the bone on the outside to compress, while the bone on the inner aspect of the mandibular angle is stretched. As in the case of the long bone fracture just described, the bone becomes electronegative, causing bone deposition on the convex side of the mandibular angle, and it becomes electropositive on the concave side of the angle, causing resorption. Use of the masseter for mastication is therefore responsible for the development of the shape of the mandibular angle. Similarly, the pull of the mylohyoid muscle on the inferior aspect of the mandibular body may be seen to produce an increase in the width of the lower jaw with growth. As one reflects on the orientation of the muscles of the face, most of the elements of facial bone growth and remodeling can be understood. Moss and Salentijn (1969) extended this idea with the notion of a *functional soft tissue matrix* around the bone being the principal determinant of facial bone growth. Harvold (1968) used these principles in the treatment of craniofacial microsomia by constructing orthopedic appliances designed to stimulate the soft tissue matrix in the desired direction.

VASCULARIZED BONE TRANSFERS

Much of the early clinical experience with vascularized bone transfer involved various types of cranioplasty (Rogers, 1930; Woolf and Walker, 1945). Ollier suggested the osteoplastic flap in 1867, but Wagner was the first to perform the procedure in 1889. Mueller and Koenig both reported transposition of vascularized cranial bone based on full-thickness scalp in 1890 (Bardenheuer, 1892). Durante (1904) transferred the outer table of the calvarium for cranioplasty based only on the periosteum. This was popularized by Watson-Jones (1933). In 1905 Huntington performed the first successful vascularized fibula interposition into a large tibial bone defect. The success of this last procedure, in what had previously been a nearly impossible clinical situation, pointed to the clear superiority of vascularized bone transfer. Unfortunately, fibula interposition could be performed only rarely as this bone was usually injured with the tibia. Unlike the nonvascularized bone graft, the vast majority of which is composed of dead bone matrix, the vascularized bone flap maintains its cellular viability. Bone flaps heal in a manner analogous to simple fracture healing. "Creeping substitution" of dead bone matrix by bone-forming cells at the periphery is not required. Moreover, vascularized bone transfers undergo less resorption than nonvascularized grafts (Cutting and McCarthy, 1983). Central resorption in a bone graft causes it to become mechanically weaker than vascularized bone transfers (Moore, Mazur, and Zehr, 1981).

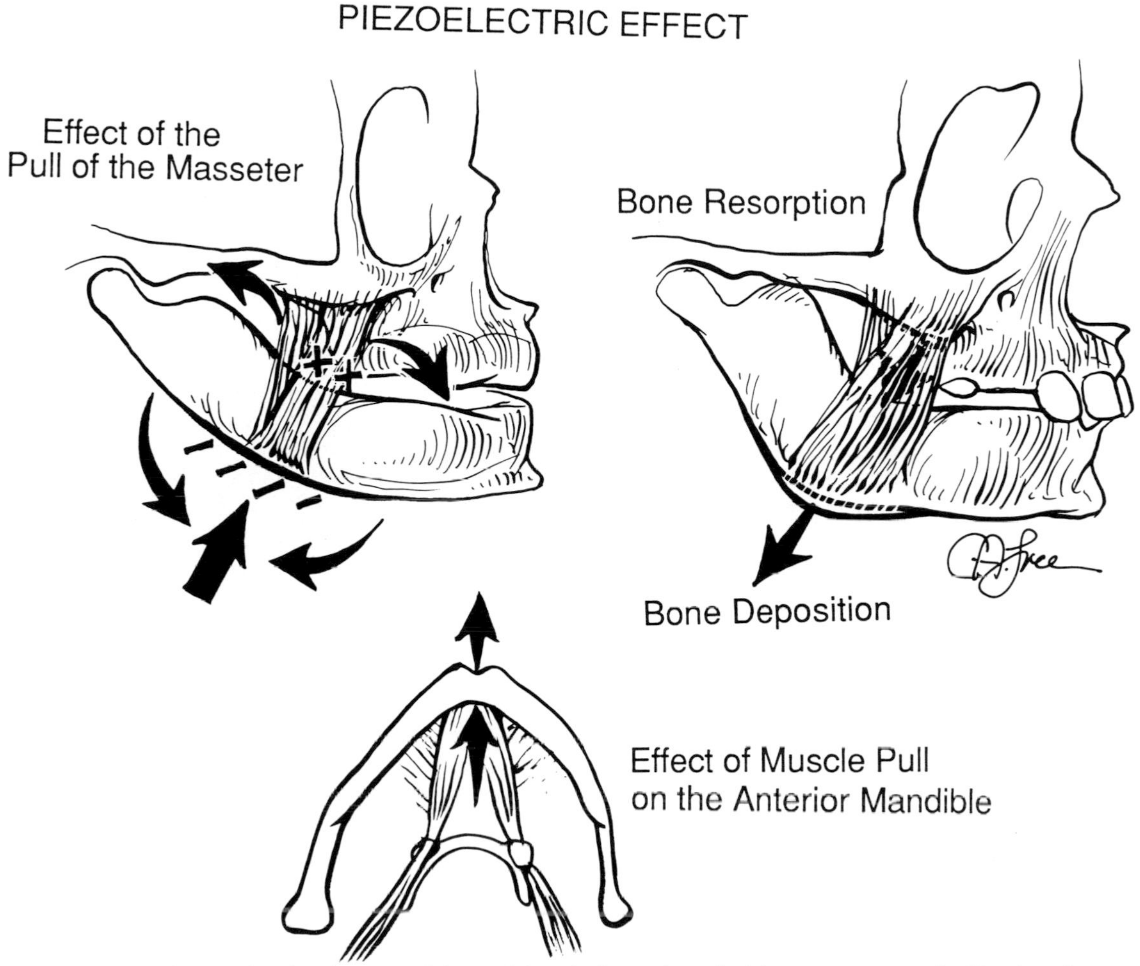

Figure 18–10. Progressive development of the gonial angle due to the pull of the masseter muscle. Muscle pull causes compression on the outer side of the future angle of the mandible, and an elongation or stretching of the bone on the opposite side of the cortex. In a manner analogous to that described in Figure 18–9, the electropositivity and negativity thus induced result in the progressive development of a mandibular angle. In like manner, the pull of the digastric and geniohyoid muscles result in the downward and forward growth of the chin point. Applying this mechanistic view to bone-muscle relationships allows one to understand bone development and predict the skeletal abnormalities that result from various pathologic neuromuscular conditions.

Experience with reconstruction of the mandible following ablative surgery for cancer demonstrates other advantages of vascularized bone reconstruction (Macomber and Shepard, 1948; Conley, 1953, 1972; McDowell and Ohlwiler, 1962; Snyder and associates, 1970; Rosen and associates, 1979; Panje and Cutting, 1980; Dufresne and associates, 1987). In 1918 Blair was the first to note the superiority of a vascularized composite bone flap in mandible reconstruction after tumor resection. As radiation therapy proved its usefulness in improving the cure rates for squamous cell cancer of the oral cavity, the difficulties of mandible reconstruction compounded. The high bacterial count in the oral cavity tends to make bone grafting of the mandible more hazardous than in other sites. Bone grafting of the mandible was well developed as a result of experience with war injuries in healthy young men. These techniques were considerably less successful in older patients with oral cavity cancer who were frequently in a poor nutritional state and for whom radiation therapy was to be administered. The poor blood supply and the ease of tissue breakdown, which occur secondary to radiation therapy, produces a recipient tissue bed unfavorable to the chances of success of a conventional bone graft. As experience with various methods of reconstructing the mandible with vascularized bone grew, the incidence of rapid primary healing increased.

The microsurgical revolution in plastic surgery has vastly expanded the potential for vascularized bone reconstruction. The number of bone donor sites in the body is, however, relatively limited. The use of muscle as a vascular carrier for a bone transfer is applicable in some situations (Rydygier, 1908; Codivilla, 1910; Davis and Taylor, 1952; Baadsgaard and Medgyesi, 1965) but often the short rotation arc severely limits a flap's versatility. Microvascular anastomosis makes transfer of any bone donor site to any recipient site possible (Ostrup and Fredrickson, 1974, 1975). In Chapters 29 and 82 specific examples of transfer of vascularized ilium, scapula, metatarsus, radius, rib, fibula, and calvarium are presented. The following section concerns itself only with the conceptual basis for such transfers.

Vascularized bone transfer raises the expectation that the transferred tissue may grow. Donski, Carwell, and Sharzer (1979) experimentally transferred a growing epiphysis using microvascular anastomoses and demonstrated continued growth in the transfer (Freeman, 1965). Clinical work with the transfer of the second metatarsal to the mandibular ramus in hemifacial microsomia demonstrated the efficacy of transfer of the growing epiphysis in humans. Antonyshyn, Cocleugh, and Anderson (1987) and LaTrenta, McCarthy, and Cutting (1987) showed that vascularized membranous bone transfers also retain their ability to grow.

Knowledge of bone blood supply is fundamental to the design and technique of vascularized bone flaps. In the development of free flaps the plastic surgery community rediscovered the work of the German anatomists of the late nineteenth century. As Manchot (1889) and Spalteholz (1893) pointed the way to the development of many cutaneous free flaps, Langer (1877) and Lexer, Kuliga, and Turk (1904) sought the vascular supply of osseous flaps. Subsequently, Johnson (1927), Trueta (1968), and Brookes (1971) focused their attention on the significance of bone blood supply in health and disease.

The long bones receive their blood supply from three principal sources: (1) the nutrient artery, (2) the periosteal vessels of the diaphysis, and (3) the metaphyseal-epiphyseal periosteal vessels (Fig. 18–11). The *nutrient artery* is the principal vascular supply of the long bone. It passes through a canal in the cortex of the bone in the mid-diaphysis and gives off ascending and descending branches that run the length of the marrow space. The vessels of the *diaphyseal periosteum* supply the outer cortex of the diaphysis directly. The last vessel set, and the supply most neglected by the plastic surgery community to date, consists of the periosteal vessels of the *metaphysis and epiphysis*. These vessels are related to the cartilaginous growth plate of the bone during its development. The periosteum of this region usually contains a vascular ring around the growth plate. Unlike the diaphyseal periosteal vessels, the metaphyseal-epiphyseal vessels deeply penetrate the cortex to supply the bone at this area of active growth. After bone growth is complete and the cartilaginous growth plate has disappeared, the penetrating periosteal vessels persist and form an anastomotic network with the nutrient artery system in the marrow space (Fig. 18–12). The importance of this network will be discussed.

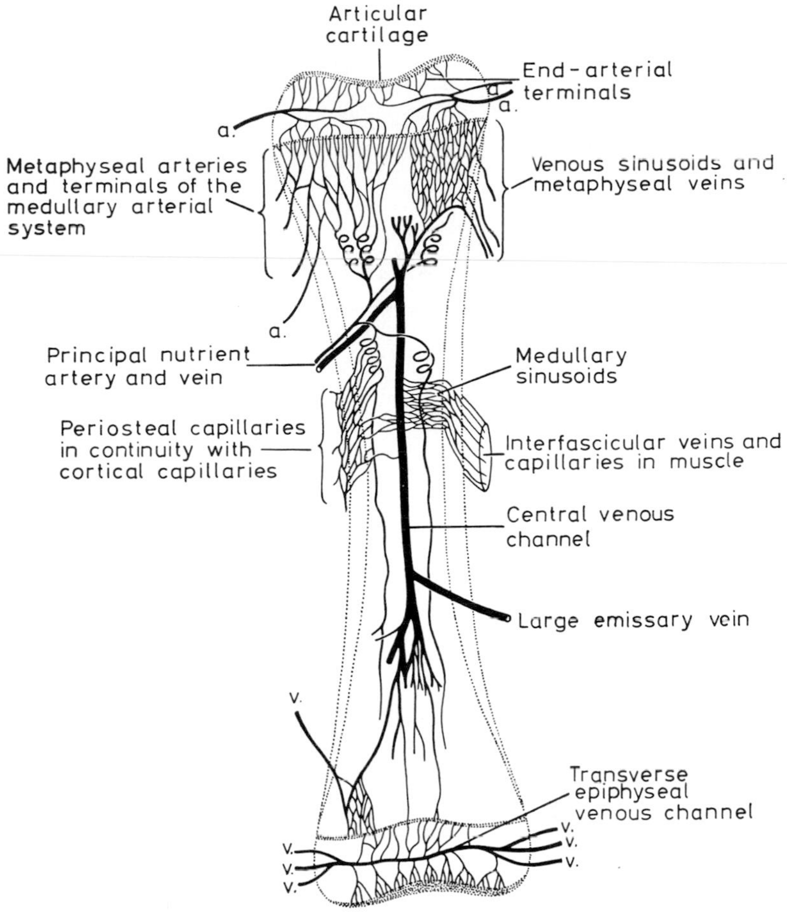

Figure 18–11. The three sources of blood supply to the long bone are illustrated. *A,* The nutrient artery provides the principal source of supply to the marrow cavity and the inner cortex. *B,* The diaphyseal periosteal vessels supply the outer cortex of the diaphysis. *C,* The metaphyseal-epiphyseal periosteal vessels penetrate the cortex of the bone in the adult and anastomose with the nutrient artery, providing adequate supply to the marrow cavity and inner cortex in cases of disruption of the nutrient artery. (From Brookes, M.: The Blood Supply to Bone. London, Butterworths, 1971.)

What is the contribution of each of the three vascular systems to the viability of the long bone? Johnson (1927) performed the pioneering work in this area. This study has been repeated and the findings extended by subsequent work (Huggins and Wiege, 1939; Rhinelander, 1968; Shim, 1968; Shim, Copp, and Patterson, 1968), most notably that of Brookes (1960) and of Trueta and Cavadius (1964). In these studies two of the three vessel systems were interrupted in each experimental group. Angiographic, radiographic, and histologic studies were performed at various times after interruption of all but one of the vessel systems. In this way the significance of each vascular supply system to the long bone was assessed. The periosteal vessels of the diaphysis supply the outer one-third to one-half of the cortex of the bone. The anastomoses through the haversian system are not adequate to perfuse the inner cortex and the marrow. As a result, most of the inner parts of the long bone become necrotic. In response the cortex on the surface thickens and the periosteal vessels proliferate. Resorption and substitution of the central necrotic bone begins. This process was not found to be complete eight months after interruption of the nutrient artery and the metaphyseal system. It is clear that a diaphyseal periosteal pedicle bone transfer produces better survival than a nonvascularized bone graft, but it does not provide sufficient vascular supply to keep most of the long bone alive.

The nutrient artery pedicle provides most of the blood supply to the bone. If all the periosteal supply is interrupted from both the diaphysis and the metaphysis, only the outer one-fourth to one-third of the cortex becomes necrotic. This fact accounts for the popularity of the free fibula transfer in extremity salvage. One criticism of the use of nutrient artery pedicled long bone transfers is that the bone segment cannot be divided and

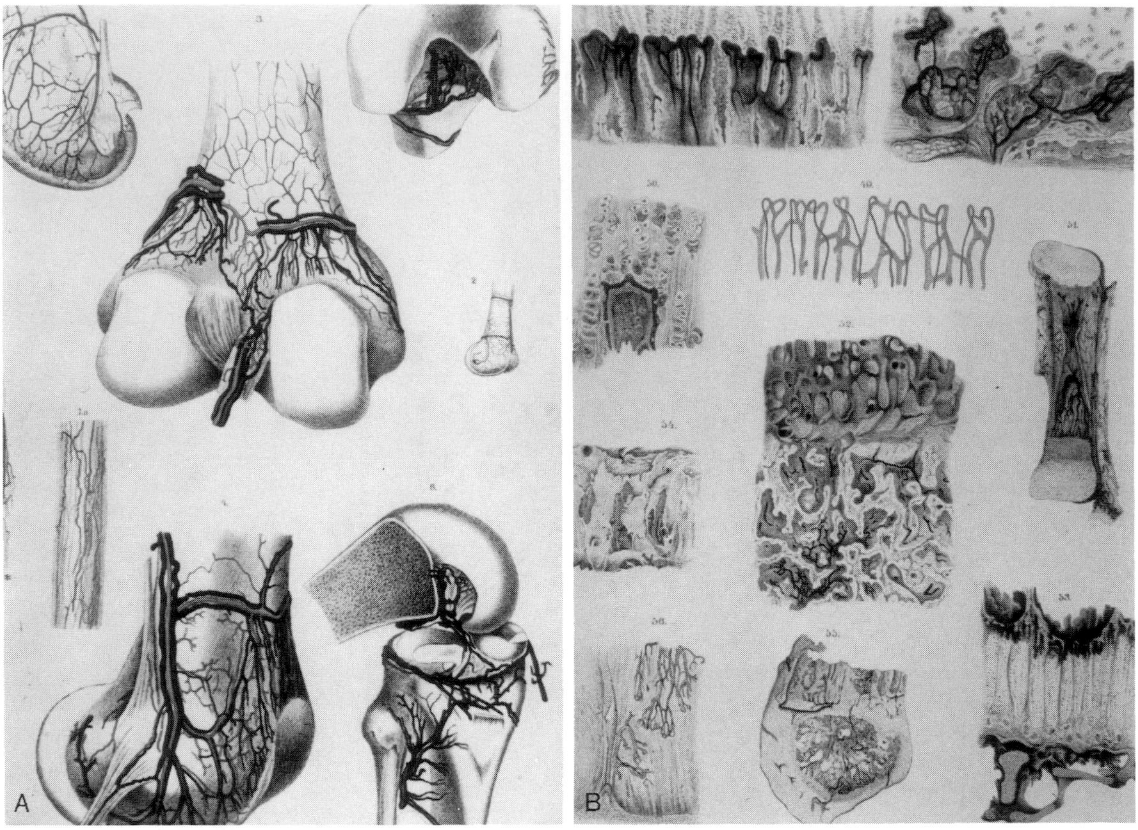

Figure 18–12. *A,* Langer's anatomic drawings of the abundant vascular supply at the distal metaphysis of the femur. *B,* Detailed microangiographic drawings of the blood supply at the cortex of the metaphysis. (From Langer, K.: Ueber das Gefaessystem der Roehrenknochen. Denkschr. Akad. Wiss. Wien, *36*:1, 1876.)

shaped, otherwise the distal bone fragment becomes devascularized. This type of bone transfer is a one-piece bone movement.

The metaphyseal-epiphyseal periosteal supply has not been adequately explored as a vascular leash for bone transfer. When pedicled only on this system, young and old animals exhibited different behavior. In young animals, in whom epiphyseal fusion had not yet occurred, the nutrient artery did not fill from the metaphyseal pedicle. *In older animals, however, the nutrient artery filled from this pedicle almost as completely as in animals in which the nutrient artery was left intact.* In those animals the histologic appearance of the marrow remained normal. More of the cortex became necrotic than in the nutrient artery pedicle group, however, with as much as the outer two-thirds of the cortex exhibiting necrosis. This is later resorbed and replaced by "creeping substitution" from within. This observation explains why a long bone fracture heals well by endosteal healing when the bone on one side is obviously without nutrient artery supply. The vessel has filled in a retrograde manner through anastomoses with the epiphyseal-metaphyseal system (Fig. 18–13).

It should be clear that bone flaps pedicled on the metaphyseal-epiphyseal periosteum will maintain most of the viability of the central part of the bone. When the transfer is pedicled on both the epiphyseal-metaphyseal and the diaphyseal periosteal systems (i.e., only the nutrient artery is divided), there is no evidence of necrosis within the bone whatever. It should be clear that a periosteally pedicled bone transfer in which careful attention has been paid to preserving the metaphyseal-epiphyseal vessels provides a well-vascularized transfer.

The blood supply to the flat or membranous bones is more variable than that of the long bones. Lexer's (Lexer, Kuliga, and Turk, 1904) microangiograms of the ilium appear in Figure 18–14. Although the bones have

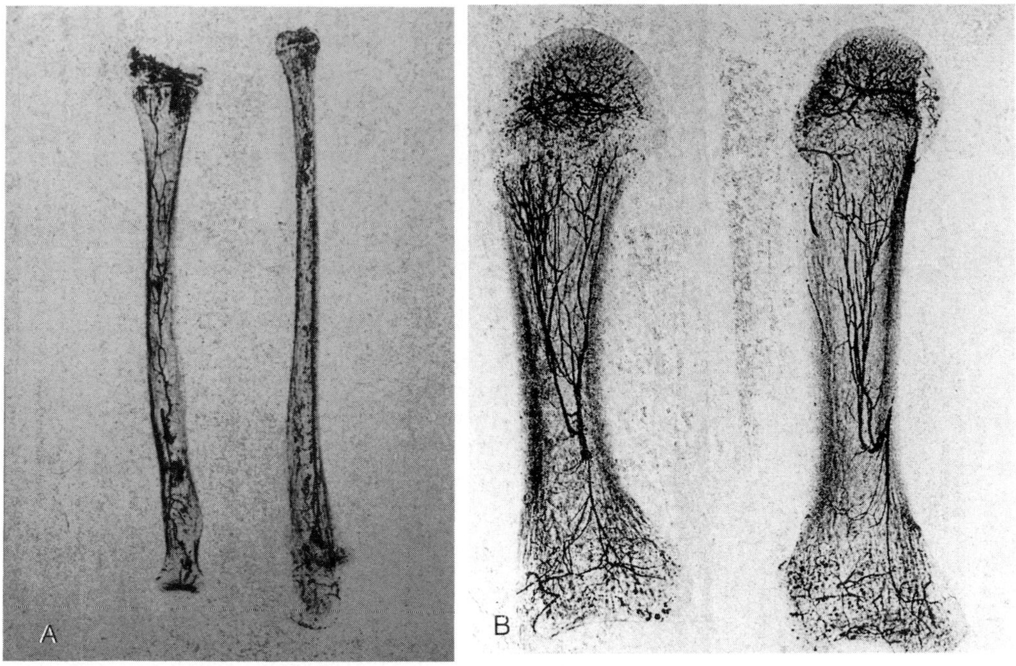

Figure 18–13. *A,* Lexer's microangiograms of the fibula. Aside from the nutrient artery, note the abundance of vessels at the metaphysis. *B,* The metatarsal again demonstrating the preponderance of cortical vessels at the metaphyses. (From Lexer, E.: Knochenbildung in Bindegewebe osteoplastischer Hernkunft. Dtsch. Z. Chir., *217*:1, 1929.)

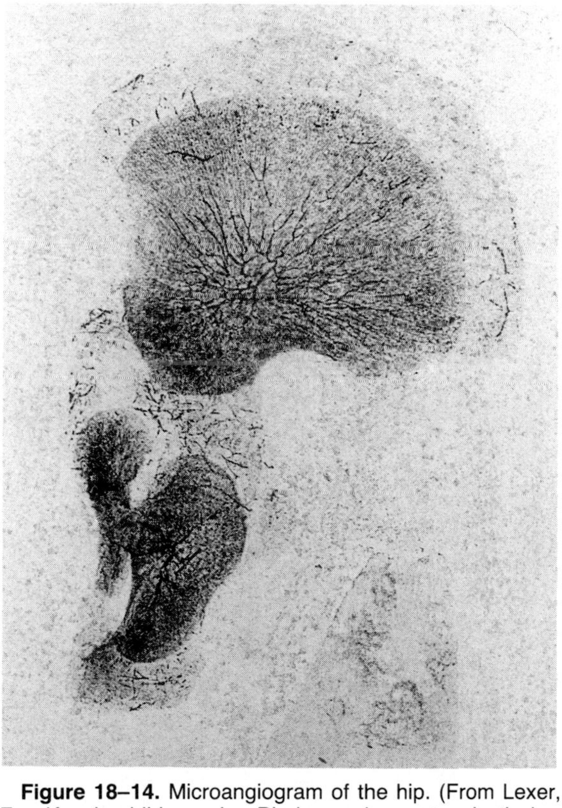

Figure 18–14. Microangiogram of the hip. (From Lexer, E.: Knochenbildung in Bindegewebe osteoplastischer Hernkunft. Dtsch. Z. Chir., *217*:1, 1929.)

nutrient arteries, they are difficult for the plastic surgeon to exploit. Periosteal pedicles are much more common. Fortunately, periosteal vessels penetrate the cortical bone much better in flat bones than in long bones (Baadsgaard and Medgyesi, 1965). In lines of fusion or primary ossification centers in these bones the penetration is particularly good, and may be shown to fill the nutrient vessel canals through anastomotic channels in a manner analogous to the metaphyseal system of long bones (Mall, 1906; Dufresne and associates, 1987). In some ways a vascular leash that includes the length of one of these fusion lines is superior to a nutrient artery pedicle. The bone can be cut on its inner surface into several pieces for shaping without interrupting the blood supply to any of the fragments. This principle is widely applied in Taylor's iliac crest free flap (Taylor, Townsend, and Corlett, 1979a,b) and in flaps using the scapular spine (Panje and Cutting, 1980; Dufresne and associates, 1987).

The blood supply of the calvarium and facial bones is derived from three sources (Figs. 18–15, 18–16) (Cutting, McCarthy, and Berenstein, 1984). Unfortunately, most of the calvarium receives its blood supply from the middle meningeal vessels. This pedicle is ex-

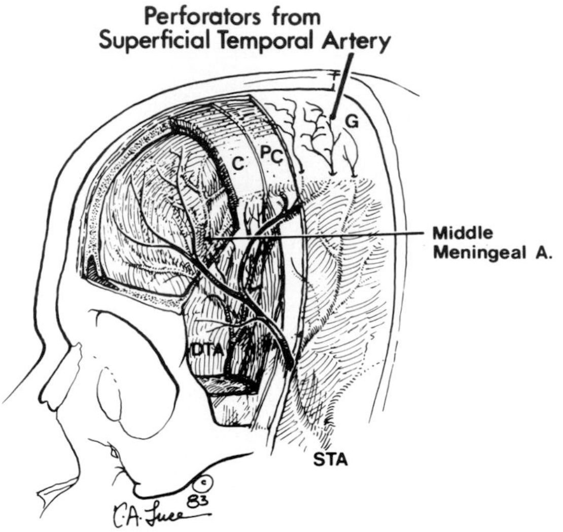

Figure 18–15. The blood supply of the calvarium. The middle meningeal artery provides most of the blood supply to the inner table of the calvarium. The deep temporal vessels under the temporalis muscle supply the squama of the temporal bone. The principal supply to the outer table of the calvaria is through the periosteum, which in turn is supplied by an anastomotic network of vessels lying above the galea-SMAS. This network is formed from the superficial temporal, occipital, posterior auricular, supraorbital, and supratrochlear arteries. (From Cutting, C. B., McCarthy, J. G., and Berenstein, A.: The blood supply of the upper craniofacial skeleton: the search for composite calvarial bone flaps. Plast. Reconstr. Surg., *74*:603, 1984.)

tremely difficult for the surgeon to exploit. The various neurovascular bundles that penetrate the bone also give vascular supply to it. There is a potential clinical application of this finding. The zygoma might be pedicled on the zygomaticofacial and zygomaticotemporal vessels retrograde through a periosteal pedicle containing those bundles. Other neurovascular bundles might be used in a similar fashion. Unfortunately the initial supposition that a rich vascular network connected the outer periosteum to the calvarium in the region of the sutures (Brookes, 1960) has not been found to be correct (Dorenbos, 1971, 1972). In fact the periosteal supply to the outer cortex of the calvarium appears to be relatively tenuous after fusion of the sutures. The broadly diffuse periosteal supply to the calvarium has more recently been used to advantage for vascularized calvarial bone transfers to unfavorable tissue beds (McCarthy and Zide, 1984; McCarthy, Cutting, and Shaw, 1987). The temporalis muscle does not vascularize the calvarium much beyond the superior temporal line. The muscle may be used as a carrier, but the amount of bone that can be transferred with it is limited. The principal vascular supply to the calvarial periosteum is derived from a rich anastomotic network of vessels lying superficial to the galea. The vessels send perforators through the galea to the periosteum (Fig. 18–16). The surgeon can dissect the scalp away from these vessels by staying in a subfollicular plane. A segment of galea with its overlying vessels is carefully left attached to the underlying bone. After the bone is elevated the galea is sutured to the bone edges to prevent shearing (Fig. 18–17). Such a pedicle may be based on the supraorbital, supratrochlear, superficial temporal, or occipital vessels. There is some dif-

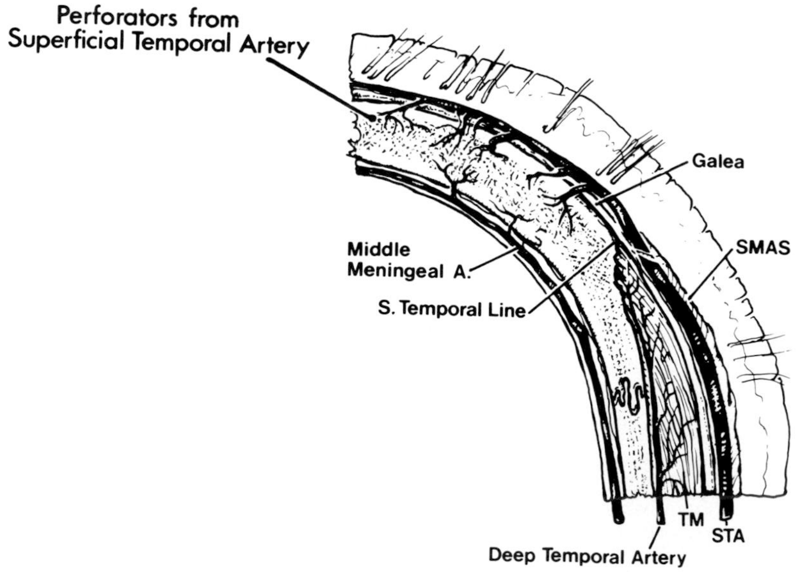

Figure 18–16. Cross-sectional view of the temporoparietal region. The superficial temporal artery sends perforators to the periosteum of the calvarium. The deep temporal artery lies below the temporalis muscle (TM). The middle meningeal artery is the source of most blood supply to the inner calvarial table. Note that it is necessary to elevate the scalp flap in a plane just below the hair follicles (subfollicular) in order to preserve the blood supply derived from the superficial temporal artery (STA). (From Cutting, C. B., McCarthy, J. G., and Berenstein, A.: The blood supply of the upper craniofacial skeleton: the search for composite calvarial bone flaps. Plast. Reconstr. Surg., *74*:603, 1984.)

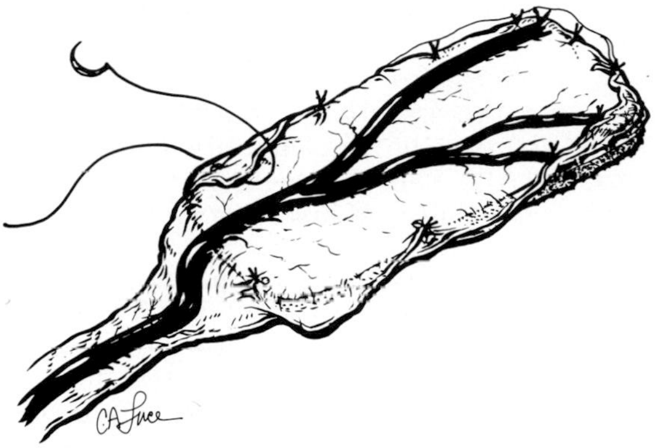

Figure 18–17. The generic calvarial bone flap. A flap of galea, including one of its overlying arteries, is developed by elevating the overlying scalp in a subfollicular plane. The outer table of the calvarium is harvested, care being taken not to divide the galeal perforators. The galea is sutured to the edges of the bone to prevent shearing or dissociation of the pedicle from the bone.

ference of opinion in the literature regarding the adequacy of the anastomotic connections within the pericranium itself. In one study (Cutting, McCarthy, and Berenstein, 1984), these connections were not thought to be adequate to ensure vascularized bone transfer, whereas another study (Casanova and associates, 1986) concluded that they are sufficient.

CLINICAL USES OF BONE TRANSFERS

Tibia

Before World War I and for many years thereafter, the tibia was used as a source of osteoperiosteal grafts of cortical and cancellous bone. The approach is made along the anteromedial surface of the tibia through an incision parallel to the tibial crest. The osteoperiosteal grafts may be removed by cutting the periosteum with a knife and removing shavings of cortex and periosteum with a chisel or gouge (Fig. 18–18). In order to fill a defect, numerous grafts must be superimposed, and the contour is rather irregular. The fact that the grafts are thin accounts for the excellent osteogenic properties of this type of graft. If the amount of bone removed is small, there is little residual defect. If, however, the amount removed is large (e.g., after the removal of a corticocancellous graft), a bone defect is produced that not only is disfiguring but also is the cause of pain and frequently secondary (pathologic) fracture.

Ilium

Nonvascularized Autografts. Over the past four decades the ilium has become a favorite source of bone grafts. It is composed almost entirely of cortical bone with an abundant supply of cancellous bone, and is of variable thickness, surrounded by two thin plates of cortex. The fact that the iliac crest is so accessible makes the removal of the graft relatively simple, and the secondary defect is usually covered. However, the morbidity that follows the removal of this graft (in terms of bleeding, ileus, pain, and limping due to muscular spasm) is great in relation to the amount of bone removed.

One of the thicker (1.3 to 1.7 cm) areas of the iliac crest is the anterior one-third between the anterior superior iliac spine and the tubercle of the crest. Posterior to this area the crest and ala become thinner until the posterior iliac spine is reached; the thinner region provides an additional source of bone.

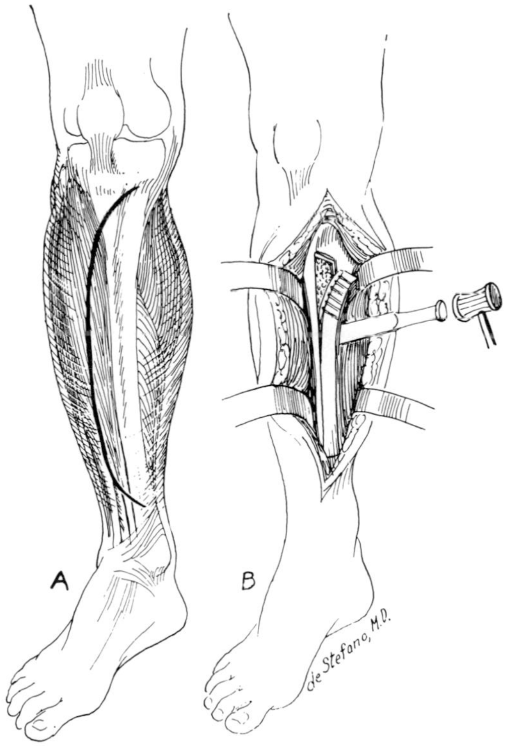

Figure 18–18. Tibial grafts. *A,* Incision for removal of the graft. *B,* Removal of the graft with an osteotome.

Technique. The incision extends through the skin and periosteum to the crest of the ilium. Just before the incision, the skin is retracted by the assistant so that the incision lies lateral to and below the crest instead of over the crest (Fig. 18–19). The periosteum is reflected and raised with a periosteal elevator (Fig. 18–20*A*). A part of the crest, the full thickness of the crest (Fig. 18–20*B*), or the inner table is exposed (Fig. 18–20*C*), depending on the amount and shape of the bone graft required. The periosteum covering the outer surface of the ala is also raised if the full thickness of the ala is required (Fig. 18–20*B*). The inner table of the ilium and adherent cancellous bone are resected when a wider surface of bone is required; the periosteum is further elevated, raising the iliac muscle with the periosteum and thus exposing a portion of the iliac fossa. By vertical sectioning of a portion of the crest between the vertical cuts, a section of the inner cortical table, with its underlying cancellous bone, may be separated and removed from the outer table (Fig. 18–20*C*). The inner surface of the ilium is exposed rather than the lateral aspect, for the periosteum is raised with greater ease over the smooth medial surface, which is roofed over the iliac muscle. The lateral aspect of the bone is uneven in the adult, serving as the area of insertion for the gluteal muscles.

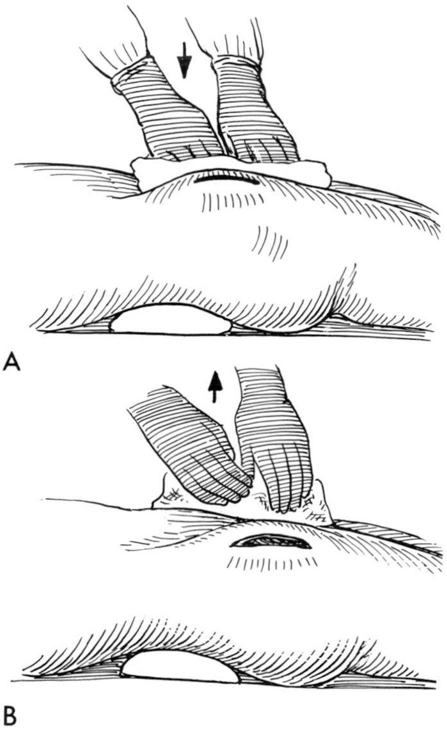

A

B

Figure 18–19. Exposure of the crest of the ilium for bone graft. *A,* The patient's hip is elevated by a sandbag to make the iliac crest prominent. The assistant presses a gauze pad against the skin just below the crest of the ilium and retracts the skin over the crest. *B,* The skin incision lies lateral to the crest of the ilium.

In the adult, when cancellous bone alone is needed, an osteotomy is made over the central portion of the iliac crest, and a wedge of cancellous bone is resected (Fig. 18–21); the outer and inner tables of the ilium are then fractured toward each other with heavy forceps in order to eliminate the resulting dead space between them. The technique does not disturb the continuity of the crest and leaves no visible deformity.

The technique advocated by Robertson and Baron (1946) can be employed when a large amount of cancellous bone is required. In this technique, the bone is sectioned below the crest of the ilium, reflecting the crest upward and preserving the origin of the abdominal muscles (Fig. 18–22). Cancellous bone is removed from the center of the bone after separation of the cortical surfaces, and the crest is replaced in its original position; cancellous chips can be removed with a gouge.

Patients experience more discomfort and difficulty in early ambulation when the full thickness of the ala is removed than when the outer table of the ilium is preserved. This inconvenience may be the result either of the extensive stripping of the lateral surface of the ilium to obtain wide exposure or of the weakening of the attachments of the gluteal musculature, the fascia lata, and the tensor of the fascia lata. The result is the so-called "gluteus gait," a persistent type of dragging limp. When the wound is being closed, care should be exercised to obtain a strong repair of the fascia lata, if divided, and an accurate apposition of the edges of the periosteum from which the abdominal and gluteal muscles arise.

Although it is occasionally necessary to remove all or part of the anterior superior iliac spine, this is likely to be attended by a palpable contour irregularity and a definite morbidity, and is better avoided. The outer edge of the crest gives attachment to the fascia lata and origin to the tensor fascia lata. Failure of repair may result in disturbances of gait, as already noted, or a "clicking" sound when the patient walks, produced

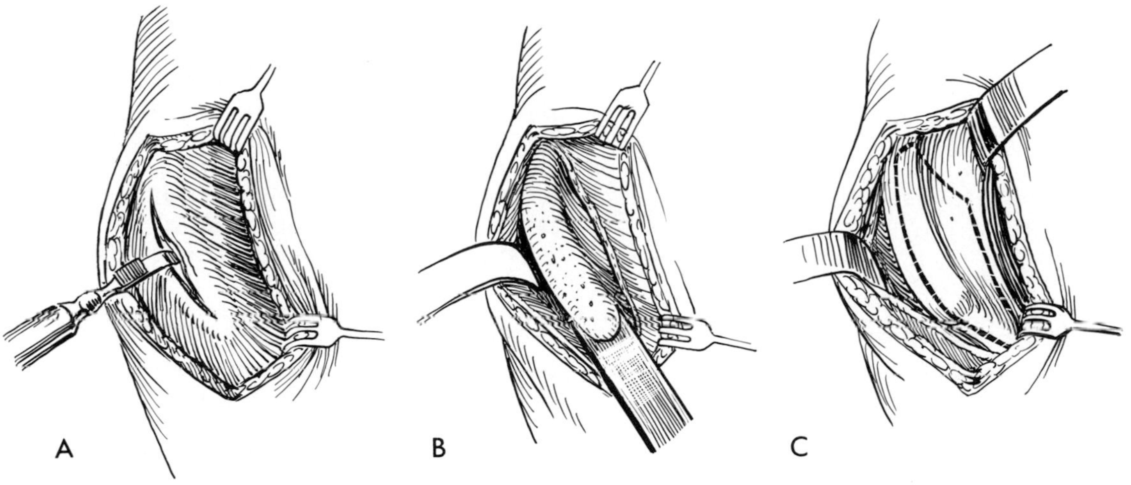

Figure 18–20. Removal of bone from the ilium. *A,* The periosteum has been incised and is being raised by an elevator. *B,* Resection of bone from the crest. *C,* Resection of bone from the inner table.

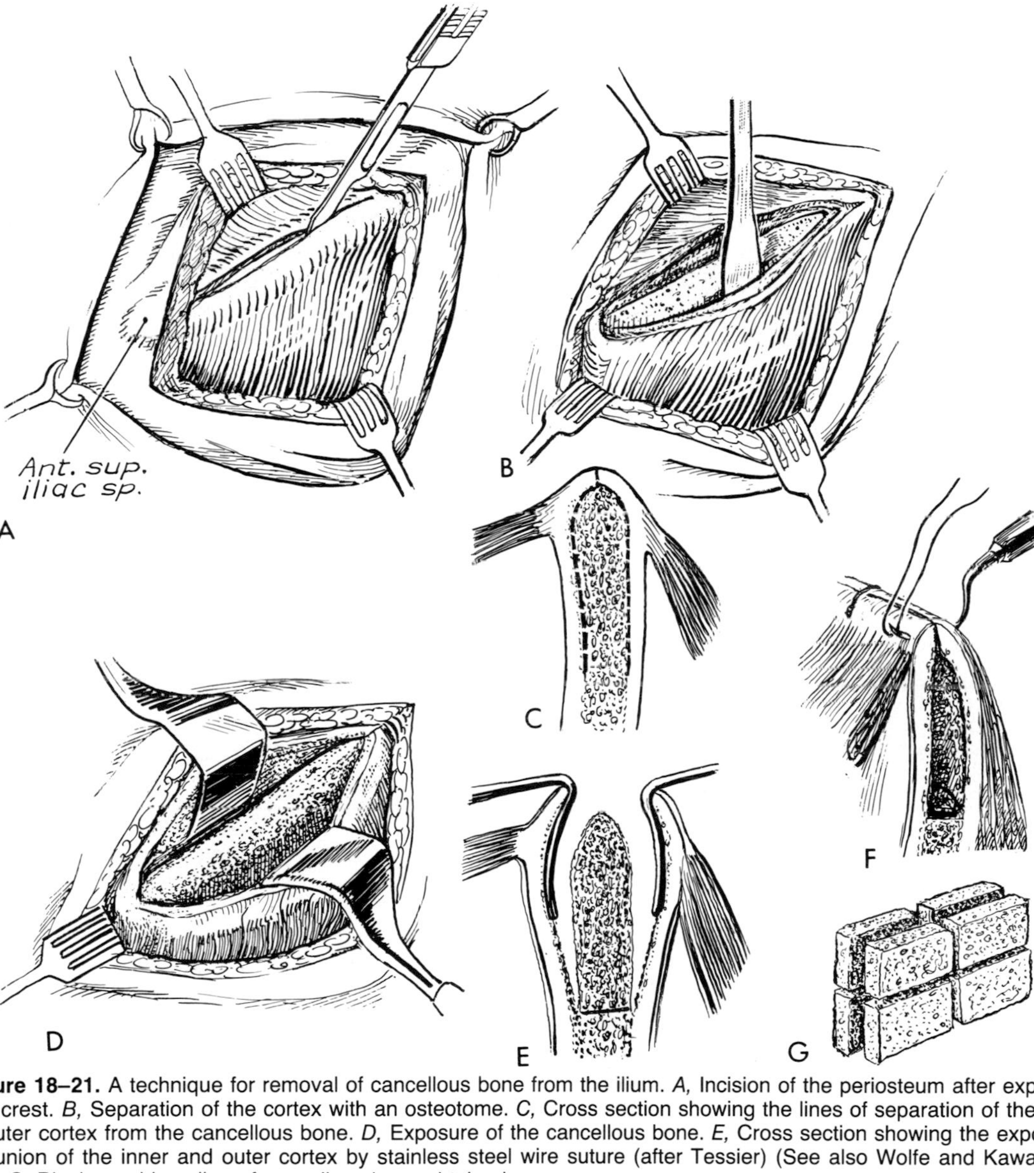

Figure 18–21. A technique for removal of cancellous bone from the ilium. *A,* Incision of the periosteum after exposure of the crest. *B,* Separation of the cortex with an osteotome. *C,* Cross section showing the lines of separation of the inner and outer cortex from the cancellous bone. *D,* Exposure of the cancellous bone. *E,* Cross section showing the exposure. *F,* Reunion of the inner and outer cortex by stainless steel wire suture (after Tessier) (See also Wolfe and Kawamoto, 1978). *G,* Blocks and lamellae of cancellous bone obtained.

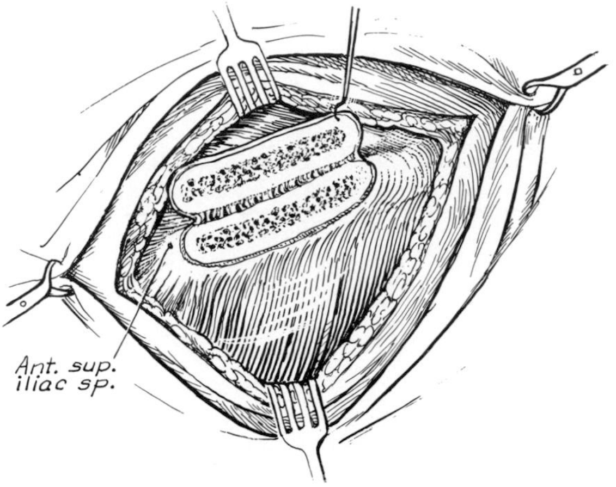

Figure 18–22. The crest of the ilium has been separated, remaining attached to the abdominal musculature. The cancellous bone is exposed.

by the fascia slipping suddenly over the greater trochanter instead of gliding smoothly over it.

The lateral femoral cutaneous nerve of the thigh, in its pelvic location, takes a retroperitoneal course on the deep surface of the iliac muscle (Fig. 18–23). It leaves the pelvis by a variable route, usually just deep to the attachment of the inguinal ligament to the anterior and superior iliac spine, but sometimes through the ligament or even across the spine itself (Ghent, 1961). The nerve is thus easily damaged in this region, producing paresthesia and hypoesthesia, which may be permanent over the lateral aspect of the thigh.

Interference with the attachment of the inguinal ligament or removal of massive grafts of the full thickness of the ilium may also lead to the formation of hernias (Oldfield, 1945; Reid, 1968).

Cancellous bone bleeds readily, and hematoma formation is common, particularly if the inner table of the bone has been exposed, since a dead space remains between the bone and the detached iliac muscle. Gelfoam soaked in thrombin solution or bone wax may be rubbed into the bleeding cancellous bone; hemorrhage from a spurting vessel is arrested by crushing the bone around the vessel. If the full thickness of the ala is removed, the dead space can be eliminated by suturing the iliac muscle to the glutei, as advised by Dingman (1950). When relatively small bone grafts are resected from the iliac crest, a pressure dressing will collapse the dead space and prevent hematoma formation. It is the authors' practice, after exposure of the inner table, to leave a drain with continuous suction to evacuate the accumulated blood. The drain is placed in such a way that it may be removed without displacing the entire dressing. Early ambulation reduces the period of discomfort and disability.

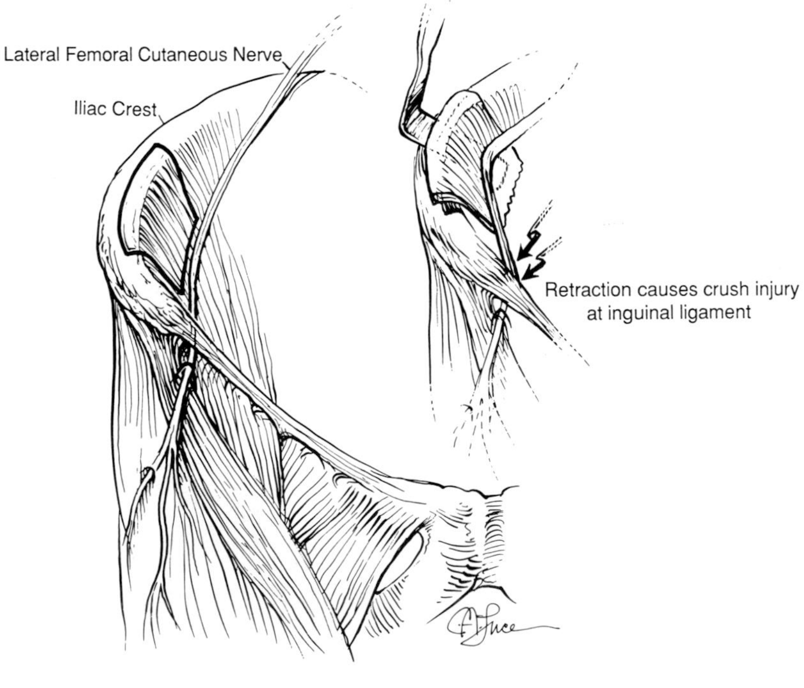

Figure 18–23. The course of the lateral femoral cutaneous nerve and a common way to injure it simply by excessive retraction.

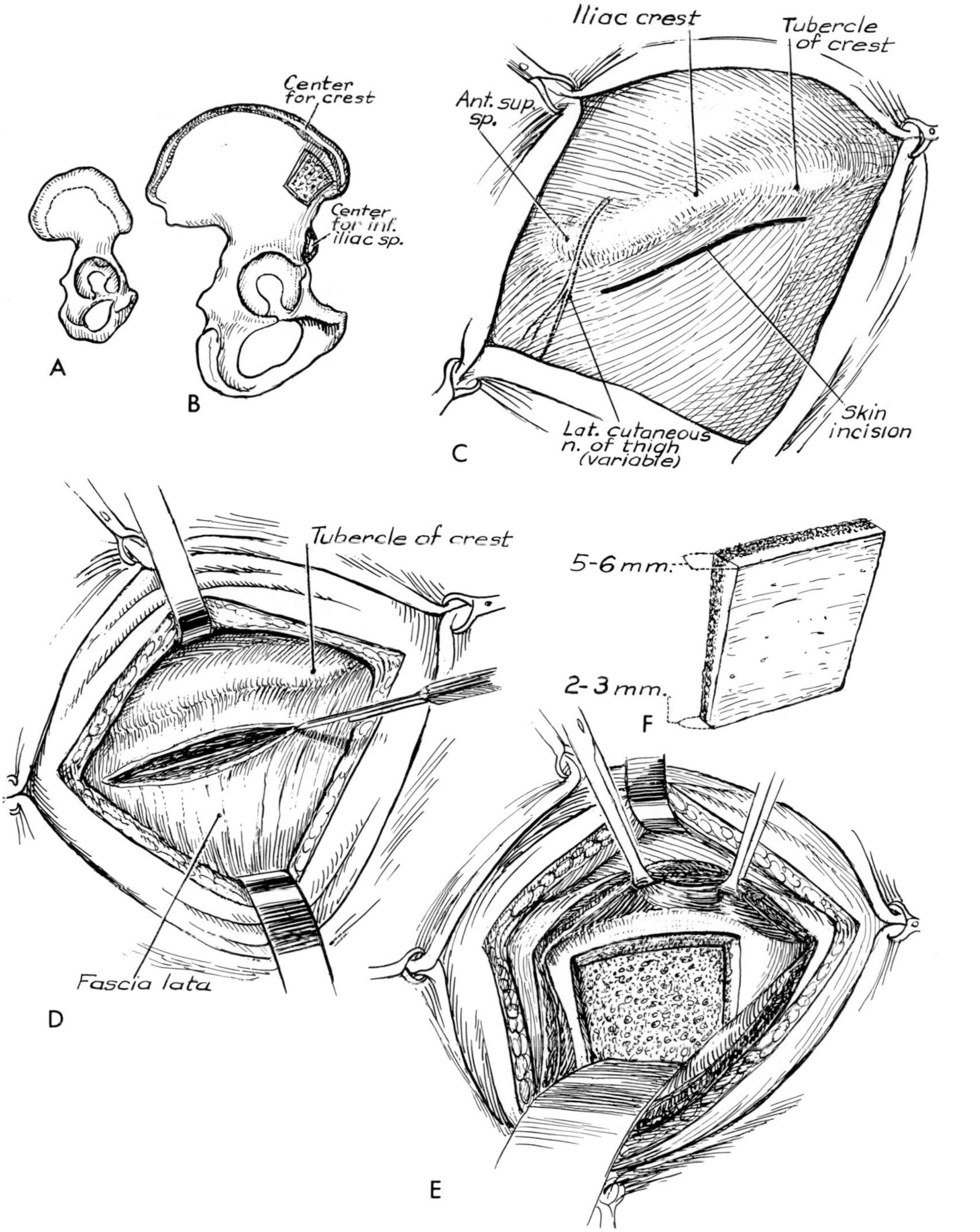

Figure 18–24. The ilium as a donor site for bone grafts in children. *A,* At birth approximately two-thirds of the ilium is ossified. The width of the cartilaginous epiphyseal crest is indicated by the dotted line. *B,* The ilium at birth. The growth centers for the iliac crest and the anteroinferior spine are indicated, as well as the site of bone graft removal. *C,* The site of the skin incision. *D,* The fascia lata and muscles are incised down to bone. *E,* The bone graft has been removed; the inner table is spared. *F,* The thickness of the bone graft removed in a 12 year old child. (From Crockford, D. A., and Converse, J. M.: The ilium as a source of bone grafts in children. Plast. Reconstr. Surg., *50*:270, 1972. Copyright 1972, The Williams & Wilkins Company, Baltimore.)

THE BUTTONHOLE INCISION FOR CANCELLOUS CHIPS. When cancellous chips are required to enhance the osteogenic processes along a line of osteotomy or to provide additional contour restoration, a short incision is made immediately behind the anterosuperior spine. Cancellous bone is abundant in this area and is resected without submitting the patient to a major operation.

Ilium as a Source of Bone Grafts in Children. Bone grafts, either in the form of corticocancellous grafts or cancellous chips, are in general use for a number of pediatric reconstructive procedures. Breine and Johanson (1966) found that in infants the tibia yields sufficient material for alveolar grafts in the cleft palate deformity. Knowledge of the various dimensions of the ilium in a child allows the surgeon to obtain a surprising amount of corticocancellous and cancellous bone (Crockford and Converse, 1972). Moreover, it is possible to secure such bone through a subepiphyseal lateral approach, without in any way disturbing the integrity of the epiphyses of the crest—a disadvantage of the previously described techniques (Crenshaw, 1963).

APPLIED ANATOMY. At birth, the crest of the ilium is composed of a thick cap of primary cartilage that forms the rims and superior part of the ala, and which sits on the ossifying part of the body of the bone (Fig. 18–24*A*). By the age of 9 years, this layer is only 1 cm in height. It is not until puberty that one or two secondary centers appear in it; they unite at 20 to 25 years of age (Brash, 1951).

Before puberty and the adolescent growth spurt, there is little difference between the pelvic bones of the sexes (Tanner, 1962). Thereafter, the characteristic changes of shape, angulation, and thickness occur, the female bone remaining thinner than that of the male (Bryce, 1915). Further information was obtained from observations made in 26 infants, children, and young adolescents in the course of bone graft removals. Fig. 18–25 shows, by transillumination, that the bone in the center of the iliac fossa is the thinnest part and may even be defective. This thin area lies posterior to a radius drawn through the tubercle of the crest, an easily identifiable landmark (Fig. 18–26, *cut 2*). As the tubercle also indicates the posterior limit of the thickest part of the crest, it is the bone between the tubercle and the anterosuperior iliac spine that forms the best source of grafts.

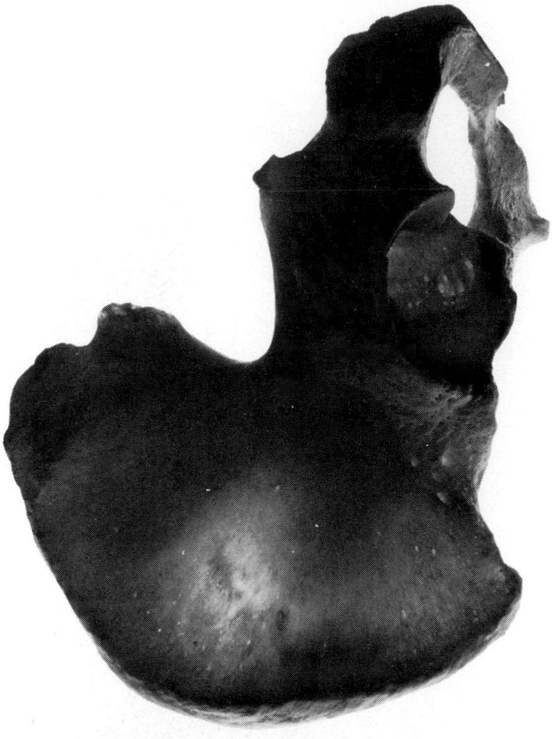

Figure 18–25. Transillumination shows that the thinnest part of the bone is in the center of the iliac fossa. (From Crockford, D. A., and Converse, J. M.: The ilium as a source of bone grafts in children. Plast Reconstr. Surg., *50*:270, 1972. Copyright 1972, The Williams & Wilkins Company, Baltimore.)

Measurements of fresh adult cadavers show that, for an "average" pelvis, the thickness of the crest 2 cm posterior to the anterior superior iliac spine is 1.5 cm; this increases to 1.7 cm through the tubercle. However, along a radius taken through the first point (Fig. 18–26, *cut 1*), the thinnest area is 0.9 cm; an equivalent figure in the line of the tubercle is 0.5 cm. As can be readily appreciated from Figure 18–26, *cut 3*, the bone becomes progressively thinner posterior to the tubercle, until the region of the sacroiliac articulation is reached. The dimensions in childhood are proportionately less. In the 9 year old, the thickest part of the crest is between 0.8 and 1.0 cm.

When a child is operated on, the immediate region of the anterosuperior iliac spine should remain inviolate, owing to its important ligamentous and muscular attachments.

The two important structures disturbed by this operation are the *fascia lata,* which is attached along the line of the crest, and the *tensor fascia lata* muscle, which originates in the anterior quarter of the lateral edge of the

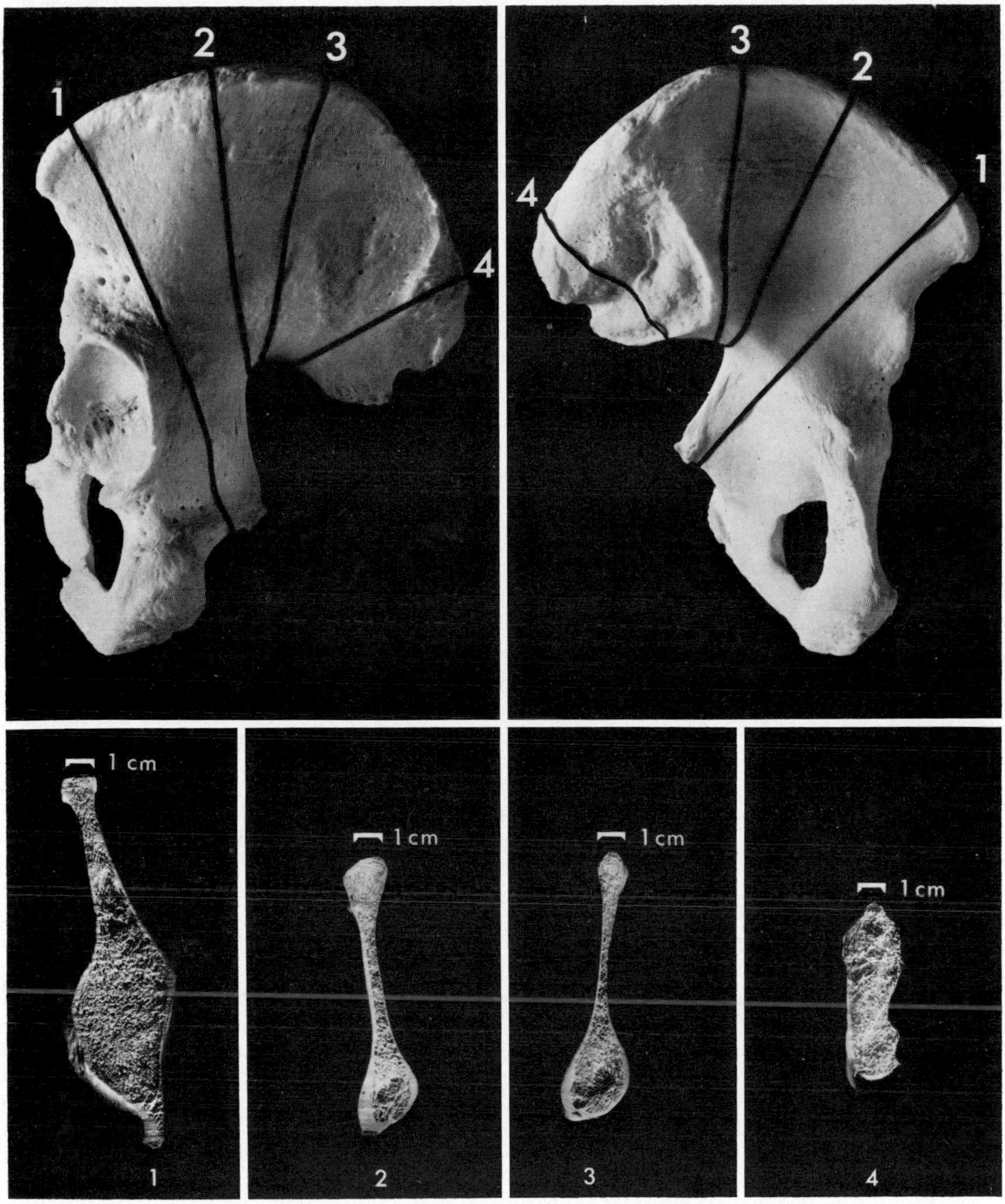

Figure 18–26. The same specimen as that in Figure 18–25. In the two top photographs, the black marker tapes show the lines of section. In the lower photographs, the cross-sectional appearance of the bone is shown—at the lines of section, looking anteriorly at each. *Cut 1,* Through the crest 2 cm posterior to the anterior superior iliac spine. *Cut 2,* Through the tubercle of the crest. *Cut 3,* Through the thinnest part of the crest. *Cut 4,* Through the posterior superior iliac spine. The photographs are all the same scale. (From Crockford, D. A., and Converse, J. M.: The ilium as a source of bone grafts in children. Plast Reconstr. Surg., *50*:270, 1972. Copyright 1972, The Williams & Wilkins Company, Baltimore.)

crest. The normal locking of the knee joint in extension is dependent on the perfect function of these two structures.

TECHNIQUE IN CHILDREN. Before draping, the pelvis is rotated 30 to 40 degrees away from the surgeon on sandbags. It is also advisable to place a sandbag under the ipsilateral shoulder to prevent excessive spinal rotation. The skin is prepared and draped in the usual fashion, leaving the anterosuperior iliac spine and the anterior half of the crest exposed.

After retraction of the skin medially by an assistant (to ensure that the final position of the scar is well clear of the iliac crest), the incision is made in the line of the crest, starting 1 to 2 cm posterior to the anterosuperior iliac spine and extending posteriorly as far as necessary. The wound is deepened through the superficial fascia to the *fascia lata,* and hemostasis is secured (see Fig. 18–24*C,D*). With a knife, an incision is made through the *fascia lata* and the underlying muscle down to the bone; the line of the incision should lie approximately 2 cm below the curve of the crest (Fig. 18–24*C,D*). The bone is exposed by subperiosteal dissection; care is taken superiorly not to disrupt the firm attachment of the periosteum to the epiphyseal line.

When hemostasis has been obtained, the corticocancellous graft or grafts required may be marked out with the corner of an osteotome, keeping at least 1 to 1.5 cm posterior to the anterior superior iliac spine and the anterior edge of the ilium. Using a curved osteotome of the required width, the surgeon can remove the grafts (Fig. 18–24*E,F*). With care, such an instrument will stay in the plane of the medulla. When sufficient graft has been obtained, a large curette or gouge may be used to harvest the cancellous bone lying between the two tables of the anterior (so far untouched) part of the ilium.

The wound should be closed in layers—*fascia lata* and muscle, Scarpa's fascia, and skin. It is rarely possible to make a comprehensive repair of the periosteum, but it cannot be too strongly emphasized that, if the *tensor fascia lata* muscle and the *fascia lata* are not thoroughly repaired, an abnormal gait may result.

Vascularized Iliac Transfers. The blood supply to the ilium has been thoroughly investigated by Taylor, Townsend, and Corlett (1979a,b) with the intention of using it as a donor site for vascularized transfer. As shown in Figure 18–14 the nutrient artery to this bone is extremely difficult to exploit (Lexer, 1929). Fortunately the iliac crest has a long apophysis along the length of its outer edge. This is also the principal site of growth of the crest. After maturation the periosteal vessels penetrate the bone extensively at this site in a manner analogous to the metaphyseal periosteal vessels of the long bone. In many ways this broad source of blood supply to the crest is far superior to a nutrient artery pedicle in that the bone may be cut and shaped with preservation of the blood supply to every part of the graft. Investigation has centered on which of the vessels provides the best source of blood supply to the periosteum. Initially the superficial circumflex iliac vessels were used in conjunction with a free groin skin flap for coverage. Taylor, Townsend, and Corlett (1979a,b) subsequently showed that the deep circumflex iliac artery that takes its origin from the external iliac artery deep to the inguinal ligament is a much better source of blood supply to the bone. In Chapter 29 the use of this free osteocutaneous flap for mandible reconstruction is described in detail.

Greater Trochanter and Olecranon

Autografts. When only a small volume of autologous bone is needed, as is often the case for many hand surgical procedures, convenient donor areas are the greater trochanter and the olecranon process. The olecranon process is especially convenient, since it can be included in the same surgical field as the hand.

An incision over the proximal end of the olecranon process is made down through periosteum. A periosteal elevator is used to expose a 1 cm square area of bone. A 4 mm osteotome is effective to transect the cortex, permitting the removal of a 1 × 1 cm section of cortical bone. Through this opening, cancellous bone can be removed with a curette. If the cortical bone is not needed, it can be replaced over the opening.

The greater trochanter is approached through a 3 to 4 cm vertical incision directly over this bony landmark. The fascia lata and tendinous insertions are split longitudinally, and with the wound retracted, periosteum is raised from the surface of the greater trochanter. An osteotome is used to remove a 1 to 2 cm square section of cortical bone, permitting access to the abundant supply of cancellous bone available in the greater trochanter, which can be removed with a curette. If the cortical bone is not required, it can be used to cover the defect. The wound is closed in layers.

Unlike the case in bone removal from the iliac crest, postoperative morbidity from using either the greater trochanter or the olecranon process is low. In the case of the trochanter, the patient may ambulate early with minimal discomfort.

Rib

Nonvascularized Autografts. Macewen (1912) was among the first to use the rib to repair a mandibular defect. In 1915 Kappis employed full-thickness rib with periosteum to cover a dural and cranial defect. The rib graft fell into disfavor principally because of the way in which it was used. When a whole rib is inserted, the only possible vascular penetration is through the cut ends of the graft and several Volkmann's canals, otherwise the rib presents only dense cortical bone on its surfaces with little chance of survival. The early work of Brown of Australia (1917) and Ballin of America (1921), both of whom suggested splitting the rib, leaving the inner portion of the rib to maintain an intact thoracic wall, made little impression. In 1928 Brown presented a ten-year "postal card" follow-up of his split rib graft cases, including the roentgenograms of one patient. In 1937 Fagarasanu split the rib in order to gain more substance.

Until 1955, no one indicated the fact that rib bone differed from other bone in its osteogenic properties, in its adaptability to fit many defects, and in its extraordinary power to regenerate repeatedly and thus provide a continuous source of autogenous bone to repair even the largest defects. Histologic studies were made on numerous cases (Longacre and deStefano, 1957). At one week (Fig. 18–27) the osteocytes are absent from the lacunae, but living osteoblasts are still present along the surface of some of the trabeculae. At two weeks (Fig. 18–28) there is rapid ingrowth of granulation tissue between the trabeculae and beginning regeneration. There are many areas of resorption of bone with beginning formation of Howship's spaces. In other areas there are living osteoblasts, some of which have already surrounded themselves with osteoid substance

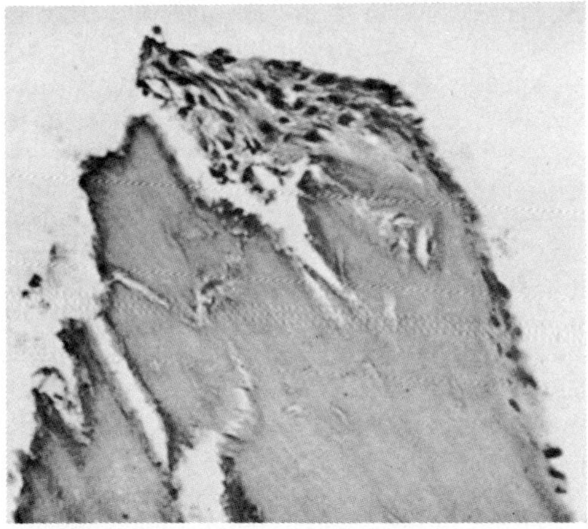

Figure 18–27. Split rib graft removed one week following insertion into a cranial defect. Note the absence of cells in the lacunae and the presence of living osteoblasts along the surface of the trabeculae.

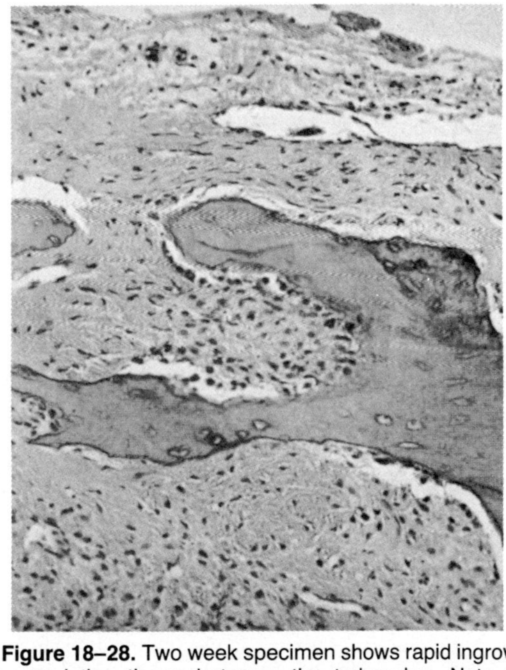

Figure 18–28. Two week specimen shows rapid ingrowth of granulation tissue between the trabeculae. Note the resorption of bone with beginning formation of Howship's spaces in certain areas. In other areas there are living osteoblasts, and some have already surrounded themselves with osteoid tissue.

(osteocytes). The five week specimen (Fig. 18–29) reveals continuing resorption along with the increase in vascularity of the granulation tissue between the trabeculae. There is evidence of active regeneration of new bone along the surfaces of most of the trabeculae. This process is most active in the neighborhood of blood vessels with the beginning of osteon formation. The six month specimen (Fig. 18–30) shows the split rib grafts attached to the skull by a layer of fibrous tissue, and between the two there is an area of newly formed bone with some areas not yet calcified. There is osteoid substance around some rather large (young) osteocytes. The remaining portion of the graft reveals reversal lines and a few areas of resorption, but for the most part the split rib graft is replaced with new bone. The studies at the end of one year (Fig. 18–31) show the graft and host skull joined by a band of tissue resembling a cranial suture. Whether this suture would close in time cannot be said, but there is new bone formation by metaplasia from stroma along the line at a slow rate (i.e., by the same mechanism as that of membranous bone formation).

Technique of Obtaining Split Rib Graft. If only a small portion of bone is required, an incision is made directly over the seventh rib anteriorly. If the defect is extensive, the posterolateral thoracoplasty approach over the seventh rib opens up a fascial plane for dissection, through which three to four full-length ribs may be removed at one sitting. Care should be taken that only alternate ribs are removed and that each rib bed is closed with a running suture.

Under endotracheal anesthesia the incision is made parallel to the seventh rib from the angle of the scapula to the anterior axillary line, cutting through the latissimus dorsi and raising the lower edge of the trapezius (Fig. 18–32*A*). The fibers of the serratus anterior are split anteriorly. On elevating the scapula, a fascial plane is opened that allows access to the full extent from the second to the tenth ribs. The periosteum is incised and carefully elevated (Fig. 18–32*B*). After the removal of each rib, the periosteum is carefully closed with a running suture of catgut, the muscle is closed in layers with figure-of-eight sutures of chromic catgut, and the skin is sutured with silk or nylon (Fig. 18–32*C*). With careful technique, perforation of the pleura should seldom occur. If it is punctured, careful closure of the wound under positive pressure is required after the introduction of a catheter with a water seal. Once the lung has expanded fully, the catheter may be removed. The ribs are split lengthwise with a Beaver blade, opening the cancellous portion and at the same time preserving the cortex as a scaffold (Fig. 18–32*D,E*). The split rib graft may now be bent and contoured to fit almost any defect (Fig. 18–33).

Vascularized Rib Transfers. The rib has a vascular supply more similar to that of flat bones than that of long bones. Daniel (1978) extensively reviewed the blood supply of the

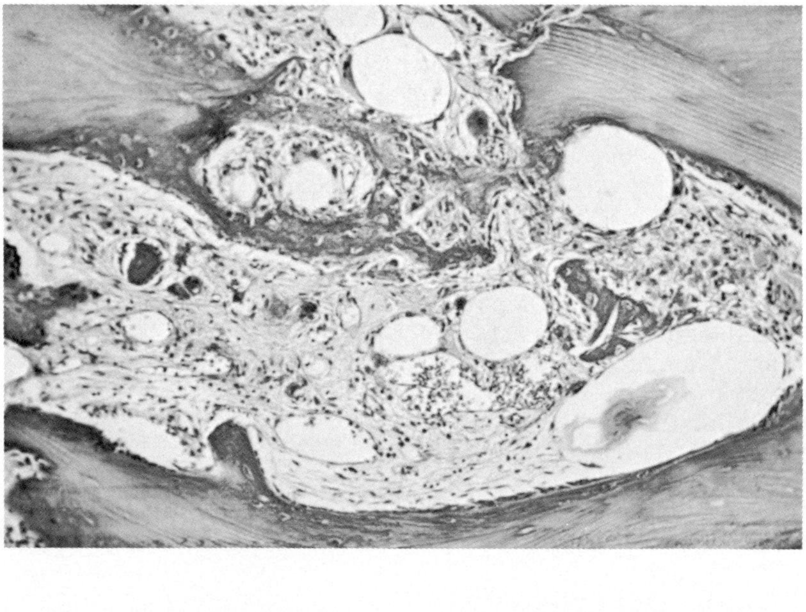

Figure 18–29. Five week specimen shows continuing resorption along with an increase in vascularity of the granulation tissue between the trabeculae. There is active regeneration of new bone along the surface of the trabeculae. This process is most active in the vicinity of blood vessels.

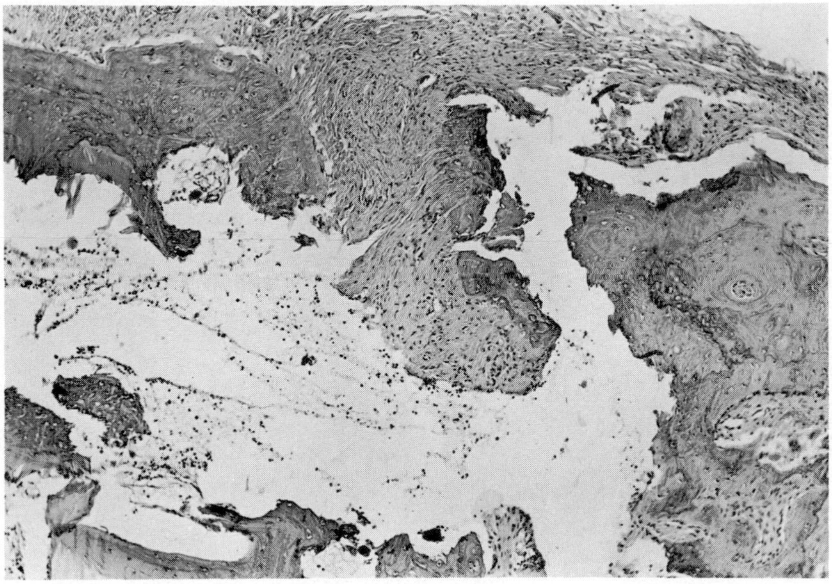

Figure 18–30. Six month biopsy shows rib graft attached to a portion of the skull. They are separated by a layer of fibrous tissue, and between the two there is an area of newly formed bone with some areas not yet calcified. There is osteoid substance around some large osteoblasts.

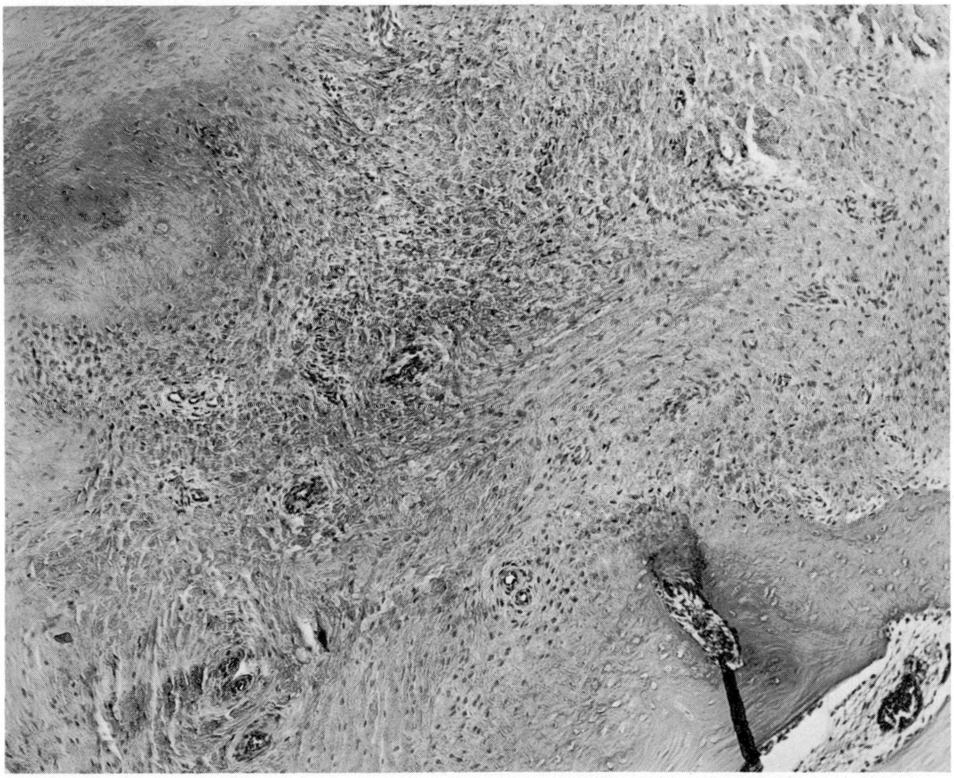

Figure 18–31. One year specimen shows the graft and host bone joined by a band of tissue resembling a cranial suture. Note that new bone is being formed by metaplasia from the stroma along the line at a slow rate (namely, by the same mechanism as membranous bone formation).

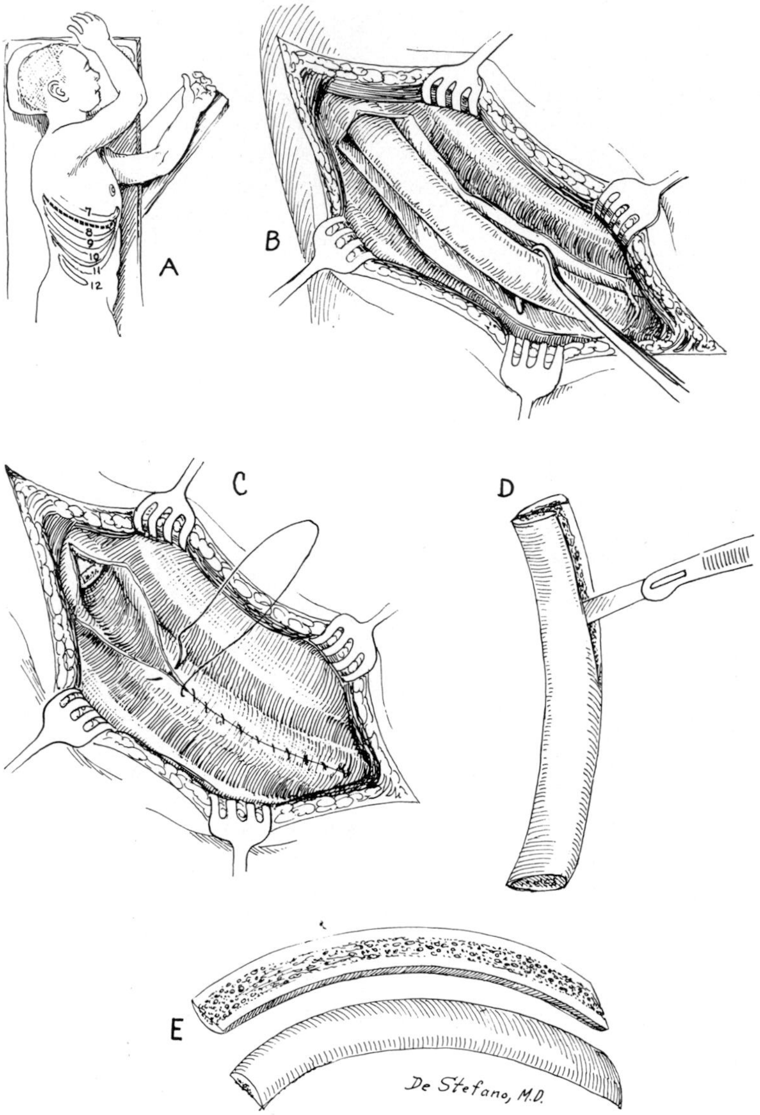

Figure 18–32. *A, B,* Removal of a full length of rib by the subperiosteal technique. The Doyen elevator is used to free the periosteum of the rib bed. *C,* Closing the periosteal bed with a running chromic catgut suture. *D, E,* Technique of splitting the rib with the #10 knife blade.

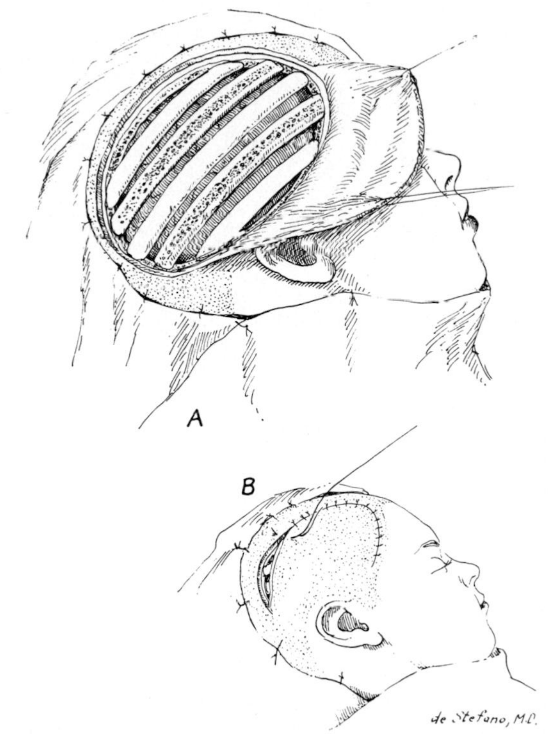

Figure 18–33. *A*, The split ribs have been contoured to fit snugly against the host skull in the reconstruction of cranial defects. *B*, The split rib grafts are secured into position within the defect under the replaced scalp flap.

rib in terms of its exploitation as a vascularized free bone transfer. Unfortunately the nutrient vessels of the rib take their origin from the posterior intercostal artery and vein, and enter the bone just short of the costovertebral junction. This dictates a deep posterior thoracotomy with disarticulation of the costovertebral junction to harvest the bone and pedicle. The vascular pedicle is also short. Ostrup and Fredrickson (1975) demonstrated the successful use of composite rib based on the nutrient vessels in a radiated bed in the dog. Daniel (1978) reported a clinical case that failed owing to a problem with the venous anastomosis.

Most of the successful clinical vascularized rib transfers depend on a periosteal pedicle. Vascularized rib is commonly used for mandible reconstruction following ablation of oral cancer. At the junction of rib and costal cartilage the penetration of the periosteal vessels appears to be somewhat superior, in a manner similar to the metaphyseal periosteal pedicle of a long bone. It is presumed that periosteal pedicles that include this region provide better bone survival. Strauch, Bloomberg, and Lewin (1971) transferred rib based on the intercostal extensions of the internal mammary artery in an experimental environment. McCullough and Fredrickson (1973) transferred vascularized rib to the mandible based on the intercostal vessels (Serafin, Villarreal-Rios, and Georgiade, 1977; Buncke and associates, 1977; Ariyan and Finseth, 1978). The most common periosteal pedicle for the rib involves carrying the rib as a composite pectoralis major osteomyocutaneous flap based on the thoracoacromial artery (see Chap. 70). Cuono and Ariyan (1980) demonstrated survival of the bone transferred to the mandible in this manner using tetracycline labeling. Cadaver injection studies of the thoracoacromial artery by Cutting (1981) did not show filling of the nutrient artery, however. The serratus anterior free flap based on the lateral thoracic artery has also been successfully used to carry rib.

Calvarium

Nonvascularized Autografts. In the adult the thickness of the calvarial bone averages 7 mm. Unfortunately the variability is large (range 3 to 12 mm). Moreover, in children the bone is thin. The youngest patient in whom the authors have been able to split the calvarium was 4 years old. This was extremely difficult and the bone happened to be unusually thick. Splitting the calvarium is not usually contemplated until the child reaches adolescent years. Pensler and McCarthy (1984) published measurements of the thickness of the calvarium in various sites in adults (Fig. 18–34, Table 18–1). It has been

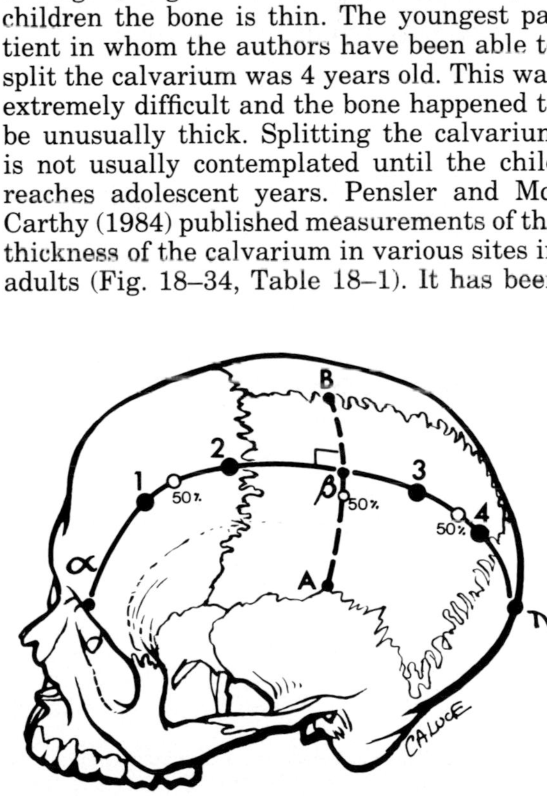

Figure 18–34. Sites of calvarial thickness measurement given in Table 18–1 (after Pensler and McCarthy, 1984).

Table 18–1. Calvarial Thickness Measurements

Variable	Number	Mean	Std. Dev.	Median	Minimum	Maximum
Rt. side 1	200	6.80	1.04	6.80	3.50	10.0
Rt. side 2	200	7.03	1.06	7.01	3.50	10.9
Rt. side 3	200	7.45	1.03	7.38	4.25	11.2
Rt. side 4	200	7.72	1.07	7.60	4.00	12.0
Left side 1	200	6.86	0.99	6.89	3.75	10.25
Left side 2	200	7.03	1.05	7.00	3.75	10.25
Left side 3	200	7.46	1.09	7.49	3.0	11.50
Left side 4	200	7.72	1.11	7.55	4.0	12.0

From Pensler, J., and McCarthy, J. G.: The calvarial donor site: an anatomic sudy in cadavers. Plast. Reconstr. Surg., *75*:648, 1984.

shown that membranous bone undergoes less resorption than endochondral bone when used in the facial region (Smith and Abramson, 1974; Zins and Whitaker, 1979).

There are multiple methods to harvest calvarial bone grafts. For some applications the bone is harvested as bone dust or multiple small shavings. Shehadi (1970) and Bakamjian and Leonard (1977) reported the use of calvarial bone dust, harvested during craniotomy, in cranioplasty. The bone dust is sprinkled on the dura and the scalp is closed. The living bone-forming cells eventually coalesce to reform the calvarium. This approach has also been applied to bone grafting the alveolus in cleft palate patients (see Chap. 55). Bone dust is harvested using an electric craniotome or preferably a brace and bit, and placed into the alveolar cleft after suitable mucoperiosteal flaps have been raised.

The two most common methods of harvesting calvarial grafts split the bone through the diploë, separating the outer and inner table (McCarthy and Zide, 1984). This achieves a doubling of the surface area at the expense of decreasing its thickness. If a relatively small graft is needed, this can be harvested by the in situ technique illustrated in Figure 18–35. Using a bur, a trough is created around the proposed graft. Applying

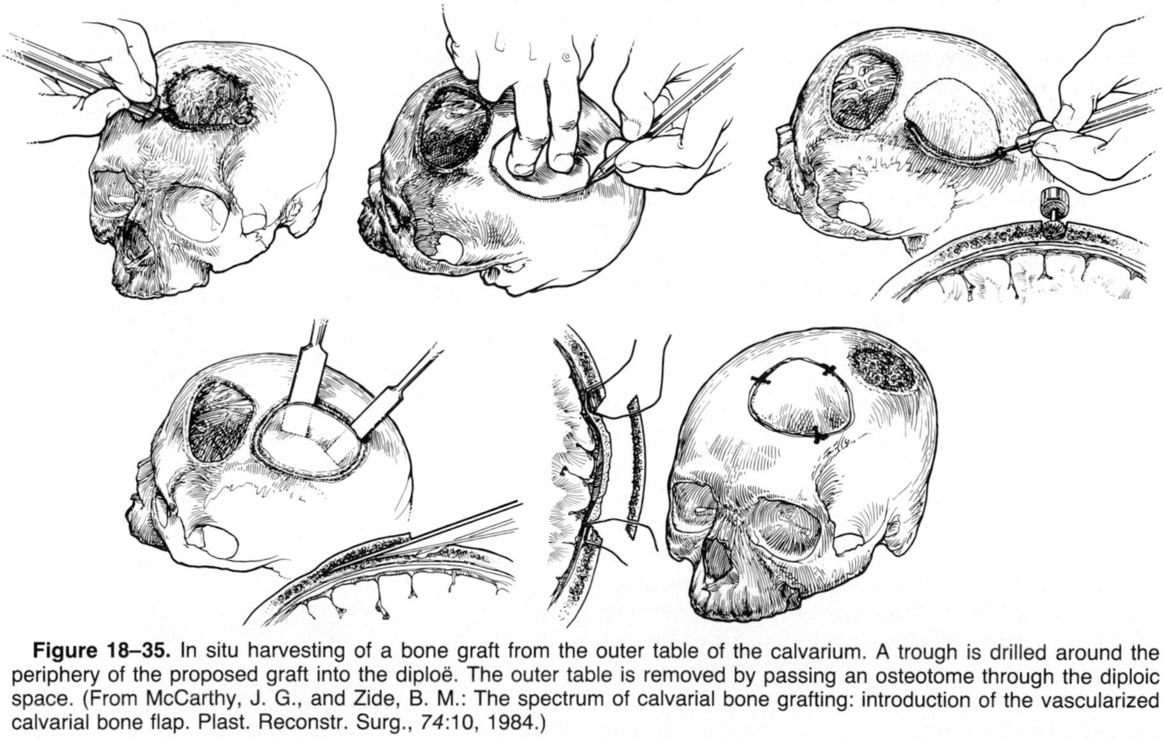

Figure 18–35. In situ harvesting of a bone graft from the outer table of the calvarium. A trough is drilled around the periphery of the proposed graft into the diploë. The outer table is removed by passing an osteotome through the diploic space. (From McCarthy, J. G., and Zide, B. M.: The spectrum of calvarial bone grafting: introduction of the vascularized calvarial bone flap. Plast. Reconstr. Surg., *74*:10, 1984.)

an osteotome to the diploic space, the surgeon can remove the outer table of the calvarium and use it as a graft. It is not uncommon to remove full-thickness bone inadvertently with this maneuver. This is often of no consequence, but dural tears and serious venous sinus hemorrhage have been reported. These complications become more frequent as the size of the desired graft increases. For this reason, when a large section of calvarial graft must be harvested, it is usually wise to perform a *formal craniotomy* and split the bone on a back table, as illustrated in Figure 18–36. A sagittal saw with a long blade is applied to the diploic space around the periphery of the excised section. The rest of the separation is performed with curved osteotomes. One of the two cortical tables is used to cover the donor site, while the other serves as the graft. With this method, large one-piece reconstructions of calvaria have been performed.

Vascularized Calvarial Transfers. As early as 1890, Mueller reported a dermo-osteoperiosteal flap incorporating bone from the outer table of the calvaria. According to Ivy (1951), early bone grafting efforts in mandibular reconstruction employed composite flaps consisting of skin, soft tissue, and bone. Bardenheuer (1892) used flaps of forehead skin and underlying bone, Rydygier (1908) a flap of skin and clavicle, and Sykoff (1900) a "sliding" or advancement bone flap. Watson-Jones (1933) described a calvarial bone flap with a pedicle incorporating the periosteum and the more proximal temporalis muscle.

In 1972, both Conley and Stricker and associates individually reported calvarial osteomuscular flaps. Vandervord, Watson, and Teasdale (1982) designed a full-thickness calvarial bone flap that was pedicled on both temporalis muscles; however, it left a significant donor defect. In 1984, McCarthy and Zide described their experience in reconstructing malar deformities with an outer table calvarial bone flap carried on a pedicle of galea, periosteum, and temporalis muscle. Later in 1984, Van der Meulen, Hauben and Vaandrager reported the use of a calvarial osteoperiosteal flap to reconstruct the zygomatic deformity in the Treacher Collins syndrome.

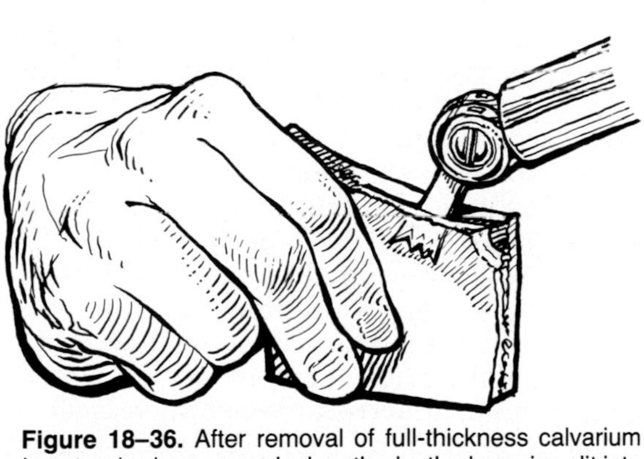

Figure 18–36. After removal of full-thickness calvarium using standard neurosurgical methods, the bone is split into two cortices. A sagittal saw is applied to the diploic space around the edges of the graft. Curved osteotomes are used to complete the separation of the two tables. Large pieces of calvarial graft may be harvested in this manner.

Anatomy. As in the design of any flap, an understanding of the regional vasculature is critical. This should include details not only of the regional soft tissue layers, but also of the three-dimensional blood supply and the osseous component of the flap. In a study of the blood supply of the calvarium conducted on fresh adult cadavers, Cutting, McCarthy, and Berenstein (1984) injected Prussian blue dye and barium sulfate (Micropaque) into the external carotid arteries. The bone was decalcified and microangiography, including thick-section histology, was performed. It was demonstrated that the superficial temporal artery, a branch of the external carotid, crosses the temporal crest and continues on the outer aspect of the galea, which is an extension of the SMAS (see Figs. 18–15, 18–16). It divides into frontal and parietal branches to irrigate the skin, subcutaneous tissue, galea, and periosteum of this region.

The above study demonstrated that the outer table of the calvaria receives its blood supply diffusely from the periosteum without any increase in concentration of penetrating vessels at the sutures. The periosteum in turn is supplied by the rich anastomotic network above the galea, which sends perforating vessels through the galea to the periosteum. There is no true axial pattern to the periosteal blood supply, and the periosteal vascular organization is irregular. In the study, perforating vessels were observed as they coursed at right angles into the periosteum; the inner table of the calvaria was predominantly supplied by the middle meningeal system.

The temporalis muscle, fan shaped and lying in the temporal fossa, is innervated by the trigeminal nerve. Testut and Jacob (1909) described the vascular supply of the temporalis muscle as being derived from three sources: branches of the superficial temporal vessels and the deep temporal vessels, two of which are branches off the internal maxillary artery (Fig. 18–37). These findings were confirmed by Casanova and associates (1986) and Antonyshyn and colleagues (1986), although their anatomic terminology varied. The deep temporal fascia (aponeurosis) invests the temporalis muscle down to the zygomatic arch and is firmly attached to the periosteum around the periphery of the temporalis muscle. The deep temporal fascia extends cephalically as the periosteum of the calvaria. The deep temporal fascia is supplied solely by one of the terminal branches of the superficial temporal artery (Abul-Hassan, Ascher, and Acland, 1986). Consequently, a bilayered flap of both fascial layers can be transferred by microvascular surgical techniques.

In the *frontoparietal region,* the soft tissue covering of the skull is composed of the following layers: skin or scalp, subcutaneous layer, galea, a subaponeurotic layer or Merkel's gap, and periosteum. In the *temporal region,* the layers can be divided as follows: skin, subcutaneous layer, temporoparietal fascia or SMAS (an extension of the galea), Merkel's gap, deep temporal fascia or temporal aponeurosis, and temporalis muscle. In an anatomic study, Casanova and associates (1986) identified a distinct layer overlying the deep temporal fascia. Termed the *innominate fascia,* it extends in the cephalic direction as the periosteum of the frontoparietal region. The superficial and deep temporal arterial systems contribute to the vascularization of the innominate fascia and temporal aponeurosis. These authors also noted a thin, areolar layer between the outer calvarial table and periosteum; it also continued beneath the temporal muscle and was termed the *subperiosteum* (Table 18–2).

Table 18–2. Soft Tissue Layers

Frontoparietal Region	Temporal Region
1. Skin/scalp	1. Skin
2. Subcutaneous	2. Subcutaneous
3. Galea	3. Superficial temporoparietal fascia/SMAS
4. Periosteum	4. Deep temporal (aponeurosis) fascia; ? innominate fascia
5.	5. Temporalis muscle
6. Subperiosteum	6. ? Subperiosteum

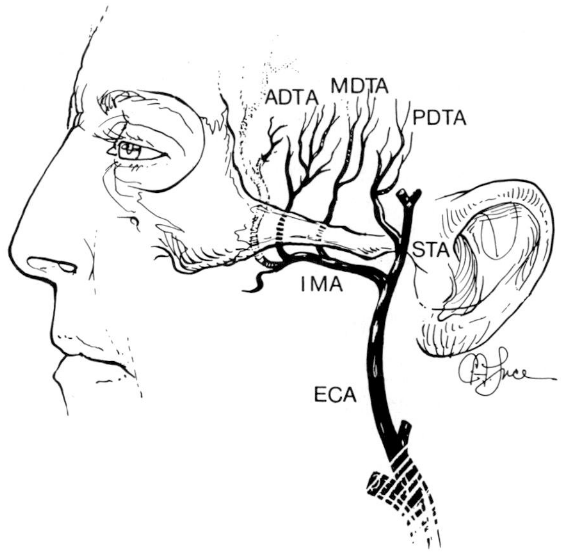

Figure 18–37. The superficial and deep temporal arterial system. The superficial temporal artery (STA) is a terminal branch of the external carotid artery (ECA), and the deep temporal artery is a branch of the internal maxillary artery (IMA). Note the terminal branches of these two systems, which make up the deep temporal artery. ADTA = anterior deep temporal artery; MDTA = middle deep temporal artery; PDTA = posterior deep temporal artery. (From McCarthy, J. G., Cutting, C. B., and Shaw, W. W.: Vascularized calvarial flaps. Clin. Plast. Surg., 14:40, 1987.)

Flap Design. There are two points of controversy in the design of vascularized calvarial flaps: (1) the plane of scalp-skin elevation and (2) the anatomic components of the pedicle. In the technique reported by McCarthy and Zide (1984), the scalp dissection was done in a subfollicular plane in order to preserve the superficial temporal vessels that course on the outer surface of the galea-SMAS. In this way the feeding vessels of the perforators of the calvarial periosteum would be preserved. In the initial report, the pedicle of the flap consisted of galea (SMAS), periosteum, and temporalis muscle, including the deep fascia or aponeurosis. At present the authors have modified the pedicle to include only the galea (and SMAS), the periosteum, and the deep temporal fascia or aponeurosis. The muscle is not included in the flap, with the result that there is minimal, if any, donor defect. The scalp dissection is still performed in a subfollicular plane in order to avoid injury to the superficial temporal vessels.

On the basis of their anatomic studies, Casanova and associates (1986) included neither the temporalis muscle nor the galea in the bone flap pedicle. It was their consensus that a pedicle of innominate fascia and deep temporal fascia (aponeurosis) provides sufficient blood supply for outer table calvarial bone flaps. However, they would include the galea in the pedicle of a full-thickness calvarial bone flap. As mentioned previously, neither group would include the temporal muscle in the flap pedicle. Antonyshyn and associates (1986) included the muscle in the flap, which was elevated in a "subgaleal" plane.

A bone donor site above the squamosal-parietal suture and behind the coronal suture is usually selected. The closer the donor site is chosen toward the vertex of the skull, the more flap mobility one will have, because the arc of rotation is greater. Flap mobility is also facilitated by transecting the zygomatic arch. In the bone-thickness studies reported by Pensler and McCarthy (1984), the optimal bone donor site is at a point approximately 2 cm posterior to the coronal suture in the parietal bone.

Advantages of Calvarial Flaps. In an experimental study, Zins and Whitaker (1983) demonstrated the increased surviving mass of membranous (calvarial) versus enchondral bone grafts. Furthermore, in an immature rabbit model, Cutting and McCarthy (1983) reported an increased surviving volume of calvarial bone after a vascularized transfer versus a traditional nonvascularized bone graft. In a rabbit model, Antonyshyn and associates (1986) compared vascularized (temporalis myo-osseous flap) and nonvascularized calvarial bone transfers. Fluorochrome labeling documented the ability of the periosteal circulation to maintain the viability of the bone and also demonstrated new osteoid formation in the calvarial bone of the flap. Necrosis of most cellular elements was observed after the transfer of nonvascularized calvarial bone grafts.

In a study from our laboratory (LaTrenta, McCarthy, and Cutting, 1987), growth of vascularized calvarial transfers was demonstrated in the immature animal (as manifested by increase in dry bone weights), although the bone transfers never attained the size and volume of the corresponding part of the adult animal.

A final advantage of calvarial flaps is that the donor bone can be harvested through the same operative field. In addition, the patient is spared the discomfort that is experienced at the rib and iliac donor sites.

Disadvantages of Calvarial Flaps. The variable thickness of the calvarial donor site is the major disadvantage of the technique and accounts for inadvertent entry into the intracranial space. This is especially a problem in the infant or younger child in whom the bone is thin. In the adult, one can estimate the probable thickness from the data listed in Table 18–1. It has been the authors' experience that calvarial thickness cannot be accurately assessed preoperatively by CT scans. Another disadvantage is that calvarial bone tends to be more brittle than iliac or rib bone.

Temporoparietal Flap. A bicoronal incision is made from ear to ear when bilateral flaps are elevated, but a more limited incision is adequate for a unilateral flap (Fig. 18–38).

The scalp-skin is elevated in a *subfollicular* plane above the SMAS and galea. This is not a natural cleavage plane, but the dissection is facilitated by keeping the hair follicles in the elevated flap under direct vision. The scalp elevation must be extensive in order to expose the temporalis muscle, temporal crest, coronal suture, potential osseous donor site, and vasculature of the superficial temporal system (Fig. 18–39).

A metal template of the osseous defect is taken and transferred to the calvarial donor site. Care must be taken to ensure that the

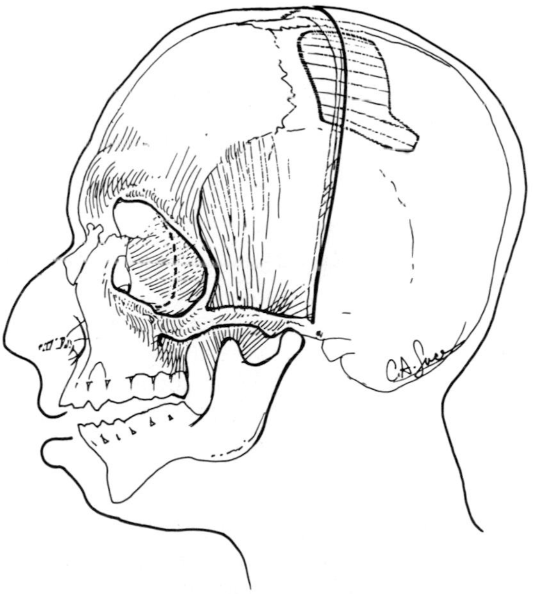

Figure 18–38. Temporoparietal flap. A coronal incision is made and the scalp is elevated in a subfollicular plane. The bone donor site is illustrated posterior to the coronal suture. (From McCarthy, J. G., Cutting, C. B., and Shaw, W. W.: Vascularized calvarial flaps. Clin. Plast. Surg., 14:42, 1987.)

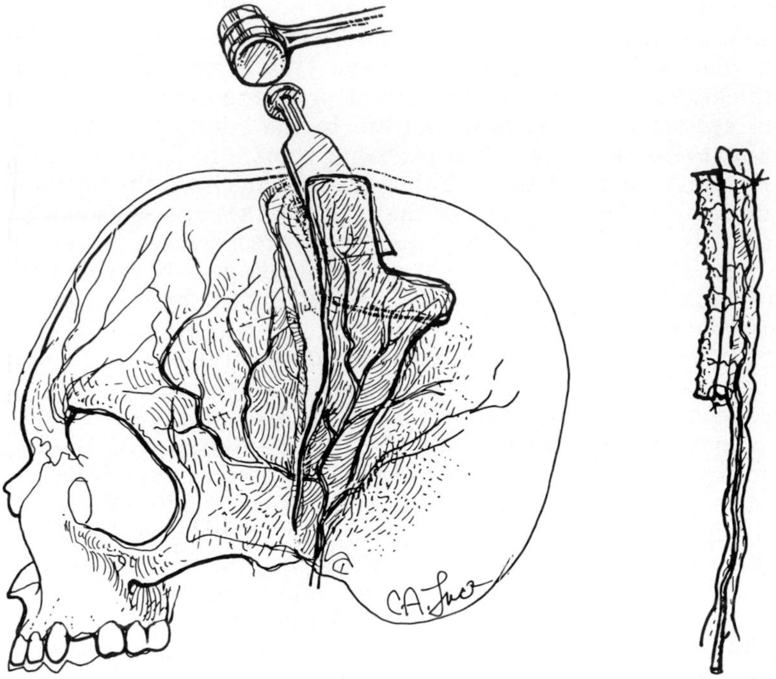

Figure 18–39. The superficial temporal arterial system is preserved along its main axis, and the outer table is harvested with a curved osteotome after a trough is created around the periphery with an air-driven bur. Inset shows the flap and pedicle. Note that sutures are passed between the overlying galea and periosteum and calvaria in order to preserve the pedicle. The pedicle consists of the galea-SMAS as well as the deep temporal fascia (aponeurosis). (From McCarthy, J. G., Cutting, C. B., and Shaw, W. W.: Vascularized calvarial flaps. Clin. Plast. Surg., 14:43, 1987.)

proposed flap pedicle provides sufficient length for transfer of the bone. It has been the authors' experience that the osseous component can be transferred as far inferiorly as the mandible.

The overlying galea and periosteum are incised with an excess 5 mm perimeter about the proposed bony component. A round, air-driven bur is employed to create a trough about the bony component. Bleeding is observed as the diploic space is entered. A curved osteotome is driven by a mallet to elevate or separate the outer table of the calvaria (Fig. 18–39).

Drill holes are placed in the bone, and sutures are passed through the holes and overlying periosteum-galea to prevent dissociation of the pedicle from the bony component.

The flap pedicle is incised, incorporating an axial component of the superficial temporal artery. This can be done under direct vision after elevation of the scalp or can be planned before the scalp incision with the Doppler flow meter. The pedicle in the temporal region includes the galea-SMAS and the underlying aponeurosis (deep temporal fascia).

The skeletal donor site can usually be managed by burring the margins of the outer table defect. Methyl methacrylate can also be used to restore the contour in the adult, but is contraindicated if the associated operation includes entry into the nose or paranasal sinuses.

If the outer and inner tables are harvested, split-thickness calvarial grafts can be removed from another site and placed in the defect.

The temporoparietal flap finds its greatest application in the reconstruction of defects of the brow and zygoma (Fig. 18–40). Additional modifications include the simultaneous application of two flaps from the same side (Fig. 18–40) and the placement of nonvascularized calvarial bone grafts below the vascularized transfer (Fig. 18–41). The bony component of the flap can also be contoured with the aid of an air-driven bur (Fig. 18–42). It is especially helpful in the one-stage reconstruction of the patient with Treacher Collins syndrome in whom a bilateral calvarial bone flap to the zygomatic complex is combined with lateral canthopexy and transposition flaps of skin and orbicularis muscle from the upper to the lower eyelids (Fig. 18–43).

Frontoparietal Flap. A more recently developed vascularized calvarial transfer is the frontoparietal flap. Through a bicoronal incision, the scalp is elevated in a subfollicular plane and the frontoparietal region is exposed (Fig. 18–44).

The donor site is identified along the mid-

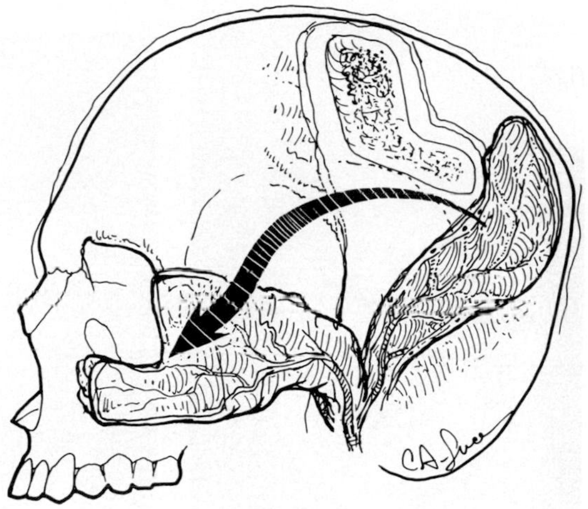

Figure 18–40. Composite flap in position to augment the zygomatic complex and lateral orbital wall. Note that a second flap can be taken from the same side when additional augmentation is required. (From McCarthy, J. G., Cutting, C. B., and Shaw, W. W.: Vascularized calvarial flaps. Clin. Plast. Surg., 14:43, 1987.)

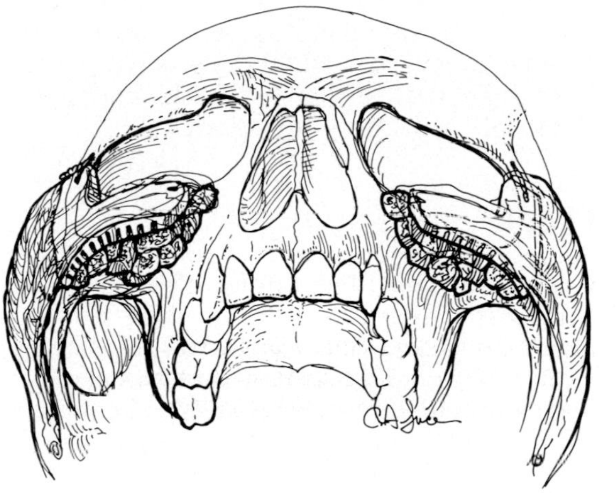

Figure 18–41. Nonvascularized calvarial bone grafts can be placed under the osseous component of the flap. (From McCarthy, J. G., Cutting, C. B., and Shaw, W. W.: Vascularized calvarial flaps. Clin. Plast. Surg., 14:44, 1987.)

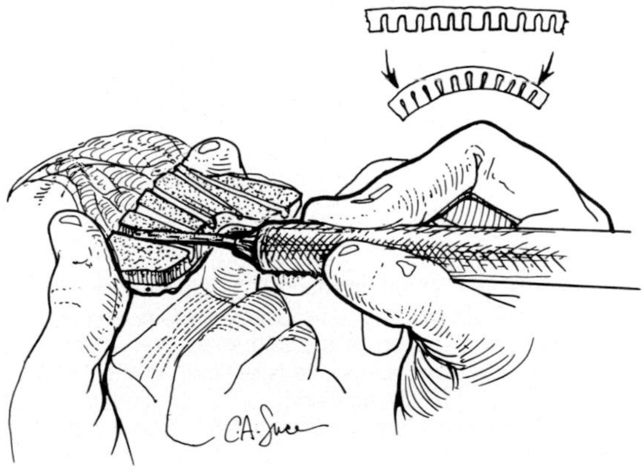

Figure 18–42. Recontouring the bony component with an air-driven bur. (From McCarthy, J. G., Cutting, C. B., and Shaw, W. W.: Vascularized calvarial flaps. Clin. Plast. Surg., 14:44, 1987.)

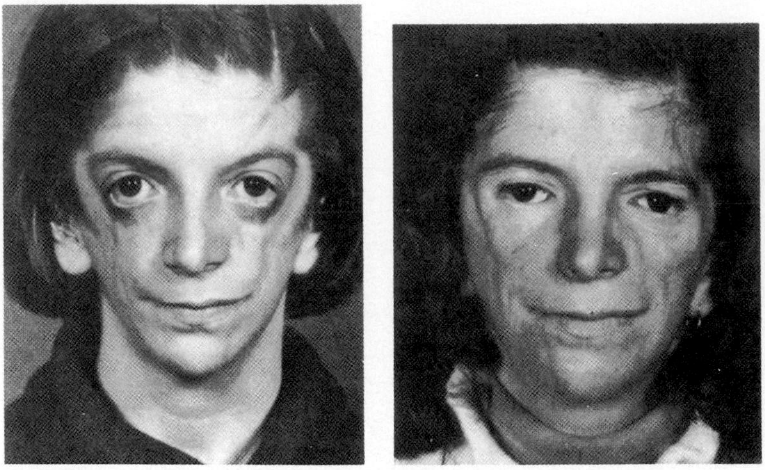

A B

Figure 18–43. Temporoparietal flap in a 27 year old woman with Treacher Collins syndrome. She had previously undergone multiple cartilage grafts to the zygomatic complex as well as lower eyelid reconstruction with residual scarring and contour irregularities. *A,* Preoperative view. *B,* Following calvarial bone flaps, bilateral external canthopexy, and reconstruction of the lower eyelids with skin–orbicularis muscle flaps from the upper eyelid. (From McCarthy, J. G., Cutting, C. B., and Shaw, W. W.: Vascularized calvarial flaps. Clin. Plast. Surg., 14:45, 1987.)

line of the frontal bone, and the overlying soft tissue is incised with a cuff extending beyond the donor bone. The outer table is harvested as previously described for the temporoparietal flap. The flap pedicle is elevated in a subperiosteal plane and incorporates at least one supratrochlear vessel (McCarthy and associates, 1987). The adjacent supraorbital vessel is divided to provide flap mobility (Fig. 18–45). The donor bone defect is managed by recontouring the margins with an air-driven bur, as described.

The flap can be used in nasal reconstruction. It provides bony skeletal support and cutaneous coverage when the overlying fascia is covered with either a full-thickness or a thick split-thickness skin graft.

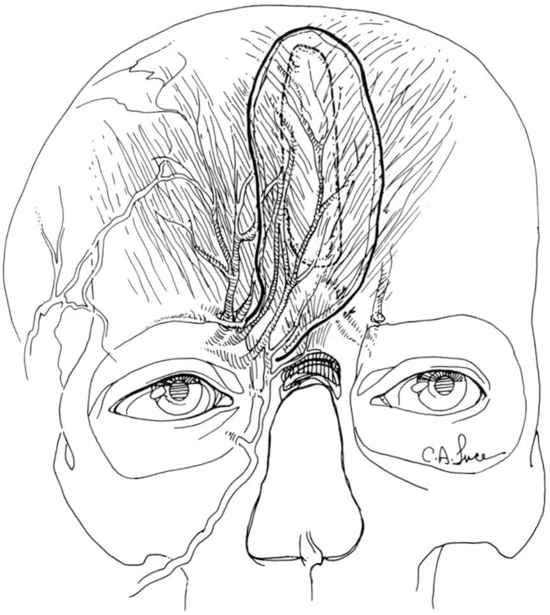

Figure 18–44. The frontoparietal flap is exposed through a bicoronal incision; the skin is elevated in a subdermal plane. Note the outline of the supratrochlear vasculature. The underlying bony donor site is outlined in the midline of the frontal bone. (From McCarthy, J. G., Cutting, C. B., and Shaw, W. W.: Vascularized calvarial flaps. Clin. Plast. Surg., 14:45, 1987.)

Fibula

Vascularized Transfers. The fibula has become the mainstay of long bone free flap donor sites (see Chap. 82). Taylor, Miller, and Ham (1975) demonstrated that the peroneal artery provided the principal blood supply to this bone. They were able to harvest the fibula in such a way that the nutrient artery and the proximal metaphyseal periosteal pedicle remained intact. Either of these sources of blood supply is adequate to ensure a well-vascularized bone transfer. In recent years the free fibula transfer has become the standard method of reconstructing a large bone gap in lower extremity trauma. The details of harvesting this flap are presented in Chapter 82 on lower extremity reconstruction.

Scapula

Vascularized Transfers. The scapula has also been used as a donor site for vascularized bone transfer. The nutrient artery enters the bone inferior to the lateral attachment of the acromion to the plate of the scapula. While it is possible to use the nutrient artery to carry

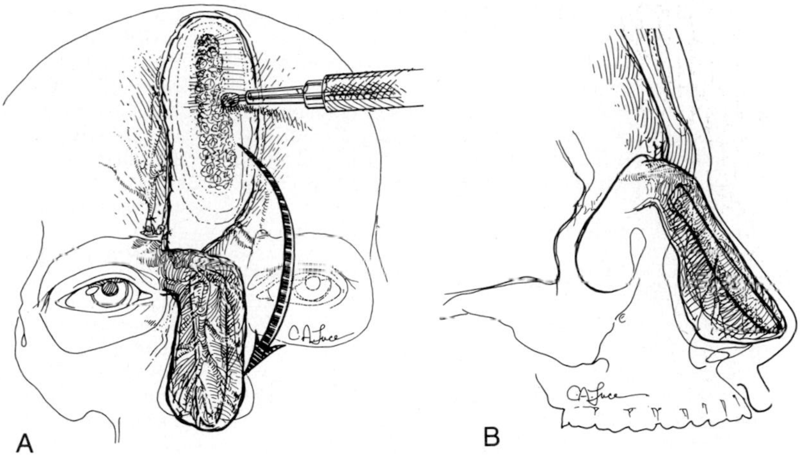

Figure 18–45. *A,* The vascularized frontoparietal bone flap is transferred to the nasal defect as indicated. The margins of the outer table frontal bone defect are contoured with a bur driven by an air drill. *B,* Lateral view of the flap in position in the nasal defect prior to coverage with a thick split-thickness or a full-thickness skin graft. (From McCarthy, J. G., Cutting, C. B., and Shaw, W. W.: Vascularized calvarial flaps. Clin. Plast. Surg., 14:46, 1987.)

the bone, most of the clinical uses of this flap harvest the scapular spine based on the muscular attachment of the trapezius, which receives its dominant vascular supply in this region from the transverse cervical artery. Owing to the broad attachment of the trapezius to the spine, with the attendant blood supply entering along its length, it is relatively easy to cut and shape the bone as indicated. This flap, as an island based on the transverse cervical artery, has been used to reconstruct small mandibular defects in one stage at the time of tumor ablation (Demergasso, 1976; Panje and Cutting, 1980; Dufresne and associates, 1987). It is also possible to use the inferolateral aspect of the plate of the scapula based on the circumflex scapular artery (Kim and associates, 1987). Swartz and associates (1986) carried this segment of bone as a composite free flap along with a parascapular flap in the reconstruction of a postmaxillectomy defect.

Metatarsus

Vascularized Transfers. The metatarsus has also found use as a vascularized bone transfer. Its greatest clinical use has been as a composite great toe to thumb transfer in cases of thumb amputation or congenital absence (May, 1981). The operative technique is described in Chapter 95. The metatarsus has also been carried as a free flap in conjunction with a dorsalis pedis flap (May, 1981). Because this small long bone can be transferred with an intact epiphysis and joint surface, growth can be expected (Donski, Carwell, and Sharzer, 1979) and it is reasonable to assume that the joint surface can be preserved. Swartz (1985) has transferred the metatarsal as a free flap in construction of the mandibular ramus in a case of congenital ankylosis of the temporomandibular joint. It is hoped that the provision of a joint surface will prevent refusion of the temporomandibular joint.

Acknowledgement: Figures 18–4 to 18–6 and 18–27 to 18–31 were supplied by the late J. J. Longacre.

REFERENCES

Abul-Hassan, H. S., Ascher, G. D., and Acland, R. D.: Surgical anatomy of blood supply of the fascial layers of the temporal region. Plast. Reconstr. Surg., *77*:17, 1986.

Adeloye, A., Kattan, K. R., and Silverman, F. N.: Thickness of the normal skull in the American blacks and whites. Am. J. Phys. Anthropol., *43*:23, 1975.

Albee, F. H.: Bone Graft Surgery. Philadelphia, W. B. Saunders Company, 1915.

Albrektsson, T.: In vivo studies of bone grafts. The possibility of vascular anastomoses in healing bone. Acta Orthop. Scand., *51*:9, 1980.

Antonyshyn, O., Cocleugh, R. G., and Anderson, C.: Growth potential in suture bone inlay grafts: a comparison of vascularized and free calvarial bone grafts. Plast. Reconstr. Surg., *79*:1, 1987.

Antonyshyn, O., Cocleugh, R. G., Hurst, L. N., and Anderson, C.: The temporalis myo-osseous flap: an experimental study. Plast. Reconstr. Surg., *77*:406, 1986.

Ariyan, S., and Finseth, F. J.: The anterior chest approach for obtaining free osteocutaneous rib grafts. Plast. Reconstr. Surg., *62*:676, 1978.

Axhausen, G.: Histologische Untersuchungen über Knochentransplantation am Menschen. Dtsch. Z. Chir., *91*:388, 1907.

Axhausen, G.: Die histologischen und klinischen Gesetze der freien Osteoplastik auf Grund von Thierversuchen. Arch. Klin. Chir., *88*:23, 1908–1909.

Baadsgaard, K., and Medgyesi, S.: Muscle pedicle bone grafts. Acta Orthop. Scand., *35*:279, 1965.

Bakamjian, V., and Leonard, A.: Bone dust cranioplasty. Plast. Reconstr. Surg., *60*:784, 1977.

Ballet, J., and Griscelli, C.: Lymphoid cell transplantation in human osteopetrosis. *In* Horton, J., Tarpley, T., and Davis, W. (Eds.): Mechanisms of Localized Bone Loss. Calcif. Tissue Abstracts (Suppl.), 1978, pp. 399–414.

Ballin, M.: A method of cranioplasty. Surg. Gynecol. Obstet., *33*:79, 1921.

Bardenheuer, B.: Vorschlage zu plastische Operationen bei chirurgischen Eingriffen der Mundhohle. Arch. Klin. Chir., *43*:32, 348, 1892.

Barth, A.: Über histologische Befunde nach Knochenimplantation. Arch. Klin. Chir., *46*:409, 1893.

Bassett, C. A. L.: Pulsing electromagnetic fields: a new method to modify cell behavior in calcified and noncalcified tissues. Calcif. Tissue Int., *34*:1, 1982.

Bassett, C. A. L., Hurley, L. A., and Stinchfield, F. E.: The fate of long-term anorganic bone implants. Transplant. Bull., *29*:51, 1962.

Becker, R. O., Bassett, C. A. L., and Bachman, C.: Bioelectric factors controlling bone structure. *In* Frost, H. (Ed.): Bone Biodynamics. Boston, Little, Brown and Company, 1964, pp. 209–232.

Black, J.: Tissue response to exogenous electromagnetic signals. Orthop. Clin. North Am., *15*:15, 1984.

Blair, V.: Surgery and Disease of the Mouth and Jaws. St. Louis, MO, C. V. Mosby Company, 1918.

Bonome, A.: Intorno alla rigenerazione del tessuto ossoe; studi sperimentali. Arch. Sci. Med., *9*:131, 1886.

Brash, J. C.: Cunningham's Textbook of Anatomy. 9th Ed. London, Oxford Medical Publications, 1951.

Breine, U., and Johanson, B.: The tibia as donor area for bone graft in infants. Influence on the longitudinal growth. Acta Chir. Scand., *131*:230, 1966.

Brighton, C. T.: Symposium on electrically induced osteogenesis. Orthop. Clin. North Am., *15*, 1984.

Brookes, M.: Sequelae of experimental partial ischemia in long bones of the rabbit. J. Anat., *94*:552, 1960.

Brookes, M.: The Blood Supply to Bone. London, Butterworths, 1971.

Brooks, D. B., Heiple, K. G., Herndon, C. H., and Powell, A. E.: Immunological factors in homogenous bone transplantation. 4. The effect of various methods of preparation and irradiation on antigenicity. J. Bone Joint Surg., *45A*:1617, 1963.

Brown, R. C.: The repair of skull defects. Med. J. Aust., *11*:409, 1917.

Brown, R. C.: Cranioplasty by split rib method. J. Coll. Surg. Austral., *1*:238, 1928.

Bryce, T.: Quain's Anatomy. 11th Ed. Vol. 14. Part I. London, Longmans, Green, & Company, 1915, p. 177.

Buncke, H. J., Furnas, D. W., Gordon, L., and Achauer, B. M.: Free osteocutaneous flap from a rib to the tibia. Plast. Reconstr. Surg., *59*:799, 1977.

Burchardt, H., and Enneking, W. F.: Transplantation of bone. Surg. Clin. North Am., *58*:403, 1978.

Burwell, R. G.: Studies in the transplantation of bones. IV. The immune responses of lymph nodes draining second set homografts of fresh cancellous bone. J. Bone Joint Surg., *44B*:688, 1962.

Burwell, R. G.: Studies in the transplantation of bone. VIII. Treated composite homograft-autografts of cancellous bone: an analysis of inductive mechanisms in bone transplantation. J. Bone Joint Surg., *48B*:532, 1968.

Burwell, R. G., Friedlaender, G. E., and Mankin, H. J.: Current perspectives and future directions: the 1983 invitational conference on osteochondral allografts. Clin. Orthop., *197*:141, 1985.

Casanova, R., Cavalcante, D., Grotting, J. C., Vasconez, L. O., and Psillakis, J. F.: The anatomic basis for vascularized outer table calvarial bone flaps. Plast. Reconstr. Surg., *78*:300, 1986.

Cestero, H. J., Jr., and Salyer, K. E.: Regenerative potential of bone and periosteum. Surg. Forum, *26*:555, 1975.

Chalmers, J.: Transplantation immunity in bone homografting. J. Bone Joint Surg., *41B*:160, 1959.

Chase, S., and Herndon, C.: The fate of autogenous and homogenous bone grafts: a historical review. J. Bone Joint Surg., *37A*:809, 1955.

Codivilla, A.: Über die Behandlung der Pseudoarthrosen und der ausgedehnten diaphysaren Continuitelstrennungen. Arch. Klin. Chir., *92*:452, 1910.

Conley, J.: A technique of immediate bone grafting in the treatment of benign and malignant tumors of the mandible and a review of seventeen consecutive cases. Cancer, *6*:568, 1953.

Conley, J.: Use of composite flaps containing bone for major repairs in the head and neck. Plast. Reconstr. Surg., *49*:522, 1972.

Crenshaw, A. H.: Campbell's Operative Orthopedics. 4th Ed. St. Louis, MO, C. V. Mosby Company, 1963, p. 57.

Crockford, D. A., and Converse, J. M.: The ilium as a source of bone grafts in children. Plast. Reconstr. Surg., *50*:270, 1972.

Cuono, C. B., and Ariyan, S.: Immediate reconstruction of a composite mandibular defect with a regional osteomyocutaneous flap. Plast. Reconstr. Surg., *65*:477, 1980.

Cutting, C. B.: Unpublished results, 1981.

Cutting, C. B., and McCarthy, J. G.: Comparison of residual osseous mass between vascularized and nonvascularized onlay bone transfers. Plast. Reconstr. Surg., *72*:672, 1983.

Cutting, C. B., McCarthy, J. G., and Berenstein, A.: The blood supply of the upper craniofacial skeleton: the search for composite calvarial bone flaps. Plast. Reconstr. Surg., *74*:603, 1984.

Daniel, R. K.: Mandibular reconstruction with free tissue transfers. Ann. Plast. Surg., *1*:346, 1978.

Davis, J., and Taylor, A.: Muscle pedicle bone grafts: experimental study. Arch. Surg., *65*:330, 1952.

Demergasso, F.: Colgajo cutaneo aislado a pediculo muscular. Nueva technica reconstructiva de cavidad oral en cancer de cabeza y cuello. Acta Soc. Cir. Rosario, *32*:27, 1976.

Dingman, R. O.: The use of iliac bone in the repair of facial and cranial defects. Plast. Reconstr. Surg., *3*:24, 1950.

Donski, P. K., Carwell, G. R., and Sharzer, L. A.: Growth in revascularized bone grafts in young puppies. Plast. Reconstr. Surg., *64*:239, 1979.

Dorenbos, J.: The blood supply of the spheno-occipital synchondrosis in the Wistar albino rat. J. Dent. Res., *50*:983, 1971.

Dorenbos, J.: The blood supply of cranial base synchondroses. Acta Morph. Neerl. Scand., *9*:380, 1972.

Dufresne, C. R., Cutting, C. B., Valauri, F., Parker, P. M., Colen, S. R., and McCarthy, J. G.: Reconstruction of mandibular and floor of mouth defects using the trapezius myocutaneous and osteomyocutaneous flaps. Plast. Reconstr. Surg., *79*:687, 1987.

Duhamel, H.: Sur le developpement et la crue des os des animaux. Mem. Acad. Roy. Sci. Paris, *55*:354, 1742.

Durante, F.: Trattato di patologia generale e speciale e terapia chirurgica. Roma Societa Editrice. Rome, Dante Alighieri, 1904.

Engström, A.: Quantitative micro- and histochemical elementary analysis. Acta Radiol. Suppl., *63*, 1946.

Engström, A.: The detection of small difference in cellular mass by historadiography and a new equipment for microradiography. Exper. Cell Res. (Suppl.), *3*:117, 1955.

Engström, A., and Amprino, R.: X-ray diffraction and x-ray absorption studies of immobilized bones. Experientia, *6*:267, 1960.

Engström, A., and Finean, J. B.: Low-angle x-ray diffraction of bone. Nature (Lond.), *171*:564, 1953.

Enlow, D. H.: Principles of Bone Remodeling. Springfield, IL, Charles C Thomas, 1963.

Enneking, W.: Immunologic aspects of bone transplantation. South. Med. J., *55*:894, 1962.

Fagarasanu, I.: Procède de cranioplastie pars des greffons costaux redoubles: Procède du "grillage protecteur." Tech. Chir. (Paris), *29*:57, 1937.

Foster, C. A., and Sherman, J.: Surgery of Facial Bone Fractures. New York, Churchill Livingstone, 1987, p. 198.

Freeman, B.: The results of epiphyseal transplants by flap and by free graft. Plast. Reconstr. Surg., *36*:227, 1965.

Friedenberg, Z. B., and Kohanim, M.: The effect of direct current on bone. Surg. Gynecol. Obstet., *126*:97, 1968.

Fukada, E., and Yasuda, I.: On the piezoelectric effect of bone. J. Phys. Soc. Japan, *10*:1158, 1957.

Gallie, W. E., and Robertson, D. E.: Transplantation of bone. J.A.M.A., *70*:1134, 1918.

Ghent, W. R.: Further studies on meralgia paraesthetica. Can. Med. Assoc. J., *85*:871, 1961.

Goldberg, V. M., and Lance, E. M.: Revascularization and accretion in transplantation. J. Bone Joint Surg., *54A*:807, 1972.

Gordon, S., and Ham, A.: Essays in Surgery. Toronto, University of Toronto Press, 1950, p. 296.

Groves, E. W. H.: Bone transplantation. J. Bone Joint Surg., *5*:185, 1917.

Ham, A. W.: Histological study of the early phases of bone repair. J. Bone Joint Surg., *12*:827, 1930.

Ham, A. W., and Gordon, S.: The origin of bone that forms in association with cancellous chips transplanted into muscle. Br. J. Plast. Surg., *5*:154, 1952.

Hancock, D.: The fate of replaced bone flaps. J. Neurosurg., *20*:983, 1963.

Hancox, M.: Survival of transplanted embryo bone grafted to chorioallantoic membrane: subsequent osteogenesis. J. Physiol., *106*:279, 1947.

Harakas, N.: Demineralized bone matrix induced osteogenesis. Clin. Orthop., *188*:239, 1984.

Harvold, E. P.: The role of function in the etiology and treatment of malocclusion. Am. J. Orthod., *54*:883, 1968.

Heine, B.: Ueber die Wiedererzeugung neuer Knochenmassen und Bildung neuer Knochen. J. Chir. Augenheilk., *24*:513, 1836.

Heinen, J.: The experimental production of ectopic cartilage and bone in the muscles of rabbits. J. Bone Joint Surg., *31A*:765, 1949.

Heppenstall, R. B.: Fracture healing. *In* Heppenstall, R. B. (Ed.): Fracture Treatment and Healing. Philadelphia, W. B. Saunders, 1980, pp. 35–64.

Heslop, B., Zeiss, I., and Nesbit, N.: Studies on transference of bone. I. A comparison of autologous and homologous bone implants with reference to osteocyte survival, osteogenesis and host reaction. Br. J. Exp. Pathol., *41*:269, 1960.

Holmes, R. E.: Bone regeneration within a coralline hydroxyapatite implant. Plast. Reconstr. Surg., *63*:626, 1979.

Holmstrand, K.: Biophysical investigations of bone transplants and bone implants; an experimental study. Acta Orthop. Scand. (Suppl.), *26*, 1957.

Holmstrand, K., Longacre, J., and deStefano, G. A.: Biophysical studies of split rib grafts in the repair of defects of the cranium. Plast. Reconstr. Surg., *26*:3, 1960.

Hoogendoorn, H. A., Renooij, W., Akkermans, L. M., Visser, W., and Wittebol, P.: Long-term study of large ceramic implants (porous hydroxyapatite) in dog femora. Clin. Orthop., *187*:281, 1984.

Horowitz, N.: Scanning and scintigraphy. *In* Powsner, E., and Raeside, D. (Eds.): Diagnostic Nuclear Medicine. New York, Grune & Stratton, 1971, pp. 501–505.

Huggins, C.: The formation of bone under the influence of epithelium of the urinary tract. Arch. Surg., *22*:377, 1931.

Huggins, C., and Wiege, E.: The effect on the bone marrow of disruption of the nutrient artery and vein. Ann. Surg., *110*:940, 1939.

Huntington, T.: Case of bone transference. Ann. Surg., *41*:249, 1905.

Ivy, R. H.: Bone grafting for restoration of defects of the mandible. Plast. Reconstr. Surg., *7*:333, 1951.

Johnson, R.: A physiological study of the blood supply of the diaphysis. J. Bone Joint Surg., *9*:153, 1927.

Kappis, A.: Zur Deckung von Schadeldefekten. Zentralbl. Chir., *42*:897, 1915.

Kazanjian, V.: Bone transplanting to the mandible. Am. J. Surg., *83*:633, 1952.

Kim, P. S., Gottlieb, J. R., Harris, G. D., Nagle, D. J., and Lewis, V. L.: The dorsal thoracic fascia: anatomic significance with clinical applications in reconstructive microsurgery. Plast. Reconstr. Surg., *79*:72, 1987.

Koch, J.: The laws of bone architecture. Am. J. Anat., *21*:177, 1917.

Koekenberg, L.: Vascularization in the Healing of Fractures. Springfield, IL, Charles C Thomas, 1963.

Koenig, F.: Der knocherne Ersatz grosser Schädeldefekte. Zentralbl. Chir., *17*:65, 1890.

Langer, K.: Ueber das Gefaessystem der Roehrenknochen. Denkschr. Akad. Wiss. Wien, *36*:1, 1876.

Langer, K.: Über die Blutgefasse der Knochen des Schädeldaches und der harten Hirnhaut. Denkschr. Akad. Wiss. Wien, *37*:217, 1877.

LaTrenta, G. S., McCarthy, J. G., and Cutting, C. B.: The growth of vascularized onlay bone transfers. Ann. Plast. Surg., *18*:511, 1987.

Leriche, R., and Policard, A.: La Physiologie Normale et Pathologique de l'Os. St. Louis, MO, C. V. Mosby Company, 1928.

Lexer, E.: Knochenbildung in Bindegewebe osteoplastischer Hernkunft. Dtsch. Z. Chir., *217*:1, 1929.

Lexer, E., Kuliga, and Turk, W.: Untersuchungen über Knochenarterien. Berlin, Hirschwald, 1904.

Longacre, J., and deStefano, G. A.: Further observations of the behavior of autogenous split-rib grafts in reconstruction of extensive defects of the cranium and face. Plast. Reconstr. Surg., *20*:281, 1957.

Macewen, W.: The Growth of Bone. Glasgow, J. Maclehose & Sons, 1912.

Macomber, W., and Shepard, R.: Mandibular bone grafts. Plast. Reconstr. Surg., *3*:570, 1948.

Mall, F.: On ossification centers in human embryos less than one hundred days old. Am. J. Anat., *5*:433, 1906.

Manchot, C.: Die Hautarterien des menschichen Körpers. Leipzig, F. C. W. Vogel, 1889.

Marks, S. C., Jr.: Congenital osteopetrotic mutations as

probes of the origin, structure and function of osteoclasts. Clin. Orthop., *189*:239, 1984.

Mathews, J.: Bone structure and ultrastructure. *In* Urist, M. (Ed.): Fundamental and Clinical Physiology of Bone. Philadelphia, J. B. Lippincott Company, 1980.

May, J. W., Jr.: Aesthetic and functional thumb reconstruction: great toe to hand transfer. Clin. Plast. Surg., *8*:357, 1981.

McCarthy, J. G., Cutting, C. B., and Shaw, W. W.: Vascularized calvarial flaps. Clin. Plast. Surg., *14*:37, 1987.

McCarthy, J. G., Lorencz, Z. P., Cutting, C., and Rachesky, M.: The median forehead flap revisited: the blood supply. Plast. Reconstr. Surg., *76*:866, 1985.

McCarthy, J. G., and Zide, B. M.: The spectrum of calvarial bone grafting: introduction of the vascularized calvarial bone flap. Plast. Reconstr. Surg., *74*:10, 1984.

McCullough, D., and Fredrickson, J. M.: Neovascularized rib grafts to reconstruct mandibular defects. Can. J. Otolaryngol., *2*:96, 1973.

McDowell, F., and Ohlwiler, D.: Mandibular resection and replacement. Internat. Abstrs. Surg., *115*:103, 1962.

McLean, F., and Urist, M.: Bone: An Introduction to the Physiology of Skeletal Tissue. Chicago, University of Chicago Press, 1961.

Meyer, H. von: Die Architectur der Spongiosa. Arch. Anat. Physiol., *34*:615, 1867.

Milch, R., Rall, D., and Tobie, J.: Bone localization of the tetracyclines. J. Natl. Cancer Inst., *19*:87, 1957.

Milhaud, G., Labat, M., Graf, B., and Thillard, M.: Relation between the thymus and osteopetrosis. *In* Copp, D. H., and Talmage, R. (Eds.): Endocrinology of Calcium Metabolism. Amsterdam, Excerpta Medica, 1978, p. 143.

Moore, J., Mazur, J., and Zehr, D.: Biomechanical and histologic comparison of vascularized and conventional autogenous bone grafts. *In* Abstracts of the Plastic Surgery Research Council Meeting, May 21, 1981, Springfield, IL.

Moss, M., and Salentijn, L.: The primary role of the functional matrices in facial growth. Am. J. Orthod., *55*:566, 1969.

Mowlem, R.: Cancellous chip bone grafts: report on 75 cases. Lancet, *2*:746, 1944.

Mowlem, R.: Bone grafting. Br. J. Plast. Surg., *16*:293, 1963.

Mueller, W.: Zur frage der temporarem Schadelresektion an stelle der Trepanation. Zentralbl. Chir., *17*:65, 1890.

Mulholland, M., and Pritchard, J.: The fracture gap. J. Anat. (Lond.), *93*:590P, 1959.

Mulliken, J. B., and Glowacki, J.: Induced osteogenesis for repair and construction in the craniofacial region. Plast. Reconstr. Surg., *65*:553, 1980.

Neuman, W.: Bone material and calcification mechanisms. *In* Urist, M. (Ed.): Fundamental and Clinical Physiology of Bone. Philadelphia, J. B. Lippincott Company, 1980.

Oikarinen, J., and Korhonen, L. K.: The bone inductive capacity of various bone transplanting materials used for treatment of experimental bone defects. Clin. Orthop., *140*:208, 1979.

Oklund, S. A., Prolo, D. J., Gutierrez, R. V., and King, S. E.: Quantitative comparisons of healing in cranial fresh autografts, frozen autografts, and processed autografts and allografts in canine skull defects. Clin. Orthop., *205*:269, 1985.

Oldfield, M.: Iliac hernia after bone grafting. Lancet, *1*:810, 1945.

Ollier, L.: Traite experimental et clinique de la regeneration des os et de la production artificielle du tissu osseux. Paris, P. Masson et Fils, 1867.

Ostrup, L. T., and Fredrickson, J.: Distant transfer of a free living bone graft by microvascular anastomoses. Plast. Reconstr. Surg., *54*:274, 1974.

Ostrup, L. T., and Fredrickson, J.: Reconstruction of mandibular defects after radiation using a free living bone graft transferred by microvascular anastomoses. Plast. Reconstr. Surg., *55*:563, 1975.

Panje, W., and Cutting, C.: Trapezius osteomyocutaneous island flap for reconstruction of the anterior floor of the mouth and the mandible. Head Neck Surg., *3*:66, 1980.

Peltier, L. F.: The classic. The growth of bone. Chapter III. Osteogenic power of bone bereft of periosteum. William Macewen, F. R. S. Clin. Orthop., *174*:5, 1983.

Pensler, J., and McCarthy, J. G.: The calvarial donor site: an anatomic study in cadavers. Plast. Reconstr. Surg., *75*:648, 1984.

Phemister, D.: The fate of transplanted bone and regenerative power of its various constituents. Surg. Gynecol. Obstet., *19*:303, 1914.

Pollack, S. R.: Bioelectrical properties of bone: endogenous electrical signals. Orthop. Clin. North Am., *15*:3, 1984.

Pritchard, J.: Repair of fractures of the parietal bones in rats. J. Anat. (Lond.), *80*:55, 1946.

Prolo, D. J., and Rodrigo, J. J.: Contemporary bone graft physiology and surgery. Clin. Orthop., *200*:322, 1985.

Ray, R. D.: Vascularization of bone grafts and implants. Clin. Orthop., *87*:43, 1972.

Reid, R.: Hernia through an iliac bone graft donor site. Case report. J. Bone Joint Surg., *50A*:757, 1968.

Rhinelander, F. W.: The normal microcirculation of diaphyseal cortex and its response to fracture. J. Bone Joint Surg., *50A*:784, 1968.

Rhinelander, F. W.: Tibial blood supply in relation to fracture healing. Clin. Orthop., *105*:34, 1974.

Ritsila, V., Alhopuro, S., and Rintala, A.: Bone formation with free periosteum. Scand. J. Plast. Reconstr. Surg., *6*:51, 1972.

Robertson, I., and Baron, J.: A method of treatment of chronic infective osteitis. J. Bone Joint Surg., *28*:19, 1946.

Robison, R.: The Significance of Phosphoric Esters in Metabolism. New York, New York University Press, 1932.

Rogers, L.: The history of craniotomy. Ann. Med. Hist., *2*:495, 1930.

Rosen, I. B., Bell, M. S., Barron, P. T., Zuker, R. M., and Manktelow, R. T.: Use of microvascular flaps including free osteocutaneous flaps in reconstruction after composite resection for radiation-recurrent oral cancer. Am. J. Surg., *138*:544, 1979.

Roux, W.: Das Gesetz der Transformation der Knochen. Berl. Klin. Wchschr., *30*:509, 533, 557, 1893.

Rydygier, L. R.: Zum osteoplastischen Ersatz nach Unterkieferresektion. Zentralbl. Chir., *35*:1321, 1908.

Sato, K. and Urist, M.: Induced regeneration of calvaria by bone morphogenetic protein (BMP) in dogs. Clin. Orthop., *197*:301, 1985.

Serafin, D., Villarreal-Rios, A., and Georgiade, N. G.: A rib-containing free flap to reconstruct mandibular defects. Br. J. Plast. Surg., *30*:263, 1977.

Shehadi, S.: Skull reconstruction with bone dust. Br. J. Plast. Surg., *23*:227, 1970.

Shim, S. S.: Physiology of blood circulation of bone. J. Bone Joint Surg., *50A*:812, 1968.

Shim, S. S., Copp, D. H., and Patterson, F. P.: Measurement of the rate and distribution of the nutrient and other arterial blood supply in long bones of the rabbit. J. Bone Joint Surg., *50B*:178, 1968.

Skoog, T.: The use of periosteum and Surgicel for bone restoration in congenital clefts of the maxilla. Scand. J. Plast. Reconstr. Surg., *1*:113, 1967.

Smith, J. D., and Abramson, M.: Membranous versus endochondrial bone autografts. Arch. Otolaryngol., *99*:203, 1974.

Snyder, C. C., Bateman, J. M., Davis, C. W., and Warden, G. D.: Mandibulo-facial restoration with live osteocutaneous flaps. Plast. Reconstr. Surg., *45*:14, 1970.

Spalteholz, W.: Die Vertheilung der Blutgefässe in der Haut. Arch. Anat. Entwcklngsgesch., *1*, 1893.

Stein, I., and Shapiro, B.: Applications of radionuclides in the evaluation of bone disorders. *In* Goswitz, F., Andrews, G., and Viamonte, M. (Eds.): Clinical Uses of Radionuclides. Springfield, VA, National Technical Information Service, 1971, pp. 162–201.

Strauch, B., Bloomberg, A. E., and Lewin, M. L.: An experimental approach to mandibular replacement: island composite vascular rib grafts. Br. J. Plast. Surg., *24*:334, 1971.

Stricker, M., Montaut, J., Hepner, H., and Flot, F.: Osteotomies du crane et de la face. Ann. Chir. Plast., *17*:233, 1972.

Stringa, G.: Studies in the vascularization bone grafts. J. Bone Joint Surg., *39B*:3955, 1957.

Swartz, W.: Personal communication, 1985.

Swartz, W. M., Banis, J. C., Newton, E. D., Ramasastry, S., Jones, N. F., and Acland, R.: The osteocutaneous scapular flap for mandibular and maxillary reconstruction. Plast. Reconstr. Surg., *77*:530, 1986.

Sykoff, W.: Zur Frage der Knochenplastik am Unterkiefer. Zentralbl. Chir, *27*:881, 1900.

Tanner, J. M.: Growth at Adolescence. 2nd Ed. Oxford, Blackwell Scientific Publications, 1962, p. 45.

Taylor, G. I., Miller, G. D. H., and Ham, F. J.: The free vascularized bone graft. Plast. Reconstr. Surg., *55*:533, 1975.

Taylor, G. I., Townsend, P., and Corlett, R.: Superiority of the deep circumflex iliac vessels as the supply for free groin flaps. Experimental work. Plast. Reconstr. Surg., *64*:595, 1979a.

Taylor, G. I., Townsend, P., and Corlett, R.: Superiority of the deep circumflex iliac vessels as the supply for free groin flaps. Clinical work. Plast. Reconstr. Surg., *64*:745, 1979b.

Testut, L., and Jacob, O.: Traite D'Anatomie. Paris, Octobe Doin, 1909.

Triffitt, J.: The organic matrix of bone tissue. *In* Urist, M. (Ed.): Fundamental and Clinical Physiology of Bone. Philadelphia, J. B. Lippincott Company, 1980.

Trueta, J.: The role of vessels in osteogenesis. J. Bone Joint Surg., *45B*:402, 1963.

Trueta, J.: Studies in the Development and Decay of the Human Frame. Philadelphia, W. B. Saunders Company, 1968.

Trueta, J., and Cavadius, A.: A study of the blood supply of the long bones. Surg. Gynecol. Obstet., *118*:485, 1964.

Urist, M.: Bone transplants and implants. *In* Urist, M. (Ed.): Fundamental and Clinical Physiology of Bone. Philadelphia, J. B. Lippincott Company, 1980.

Urist, M., and McLean, F.: Osteogenetic potency and new bone formation by induction in transplants to the anterior chamber of the eye. J. Bone Joint Surg., *34A*:443, 1952.

Urist, M. J., Urist, J. M., Jr., Dubuc, F. L., and Strates, B. S.: Quantitation of new bone formation in intramuscular implants of bone matrix in rabbits. Clin. Orthop., *68*:279, 1970.

Van der Meulen, J. C. H., Hauben, D. J., Vaandrager, J. M., and Birgenhager-Frankel, D. H.: The use of a temporal osteoperiosteal flap for the reconstruction of malar hypoplasia in Treacher Collins syndrome. Plast. Reconstr. Surg., *74*:687, 1984.

Vandervord, J. G., Watson, J. D., and Teasdale, G. M.: Forehead reconstruction using a bi-pedicled bone flap. Br. J. Plast. Surg., *35*:75, 1982.

Van Meekren, J.: Observationes Medicochirurgicae. Amsterdam, Henrici & T. Bloom, 1682.

Wagner, W.: Die temporare Resektion des Schadeldaches an Stelle der Trepanation. Zentralbl. Chir., *16*:833, 1889.

Walker, D. G.: Spleen cells transmit osteopetrosis in mice. Science, *190*:785, 1975.

Watson-Jones, R.: The repair of skull defects by a new pedicle bone graft operation. Br. Med. J., *1*:780, 1933.

Wlodarski, K., Hancox, N., and Brooks, B.: The influence of cortisone on the implantation site on bone and cartilage induction in various animals. J. Bone Joint Surg., *55B*:595, 1973.

Wolfe, S. A., and Kawamoto, H. K.: Taking the iliac bone graft. J. Bone Joint Surg., *60A*:411, 1978.

Wolff, J.: Uber die innere Architectur der Knochen und ihre Bedeutung fur die Frage vom Knochenwachstum. Arch. Pathol. Anat., *50*:389, 1870.

Wolff, J.: Über die Theorie des Knochenschwindes durch vermehrte Druck und der Knochenanbildung durch Druckenlastung. Arch. Klin. Chir., *42*:302, 1892.

Wolff, J.: Die Lehre der funktioneller Knochengestalt. Arch. Pathol. Anat., *155*:256, 1895.

Woolf, J., and Walker, A.: Cranioplasty: collective review. Int. Abstr. Surg., *81*:1, 1945.

Yabe, H., and Hanaoka, H.: Investigation of the origin of the osteoclast by use of transplantation on chick chorioallantoic membrane. Clin. Orthop., *197*:255, 1985.

Young, R.: The control of cell specialization in bone. *In* Robinson, R. (Ed.): The Healing of Osseous Tissue. Washington, DC, National Academy of Science, 1967.

Zeiss, I., Nesbit, N., and Heslop, B.: Studies on transference of bone. II. Vascularization of autologous and homologous implants of cortical bone in rats. Br. J. Exp. Pathol., *41*:345, 1960.

Zins, J., and Whitaker, L.: Membranous versus endochondral bone autografts: implications for craniofacial reconstruction. Surg. Forum, *30*:521, 1979.

Zins, J., and Whitaker, L.: Membranous versus endochondral bone: implications for craniofacial reconstruction. Plast. Reconstr. Surg., *72*:778, 1983.

19

Julia K. Terzis
Kevin L. Smith

Repair and Grafting of the Peripheral Nerve

Over the past two decades the therapeutic approach toward the patient with a peripheral nerve injury has significantly changed. Facilitated by new technologies of intraoperative electrodiagnosis, by better magnification, and by increased understanding of peripheral nerve structure and function, reconstructive surgery is being optimized. In the case of proximal injury, early nerve repair has helped to circumvent denervation atrophy of the distal muscles for better functional results.

Awareness of fascicular anatomy has made nerve repair more precise, and an appreciation of the detrimental effects of tension at the site of nerve repair has made nerve grafting commonplace. Development of biochemical, histochemical, and immunochemical markers will allow the surgeon to define motor and sensory units within nerve fascicles; improved results will follow from better identification of the topographic anatomy of the nerve.

Knowledge of the patterns of sensory recovery has led to sophisticated postoperative programs of sensory reeducation that make possible more functional use.

HISTORICAL BACKGROUND

The first written description of the peripheral nervous system is found in the writings of Hippocrates (460–370 B.C.) although it is not certain that he differentiated between tendons and nerves (hence, the term *aponeurosis*). Galen (A.D. 130–200) was the first to study the effects of transections of the peripheral nerves. He noted decreased sensibility after transection of some nerves and decreased muscle power with others. He took pride in relating the story of his discovery that the recurrent laryngeal nerves controlled the voice, and these nerves are still known as Galen's (Majno, 1975). Scholars of the Sushruta would argue that the vagus, glossopharyngeal, and recurrent laryngeal nerves and their functions were described several centuries earlier (circa 1000 B.C.) (Majno, 1975). The first record of nerve suture was not until the thirteenth century and made by William of Saliceto (circa 1210–1277) at Bologna. The sixteenth to the nineteenth centuries yielded more information about the nerve fibers themselves: their excitable nature by Glisson (1597–1677); the microscopic structure–an early preparation by van Leewenhoek (1632–1723); the axon and myelin sheath that made up the nerve fiber by Fontana (1730–1805). Function was elucidated by Galvani (1737–1798) in frog experiments showing that nerve fibers responded to electrical stimulation. Anatomic organization was appreciated by Bell (1774–1842), who recognized that motor nerves were associated with the ventral spinal roots, and by Magendie (1783–1855), who determined that sensory function was localized in the dorsal roots. Myelinated and unmyelinated ("fiber of Remak") nerve fibers were differentiated by Remak (1815–1855) in his work with rabbit embryos, and a contemporary, von Purkinje (1787–1869), elucidated the connection between neurons and axons (Clarke and O'Malley, 1968; McHenry, 1969; Bradley, 1974).

As early as 1828 experiments were performed that surgically manipulated nerves. Flourens reportedly transposed the nerves of the flexors and extensors in the wing of the rooster (Wilgis, 1982). In 1839 Schwann published his findings regarding the structure of the cell that bears his name (Causay, 1960).

One of the earliest reports of nerve repair was by Paget (1847), describing an 11 year old patient who sustained a median nerve laceration that was primarily sutured and who demonstrated a complete recovery (Wilgis, 1982).

A milestone in the understanding of nerve injury was reached in 1850 with the publication of the findings of Waller. This study of the glossopharyngeal and hypoglossal nerves of the frog showed degenerative changes distal to the level of nerve injury, and orderly progression of regenerating axons down the preserved nerve fiber. Waller noted that regeneration was more rapid in the young and was not hastened by galvanic stimulation. From these experiments he concluded that the nerve cell functioned as a trophic center and was responsible for the maintenance of the peripheral nerve fiber (Waller, 1850; Boyes, 1976).

Conduction velocities of nerves were measured by von Helmholtz and Duchenne. They applied electrophysiologic principles to the clinical situation, and added considerably to the knowledge of nerve function and dysfunction on clinical parameters. Biochemical manipulations of nerve transmission followed, pioneered by the studies of neuromuscular blockade with curare performed by Bernard (Clarke and O'Malley, 1968; McHenry, 1969; Bradley, 1974).

Shortly thereafter, a student of Bernard, Mitchell, published the first description of causalgia (1864), which was expanded to become what is now a classic text: *Injuries of Nerves and their Consequences* (Mitchell, 1872).

While clinicians began to appreciate the consequences of nerve injury, basic scientists defined the structure of the nervous system. Golgi and Cajal shared the 1906 Nobel Prize for their work demonstrating the nervous system to be a continuous neural network composed of individual nerve cells with functional connections (Daniel and Terzis, 1977a).

Sherrington named the functional connections "synapses" and developed the modern concept of the functional organization of the nervous system, which relies on the integration of innumerable independent, discrete nerve cells through the "synapses" (Sherrington, 1906).

Independently, Hoffman and Tinel reported similar accounts of tingling sensations perceived by patients at increasingly distal points along the trunk of a regenerating nerve. To Tinel, the tingling sensations were felt to represent ". . . the presence of young axons in the process of growing." While both papers were published in 1915 (Hoffman in March, Tinel in October), this familiar sign of nerve regeneration bears Tinel's name (Clark, 1983).

Another Nobel Prize was shared in 1944 by Erlanger and Gasser for their research relating to the highly differentiated functions of single nerve fibers and their interrelations, studies providing much understanding of the compound action potential, nerve fiber conduction, and the refractory period of nerves. Using these concepts, Hodes, Larrabee, and German (1948) developed the application of electrophysiology for clinical nerve testing.

The foundation of the current science of peripheral nerve surgery was probably laid by Seddon. With innumerable battle casualties, he studied and reported on multiple traumatic injuries over all levels of the peripheral nerve (Seddon, 1948). In addition, he pioneered nerve grafting techniques (Seddon, 1963), studied the effects of ischemia on the peripheral nerve (Seddon and Holmes, 1945), and measured the rates of nerve regeneration following repair (Seddon, Medawar, and Smith, 1943).

Contemporary milestones are being reached with the research of Sunderland (1945b, 1952, 1953, 1968; Sunderland, Lavarack, and Ray, 1947, 1949), Millesi (1981a, 1984; Millesi, Meissl, and Berger, 1972, 1976), and Terzis (Terzis, Faibisoff, and Williams, 1974, 1975; Williams and Terzis, 1976; Dykes and Terzis, 1979; Terzis and Dykes, 1980) regarding the management of peripheral nerve injuries and the technical considerations of their repair. These technical advances have been associated with the advances in basic sciences that have better delineated the role of the Schwann cell, the neural response to injury, axonal growth and transport, and axonal response to changes of local environment.

PERIPHERAL NERVE COMPOSITION

The peripheral nervous system is a complex, composite structure of cell bodies (neurons), supportive connective tissue and cellular elements, and end organs. It is designed to receive and relay input from the environment to the central nervous system, and effect changes in the environment by relay of sympathetic and autonomic outflow (Fig. 19–1). In this manner the central nervous system connects to the periphery, with incoming afferent fibers predominantly received in the dorsal spinal roots and outgoing efferent motor fibers originating within the ventral horns of the spinal cord. The neurons interface with one another by multiple cytoplasmic extensions, the dendrites, and each neuron generally sends a single axon to the periphery. Bundles of the axons make up the spinal roots (dorsal and ventral), which join at a point distal to the sensory ganglion. The union of the two roots marks the most proximal extent of the spinal nerves, which contain mixed populations of sensory and motor fibers. Afferent fibers terminate at the peripheral sensory receptors; the density of the fibers is directly proportional to the areas of greatest sensory input. Efferent fibers terminate at the motor end plates of the extrafusal and intrafusal muscle fibers. A bimodal population of myelinated efferent fibers exists: the large fibers innervating the extrafusal fibers, and the small, the intrafusal fibers. In addition, the spinal efferent outflow includes myelinated autonomic fibers that provide motor innervation to the blood vessels and epidermal appendages.

Nerve fibers, efferent or afferent, travel in bundles termed "fascicles" (the term "funicle" is no longer in use) bound by supportive connective tissues. Study of nerve cross sections shows the proportion of connective tissue to vary in area from 25 to 85 per cent (Sunderland and Bradley, 1949; Slingluff, Terzis, and Edgerton, 1987). This proportion varies from nerve to nerve and from proximal to distal. Sunderland (1968) noted a greater proportion of connective tissue stroma at points where nerves cross joints or where there are relatively greater numbers of smaller fascicles. He also pointed out that the connective tissue elements are largely re-

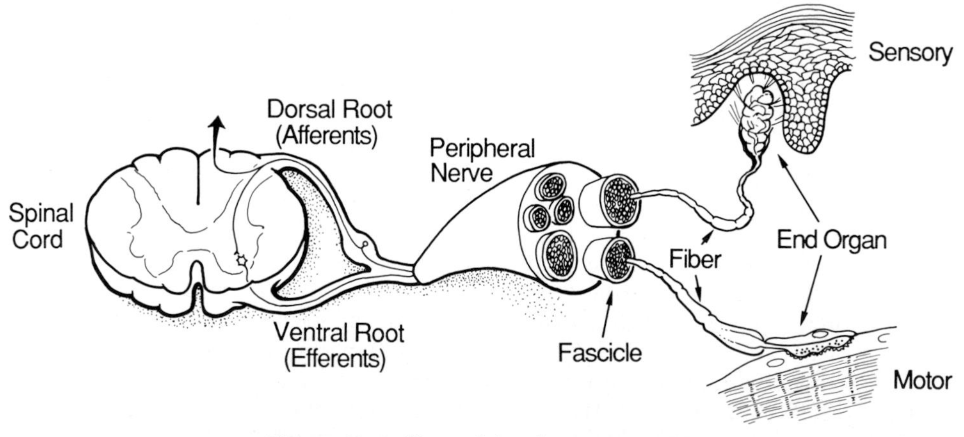

Figure 19–1. The peripheral nervous system.

sponsible for the tensile strength of any nerve fascicle. At the level of the brachial plexus, connective tissue elements account for 57 to 85 per cent of the cross sectional area (Slingluff, Terzis, and Edgerton, 1987).

An important cause of variability in the relative proportions of connective tissue is fascicular plexus formation and fascicular branching (Fig. 19–2). Early work by Sunderland (1945, 1968; Sunderland, Marshall, and Swaney, 1959) using histologic techniques to trace nerve fibers, and later "labeling" by proximal fascicular transection and distal tracing of wallerian degeneration, led to the conclusion that nerve fibers did not demonstrate a predictable fascicular localization. These findings stimulated 30 years of pessimism regarding peripheral nerve surgery. Many surgeons, believing that it was not possible to identify or "match" nerve fascicles, accepted less than optimal nerve reconstruction results and avoided intraneural dissection and proximal nerve grafting.

Within the last decade, findings by Slingluff, Terzis and Edgerton (1987), Jabaley, Wallace, and Heckler (1980), Schady and associates (1983), Ueyama (1978), Bonnel (1981, 1985), and others have better defined the internal topographic anatomy of peripheral nerves. Plexus formation and fascicular interchange do occur, but not to a degree that would preclude intraneural dissection, fascicular repair, or interfascicular nerve interposition grafting.

Schady and associates (1983), in studies on awake patients that used intraneural microstimulation combined with microneurography, noted the degree of fascicular segregation proximally and distally between motor and sensory fascicles. The results revealed that despite a highly variable fascicular pattern, there remained a high degree of efferent and afferent segregation with fascicles of essentially pure motor or sensory axons. In the median nerve at the level of the upper arm, 20 to 40 per cent of fascicles appeared to project to the skin. However, these projections did not follow typical cutaneous dermatomes, and there appeared to be overlap of cutaneous territories between the fascicles. Similar overlap has been shown in the greater auricular nerve of the rabbit by Terzis (1981) and in the macaque monkey by Denny-Brown, Kirk, and Yanagisawa (1973). Extensive redistribution of the nerve fibers must take place within fascicles proximally to account for the generally observed overlap of three to five dermatomes in each fascicular territory (Dykes and Terzis, 1981; Schady and associates, 1983).

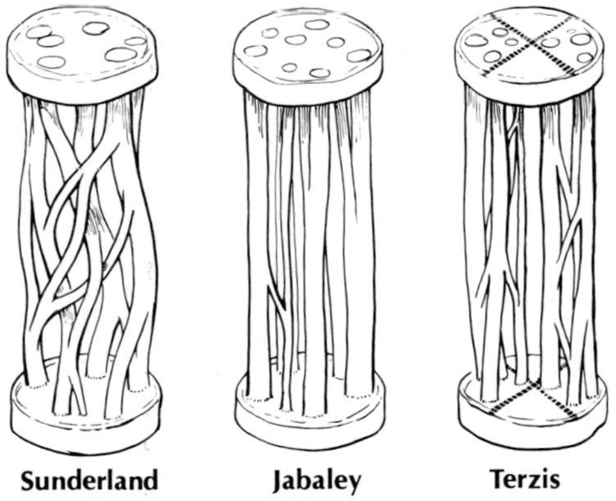

Figure 19–2. The internal topographic anatomy of the peripheral nerve with emphasis on fascicular organization. Note the variable patterns. (Modified from Terzis.)

It was speculated by Schady and associates (1983) that interfascicular communications do not serve the purpose of translating groupings of spinal roots into innervation patterns at the terminal branch level, but may serve the protective benefit of redundancy. Double representation of target tissue is obviously advantageous in cases of partial nerve injury, and explains the frequently small deficit in partial injuries of proximal nerves.

The most extensive study of plexus topographic anatomy performed by Slingluff, Terzis, and Edgerton (1987) examined the nerves at 0.5 to 1 mm intervals. They determined that fascicles in the plexus traveled only an average of 5 mm without branching or joining a neighboring fascicle. However, fascicle groups representing brachial plexus branches remained cohesive for lengths of up to 25 mm, and certain regions are characteristically monofascicular: the spinal nerves, the anterior and posterior divisions of the upper trunk, and the origins of the suprascapular and musculocutaneous nerves. The posterior division of the lower trunk is typically bifascicular. Several branches were identified as being purely motor (or nearly so) and together they make up nearly 30 per cent of the brachial plexus neural tissue. These branches are the dorsal scapular, long thoracic, subscapular, suprascapular, pectoralis, axillary (82 per cent muscular), thoracodorsal, and radial (77 per cent muscular). Thus, almost 85 per

Table 19–1. Classification of Peripheral Nerve Fibers

Group	Diameter (μ)	Conduction Velocity (m/sec)	Function
A (α, β, γ, δ)	2.5–22	15–100	Myelinated somatic afferent and efferent
B	3	3–15	Myelinated preganglionic autonomic (visceral)
C	0.2–1.5	0.3–1.6	Unmyelinated somatic afferent and autonomic postganglionic efferent (pain, pilomotor, sudomotor, and vasomotor)

*After Daniel, R. K., and Terzis, J. K.: Structure and function of the peripheral nerves. *In* Daniel, R. K., and Terzis, J. K. (Eds.): Reconstructive Microsurgery. Boston, Little, Brown & Company, 1977b.

cent of the posterior cord is motor. Seventy-five per cent of the axons are contributed by C6, C7, and C8. Twenty-two per cent supply the median nerve, 21 per cent the radial nerve, and 14 per cent the ulnar nerve.

There are several indeterminate zones with poor localization of fascicle groups, such as at the upper trunk at the formation of the divisions and at the origin of the suprascapular nerve, and the lower trunk as it forms the medial cord and the posterior cord between the posterior divisions and the axillary nerve origin (Slingluff, Terzis, and Edgerton, 1987). Knowledge of the origin of the neural supply of the plexus branches (i.e., C5, C6, C7, C8, or T1) allows the surgeon to bypass the "gray zones" by grafting, and to achieve satisfactory results in patients previously considered inoperable.

In 1894 Sherrington published his first work on the composition of peripheral nerves. He determined that larger afferent fibers were to be found in nerves to muscles than in those to skin. Later, with Eccles (Eccles and Sherrington, 1930), two distinct motor nerve populations were found in the peripheral nerves. Large and small fibers were named "alpha" and "gamma," respectively. The alpha population was subsequently determined to be the large, fast-conducting axons that innervate large skeletal muscle fibers (extrafusal) (Burke, 1980), and gamma fibers were found to terminate on the intrafusal muscle fibers within muscle spindles (Leskell, 1945). Sherrington and Eccles had thought that the smaller gamma fibers supplied small motor units in the extrafusal muscle (Kennedy, Poppele, and Quick, 1980). In a review by Matthews (1972), beta fibers, intermediate in size and conduction velocity between alpha and gamma, were identified. The beta population was seen to innervate both extrafusal and intrafusal fibers.

Another classification of peripheral afferent fibers still in use today is by Lloyd (1943) and is based largely on fiber size. The largest fibers (12 to 22 μ) are assigned to Group I, intermediate (6 to 11 μ) to Group II, small (1 to 5 μ) to Group III, and unmyelinated to Group IV.

In a more complete classification system, Erlanger and Gasser (1937; Gasser and Grundfest, 1939) included all types of peripheral nerve fibers and divided them as a function of fiber diameter and conduction velocity. The myelinated fibers were designated A and B, and unmyelinated fibers, C (Table 19–1). The A fibers include all somatic myelinated fibers, afferent and efferent, and can be divided into subgroups alpha, beta, gamma, and delta (in descending order of size). B fibers include only the visceral nerves (e.g., vagus and white rami communicantes), and Group C unmyelinated fibers are both somatic afferent and autonomic efferent (McIntyre, 1980). This is the classification system preferred by the authors.

Cellular Morphology

The functional unit of the nervous system upon which all structures are dependent is the *neuron*, or cell body (soma) (Fig. 19–3). The neuron has many intracellular structures in common with other cells of the body, but it also has several very specialized characteristics. Each cell body has a large surface area with extensions for reception, conduction, and transmission of nerve impulses. With the exception of the axon hillock (the cytoplasmic extension that gives rise to the axon), the entire surface area of the neuron is covered with a variety of synaptic terminals, or *boutons*, the variety of which is appreciated only by electron microscopy (Conradi, 1969; McLaughlin, 1972). Cytoplasmic extensions, specialized for receptive function, are known

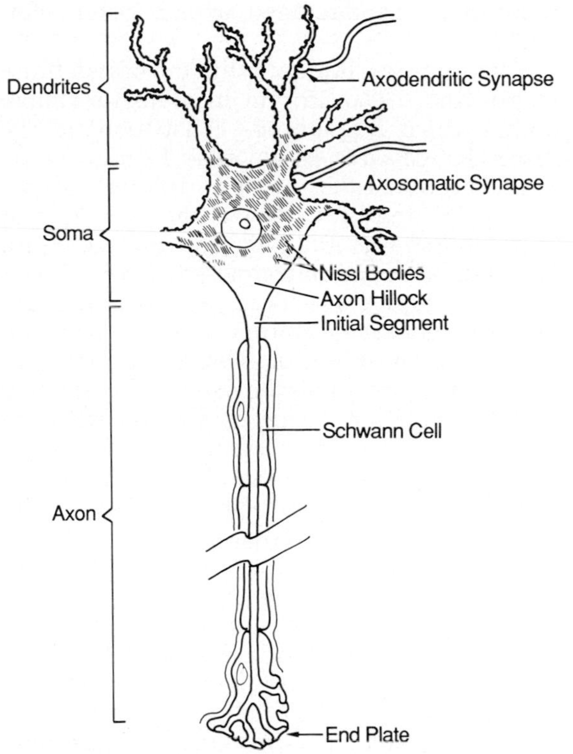

Figure 19–3. The components of the neuron.

as *dendrites.* Most neurons have one axon without collaterals, but alpha motor neurons give off one or more axon collaterals. The collaterals terminate on Renshaw interneurons or can end directly on other alpha motor neurons. These interconnections produce recurrent inhibitions of motor neurons that regulate the entire afferent system (Burke, 1980).

A neuron contains within its cytoplasm a single nucleus that is round and pale, and contains one or more nucleoli. Prominent features are the Golgi apparatus and mitochondria. Although the Golgi vesicles appear within the axon cylinder, prominent mitochondria are seen at the axonal and dendritic endings and are also scattered along the axon. These probably represent the sources of energy for neural impulse transmission (Peacock, 1984). Basophilic *Nissl bodies* (or chromophil substance) are found within the *soma* (neural cytoplasm) and they represent rough endoplasmic reticulum with polyribosomes.

Neurons of the peripheral nervous system are both unipolar and multipolar. Sensory nerve cells, located in the dorsal root ganglia, are unipolar, with one process leaving the cell body and subsequently dividing into two, a dendrite and an axon. The "dendrite" of the sensory nerve, efferent from the sensory receptors, is structurally similar to an axon and by convention is referred to by that term. Alpha motor neurons are examples of multipolar cells, usually with one axon and several dendrites.

The *axon* is a generally cylindric extension of the neurite that arises at the funnel-shaped *axon hillock*. It is bounded by the axolemma, which is a specialized trilaminar random mosaic of protein molecules floating within a fluid matrix of highly mobile phospholipid molecules, 7 to 8 mm in thickness (Thomas and Ochoa, 1984). The hillock is devoid of Nissl substance but there is a dense layer of granular substance approximately 200 A below its cell membrane (Palay and associates, 1968; Peters and Vaughan, 1970). Within the hillock there is a confluence of microtubules that exhibit clustering and crosslinkage (Daniel and Terzis, 1977b). The junction between the cell body hillock and the axon is termed the *initial segment*; it is short, narrow, and devoid of myelin (Peters and Vaughan, 1970; Thomas, Landon, and King, 1984). It is possible that this zone is the area at which nerve impulses are initiated (Mira, 1981a). Other sites without myelination, e.g., the nodes of Ranvier, also appear to exhibit the same dense, granular layer below the axolemma and are known to be responsible for the propagation of the action potential (Elfvin, 1961). Support is lent by the observation that sensory neurons do not show the dense layer at the axon hillock, nor are any impulses generated from that point (Daniel and Terzis, 1977b). The nerve fiber becomes myelinated abruptly beyond the axon hillock, greatly increases in diameter, and continues this size until the axon terminates at the end organ (Thomas, Landon, and King, 1984).

The axolemma is a highly specialized membrane that is able to maintain a resting potential across its entire thickness by selectively altering the intra- and extracellular concentrations of monovalent ions (Barchi, 1980). This process appears to be energy dependent and is associated with a sodium-potassium-ATPase pump. Freeze fracture electron microscopic studies have revealed dense concentrations of particles (1200/μm) within the axolemma (Schnapp and Mugnaini, 1978). Rosenbluth (1976) suggested that these particles correspond to membrane sodium channels and may be associated with ATPase activity; he also believed that these particles are synthesized within the cell body and actively transported to sites along the axolemma, with clusters deposited at the nodes of Ranvier—the sites of membrane depolarization and repolarization in myelinated axons. In a resting state, the axolemma maintains a high intracellular concentration of potassium (approximately 110 mmol) and a high extracellular concentration of sodium (approximately 130 mmol) (Barchi, 1980), but without energy input (ATP) the gradient would gradually fall to zero. The electrochemical gradient endows the neuron and axon with the property of excitability. As a reaction to specific stimuli, ion flux is created along the axon, and an action potential is initiated and propagated; the latter can proceed to trigger a muscle twitch or somesthetic impulse.

Within the axon cylinder is the axoplasm, which is structurally much less complex than its parent neuron. The principal structures within are microfilaments, neurotubules, and microtubules suspended in an amorphous matrix similar to that of cytoplasm. However, the primary difference between the axon and the cell body cytoplasm is the relative lack of organelles in the axoplasm. The axon lacks any of the structures associated with protein synthesis or assembly, namely, ribosomes, rough endoplasmic reticulum, and Golgi vesicles. Because of their absence, the axon must be dependent on the neuron structures (Thomas, Landon, and King, 1984) or the satellite cells for maintenance.

The smallest axoplasmic components are the microfilaments, which are thought to be paired helical chains of actin. The microfilaments are generally confined to the cortical zone near the axolemma, and their contractile actin proteins may play a role in the mechanism of intra-axonal transport (Elfvin, 1961).

Larger and more prevalent within the axoplasm are the neurofilaments (8 to 11 mm in diameter), linked into an irregular polygonal lattice by less dense filaments. These filaments occupy the area within the axoplasm not occupied by other organelles. Neurofilaments are composed of three proteins of 68,000 to 200,000 molecular weight and are shown to be readily digested by intrinsic axonal calcium-activated protease (Schlaepfer and Hasler, 1979). This mechanism may account for the rapid disappearance of neurofilaments in damaged axons (Schlaepfer, 1983).

Microtubules, hollow cylinders of indefinite length and 23 to 25 mm in diameter, make up the third filamentous constituent of the axon. Composed of 13 globular 4 μm subunits of the protein tubulin, these tubules are arranged in longitudinal orientation, singly or parallel (Schmitt and Samson, 1968). Tubulin is a diameric protein composed of two similar subunits, alpha and beta. Microtubules are helically arranged chains of alternating alpha and beta subunits. The numbers of microtubules vary along the axon and it appears that the number increases directly with axonal mass. Terminal axon branches have been observed to have ten times more microtubules than the more proximal axon segments (Zenker and Hohberg, 1973).

Microtubule density and number also vary between classes of nerves, with unmyelinated axons possessing five times the number of microtubules per unit cross sectional area than large myelinated fibers (Friede and Samorajski, 1970).

The most common site of dense microtubule groupings is within the initial segment (Palay and associates, 1968), within the dorsal root ganglia (Lieberman, 1976), at the nodes of Ranvier where they form palisades around other intra-axonal organelles (Landon and Hall, 1976), and in the internodal segments of large Group A fibers where they are arranged in regular fashion. In all the above cases the microtubules are arranged along the long axis of the nerve fiber. It has been observed that there are populations of circumferentially oriented microtubules in the nodal axon that may function to maintain the shape of the node (Mohammed, Landon, and Love, 1983).

With the filamentous structures in the axoplasm, there exists a variety of organelles including mitochondria, smooth endoplasmic reticulum, lysosomes, and vesicles. Mitochondria vary in number in an inverse ratio to the axonal cross sectional area (Berthold, 1968a). They are often associated with one or more microtubules, and many observers have reported both distal and proximal transport of the mitochondria along the axonal cylinder (Zelena, 1968; Cooper and Smith, 1974; Droz, Rambourg, and Koenig, 1975; Forman, Padjen, and Siggins, 1977). Microcinematography has also documented a rapid saltatory side to side motion of the mitochondria (Droz, 1981).

The smooth endoplasmic reticulum exists as a three-dimensional dynamic network of intra-axonal conduits that appear to coalesce, disperse, and give rise to secretory vesicles along the axon. This pattern includes the synaptic regional specializations such as subaxolemmal sacs or locally flattened expansions. The smooth endoplasmic reticulum forms a continuous network from the cell body to the distal termination of the axon. Although radioautographs have demonstrated that the smooth endoplasmic reticulum is associated with transport of materials along the axon, it does not appear that the reticulum is itself transported (Ellisman and Lindsey, 1983).

The remaining axoplasmic structures are the secretory vesicles and secondary lysosomes. The vesicles range in size from 40 to 100 μm and they can be found along any point of the axon (Berthold, 1978). As with many of the other organelles, the concentrations of vesicles are found at the nodes of Ranvier and within the nerve terminal (Landon and Hall, 1976). These vesicles are believed to be involved in the transport of catecholamines (Thomas, Landon, and King, 1984).

"Coated" vesicles, found commonly at the neuromuscular junctions, appear to be involved in the recycling of synaptic vesicle membrane from the axolemma to the endoplasmic reticulum (Heuser and Reese, 1973; Holtzman, 1977). "Dense-cored" vesicles, seen in postganglionic unmyelinated autonomic fibers, also appear to play a role in the storage and release of catecholamines. Lysosomes are observed, usually near the nodes of Ranvier, and are seen to accumulate during wallerian degeneration after injury (Webster, 1962; Holtzman and Novikoff, 1965).

Axoplasmic Transport

From a study of the axon and the neuron cell body, it is apparent that the former relies on the latter for the synthesis and assembly of protein macromolecules. These molecules are transported "down" the axon (somatofugal or anterograde flow) and others are transported "up" the axon (somatopedal or retrograde flow) concurrently at a variety of rates (Zelena, 1968; Lubinska and Niemerko, 1971; Courand and DiGiamberardino, 1981; Lasek, 1982). Not all substances are derived from the neuron cell body, however, as it appears that some trophic substances are imbibed from the adjacent Schwann cells (Droz, 1981) and end organs.

After severance of a nerve, the distal stump ceases to be able to transmit impulses. Synaptic transmission and nerve terminal function are also dependent on an intact peripheral nerve. This finding infers that the break in connection between the axon and neuron leads to the depletion or loss of some property vitally necessary for normal function (Daniel and Terzis, 1977b). Motor nerve severance is followed within days by muscle synaptic dysfunction and failure of transmission (Gutmann, 1964; Guth, 1968; Drachman, 1974), and the same occurs in denervated sensory terminals (Guth, 1971).

Axoplasmic transport does not proceed at a single rate. Radiochemical and histochemical techniques have documented axoplasmic transport at various rates from slow (0.25 to 1 mm per day) (Tytell and associates, 1981) to fast (up to 468 mm per day) (Koshima and Harii, 1984). Slow axoplasmic transport appears to be the bulk movement of a coherent neurotubule-neurofilament network along the axon in a proximodistal direction. A second slow-moving component, moving at a slightly faster rate of 2 to 4 mm per day, is composed of actin microfilaments and their complexed proteins and multiple soluble enzymes such as the glycolytic enzymes (DiGiamberardino and associates, 1973; Wilson and Stone, 1979). The slow anterograde transport rate is equivalent to the velocity of outgrowth of axonal sprouts in developing and regenerating neural tissue (Wilson and Stone, 1979; Pleasure, 1980).

Day to day maintenance of axon terminals cannot be served by the cell body solely by this mode of slow transport. The axon also exhibits a method of fast transport of molecules that is energy dependent and ATP utilizing (Grafstein and Forman, 1980), and appears to be able to act without an intact neuron (Lubinska, 1964; Ochs, 1972, 1977; Lasek, 1982). The packaging of materials for transport still occurs in the cell body (in rough endoplasmic reticulum and the Golgi apparatus) and, if transport is blocked, these components collect in the cell (Gross and Kreutzberg, 1978; Ribak, Vaughn, and Saito, 1978). The fast transport system is responsible for the conveyance of axoplasmic particulate, including mitochondria and neuro-transmitted storage vesicles, and enzymes such as acetylcholinesterases and axolemmal constituents (Droz and associates, 1979; Courand and DiGiamberardino, 1981; Griffin and associates, 1981). There is no difference in the rate or materials transported between sensory and motor axons (Ochs, 1972; Barker, Neale, and Gainer, 1976).

Fast axoplasmic transport requires energy in the form of high energy phosphate compounds; therefore, it is necessary for the neuron to be adequately oxygenated. Any interruption of mitochondrial oxidative phosphorylation causes axoplasmic flow to cease (Leone and Ochs, 1978). Colchicine, the vinca alkaloids (vincristine and vinblastine), and any other drug that causes microtubular dissolution also interrupt fast axonal transport (Goldman, Kim, and Schwartz, 1976; Green and associates, 1977).

Actin microfilaments do not appear necessary for fast transport, as cytochalasin B, an inhibitor of microfilament formation, does not block transport (Banks, Mayor, and Mraz, 1973); neither do the sodium channel inactivators, such as tetrodotoxin, which destroys the axonal membrane's ability to conduct an action potential (Ochs and Worth, 1975).

In addition to somatofugal (anterograde) fast and slow transport, a concurrent somatopedal (retrograde) flow exists. First demonstrated by Lubinska (1964; Lubinska and Niemierko, 1971), it has come to light that the retrograde transport system is a very important mechanism for recycling of the intra-axonal proteins and neurotransmitters (Pleasure, 1980), but (possibly more important) the somatopedal flow transmits extraneural material (accumulated by active endocytosis) from the nerve endings to the neuron, providing a mechanism for trophic influence upon neurons by end organs (Price, 1974; Olsson, Forsberg, and Kristensson, 1978). Exogenous nerve growth factor, released by a variety of tissues innervated by motor and sensory fibers (Murphy and associates, 1977; Ebendal and associates, 1980; Harper and associates, 1980), is taken up by the axolemmal and nerve terminal high affinity receptors (Dumas, Schwab, and Thoenen, 1979) and is transported to the neuron, where it has been shown to stimulate cell metabolism (Thoenen and associates, 1971). Retrograde transport also provides a pathway to the neuron and ultimately the central nervous system for many pathogens and toxins. A case in point is the transmission of herpes simplex virus along the axon to infect the spinal cord.

One mechanism postulated to be responsible for axoplasmic transport is similar to the sliding filament theory of muscle contraction. Movement could be generated by interactions between actin and myosin and the stationary microtubule-neurofilament network of the axoplasm. The observation that heterogeneous molecules are all carried down the axon at constant rates—slow or fast—suggests that the mechanism is based on a common transport "carrier." The "carrier" may be a microfilament system that moves down the microtubule network by alternate binding and release (Fig. 19–4). Indirect evidence to support this theory is provided by the observation that axon transport is halted by any substance that causes microtubular disaggregation, and the fact that dense microtubules have been identified that crosslink transported organelles and the microtubule-neurofilament network (Ochs, 1971, 1982, 1984; Ochs and Hollingsworth, 1971; Smith, Jarlfors, and Cameron, 1975; Hanson and Edström, 1978; Tsukita and Ishikawa, 1980).

This mechanism for axoplasmic transport does require energy in the form of ATP utilized by the Ca^{++}-Mg^{++}-ATPase associated with the transport filaments. As long as oxidative metabolism is maintained to provide ATP, transport continues. Anoxia, produced by nitrogen, sodium azide, or cyanide, produces a block of fast axoplasmic transport within 15 minutes (Ochs and Hollingsworth, 1971).

Nerve Conduction

Nerves transmit information in two ways: first, slowly by physical movement of molecules utilizing axoplasmic transport as described above, and second, quickly by the initiation and propagation of electrical currents generated across the cell membrane. The unique resting membrane potential of the peripheral nerve axon maintains an electrical gradient of approximately -70 mV by active partitioning of the sodium and potassium molecules (sodium extracellular) (Barchi, 1980). This mechanism is facilitated by the selective permeability to small charged ions through channels that seem to be capable of variable "gating" (Armstrong, 1975). Elec-

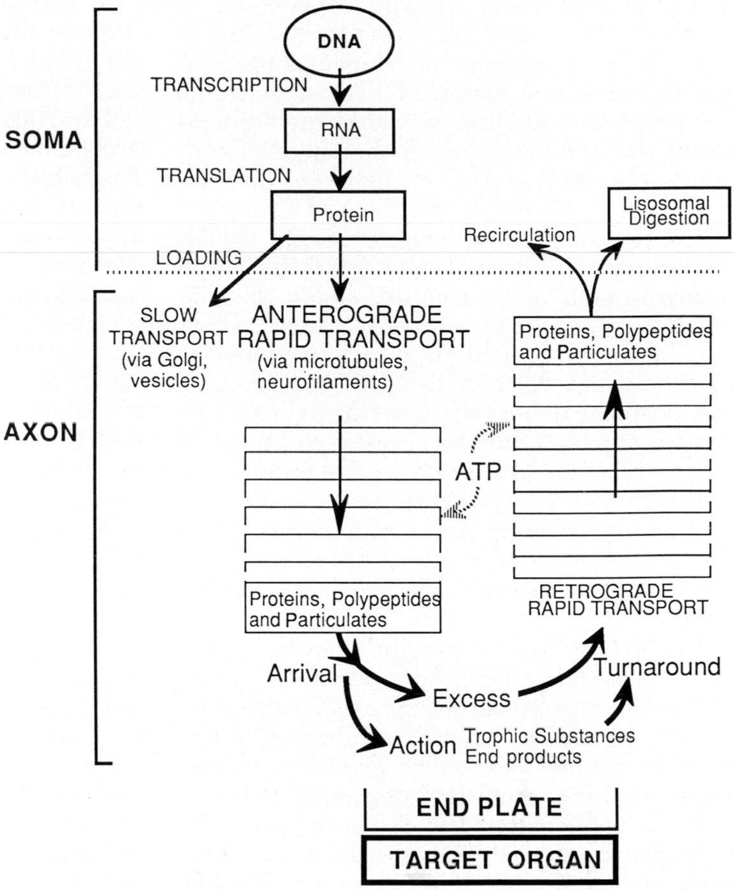

Figure 19–4. Mechanism of axoplasmic transport.

trical signals are generated by changes in the membrane permeability to ions (i.e., opening and closing gates) and by allowing the ions to follow the electrochemical gradient and pour through the membrane, creating an electrical flux. With each current impulse (action potential or localized potential), sodium rushes into the cell, and at a slightly slower rate potassium leaves the axoplasm. Energy, driving the sodium-potassium ATPase pump, restores the membrane potential by pumping sodium out of the intracellular space. Potassium passively flows back in, driven by the changing electrochemical gradient.

Depolarization of axons can generate two types of signals: localized potentials and action potentials. Localized potentials, which travel over only short distances, play a role in the functional integration between individual cells, especially at the cell-cell junctions and sensory endings. The action potential is a conducted impulse that obeys the "all or none" law (Daniel and Terzis, 1977b), which is propagated the entire length of the axon without decrement. In unmyelinated fibers, propagation is by longitudinal spread of current. Any local depolarization of the axolemma results in an explosive depolarization spike that creates in the surrounding membrane other depolarizing currents, depolarization spikes, and so on along the axon (Sebille, 1981). After each localized depolarization a period of recovery occurs, the absolute refractory period, when there is insufficient sodium conductance available to generate another action potential. During this period of repolarization, the membrane resting potential is restored. The refractory period ensures that the action potential is propagated unidirectionally, and the length of this period determines the minimal amount of time that must elapse before successive action potentials.

For any given membrane, the conduction velocity is determined by the specific membrane's resistivity (a constant) and by the fraction of the total current of an action potential that flows radially as opposed to axially. Since radial resistance is due almost entirely to membrane resistance, and axial resistance is a function of both axoplasmic conductivity and cross sectional area, essentially the only variable in the speed of conduction is the diameter of the axon. Conduction velocity therefore increases as a function of the square of the diameter (Barchi, 1980). Experimentally it has been proved that large unmyelinated fibers conduct faster than do small (Burrows and associates, 1965). However, in order to achieve sufficient increases in conduction velocity to fulfill the needs of the peripheral nervous system, axons of titanic diameter would be necessary and would create severe space problems, leaving room for little else except nerve fibers within the human form. Owing to size constraints in the human, unmyelinated axons are limited to a conduction of about 1 m per sec (Barchi, 1980).

The evolution of a myelin sheath, a high resistance, low capacitance insulator, overcame these space limitation considerations by allowing greatly increased conduction velocities in smaller axons. The myelin sheath is produced by a complex interaction between the nerve axon and the Schwann cell. The myelin insulation divides the axon into short regions (1 to 2 mm) (Napolitano and Scallen, 1969; Rydinack and Berthold, 1983) capable of depolarization, and longer regions (16 to 19 mm) (Bunge, Williams, and Wood, 1982) unable to generate an action potential. The nerve impulse is propagated by jumping from one myelin-free area (*node of Ranvier*) to the next in a process known as *saltatory conduction*. Most current flow in the "myelinated" nerves is in an antegrade fashion within the axon, and exits out the next node of Ranvier, with no evidence of membrane excitation within the internodal region (Huxley and Stämpfli, 1949). Saltation allows for much faster conduction velocity, up to approximately 70 m per sec (Thomas, Landon, and King, 1984).

The Schwann Cell

The Schwann cell is the neuronal satellite cell of the peripheral nervous system, and all axons are ensheathed to varying degrees by these cells, which produce myelin. The cells, which are neuroectodermally derived (neural crest and possibly neural tube), grow with or slightly ahead of the neurites that arise from the primitive dorsal root ganglia and ventral horn neurons (Gamble, 1976). Each Schwann cell initially has multiple bundles of immature axons within its cytoplasm (Dunn, 1970). The Schwann cells then continue to divide by mitosis until there is a 1:1 ratio between axons and Schwann cells for those axons destined to become myelinated (Friede and Samorajski, 1968; Webster, Martin, and O'Connell, 1973). For those axons destined to remain unmyelinated (50 to 80 per cent of the average nerve fiber (Ochoa, 1976), groups of eight to 15 axons eventually come to lie within individual longitudinal enfoldings of the Schwann cell membrane (Thomas, Landon, and King, 1984).

What determines the selection of fibers for myelination is not entirely known. It is related to axon caliber (Fraher, 1972) and may involve some trophic influence on the Schwann cell by the axon (Aguayo and associates, 1976). Maintenance of the Schwann cell certainly requires trophic input from the axon (Weinberg and Spencer, 1978), and vice versa.

When an axon becomes myelinated, the envaginating Schwann cell lays down many layers of specialized cell membrane by spiraling around the axon perimeter. The myelin sheath is a proteophospholipid multilayered spiral of compacted apposed cell membranes that have extruded the Schwann cell cytoplasm from within (Geren, 1954).

The thickness of the myelin layer varies with the diameter of the ensheathed axon; larger fibers have thicker sheaths (Yates, Bouchard, and Wherrett, 1976; Thomas, Landon, and King, 1984). For a given axon diameter, motor nerves have a thicker sheath than do sensory nerves (Williams and Wendell-Smith, 1971). Despite the fact that there is a difference in conduction velocities between large and small nerve fibers, it does not seem that the thickness of the myelin sheath and its passive properties as an electrical insulator are responsible. The difference most likely resides in variations of conductance between one node of Ranvier and another (Jack, 1976).

Whether myelinated or unmyelinated, any axon is ensheathed along its entire length from the ventral or dorsal roots to the distal axon termination. For unmyelinated axons, the Schwann cells form branching and anastomosing cords of cells (Gasser, 1955; Aguayo and associates, 1976) with an internuclear distance of 200 to 500 μm (Carlsen and Behse, 1980). The boundaries of adjacent Schwann cells in unmyelinated fibers are indistinct owing to the presence of numerous cytoplasmic interdigitations (Eames and Gamble, 1970; Carlsen, Knappeis, and Behse, 1974). Although frequent *puncta adherentia* are seen, they cannot be assumed to be areas of specialized intracellular contact between each adjacent Schwann cell (Ochoa, 1976).

The Schwann cell observed in unmyelinated fibers contains the usual complement of intracellular organelles, but peculiar to the Schwann cell is the elaboration of a basal lamina that surrounds the axon and is continuous across cell junctions to isolate the nerve axon from its surrounding environment. The elaboration of the basal lamina by the Schwann cell is another example of trophic dependence on innervation. Without the axon, no basal lamina is produced (Bunge, Williams, and Wood, 1982; Bunge and Bunge, 1984).

Like the unmyelinated axon, the myelinated axon is covered by a cord of Schwann cells. However, this is not a continuous tube along the whole length of the axon but is segmented as noted above. Each segment consists of a single Schwann cell, and in the space between the cells, the node of Ranvier, there is a specialized elaboration of both the axon and the two adjacent Schwann cells. The myelinated axon is capable of depolarization only at the nodes. Conduction proceeds by sequential activation of successive nodes without depolarization of the intervening internode. Local currents spread within the axon in an antegrade fashion and exit through the low resistance pathway provided by the node. Owing to the passive membrane properties of the insulating myelin, the internode is not depolarized (Barchi, 1980). By saltatory conduction, velocity is maximized.

The ultrastructure of the node of Ranvier reveals that the entire paranodal region, the adjacent Schwann cell membranes and the nodal axon, should be considered a single functional unit with contributions from each component (Fig. 19–5) (Williams and Landon, 1963; Landon and Williams, 1963). The axolemma at this level is lined with an electron-dense granular layer similar to that at the initial segment (Elfvin, 1961). It has been suggested that this area of density represents voltage-sensitive ionic channels, a theory based on electron microscopy (Kristol, Sandri, and Akert, 1978), current fluctuation studies (Sigworth, 1980), and current gating studies (Chiu, 1980).

The axon at the node of Ranvier also shows variations unique to this area. The number of mitochondria in the nodal axon is five times higher than elsewhere (Berthold, 1968b), and the lamellated autophagic vesicles, smooth endoplasmic reticulum, glycogen granules, and lysosome-like granules are found in greater abundance at this site (Thomas, Landon, and King, 1984). In addition, there is an overall narrowing of the axon "cylinder" at the nodal region (Hess and Young, 1952).

The juxtanodal myelin and Schwann cell terminate at the node by forming a series of loops containing cytoplasm with a large number of mitochondria (Hess and Young, 1952; Berthold and Skoglund, 1967). Outside the myelin the Schwann cell forms a finger-like

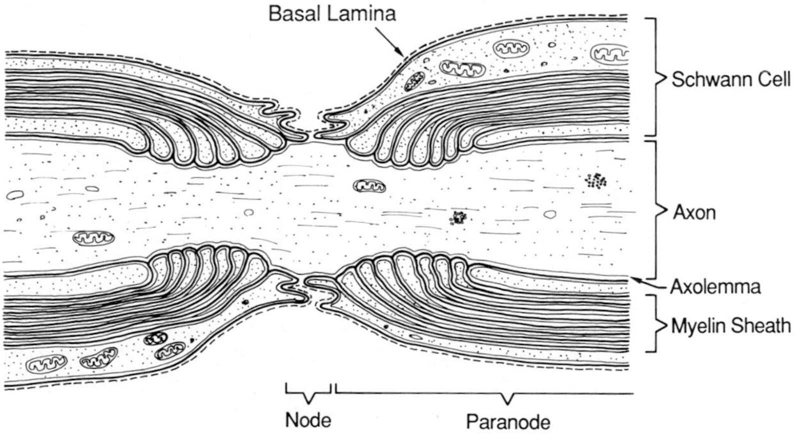

Figure 19–5. The ultrastructure of the node of Ranvier.

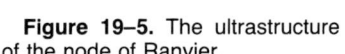

projecting cytoplasmic collar that also contains numerous mitochondria (Asbury, 1975). The nodal processes constitute a specialized form of contact between the axon and the Schwann cell, and it has been suggested that the finger-like projections serve as the site for metabolic and ionic exchange between the axon and Schwann cell (Williams and Landon, 1964; Kristensson and Olsson, 1973).

The annular space around the nodal axon, delimited by the axolemma, the adjacent Schwann cells, and the continuous basement membrane, is defined as the perinodal space (Thomas, Landon, and King, 1984), and contains a material of moderate electron density with a mottled appearance (Berthold, 1968) known as "gap substance" (Landon and Williams, 1963). It has been demonstrated that this substance contains glycosaminoglycans having cation exchange and binding properties similar to those of ion exchange resins (Landon and Langley, 1971; Langley, 1971). The "gap substance" could maintain an ionically inactive pool of sodium ions close to the nodal axolemma, and also retard diffusion of other cations away from the axon (Langley and Landon, 1967; Landon and Hall, 1976).

This complex paranodal apparatus, therefore, apparently functions to provide a source of high energy compounds and an ion pool sufficient to maintain the repolarization of the nodal axolemma, facilitating high frequency impulse transmission (Landon, 1981).

The internodal axon is far less complex. The general organization of the axon and Schwann cell is as described above, the Schwann cell providing a multilamellated myelin coat for the axon. The adaxonal Schwann cell (the innermost portion) makes almost one complete turn around the axon. The myelin in the first turn is only semicompact, and the slender band of remaining cytoplasm contains only an occasional lysosome or mitochondrium (Thomas, Landon, and King, 1984). Except where the periaxonal space is sealed at the proximal and distal ends of the adaxonal Schwann cell (immediately adjacent to the nodes) by close approximation to the axolemma, no specialized interconnections are apparent (Thomas, Landon, and King, 1984). As the Schwann cell completes the first revolution around the axon, a tight junction completes the segregation of the periaxonal space. At this site the densely compacted cell membrane extrudes its cytoplasm and begins the spiral enfolding of the axon. At the completion of the spiral, the myelin sheath is sealed from the abaxonal Schwann cell (the outermost turn) by another tight junction. The bulk of the cytoplasm, cell nucleus and organelles are contained herein.

Longitudinal sections of the internodal axon and myelin sheath reveal regular interruptions in the myelin. It appears that the periodic line of each myelin lamella is divided and forms a pocket that encloses a small amount of cytoplasm. Each pocket overlaps with the next from abaxonal cytoplasm to the adaxonal sheath. Reconstructions from electron microscopy suggest that these are continuous tubules that connect the innermost and outermost portions of the cell (Hall and Williams, 1970; Ghabriel and Allt, 1979a,b). Although these were originally considered to be artifacts, it is now speculated that these Schmidt-Lanterman incisures are the route by which various metabolites and ions pass between the two parts of the cell (Rawlins, 1973; Ghabriel and Allt, 1981), and they may even possess pulsatile flow of cytoplasm.

Connective Tissue Elements

The peripheral nerves are associated with three separate and distinct supportive tissue sheaths, the *endoneurium, perineurium*, and *epineurium*, divisions suggested in the classic study by Key and Retzius (1986). Since that time, the fine structure and function of the connective tissue sheaths have been the subject of intense investigation and it is now well demonstrated that the sheaths provide multiple mechanical and physiologic functions.

At the level of the peripheral nerve fiber (the axon–Schwann cell complex), many fibers are brought together in a densely packed bundle, the fascicle (Fig. 19–6). Within this fascicle, the nerve fibers are packed in a mucopolysaccharide ground substance with longitudinally oriented collagen fibrils and smaller reticulin fibers (Thomas, 1963; Gamble and Eames, 1964). The principal cellular component of this structure is the fibroblast and it is responsible for collagen synthesis. The cells, collagen, reticulin, and the ground substance are referred to as the *endoneurium* (Thomas and Olsson, 1984). Mast cells and macrophages are occasionally found within the endoneurium and are probably of hematogenous origin (Olsson, 1971; Oldfors, 1980).

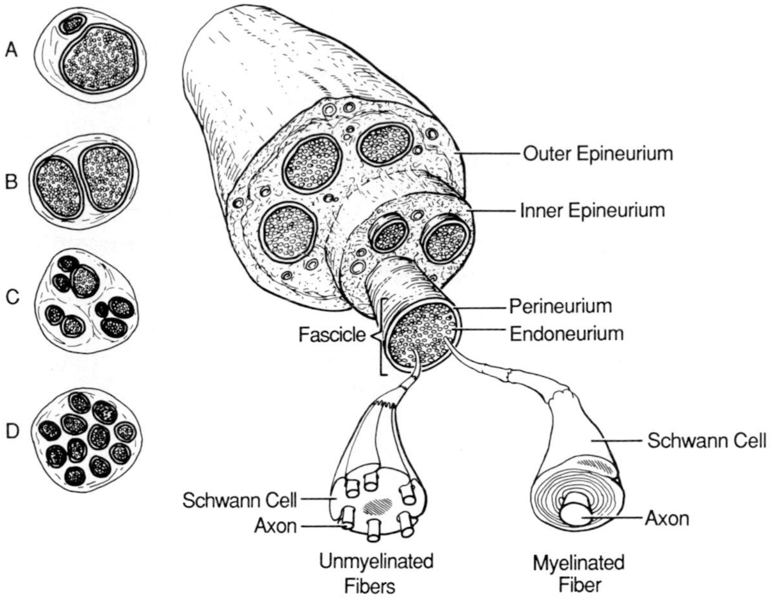

Figure 19–6. The connective tissue elements of the peripheral nerve and the basic patterns of intraneural structure. *A*, Monofascicular; *B*, oligofascicular; *C*, polyfascicular with group arrangement; *D*, polyfascicular with no identifiable group pattern.

The next level of organization is the *perineurium*, which is the connective tissue condensation around individual nerve fascicles. This layer is more organized than the endoneurium, and consists of inner layers of lamellated, squama-like cells and an outer layer of collagen fibers condensed into a dense lattice of longitudinal, circumferential, and oblique bundles (Thomas, 1963; Thomas and Olsson, 1984). In between each lamella of cells there are longitudinal bundles of collagen and elastic fibrils and occasional fibroblasts (Mira, 1981a).

The cellular layer is composed of multiple concentric sleeves of cells, the number of layers of which vary directly with the fascicular diameter. Up to 15 layers have been described in human nerves (Shanthaveerppa and Bourne, 1962, 1963a). These flattened cells have a basement membrane on both sides that may reach up to 0.5 μm in thickness (Gamble and Eames, 1964). The cytoplasm is metabolically active, with the mitochondria and endoplasmic reticulum located near the discoid nucleus. There are many pinocytotic vesicles that open on both sides of the membrane (Cravioto, 1966), and the scanty cytoplasm is full of glycogen granules (Shanthaveerppa and Bourne, 1963a; Waggener, Bunn, and Beggr, 1965; Cravioto, 1966). The cells form a confluent sheet and are linked by either interdigitation or multiple tight junctions (zonulae occludentes) (Thomas and Jones, 1967; Reale, Luciano, and Spitznas, 1975).

The perineurium is traversed by blood vessels that connect the vascular network of the epineurium with that of the endoneurium. The vessels carry sleeves of perineurial cells for some distance into the endoneurium, but they do not come into close contact with the vessels. A terminal opening provides a communication between the endoneurial and epineurial connective tissue spaces (Burkel, 1967).

Just before any site of fascicular branching, the perineurium partitions the fascicle. The perineurial sheath follows the branches to the periphery, where it may eventually be reduced to a single cell layer (the sheath of Henle). At the termination of the branches, the perineurium can extend to ensheath muscle spindles and the encapsulated end organs (Shanthaveerppa and Bourne, 1963b). However, at motor end plates the tube is open-ended and does not directly contact the neuromuscular junction (Saito and Zacks, 1969).

The perineurium is a specialized structure that provides active transport of materials across the perineurial cells by the pinocytotic vesicles (Waggener, Bunn, and Beggr, 1965). This is a mechanism for transport of substances to the fascicles, but Allt (1972) proposed that this pinocytotic transport may work as well in reverse, i.e., to transport proteins out of the endoneurium, especially in conditions of edema of the peripheral nerves. It is also a diffusion barrier that acts as the "blood nerve" barrier much as the pia arachnoid mater with which it becomes contiguous at the spinal angle (Allt, 1972). This barrier facilitates the regulation of the internal milieu of the fascicles and serves a protective function by excluding macromolecules such as toxins, antigens, and viruses that are disease producing (Waggener, Bunn, and Beggr, 1965).

The perineurium furnishes the strong "skeletal" support for the enclosed neural tissue and is the primary contributor to the tensile strength of the peripheral nerve. This layer also maintains positive pressure, which is necessary for the maintenance of endoneurial fluid pressure (Shanes, 1953; Daniel and Terzis, 1977b). There is a pressure differential of 2 to 20 mm Hg between the endoneurial arteriolar and venular ends of the capillary plexus. The hydrostatic pressure gradient generates a protein-free capillary filtrate and is augmented by the osmotic pressure of the endoneurial environment (Low, 1984). As there are no lymphatics within the endoneurium (Nukada, Pollock, and Allpress, 1981), the perineurial pressure is necessary to counteract these forces and to promote centrifugal flow toward the open-ended perineurium where the excess endoneurial fluid may gain access to epineurial lymphatic drainage (Malmgren and Olsson, 1980; Nukada, Pollock, and Allpress, 1981; Low, 1984).

The final supportive ensheathment of the peripheral nerve is the *epineurium*. This is a loose outer sheath that comprises the perifascicular and interfascicular connective tissue around and between the nerve fascicles. Its outer layers are continuous with the mesoneurium, the suspensory mesentery of the peripheral nerve that arises from the areolar connective tissue of the underlying fascia. The innermost layers blend with the perineurium (Sunderland, 1965). It is a structure that functionally can be considered to have two components, one that circumferentially encircles each fascicle and extends between them—the "inner" or "internal" epineurium—and the other epineurium that encircles the entire nerve trunk—the "outer" or "external" epineurium (Fig. 19–6).

The epineurium is a vascular structure, since it carries the nutrient blood vessels that supply the capillary plexus of the nerve. Lymphatics are also found in this layer. The lymphatic drainage accompanies the arterial supply and venous drainage of the nerve, and ultimately is collected in the regional lymph nodes (Sunderland, 1965).

The collagen fibrils, admixed with sparse elastin, are oriented parallel to the nerve in the longitudinal axis, and occasionally have a shallow spiral orientation (Thomas, 1963; Gamble and Eames, 1964). Within this matrix there are also fibroblasts, a few mast cells, and variable amounts of fat (Sunderland, 1945a). The fat may serve a protective function in cushioning the fascicles against injury by compression. As noted before, greater amounts of epineural connective tissue exist where the number of fascicles is greatest, and it is also thicker in areas where nerves cross joints. In general, the peripheral nerve lies loosely in its bed except where it is tethered by entering vessels or by its branches.

There are three basic patterns of intraneural architecture that can be recognized. Peripheral nerves that contain one large fascicle are termed *monofascicular*. Those that contain a few large fascicles are termed *oligofascicular*. Those that have many fascicles of different sizes are considered *polyfascicular*, and these fascicles may or may not be in identifiable group patterns (see Fig. 19–6).

Vascular Supply

As discussed above, nerve cells require a continuous and adequate supply of oxygen for aerobic metabolism to maintain normal function. After transection of a nerve axon, the distal part may remain excitable for a few days provided the blood supply is sufficient. In contrast, complete ischemia is followed by rapid deterioration of function within hours (Lundborg, 1977). Since the nerve is so susceptible to ischemia, it has developed a dynamic vascular plexus in all layers with well-developed collaterals between layers and between different segments of the nerve. This is accomplished by two integrated but functionally independent systems, the *extrinsic* and *intrinsic*.

Early studies of the blood vessels to the peripheral nerve (arteriae nervorum) concentrated on identifying their sources of supply by studying vascular patency under various conditions and the distribution of the intraneural branches (Adams, 1942; Sunderland, 1945a, 1968; Lundborg, 1970) (Fig. 19–7). The *extrinsic* system is composed of segmentally arranged vessels that vary in size and generally originate from neighboring large arteries and veins. In addition, considerable blood supply can originate from muscular perforators and periosteal vessels. As the nutrient vessels reach the epineurium, they ramify within the epineurium and supply the intraneural plexus through ascending and descending branches. (As defined by Bell and Weddell (1984b) "intraneural" refers to those vessels contained in all layers of the nerve: epi-, peri-, and endoneurium.)

Emerging veins of the extrinsic system are usually paired with the arteries. In situ, the arteries and veins appear tortuous or coiled and exhibit a "reserve in length" that allows the nerve significant freedom of movement before the vessels are stretched (Lundborg, 1979). The intraneural vessels of the epineurium are sympathetically innervated, and the nerve fibers travel closely with the nutrient vessels (Lundborg, 1970; Bell and Weddell, 1984a, b).

Most studies of the structure and function of the intraneural microvasculature have been performed in animals. Lundborg (1979) demonstrated the vascular similarities between animal and man and believed the experimental models to be applicable to human nerves.

The *intrinsic* vascular system begins at the points of branching of the extrinsic nutrient vessels. The branches run longitudinally within the epineurium and form part of an extensive vascular plexus with venular characteristics. In these vessels the blood flow shows no predominant pattern, and opposite flow directions have been documented to occur simultaneously at different points along the same vessel (Morgan, Reisman, and Wilgis, 1983). Anastomoses are common between arterioles, between venules, and between arterioles and venules. The vascular plexus of the epineurium is a highly adaptable system, able to reroute large volumes of blood on demand (Bell and Weddell, 1984a).

A similar organizational system is found in the perineurial vessels. There are multiple longitudinal vessels with numerous anastomoses with each other and with the underlying capillary plexus of the endoneurium. These connecting vessels often pursue an oblique course through the cellular perineurium and carry with them a sleeve of perineurial cells (Burkel, 1967; Olsson, 1984).

The endoneurial capillary plexus forms what Lundborg described as a "longitudinal basket formation" (Lundborg, 1979) that lies just beneath the perineurial cellular layers. The endoneurial vessels frequently anastomose, but under normal conditions only part of the vascular bed is functioning at any one time. In vital experiments, complete perfu-

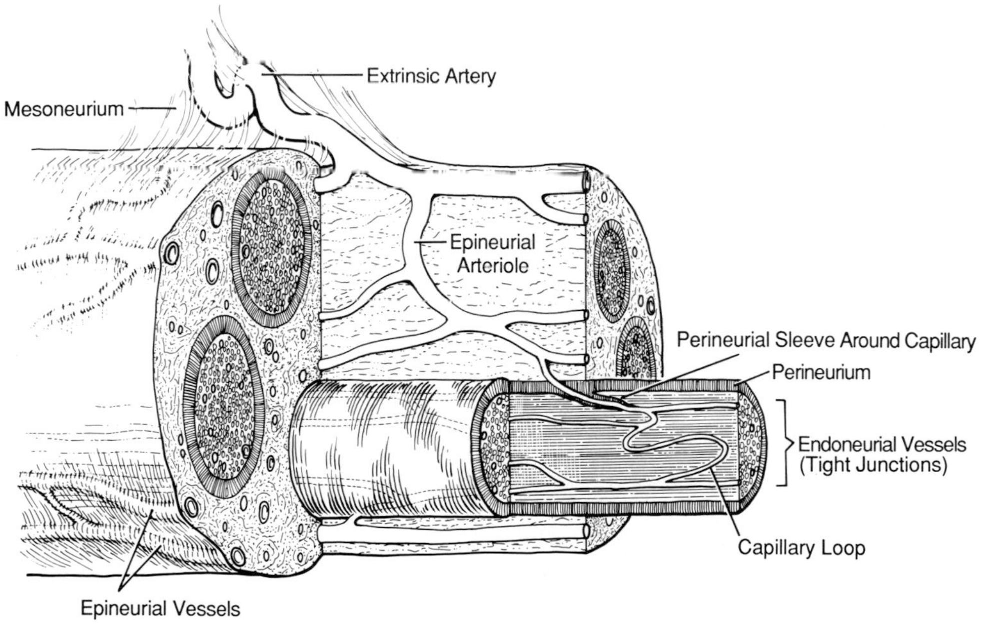

Figure 19–7. The vascular system of the peripheral nerve.

sion is observed only during periods of stress such as slight mechanical trauma or when warm saline is applied to the nerve (Lundborg, 1977).

The perineurial and endoneurial vessels form a fascicular plexus that can be separated from the epineurial vessels and can function essentially as a nerve trunk in miniature. The tough perineurium provides significant protection from external trauma, allowing each fascicle within a peripheral nerve to be gently mobilized for considerable distances without fear of ischemia (Rydevik, Lundborg, and Nordborg, 1976). In fact, vital microscopic studies by Lundborg (1977) demonstrated that the entire rabbit sciatic-tibial nerve could be mobilized by dividing all except the proximal and distal nutrient vessels (entire length 15 cm) with no detrimental effects on microvascular flow, provided the longitudinal epineurial vessels remained undamaged. The microvascular flow was impaired, however, when the nerve trunk was stretched. Elongation of 8 per cent slowed venular flow, and all flow was halted when the nerve reached an elongation of 15 per cent (Lundborg and Rydevik, 1973).

The ultrastructure of epineurial and endoneurial vessels differs. The endothelial cells that make up the epineurial vessels have cell junctions of the open variety that allow extravasation of protein macromolecules (Palade, Simionescu, and Simionescu, 1979). Fenestrated capillaries have also been identified in the epineurial microvasculature (Olsson and Reese, 1971). Small amounts of circulating serum proteins can diffuse out into the epineurium and close to the perineurium, but cannot pass through the impermeable perineurium. The endoneurial endothelial cells possess tight junctions between adjacent cells, similar to those in the brain parenchyma, which prevent the extravasation of proteins within the endoneurial space (Reese and Karnovsky, 1967). These vessels, together with the perineurium, create the blood-nerve barrier.

Strong alkaline phosphatase activity has been demonstrated in the endothelial cells of endoneurial arterioles. Associated with pinocytotic vesicles the alkaline phosphatase activity suggests the presence of an active transport function. It was postulated by Bell and Weddell (1984b) that the pinocytotic vesicles may provide a means by which the intrafascicular ionic and osmotic milieu can be sampled and the regional blood flow can be adjusted accordingly in the absence of direct arteriolar sympathetic innervation.

The intrafascicular vascular network is composed of capillaries that are larger in caliber than ordinary capillaries, a property that makes the intrafascicular potential vascular volume as large as that in high metabolic demand tissues such as muscle. This capacity, an "in situ reservoir," in addition to the ability to reroute large volumes of blood through ample conduits and the specialized transport pinocytotic vesicles quickly, suggests that the vascular bed of the nerve fascicle is as important in maintaining the intraneural environment as it is in providing oxygen and nutrients (Morgan, Reisman, and Wilgis, 1983).

PERIPHERAL NERVE END ORGANS

Sensory Receptors

Review of the literature, especially that regarding cutaneous sensibility, is fraught with confusion and inconsistency. Complex schemes to explain the organization of the peripheral receptor system were often based on observations of cutaneous structures that more often than not proved to be artifact.

With the advent of electron microscopy, some consistent observations could finally be drawn regarding the structure of receptors. It was Chouchkov (1978) who first recognized that only two basic types of receptors (unencapsulated and encapsulated) could be found. He later subdivided the encapsulated endings according to the function of the organization of the Schwann cell component of the capsule. With electron micrography and precise neurohistology, coupled with single-unit electrodiagnosis, accurate relationships between the peripheral sensory receptors and their innervation have been drawn (Cauna, 1954; McIntyre, 1980; Mountcastle, 1980).

Sensory receptors can now be classified either by function, by structure, by a combination of these, or by anatomic localization. Receptors can be mechanoreceptors, thermoreceptors, or nociceptors (McIntyre, 1980; Mountcastle, 1980; Darian-Smith, 1984). They can be composed of free nerve endings or encapsulated endings, or can be located in glabrous skin, mucocutaneous skin (without hair follicles or dermal papillae), hairy skin, or muscles or joints (Dellon, 1981; Darian-Smith, 1984).

The afferent fibers that subserve peripheral sensibility have been identified to be primarily from Groups A and C categories as defined by Erlanger and Gasser (1937) (see Table 19–1). The Group A beta fibers are correlated with touch; the Group A delta fibers with cooling, pricking pain and tickle; and the Group C fibers with warming, burning pain and itch. The "touch" sensory function is further differentiated into touch-pressure, contact, and flutter-vibration (Mountcastle, 1980). The ratio of A fibers to C fibers in peripheral nerves varies from 1:1, in areas of the face and hand, to 1:5 in nerves innervating proximal parts (Ranson and associates, 1935). The perception of stimulus intensity is encoded by the discharge frequency of a given receptor and the number of receptors activated. A stronger stimulus generates a correspondingly greater frequency of receptor discharge and stimulates a greater number of receptors. These two parameters are then centrally "processed" to quantitate stimulus (Martin, 1985).

Each receptor possesses different sensitivity and adaptive properties based on their response to continuous monotonic stimulation (Fig. 19–8). Adaptation refers to the afferent output of the receptor, and the latter can be either quickly adapting or slowly adapting. Quickly adapting receptors produce impulses that gradually decrease to zero or to a baseline value in response to a constant unvarying stimulus, whereas slowly adapting receptors continue their pulse response throughout the duration of the stimulus. If a mechanical stimulus changes in magnitude (increases or decreases), the quickly adapting receptor responds to the changing stimulus by another single-discharge pulse, and the slowly adapting receptors respond by a change in frequency of output (Mountcastle, 1980). There are two classes of slowly adapting receptors that are distinguished on the basis of their patterns of discharge and also by differences in receptive field. Type I receptors have little or no spontaneous discharge in the resting state and have two phases of response (dynamic and static) during monotonic stimulation. During the dynamic phase, Type I (SA I) receptors respond with a high rate of discharge (up to 1500 per sec). The static phase begins with the end of active receptor displacement and is marked with an exponential fall in frequency of discharge followed by a slow decrease in rate, until an irregular (but low) rate of discharge is maintained for the duration of the stimulus. SA I receptors are also most sensitive to vertical displacement and have less response to skin stretch (Iggo and Muir, 1969; Ruch, 1979; Mountcastle, 1980).

Slowly adapting Type II receptors (SA II) maintain a slow regular discharge in the absence of stimulation. The maximal frequency of output of the SA II receptors is lower than the SA I (up to 300 per sec) during the dynamic phase of monotonic stimulation, and the static phase has a regular rate of discharge that remains above baseline. The SA II receptors appear to be more sensitive to stretch than to vertical displacement (Iggo and Muir, 1969; Chambers and associates,

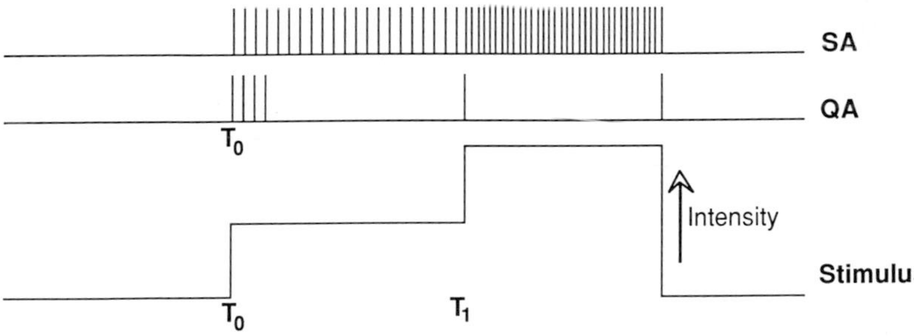

Figure 19–8. Characteristics of slowly adapting (SA) and quickly adapting (QA) receptors. A constant stimulus is applied to the skin at time zero (T_0). The QA receptor briefly discharges during the acceleration phase of the stimulus but fails to respond after movement ceases. At T_1, the intensity of the stimulus is increased and the QA receptor responds with another volley of discharges as it does on termination of the stimulus. The SA receptor discharges for the duration of the initial stimulus and increases the frequency of discharge with greater intensity. While SA receptors respond throughout the duration of a stimulus, QA receptors respond only to acceleration, i.e., to movement and transient stimuli. (After Dykes, R. W.: Sensory receptors. *In* Daniel, R. K., and Terzis, J. K. (Eds.): Reconstructive Microsurgery. Boston, Little, Brown & Company, 1977.)

1972; Ruch, 1979; Mountcastle, 1980). Owing to the steady rate of response during the static phase, SA II receptors can provide more sensory information about pressure and position than the irregular SA I receptors. SA I receptors, however, have much shorter recovery cycles than SA II receptors (40 to 50 msec for SA I versus 100 msec for SA II) (Burgess and Perl, 1973). Changes in the frequency of impulses generated during the static phase for both SA I and SA II receptors may result from mechanical and chemical changes of the end organ. There is not only a progressive decrease in tension within the receptor (shown best in the muscle spindle), but also a local change in the ionic environment at the level of the end organ (Lippold, Nicholls, and Redfearn, 1960; Husmark and Ottoson, 1970, 1971a,b).

GLABROUS SKIN RECEPTORS

Glabrous (nonhairy) skin of humans has the highest peripheral innervation density and is represented by one of the largest areas of the sensory homunculus (Fig. 19–9). The important structural features of glabrous skin that relate to its innervation are the relative thickness of the epidermis and the pattern of ridges. These are the papillary ridge or "fingerprint" on the surface of the skin and the complementary ridge on the underside of the epidermal layer that projects into the dermis (the intermediate ridge). Both structures influence the mechanical deformation of the skin surface and thereby modulate tactile sensitivity (Darian-Smith, 1984). Peripheral nerves branch beneath the glabrous skin and form a subdermal plexus from which further branchings ascend to form a subpapillary plexus. Containing both myelinated and unmyelinated fibers (Groups A and C), these networks innervate the specific end organs of glabrous skin and also terminate as free nerve endings. Three encapsulated receptors have been identified in glabrous skin, two of which are quickly adapting (Meissner's and Pacini's corpuscles) and one of which is the Type I slowly adapting group (the Merkel cell–neurite complex). Analysis of afferent impulses has also demonstrated the existence of an SA II type receptor by virtue of identification of the characteristic SA II output (Johansson, 1978; McIntyre, 1980). The source of the afferent impulses is the Ruffini complex, but unfortunately this elusive receptor is seen only occasionally in glabrous skin. No other end organ has been identified that could be responsible for the SA II output of glabrous skin.

Within the dermal papillae of the skin is the end organ, *Meissner's corpuscle* (Fig. 19–10). This corpuscle is the terminal ending of several Group A beta fibers encapsulated by

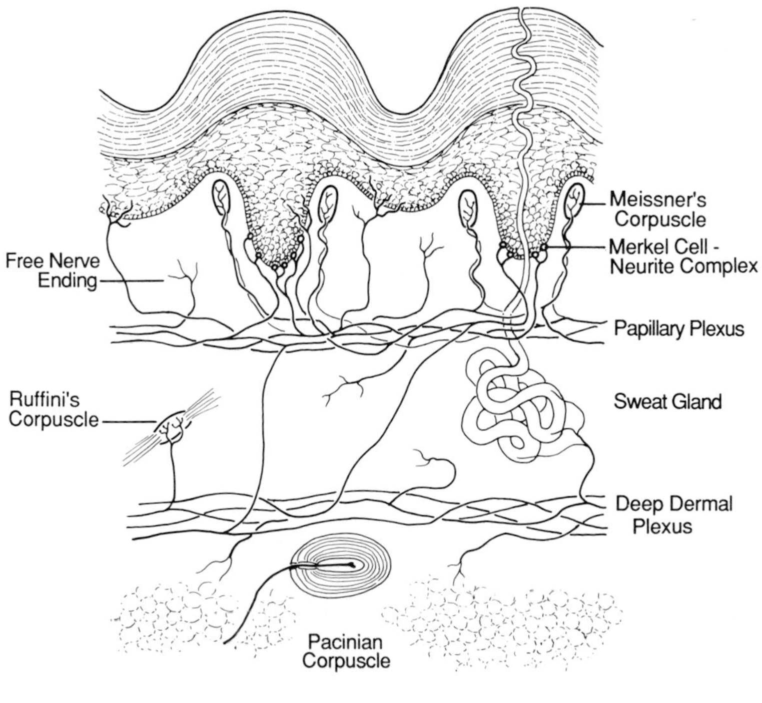

Figure 19–9. Glabrous skin receptors.

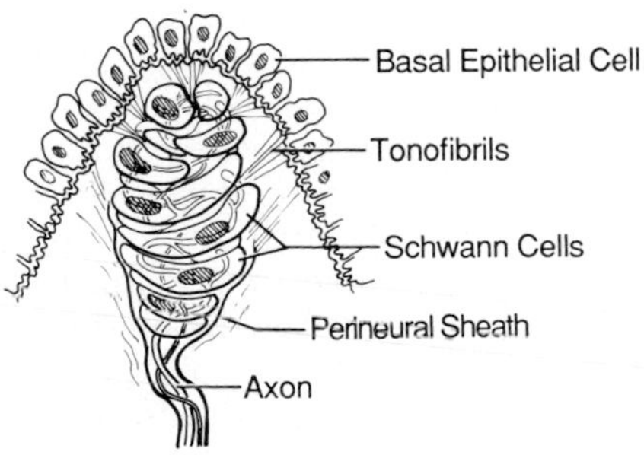

Figure 19–10. Composition of Meissner's corpuscle.

what appear to be modified Schwann cells folded into multiple lamellae. The nerve endings flatten into plates interleaved with the flattened lamellar cells (Cauna, 1956; Cauna and Ross, 1960; Iggo, 1977). Fine collagen fibrils extend from the lamellar cells and are attached to the surrounding basal layer of the epidermis by semidesmosomes (Andres and von Düring, 1973). This arrangement provides a mechanical linkage between the skin and the corpuscle, and explains how skin stimuli are transferred to the more central nerve endings of the multilamellated structure (Darian-Smith, 1984). The multiple innervating fibers, two or three entering from the base of the corpuscle and the others entering from the sides and top, provide receptive field overlap, not seen in the Merkel cell–neurite complex (Dellon, 1981).

The sensory modality subserved by this quickly adapting structure is low frequency flutter-vibration and moving touch (Talbot and associates, 1968). Under sustained pressure an impulse is produced only at the onset, removal, or change of magnitude of the stimulus; hence, this is a velocity or acceleration sensor and it is "tuned" to receive optimal vibrations of 30 to 40 Hz (Mountcastle, 1980).

Another encapsulated end organ found in glabrous skin is the *pacinian corpuscle* (Fig. 19–11), which is sufficiently large to be detected by the naked eye (from 0.5 × 1.00 mm to 1.0 × 4.0 mm). It therefore was the first anatomic structure associated with cutaneous sensation. First incorrectly identified as a pressure sensor (Winkleman, 1960; Sunderland, 1968), this quickly adapting structure provides the basis for the sensation of high frequency vibrations and moving touch (Talbot and associates, 1968). The pacinian corpuscle lies in the deep dermis and subcutaneous tissue, is innervated by a single Group A beta fiber, and exists singly or multiply. The axon terminus enters the corpuscle and shortly loses its myelin sheath. The terminal two nodes of Ranvier are intracorpuscular. Distal to the last node, the unmyelinated axon thickens and is filled with multiple mitochondria, neurofilaments, and neurotubules. An inner core, divided in halves by a cleft, surrounds the nerve ending and its multiple processes with up to 60 layers of concentric lamellar cells, each with its own basal lamina. The outer capsule of another 20 to 30 more lamellae is separated from the inner core by a subcapsular space filled with amorphous ground substance. The outer capsule is contiguous with the perineural sheath of the afferent nerve (Lowenstein, 1960; Andres and von Düring, 1973; Darian-Smith, 1984). Acting as a filtered transducer, the capsule acts to dampen low frequency vibra-

Figure 19–11. Pacinian corpuscle.

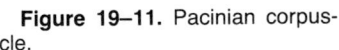

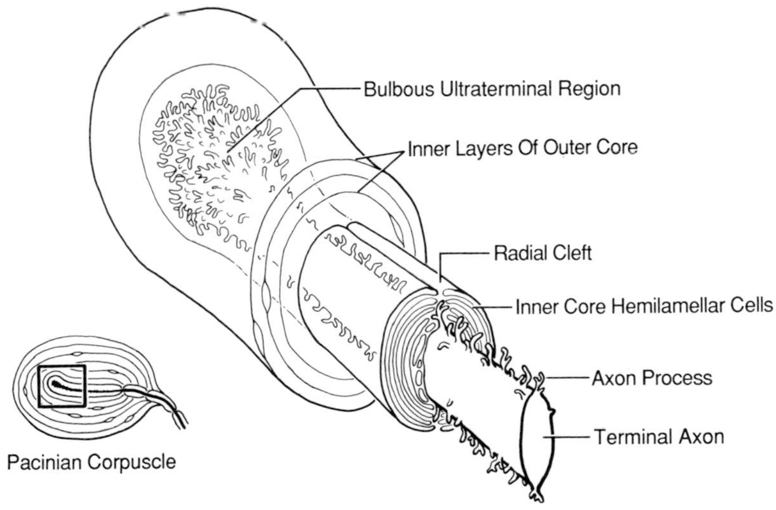

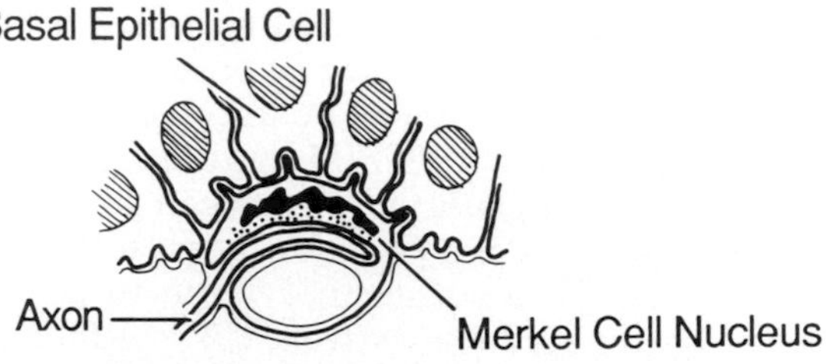

Figure 19–12. Merkel cell–neurite complex.

tions from the central end organ, virtually eliminating any vibration less than 100 Hz (Iggo, 1977). The pacinian corpuscle is maximally responsive at 250 to 300 Hz (Mountcastle, 1980). The recovery cycle for this receptor is extremely short (5 to 6 msec) and there is virtually no fatigue with repetitive stimulation (Burgess and Perl, 1973). Of the estimated 2000 pacinian corpuscles in human skin, over one-third are in the digits and over 100 in a single finger (Sinclair, 1981).

The *Merkel cell–neurite* complex is found at the dermal-epidermal junction of the intermediate ridges that project into the dermis (Fig. 19–12). Groups of five or ten such complexes are interspersed among the basal layer cells. The afferent Group A beta fiber ends in a spray of terminals, each of which is enclosed by a specialized epithelial cell with clear cytoplasm that is possibly of neural crest derivation–the Merkel cell (Munger, 1965; Darian-Smith, 1984). One Merkel cell–neurite complex may receive more than one terminal, and a given fiber may supply more than one complex (Sinclair, 1981). A characteristic of the Merkel cell–neurite complex is the presence of multiple cytoplasmic processes that contain microvilli and lie between the cells of the adjacent epidermis (Andres and von Düring, 1973).

This end organ complex is slowly adapting and exhibits both a dynamic phase and a static phase output to the continuous stimulation. During the dynamic phase, the receptor responds to both the velocity and magnitude of the stimulus with a high impulse rate of up to 1500 per sec. The Merkel cell–neurite complex is a slowly adapting mechanoreceptor of the Type I variety (see above). This adaptive character endows this receptor with the ability to subserve the sensory modality of constant touch or pressure, and is largely responsible for tactile gnosis of static objects (Dellon, 1981). The discharge frequency of the Merkel cell–neurite complex is temperature dependent. Cooling the skin causes receptor excitation, and warming inhibits discharge (McIntyre, 1980).

Although rarely found, the putative SA II receptor of glabrous skin is the *Ruffini end organ* (Fig. 19–13). This encapsulated end organ is spindle shaped in configuration and is found at many levels within the dermis. The receptor is made up of the terminal unmyelinated branch of a Group A beta fiber ensheathed by a specialized endoneural cell. Collagenous fibers emanating from the subcutaneous and dermal layers enter the thin capsule that surrounds the central nerve terminals to interdigitate with the terminals of the receptor core.

An amorphous fluid ground substance (similar to that within the meissnerian and pacinian corpuscles) is found surrounding the core terminals. Like Meissner's corpuscle, the collagen fibrils entering the Ruffini ending serve as a mechanical link to the surrounding dermal and subdermal collagen (Andres and von Düring, 1973; Iggo, 1977). Each Ruffini ending is innervated by a single myelinated axon and the latter may innervate several adjacent endings (Darian-Smith, 1984).

The Ruffini endings are examples of slowly adapting Type II receptors, which show a continuous background discharge in the absence of mechanical stimulation, increasing the frequency of discharge with stimulation. During unvarying stimulation, discharge frequency declines to a plateau that is above baseline and maintains a regular low frequency output for the duration of the stimulus. As SA I receptors, the baseline background discharge of the SA II receptors is altered by skin cooling (excitation) or warm-

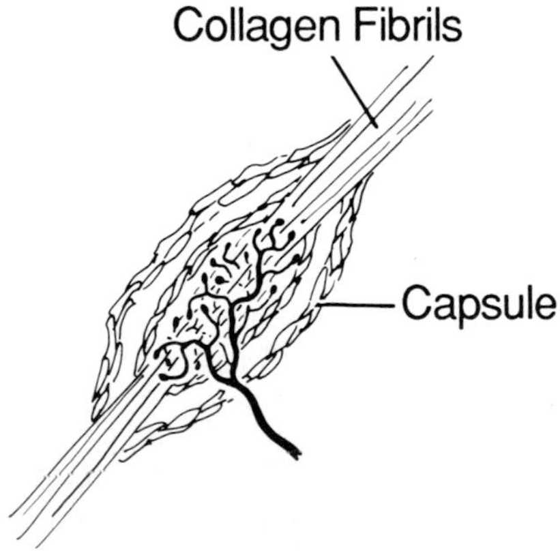

Figure 19–13. Ruffini end organ.

ing (inhibition). Overall it plays a role in the touch-pressure sensory function as a velocity and position detector (Merzenich and Harrington, 1969; Chambers and associates, 1972; Andres and von Düring, 1973; Mountcastle, 1980). Ruffini endings respond maximally to skin stretch and less well to direct vertical displacement. A secondary role as a thermoreceptor may be played by the Ruffini complex because of the temperature dependence of the continuous regular background discharge.

In addition to the four named end organs, there are numerous poorly defined free nerve endings in glabrous skin that are assumed to be responsible for the sensations of cold and warmth, the nociceptive response of pain, and the vague sensations of itch and tickle. These bare nerve endings appear to be slowly adaptive and are A delta and C fibers (Mountcastle, 1980).

Although it is likely that these free nerve endings are specialized to receive specific sensory stimuli, current investigative techniques are limited and the free nerve endings appear to be a relatively homogenous population (Dykes, 1977). Two free nerve ending configurations (short-thick and long-thin) have been identified by Macintosh (1975) that project into the stratum granulosum of glabrous skin. Free nerve endings can be found throughout the basal layer of the epidermis, the deeper aspect of the dermis, and the underlying connective tissue layers (McIntyre, 1980).

Iggo (1959, 1969) developed techniques for single-unit recording of A delta and C fibers, and since that time it has been possible to determine that specific receptors for cold and warmth exist despite lack of anatomic differentiation. Hensel and Boman (1960; Hensel, 1973) confirmed these findings by identifying a small myelinated fiber (A delta) associated with cold sensation, and Darian-Smith and Dykes (1971) identified unmyelinated fibers (C) as those associated with warmth reception. Both cold and warm receptors have a temperature-dependent continuous discharge and are slowly adapting. Receptive fields are small (approximately 1 mm), and the high sensitivity of the receptors of the human hand allows temperature differentiation of increments as small as 0.05°C (McIntyre, 1980). There are small A delta fibers that respond with the sensation of itch or tickle (Burgess, Petit, and Warren, 1968), and two classes of fibers that are nociceptive, responding to mechanical or thermal stimuli. Each class of fibers has myelinated (A delta) fibers as well as unmyelinated (C) fibers. All these receptors, which are free nerve endings, have high thresholds and do not generate impulses with less than noxious stimuli (Dykes, 1975; Ruch, 1979; McIntyre, 1980). In glabrous skin there are occasionally A delta free nerve endings that serve as mechanoreceptors (Schmidt, 1981).

HAIRY SKIN RECEPTORS

Hairy skin (Fig. 19–14) shares many of the characteristics of glabrous skin. There is essentially no difference between hair-bearing and smooth skin in terms of the location and function of the A delta and C fiber free nerve endings. Pacinian corpuscles reside in the same deep dermal locations and have identical sensory capabilities. The Merkel cell–neurite complex is also found in the basilar epidermis, clusters in "touch spots," "haarscheibe," or "Pinkus corpuscles" (Sinclair, 1981). These specialized epidermal structures are 0.2 to 0.5 mm in diameter. Elevated slightly above the surrounding skin, they serve a single fiber and its multiple Merkel cell–neurite complexes (Darian-Smith, 1984). Ruffini's end organs are found in abundance in hairy skin and occur separately at varying levels of the dermis and subdermal tissue.

The hair itself is a specialized component of the cutaneous receptor mechanism, and there are several distinct nerve structures that innervate each hair follicle, differentiated on the basis of dynamic sensitivity, conduction velocity, and extent of receptive field (Fig. 19–13). Extensive branching occurs in the A beta fibers, which innervate the hair follicles so that one nerve innervates multiple follicles and one follicle is innervated by multiple nerves (Iggo, 1977). Human hair does not seem to have the complexity of innervation seen in the animal models, where there is a functional specificity of vibrissae, down hair (pelage), or guard hairs. There are only three types of endings associated with hair follicles in human skin.

The common hair follicle of the human (pelage) is innervated by several myelinated fibers that encircle the follicle just below the sebaceous gland. As the fibers branch within the dermal sheath of the follicle, they lose their myelin sheath, become spindle shaped

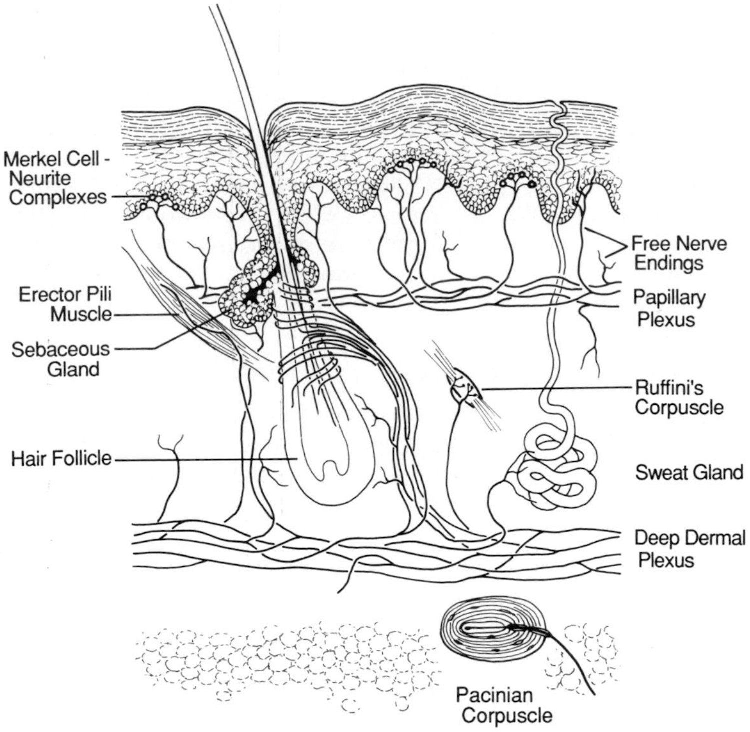

Figure 19–14. Hairy skin receptors.

or lanceolate, and proceed along the basal lamina. The inner surface of each nerve terminal contacts the basal lamina of the follicle, and the outer surface is ensheathed by a Schwann cell. The nerve terminal at this junction is filled with multiple mitochondria, vesicles, neurotubules, and filaments (Darian-Smith, 1984). Another cluster of spindle-like nerve endings is found just deep to the sebaceous gland and is supplied by myelinated fibers that ascend along the hair shaft. These nerve endings are totally ensheathed by Schwann cells and they form a semicircular cluster (Cauna, 1976). Also associated with hair follicles is an unmyelinated fiber that ascends along the entire follicle and ends in a "spray" within the basal lamina of the epidermis, known as papillary endings (Andres and von Düring, 1973; Cauna, 1976; Dykes, 1977).

Hair movement is transmitted to these receptors and is augmented by the lever action of the dermal fulcrum on the follicle. The impulse is transient as the receptor complex is quickly adapting and responds to vibratory or moving stimulus. The receptor is the functional analogue of Meissner's corpuscle in glabrous skin (Dellon, 1981). Maximal stimulation occurs at vibrations of 30 to 40 Hz as well (Mountcastle, 1980).

MUCOCUTANEOUS RECEPTORS

The transitional zones between hairy skin and true mucous membranes possess sensory end organs not seen in either glabrous or hairy skin. This category of transitional, or mucocutaneous, skin includes such structures as the glans penis and clitoris, lip, eyelid, and perianal region. They have a glomerular corpuscle distinct from the corpuscles found in glabrous or hairy skin. The terminal neurite complex of this receptor resembles a tangled skein of yarn. This ending is not encapsulated and has been variously designated the *Krause end bulb*, the genital end bulb, Dogiel's end bulb, and the mucocutaneous end organ of Winkleman. The preferred nomenclature is the genital end bulb. Otherwise these regions of skin are richly innervated with free nerve endings, meissnerian corpuscles, ruffinian corpuscles, and pacinian corpuscles (Winkleman, 1960; Grossman and Hattis, 1967; MacDonald and Schmitt, 1979; Dellon, 1981; Sinclair, 1981; Halata, 1984). The Merkel cell–neurite complex has been identified but in only four of several thousand sections of the human glans penis and prepuce in one study (Halata, 1984), and has not been found in the lingual mucosa. It probably is common in the lips and buccal mucosa.

Much confusion has arisen regarding the so-called "Krause end bulb," especially since Krause identified two structures morphologically different and called both "end bulbs" (Sinclair, 1981). It is apparent, however, that there are several encapsulated morphologic variations of Meissner's corpuscle, presumably owing to the variability of the dermal architecture (Dellon, 1981). Originally described as a cold receptor (Sunderland, 1968; Andres and von Düring, 1973), the mucocutaneous Krause end bulb is probably a Meissner's corpuscle variant with no apparent functional difference that would warrant differentiation from Meissner's corpuscle proper (Chauchov, 1981).

Free nerve endings are by far the most common receptor of genital skin, followed by the genital corpuscle and the pacinian corpuscle in ratios of 100:10:1, respectively (Halata, 1984). No functional correlations have yet been made from single-unit studies, and therefore the sensory modality subserved by these structures can only be theorized on the basis of their morphologic analogues in glabrous and hairy skin.

MUSCULAR AND SKELETAL RECEPTORS

Regarding the clinical classification of sensory modalities, the muscular and skeletal (primarily tendon and joint) sensory receptors make up that category of nerves and receptors anatomically defined as "deep sensibility" (proprioception [position sense] and muscle stretch and tension) (Skoglund, 1973). There are several types of sensory receptors that subserve these functions in muscles, tendons, and joints. These are the muscle spindles (two types), the Golgi tendon organs, the encapsulated joint receptors (pacinian, paciniform, and Golgi-Mazzoni corpuscles), the Ruffini endings (which resemble the Golgi tendon organs), and the nociceptive free nerve endings (Skoglund, 1973; Ruch, 1979; Kennedy, Poppele, and Quick, 1980; Kuffler, Nicholls, and Martin, 1984).

The muscle spindle is a fusiform encapsulated receptor found within skeletal muscle (Fig. 19–15). Enclosed by the multilayered capsule are several specialized muscle fibers (intrafusal) that are innervated by gamma efferent fibers (fusimotor). Several of the longer intrafusal fibers extend beyond the capsule and insert on intramuscular connective tissue or tendon. Two configurations of intrafusal nuclei differentiate two types of spindles. Those with a thickening in the equatorial region possess a tight grouping of round vesicular nuclei, the "nuclear bag" fibers. There are also thin cylindric fibers that have a central row of nuclei, the "nuclear chain" fibers (Barker, 1974; Kennedy, Poppele, and Quick, 1980; Kuffler, Nicholls, and Martin, 1984).

The terminal endings of the sensory afferents enter the muscle spindle through the capsule (the perineurium of the nerve becomes confluent with the capsule) and are of two types: the heavily myelinated, large, fast-conducting Type I alpha fibers and the myelinated Type I beta fibers. The receptor endings of the A alpha fibers (primary endings) surround the intrafusal fibers at the nuclear bag or chain with a series of annulospiral terminals. Schwann cells ensheath the terminals except where they lie on the surface of the muscle fibers in shallow grooves, and the Schwann cells and muscles share a common basement membrane (Barker, 1974;

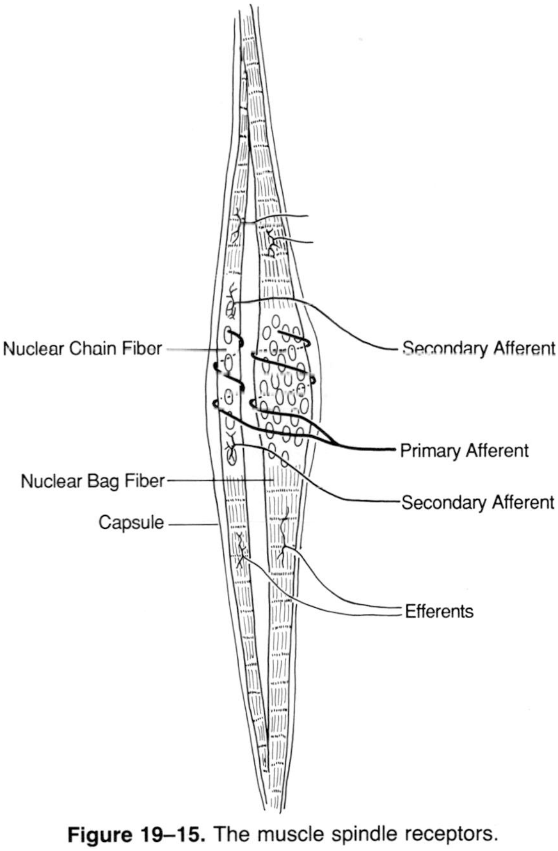

Figure 19–15. The muscle spindle receptors.

Kennedy, Poppele, and Quick, 1980). This arrangement is reminiscent of the terminal ending of the hair follicle. The secondary afferent (A beta) fibers are smaller than the primary and are usually located on both sides of the primary endings. The secondary terminus appears as a fine spiral of delicate axons that encircle the intrafusal muscle fibers and occasionally end in a terminal spray. Free nerve endings, which have also been identified within muscle spindles, are of the C fiber class (Barker, 1974; Kennedy, Poppele, and Quick, 1980).

The primary afferent is more sensitive to dynamic stretch than the secondary (Cooper, 1961). The primary receptor exhibits a much greater frequency of impulse during the acceleration phase of stretch or during the development of tension than the secondary receptor, and this slowly adapting receptor decreases its frequency of impulse during the static phase. The secondary receptors are little affected during the dynamic phase of stretch but maintain a regular discharge during the static phase (Hunt, 1974; Kennedy, Poppele, and Quick, 1980; Kuffler, Nicholls, and Martin, 1984). Consequently, the primary afferent is especially sensitive to vibratory stimulation with response characteristics that are a function of both intrafusal stretch (tension) and frequency of vibration (Hunt, 1974; Kennedy, Poppele, and Quick, 1980).

Unlike any other receptors, the muscle spindle is subject to centrifugal control by virtue of the gamma efferent fusimotor fibers. Since the intrafusal fibers lie in parallel with extrafusal muscle fibers, contraction (shortening) of the intrafusal fiber is perceived as a reduction of tension or shortening of the surrounding muscle mass. The converse is also true. Therefore, the intrafusal fiber serves to modulate the sensory reception by maintenance of a constant range of spindle length to allow the spindle to perform over a wide range of muscle length (Barker, 1974; Kennedy, Poppele, and Quick, 1980; Kuffler, Nicholls, and Martin, 1984). Through this mechanism, the muscular afferents play a role in kinesthesia (proprioception) by the central processing of afferent and efferent muscle spindle signals (Matthews, 1977; McCloskey and associates, 1983). In fact, position sense remains intact even with neural blockade or surgical removal of the joint capsule and its innervating structures (Grigg, Finerman, and Riley, 1973). However, this finding has been repudiated by other studies (Moberg, 1983).

The *Golgi tendon organ* is found within the tendinous structures and ligaments. This slowly adapting receptor is structurally similar to the Ruffini endings and has the same SA II characteristics, making possible continuous feedback as a function of tendon tension (Ruch, 1979). The capsule of the Golgi tendon organ is continuous with the perineurium of the afferent I-beta fiber. Like the Ruffini ending, it is not as elaborate as other encapsulated endings. The Golgi organs respond in a linear fashion with maximal output frequencies at times of maximal tension (Skoglund, 1973).

Ruffini endings are found in abundance throughout the joint capsule in an apparently random distribution. There is no morphologic difference between them and the cutaneous receptor, and the functional characteristics are also similar. This slowly adapting (SA II) receptor is an important proprioceptive organ and there are three populations found in joint capsules differentiated by their position-related output. All Ruffini endings maintain constant baseline output but each population responds maximally at a different joint position. One population responds maximally at extremes of flexion and another at extremes of extension (Fig. 19–16). These are termed single-ended receptors. The third population responds best through the middle of the range of motion of the joint and is considered bimodal. The bimodal receptor maintains a baseline output when its joint is 50 per cent flexed. It increases frequency of impulse with increased flexion and decreases frequency with decreased flexion. The receptor characteristics provide sensitive proprioceptive feedback (Boyd and Roberts, 1953; Skoglund, 1973).

Three quickly adapting receptors have been identified within joint capsules and the surrounding periosteum: the pacinian corpuscles, the paciniform corpuscles, and the Golgi-Mazzoni receptors. The pacinian corpuscles do not differ in morphology or function from those of the cutaneous regions and are distributed throughout the capsular structures. Paciniform corpuscles differ as there are only two to six lamellae in the outer capsule. These receptors are often found in ligamentous structures, joint capsules, and interosseus membranes; they are quickly adapting and

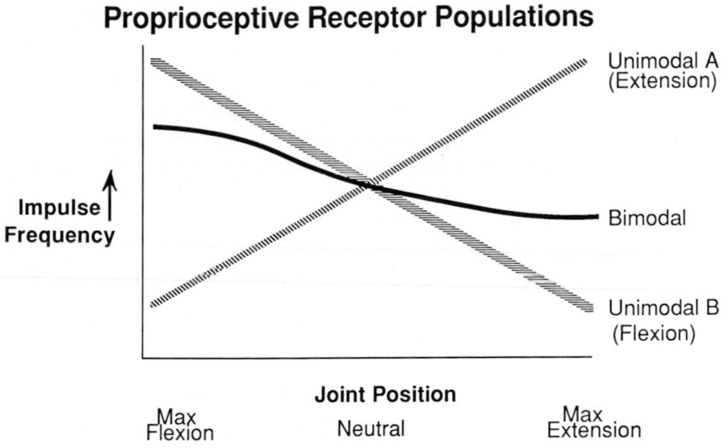

Figure 19–16. Types of responses of the proprioceptive receptors.

have a low threshold. The paciniform corpuscles, like their larger relative, are acceleration or vibratory sensors (Barker, 1974; Ruch, 1979).

The last encapsulated ending, found in the periosteum adjacent to joints, is the Golgi-Mazzoni receptor, a quickly adapting vibratory receptor (maximal response under 200 Hz) that seems to act like the pacinian and paciniform corpuscles. The Golgi-Mazzoni receptor is smaller than the pacinian corpuscle and its receptor ending is encapsulated by two ellipsoidal caps. The lamellae are densely packed and there is little interposed connective tissue (Skoglund, 1973; Ruch, 1979).

Free nerve endings of group C fibers, which are presumably nociceptive, are also found within the joint capsules, ligaments, and occasionally within muscle spindles and tendons (Ruch, 1979).

Motor End Organs

The term "motor unit" was first used by Sherrington in 1929 and was defined as ". . . an individual nerve fibre with the bunch of muscle-fibres it activates" (Sherrington, 1980), and this definition remains workable today. This definition includes the alpha motor neuron, its group A-alpha or -beta axon, and the extrafusal (and intrafusal with beta axon) muscle fibers that it innervates. Each axon innervates several muscle fibers, but only one axon innervates each fiber. In the case of beta axons, these innervate both intra- and extrafusal fibers, but they are relatively rarely found (Burke, 1980). The gamma motor neurons were discussed above with the muscle spindle.

The general features of the motor end plate, the terminal structure of efferent axons, is as follows: the myelinated A-alpha fiber approaches the muscle fiber it is to innervate and forms a divergent "spray" of unmyelinated axons that spread over the muscle fiber. Each terminal axon branch lies embedded in a trough in the muscle fiber with a synaptic cleft separating the nerve from the muscle, which is approximately 50 mm in width. The entire end plate (consisting of all the terminal fibers) is covered by a Schwann cell membrane isolating it from the surrounding connective tissue. Each terminal ending is filled with mitochondria and numerous vesicles shown to contain acetylcholine. In short, axon depolarization releases the transmitter agent (acetylcholine) and the innervated muscle fiber contracts. Each motor axon (A-alpha) innervates from 10 to 100 individual muscle fibers, all of which make up the motor unit (Nastuk, 1980; McCloskey and associates, 1983; Moberg, 1983).

PERIPHERAL NERVE INJURY

The causes of peripheral nerve dysfunction are extremely diverse and most are beyond the scope of the peripheral nerve surgeon. In order to assess the extent of injury and prognosis, it is important for the surgeon to understand changes that affect the nerve cell, axon, and target organ; the potential for reversibility; and the possibilities for surgery to improve the patient's condition (Mira, 1981b).

As a result of the retrospective analysis of their vast experience in the treatment of patients with peripheral nerve injuries, both

Seddon (1948) and Sunderland (1968) developed schemes of classification of nerve injuries based on the disrupted internal structures of the peripheral nerve. It was apparent to each that the prognosis for functional return was highly correlated with the degree of intraneural disruption.

The classification scheme devised by Seddon (1948) is the least complicated and the most commonly used today. *Neurapraxia* is the mildest form of nerve injury and denotes a localized conduction block along a nerve. Axonal continuity is maintained, and nerve conduction proximal and distal to the lesion is preserved. Recovery is rapid and impulse conduction (return of function) is complete within weeks (Simpson, 1970; Spencer, 1977; Horn and Crumley, 1984; Costaldo and Ochoa, 1984).

The next category, *axonotmesis*, is more serious, and denotes sufficient damage to disrupt the continuity of axons within the connective tissue of the peripheral nerve. Not only is there complete conduction block, but distal axon degeneration also follows the injury. Prognosis remains good because of the continuity of the supportive connective tissue, satellite cells, and basement membrane (Simpson, 1970; Spencer, 1977; Horn and Crumley, 1984; Costaldo and Ochoa, 1984).

The most severe injury occurs in *neurotmesis*. Complete anatomic severance of the peripheral nerve occurs and no recovery is expected without surgical coaptation of the ends of the fibers. There is distal degeneration, as well as some degree of proximal degeneration (Simpson, 1970).

The classification system developed by Sunderland (1968) is similar to that of Seddon; however, emphasis is placed on the importance of the fascicular structure of the nerve, and the categories are expanded to five (Sunderland, 1968) (Fig. 19–17).

The Sunderland *first degree injury* is iden-

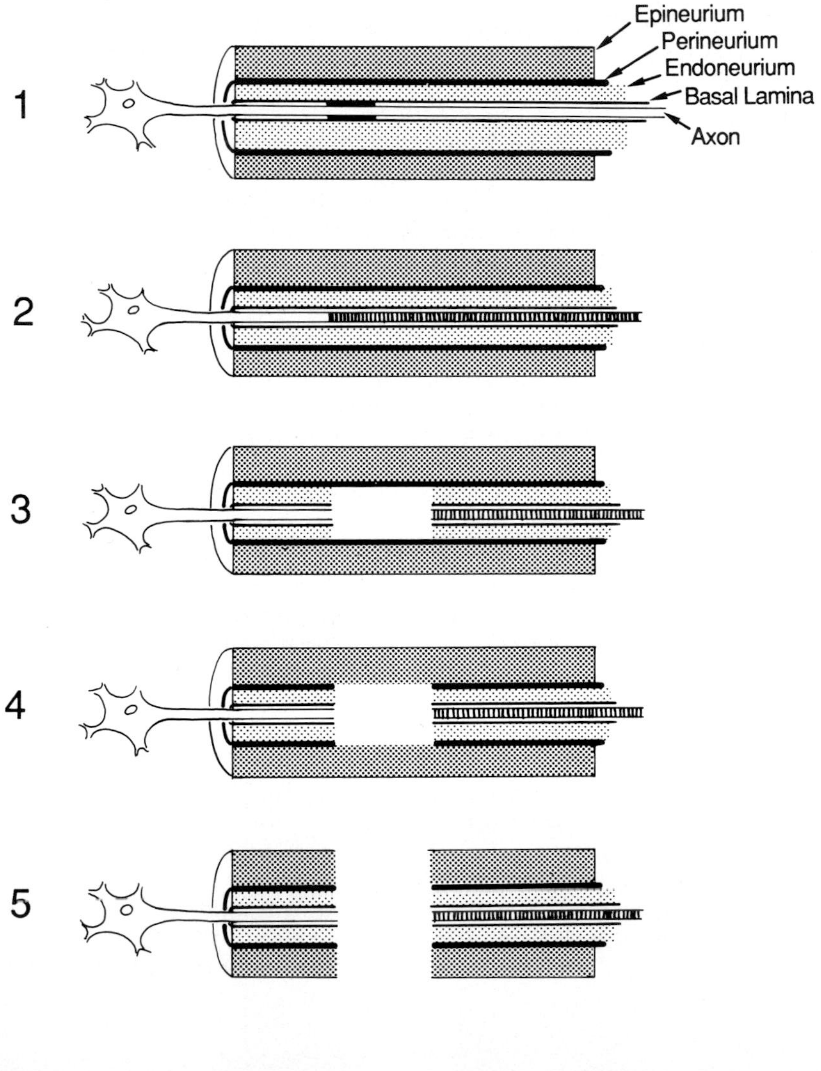

Figure 19–17. Sunderland's classification of nerve injury (see text for details).

tical to the neurapraxia injury of Seddon. Local conduction block occurs but the supportive structures and axons remain intact. *Second degree injury* is the equivalent of the axonotmetic injury. The axon is either severed or severely damaged and distal degeneration follows. The supportive structures remain intact. Seddon's third category, neurotmesis, includes the third, fourth, and fifth degree injuries of Sunderland. In the *third degree injury*, nerve fibers are severed along with their endoneurial covering but the perineurium remains intact. Regeneration occurs but the reinnervation of target organs is haphazard owing to intrafascicular mixing of growing axons. The *fourth degree injury* is more severe because the perineurium is disrupted and there is extensive damage to the endoneurial architecture. The continuity of the nerve trunk is maintained by a reasonably intact epineurium, and scarring is far more extensive than in the previous degrees of injury. There is extensive interfascicular mixing of growing axons. The *fifth degree injury* denotes complete disruption of the nerve trunk with little hope of spontaneous recovery of function (Sunderland, 1968; Spencer, 1977).

Sunderland was quick to point out that except in the most severe (fourth and fifth degree) nerve injuries, any given nerve injury contains elements from all the categories of injury, and the mixed lesions explain the often confusing array of clinical findings (Sunderland, 1968). It is not at all uncommon to see all five degrees of injury incurred by the nerves of a brachial plexus.

The effects of denervation on the end organ, be it sensory or motor, are manifold. In all cases the terminal axon degenerates as a normal consequence of wallerian degeneration. The supporting structures of the axon terminal degenerate to varying degrees, depending on the life cycle of the involved structure. When complete degeneration occurs, there is no potential for regeneration. These structures are lost to potential reinnervation. On the other hand, when only supporting structures become atrophic, reinnervation restores function to variable degrees, depending on many factors such as time and scar. The end organ retains its capacity for reinnervation for many years, and after proper nerve reconstruction and subsequent axon growth, function is limited only by the condition of the end organ and the precision of the reconstruction.

Denervation presents as insensitivity of the supplied receptor field or as paralysis of the involved motor units. Denervated muscles can be stimulated to function electrically and they spontaneously produce fibrillation potentials, the latter being an important diagnostic parameter.

Direct muscle stimulation can prevent some of the denervation changes seen, such as denervation hypersensitivity, lowered membrane potentials and increased capacitance, and fibrillations (Lomo and Rosenthal, 1972; Purves and Sakmann, 1974; Lomo and Westgaard, 1975a,b; Westgaard, 1975). Methods of intermittent trains of stimulation are useful to improve the results of reconstructive surgery for the injured nerve.

PERIPHERAL NERVE REGENERATION

Neuron and Proximal Axon

As a consequence of any severe injury to a peripheral nerve there is a predictable sequence of distal (wallerian) and proximal axonal degeneration, the extent of which depends on the severity of the injury. If the injury does not lead to neuronal death, a sequence of regeneration proceeds, which may be abortive or may result in effective functional restoration (Fig. 19–18). Degeneration occurs in injuries sufficient to disrupt axonal continuity. Wallerian degeneration of the distal nerve consists of fragmentation of axons and surrounding myelin from the point of axonal separation to the nerve terminal ending (Selzer, 1980; Thomas, Landon, and King, 1984).

Proximal to the axonal disruption, the axon undergoes limited degeneration up to the last preserved internode. The axonal degeneration is similar to that observed in the distal stump (Lubinska, 1961). The neuron exhibits central chromatolysis, and this represents the metabolic preparation for a shift from maintenance of nerve conduction to a regenerative mode geared to generate structural proteins. To this end, there is a reduction in the effectiveness of synaptic transmission, and the afferent boutons appear to retract from the neuronal cell membrane (Selzer, 1980). As regeneration proceeds, neuronal RNA content increases followed by increased synthesis of proteins, including glycolytic and respiratory enzymes and neuronal lipoproteins necessary

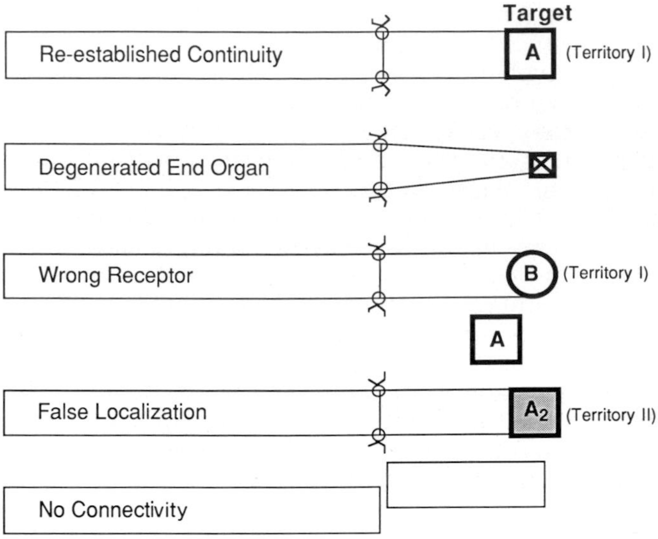

Figure 19–18. Potential outcomes of axonal regeneration.

for axonal membrane synthesis (Brattgard, Edstrom, and Hyden, 1957; Watson, 1968; Lieberman, 1971; Selzer, 1980). Tubulin, the constituent protein in neurofilaments and neurotubules, is also synthesized at a greater rate after axotomy (Lasek and Hoffman, 1976), and transmitter substances fall in concentration (Selzer, 1980).

After careful histologic observations of silver-stained nerve fibers following injury, Cajal started the modern era in nerve regeneration research by proving that nerve regeneration occurs by outgrowth from the proximal stump and not by autoregeneration of the degenerated distal nerve (Ramon and Cajal, 1928). After a variable latent period of up to 24 hours after injury, the proximal cut axon tip bulges into a growth cone (Fig. 19–19). Anterograde growth occurs by advancement of the tip in conjunction with the sprouting of collaterals from the growth cone, as well as from nodes of Ranvier up to several segments proximal to the axon tip (Matson, 1950; Grafstein and McQuarrie, 1978; Forman and Berenberg, 1978). By the end of the first 24 hours a few sprouts have reached the area of injury, and penetration of the developing scar at the site of injury proceeds from the second or third day. Accompanying the axonal sprouts out of the proximal stump are Schwann cells derived from the replication of the terminal satellite cells (Spencer, 1977).

The growth cone is a region of axoplasmic enlargement at the tip of the proximal disrupted axon. By histologic and electron microscopic parameters it resembles the structure of growing axons in the embryo and in tissue culture. The growth cone is rich with smooth endoplasmic reticulum, microtubules, microfilaments, large mitochondria, lysosomes, and other vacuolar and vesicular structures of unknown significance. There are internal actin filaments and myosin, and the membrane elaborates numerous filopodia that protrude and retract in an ameboid fashion (Tennyson, 1970; Yamada, Spooner, and Wessells, 1971; Bunge, 1973; Selzer, 1980; Letourneau, 1981).

Anterograde motion appears to be produced in part by this random filopodial protrusion. When a suitably adhesive substratum is "sensed" by the filopodium (i.e., a Schwann cell membrane), adherence occurs. Through a transmembrane event, internal actin filaments are stabilized, and when retraction occurs the growth cone is pulled forward. The axon and its contents are then propelled into the attached filopodium, and the axon is lengthened in that direction (Weiss, 1941, 1944a; Letourneau, 1975; Bunge and Bunge, 1984). Many filopodia from one axon can progress down the nerve fiber in this manner, or they may branch or grow back on themselves in an arbitrary fashion. When one sprout establishes contact with the target organ, the other sprouts degenerate and the single axon matures (Spencer, 1977; Bunge and Bunge, 1984). This single axon is enfolded by Schwann cells proximal to distal, and only a few axons are seen to enter old endoneurial sheaths. Most regenerating sprouts move along new Schwann cell interfaces. Myelination is predetermined by the parent axon and not by the end organ (Cabaud, Rodkey, and Nemeth, 1982).

A second factor in axonal growth and guidance may be tropic (guiding) or trophic (nutrient) factors. The growth cone possesses a high endocytotic activity and there is rapid internalization of exogenous materials, which are retrogradely transported to the cell body (Bunge, 1977). Cell membrane is removed from the growing tip by endocytotic vacuolization, and it is constantly replaced by packages of membrane from the neuronal cell body (Bunge and Bunge, 1984). By this mechanism the growth cone is possibly stimulated to "follow" the concentration gradient of trophic or tropic substances. The importance of the retrogradely transported substances is indirectly borne out by the objective evidence that fast retrograde transport rates accelerate during the early phases of regeneration and gradually return to normal as regeneration is completed (Ochs, 1976; Bisby, 1980).

The direction of growth and the shape of the growth cone are influenced by mechanical factors along its path. Impenetrable scar

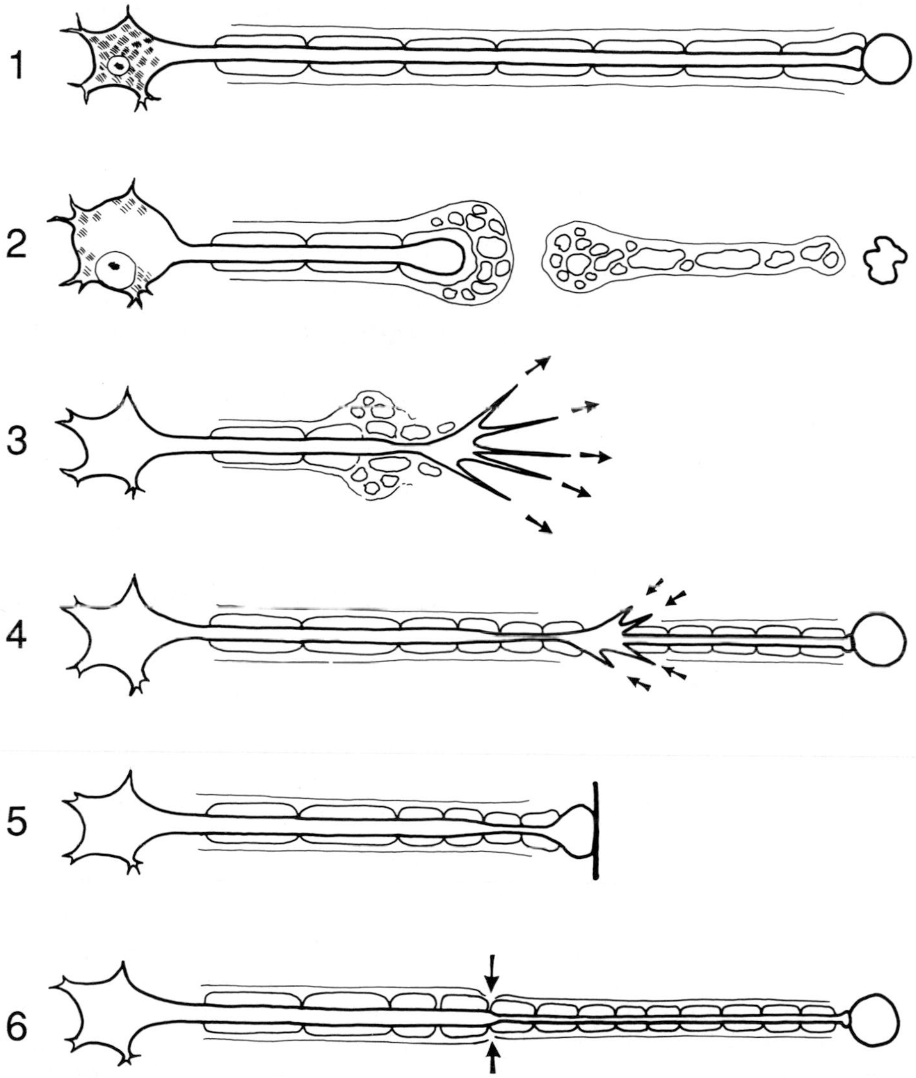

Figure 19–19. Peripheral nerve degeneration and regeneration. 1, Intact nerve. 2, Axonal degeneration (partial) and distal wallerian degeneration after division. 3, Outgrowth from the proximal stump with a growth cone at the proximal cut end. Note the regenerating sprouts. 4, Regeneration and successful target contact of one axonal sprout; redundant sprouts undergo the dying-back process. 5, A terminal bulb forms if an insurmountable obstruction is encountered. 6, Compression by scar at the coaptation site results in abnormalities in axonal caliber and internodal distance.

causes a change in the direction of growth of the advancing axon or causes it to branch (Weiss, 1944a; Bunge and Bunge, 1984). There is some evidence, however, that the growth cone is capable of elaboration of proteases (plasminogen activators), which may enhance the ability of the growth cone to burrow through tissue (Krystosek and Seeds, 1981). Ideally, with no scar to surmount, the advancing axon will grow to the distal stump where the longitudinally arranged Schwann cells will help to guide the axon to the appropriate end organ.

Distal Axon

During wallerian degeneration, pleuripotential Schwann cells assume the dual role of degradation of myelin and axonal debris, and they proliferate within the basal lamina of the remaining endoneurial connective tissue sheath (Satinsky, Pepe, and Liu, 1964). As they proliferate they become densely packed in longitudinal rows histologically recognized as the bands of Büngner. They are ready to accept axon buds and remyelinate the advancing regenerating axons (Selzer, 1980; Thomas, Landon, and King, 1984). Unfortunately, beginning between 28 and 35 days after a nerve lesion (during a period of active regeneration), there is a deposition of an additional layer of endoneurial collagen. This narrows the potential space available for axonal growth. Despite the peripheral migration of the Schwann cells to open the center of the endoneurial cylinder for axonal growth, the ultimate diameter of the regenerated axon is decreased (Thomas, 1964). The overall number of Schwann cells per unit length is increased, and after remyelination of the regenerated axon this is reflected in a decreased internodal length (Cragg and Thomas, 1964; Thomas, Landon, and King, 1984).

Since the connective tissue elements of the distal nerve fiber are dependent on the presence of an intact axon to maintain anatomic, metabolic, and functional integrity, failure of regeneration of a nerve eventually leads to irreversible shrinkage of the distal endoneurial tube. Within two years, the cross sectional area of the empty endoneurial sheath will be only 1 per cent of its normal size. The blood supply of the distal nerve fiber also undergoes contraction and reexpands following regeneration of the nerve. Even after optimal axonal regeneration, the blood supply never exceeds 60 to 80 per cent of its original cross sectional area (Sunderland and Bradley, 1950; Ducker, Kempe, and Hayes, 1969).

On the average, a regenerating axon grows through a scar at a rate of approximately 0.25 mm per day, and after the axonal sprouts reach the distal endoneurial tube, growth continues at 1.0 to 8.5 mm per day, depending on multiple factors. The rates of nerve regeneration are inversely proportional to the distance from the cell body as observed by a progressing Tinel's sign (Tinel, 1971). Reported regeneration rates are 8.5+ mm per day in the upper arm, 6 mm per day in the proximal forearm, 1 to 2 mm per day at the wrist, and 1 to 1.5 mm per day in the hand. These high rates of regeneration were observed in second degree crush injuries in humans (Sunderland, 1968). In each instance, the nerve was regenerating under ideal conditions. On the average, nerve regeneration proceeds through nonvascularized nerve grafts at 3 to 4 mm per day (Terzis, 1988).

Relationship to Degree of Injury

At the microscopic, single-axon level, a second degree (axonotmetic) nerve injury results in wallerian degeneration and proximal axonal reaction. As degeneration proceeds, the proximal axon stump develops a growth cone and sprouts with up to 25 filopodia (Thomas, Landon, and King, 1984). Since the second degree injuries do not disrupt the endoneurial tubes bound by a relatively nondistensible basal lamina, the sprouts are "guided" forward through the site of injury. After the first sprout reaches the target organ of the nerve, the remaining sprouts degenerate (the dying-back process) and only one sprout survives to mature within the endoneurial cylinder (Denny-Brown and Brenner, 1944). The new population of longitudinally arranged Schwann cells enfold the regenerating axon in a proximal to distal direction (Cabaud, Rodkey, and Nemeth, 1982; Peacock, 1984). Since the continuity of the basal lamina maintains the endoneurial tube integrity, the old tube is utilized and there is no chance of misrouting. End organ specificity is thus maintained (Horch, 1979). When an injury results in disruption of the basal lamina (third degree injury), there is no longer the regenerative specificity that is possible with second degree injuries. Neighboring regenerating axons are able to intermix and misrouting can occur. An axon enters its native endoneurial tube only as a random event. The greater the disruption, the lower is the likelihood of end organ specific regeneration. By definition, fascicular integrity is maintained, although there may be a large gap between the proximal and distal axonal stumps with significant interposed scar (see neuroma-in-continuity). If regeneration occurs spontaneously, the prognosis depends on the level of the lesion and the proximity of the nerve to its target organs. For any given fascicle, the closer it is to its terminal branching, the greater is the axonal homogeneity within the fascicle. A distal injury, therefore, can regenerate and a reasonable functional return can be expected. In a proximal nerve fascicle, there is much less heterogeneity. Proximal fascicles have a much lower cross sectional area devoted to any single target, and the fibers supplying the distal musculature and sensory end organs are scattered throughout the proximal nerve trunk (Daniel and Terzis, 1977). Consequently, random regeneration is less likely to produce function.

When a fourth degree injury occurs, the proximal and distal stumps behave in the same fashion as the lesser injured nerves. The fascicular disruption that defines this injury allows greater stump retraction proximally and distally. However, the intact epineurium limits the extent and confines the interposed scar. Budding axons become entangled in the scar and few succeed in bridging the gap between the stumps. The few sprouts that find their way to the degenerating distal stump lengthen, mature, and remyelinate but distal functional connectivity is haphazard (Ducker, Kempe, and Hayes, 1969; Mira, 1981b; Cabaud, Rodkey, and Nemeth, 1982). These lesions are clinically detected as neuroma-in-continuity masses of misdirected axons entangled within the scar confined by the epineurium. Some budding axons can follow perineurial and epineurial blood vessels and "escape" the nerve trunk to become a lateral neuroma (Daniel and Terzis, 1977b).

Fifth degree neurotmetic injuries result in separation of the entire proximal and distal stumps. The normal regenerative pattern of the proximal stump proceeds, but growth cones and their accompanying Schwann cells grow into the random scar tissue separating the ends. The more disoriented the substratum, the more the growth cone sprouts will branch. Miniature fascicles in random orientation, embedded in dense connective tissue scar, are the result—an amputation neuroma (Weiss, 1944a; Spencer, 1977). It is virtually impossible for a fifth degree lesion to regenerate without some form of directional guidance to the distal stump.

Influencing Factors

The foundation upon which peripheral nerve surgery is built is based on the principles that facilitate the natural regenerative process of the nerve. It is recognized that the quality and speed of regeneration of a nerve is improved when there is a minimal amount of scar tissue within the gap. A better prognosis for the return of function is found if the regenerating axons enter their native endoneurial tube so that they can be guided back toward the proper target organ (appropriate topographic orientation) (Selzer, 1980). Thus, three "mechanical" factors, as well as the amount of time allowed to elapse between injury and repair, are to some degree under the control of the surgeon. Other factors such as the age of the patient, the type of nerve, the level of the nerve injury, the cause of the injury, and the associated injuries affect the functional outcome after nerve reconstruction but cannot yet be manipulated.

Mechanical Factors. In general, the natural wound-healing mechanism of the body, cicatrization, runs counter to what would be in the best interest of nerve healing and subsequent regeneration. Scar formation between the proximal and distal ends of a coapted nerve physically blocks the forward growth of the axons and causes the nerve growth cone to branch, divert, turn back, or terminate. Axons and Schwann cells have the tendency to align themselves along linear structures; therefore, the confusing substratum of an interposed scar creates a tangled mass of misdirected fibers, few of which reach the distal stump. Under satisfactory conditions following nerve transection and coaptation, Cajal estimated that only one-sixth or one-seventh of the sprouting axons in the adult reached the distal stump and went on to grow distally; a higher percentage was observed in young patients (Weiss, 1944a).

Only part of the problem of functional reconstruction lies in the avoidance of neuroma formation by scar-free coaptation with a negligible gap. Discrepancies in the intraneural topography between proximal and distal stumps lead to axons being misdirected or lost in the interfascicular, epineurial connective tissue and missing the distal endoneurial tubes (Daniel and Terzis, 1977b). In suture coaptation following injury, the absence of perineurium and subsequent loss of fascicular structure, as well as local swelling and technically imprecise repair, increase the tissue disarray and topographic disorientation. Even when debridement is required and there is no longer an exact fascicular match, orientation can be maintained since fascicular groupings in each quadrant reliably carry homogeneous axon populations.

During wallerian degeneration and proximal axonal regeneration, collagen fibrils are deposited externally to the persisting basal lamina tubes—especially near the site of axonal severance. Deposition continues until regeneration is complete (Thomas, 1964; Thomas, Landon, and King, 1984). The more time it takes for the distal nerve stump to become reinnervated, the more collagen is laid down, and consequently the thickened endoneurial tube decreases in internal diameter (Holmes and Young, 1944). Not only does the thickening decrease the available potential area for axonal reentry, but the thickened tubes create a local constriction of the growing axon. This restricts ultimate axonal diameter and leads to a permanent reduction in axonal size and myelin thickness (Weiss and Taylor, 1944b; Holmes and Young, 1944). If a healthy vascular bed is not maintained or created, the satellite cells and support structures of the regenerating nerve suffer an ischemic insult, and increased collagen deposition results. The character of the collagen deposited under conditions of ischemia is consistent with the type of collagen found in dense mineralized tissue scar. There are increased hydroxylysino-hydroxynorleucine crosslinkages, and this type of collagen matrix presents a greater obstacle to axonal regeneration than that found in nonischemic nerve (Starkweather and associates, 1978).

Effect of Delay Before Repair. When the effects of the passage of time on nerve regeneration are considered, it is understood that the regenerative capacity of the cell body and proximal stump is maintained as long as cell death does not occur (Sunderland, 1968). Time, therefore, assumes importance only as regards the distal nerve and target organs. Clinical studies have documented that functional regeneration can occur after late secondary reconstruction, and anecdotal reports document functional recovery as late as 22 years after denervation (Madden and Peacock, 1971), even in the face of irreversible muscle changes by three years (Bowden and Gutmann, 1944).

Within the first four days after injury, there remains sufficient independent functional and structural integrity in the distal nerve stump for electrical stimulation to allow fascicular identification (Daniel and Terzis, 1977b). The distal stump then fails and degeneration proceeds. Collagen, laid down within the endoneurium, progressively shrinks the Schwann cell tubes, making it increasingly more difficult for the regenerating axons to reenter the distal stump, and making it impossible for maturing axons to achieve their preinjury diameter (Weiss and Taylor, 1944b; Holmes and Young, 1944).

Age. Although the reasons are still not well understood, there is little question that a younger patient achieves a much better functional recovery after nerve repair and subsequent regeneration than an older patient (Souttar, 1945; Bristow, 1947; Önne, 1962; Lindsay, Walker, and Farmer, 1962; McEwan, 1962; Schut, 1972). Many possible mechanisms have been suggested to explain this observation. In the periphery, the decreased rates and extent of degeneration of the distal axon and end organ, or increased axonal regeneration and reinnervation (quality and quantity), may lead to the improved results seen in the young. Centrally, young people may be better able to adapt to any peripheral deficit that results from axonal disorganization (Terzis and Breidenbach, 1984) by increased plasticity.

Studies have demonstrated that the rates of nerve regeneration are age related. Rates decline with increasing age and may be due to differences in the velocity of slow axonal transport between young and old patients (Black and Lasek, 1979). In addition, the mechanism that enables growing axons to select appropriate target organs (tropic or trophic) appears to operate over greater distances in young animals (Selzer, 1980).

In a study of recovery of sensibility, Önne (1962) reported that recovered two-point discrimination (2pd) in millimeters was approximately the same as the patient's age, up to 20 years of age. For patients aged 20 to 31, regained 2pd was variable but tended to be poor. In older patients there was uniformly poor return of function, with 2pd rarely below 30 mm. Young, Wray, and Weeks (1981), in a randomized prospective study of digital nerve repairs, also showed that age was a factor in the quality of regeneration. Eighty per cent of patients under 20 years of age attained a functional 2pd after repair, but no patient over 40 achieved more than protective sensation. Using a plastic ridge device, Poppen and associates (1979) were able to document that only children under the age of 13 years consistently achieved a return of fine sensibility after nerve repair.

In the assumption that there were age-related differences in return of function after peripheral nerve repair, several studies were designed to seek an objective reason. Using adult and baby monkeys, Almquist, Smith, and Fry (1983) measured nerve conduction velocities and studied total axon counts in regenerated axons as well as the degree of myelination, the axonal size, and the internal structure of the regenerated axons. No physiologic or morphologic difference was found between nerves sutured in young and those in old monkeys (Almquist, Smith, and Fry, 1983). Nerve conduction velocity after nerve repair in humans also did not correlate with the better 2pd observed in younger patients (Almquist and Eeg-Olofsson, 1970). On the other hand, examination of receptor density (Meissner's corpuscles) in humans showed significant differences between young and old patients. There was a greater than fourfold decrease in the density of Meissner's corpuscles in the fingertips of normal cadavers from the first to the eighth decade (Ridley, 1968).

No difference is apparent in the regenerative behavior of young and old axons, and the consistently better functional return in the young may be due to greater cortical plasticity (Almquist and Eeg-Olofsson, 1970; Guth, 1974). In essence, cortical plasticity suggests an ability to relearn or reorganize the spatially disrupted input at the level of the cerebral cortex, and to partially overcome inexact peripheral nerve regeneration (Dykes, 1984). Since the younger patient has a greater capacity to adapt to the altered input than the old by reeducation, functional recovery of sensation is superior. The young patient also has a greater capacity to substitute and modify muscles to compensate, and therefore achieve a better functional motor result (Brown, 1972a).

Type of Nerve. It is attractive to consider that repair of a "pure" sensory or a "pure" motor nerve would achieve a higher degree of functional recovery than would a "mixed" nerve, as some authors have reported (Brown, 1972a). However, any nerve is far from being functionally uniform. More than 50 per cent of the fibers of the deep "motor" branch of the ulnar nerve were found to be sensory, including muscle afferents, joint afferents, and receptor fibers from the skin and deep subcutaneous tissue of the hand. Likewise, sensory nerves carry sympathetic motor fibers for the vasa vasorum, piloerecti, and so forth (Daniel and Terzis, 1977b). At the fascicular level, microcoaptation of the heterogeneous mixes of axons presents the same problem as coaptation of a nerve trunk in terms of topographic orientation. Random axonal reentry almost precludes exact target organ specificity, and axons are "wasted" by growth down to unrelated sensory or motor terminals.

Level of Injury. This factor is by far one of the most important for predicting the return of function after nerve repair. Proximal injuries in general carry a worse prognosis than distal injuries, for many reasons. First, since the axon is an extension of the neuron, a proximal injury actually injures a greater percentage of the total mass of the cell. Regenerative demands are far higher on the neuron for both metabolic needs and the time required for regeneration (Torvik and Skjörten, 1971; Brown, 1972a). Perhaps in proximal injury the greater percentage of total cell mass damaged and the higher regenerative demand are the cause of more intense retrograde reaction and a greater likelihood of neuron death. Second, the more proximal the level of axonal disruption, the farther is the distance to the target organ. This lesion requires a greater length of time for axonal regrowth and maturation, and during this time a greater amount of distal nerve and target organ degeneration occurs (Gutman and Gutman, 1942; Brown, 1972a; Daniel and Terzis, 1977b), increasing the potential for irreversible change (Torvik and Skjörten, 1971).

Intraneural topography again plays an important role in the quality of regeneration and is closely related to the level of injury.

In a proximal nerve trunk, electrophysiologic studies show that motor and sensory axons are randomly distributed throughout the fascicular network. Axonal homogeneity increases as the nerve proceeds distally and approaches the target organs (Sunderland, 1968). In the case of proximal musculature, there is no doubt that functional recovery is much higher after repair of a proximal nerve lesion than is the recovery of a distal muscle. Not only is there a greater cross sectional area of the nerve occupied by the corresponding fibers, but the axons supplying the proximal musculature are more localized at the suture line than those of the distal muscles (Daniel and Terzis, 1977b). The difficulty lies not in inadequate regenerative response, but in the greater randomness with which motor axons reform connections with distal muscles (Weiss and Hoag, 1946).

In a high upper extremity nerve lesion, the proximal muscles uniformly achieve a better functional return than the distal muscles. This finding is partly explained by the fact that the proximal muscles function in simple flexion and extension movements, and several muscles function in parallel to perform the same motion. Imprecise reinnervation is better tolerated in these "all-or-none" gross motor movements than in the finely coordinated, precise, independent, and small intrinsic muscles of the hand (Daniel and Terzis, 1977b). Since axonal localization improves as the nerve proceeds distally and there is greater fascicular homogeneity, this helps to explain the common clinical observation that the prognosis for return of function is better in the more peripheral nerve injuries (Kirklin, Murphy, and Berkson, 1949; Shaffer and Cleveland, 1950; Oester and Davis, 1956; Yahr and Beebe, 1956; Omer, 1974).

Cause of Nerve Injury and Associated Injuries. The cause of nerve injury is of considerable importance if one is to estimate the regenerative capacity of a nerve and the prognosis for reconstruction. The less a nerve is traumatized, the greater is the likelihood of a successful functional recovery. In the minimal trauma situation, such as a guillotine cut of a nerve, localized damage to the nerve and satellite support structures is the result, with only minimal longitudinal extension of the injury, either proximal or distal. A severe injury is frequently extensive and possibly on multiple levels, and results from direct injury, traction, and ischemia. Devitalized tissue, nerve contusion, and hematoma increase scarring around and within the affected nerve trunk, producing a poor nutrient bed for subsequent regeneration. Severe proximal injuries further compromise functional recovery owing to the higher number of central cells that die, leaving a reduced regenerating axon population.

When a nerve injury is severe, such as in the case of high velocity missile or shotgun blasts, extensive longitudinal involvement is apparent and repair requires careful resection of the injured nerve. It is obviously imperative that the entire length of the involved nerve be examined directly or indirectly with electrodiagnostic techniques to avoid missing a previously undiagnosed multilevel nerve injury.

The condition of the associated tissues—skin, bone, joint, and vascular system—indirectly affects the quality of nerve regeneration. Any concomitant injury must be addressed before nerve repair is undertaken. It is often the associated injury that dictates the timing of repair, and neurorrhaphy should not be performed in a limb without adequate skin cover, skeletal stability with supple joints, and vascular sufficiency. Infection should be aggressively treated, and procedures that would not routinely be performed, such as flap coverage and internal or external bone fixation, are definitely indicated if they are likely to facilitate earlier nerve reconstruction.

Trophic Influence. There is no question that the peripheral nervous system possesses a remarkable potential for regeneration, but the functional significance of this depends on the ability of the axon to reinnervate the appropriate target tissue. To find its original end organ, the regenerating axon requires positive directional guidance as well as the absence of mechanical handicaps.

It has been repeatedly shown that the peripheral nervous system of lower animals (including salamanders, crayfish, and fish) is able to preferentially reinnervate a muscle by its original nerve fibers with restoration of function indistinguishable from normal (Sperry, 1950; Daniel and Terzis, 1977b; Ely and Velez, 1982). This specificity of reinnervation is also seen in cutaneous sensory innervation. It has been demonstrated that when a patch of skin is transplanted from ventral to dorsal (or vice versa) in a young tadpole, anomalous wiping responses develop in the adult frog (Miner, 1956). This is attributed to the ability of the axons to reroute themselves and reinnervate the original target organs despite the altered locale (Sklar and Hunt, 1973; Bloom and Tompkins, 1976; Heidemann, 1977). Unfortunately, mammals do not have this uncanny ability. Poor functional results are not secondary to an inadequate regenerative response, but are due to greater randomness of connectivity with target organs when these are separated by great distances (Weiss and Hoag, 1946; Selzer, 1980).

Mammalian studies have implied that regenerating cutaneous nerves can find their way back to the appropriate types of receptors over short distances. Examination of regenerating sural nerves of the cat revealed that control and regenerated nerves had almost identical response properties, specificity, response dynamics, conduction velocities, and central connectivity (Burgess and Horch, 1973). All identifiable fibers reinnervated the same type of mechanoreceptor that was their normal end organ. Similarly, all the identifiable mechanoreceptors were reinnervated by the appropriate nerve fibers. In a similar experimental model modified by destruction of the cutaneous mechanoreceptors supplied by the nerve, it was possible to show that regenerating axons returned preferentially to other sites with viable mechanoreceptors. Areas of receptor destruction were then randomly innervated (Horch, 1982). These studies strongly suggested that it is not the distal endoneurial tubule that dictates entirely the destiny of the regenerating axon, but that it is more likely that viable end organs influence the regeneration of the nerve. Under this assumption, some theories of nerve regeneration have turned away from mechanical "contact" guidance as the sole factor for axonal direction (Weiss and Taylor, 1943, 1944a) and returned to the concept of "neurotrophism" suggested by Forssman in 1898, in which the nerve is attracted to the distal stump; it could therefore regenerate and find its appropriate target.

With the serendipitous discovery of a humoral factor that produced a stimulatory effect on sympathetic and sensory ganglia, it was recognized that tissues could attract growing axons (Levi-Montalcini, 1982). Identification and purification of a diffusible protein macromolecule by Cohen (1959) enabled in vivo and in vitro examination of the role of this substance named *nerve growth factor (NGF)*. Since that time, it has been demonstrated that NGF plays a role of paramount importance in the development, maintenance, and regeneration of sympathetic and sensory nerves (Thoenen and Barde, 1980). It is released by tissues innervated by sympathetic and sensory axons (Ebendal and associates, 1980; Harper and associates, 1980) and there are high affinity receptors specific for NGF present on the nerve membranes (Dumas, Schwab, and Thoenen, 1979). NGF, bound to the nerve cell membrane, is internalized and transported in a retrograde fashion to the cell body, where it affects neuronal metabolism (Thoenen and associates, 1971; Stockel, Paravicini, and Thoenen, 1974). It exhibits a stimulatory effect on the growth of axons (Bjerre and associates, 1975); it can prevent the retrograde axonal reaction following severance of an axon and prevent subsequent cell death (Nja and Purves, 1978; Hamburger, Brunso-Bechtold, and Yip, 1981). Concentration gradients of NGF can guide growth cones in culture (Letourneau, 1978; Gundersen and Barrett, 1980) and in vivo (Menesini-Chen, Chen, and Levi-Montalcini, 1978; Gundersen and Barrett, 1979), and may possibly play a significant role in the guidance of regenerating axons to their target organs. More recently, other protein macromolecules have been identified. One is associated with motor nerves and is similar to NGF in composition and function (*motor or MNGF*) (Slack, Hopkins, and Pockett, 1983), and another appears to be produced in degenerating nerve stumps (Edwards and associates, 1984). Other factors seem to facilitate the actions of NGF and MNGF (Berg, 1984). These neurotrophic factors may be humoral or substrate bound (Varon and Bunge, 1978; Varon and Adler, 1980).

Berg (1984) suggested that there are four major actions of humoral or substrate-bound neurotrophic factors: (1) neuronal survival factors that prevent death in dissociated cell culture; (2) neurite extension factors that promote axonal sprouting; (3) substrate adhesion/neurite promoting factors that appear to augment cellular adherence and facilitate the actions of other factors; and (4) developmental factors that influence neuronal differentiation and guide neuronal development in culture. These actions are not mutually exclusive, and a single neurotrophic factor may function in several categories.

Although proof is not available, substantial

circumstantial evidence exists that mammalian axons can select appropriate targets at close range, and the mechanism involved appears to include specific recognition of a target organ by the growing axon. The specificity of target recognition appears to operate over greater distances in younger animals than in older ones, and this is consistent with the common clinical observation that the recovery of nerve function is better in the young (Omer, 1974). The prognosis for functional recovery is also better if the nerve injury is more peripheral and closer to the target organ (Zachary and Holmes, 1946; Oester and Davis, 1956; Yahr and Beebe, 1956). Schwann cells also seem to have the capacity to attract regenerating axons by a chemotactic mechanism (Politis, Ederle, and Spencer, 1981), as does the distal stump of a transected nerve trunk.

In multiple studies examining the regeneration of nerves across chambers of various design and materials, investigators have demonstrated neurotrophism. Lundborg and associates (1982) separated proximal and distal nerve stumps by a mesothelial chamber and showed that the fluid that collected within contained trophic activity for cultured sensory neurons. Seckel and colleagues (1984) showed the importance of the distal nerve stump as a source of neurotrophic factors by demonstrating failure of regeneration across a gap when the distal stump was absent or was at a distance greater than 10 mm from the proximal stump. Likewise, in "multiple choice" experiments (chambers configured in a "Y"), Williams and associates (1984), Politis (1985), and Mackinnon and colleagues (1986) demonstrated that regenerating nerve fibers selectively grew down the limb of the "Y" that contained the distal nerve stump, presumably following the concentration gradient of trophic factors. Using the same model, Longo and associates (1983) added antiserum to NGF and demonstrated that regenerative specificity was maintained without the presence of NGF. Therefore, it was presumed that the neurotrophic factors were substances other than NGF.

In a primate model, Mackinnon and colleagues (1985a) showed regeneration through a vascularized mesothelial chamber over a distance of 3 cm. In this and all other models, nerve fiber diameter and subsequent myelination matured with time. The regenerating axons grouped into multiple small "minifascicles," each delineated by a distinct perineurial layer (Mackinnon, Hudson, and Hunter, 1985). As suggested by Morris, Hudson, and Weddell (1972), these small fascicles represented individual functional units, compartmentalized in an attempt by the regenerating nerve to reconstitute its own endoneurial environment.

It is now evident through the discovery of neurotrophic influence in regeneration that the role of the distal nerve fiber is much more important than simply that of a conduit to the periphery for growing axons, and that end organs are much more than passive targets.

Reinnervation

In nerve regeneration, outgrowth of the axon is only the first step in a series of developments leading to restoration of a mature functional system. After bridging the site of nerve injury (or repair), the axon sprout reaches the distal stump that, by the process of wallerian degeneration, has been prepared to accept the sprout. The sprout then grows along the bands of Büngner toward the periphery, following fascicles but also able to traverse the plexiform fascicular interconnections from one to another. However, even entry into an axon's native fascicle does not ensure ultimate arrival at its native end organ. When the growing axon reaches an end organ (if it is of the appropriate class), connectivity occurs and maturation follows (Gutman and Young, 1944). Maturation progresses from proximal to distal with first an increase of axonal diameter, followed by myelination (Gutman and Sanders, 1943). Myelination proceeds in the identical fashion observed during embryogenesis. In myelinated fibers the membranes wrap around the axon to form the characteristic spiral, and in unmyelinated fibers the Schwann cell is invaginated by multiple axons. The final diameter of the mature regenerated axon is rarely normal and is usually smaller with a thinner myelin sheath (Mira, 1981b). When a regenerating nerve fiber grows through a localized constriction, the segment of the axon distal to the constriction never regains its previous size or thickness of myelin sheath (Weiss and Taylor, 1944b). Therefore, scar developing in the regenerating nerve's bed represents an obstacle to both longitudinal growth and growth in diameter during maturation (Mira, 1981b).

REINNERVATION OF MOTOR UNITS

Only motor neurons have the capacity to recreate neuromuscular junctions. When a regenerating motor axon reaches a denervated muscle, reinnervation generally occurs at the old motor end plates, possibly because of a trophic attraction of the growth bulb for the old junctional contact (Rosenthal, 1977; Brown, Holland, and Hopkins, 1981). Reinnervation of contiguous muscle fibers by collateral sprouting of the first axons to reestablish neuromuscular junctions produces a topographic redistribution of the motor unit (Mira, 1987). Reinnervated muscle units are histochemically uniform. This finding is based on the assumption that the individual muscle fibers undergo a conversion from one type to another, depending on the reinnervating motor neuron (Kugelberg, Edström, and Abbruzzese, 1970). This change occurs by approximately two weeks after reinnervation. Overall, the range of physiologic properties and muscle fiber types over the entire reinnervated muscle is normal, with heterogeneous mixtures of "type S" (slowly contracting, fatigue-resistant, small force units); "type FR" (moderate force, fast contracting, fatigue-resistant units); and "type FS" (large force, fast contracting, fatigue-sensitive units). Instead of a random "mosaic" distribution of the motor units as seen in normal muscle, reinnervated muscle shows clusters of commonly innervated fibers and smaller motor units (Mira, 1987). When only a few regenerating axons reach the denervated muscle, the "adoption phenomenon" occurs, in which axons can multiply sprout to reinnervate many surrounding end plates and salvage some function. This type of neurotization of many end plates by relatively few axons forms giant motor units with greatly expanded territories (Burke, 1980).

Recovery of motor function does not occur immediately upon reestablishment of a neuromuscular junction. Studies by Gutman and Young (1944) showed an 18 day delay before nerve stimulation would produce contraction, and an additional five days before functional reflex activity occurred. Recovery of useful function best correlates with the return of gamma efferent control of the intrafusal fibers but, as with any axonotmetic or neurotmetic lesion, gamma reinnervation is haphazard. The distortion in feedback control that results might be manifest clinically by imprecision of movement, which would tend to downgrade even a satisfactory recovery of contraction. Furthermore, residual motor deficits can result from wasted regeneration (lack of peripheral connectivity), or from lack of specificity of reinnervation. The latter can result in inappropriate connectivity giving rise to antagonistic synkinetic contractions (appropriate target class—incorrect field) or dilution of the effectiveness of contraction through sparse reinnervation of several parallel muscles.

All the above schemata for motor neuron regeneration and muscular reinnervation depend on the condition of the muscle at the time reinnervation is achieved. During the period of denervation the muscle must be kept in optimal condition through physical therapy and electrical stimulation. Any denervation atrophy is harmful to a muscle, because progressive thickening of connective tissue elements within the muscle hinders nerve regrowth and end plate reformation. By two years, without adjunctive therapy, skeletal muscle is probably beyond satisfactory functional recovery (Ducker, 1972).

REINNERVATION OF SENSORY MECHANORECEPTORS

As with regeneration of motor fibers, the axons responsible for the conveyance of sensory modalities sprout from the proximal nerve stump, traverse the area of injury, and grow down Schwann cell linear tubes to the periphery, where reinnervation of degenerating end organs by submodality-specific axons occurs. Owing to the haphazard nature of axonal regeneration in axonotmetic and neurotmetic injuries, this pattern of regeneration can result in a significant alteration in the central input of peripheral information as the receptive fields are altered (Dellon, 1981). It is only in crush injuries, where basal membranes remain intact, that receptive fields remain undisturbed after regeneration and normal sensibility is restored.

The conclusions drawn from multiple studies, mostly using a skin graft model, resulted in the rejection of the early hypothesis of de novo generation of sensory end organs (Terzis, 1979), and it is now evident that regenerating axons grow into denervated sensory receptors and reestablish functional end organs (Ridley, 1970; Orgel, Aguayo, and Williams, 1972; Dellon, 1981). The quality of regeneration, of course, depends on the condition of the end organ at the time of reinnervation, and not on the seemingly unlimited regenerative capacity of the severed peripheral nerve (Terzis, 1979). The outside time limit of reversible degeneration of sensory end organs is not known, but probably the Merkel cell–neurite complex is irreversibly damaged first, with complete disappearance of touch domes in the cat by 35 days after nerve transection (Burgess and associates, 1974). Although this is not documented in primates or humans, Merkel cell–neurite complexes probably degenerate faster than Meissner's corpuscles, which are seen to maintain a distinct lamellar structure for four months after denervation (Dellon, Witebsky, and Terrill, 1975). The corpuscular size and general architecture are maintained for approximately six months, following which there is progressive collapse of the lamellae and decreasing size, probably rendering the end organ incapable of full reinnervation (Dellon, 1981). On the other hand, the pacinian corpuscle appears to be relatively stable, identifiable, and structurally intact after 400 days of denervation (Glees, Mohiuddin, and Smith, 1949). The clinical impression that there is little return of functional sensation following sensory nerve repair longer than six months after injury (Önne, 1962; Honner, Fragiadakis, and Lamb, 1970; Poppen and associates, 1979) is supported by these morphologic studies.

When sprouting axons reach the area of denervated receptors, preexisting Schwann cell tubes and trophic factors help to guide submodality-specific axons to their appropriate targets. Skin grafting and crossinnervation studies have shown that the major determinants of the quality of sensory recovery are factors intrinsic to the territory or graft, and are not necessarily dependent on the regenerating axons. In these studies, reinnervation of glabrous skin, with nerves from hairy skin and vice versa, showed specificity in adaptation characteristics. Slowly adapting fibers innervated slowly adapting receptors, and quickly adapting fibers innervated quickly adapting receptors, regardless of their native end organ.

Recovery of sensibility occurs in a repeatable order sequence that correlates with the observed morphology of nerve fibers and reinnervated receptors (Dellon, 1981). According to Dellon (1981), it is generally agreed that perception, pain, and temperature precede the return of touch, and that touch submodalities also recover in an orderly sequence, beginning with perception of 30 cycles per second (cps) frequencies, followed by moving touch, by constant touch, and finally by perception of a 256 cps stimulus.

Initial recovery is a function of nerve fiber size. Since all axons sprout and grow as thin unmyelinated fibers before they mature, it is understandable that the small unmyelinated C fibers and thinly myelinated A delta fibers responsible for pain and temperature (which require no end organ) recover first. The recovery of touch submodalities follows and is dependent on establishment of end organ reinnervation and subsequent fiber maturation.

Terzis (1981b) hypothesized that part of the reason for the temporal dissociation of recovery of touch submodalities lies in the intrinsic design of the fiber-receptor systems. In Meissner's corpuscle, which is subserved by multiple nerve fibers (three to nine axons per receptor), there is a statistically higher probability that reinnervation by a quickly adapting fiber will occur than in a singly innervated pacinian corpuscle. Hence, 30 cps sensibility precedes 256 cps sensibility. The Merkel cell–neurite complex, with an axon-to-corpuscle ratio of less than one, should reinnervate even more slowly than the pacinian corpuscle on the basis of this statistical argument. But, since receptor density for this slowly adapting end organ is much higher, this probably shortens the reinnervation delay. Alternatively, recovery of sensibility may be solely dependent on fiber-receptor maturation and threshold recovery, not reinnervation (Dellon, 1981).

The capacity for reinnervation is also affected by axonal morphology and quantity after regeneration. In studies of reinnervated skin grafts, it was found that there was an alteration in counts of myelinated and unmyelinated fibers with a decrease in the total number of myelinated fibers, and an increase in the total number, both relatively and absolutely, of unmyelinated fibers (Orgel, Aguayo, and Williams, 1972; Almquist, Smith, and Fry, 1983). This imbalance in fiber population persisted for at least 15 months, and perhaps it is this that gives rise to some of the altered sensory perceptions after skin grafting or nerve repair.

After successful regeneration of nerve and reinnervation of sensory end organs, functional recovery depends on the ability of the patient to interpret the sensory input. The localization of a stimulus applied to the skin therefore depends on the orderly projection of cutaneous nerves to central integrating areas. There are three potential fates for axons that successfully bridge a site of nerve repair. First, the axon can reestablish continuity with the proper end organ in the appropriate territory and achieve axonal satisfaction. Second, the axon can be misdirected and achieve reinnervation of an appropriate target that resides in an improper territory, or it may reinnervate the wrong receptor in the appropriate receptive field (false localization and axonal disorganization). Third, the axon can be frustrated in its regenerative attempts and achieve connectivity with a degenerated end organ or no connectivity at all (axonal frustration) (Fig. 19–19). All outcomes except reinnervation of the right receptor in the right field cause the cortex to receive a confusing volley of impulses that may or may not be recognizable. Another cause of sensory deficiency, in addition to faulty localization and faulty input, is inadequacy of input caused by insufficient axonal regeneration or insufficient receptor density. The former may result from several factors including the level of the injury, the vascularity, and the amount of scar. Receptor density is a function of age (it decreases with increasing age) (Ridley, 1968), of irreversible end organ degeneration, of receptor death due to an ischemic insult (e.g., replantation), or of an intrinsic deficiency in transplanted tissues (skin grafts). Altered sensory input may also occur from permanent changes in electrophysiologic properties after nerve regeneration. The conduction velocity and amplitude of action potential never return to normal and remain 20 to 40 per cent below control values (Mira, 1981b).

Central Plasticity

After anomalous nerve regeneration, there is a variable facility to reorganize afferent and efferent impulses in order to reeducate the cortex to the novel sensory input or to refine crude motor movements. The ability to "repair" incorrect central connections decreases phylogenetically and ontogenetically, and within each species decreases with increasing age. Exacting regeneration occurs consistently following nerve injuries in some adult fish and amphibians, but comparable regeneration is seen only in embryologic stages of higher vertebrates (Grinnell, 1977). Experiments with monkeys showed some degree of cortical reorganization after median nerve transection and repair, but an abnormality in cortical organization of spatial information persisted. To Dykes (1984), this suggested that spatial information was significantly downgraded or disorganized after nerve repair and regeneration, and was permanent. Patients could perceive individual sensory submodalities, but tactile gnosis, requiring pattern recognition, was lost. There is no apparent basic difference, per se, in the mechanism or capacity of regeneration in lower animals, but there is a greater ability for cortical reorganization than spontaneously occurs in humans. Hence, functional results of nerve repair in lower animals are consistently better. The implication, therefore, is that the somatosensory cortex (and possibly the motor cortex) is not "hard wired" but is capable of being dynamically reorganized within cytoarchetectonic boundaries, and of adapting to altered input and modifying output (Dykes, 1984).

Dellon (1981), taking the hypothesis of central plasticity one step further, felt that, if spatial pattern recognition was altered but sensory input was present, careful reeducation of the patient could "reprogram" cortical "software" and improve sensibility. Perhaps in this way biofeedback training can improve motor precision.

Neuroma Formation

When an axon is severed and unable to reestablish continuity with its distal counterpart, a neuroma forms. This process begins at the proximal stump by the sprouting of axons from the growth cones and the proliferation of Schwann cells after the neuron has recovered from the retrograde reaction. Fibroblastic proliferation, encouraged by blood clot, foreign body, or necrotic debris, occurs between the proximal and distal stumps and impedes the regenerating axons and Schwann cells. The regenerating fibers haphazardly grow and branch, and abundant, irregular ramifications of axons are created in their abortive attempt to reach their end organs (Williams and Terzis, 1976).

The overall configuration of a neuroma depends largely on the characteristics of the local environment. Since fibers have no intrinsic tendency to branch, the more confused and dense the substratum, the more profuse is the branching. If the scar tissue at the proximal stump is diffuse and radiates into the surrounding tissues, the growing axons and proliferating Schwann cells follow. If the scar has tightly capped the proximal stump, the entrapped fibers circle within, forming whorls, and in some instances the axons turn back on themselves and form irregular spirals within the substance of the proximal stump. The regenerating axons are not seen to stop short but continue to proliferate without apparent direction, giving rise to the bulging clinically observed (Weiss, 1944a). The indefinite proliferation is probably halted by crowding (Mathews and Osterholm, 1972). The quality of blood supply to the nerve stump does not appear to alter neuroma formation (Petropoulos and Stefanko, 1961a), but the presence of infection, foreign body, or repeated irritation from pressure or friction tends to increase the size (Herndon, 1982). Since it has been shown that fibroblasts secrete nerve growth factor, a high local concentration of trophic substance could contribute to the disarray of regenerating axons and the apparent lack of directional guidance.

A neuroma can be classified as a *terminal bulb* or a *neuroma-in-continuity*. A terminal bulb neuroma results when a nerve is completely severed and it is typically observed in amputation stumps. A neuroma-in-continuity is the result of partial severance of a nerve, or of a crushing or traction injury in which all or part of the epineurium and perineurium remain intact. A neuroma-in-continuity can be further subdivided into categories as a function of the integrity of the supportive structures. If the perineurium is intact, the neuroma is completely contained within the confines of the nerve sheath and it usually forms a fusiform "spindle" neuroma (an occasional axon can escape the fascicle by growing out along a perineurial vessel). When the perineurium of some of the fascicles is divided, the neuroma grows to the side of the intact fascicles and forms a lateral neuroma (Herndon, 1982; Omer, 1987; Williams, 1987). Because most nerve injuries are partial and do not completely sever the nerve, the majority of neuromas are in continuity (Kline and Nulson, 1972).

It is estimated that as few as 2 per cent (Wilson, 1981) or as many as 30 per cent (Herndon, 1982) of neuromas are painful, but there is no reliable way to predict which will be so. There is no direct relationship between neuroma size and configuration and the presence of symptoms (Madden and Peacock, 1971). Painful neuromas tend to be large and soft, and asymptomatic neuromas are likely to have a firm, fibrous outer "capsule" and be of smaller size. Perhaps the small unmyelinated nerve fibers, reported to be the source of neuroma pain, are protected by the firm scar around asymptomatic neuromas (Wilson, 1981). Some nerves, such as the superficial sensory branch of the radial nerve, appear to have a predisposition to painful neuroma formation—a fact accounted for by the unique anatomic tethering of the nerve and the necessity for a large excursion of the nerve during wrist motion (Dellon and Mackinnon, 1984).

The formation of neuromas does appear to be under some degree of surgical control. By changing the microenvironment of nerve stumps, the amount of axonal proliferation can be manipulated, and under the right circumstances the likelihood of a painful neuroma developing can be lessened. The most successful methods of altering the stump environment have involved transplanting the nerve into muscle or bone (Petropoulos and Stefanko, 1961b; Mass and associates, 1984; Goldstein and Sturim, 1985; Mackinnon and associates, 1985b; Dellon and Mackinnon, 1986; Wood and Mudge, 1987). Implantation into a normally innervated muscle seems to inhibit the ability of the nerve to regenerate. Perhaps the innervated muscle produces an inhibitory protein that prevents superinnervation, or the trophic stimulus for regeneration is absent in the new location in muscle or bone.

In the distal stump an analogous nodule grows, but it lacks a neural component. After wallerian degeneration, the Schwann cell and connective tissue elements proliferate and give rise to a glioma—always smaller than its neuroma counterpart (Herndon, 1982).

ELECTRODIAGNOSIS

Electrodiagnosis refers to the observation and interpretation of the electrical signals derived from depolarization and repolarization of the peripheral nerves. These action potentials can be produced by voluntary muscle contractions or evoked by electrical stimulation. Recordings can be obtained by using surface or needle electrodes, each having specific indications. The electrodiagnostic examination consists of two parts: (1) motor and sensory nerve conduction velocity studies and (2) needle electrode examination. By convention, conduction studies are referred to as *NCV (nerve conduction velocity)* and *needle electrode studies* as *EMG (electromyograms)* (Bralliar, 1981; Van Beek, Massac, and Smith, 1986). Recently, a third study, the *somatosensory evoked potentials (SEP)*, has become popular and should be included.

Nerve Conduction Velocity (NCV)

Electrical stimulation of a nerve elicits an evoked depolarization potential that travels along axonal membranes orthodromically and antidromically. Both sensory and motor nerves can be studied but different techniques are used. Motor conduction velocity determination requires that recording electrodes be placed over the appropriate muscle, and a supramaximal stimulus is applied at two points along the appropriate nerve. The time it takes from stimulation for a muscle action potential to occur is largely dependent on conduction velocity. NCV is calculated as the difference in time to produce a response between a proximal stimulus and the distal stimulus divided by the distance between the two points. The time it takes for production of an action potential from a distal site near the muscle belly (the distal motor latency) is remarkably constant and takes into account NCV, the lag time for transmission of a stimulus across the motor end plate. Sensory NCV can be determined orthodromically or antidromically and does not require the determination of nerve-receptor latency. Owing to the much smaller amplitude of the sensory action potential, signal averaging techniques are often required to record the evoked response above the background "noise" (Howard, 1972; Bradley, 1974; Bralliar, 1981; Van Beek, Massac, and Smith, 1986; Schwartz, Iyer, and Kutz, 1986).

Normal NCV for most nerves is 50 to 70 m per sec (Bradley, 1974), but there are normal physiologic variations to be taken into account. Infants have NCV of only 20 to 30 m per sec and do not reach the adult range until ages 3 to 5 years. After 30 years of age, NCV slows by approximately 10 per cent up to the 80th year (Bradley, 1974).

Temperature also affects NCV. For every drop of 1°C in temperature there is a 2.4 m per sec fall in NCV (Abramson and associates, 1966). Variations in stimulus amplitude, apparatus inconsistencies, electrode malposition, and measurement errors probably result in a day to day variation of approximately 5 per cent (Bradley, 1974).

Interpretation of NCV after peripheral nerve injury depends on the time that has elapsed since the injury as well as the severity of the injury. If a nerve is completely transected or suffers damage sufficient to cause wallerian degeneration (second degree injury and above), there is no transmission across the lesion. This is observed immediately after injury. However, the axons of the distal nerve segment remain electrically excitable for up to 96 hours after the injury; therefore, stimulation will produce an evoked potential until wallerian degeneration is complete. Serial examinations during the first 96 hours after injury reveal a progressive loss of the amplitude of the evoked potential, and by 48 hours the amplitude decreases by as much as 90 per cent owing to axonal loss. NCV remains within 20 per cent of normal until conduction ceases. If spontaneous regeneration occurs or if there is successful nerve reconstruction, nerve conduction will return after distal axonal connectivity, and velocity, initially slow, will gradually rise to 60 to 80 per cent of normal (Howard, 1972; Bradley, 1974; Mira, 1981b). Proximal to a nerve lesion, conduction velocity is reduced and does not recover unless regeneration occurs. In the cat, within one to two months, NCV is reduced by 20 per cent after large motor nerve transections. If reinnervation does not occur, NCV progressively declines to 35 to 40 per cent of normal by four months (Gilliatt, 1980).

Compression neuropathies are ideally suited to evaluation by NCV measurements. The site of nerve compression can be readily localized by the focal slowing created by the injury. By studying the entire course of a nerve several focal lesions can be identified in the "multiple crush" syndromes (Bradley, 1974).

One of the major drawbacks in the clinical application of NCV measurements is the inability to study any but the largest, fastest conducting axons. For example, in some small fiber neuropathies, marked analgesia results from loss of group C and A delta fibers but no changes in the NCV are apparent. As long as some high conduction velocity axons remain functional, there is no apparent slowing (Bradley, 1974). Currently, attempts are being made to correlate severity of compression injury (i.e., percentage of axons injured) with integrated area measurements of the action potential wave form (Olney and Miller, 1984). These studies will also be able to analyze the heterogeneity of any given nerve. The greater the heterogeneity, the greater is the diversity of conduction velocities that broadens the compound action potential wave form (Publicover and Terzis, 1987). Computed signal processing based on time domain analysis and frequency domain analysis may help to uncover this buried information (Schwartz, Iyer, and Kutz, 1986).

In the clinical situation in which a nerve is being serially examined after microreconstruction, no significant correlations can be drawn between NCV, amplitude measurements, and recovery of 2pd vibration sensibility or threshold. Therefore, the NCV has no predictive value. The diagnostic value becomes more apparent during the evaluation of brachial plexus trauma. If the NCV can be measured for a nerve that supplies an anesthetic region of an injured arm, the lesion proximal to the sensory ganglion (preganglionic) can be localized. Since the cell bodies are found in the sensory ganglion, a preganglionic injury does not lead to wallerian degeneration, and nerve conduction is maintained (Howard, 1972).

Needle Electromyography

Electromyography (EMG) specifically refers to the recording and measurement of muscle action potentials produced by the depolarization and repolarization of a small group of muscle fibers isolated by the tip of the needle electrode. Because normal muscle function is dependent on normal innervation, the condition of a peripheral motor nerve is reflected in the activity of its motor unit (Bralliar, 1981). The needle electrodes should be skillfully placed within the muscle fibers to be studied with the needle bevel in contact with only a few motor units. In this way, the needle electrodes pick up only localized activity, in contrast to the mass action (compound action potential) recorded by the surface electrode used in testing for NCV (Rainbault, 1981).

Except for the current of injury, produced by the insertion of the recording needle, a normal muscle shows no activity while at rest. Voluntary contraction breaks this electrical silence with volleys of action potentials representing the activity of the single motor unit being measured. Weak contraction evokes action potentials 8 to 12 msec in duration and anywhere from 200 to 800 mV in amplitude. Moderate contraction produces more action potentials, and strong voluntary contraction produces action potentials that completely obliterate the baseline. The latter is known as a "full interference pattern" (Bradley, 1974; Rainbault, 1981).

After nerve injury, there is an absence or a decrease in motor unit action potentials with attempted voluntary contraction. The denervated muscle begins to show abnormalities and spontaneous activity, depending on the length of time it takes for wallerian degeneration of its nerve to reach the motor end plate. If a muscle is in close proximity to the level of nerve injury, the abnormalities may appear within five days of the injury. Generally, abnormal activity evoked by the current of injury upon electrode insertion appears between eight and 14 days. Spontaneous fibrillations usually are not seen until two to four weeks after injury. The more distal muscles are the last to exhibit fibrillation potentials (Howard, 1972).

Fibrillation potentials are the single most important diagnostic finding of EMG since they indicate denervation, partial or complete. Fibrillations are low amplitude (less than 200 mV), short duration (less than 2 msec) rhythmic twitches that occur between 1 and 10 times per second, and probably are due to spontaneous discharge of single presynaptic terminals of degenerating nerves. If a muscle is completely denervated, fibrillation potentials usually disappear within one year. A partially denervated muscle can exhibit fibrillations indefinitely. Positive sharp waves are also occasionally noted on an EMG of denervated muscle. The wave forms are thought by most investigators to represent fibrillations that approach but do not propagate beyond the needle electrode (Howard, 1972; Bradley, 1974; Bralliar, 1981). The presence of fibrillation potentials confirms that the muscle is still living and theoretically capable of reinnervation (Rainbault, 1981).

Reinnervation of skeletal muscle also shows characteristic EMG changes, and can be assessed by the relative disappearance of fibrillation potentials and the simultaneous appearance of polyphasic potentials. Polyphasic potentials, thought to be a sign of muscle fiber asynchrony, are characteristically of small amplitude (100 to 500 mV) and are less than 5 msec in duration. These diphasic, triphasic, or polyphasic peaks are thought to result from muscular reinnervation by terminal axonal branching with the expansion of the motor unit territory. Produced by voluntary contraction, they are likely to precede any clinical evidence of motor return. Maximal voluntary contraction in a partially innervated (or partially denervated) muscle produces an incomplete interference pattern, recognized by incomplete obliteration of the baseline. As with the advancing Tinel sign, the presence of polyphasic potentials documents reinnervation, but does not guarantee that the reinnervation will progress and produce functional reinnervation (Howard, 1972; Bradley, 1974; Bralliar, 1981; Schwartz, Iyer, and Kutz, 1980). If the polyphasic potentials gradually reduce in pattern and in length of latency over several serial examinations, this can be taken as a sign that the muscle is returning to normal innervation levels.

Somatosensory Evoked Potentials (SEP)

Electromyographic and NCV measurements are necessarily limited to the study of nerves distal to the spinal roots. In high plexus lesions there are anatomic limitations to stimulation and recording at the proximal extent of the nerves. For motor nerves, the presence or absence of wallerian degeneration of the most proximal axons indicates the state of the neuron. If degeneration is present, it is likely that root avulsion from the spinal cord has occurred and probably no meaningful regeneration is possible. Injury to the preganglionic dorsal root does not alter the NCV of the sensory axons owing to the integrity of the cell bodies in the dorsal ganglion. Before the development of SEP it was virtually impossible to study the preganglionic dorsal roots.

In 1947 Dawson observed that distal stimulation (just above motor threshold) evoked orthodromic potentials that could be recorded by skin surface electrodes beyond the level of the nerve roots and cervical spine and up to the somatosensory cortex. The technique requires somewhat sophisticated signal averaging to record the amplitudes. Cortical responses can now be compared with analogous responses from the uninvolved arm. Determination of the degree of signal attenuation can be made, and this is directly proportional to the extent of pre- and postganglionic injury. The presence of SEP testifies to the integrity of at least part of the preganglionic sensory tract (Rainbault, 1981). Evaluation of regeneration can also be made by documenting the reappearance of the SEP (Rainbault, 1981).

Clinical electroneurography, including EMG, NCV, and SEP, offers important adjunctive information to the microsurgeon provided that the tests are carried out by experienced individuals. The most valuable information that can be obtained is reviewed as follows (Lister, 1981).

1. First degree injuries (neurapraxia) can be differentiated from second to fifth degree injuries by the presence or absence of evoked action potentials distal to the lesion, provided sufficient time has elapsed for wallerian degeneration to take place (48 to 72 hours).
2. Muscle denervation can be proved by the appearance of fibrillation potentials (two to four weeks after injury).
3. The site of nerve injury can be localized by documenting focal slowing (compression syndromes) or by identifying the site at which orthodromic stimulation is lost.
4. Persistent sensory nerve action potentials (SNAP) in an anesthetic area localize the nerve lesion to a preganglionic level in the dorsal root.
5. SEP assesses the continuity of the afferent pathway to the level of the cerebral cortex.
6. Muscular reinnervation potentials (polyphasics) can be observed before clinical evidence of return of muscle function, and their disappearance with replacement by more normal action potentials parallels the return of normal innervation patterns.

Intraoperative Diagnosis and Fascicle Identification

When the microsurgeon prepares for operative reconstruction of a peripheral nerve lesion, he arms himself with all the diagnostic information available, using physical diagnosis of the level of injury and functional deficit, as well as assessment of the involved nerve or nerves with EMG, NCV, and SEP. For brachial plexus lesions, cervical myelography has documented the presence or absence of a meningocele to determine the physical status of the nerve roots. Despite all this information, unequivocal treatment options are present only in a nerve that is completely transected physically or functionally. More precise diagnostic techniques are necessary to demonstrate function at the fascicular level, and to identify major motor and sensory fascicles and facilitate appropriate coaptation. Since most nerve injuries are partial (Kline and Nulson, 1972; Kline, 1982), it is important to be able to determine which fascicles traverse the neuroma-in-continuity, in order to avoid inadvertent damage and downgrade of function.

Numerous elaborate techniques of intraoperative nerve recording and stimulation have been developed and do not differ in principle from the basic EMG, NCV, or SEP (Terzis, Dykes, and Hakstian, 1976). In all instances, intraoperative electrodiagnostic techniques involve the stimulation of a nerve or nerve fascicle and subsequent recording of a response. This can be either an orthodromic or an antidromic action potential or the appearance of a muscle twitch. In the intraoperative use of SEP, major nerves or individual fascicles can be stimulated and identified by the cortical response. Transskull motor area stimulation can also be recorded directly from the cervical root or peripheral nerve.

At exploration, the exposed neuroma-in-continuity offers little information by its gross appearance about the presence or absence of intact fascicles that pass through the lesion. Owing to the marked alterations in fascicular topography, fascicles that enter the neuroma often exit in a different position and can have a different functional make-up. It is necessary, therefore, to have an objective means to identify intact fascicles and assess the damage to others. To this end, Williams and Terzis (1976) devised a technique of recording the electrical activity of single fascicles to assess axonal integrity intraoperatively. After surgical exposure of all fascicles proximal and distal to a neuroma-in-continuity, two pairs of fine platinum electrodes are used to stimulate and record evoked responses and NCV. The amplitude and shape of the action potential wave form are measured. On the basis of these findings, individual fascicles are left alone, neurolysed, or divided and reconstructed as necessary. Intact motor fascicles often produce muscle contraction, which eases interpretation. However, when regenerating axons have not yet reached the target organ, recording techniques are needed to assess the quality of regeneration and the potential for successful reinnervation (Kline, 1982). A dilemma arises if the tested fascicle within a neuroma-in-continuity has some function. Fascicles demonstrating an NCV less than 10 to 20 m per sec or amplitudes of less than 25 to 30 per cent of normal should be considered unfavorable, and resection followed by reconstruction is indicated (Van Beek, Massac, and Smith, 1986).

Under conditions of "wake-up" anesthesia (Hall, Levine, and Sudhir, 1978), electrical fascicle stimulation can be used to map the proximal stump after nerve transection. With a patient "awake," individual fascicles can be stimulated (0.5 to 2 mA). The patient is asked to identify where the stimulus is perceived (e.g., "index" or "thumb" for lesions of the median nerve) and silent fascicles are presumed to be motor. Distal fascicles are identified by stimulation if the injury is acute and wallerian degeneration is incomplete (within 100 hours). Dissection of fascicles toward the periphery is necessary to identify the target if stimulation fails. This technique has been used successfully for nerve lesions up to the proximal forearm and distal arm (Hakstian, 1968; Gaul, 1986).

Intraoperative electrodiagnostic techniques outwardly appear too technical, or too cumbersome and time consuming, to warrant common use (Van Beek and associates, 1983). In contrast, simple electrical stimulation by commercially available disposable nerve stimulators can quickly produce useful information concerning sensory-motor differentiation by observing distal motor contraction (Terzis, 1979) or by producing orthodromic sensory stimulation that is localized by the awake patient (Gaul, 1986).

Histochemical Fascicle Identification

On the basis of the fact that motor axons are derived from cholinergic neurons, they can be differentiated from sensory axons by the presence of acetylcholine and its associated enzymes. Utilizing acetylcholinesterase activity, motor axons can be satisfactorily identified (Gruber and Zenker, 1973; Gruber and associates, 1976). Requiring 24 to 36 hours of incubation, the study technique necessitates a two-stage nerve repair that is hardly ideal. More rapid analysis is needed for chemical identification to be clinically feasible.

Carbonic anhydrase (CA) histochemistry may provide timely results that can be used at the same surgical procedure. Accomplished within three to four hours of harvesting nerve stump specimens, the CA study shows preferential staining of sensory axons (Riley and Lang, 1984; Carson and Terzis, 1985). The evaluation of chronic nerve lesions has not shown such successful results. Staining characteristics are more difficult to interpret and there is no activity apparent in the distal stumps (Carson and Terzis, 1985). Acute examination of the distal stump may be clinically applicable, as CA staining persisted for at least 24 hours in a severed distal stump and may remain up to 48 hours after transection (Riley and Lang, 1984).

A third technique with an even shorter completion time uses a radiobiochemical assay of choline acetylase activity. Produced in the cell body and transported down the axon, choline acetylase is found to be eight times higher in motor than in sensory fascicles. Each proximal stump fascicle can therefore be identified as predominantly motor or sensory on the basis of activity counts. As in all other histochemical techniques, acetylase activity is lost in the distal axon within 96 hours of transection, which limits the use of this test to within three days of the acute injury.

Although academically interesting, fascicle identification by chemical means has yet to prove its practical efficacy in the routine treatment of peripheral nerve injuries. Until unique staining characteristics can be identified that distinguish sensory from motor axons in the degenerated state, the clinical applicability remains questionable.

RECONSTRUCTION

Many factors, both biologic and surgical, influence the quality of functional return after a nerve injury. Surgeons historically have avoided manipulations of the stump of a transected nerve because it was feared that this would lead to convulsions. Moving away from this tradition, Hueter in 1873 achieved end to end coaptation of nerve stumps by placing sutures in the epineurium. This technique was to become the standard method of repair (Millesi, 1981a). Suggested in 1917 by Langley and Hashimoto, perineurial or fascicular repair achieved limited use but did not become popular (Millesi, 1981a). Little change occurred in the state of peripheral nerve surgery, and by the mid-1940's pessimism generally pervaded the attitude of the surgeons. Poor results from initial attempts at nerve grafting led surgeons to attempt repair at all costs. Extreme tension at the site of coaptation was often the result, and when the suture line did not fail, functional return was poor. Frequent wound infections in the preantibiotic era prevented successful repair by causing undue delays, by increasing necessary nerve stump debridement, or by producing infectious breakdown of the coaptations. Simple end to end coaptation was thought to be adequate and "nature" was expected to ensure functional reinnervation (Sunderland, 1981).

When antibiotics became available, an increased knowledge of intraneural topography revealed that simple end to end coaptation without attention to fascicular alignment would result in less than maximal functional return (Sunderland, 1981).

Attempts to facilitate axonal regeneration by reduction of scar tissue at the coaptation led several investigators to resurrect the entubulation techniques of the years 1910 to 1920. Nerve stumps were placed without sutures into tubes constructed of various materials such as artery, vein, preserved dura, fascia, rubber, parchment, and tantalum (Weiss, 1944a,b), but none of these methods was generally adopted. Conventional suture coaptations were also wrapped with materials such as tantalum foil to reduce fibroblastic infiltration between the stumps (Spurling, 1944). A recent resurgence of these techniques has reflected new interest in chemotrophic guidance. It is proposed that reestablishment of a closed environment between the stumps may provide an optimal milieu for axonal growth cones to find their appropriate distal endoneurial pathway (Lundborg and associates, 1982; Longo and associates, 1983; Restrepo and associates, 1983; Seckel and associates, 1984; Mackinnon and associates, 1985a; Restrepo and associates, 1985; Mackinnon and associates, 1986). Clinical relevance has yet to be proved, however.

In 1964 reports first appeared describing the use of the microscope to perform epineurial repairs (Kline and Hayes, 1964; Smith, 1964). These techniques continue to be refined. Higher magnification and microsurgical techniques allow precise manipulation of the nerve without injury to the delicate structure. Optimal alignment can be obtained on the fascicular level, but attempts to achieve precise axon to axon coaptation are still frustrated. The fine microstructure of the peripheral fiber will probably always prevent this type of axonal level of repair. Greater understanding of fascicular topography in recent times has made possible improved fascicular matching and has lessened wasteful regeneration.

The surgeon is still unable to control many of the factors that influence the outcome of peripheral nerve reconstruction: the age of the patient, the type of nerve, the level and extent of injury, and the associated injuries. The surgeon, however, controls a few important variables: (1) the timing of the repair, (2) the type of repair and the skill with which it is executed, and (3) the pre-, peri-, and postoperative management of each patient. The timing of the nerve repair depends on all the factors that are not under the surgeon's control. On too many occasions the choice has already been made for the surgeon because of late referral. The type of repair that is best is still the subject of considerable debate.

As noted by Jabaley (1984), the "ideal" nerve repair would use no sutures. Alignment of fascicles would be perfect (at the axonal level) and stumps would be bonded with a noninflammatory tissue glue. No epineurium or soft tissue would be interposed between the stump ends, and perfect coaptation would preclude tension. The nerve would heal in a viable vascular bed without foreign body reaction. Although this ideal situation is not possible today, these principles should remain the goal to strive for. Pre-, peri-, and postoperative care should focus on the facilitation of nerve regeneration by maintenance of the target organs and the quality of the involved extremity. Objectives of nonsurgical care should include the relief of discomfort, the protection of anesthetic areas of skin from injury, the avoidance of deforming posture by appropriate splinting, the maintenance of mobility of tendons and joints, and the protection of the nerve reconstruction. Therapeutic modalities include massage, edema control, skin care, splinting, and regular physiotherapy (with muscle stimulation and biofeedback) (Chiu and Ishii, 1986).

Timing

Reconstruction of the peripheral nerve has spawned many controversies, not the least of which concerns the appropriate time allowed to lapse between injury and surgical repair. Logical arguments supporting two quite contradictory points of view abound in the literature. On one hand, there exists the premise that it is never too late to perform a nerve repair; on the other there is the philosophy that the sooner the repair is performed, the better will be the chance of success (Brown, 1972a). Depending on the characteristics of the lesion with which the surgeon is faced, both views can be correct. The whole basis of the controversy stems, unfortunately, from the comparison of data on functional recovery from nerve lesions that were very different.

Retrospective analysis of the results of nerve repair subsequent to combat injury (Zachary and Holmes, 1946; Woodhall, 1947; Morgan, Reisman, and Wilgis, 1983) showed generally poor results from primary repair, but experimental and clinical evidence argues favorably for primary repair provided that the injuries are clean, simple lacerations (Brown, 1972a; Van Beek, Glover, and Zook, 1975; Horn and Crumley, 1984; Peacock, 1984). Generally, the bias toward secondary suture for war wounds stems from the severity of the injuries incurred, and the experience should not be extended to apply to all nerve injuries. A meticulously executed primary nerve repair is doomed to failure if it has been performed on nonviable nerve (Buncke, 1972), and in cases of severe injury secondary repair is indicated in order to better delineate viable and nonviable tissue.

There are no absolute rules with regard to the timing of nerve repair, and decisions should be made after consideration of the nature of the injury, the condition of the patient, and the status of associated injuries. Nerve injuries can be divided into two broad categories that help to dictate timing. First, there are the suspected transections. These should be handled with primary reconstruction if all conditions permit. Second, there are the nerve lesions that are expected to be in continuity, or those injuries that are multilevel or markedly contused. For these, secondary repair is mandatory (Kline and Hackett, 1975; Daniel and Terzis, 1977b; Millesi, 1981a; Kline, 1982). By definition, primary repair is that which is done up to 48 hours after injury. Early secondary repairs are accomplished within the first three to six weeks following injury, and late secondary repairs are those performed after three months.

In the case of sharply transected nerves, Grabb (1968) and Kline and Hackett (1975) demonstrated a higher grade of motor reinnervation in primarily sutured nerves than in those repaired secondarily. Other authors (Sakellarides, 1962; Ducker, 1972; Horn and Crumley, 1984) have also supported primary repair in guillotine transections of all nerves, provided that the limits of injury can be defined. Advantages of early primary repair include the ability to identify fascicles by electrical stimulation, and the limitation of stump retraction and scar formation. If nerve exploration is delayed beyond four days, electrical stimulation of the distal motor axons will not elicit contraction because of wallerian degeneration. If the wound is contaminated or a soft tissue deficit complicates the reconstruction, or if fractures exist that require stabilization, nerve reconstruction should be delayed until a clean, stable wound can be assured. Failure of primary repair made under poor conditions probably condemns the patient to a worse functional result than if a secondary repair is performed under satisfactory conditions.

Ducker (1972) favored a short but definitive delay in nerve suture in consideration of the metabolic response of the cell body following trauma. The retrograde reaction takes three to four days to initiate, and peak metabolic response is seen at two to three weeks during the subacute phase after injury. Thus, the reparative powers of the neuron are not optimal acutely, but peak after a short period. This view was echoed by Kleinert and Griffin (1973). Horn and Crumley (1984) advocated a longer delay for complex nerve lesions, considering that three to five weeks is advisable because (1) the state of the nerve can better be defined in relation to the surrounding tissues; (2) intraneural scarring is more apparent in both the proximal and distal stumps, and this facilitates more accurate debridement; (3) the epineurium is thicker at this time, yielding a more secure repair; and (4) surgery can be planned to proceed in an unhurried elective manner. Holmes and Young (1944) reported that a two to three week delay of primary nerve suture allowed a better chance for recovery. Of the six factors that they believed affected the success of secondary suture, two improved during the initial two weeks after injury. The proximal stump was better able to send out new fibers, and the distal stump, through proliferation of Schwann cells, was better able to accept them. However, the four remaining factors lead to reduced success with the passage of time: (1) the longer the delay, the greater is the distal endoneurial tube shrinkage, which prejudices successful reentry; (2) successful reconnection with the periphery may be prejudiced by the shrinkage of the Schwann tubes; (3) prolonged delay in nerve repair may affect maturation of remaining regenerating axons so that they may never attain preinjury diameters; and (4) the longer the period of denervation, the greater is the atrophy of the end organs. Reinnervation is therefore made more difficult.

As a result of studying ultrastructural changes after peripheral nerve transection and repair, Cabaud, Rodkey, and Nemeth (1982) were impressed that fibrosis of the distal endoneurial space could preclude satisfactory regeneration, and that the critical period within which nerve regeneration should occur was four to six weeks after injury. The investigation by Guelinckx and associates (1985) indirectly supported the necessity of early reconstruction. Under optimal conditions, the functional results of nerve suture, performed by skilled surgeons, are no different between primary and early secondary repair (Önne, 1962). Both Poppen and colleagues (1979) and Millesi (1981b) reported results of nerve suture and grafting, and found no significant functional difference between nerves repaired acutely and those reconstructed within six months. In both instances, however, the results of nerve reconstruction after six months were poor. In rabbits, epineurial technique was used to repair peroneal nerves after delays of up to 12 months. Uniformly, poorer quality reinnervation (as demonstrated by fibrillation potentials) and poorer functional results (toe spread) were directly related to the length of time that elapsed before repair. Increased, irreversible degenerative muscle changes in both the end plate and muscle fibers were also related to increased periods of denervation. In this example, both functional and morphologic considerations support early reconstruction (Richter, 1982).

There are occasions, however, when a surgeon is forced to wait, or when it is prudent to do so. For instance, when a nerve injury is due to a bullet wound, the bullet is unlikely to have transected the nerve, even if there is complete loss of function. In most cases the surgeon faces a neuroma-in-continuity, and a more satisfactory recovery is achieved by secondary exploration and repair. Since no surgical reconstruction is better than an intact fascicle, time should be allowed to elapse for the resolution of first and second degree, and possibly third degree, injuries. For low velocity bullets, eight to ten weeks are probably sufficient; for high velocity bullets, 12 to 16 weeks are indicated to allow differentiation between intact and injured fascicles of the neuroma (Kline, 1982; McQuarrie, 1986). The same waiting period (eight to 16 weeks) is also allocated for nontransecting blunt injuries or stretch injuries (Buncke, 1972; Kline and Judice, 1983). Most clinical observations have been derived from anecdotal or uncontrolled studies on the repair of nerve injuries, and both good and poor results are claimed after both primary and secondary repairs. Reconciliation of these conflicting results is not easy and the surgeon need only realize that a certain degree of effective regeneration can follow either course (Peacock, 1984). The great advantage of primary repair is the saving of time (Millesi, 1981a). The great disadvantage is the inability to detect the precise extent of neural injury. If repair is performed under these circumstances (undetected injury) and some function returns with time, the surgeon is then faced with the decision whether to reoperate in hopes of a greater return or whether to wait for improvement that is likely not to occur.

Delay and secondary repair can be advantageous because surgery can be electively planned, the operating team is likely to be unfatigued, and proper facilities can be made available. Time is a factor that should not be taken lightly. As the surgeon waits, irreversible degenerative changes proceed. Considering all options, a primary repair should be done if the damage to all neural elements can be identified, if contamination and associated trauma are minimal, and if a well-trained surgical team is available. If these optimal conditions are not met, secondary repair should be performed with a pneumatic tourniquet. The tourniquet should be inflated after exsanguination of the extremity and should be maintained throughout the exploration of the nerve lesion, preparation of the nerve ends, interfascicular dissection, and fascicular identification. A bloodless field is not necessary for the actual nerve repair or reconstruction. It is necessary that the tourniquet be deflated and sufficient time allowed to elapse before intraoperative stimulation is performed. In most instances, the entire preliminary nerve dissection can be accomplished within the two hour time limit imposed for tourniquet ischemia. For simple nerve repairs, the procedure can usually be completed within that time. For complicated cases and those that require grafting, the preliminary dissections can be completed and the tourniquet released. While one team of surgeons achieves hemostasis, a second team can use the opportunity to harvest nerve grafts. A second tourniquet inflation is then possible, if needed, to place the grafts or complete the repair. In any event, it is absolutely necessary that meticulous hemostasis be obtained before the wound is closed.

At the outset of nerve exploration, wide exposure, proximal and distal, is essential. No attempt is made to manipulate the injured nerve, and dissections are carried out from uninjured to injured areas. Tissues are retracted away from the nerve, and in this way complete exposure is obtained with the nerve and mesoneurium intact. Rotational displacement, causative agents, or scarring can be appreciated at this time under high magnification and the surgeon has the opportunity to determine the exact orientation of the nerve. Upon completion of exploration of the lesion, two orienting sutures are placed proximally and distally on the normal portion of the nerve as it lies in situ. These are placed at 12 and 6 o'clock positions with the tails cut at different lengths, and are critical in avoiding rotational deformities during subsequent mobilization. During the microsurgical manipulation of the nerve, the field should be kept moist at all times with saline solution. During an especially long reconstruction it is probably appropriate to use an antibiotic-containing solution.

The dissection is always started from the normal portion of the nerve and it proceeds in the direction of the lesion. By definition, the lesion in continuity is bridged by fascicles that are functionally intact; therefore, a priority is to avoid injury to these. Dissection is begun by making a longitudinal incision proximally in the normal-appearing epineurium. Using a diamond knife or microscissors, the epineurium is dissected off in a direction toward the lesion. Normal epineurium is off-white in color, contains longitudinally oriented vessels, and is composed of several layers of loose connective tissue.

As the lesion is approached, the epineurium becomes thickened and eventually cannot be distinguished from the entrapping scar. The epineurectomy is stopped at this point and repeated on the distal stump. After the epineurium is resected, the intraneural dissection is initiated proximally if indicated. If the extent of the scar resides in the resected epineurium, as in cases of compression neuropathy, dissection is stopped. In this instance, a total external neurolysis has been performed by epineurectomy (Frykman, Adams, and Bowen, 1981) and success is apparent as the intraneural contents balloon out.

If scar is observed binding the fascicles within the inner epineurium, an internal neurolysis or interfascicular neurolysis (Brown, 1972b; Frykman, Adams, and Bowen, 1981) is performed. Fascicular groups are carefully isolated, making sure to observe and maintain the integrity of the perineurium, which is normally glistening white and devoid of blood vessels. Millesi (1975a) stated that "septa" separate the various fascicular groups, and during interfascicular dissection the inner epineurial planes can be easily opened in a longitudinal direction, which allows the fascicles to unfold from each other. As the lesion is reached, fascicles that do not contribute to the neuroma can be carefully dissected through the lesion into the distal stump. Every effort should be made to preserve the intact fascicles so that remaining function can be spared. The fascicles that contribute to the neuroma are resected and continuity is reestablished by end to end coaptation or by grafting as necessary (Kline, 1982).

In neurolysis procedures performed at proximal levels (the brachial and sacral plexus), the intraneural organization of the nerves is quite different. The amount of intraneural connective tissue is much less proximally than distally and the bands of Fontana, which are characteristic of the perineurium in normal peripheral nerve, are not so distinct (Terzis, 1979). If scar is present, intraneural dissection is difficult. Consequently, intraneural neurolysis at the plexus level carries a high risk of neural injury. When indicated, brachial plexus neurolysis results in recovery of useful function in 96 per cent of patients (Millesi, 1987b).

The treatment of the lesion-in-continuity can be facilitated if the technique of intraoperative single fascicle recording is available (Williams and Terzis, 1976; Van Beek and associates, 1983). If not, the surgeon must rely solely on magnification to preserve the integrity of intact bundles.

Of the two types of neurolysis, internal (or interfascicular) and external, the former has been shown to be efficacious. Although there are no clear guidelines in the literature for neurolysis (Frykman, Adams, and Bowen, 1981), several series demonstrated significant functional improvement when peripheral nerves were released from entrapping scar (Brown, 1972a,b; Kline and Nulson, 1972; Frykman, Adams, and Bowen, 1981; Millesi, 1987b). Dellon (1987a,b) demonstrated sensorimotor improvement in 80 per cent of 84 nerves by internal neurolysis in patients with diabetic peripheral neuropathy, an affliction previously thought to be incurable. Neurolysis, combined with the application of a Silastic envelope for ulnar nerve entrapment at the elbow, achieved clinical relief in 64 per cent, but only 45 per cent showed improved motor conduction velocities (Benoit and associates, 1987). However, the Silastic wrap appears to be superfluous to the already standard operation for ulnar entrapment (Hardy, 1987). Internal neurolysis is not without complication and it actually represents an additional intraneural insult that may produce scar after the procedure. Therefore, it is recommended that internal neurolysis be carried out only when it is thought that the preoperative intraneural fibrosis is more severe than the scarring that can be induced by the surgical procedure (Rydevik, Lundborg, and Nordborg, 1976).

Epineurial Repair

Epineurial repair (Fig. 19–20) is the conventional method of surgical coaptation of peripheral nerves and is used by most surgeons dealing with nerve injuries (Braun, 1982). Its advantage lies in the short execution time, its simplicity, and the need for only minimal magnification. The intraneural contents are undisturbed and there is no intraneural suture foreign body. The technique is applicable in primary and secondary repairs, and it is easy to perform. In contrast, the technique of epineurial repair, in spite of optimal fascicular alignment, allows considerable disorganization at the site of coaptation (Lehman and Hayes, 1967; Kutz, Shealy, and Lubbers, 1981).

A standard epineurial repair is applied to the completely transected nerve. Adequate exposure is achieved under tourniquet control as is done for the lesion-in-continuity. Dissection is always carried from the normal nerve toward the transected stump. The nerve is mobilized proximally and distally to achieve a tension-free repair. Nerves, like vessels, retract on severance. After a sharp cut of a nerve a gap of 10 to 15 mm is created, and mobilization can be achieved by gently lifting the nerve and cutting the suspending mesoneurium.

The initial difficult step is the surgical transection of the nerve. Neurotomes with nerve-holding forceps or a razor blade with a wetted tongue depressor platform are used to achieve a flush face for the cut and to maintain uniform fascicle length (Braun, 1982). Cutting nerve stumps with scissors produces more severe crush changes in nerve structures than does transection with a knife (Mayer, 1980). The nerve is sectioned at intervals of 1 mm until the fascicular pattern is identified and it is relatively free of scar.

Upon transecting a nerve or fascicle, axoplasmic outflow from the cut end "mushrooms" under positive intraperineural pressure. The amount of mushrooming is directly proportional to the time interval between section and repair. Contact between proximal and distal stumps arrests additional mushrooming. In excess, the mushrooming interferes with accurate coaptation; therefore, as a rule, nerves should not be cut until the last possible moment when the surgeon is prepared to perform the microcoaptation.

After the nerve ends are lying without tension opposite each other, the magnification is increased to 16 × and 10–0 nylon sutures

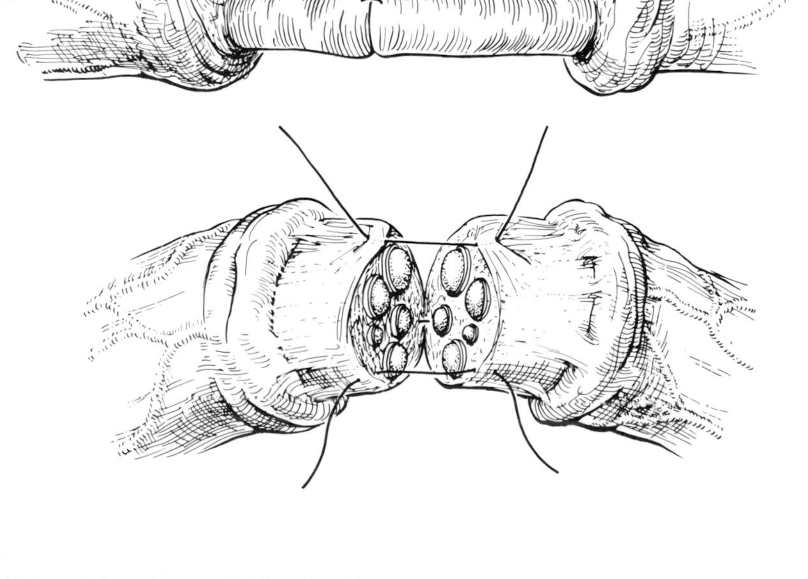

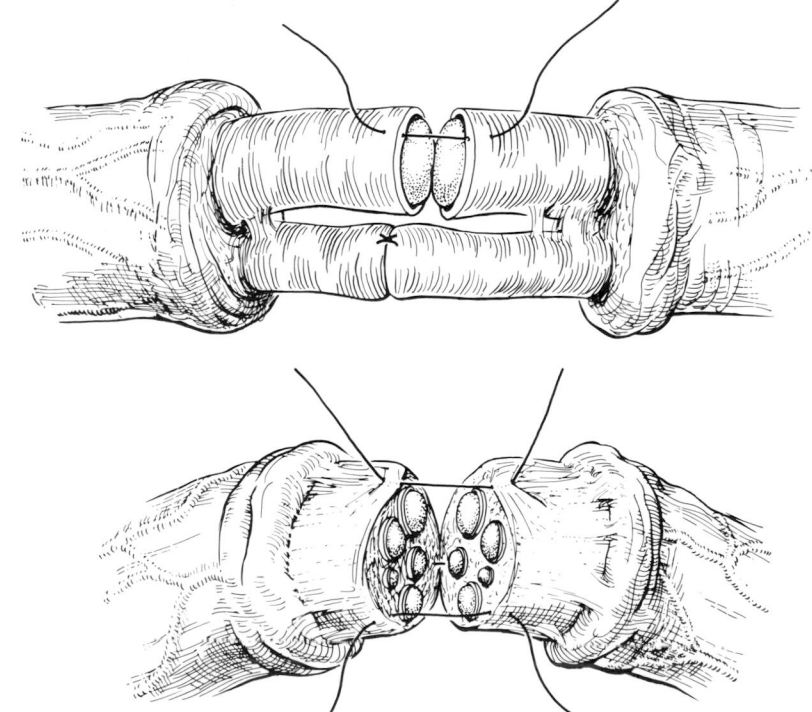

Figure 19–20. Types of nerve repair. *Upper*, perineurial (fascicular). *Lower*, epineurial.

are carefully placed in the epineurium. Before placement of the first suture, fascicular bundles are matched by necessary reorientation of the stumps, and all surface features (longitudinal vessels, position of the mesoneurium) are used to achieve exact coaptation. The suture tails are left long initially to facilitate rotation of the nerve for posterior wall coaptation. A minimal number of sutures is used to complete the microcoaptation, depending on the size of the nerve. Usually eight to ten sutures are necessary for a distal median nerve, six to eight for the ulnar, and two for a cleanly severed digital nerve. Buckling of the nerve ends caused by inappropriately large suture "bites" should be avoided since this leads to wasteful regeneration and neuroma formation.

If the gap is so large that the first 10–0 nylon suture cannot hold the stumps in apposition, one or two guide sutures no larger than 8–0 nylon can be used. These may be left or replaced with 10–0 nylon at the completion of the procedure. If 8–0 nylon suture is inadequate to maintain coaptation, the tension is considered excessive, and grafting (or transposition, in the case of the ulnar nerve at the elbow) should be performed. If a nerve gap exceeds 2.5 cm after mobilization, nerve grafting is indicated (Terzis, Faibisoff, and Williams, 1975).

The greatest pitfall of the accurately performed epineurial repair is lack of accurate coaptation of the corresponding fascicles (Kutz, Shealy, and Lubbers, 1981). Even slight tension can create a significant gap between the fascicle ends. Several investigators have documented that gapping, overriding, buckling, and straddling of the fascicles occur and are the leading causes of failure (Edsage, 1964; Bora, Pleasure, and Didizian, 1976; Matthews, 1977). Even though numerous reports in the literature have shown no differences of regeneration and functional recovery whether epineurial or perineurial (or fascicular) sutures are used (Cabaud and associates, 1976; Cabaud, Rodkey, and McCarroll, 1980; Kline, Hudson, and Bratton, 1981; Orgel, 1987), epineurial suture remains the standard by which all other methods are judged.

Perineurial (Fascicular) Repair

Perineurial or fascicular repair (Fig. 19–20) implies the surgical manipulation of corresponding fascicles in the proximal and distal stumps to achieve optimal alignment. Perhaps the greatest difficulty in this technique is deciding which fascicles in the proximal stump should coapt with which fascicles in the distal stump. Knowledge of fascicular topography facilitates the selection, and the farther distal the injury is incurred, the easier is the choice owing to progressively increasing fascicular homogeneity in the more distal portion of a peripheral nerve (Daniel and Terzis, 1977c). Techniques of intraoperative electrodiagnosis and histochemical identification, as previously reviewed, can aid this determination.

Surgical exposure is obtained as described before. The epineurium is stripped away to expose the underlying fascicles embedded in the inner epineurium. Careful maps are drawn of the proximal and distal stumps, and fascicles are matched. Under high magnification, sutures are placed into the inner epineurium, which is adherent to the perineurium, and microcoaptation is performed. Care is taken to avoid placing a suture within the endoneurium and to avoid a rotational deformity. Usually only two sutures are required to complete each coaptation. Any number of fascicles can be coapted in this manner, but each carries the potential of further intraneural foreign suture material and subsequent fibrosis.

Group fascicle coaptation expedites this technique. In lieu of dissecting out each fascicle and performing individual perineurial repairs, groups of fascicles are coapted. The most frequent indication for perineurial repair is the reconstruction of partially severed nerves. The greatest disadvantage lies in the promotion of intraneural fibrosis by increased dissection and foreign material. In addition, the technique is far more tedious and time consuming (Kutz, Shealy, and Lubbers, 1981; Urbaniak, 1982; Orgel, 1987).

Effect of Tension

When presented with a nerve defect that precludes end to end stump coaptation without tension, the surgeon faces a dilemma. Should the nerve defect be bridged by extensive mobilization of the nerve with as much stretch as necessary and repaired under tension, or should the defect be bridged with a nerve graft, forcing the axons to cross two coaptations (Fig. 19–21)?

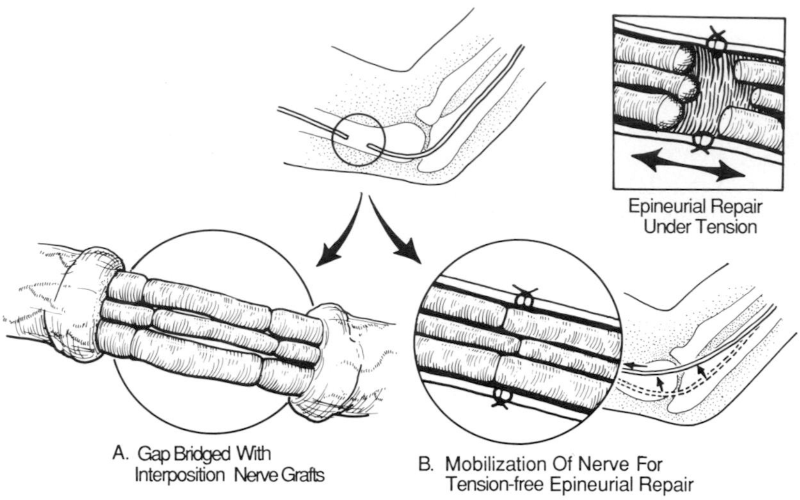

Figure 19–21. The role of tension in nerve repair. This factor can be overcome by nerve grafting or by mobilization of the injured nerve.

Tension at the site of coaptation invites connective tissue proliferation with subsequent scar formation. As scar tissue matures, it has the tendency to constrict, thereby compressing any regenerating axons (Daniel and Terzis, 1977c). If the joints are flexed to permit reduction of the nerve defect, a second traction lesion is produced as the joints are later mobilized. Even if regenerating axons manage to cross the suture line, they fail to achieve functional reinnervation in all cases (Highet and Holmes, 1943; Highet and Sanders, 1943). These studies showed that postoperative stretching of a sutured nerve does not result in its permanent elongation; instead, repetitive traction stresses are inflicted on the repaired nerve.

Millesi (1975b) studied the effects of tension on 252 nerve repairs in 146 animals, and observed that connective tissue proliferation and the length of the resulting scar between the two ends of the coapted nerve were directly related to the amount of tension. The major source of connective tissue outgrowth was the epineurium, and the proliferation of scar began at the suture line and displaced the sutures inward. As evidenced by the centroneural displacement of the sutures, the cross sectional area available for regeneration was diminished and scar tissue secondarily interfered with nerve regeneration. A coaptation without tension involved little risk of scar formation, as connective tissue invasion was seen only in repairs performed under tension. Experimental measurements of nerve conduction velocity (NCV) and the amplitude of evoked response showed similar findings, with severe drops in amplitude and NCV in the repairs subject to tension as compared with tension-free controls.

On the basis of these findings, placement of a nerve graft is believed to be indicated for any nerve defect exceeding 2.0 to 2.5 cm (Daniel and Terzis, 1977a; Terzis and Strauch, 1978; Millesi, 1981b; Moneim, 1982; Millesi, 1987a).

Nerve Grafting

Nerve exposure is performed in the usual fashion. If the decision to place nerve grafts (Fig. 19–21) has been made preoperatively, one surgical team can harvest the nerve graft at the same time that the second team prepares the recipient nerve. Dissection of the injured nerve always proceeds toward the lesion, proximally and distally. Under high magnification, the epineurectomy is performed and fascicular groups are dissected free. Regardless of the method by which the nerve fascicle is deemed healthy, be it by direct vision or by electrodiagnostic techniques, it is a safe principle to resect the nerve until no doubt exists about its viability and absence of injury. Fascicular groups are transected routinely at various intervals, thereby avoiding coaptations at the same level. This maneuver increases the stability of the repairs and maximizes regeneration. At the completion of the dissection, an intraoperative drawing is produced that can be compared with available topographic maps. The distal stump is prepared in the same fashion with identification by electrical stimulation or dissection (Daniel and Terzis, 1977a; Millesi, 1977, 1987a).

Grafts are chosen as indicated. The first choice is the sural nerve and the second is the medial antebrachial cutaneous nerve (Millesi, 1977). Other choices for autografts include the superficial radial nerve, the lateral antebrachial cutaneous nerve, and the lateral and posterior nerves of the thigh (Chiu and Ishii, 1986; Millesi, 1987a). For short defects, such as in the digital nerve, the most distal, sensory portion of the posterior interosseous nerve is readily available and is a satisfactory size match.

The grafts are cut slightly longer than the defect with the joints of the affected extremity fully extended, thus avoiding tension. Epineurectomy is not necessary since no proliferation occurs until the graft is revascularized; by that time, fascicular alignment has occurred and regeneration is under way (Millesi, 1977). Since no tension will stress the coaptation, the graft will adhere to the fascicle by fibrin clots and one or two (10–0 to 12–0) nylon sutures. Each suture is carefully placed in the inner epineurium and outer perineurium of the fascicle and the epineurium of the nerve graft (Daniel and Terzis, 1977c). Polarity of the graft is not important (Stromberg, Vlastou, and Earle, 1979; Millesi, 1987a).

Consistently satisfactory results achieved by the technique of interposition grafting have been shown repeatedly and are superior to suturing under tension (Rodkey, Cabaud, and McCarroll, 1980; Millesi, 1977, 1981b; Moneim, 1982). In the median nerve, useful motor recovery was achieved in 82 per cent and protective sensibility was restored in 42 of 43 patients. Sixteen of 16 radial nerve reconstructions achieved functional motor restoration and 44 of 44 patients with ulnar lesions showed some evidence of motor restoration (Millesi, Meissl, and Berger, 1976).

For reconstruction of the distal median nerve, five or six grafts are needed. For defects of the ulnar and radial nerves, each requires four or five grafts. The length of the nerve graft is of no consequence if the bed in which it lies is adequate to provide revascularization along the entire graft length (Seddon, 1963). Nerve grafts are revascularized by direct ingrowth instead of by growth from the transected ends. Therefore, graft diameter is the most important component in survival; if it is too large, central necrosis will occur before revascularization and degeneration will result (Smith, 1986). It is especially important for grafts but also for all nerve repairs that the nerves should lie in a well-vascularized viable bed. There should be no hematoma, foreign body, or devitalized tissue to induce scar formation. Nerve grafts should be spread apart to obtain maximal revascularization and should not be placed together as a "cable" (Torlov and Epstein, 1945).

Nerve Bed

In order to maximize regenerative potential, care must be taken to return the repaired or reconstructed nerve to a healthy vascularized bed (Smith, 1966a,b). Localized devascularization compromises the results of nerve repair because of intraneurial deposition of collagen (Starkweather and associates, 1978). Conversely, improved results of nerve regeneration have been demonstrated as attention is directed to the repair of concomitant vascular injuries at the time of nerve repair (Leclercq and associates, 1985). In severe diffuse injuries the scarring is likely to be extensive, and it is frequently necessary to bring new blood supply into the area of reconstruction by flap transfer or free tissue transfer (Terzis, 1979). For example, in the devascularized bed of a postirradiation plexitis, new vascular supply can be transferred to the nerves and nerve bed by free omental transfer (Clodius, Uhlschmid, and Hess, 1987), muscle flap transposition, or free muscle transfer.

Vascularized Nerve Grafts

When extensive nerve grafting is necessary or when the recipient bed is poorly vascularized, vascularized nerve grafting is indicated. Theoretically, the vascularized graft has an assured immediate blood supply. This avoids any period of revascularization and may limit the amount of intraneural fibrosis secondary to ischemia. Second, assured vascularization may promote more rapid axonal regeneration and consequently improve overall reinnervation (Breidenbach and Terzis, 1987). The technique has advantages, especially for the reconstruction of large proximal nerves using thick grafts in scarred beds (Townsend and

Taylor, 1984). Experimental evidence supports the clinical impression that regeneration proceeds at a faster rate and with better quality in vascularized nerve grafts than in conventional nonvascularized grafts (Koshima and Harii, 1985; Restrepo and associates, 1985; Bonney and associates, 1987). Clinical experience has also proved the feasibility of the technique (Terzis and Breidenbach, 1984; Gu and associates, 1985; Breidenbach and Terzis, 1987). Advancement of Tinel's sign over vascularized nerve grafts has been seen to progress at 7 to 12 mm per day compared with the 3 to 4 mm per day rate seen in conventional grafts (Terzis, 1988).

Free vascular nerve transfer brought with it the need to reclassify the blood supply to nerves. In terms of the configuration of the dominant vascular pedicle, three vascular patterns can be described. There may be no dominant pedicle (Type I), one dominant vessel (Type II), or multiple dominant vessels (Type III). Type II nerves with one dominant vessel are most amenable to free transfers. Type III nerves may be transferred, but would require multiple microanastomoses or the sacrifice of a major vessel. For nerves in which the dominant vascular supply does not run the greater part of the nerve length, the nerve may be cut and folded in such a fashion as to construct "cables." Care taken to maintain the continuity of the epineurium ensures blood supply via the epineurial system (Terzis and Breidenbach, 1984).

Suitable nerves that may be used for vascularized nerve grafts are the superficial radial, the ulnar, the sural, the anterior tibial, the superficial peroneal, and the saphenous (Terzis and Breidenbach, 1987). The ulnar nerve may be transferred as either a pedicle graft (Louis and Eckenrode, 1986) or a free transfer. The ulnar nerve is the ideal graft for severe injuries of the brachial plexus with C8–T1 root avulsions. The minimal functional return, which follows reconstruction of the ulnar nerve, can be easily sacrificed for improved axillary, musculocutaneous, and median nerve recovery, using the ulnar nerve as a vascularized graft (Breidenbach and Terzis, 1987).

With the wide choice of vascularized nerve grafts and the available technical expertise, the indications must now be clarified. The question that needs to be answered is whether a vascularized nerve graft is superior to a nonvascularized nerve graft in a normal bed (Terzis and Breidenbach, 1987).

Postoperative Care

In order to maximize the functional recovery after nerve repair or grafting, it is imperative that the coaptations remain protected for at least seven to ten days postoperatively. This time period begins at the completion of the placement of the last suture by avoidance of unnecessary manipulation of the coaptation. Care is taken in wound closure, and even gentle washing of the skin over the repair is avoided. Plaster immobilization is maintained for seven to ten days and the skin sutures are removed at two weeks. After immobilization the patient begins intensive physiotherapy and direct or indirect muscle stimulation. The patient is seen for evaluation at one, three, six, nine, and 12 months and yearly thereafter. Electromyographic and NCV studies are performed every three months.

After the results of testing are received, the patient is extensively reexamined. Progression of a Tinel's sign is charted and sensibility studies are performed as outlined. Returning muscle bulk is measured and accurate measurements are charted. Strength is also evaluated by Jaymar and pinch meters as indicated.

If there is no evidence of nerve regeneration, usually noted by lack of progression of the Tinel's sign, the sites of nerve coaptation should be explored in a timely fashion (within six months). Although there may be a weak distal Tinel's sign, the site of punctum maximum will reveal the most distal extent of regeneration for most axons. If this is found at the site of coaptation, it can be assumed that the axon sprouts could not cross the repair. This finding could result from disruption of the coaptation, inadequate proximal or distal debridement, or the presence of a constricting scar. If nerve grafting has been performed, each coaptation is at risk for these complications and there is a remote possibility of graft necrosis.

At reexploration for the above, the site of coaptation should be approached as if it were a neuroma-in-continuity, and an internal neurolysis should be performed to assist the identification of any intact, regenerating fascicles that may be bound in scar. Complete disruption or scar interposition necessitates recoaptation or regrafting. Partial failures are treated by debridement, recoaptation, or regrafting of the involved fascicles.

One of the most difficult decisions that faces the surgeon arises when, after surgery, the patient achieves only a partial return of function. It must be determined whether the functional deficiency results from a technically correctable problem, such as partial regeneration secondary to scar and external compression, or whether the deficiency is due to uncontrolled “wasteful” regeneration. Clinical evidence of the quality of regeneration, such as the residual Tinel's sign and the level of the punctum maximum, are extremely important in this determination. As in complete failure, a punctum maximum that lies at the level of nerve coaptation suggests that there is a greater regenerative potential in the proximal stump. Reconstruction is indicated, with care taken not to downgrade function if possible. Absence of a Tinel's sign after complete proximal to distal progression suggests near-complete regeneration with “satisfaction” of the axon sprouts. This situation probably cannot be improved by exploration and is best approached by intensive rehabilitation and reeducation.

When pain accompanies a partial return of function, owing to neuroma formation at the site of coaptation, the surgeon should be more aggressive about exploration and further reconstruction. Restoration of nerve continuity by coaptation or grafting appears to be one of the best methods of treating a painful neuroma and it increases the chances of improved functional restoration (Millesi, 1986; Terzis, 1988).

REFERENCES

Abramson, D. I., Chu, L. S. W., Tuck, S. Jr., Lee, S. W., Richardson, G., and Levin, M.: Effect of tissue temperatures and blood flow on motor nerve conduction velocity. J.A.M.A., *198*:1082, 1966.

Adams, F.: The Genuine Works of Hippocrates. New York, William Wood & Company, 1849.

Adams, W. E.: The blood supply of nerves. I. Historical review. J. Anat., *76*:323, 1942.

Aguayo, A. J., Bray, G. M., Terry, L. C., and Sweezey, E.: Three-dimensional analysis of unmyelinated fiber in normal and pathologic autonomic nerves. J. Neuropathol. Exp. Neurol., *35*:136, 1976.

Aguayo, A. J., Epps, J., Charron, L., and Bray, G. M.: Multipotentiality of Schwann cells in cross-anastomosed and grafted myelinated and unmyelinated nerves: quantitative microscopy and autoradiography. Brain Res., *104*:1, 1976.

Allt, G.: Involvement of the perineurium in experimental allergic neuritis: electron microscopic observations. Acta Neuropathol., *20*:139, 1972.

Almquist, E. E., and Eeg-Olofsson, O.: Sensory-nerve conduction velocity and two-point discrimination in sutured nerves. J. Bone Joint Surg., *52A*:791, 1970.

Almquist, E. E., Smith, O. A., and Fry, L.: Nerve conduction velocity, microscopic, and electron microscopy studies comparing repaired adult and baby monkey median nerves. J. Hand Surg., *8*:406, 1983.

Andres, K. H., and von Düring, M.: Morphology of cutaneous receptors. *In* Iggo, A. (Ed.): Handbook of Sensory Physiology. Vol. II. Somatosensory System. Berlin, Springer-Verlag, 1973, pp. 3–28.

Armstrong, C. M.: Ionic pores, gates and gating currents. Q. Rev. Biophys., *7*:179, 1975.

Asbury, A. K.: The biology of Schwann cells. *In* Dyck, P. J., Thomas, P. K., and Lambert, E. W. (Eds.): Peripheral Neuropathy. Chap. 11. Toronto, W. B. Saunders Company, 1975.

Banks, P., Mayor, D., and Mraz, P.: Cytochalasin B and the intra-axonal movement of noradrenaline storage vesicles. Brain Res., *49*:417, 1973.

Barchi, R. L.: Excitation and conduction in nerve. *In* Sumner, A. J. (Ed.): The Physiology of Peripheral Nerve Disease. Philadelphia, W. B. Saunders Company, 1980.

Barker, D.: The morphology of muscle receptors. *In* Hunt, C. C. (Ed.): Handbook of Sensory Physiology. Vol. 3. Part 2. Muscle Receptors. Berlin, Springer-Verlag, 1974, pp. 1–90.

Barker, J. L., Neale, J. H., and Gainer, H.: Rapidly transported proteins in sensory, motor and sympathetic nerves of the isolated frog nervous system. Brain Res., *105*:497, 1976.

Bell, M. A., and Weddell, A. G.: A morphometric study of intrafascicular vessels of mammalian sciatic nerve. Muscle Nerve, *7*:524, 1984a.

Bell, M. A., and Weddell, A. G.: A descriptive study of the blood vessels of the sciatic nerve in the rat, man and other mammals. Brain, *107*:871, 1984b.

Bennet, G. C., and Harrold, A. J.: Prognosis and early management of birth injuries to the brachial plexus. Br. Med. J., *1*:1520, 1976.

Benoit, B. G., Preston, D. N., Atack, D. M., and Da Silva, V. F.: Neurolysis combined with the application of a Silastic envelope for ulnar nerve entrapment at the elbow. Neurosurgery, *20*:594, 1987.

Berg, D. K.: New neuronal growth factors. Annu. Rev. Neurosci., *7*:149, 1984.

Berthold, C. H.: Ultrastructure of the node-paranode region of mature feline ventral lumbar spinal-root fibres. Acta Soc. Med. Ups., (Suppl.)*9*:37, 1968a.

Berthold, C. H.: Ultrastructure of postnatally developing feline peripheral nodes of Ranvier. Acta Soc. Med. Ups., *73*:145, 1968b.

Berthold, C. H.: Morphology of normal peripheral axons. *In* Waxman, S. G. (Ed.): Physiology and Pathobiology of Axons. New York, Raven Press, 1978.

Berthold, C. H., and Skoglund, S.: Histochemical and ultrastructural demonstration of mitochondria in the paranodal region of developing feline spinal roots and nerves. Acta Soc. Med. Ups., *72*:37, 1967.

Bisby, M.: Changes in the composition of labeled protein transported by motor axons during their regeneration. J. Neurobiol., *11*:435, 1980.

Bjerre, B., Bjorklund, A., Mobley, W., and Rosengren, E.: Short and long-term effects of nerve growth factor on the sympathetic nervous system in the adult mouse. Brain Res., *94*:263, 1975.

Black, M. M., and Lasek, R. J.: Slowing of the rate of axonal regeneration during growth and maturation. Exp. Neurol., *63*:108, 1979.

Bloom, E. M., and Tompkins, R.: Selective reinnervation in skin rotation grafts in *Rana pipiens*. J. Exp. Zool., *195*:237, 1976.

Bonnel, F.: Fascicular organization of the peripheral nerves. Intl. J. Microsurg., *3*:85, 1981.

Bonnel, F.: Histologic structure of the ulnar nerve in the hand. J. Hand Surg., *10A*:264, 1985.

Bonney, G., Birch, R., Jamieson, A. M., and Eames, R. A.: Experience with vascularized nerve grafts. *In* Terzis, J. K. (Ed.): Microreconstruction of Nerve Injuries. Philadelphia, W. B. Saunders Company, 1987, pp. 403–414.

Bora, F. W., Jr., Pleasure, D. E., and Didizian, N. A.: A study of nerve regeneration and neuroma formation after nerve suture by various techniques. J. Hand Surg., *1*:138, 1976.

Bowden, R. E. M., and Gutmann, E.: Denervation and reinnervation of human voluntary muscle. Brain, *67*:273, 1944.

Boyd, I. A., and Roberts, T. D. M.: Proprioceptive discharges from stretch receptors in the knee joint of the cat. J. Physiol. (Lond.), *122*:38, 1953.

Boyes, J. H.: On the Shoulders of Giants. Notable Names in Hand Surgery. Philadelphia, J. B. Lippincott Company, 1976.

Bradley, W. G.: Disorders of Peripheral Nerves. Oxford, Blackwell Scientific Publications, 1974.

Bralliar, F.: Electromyography: its use and misuse in peripheral nerve injuries. Orthop. Clin. North Am., *12*:229, 1981.

Brattgard, S. O., Edstrom, J. E., and Hyden, H.: The chemical changes in regenerating neurons. J. Neurochem., *1*:316, 1957.

Braun, R. M.: Epineurial nerve suture. Clin. Orthop., *163*:50, 1982.

Breidenbach, W. C., and Terzis, J. K.: The blood supply of vascularized nerve grafts. J. Reconstr. Microsurg., *3*:43, 1986.

Breidenbach, W. C., and Terzis, J. K.: Vascularized nerve grafts: an experimental and clinical review. Ann. Plast. Surg., *18*:137, 1987.

Bristow, W. R.: Injuries of peripheral nerves in two world wars. Br. J. Surg., *34*:333, 1947.

Brown, B. A.: Internal neurolysis in traumatic peripheral nerve lesions in continuity. Surg. Clin. North Am., *52*:1167, 1972b.

Brown, M. C., Holland, R. L., and Hopkins, W. G.: Motor nerve sprouting. Annu. Rev. Neurosci., *4*:17, 1981.

Brown, P. W.: Factors influencing the success of the surgical repair of peripheral nerves. Surg. Clin. North Am., *52*:1137, 1972a.

Buncke, H. J.: Digital nerve repairs. Surg. Clin. North Am., *52*:1267, 1972.

Bunge, M. B.: Fine structure of nerve fibers and growth cones of isolated sympathetic neurons in culture. J. Cell Biol., *56*:713, 1973.

Bunge, M. B.: Initial endocytosis of peroxidase or ferritin by growth cones of cultured nerve cells. J. Neurocytol., *6*:407, 1977.

Bunge, M. B., Williams, A. K., and Wood, P. M.: Neuron–Schwann cell interaction in basal lamina formation. Dev. Biol., *99*:449, 1982.

Bunge, R. P., and Bunge, M. B.: Tissue culture observations relating to peripheral nerve development, regeneration, and disease. *In* Dyck, P. J., Thomas, P. K., Lambert, E. H., and Bunge, R. (Eds.): Peripheral Neuropathy. 2nd Ed. Philadelphia, W. B. Saunders, 1984, pp. 378–399.

Burgess, P. R., English, K. B., Horch, K. W., and Stensaas, L. J.: Patterning in the regeneration of type I cutaneous receptors. J. Physiol., *236*:57, 1974.

Burgess, P. R., and Horch, K. W.: Specific regeneration of cutaneous fibers in the cat. J. Neurophysiol., *36*:101, 1973.

Burgess, P. R., and Perl, E. R.: Cutaneous mechanoreceptors and nociceptors. *In* Iggo, A. (Ed.): Handbook of Sensory Physiology. Vol. 2. Somatosensory System. Berlin, Springer-Verlag, 1973, pp. 29–78.

Burgess, P. R., Petit, D., and Warren, R. M.: Receptor types in cat hairy skin supplied by myelinated fibers. J. Neurophysiol., *31*:833, 1968.

Burke, R. E.: Motor units in mammalian muscle. *In* Sumner, A. J. (Ed.): The Physiology of Peripheral Nerve Disease. Philadelphia, W. B. Saunders Company, 1980, pp. 133–194.

Burkel, W. E.: The histological fine structure of perineurium. Anat. Rec., *158*:177, 1967.

Burrows, T. M., Campbell, I. A., Howe, E. J., and Young, J. Z.: Conduction velocity and diameter of nerve fibers of cephalopods. J. Physiol., *179*:39P, 1965.

Cabaud, H. E., Rodkey, W. G., and McCarroll, H. R.: Peripheral nerve injuries: studies in higher nonhuman primates. J. Hand Surg., *5*:201, 1980.

Cabaud, H. E., Rodkey, W. G., McCarroll, H. R., Mutz, S. B., and Niebauer, J. J.: Epineurial and perineurial fascicular nerve repairs: a critical comparison. J. Hand Surg., *1*:131, 1976.

Cabaud, H. E., Rodkey, W. G., and Nemeth, T. J.: Progressive ultrastructural changes after peripheral nerve transection and repair. J. Hand Surg., *7A*:353, 1982.

Carlsen, F., and Behse, F.: Three-dimensional analysis of Schwann cells associated with unmyelinated nerve fibres in human sural nerve. J. Anat., *130*:545, 1980.

Carlsen, F., Knappeis, G. G., and Behse, F.: Schwann cell length in unmyelinated fibres of human sural nerve. J. Anat., *117*:463, 1974.

Carson, K. A., and Terzis, J. K.: Carbonic anhydrase histochemistry: A potential diagnostic method for peripheral nerve repair. Clin. Plast. Surg., *12*:227, 1985.

Cauna, N.: Nature and functions of the papillary ridges of the digital skin. Anat. Rec., *119*:449, 1954.

Cauna, N.: Nerve supply and nerve endings in Meissner's corpuscles. Am. J. Anat., *99*:315, 1956.

Cauna, N.: Morphological basis of sensation in hairy skin. Prog. Brain Res., *43*:35, 1976.

Cauna, N., and Ross, L. L.: The fine structure of Meissner's touch corpuscles of human fingers. J. Cell Biol., *8*:467, 1960.

Causay, G.: The Cell of Schwann. Edinburgh, Livingstone, 1960.

Chambers, M. R., Andres, K. H., Düring, M. von, and Iggo, A.: The structure and function of the slowly adapting type II mechanoreceptor in hairy skin. Q. J. Exp. Physiol. Cogn. Med. Sci., *57*:417, 1972.

Chauchov, C. N.: Further observations of the fine structure of Meissner's corpuscles in human digital skin and rectum. Z. Mikrosk. Anat. Forsch. Leipzig, 87:33, 1973, cited in Sinclair, D. (Ed.): Mechanisms of Cutaneous Sensation. Oxford, Oxford University Press, 1981.

Chen, H. I., Granger, H. J., and Taylor, A. E.: Interaction of capillary, interstitial and lymphatic forces in the canine hindpaw. Circ. Res., *39*:245, 1976.

Chiu, D. T. W., and Ishii, C.: Management of peripheral nerve injuries. Orthop. Clin. North Am., *17*:365, 1986.

Chiu, S. Y.: Asymmetry currents in the mammalian myelinated nerve. J. Physiol., *309*:499, 1980.

Chouchkov, C.: Cutaneous receptors. Adv. Anat. Embryol. Cell Biol., *54*:3, 1978.

Clark, D.: Jules Tinel and Tinel's sign. Clin. Plast. Surg., *10*:627, 1983.

Clarke, E., and O'Malley, C. D. (Eds.): The Human Brain and Spinal Cord. A Historical Study Illustrated by Writings from Antiquity to the Twentieth Century. Berkeley, University of California Press, 1968.

Clodius, L., Uhlschmid, G., and Hess, K.: Irradiation plexitis of the branchial plexus. *In* Terzis, J. K. (Ed.): Microreconstruction of Nerve Injuries. Philadelphia, W. B. Saunders Company, 1987, pp. 455–462.

Cohen, S.: Purification and metabolic effects of a nerve growth promoting protein from snake venom. J. Biol. Chem., *234*:1129, 1959.

Conradi, S.: On motoneuron synaptology in adult cats. Acta Physiol. Scand. (Suppl.), *332*:1, 1969.

Cooper, P. D., and Smith, R. S.: The movement of optically detectable organelles in myelinated axons of *Xenopus laevis*. J. Physiol., *242*:77, 1974.

Cooper, S.: The responses of the primary and secondary endings of muscle spindles with motor innervation during applied stretch. Q. J. Exp. Physiol., *46*:389, 1961.

Costaldo, J. E., and Ochoa, J. L.: Mechanical injury of peripheral nerves, fine structure and dysfunction. Clin. Plast. Surg., *11*:9, 1984.

Courand, J. Y., and DiGiamberardino, L.: Axonal transport of the molecular forms of acetylcholinesterase in normal and regenerating peripheral nerves. Intl. J. Microsurg., *3*:133, 1981.

Cragg, B. G., and Thomas, P. K.: The conduction velocity of regenerated peripheral nerve fibres. J. Physiol. (Lond.), *171*:164, 1964.

Cravioto, H.: The perineurium as a diffusion barrier. Ultrastructural correlates. Bull. Los Angeles Neurol. Soc., *31*:196, 1966.

Daniel, R. K., and Terzis, J. K.: Reconstructive Microsurgery. Boston, Little, Brown & Company, 1977a.

Daniel, R. K., and Terzis, J. K.: Structure and function of the peripheral nerves. *In* Daniel, R. K. and Terzis, J. K. (Eds.): Reconstructive Microsurgery. Boston, Little, Brown & Company, 1977b.

Daniel, R. K., and Terzis, J. K.: Principles, practices, and techniques of peripheral nerve surgery. *In* Daniel, R. K., and Terzis, J. K. (Eds.): Reconstructive Microsurgery. Boston, Little, Brown & Company, 1977c, pp. 387–429.

Daniel, R. K., Terzis, J. K., and Schwarz, G.: Neurovascular free flaps. A preliminary report. Plast. Reconstr. Surg., *56*:13, 1975.

Darian-Smith, I.: The sense of touch: performance and peripheral neural processes. *In* Geiger, S. R., and Darian-Smith, I. (Eds.): Sensory Processes. Handbook of Physiology. Section 1. The Nervous System. Vol. III, Part 2. Bethesda, MD, American Physiological Society, 1984.

Darian-Smith, I., and Dykes, R. W.: Peripheral neural mechanisms of thermal sensation. *In* Dubner, R., and Kawamura, Y. (Eds.): Oral-Facial Sensory and Motor Mechanisms. New York, Plenum Publishers, 1971, pp. 7–22.

Dawson, G. D.: Cerebral responses to electrical stimulation of peripheral nerves in man. J. Neurol. Neurosurg. Psychiatry, *10*:134, 1947.

Dellon, A. L.: Evaluation of Sensibility and Reeducation of Sensation in the Hand. Baltimore, Williams & Wilkins Company, 1981.

Dellon, A. L.: Improved sensorimotor function in diabetic upper and lower extremities by internal neurolysis. Presented at the American Association of Plastic Surgeons, Nashville, TN, 1987a.

Dellon, A. L.: Personal communication to Kevin L. Smith, 1987b.

Dellon, A. L., and Mackinnon, S. E.: Susceptibility of the superficial sensory branch of the radial nerve to form painful neuromas. J. Hand Surg., *9B*:42, 1984.

Dellon, A. L., and Mackinnon, S. E.: Treatment of the painful neuroma by neuroma resection and muscle implantation. Plast. Reconstr. Surg., *77*:427, 1986.

Dellon, A. L., Witebsky, F. G., and Terrill, R. E.: The denervated Meissner corpuscle: a sequential histologic study after nerve division in the rhesus monkey. Plast. Reconstr. Surg., *56*:182, 1975.

Denny-Brown, D., and Brenner, C.: The effect of percussion of nerve. J. Neurol. Neurosurg. Psychiatry, *7*:76, 1944.

Denny-Brown, D., Kirk, E. J., and Yanagisawa, N.: The tract of Lissauer in relation to sensory transmission in the dorsal horn of spinal cord in the macaque monkey. J. Comp. Neurol., *151*:175, 1973.

DiGiamberardino, L. D., Bennett, G., Koenig, H. L., and Droz, B.: Axonal migration of protein and glycoprotein to nerve endings. III. Cell fraction analysis of chicken ciliary ganglion after intracerebral injection of labeled precursors of proteins and glycoproteins. Brain Res., *60*:147, 1973.

Doi, K., Kuwata, N., Kawakami, F., Tamaru, K., and Kawai, O.: The free vascularized sural nerve graft. Microsurgery, *5*:175, 1984.

Drachman, D. B.: Trophic functions of the neuron. Ann. NY Acad. Sci., *228*:160, 1974.

Droz, B.: Axonal transport in peripheral nerves. Int. J. Microsurg., *3*:93, 1981.

Droz, B., Koenig, H., DiGiamberardino, L., Courand, J. Y., and Souyri, F.: The importance of axonal transport and endoplasmic reticulum in the function of the cholinergic synapse in normal and pathological conditions. *In* Tucek, S. (Ed.): The Cholinergic Synapse. Progress in Brain Research. Amsterdam, Elsevier, 1979.

Droz, B., Rambourg, A., and Koenig, H. L.: The smooth endoplasmic reticulum: structure and role in the renewal of axon membrane and synaptic vesicles by fast axonal transport. Brain Res., *93*:1, 1975.

Ducker, T. B.: Metabolic factors in surgery of peripheral nerves. Surg. Clin. North Am., *52*:1109, 1972.

Ducker, T. B., Kempe, L. G., and Hayes, G. J.: The metabolic background for peripheral nerve surgery. J. Neurosurg., *30*:270, 1969.

Dumas, M., Schwab, M. E., and Thoenen, H.: Retrograde axonal transport of specific macromolecules as a tool for characterizing nerve terminal membranes. J. Neurobiol., *10*:179, 1979.

Dunn, J. S.: Developing myelin in human peripheral nerve. Scott. Med. J., *15*:108, 1970.

Dykes, R. W.: Nociception. Brain Res., *99*:229, 1975.

Dykes, R. W.: Sensory receptors. *In* Daniel, R. K., and Terzis, J. K. (Eds.): Reconstructive Microsurgery. Boston, Little, Brown & Company, 1977, p. 320.

Dykes, R. W.: Central consequences of peripheral nerve injuries. Ann. Plast. Surg., *13*:412, 1984.

Dykes, R. W., and Terzis, J. K.: Reinnervation of glabrous skin in baboons: properties of cutaneous mechanoreceptors subsequent to nerve crush. J. Neurophysiol., *42*:1461, 1979.

Dykes, R. W., and Terzis, J. K.: Spinal nerve distributions in the upper limb: the organization of the dermatome and afferent myotome. Philos. Trans. R. Soc. Lond. (Biol.), *293*:509, 1981.

Eames, R. A., and Gamble, H. J.: Schwann cell relationships in normal human cutaneous nerves. J. Anat., *106*:417, 1970.

Ebendal, T., Olson, L., Seiger, A., and Hedlund, K.-O.: Nerve growth factors in the rat iris. Nature, *286*:25, 1980.

Eccles, J. C., and Sherrington, C. S.: Numbers and contraction values of individual motor units examined in some muscles of the limb. Proc. R. Soc. Lond. (Biol.), *106*:326, 1930.

Edsage, S.: Peripheral nerve suture. A technique for improved intraneural topography. Acta Chir. Scand. (Suppl.), *331*:1, 1964.

Edwards, P. M., Van der Zee, C. E., Verhaagen, J., Schotman, P., Jennekens, F. G., and Gispen, W. H.: Evidence that the neurotrophic actions of α-MSH may derive from its ability to mimic the actions of a peptide formed in degenerating nerve stumps. J. Neurol. Sci., *64*:333, 1984.

Elfvin, L. G.: The ultrastructure of the nodes of Ranvier in cat sympathetic nerve fibers. J. Ultrastruct. Res., *5*:374, 1961.

Ellisman, M. H., and Lindsey, J. D.: The axoplasmic reticulum within myelinated axons is not transported rapidly. J. Neurocytol., *12*:393, 1983.

Ely, P., and Velez, S. J.: Regeneration of specific neuromuscular connections in the crayfish. I. Pattern of connections and synaptic strength. J. Neurophysiol., *47*:656, 1982.

Erlanger, J., and Gasser, H. S.: Electrical Signs of Nervous Activity. Philadelphia, University of Pennsylvania Press, 1937.

Finean, J. B.: X-ray diffraction studies of the myelin sheath in peripheral and central nerve fibers. Exp. Cell Res. (Suppl.), *5*:18, 1958.

Flynn, J. E., and Flynn, W. F.: Median and ulnar nerve injuries: a long range study with evaluation of the Ninhydrin test, sensory and motor return. Ann. Surg., *156*:1002, 1962.

Forman, D. S., and Berenberg, R. A.: Regeneration of motor axons in the rat sciatic nerve studied by labeling with axonally transported radioactive proteins. Brain Res., *156*:213, 1978.

Forman, D. S., Padjen, A. L., and Siggins, G. R.: Axonal transport of organelles visualized by light microscopy; cinematographic and computer analysis. Brain Res., *136*:197, 1977.

Forssman, J.: Ueber die Ursachen, welche die Wachstumsrichtung der peripheren Nerven fasern bei der Regeneration bestimmen. Beitr. Pathol. Anat., *24*:55, 1898.

Fraher, J. P.: A quantitative study of anterior root fibers during early myelination. J. Anat., *112*:99, 1972.

Friede, R. L., and Samorajski, T.: Myelin formation in the sciatic nerve of the rat. A quantitative electron microscopic, histochemical and radioautographic study. J. Neuropathol. Exp. Neurol., *27*:546, 1968.

Friede, R. L., and Samorajski, T.: Axon caliber related to neurofilaments and microtubules in sciatic nerve fibers of rats and mice. Anat. Rec., *167*:379, 1970.

Frykman, G. K., Adams, J., and Bowen, W. W.: Neurolysis. Orthop. Clin. North Am., *12*:325, 1981.

Gairus, F. W., and Aitcheson, J.: A preliminary study of the multiplicity of nerve endings in the human gum. Dent. Pract., *70*:180, 1950.

Gamble, H. J.: Spinal and cranial nerve roots. *In* Landon, D. N. (Ed.): The Peripheral Nerve. London, Chapman & Hall, 1976, pp. 330–354.

Gamble, H. J., and Eames, R. A.: An electron microscope study of the connective tissues of human peripheral nerve. J. Anat., *98*:655, 1964.

Gasser, H. S.: Properties of dorsal root unmedullated fibers on two sides of the ganglion. J. Gen. Physiol., *38*:709, 1955.

Gasser, H. S., and Grundfest, H.: Axon characters in relation to the spike dimensions and conduction velocity in mammalian A. fibers. Am. J. Physiol., *127*:393, 1939.

Gaul, J. S., Jr.: Electrical fascicle identification as an adjunct to nerve repair. Hand Clin., *2*:709, 1986.

Geren, B. B.: The formation from the Schwann cell surface of myelin. Exp. Cell Res., *7*:558, 1954.

Ghabriel, M. N., and Allt, G.: The role of Schmidt-Lanterman incisures in wallerian degeneration. I. A quantitative teased fibre study. Acta Neuropathol., *48*:83, 1979a.

Ghabriel, M. N., and Allt, G.: The role of Schmidt-Lanterman incisures in wallerian degeneration. II. An electron microscopic study. Acta Neuropathol., *48*:95, 1979b.

Ghabriel, M. N., and Allt, G.: Incisures of Schmidt-Lanterman. Prog. Neurobiol., *17*:25, 1981.

Gilbert, A.: Vascularized sural nerve graft. *In* Terzis, J. K. (Ed.): Microreconstruction of Nerve Injuries. Philadelphia, W. B. Saunders Company, 1987, pp. 117–126.

Gilliatt, R. W.: Chronic nerve compression and entrapment. *In* Sumner, A. J. (Ed.): The Physiology of Peripheral Nerve Disease. Philadelphia, W. B. Saunders Company, 1980, pp. 316–339.

Glees, P., Mohiuddin, A., and Smith, A. G.: Transplantation of pacinian bodies in the brain and thigh of the cat. Acta Anat., *7*:213, 1949.

Goldman, J. E., Kim, K. S., and Schwartz, J. H.: Axonal transport of (3H) serotonin in an identified neuron of *Aplysia californica*. J. Cell Biol., *70*:304, 1976.

Goldstein, S. A., and Sturim, H. S.: Intraosseous nerve transposition for treatment of painful neuromas. J. Hand Surg., *10A*:270, 1985.

Grabb, W. C.: Median and ulnar nerve suture. An experimental study comparing primary and secondary repair in monkeys. J. Bone Joint Surg., *50A*:964, 1968.

Grafstein, B., and Forman, D. S.: Intracellular transport in neurons. Physiol. Rev., *60*:1167, 1980.

Grafstein, B., and McQuarrie, I. G.: Role of the nerve cell body in axonal regeneration. *In* Cotman, C. W. (Ed.): Neuronal Plasticity. New York, Raven Press, 1978, pp. 155–195.

Green, L. S., Donoso, J. A., Heller-Bettinger, I. E., and Samson, F. E.: Axonal transport disturbances in vincristine-induced peripheral neuropathy. Ann. Neurol., *1*:255, 1977.

Griffin, J. W., Price, D. L., Drachman, D. B., and Morris, J.: Incorporation of axonally transported glycoproteins into axolemma during nerve regeneration. J. Cell Biol., *88*:205, 1981.

Grigg, P., Finerman, G. A., and Riley, L. H.: Joint position sense after total hip replacement. J. Bone Joint Surg., *55A*:1016, 1973.

Grinnell, A. D.: Specificity of neurons and their interconnections. *In* Brookhart, J. M., Mountcastle, V. B., and

Kandel, E. R. (Eds.): Handbook of Physiology. Section I: The Nervous System, Vol. I: Cellular Biology of Neurons. Part 2. Bethesda, MD, American Physiological Society, 1977, pp. 803–853.

Gross, G. W., and Kreutzberg, G. W.: Rapid axoplasmic transport in the olfactory nerve of the pike. I. Basic transport parameters for proteins and amino acids. Brain Res., *139*:65, 1978.

Grossman, R. C., and Hattis, B. F.: Oral Mucosal Sensory Innervation and Sensory Experience, A review. *In* Bosma, J. F. (Ed.): Symposium on Oral Sensation and Perception. Springfield, IL, Charles C Thomas, 1967, pp. 5–62.

Gruber, H., Freilinger, G., Holle, H., and Mandl, H.: Identification of motor and sensory funiculi in cut nerves and their selective reunion. Br. J. Plast. Surg., *29*:70, 1976.

Gruber, H., and Zenker, W.: Actylcholinesterase: histochemical differentiation between motor and sensory nerve fibres. Brain Res., *51*:207, 1973.

Gu, Y-D, Wu, M-M, Zheng, Y-L, Li, H-R, and Xu, Y-N: Arterialized venous free sural nerve grafting. Ann. Plast. Surg., *15*:332, 1985.

Guelinckx, P. J., Boeckx, W. D., Dom, R., and Gruwez, J. A.: Nerve fiber planimetry in acute and chronic nerve lesions and in nerve lesions in continuity. Plast. Reconstr. Surg., *76*:499, 1985.

Gundersen, R. W., and Barrett, J. N.: Neuronal chemotaxis: chick dorsal-root axons turn toward high-concentration of nerve growth factor. Science, *206*:1079, 1979.

Gundersen, R. W., and Barrett, J. N.: Characterization of the turning response of dorsal root neurites towards nerve growth factor. J. Cell Biol., *87*:546, 1980.

Guth, L.: "Trophic" influences of nerve on muscle. Physiol. Rev., *48*:645, 1968.

Guth, L.: Degeneration and regeneration of taste buds. *In* Beidler, L. M. (Ed.): Handbook of Sensory Physiology. Vol. 4. Chemical Senses, Part 2. Taste. Berlin, Springer-Verlag, 1971, p. 63.

Guth, L.: Axonal regeneration and functional plasticity in the central nervous system. Exp. Neurol., *45*:606, 1974.

Gutman, E., and Gutman, L.: Factors affecting recovery of sensory function after nerve lesions. J. Neurol. Neurosurg. Psychiatry, *5*:117, 1942.

Gutman, E., and Sanders, F. K.: Recovery of fiber numbers and diameters in the regeneration of peripheral nerves. J. Physiol., *101*:489, 1943.

Gutman, E., and Young, J. Z.: The reinnervation of muscle after various periods of atrophy. J. Anat. (Lond.), *78*:15, 1944.

Gutmann, E.: Neurotrophic relations in the regeneration process. Prog. Brain Res., *13*:72, 1964.

Guyton, A. C., Prather, J. W., Scheel, K., and McGehee, J.: Interstitial fluid pressure. IV. Its effect on fluid movement through the capillary wall. Circ. Res., *19*:1022, 1966.

Hakstian, R. W.: Funicular orientation by direct stimulation: an aid to peripheral nerve repair. J. Bone Joint Surg., *50A*:1178, 1968.

Halata, Z.: The sensory innervation of the skin of the glans penis and prepuce in man (an ultrastructural study). *In* Hamann, W., and Iggo, A. (Eds.): The International Symposium on Sensory Receptor Mechanisms. Proceedings of the Sept. 11–13, 1983 Symposium, Hong Kong. Singapore, World Scientific Publ. Company, 1984.

Hall, J. E., Levine, C. R., and Sudhir, K. G.: Intraoperative awakening to monitor spinal cord function during Harrington instrumentation and spine fusion. J. Bone Joint Surg., *60A*:533, 1978.

Hall, S. M., and Williams, P. L.: Studies on the "incisures" of Schmidt and Lanterman. J. Cell Sci., *6*:767, 1970.

Hamburger, V., Brunso-Bechtold, J. K., and Yip, J. W.: Neuronal death in the spinal ganglia of the chick embryo and its reduction by nerve growth factor. J. Neurosci., *1*:60, 1981.

Hanson, M., and Edström, A.: Mitosis inhibitors and axonal transport. Int. Rev. Cytol. (Suppl.), *7*:373, 1978.

Hardy, R. W.: Invited comment on Benoit, B. G., et al: Neurolysis combined with the application of Silastic envelope for ulnar nerve entrapment at the elbow. Neurosurgery, *20*:594, 1987.

Hargens, A. R., Romine, J. S., Sipe, J. C., Evans, K. L., Mubarak, S. J., and Akeson, W. H.: Peripheral nerve conduction block by high muscle compartment pressure. J. Bone Joint Surg., *61A*:192, 1979.

Harper, G. P., Al-Saffar, A. M., Pearce, F. L., and Vernon, C. A.: The production of nerve growth factor *in vitro* by tissues of the mouse, rat, and embryonic chick. Dev. Biol., *77*:379, 1980.

Heidemann, M. K.: Neurophysiological and behavioral evidence for selective reinnervation in skin-grafted *Rana pipiens*. Proc. Natl. Acad. Sci. U.S.A., *74*:5749, 1977.

Hensel, H.: Cutaneous thermoreceptors. *In* Iggo, A. (Ed.): Handbook of Sensory Physiology. Vol. II. Somatosensory System. Berlin, Springer-Verlag, 1973, pp. 79–110.

Hensel, H., and Boman, K. A.: Afferent impulses in cutaneous sensory nerves in human subjects. J. Neurophysiol., *23*:564, 1960.

Herndon, J. H.: Neuromas. *In* Green, D. P. (Ed.): Operative Hand Surgery. New York, Churchill Livingstone, 1982, pp. 939–955.

Hess, A., and Young, J. Z.: The nodes of Ranvier. Proc. R. Soc. Lond. (Biol.), *140*:301, 1952.

Heuser, J. E., and Reese, T. E.: Evidence for the recycling of synaptic vesicle membrane during transmitter release at the frog neuromuscular junction. J. Cell Biol., *57*:315, 1973.

Highet, W. B., and Holmes, W.: Traction injuries to the lateral popliteal nerve and fraction injuries to peripheral nerves after suture. Br. J. Surg., *30*:212, 1943.

Highet, W. B., and Sanders, F. K.: The effect of stretching nerves after suture. Br. J. Surg., *30*:355, 1943.

Hodes, R., Larrabee, M. G., and German, W.: The human electromyogram in response to nerve stimulation and the conduction velocity of motor axons. Arch. Neurol. Psychiatry, *60*:340, 1948.

Holmes, W., and Young, J. Z.: Nerve regeneration after immediate and delayed suture. J. Anat., *77*:63, 1944.

Holtzman, E.: The origin and fate of secretory packages, especially synaptic vesicles. Neuroscience, *2*:327, 1977.

Holtzman, E., and Novikoff, A. B.: Lysosomes in the rat sciatic nerve following crush. J. Cell Biol., *27*:651, 1965.

Honner, R., Fragiadakis, E. G., and Lamb, D. W.: An investigation of the factors affecting the results of digital nerve division. Hand, *2*:21, 1970.

Horch, K.: Guidance of regrowing sensory axons after cutaneous nerve lesions in the rat. J. Neurophysiol., *42*:1437, 1979.

Horch, K.: The influence of mechanoreceptor structures on regenerating sensory axons after cutaneous nerve transection in the cat. Neurosci. Ltrs., *32*:281, 1982.

Horn, K. L., and Crumley, R. L.: The physiology of nerve

injury and repair. Otolaryngol. Clin. North Am., *17*:321, 1984.
Howard, F. M.: Electromyography and conduction studies in peripheral nerve injuries. Surg. Clin. North Am., *52*:1343, 1972.
Hunt, C. C.: The physiology of muscle receptors. *In* Hunt, C. C. (Ed.): Handbook of Sensory Physiology. Vol. 3. Part 2. Muscle Receptors. Berlin, Springer Verlag, 1974, pp. 191–234.
Husmark, I., and Ottoson, D.: Relation between tension and sensory response of the isolated frog muscle spindle during stretch. Acta Physiol. Scand., *79*:321, 1970.
Husmark, I., and Ottoson, D.: The contribution of mechanical factors to the early adaptation of the spindle response. J. Physiol. (Lond.), *212*:577, 1971a.
Husmark, I., and Ottoson, D.: Is the adaptation of the muscle spindle of ionic origin? Acta Physiol. Scand., *81*:138, 1971b.
Huxley, A. F., and Stämpfli, R.: Evidence for saltatory conduction in peripheral myelinated nerve fibers. J. Physiol., *108*:315, 1949.
Iggo, A.: Cutaneous heat and cold receptors with slowly conducting (c) afferent fibers. Q. J. Exp. Physiol., *44*:362, 1959.
Iggo, A.: Cutaneous thermoreceptors in primates and sub-primates. J. Physiol. (Lond.), *200*:403, 1969.
Iggo, A.: Cutaneous and subcutaneous sense organs. Br. Med. Bull., *33*:97, 1977.
Iggo, A., and Muir, A. R.: The structure and function of slowly adapting touch corpuscle in hairy skin. J. Physiol., *200*:763, 1969.
Jabaley, M. E.: Technical aspects of peripheral nerve repair. J. Hand Surg., *9B*:14, 1984.
Jabaley, M. E., Wallace, W. H., and Heckler, F. R.: Internal topography of major nerves of the forearm and hand: a current view. J. Hand Surg., *5*:1, 1980.
Jack, J. J. B.: Electrophysiological properties of peripheral nerve. *In* Landor, D. N. (Ed.): The Peripheral Nerve. London, Chapman & Hall, 1976, pp. 740–818.
Johansson, R. S.: Tactile sensibility in the human hand: receptive field characteristics of mechanoreceptive units in the glabrous skin area. J. Physiol. (Lond.), *281*:101, 1978.
Kennedy, W. R., Poppele, R. E., and Quick, D. C.: Mammalian muscle spindles. *In* Sumner, A. J. (Ed.): The Physiology of Peripheral Nerve Disease. Philadelphia, W. B. Saunders Company, 1980, pp. 74–132.
Key, A., and Retzius, G.: Studien in der Anatomie des Nervensystems und des Bindegewebes. Stockholm, Samson & Wallin, 1986.
Kirklin, J. W., Murphy, F., and Berkson, J.: Suture of peripheral nerves. Factors affecting prognosis. Surg. Gynecol. Obstet., *88*:719, 1949.
Kleinert, H. E., and Griffin, J. M.: Technique of nerve anastomosis. Orthop. Clin. North Am., *4*:907, 1973.
Kline, D. G.: Timing for exploration of nerve lesions and evaluation of the neuroma-in-continuity. Clin. Orthop., *163*:42, 1982.
Kline, D. G., and Hackett, E. R.: Reappraisal of timing for exploration of civilian peripheral nerve injuries. Surgery, *78*:54, 1975.
Kline, D. G., and Hayes, G. J.: The use of a resorbable wrapper for peripheral nerve repair. Experimental studies in chimpanzees. J. Neurosurg., *21*:737, 1964.
Kline, D. G., Hudson, A. R., and Bratton, B. R.: Experimental study of fascicular nerve repair with and without epineurial closure. J. Neurosurg., *54*:513, 1981.
Kline, D. G., and Judice, D. J.: Operative management of selective brachial plexus lesions. J. Neurosurg., *58*:631, 1983.
Kline, D. G., and Nulson, F. E.: The neuroma in continuity. Its preoperative and operative management. Surg. Clin. North Am., *52*:1189, 1972.
Knibestol, M., and Vallbo, A. B.: Single unit analysis of mechanoreceptor activity from the human glabrous skin. Acta. Physiol. Scand., *80*:178, 1970.
Korthals, J. K., and Wisniewski, H. M.: Peripheral nerve ischemia. Part I. Experimental model. J. Neurol. Sci., *24*:65, 1975.
Koshima, I., and Harii, K.: Experimental study of vascularized nerve grafts: multifactorial analyses of axonal regeneration of nerves transplanted into an acute burn wound. J. Hand Surg., *10A*:64, 1985.
Koshima, I., and Harii, K.: Experimental analysis of axoplasmic transport and its significance for axon regeneration. Jpn. J. Plast. Reconstr. Surg., *27*:156, 1984 (abstract printed in Plast. Reconstr. Surg., *77*:172, 1986).
Kristensson, K., Lycke, E., and Sjostrand, J.: Transport of herpes simplex virus in peripheral nerves. Acta Physiol. Scand. (Suppl.), *357*:13, 1970.
Kristensson, K., and Olsson, Y.: Uptake and retrograde axonal transport of protein tracers in hypoglossal neurons. Acta Neuropathol. (Berl.), *23*:43, 1973.
Kristol, C., Sandri, C., and Akert, K.: Intramembranous particles at the nodes of Ranvier of the cat spinal cord: a morphometric study. Brain Res., *142*:391, 1978.
Krystosek, A., and Seeds, N. W.: Plasminogen activator release at the neuronal growth cone. Science, *213*:1532, 1981.
Kuffler, S. W., Nicholls, J. G., and Martin, A. R.: From Neuron to Brain, A Cellular Approach to the Function of the Nervous System. 2nd Ed. Sunderland, MA, Sinauer Associates, 1984, pp. 379–405.
Kugelberg, E., Edström, L., and Abbruzzese, M.: Mapping of motor units in experimentally reinnervated rat muscle. Interpretation of histochemical and atrophic fibre patterns in neurogenic lesions. J. Neurol. Neurosurg. Psychiatry, *33*:319, 1970.
Kutz, J. E., Shealy, G., and Lubbers, L.: Interfascicular nerve repair. Orthop. Clin. North Am., *12*:277, 1981.
Landon, D. N.: Structure of normal peripheral myelinated nerve fibers. *In* Waxman, S. G., and Ritchie, J. M. (Eds.): Demyelinating Disease: Basic and Clinical Electrophysiology. New York, Raven Press, 1981.
Landon, D. N., and Hall, S.: The myelinated nerve fiber. *In* Landon, D. N. (Ed.): The Peripheral Nerve. London, Chapman & Hall, 1976.
Landon, D. N., and Langley, O. K.: The local chemical environment of nodes of Ranvier: a study of cation binding. J. Anat., *108*:419, 1971.
Landon, D. N., and Williams, P. L.: Ultrastructure of the node of Ranvier. Nature (Lond.), *199*:575, 1963.
Langley, J. N., and Hashimoto, M.: On the suture of separate nerve bundles in a nerve trunk and on internal nerve plexus. J. Physiol. (Lond.), *51*:318, 1917.
Langley, O. K.: A comparison of the binding of Alcian blue and inorganic cations to polyanions in peripheral nerves. Histochem. J., *3*:251, 1971.
Langley, O. K., and Landon, D. N.: A light and electron histochemical approach to the node of Ranvier and myelin of peripheral nerve fibers. J. Histochem. Cytochem., *15*:722, 1967.
Lasek, R. J.: Translocation of the neuronal cytoskeleton and axonal locomotion. Philos. Trans. R. Soc. Lond. (Biol.), *299*:313, 1982.

Lasek, R. J., and Hoffman, P. N.: The neuronal cytoskeleton, axonal transport, and axonal growth. *In* Goldman, R., Pollard, T., and Rosenbaum, J. (Eds.): Cell Motility. Book C: Microtubules and Related Proteins. Cold Spring Harbor, NY, Cold Spring Harbor Laboratory, 1976, pp. 1021–1051.

Leclercq, D. C., Carlier, A. J., Khuc, T., Depierreux, L., and Lejeune, G. N.: Improvement in the results in sixty-four ulnar nerve sections associated with arterial repair. J. Hand Surg., *10A*:997, 1985.

Lehman, R. A., and Hayes, G. J.: Degeneration and regeneration in peripheral nerve. Brain, *90*:285, 1967.

Leone, J., and Ochs, S.: Anoxic block and recovery of axoplasmic transport and electrical excitability of nerve. J. Neurobiol., *9*:229, 1978.

Leskell, L.: The action potential and excitatory effects of the small ventral root fibres to skeletal muscles. Acta Physiol. Scand. (Suppl.), *10*:1, 1945.

Letourneau, P. C.: Cell-to-substratum adhesion and guidance of axonal elongation. Dev. Biol., *44*:92, 1975.

Letourneau, P. C.: Chemotactic response of nerve fiber elongation to nerve growth factor. Dev. Biol., *66*:183, 1978.

Letourneau, P. C.: Immunocytochemical evidence for colocalization in neurite growth cones of actin and myosin and their relationship to cell-substratum adhesions. Dev. Biol., *85*:113, 1981.

Levi-Montalcini, R.: Developmental neurobiology and the natural history of nerve growth factor. Annu. Rev. Neurosci., *5*:341, 1982.

Lieberman, A. R.: The axon reaction: a review of the principal features of perikaryal responses to axon injury. Int. Rev. Neurobiol., *14*:49, 1971.

Lieberman, A. R.: Sensory ganglia. *In* Landon, D. H. (Ed.): The Peripheral Nerve. London, Chapman & Hall, 1976.

Lindsay, W. K., Walker, F. G., and Farmer, A. W.: Traumatic peripheral nerve injuries in children. Results of repair. Plast. Reconstr. Surg., *30*:462, 1962.

Lippold, O. C., Nicholls, J. G., and Redfearn, J. W.: Electrical and mechanical factors in the adaptation of a mammalian muscle spindle. J. Physiol., *153*:209, 1960.

Lister, G.: The Hand: Diagnosis and Indications. 2nd Ed. Edinburgh, Churchill Livingstone, 1984.

Lloyd, D. P. C.: Neuron patterns controlling transmission of ipsilateral hind limb reflexes in cat. J. Neurophysiol., *6*:293, 1943.

Lomo, T., and Rosenthal, J.: Control of ACh sensitivity by muscle activity in the rat. J. Physiol. (Lond.), *221*:493, 1972.

Lomo, T., and Westgaard, R. H.: Control of ACh sensitivity in rat muscle fibers. Cold Spring Harbor Symp. Quant. Biol., *40*:263, 1975a.

Lomo, T., and Westgaard, R. H.: Further studies on the control of ACh sensitivity by muscle activity in the rat. J. Physiol. (Lond.), *252*:603, 1975b.

Longo, F. M., Skaper, S. D., Manthorpe, M., Williams, L. R., Lundborg, G., and Varon, S.: Temporal changes of neuronotrophic activities accumulating *in vivo* within nerve regeneration chambers. Exp. Neurol., *81*:756, 1983.

Louis, D. S., and Eckenrode, J. F.: Autogenous nerve pedicle graft in the forearm. J. Hand Surg., *11A*:703, 1986.

Low, P. A.: Endoneurial fluid pressure and microenvironment of nerve. *In* Dyck, P. J., Thomas, P. K., Lambert, E. H., and Bunge, R. P. (Eds.): Peripheral Neuropathy. 2nd Ed. Philadelphia, W. B. Saunders Company, 1984, pp. 599–617.

Lowenstein, W. R.: Biological transducers. Sci. Am., *203*:98, 1960.

Lubinska, L.: Demyelination and remyelination in the proximal parts of regenerating nerve fibers. J. Comp. Neurol., *117*:275, 1961.

Lubinska, L.: Axoplasmic streaming in regenerating and in normal fibers. Prog. Brain Res., *13*:1, 1964.

Lubinska, L., and Niemierko, S.: Velocity and intensity of bidirectional migration of acetylcholinesterase in transected nerves. Brain Res., *27*:329, 1971.

Lundborg, G.: Ischemic nerve injury. Experimental studies on intraneural microvascular pathophysiology and nerve function in a limb, subjected to temporary circulatory arrest. Scand. J. Plast. Reconstr. Surg. (Suppl.), *6*:1, 1970.

Lundborg, G.: Intraneural microvascular pathophysiology as related to ischemia and nerve injury. *In* Daniel, R. K., and Terzis, J. K. (Eds.): Reconstructive Microsurgery. Boston, Little, Brown & Company, 1977, p. 334.

Lundborg, G.: The intrinsic vascularization of human peripheral nerves: structural and functional aspects. J. Hand. Surg., *4*:34, 1979.

Lundborg, G., Dahlin, L-B., Danielsen, N., Hansson, H-A., Johannesson, A., et al.: Nerve regeneration across an extended gap: a neurobiological view of nerve repair and the possible involvement of neuronotrophic factors. J. Hand Surg., *7*:580, 1982.

Lundborg, G., and Rydevik, B.: Effects of stretching the tibial nerve of the rabbit. A preliminary study of the intraneural circulation and the barrier function of the perineurium. J. Bone Joint Surg., *55B*:390, 1973.

MacDonald, D. M., and Schmitt, D.: Ultrastructure of the human mucocutaneous end organ. J. Invest. Dermatol., *72*:181, 1979.

Macintosh, S. R.: Observations on the structure and innervation of the rat snout. J. Anat., *119*:537, 1975.

Mackinnon, S. E., Dellon, A. L., Hudson, A. R., and Hunter, D. A.: Nerve regeneration through a pseudosynovial sheath in a private model. Plast. Reconstr. Surg., *75*:833, 1985a.

Mackinnon, S. E., Dellon, A. L., Hudson, A. R., and Hunter, D. A.: Alteration of neuroma formation by manipulation of its microenvironment. Plast. Reconstr. Surg., *76*:345, 1985b.

Mackinnon, S. E., Dellon, A. L., Lundborg, G., Hudson, A., and Hunter, D. A.: A study of neurotropism in a primate model. J. Hand Surg., *11A*:888, 1986.

Mackinnon, S. E., Hudson, A. R., and Hunter, D. A.: Histologic assessment of nerve regeneration in the rat. Plast. Reconstr. Surg., *75*:384, 1985.

Madden, J. W., and Peacock, E. E., Jr.: Some thoughts on repair of peripheral nerves. South. Med. J., *64*:17, 1971.

Majno, G.: The Healing Hand: Man and Wound in the Ancient World. Cambridge, MA, Harvard University Press, 1975.

Malmgren, L. T., and Olsson, Y.: Differences between the peripheral and central nervous system in permeability to sodium fluorescein. J. Comp. Neurol., *191*:103, 1980.

Martin, J. H.: Receptor physiology and submodality coding in the somatic sensory system. *In* Kandel, E. R., and Schwartz, J. H. (Eds.): Principles of Neural Science. 2nd Ed. New York, Elsevier, 1985, pp. 287–300.

Mass, D. P., Ciano, M. C., Tortosa, R., Newmeyer, W. L.,

and Kilgore, E. S., Jr.: Treatment of painful hand neuromas by their transfer into bone. Plast. Reconstr. Surg., *74*:182, 1984.

Mathews, G. J., and Osterholm, J. L.: Painful traumatic neuromas. Surg. Clin. North Am., *52*:1313, 1972.

Matson, D. D.: Early neurolysis in the treatment of injury of the peripheral nerves due to faulty injection of antibiotics. N. Engl. J. Med., *242*:973, 1950.

Matthews, P. B.: Mammalian Muscle Receptors and Their Central Actions. Baltimore, Williams & Wilkins Company, 1972.

Matthews, P. B.: Muscle afferents and kinaesthesia. Br. Med. Bull., *33*:137, 1977.

May, R. M.: The relation of nerves to degenerating and regenerating taste buds. J. Exp. Zool., *42*:371, 1925.

Mayer, V. E.: The surgical cut-surface of peripheral nerves. Int. J. Microsurg., *2*:187, 1980.

McCloskey, D. I., Cross, M. J., Honner, R., and Potter, E. K.: Sensory effects of pulling or vibrating exposed tendons in man. Brain, *106*:21, 1983.

McEwan, L. E.: Median and ulnar nerve injuries. Aust. N.Z. J. Surg., *32*:89, 1962.

McHenry, L. C., Jr. (Ed.): Garrison's History of Neurology. Springfield, IL, Charles C Thomas, 1969.

McIntyre, A. K.: Cutaneous receptors. *In* Sumner, A. J. (Ed.): The Physiology of Peripheral Nerve Disease. Philadelphia, W. B. Saunders Company, 1980, pp. 41–73.

McLaughlin, B. J.: The fine structure of neurons and synapses in the motor nuclei of the cat spinal cord. J. Comp. Neurol., *144*:429, 1972.

McQuarrie, I. G.: Peripheral nerve surgery—today and looking ahead. Clin. Plast. Surg., *13*:255, 1986.

Menesini-Chen, M. G., Chen, J. S., and Levi-Montalcini, R.: Sympathetic nerve fibers in growth in the central nervous system of neonatal rodent upon intracerebral NGF injections. Arch. Ital. Biol., *116*:53, 1978.

Merzenich, M. M., and Harrington, T.: The sense of flutter-vibration evoked by stimulation of the hairy skin of primates: comparison of human sensory capacity with responses of mechanoreceptive afferents innervating the hairy skin of monkeys. Exp. Brain Res., *9*:236, 1969.

Miller, M. R., Ralston, H. J., and Kasahara, M.: The pattern of cutaneous innervation of the human hand. Am. J. Anat., *102*:183, 1958.

Millesi, H.: Personal communication to Julia K. Terzis, 1975a.

Millesi, H.: Treatment of nerve lesions by fascicular free nerve grafts. *In* Michon, J., and Moberg, E. (Eds.): Traumatic Nerve Lesions. Edinburgh, Churchill Livingstone, 1975b.

Millesi, H.: Fascicular nerve repair and interfascicular nerve grafting. *In* Daniel, R. K., and Terzis, J. K. (Eds.): Reconstructive Microsurgery. Boston, Little, Brown & Company, 1977, pp. 430–442.

Millesi, H.: Reappraisal of nerve repair. Surg. Clin. North Am., *61*:321, 1981a.

Millesi, H.: Interfascicular nerve grafting. Orthop. Clin. North Am., *12*:287, 1981b.

Millesi, H.: Nerve grafting. Clin. Plast. Surg., *11*:105, 1984.

Millesi, H.: Complications following secondary or reconstructive nerve repair. *In* Boswick, J. A. (Ed.): Complications in Hand Surgery. Philadelphia, W. B. Saunders Company, 1986, pp. 116–122.

Millesi, H.: Nerve grafting. *In* Terzis, J. K. (Ed.): Microreconstruction of Nerve Injuries. Philadelphia, W. B. Saunders Company, 1987a, pp. 223–237.

Millesi, H.: Brachial plexus injuries: management and results. *In* Terzis, J. K. (Ed.): Microreconstruction of Nerve Injuries. Philadelphia, W. B. Saunders Company, 1987b, pp. 347–360.

Millesi, H., Meissl, G., and Berger, A.: The interfascicular nerve—grafting of the median and ulnar nerves. J. Bone Joint Surg., *54A*:727, 1972.

Millesi, H., Meissl, G., and Berger, A.: Further experience with interfascicular grafting of median, ulnar, and radial nerves. J. Bone Joint Surg., *58A*:209, 1976.

Miner, N.: Integumental specification of sensory fibers in the development of cutaneous local sign. J. Comp. Neurol., *105*:161, 1956.

Mira, J. C.: The normal peripheral nerve. Int. J. Microsurg., *3*:77, 1981a.

Mira, J. C.: Degeneration and regeneration of peripheral nerves: ultrastructural and electrophysiological observations. Quantitative aspects and muscle changes during reinnervation. Int. J. Microsurg., *3*:102, 1981b.

Mira, J. C.: Effects of repeated denervation on muscle reinnervation. *In* Terzis, J. K. (Ed.): Microreconstruction of Nerve Injuries. Philadelphia, W. B. Saunders Company, 1987, pp. 69–82.

Mitchell, S. W.: Injuries of Nerves and Their Consequences. Philadelphia, J. B. Lippincott & Company, 1872 (reprinted by the American Academy of Neurology, New York, Dover Publications, 1965).

Moberg, E.: The role of cutaneous afferents in position sense, kinaesthesia and motor function of the hand. Brain, *106*:1, 1983.

Mohammed, U. H. M., Landon, D. M., and Love, S.: Ultrastructural morphometry of frog nodes of Ranvier. J. Anat., *137*:322, 1983.

Moneim, M. S.: Interfascicular nerve grafting. Clin. Orthop. *163*:65, 1982.

Morgan, R. F., Reisman, N. R., and Wilgis, E. F. S.: Anatomic localization of sympathetic nerves in the hand. J. Hand. Surg., *8*:283, 1983.

Morris, J. H., Hudson, A. R., and Weddell, G.: A study of degeneration and regeneration in the divided rat sciatic nerve based on electron microscopy. IV. Changes in fascicular microtopography, perineurium, and endoneurial fibroblasts. Z. Zellforsch. Mikrosk. Anat., *124*:165, 1972.

Mountcastle, V. B.: Sensory receptors and neural encoding: introduction to sensory processes. *In* Mountcastle, V. B. (Ed.): Medical Physiology. 14th Ed. Vol. 1. St. Louis, C. V. Mosby Company, 1980, p. 327.

Munger, B. L.: The intraepidermal innervation of the snout skin of the opossum. J. Cell Biol., *26*:79, 1965.

Murphy, R. A., Singer, R. H., Saide, J. D., Pantazis, N. J., Blanchard, M. H., et al.: Synthesis and secretion of a high molecular weight form of nerve growth factor by skeletal muscle cells in culture. Proc. Natl. Acad. Sci. U.S.A., *74*:4496, 1977.

Napolitano, L., and Scallen, T. J.: Observations on the fine structure of peripheral nerve myelin. Anat. Rec., *163*:1, 1969.

Nastuk, W. L.: Neuromuscular transmission. *In* Mountcastle, V. B. (Ed.): Medical Physiology. Vol. I. 14th Ed. St. Louis, C. V. Mosby Company, 1980, pp. 151–183.

Nichols, P. C., Dyck, P. J., and Miller, D. R.: Experimental hypertrophic neuropathy change in fascicular area and fiber spectrum after acute crush injury. Proc. Mayo Clin., *43*:297, 1968.

Nickel, V. L., Perry, J., Garrett, A., and Heppenstall, M.: The halo. A spinal skeletal traction fixation device. J. Bone Joint Surg., *50A*:1400, 1968.

Nja, A., and Purves, D.: The effects of nerve growth

factor and its antiserum on synapses in the superior cervical ganglion of the guinea-pig. J. Physiol. (Lond.), *277*:55, 1978.

Nukada, H., Pollock, M., and Allpress, S.: Experimental cold injury to peripheral nerve. Brain, *104*:779, 1981.

Ochoa, J.: The unmyelinated nerve fiber. *In* Landon, D. N. (Ed.): The Peripheral Nerve. London, Chapman & Hall, 1976, pp. 106–158.

Ochs, S.: Characteristics and a model for fast axoplasmic transport in nerve. J. Neurobiol., *2*:331, 1971.

Ochs, S.: Fast transport of materials in mammalian nerve fibers. Science, *176*:252, 1972.

Ochs, S.: Fast axoplasmic transport in the fibers of chromatolysed neurones. J. Physiol. (Lond.), *255*:249, 1976.

Ochs, S.: Axoplasmic transport in peripheral nerve and hypothalamoneurohypophyseal systems. Adv. Exp. Med. Biol., *87*:13, 1977.

Ochs, S.: Axoplasmic Transport and its Relation to Other Nerve Function. New York, John Wiley & Sons, 1982.

Ochs, S.: Basic properties of axoplasmic transport. *In* Dyck, P. J., Thomas, P. K., Lambert, E. H., and Bunge, R. (Eds.): Peripheral Neuropathy. Philadelphia, W. B. Saunders Company, 1984, pp. 453–476.

Ochs, S., and Hollingsworth, D.: Dependence of fast axoplasmic transport in nerve on oxidative metabolism. J. Neurochem., *18*:107, 1971.

Ochs, S., and Worth, R.: Batrachotoxin block of fast axoplasmic transport in mammalian nerve fibers. Science, *187*:1087, 1975.

Oester, Y. T., and Davis, L.: Recovery of sensory function. *In* Woodhall, B., and Beebe, G. W. (Eds.): Peripheral Nerve Regeneration—A Follow-up Study of 3656 World War II Injuries. Washington, U.S. Govt. Printing Office, 1956, VA Medical Monograph, Chap. 5.

Oldfors, A.: Macrophages in peripheral nerves. An ultrastructural and histochemical study on rats. Acta Neuropathol. Berl., *49*:43, 1980.

Olney, R. K., and Miller, R. G.: Conduction block in compression neuropathy: recognition and quantification. Muscle Nerve, *7*:662, 1984.

Olsson, T. P., Forsberg, I., and Kristensson, K.: Uptake and retrograde axonal transport of horseradish peroxidase in regenerating facial motor neurons of the mouse. J. Neurocytol., *7*:323, 1978.

Olsson, Y.: Topographical differences in the vascular permeability of the peripheral nervous system. Acta Neuropathol., *10*:26, 1968a.

Olsson, Y.: Mast cells in the nervous system. Int. Rev. Cytol., *24*:27, 1968b.

Olsson, Y.: Mast cells in human peripheral nerves. Acta Neurol. Scand., *47*:357, 1971.

Olsson, Y.: Vascular permeability in the peripheral nervous system. *In* Dyck, P. J., Thomas, P. K., Lambert, E. H., and Bunge, R. (Eds.): Peripheral Neuropathy. Philadelphia, W. B. Saunders Company, 1984, pp. 579–597.

Olsson, Y., and Reese, T. S.: Permeability of vasa nervorum and perineurium in mouse sciatic nerve studied by fluorescence and electron microscopy. J. Neuropathol. Exp. Neurol., *30*:105, 1971.

Omer, G. E.: Injuries to nerves of the upper extremity. J. Bone Joint Surg., *56A*:1615, 1974.

Omer, G. E.: Management techniques for the painful upper extremity. *In* Terzis, J. K. (Ed.): Microreconstruction of Nerve Injuries. Philadelphia, W. B. Saunders Company, 1987, pp. 145–159.

Önne, L.: Recovery of sensibility and sudomotor activity in the hand after nerve suture. Acta Chir. Scand. (Suppl.), *300*:1, 1962.

Orgel, M., Aguayo, A., and Williams, H. B.: Sensory nerve regeneration: an experimental study of skin grafts in the rabbit. J. Anat., *111*:121, 1972.

Orgel, M. G.: Epineurial versus perineurial repair of peripheral nerves. *In* Terzis, J. K. (Ed.): Microreconstruction of Nerve Injuries. Philadelphia, W. B. Saunders Company, 1987, pp. 97–100.

Palade, G. E., Simionescu, M., and Simionescu, N.: Structural aspects of the permeability of the microvascular endothelium. Acta Physiol. Scand. (Suppl.), *463*:11, 1979.

Palay, S. L., Sotelo, C., Peters, A., and Orkand, P. M.: The axon hillock and the initial segment. J. Cell Biol., *38*:193, 1968.

Peacock, E. E., Jr.: Repair of peripheral nerves. *In* Peacock, E. E., Jr. (Ed.): Wound Repair. 3rd Ed. Philadelphia, W. B. Saunders Company, 1984, pp. 363–394.

Peters, A., and Vaughan, J. E.: Morphology and development in the myelin sheath. *In* Davison, A., and Peters, A. (Eds.): Myelination. Springfield, IL, Charles C Thomas, 1970.

Petropoulos, P. G., and Stefanko, S.: Experimental studies of post-traumatic neuromas under various physiologic conditions. J. Surg. Res., *1*:235, 1961a.

Petropoulos, P. G., and Stefanko, S.: Experimental observations on the prevention of neuroma formation. J. Surg. Res., *1*:241, 1961b.

Pleasure, D.: Axoplasmic transport. *In* Sumner, A. J. (Ed.): The Physiology of Peripheral Nerve Disease. Philadelphia, W. B. Saunders Company, 1980, pp. 221–237.

Pockett, S., and Slack, J. R.: Source of the stimulus for nerve terminal sprouting in partially denervated muscle. Neuroscience, *7*:3173, 1982.

Politis, M. J.: Specificity in mammalian peripheral nerve regeneration at the level of the nerve trunk. Brain Res., *328*:271, 1985.

Politis, M. J., Ederle, K., and Spencer, P. S.: Do Schwann cells guide regenerating axons by chemotaxis? Trans. Am. Soc. Neurochem., *12*:247, 1981.

Poppen, N. K., McCarroll, H. R., Jr., Doyle, J. R., and Niebauer, J. J.: Recovery of sensibility after suture of digital nerves. J. Hand Surg., *4*:212, 1979.

Price, D. L.: Trophic functions of the neuron. VI. Other trophic systems. The influence of the periphery on spinal motor neurons. Ann. N.Y. Acad. Sci., *228*:355, 1974.

Publicover, N. G., and Terzis, J. K.: Physiologic assessment of nerve injuries. *In* Terzis, J. K. (Ed.): Microreconstruction of Nerve Injuries. Philadelphia, W. B. Saunders Company, 1987, pp. 83–95.

Purves, D., and Sakmann, B.: The effect of contractile activity on fibrillation and extrajunctional acetylcholine-sensitivity in rat muscle maintained in organ culture. J. Physiol. (Lond.), *237*:157, 1974.

Rainbault, J.: Contribution of clinical neurophysiology in the studies of lesions and regeneration of peripheral nerves. Int. J. Microsurg., *3*:161, 1981.

Ramon, Y., and Cajal, S.: Degeneration and Regeneration of the Nervous System. Vol. 1. London, Oxford University Press, 1928.

Ranson, S. W., Droegemueller, W. H., Davenport, H. K., and Fisher, C.: Number, size, and myelination of the sensory fibers in the cerebrospinal nerves. Res. Pull. Assoc. Res. Nerv. Ment. Dis., *15*:3, 1935.

Rawlins, F. A.: A time-sequence autoradiographic study of the in vivo incorporation of (1,2,-3H) cholesterol into peripheral nerve myelin. J. Cell Biol., *58*:42, 1973.

Reale, E., Luciano, L., and Spitznas, M.: Freeze-fracture faces of the perineurial sheath of the rabbit sciatic nerve. J. Neurocytol., *4*:261, 1975.

Reese, T. S., and Karnovsky, M. J.: Fine structural localization of a blood-brain barrier to exogenous peroxidase. J. Cell Biol., *34*:207, 1967.

Restrepo, Y., Merle, M., Michon, J., Folliguet, B., and Barrat, E.: Free vascularized nerve grafts: an experimental study in the rabbit. Microsurgery, *6*:78, 1985.

Restrepo, Y., Merle, M., Michon, J., Folliguet, B., and Petry, D.: Fascicular nerve graft using an empty perineurial tube: an experimental study in the rabbit. Microsurgery, *4*:105, 1983.

Restrepo, Y., Merle, M., Petry, D., and Michon, J.: Empty perineurial tube graft used to repair a digital nerve: a first case report. Microsurgery, *6*:73, 1985.

Ribak, C. E., Vaughn, J. E., and Saito, K.: Immunocytochemical localization of glutamic acid decarboxylase in neuronal somata following colchicine inhibition of axonal transport. Brain Res., *140*:315, 1978.

Richter, H.: Impairment of motor recovery after late nerve suture: experimental study in the rabbit. Parts I and II. Neurosurgery, *10*:70, 1982.

Ridley, A.: Silver staining of the innervation of Meissner corpuscles in peripheral neuropathy. Brain, *91*:539, 1968.

Ridley, A.: A biopsy study of the innervation of forearm skin grafted to the finger tip. Brain, *93*:547, 1970.

Riley, D. A., and Lang, D. H.: Carbonic anhydrase activity of human peripheral nerves: a possible histochemical aid to nerve repair. J. Hand Surg., *9A*:112, 1984.

Rodkey, W. G., Cabaud, H. E., and McCarroll, H. R., Jr.: Neurorrhaphy after loss of a nerve segment: comparison of epineurial suture under tension versus multiple nerve grafts. J. Hand Surg., *5*:366, 1980.

Rosenbluth, J.: Intramembranous particle distribution at the node of Ranvier and adjacent axolemma in myelinated axons of the frog brain. J. Neurocytol., *5*:731, 1976.

Rosenthal, J.: Trophic interactions of neurons. *In* Bookhart, J. M., and Mountcastle, V. B. (Eds.): Handbook of Physiology. Section 1: The Nervous System. Vol. I. Cellular Biology of Neurons, Part 2. Bethesda, MD, American Physiological Society, 1977, pp. 775–801.

Ruch, T. C.: Somatic sensation: receptors and their axons. *In* Ruch, T., and Patton, H. D. (Eds.): Physiology and Biophysics. The Brain and Neural Function. 20th Ed. Philadelphia, W. B. Saunders Company, 1979, pp. 157–200.

Rydevik, B., Lundborg, G., and Nordborg, C.: Intraneural tissue reactions induced by internal neurolysis. Scand. J. Plast. Reconstr. Surg., *10*:3, 1976.

Rydinack, M., and Berthold, C.-H.: Electron microscopic serial sections analysis of nodes of Ranvier in lumbar spinal roots of the cat. A morphometric study of nodal compartments in fibers of different sizes. J. Neurophysiol., *12*:537, 1983.

Saito, A., and Zacks, S. I.: Ultrastructure of Schwann and perineurial sheaths at the mouse neuromuscular junction. Anat. Rec., *164*:379, 1969.

Sakellarides, H.: A follow-up study of 172 peripheral nerve injuries in the upper extremity in civilians. J. Bone Joint Surg., *44A*:1, 1962.

Satinsky, D., Pepe, F. A., and Liu, C. N.: The neurilemma cell in peripheral nerve degeneration and regeneration. Exp. Neurol., *9*:441, 1964.

Schady, W., Ochoa, J. L., Torebjörk, H. E., and Chen, L. S.: Peripheral projections of fascicles in the human median nerve. Brain, *106*:745, 1983.

Schlaepfer, W. W.: Neurofilaments and the axonal cytoskeleton as determinants of stability and growth in regenerating axons. *In* Kao, C. C., Bunge, R. P., and Reiter, P. J. (Eds.): Spinal Cord Reconstruction. New York, Raven Press, 1983.

Schlaepfer, W. W., and Hasler, M. B.: Characterization of the calcium-induced disruption of neurofilaments in rat peripheral nerve. Brain Res., *168*:299, 1979.

Schmidt, R. F.: Somatovisceral sensibility. *In* Schmidt, R. F. (Ed.): Fundamentals of Sensory Physiology. New York, Springer-Verlag, 1981, pp. 81–123.

Schmitt, F. O., and Samson, F. E.: Neuronal fibrous proteins. Neurosci. Res. Program Bull., *6*:145, 1968.

Schnapp, B., and Mugnaini, E.: Membrane architecture of myelinated fibers as seen by freeze-fracture. *In* Waxman, S. G. (Ed.): Physiology and Pathology of Axons. New York, Raven Press, 1978.

Schut, L.: Nerve injuries in children. Surg. Clin. North Am., *52*:1307, 1972.

Schwartz, J. H.: Axonal transport: components, mechanisms and specificity. Annu. Rev. Neurosci., *2*:467, 1978.

Schwartz, K. S., Iyer, V., and Kutz, J. E.: Automated analysis of peripheral nerve regeneration. Clin. Plast. Surg., *13*:419, 1986.

Sebille, A.: Electrophysiology of nerve and muscle. Int. J. Microsurg., *3*:99, 1981.

Seckel, B. R., Chiu, T. H., Nyilas, E., and Sidman, R. L.: Nerve regeneration through synthetic biodegradable nerve guides: regulation by the target organ. Plast. Reconstr. Surg., *74*:173, 1984.

Seddon, H. J.: War injuries of peripheral nerves in wounds of the extremities. Br. J. Surg. (War Surgery Suppl.), *2*:325, 1948.

Seddon, H. J.: Nerve grafting. J. Bone Joint Surg., *45B*:447, 1963.

Seddon, H. J., and Holmes, W.: Ischemic damage in the peripheral stump of a divided nerve. Br. J. Surg., *32*:389, 1945.

Seddon, H. J., Medawar, P. B., and Smith, H.: Rate of regeneration of peripheral nerves in man. J. Physiol. (Lond.), *102*:191, 1943.

Selzer, M. E.: Regeneration of peripheral nerve. *In* Sumner, A. J. (Ed.): The Physiology of Peripheral Nerve Disease. Philadelphia, W. B. Saunders Company, 1980, pp. 358–431.

Shaffer, J. M., and Cleveland, F.: Delayed suture of sensory nerves of the hand. Ann. Surg., *131*:556, 1950.

Shanes, A. M.: Effects of sheath removal on bullfrog nerve. J. Cell Comp. Physiol., *41*:305, 1953.

Shanthavcerppa, T. R., and Bourne, G. H.: The "perineurial epithelium," a metabolically active, continuous, protoplasmic cell barrier surrounding peripheral nerve fasciculi. J. Anat., *96*:527, 1962.

Shanthavcerppa, T. R., and Bourne, G. H.: The perineural epithelium: nature and significance. Nature, *199*:577, 1963a.

Shanthavcerppa, T. R., and Bourne, G. H.: New observations on the structure of the pacinian corpuscle and its relation to the perineural epithelium of peripheral nerves. Am. J. Anat., *112*:97, 1963b.

Sherrington, C. S.: On the anatomical constitution of nerves of skeletal muscles; with remarks on recurrent fibres in the ventral spinal nerve root. J. Physiol. (Lond.), *17*:211, 1894.

Sherrington, C. S.: The Integrative Action of the Nervous System. New Haven, Yale University Press, 1906.

Sherrington, C. S.: Ferrier Lecture—some functional problems attaching to convergence. Proc. R. Soc. Lond. (Biol.), *105*:332, 1929 cited in Burke, R. E.: Motor units in mammalian muscle. *In* Sumner, A. J. (Ed.): The Physiology of Peripheral Nerve Disease. Philadelphia, W. B. Saunders Company, 1980, pp. 133–194.

Sigworth, F. J.: The variance of sodium current fluctuations at the node of Ranvier. J. Physiol., *307*:97, 1980.

Simpson, J. A.: Nerve injuries, general aspects. *In* Vinken, P. J., and Bruyn, G. W. (Eds.): Handbook of Clinical Neurology. Diseases of Nerves. Part I. New York, American Elsevier Publ. Company, 1970, pp. 244–264.

Sinclair, D.: Mechanisms of Cutaneous Sensation. Oxford, Oxford University Press, 1981.

Singer, M., and Bryant, S. V.: Movements in the myelin Schwann sheath of the vertebrate axon. Nature, *21*:1148, 1969.

Singer, S. J., and Nicolson, G. L.: The fluid mosaic model of the structure of cell membranes. Science, *175*:720, 1972.

Sklar, J. H., and Hunt, R. K.: The acquisition of specificity in cutaneous sensory neurons: a reconsideration of the integumental specification hypothesis. Proc. Natl. Acad. Sci. U.S.A., *70*:3684, 1973.

Skoglund, S.: Joint receptors and kinaesthesis. *In* Iggo, A. (Ed.): Handbook of Sensory Physiology. Vol. II. Somatosensory System. Berlin, Springer Verlag, 1973, pp. 111–136.

Skou, S. J.: Enzymatic basis for active transport of Na^+ and K^+ across cell membranes. Physiol. Rev., *45*:596, 1965.

Slack, J. R., Hopkins, W. G., and Pockett, S.: Evidence for a motor nerve growth factor. Muscle Nerve, *6*:243, 1983.

Slingluff, C. L., Terzis, J. K., and Edgerton, M. T.: The quantitative microanatomy of the brachial plexus in man: reconstructive relevance. *In* Terzis, J. K. (Ed.): Microreconstruction of Nerve Injuries. Philadelphia, W. B. Saunders Company, 1987, pp. 285–324.

Smith, D. S., Jarlfors, U., and Cameron, B. F.: Morphological evidence for the participation of the microtubules in axonal transport. Ann. N.Y. Acad. Sci., *253*:472, 1975.

Smith, J. W.: Microsurgery of peripheral nerves. Plast. Reconstr. Surg., *33*:317, 1964.

Smith, J. W.: Factors influencing nerve repair. I. Blood supply of peripheral nerves. Arch. Surg., *93*:335, 1966a.

Smith, J. W.: Factors influencing nerve repair. II. Collateral circulation of peripheral nerves. Arch. Surg., *93*:433, 1966b.

Smith, J. W.: Peripheral nerve surgery—retrospective and contemporary techniques. Clin. Plast. Surg., *13*:249, 1986.

Souttar, H. S.: Nerve injuries in children. Br. Med. J., *2*:349, 1945.

Spencer, P. S.: Morphology of the injured peripheral nerve. *In* Daniel, R. K., and Terzis, J. K. (Eds.): Reconstructive Microsurgery. Boston, Little Brown & Company, 1977, pp. 342–349.

Sperry, R. W.: Myotypic specificity in teleost motoneurones. J. Comp. Neurol., *93*:277, 1950.

Spurling, R. G.: Peripheral nerve surgery—technical considerations. J. Neurosurg., *1*:149, 1944.

Starkweather, R. J., Neviaser, R. J., Adams, J. P., and Parsons, D. B.: The effect of devascularization on the regeneration of lacerated peripheral nerves: an experimental study. J. Hand Surg., *3*:163, 1978.

Stockel, K., Paravicini, U., and Thoenen, H.: Specificity of the retrograde axonal transport of nerve growth factor. Brain Res., *76*:413, 1974.

Stromberg, B. V., Vlastou, C., and Earle, A. S.: Effect of nerve graft polarity on nerve regeneration and function. J. Hand Surg., *4*:444, 1979.

Sunderland, S.: The adipose tissue of peripheral nerve. Brain, *68*:118, 1945a.

Sunderland, S.: The intraneural topography of the radial, median and ulnar nerves. Brain, *68*:243, 1945b.

Sunderland, S.: Blood supply of the sciatic nerve and its popliteal divisions in man. Arch. Neurol. Psychiatry (Chicago), *54*:283, 1945c.

Sunderland, S.: Factors influencing the course of regeneration and the quality of the recovery after nerve suture. Brain, *75*:19, 1952.

Sunderland, S.: Funicular suture and funicular exclusion in the repair of severed nerves. Br. J. Surg., *40*:580, 1953.

Sunderland, S.: The connective tissues of the peripheral nerves. Brain, *88*:841, 1965.

Sunderland, S. (Ed.): Nerves and Nerve Injuries. Edinburgh, E. & S. Livingstone, 1968.

Sunderland, S.: The anatomic foundation of peripheral nerve repair techniques. Orthop. Clin. North Am., *12*:245, 1981.

Sunderland, S., and Bradley, K. C.: The cross-sectional area of peripheral nerve trunks devoted to nerve fiber. Brain, *72*:428, 1949.

Sunderland, S., and Bradley, K. C.: Denervation atrophy of the distal stump of a severed nerve. J. Comp. Neurol., *93*:401, 1950.

Sunderland, S., Lavarack, J. O., and Ray, L. J.: The selection and use of autografts for bridging gaps in injured nerves. Brain, *70*:75, 1947.

Sunderland, S., Lavarack, J. O., and Ray, L. J.: The caliber of nerve fibers in human cutaneous nerves. J. Comp. Neurol., *91*:87, 1949.

Sunderland, S., Marshall, R. D., and Swaney, W. E.: The intraneural topography of the circumflex, musculocutaneous and obturator nerves. Brain, *82*:116, 1959.

Tackmann, W., Brennwald, J., and Nigst, H.: Sensory electroneurographic parameters and clinical recovery of sensibility in sutured human nerves. J. Neurol., *229*:195, 1983.

Talbot, W. H., Darian-Smith, I., Kornhuber, H. H., and Mountcastle, V. B.: The sense of flutter-vibration: comparison of the human capacity with response patterns of mechanoreceptive afferents from the monkey hand. J. Neurophysiol., *31*:301, 1968.

Tennyson, V. M.: The fine structure of the axon and growth cone of the dorsal root neuroblast of the rabbit embryo. J. Cell Biol., *44*:62, 1970.

Terzis, J. K.: Clinical microsurgery of the peripheral nerve: the state of the art. Clin. Plast. Surg., *6*:247, 1979.

Terzis, J. K.: Patterns of cutaneous innervation and reinnervation following nerve transection. *In* Gorio, A. (Ed.): Post-traumatic Peripheral Nerve Regeneration: Experimental Basis and Clinical Implications. New York, Raven Press, 1981a.

Terzis, J. K.: Functional aspects of cutaneous reinnervation. Ph.D. Thesis, McGill University, 1981b.

Terzis, J. K.: Unpublished observations, 1988.

Terzis, J. K., and Breidenbach, W. C.: Surgical treatment

of peripheral nerve injuries in children. *In* Serafin, D., and Georgiade, N. G. (Eds.): Pediatric Plastic Surgery. St. Louis, C. V. Mosby Company, 1984, pp. 1159–1167.

Terzis, J. K., and Breidenbach, W. C.: The anatomy of free vascularized nerve grafts. *In* Terzis, J. K. (Ed.): Microreconstruction of Nerve Injuries. Philadelphia, W. B. Saunders Company, 1987, pp. 101–116.

Terzis, J. K., and Dykes, R. W.: Reinnervation of glabrous skin in baboons: properties of cutaneous mechanoreceptors subsequent to nerve transection. J. Neurophysiol., *44*:1214, 1980.

Terzis, J. K., Dykes, R. W., and Hakstian, R. W.: Electrophysiological recordings in peripheral nerve surgery: A review. J. Hand Surg., *1*:52, 1976.

Terzis, J. K., Faibisoff, B., and Williams, H. B.: A diamond knife for microsurgical repair of peripheral nerves. Plast. Reconstr. Surg., *54*:102, 1974.

Terzis, J. K., Faibisoff, B., and Williams, H. B.: The nerve gap: suture under tension versus graft. Plast. Reconstr. Surg., *56*:166, 1975.

Terzis, J. K., Liberson, W. T., and Levine, R.: Obstetric brachial plexus palsy. Hand Clin., *2*:773, 1986.

Terzis, J. K., and Strauch, B.: Microsurgery of the peripheral nerve: a physiological approach. Clin. Orthop., *133*:39, 1978.

Thoenen, H., Angeletti, P. U., Levi-Montalcini, R., and Kettler, R.: Selective induction by nerve growth factor of tyrosine hydroxylase and dopamine-β-hydroxylase in rat superior cervical ganglion by nerve growth factors. Proc. Natl. Acad. Sci. U.S.A., *68*:1598, 1971.

Thoenen, H., and Barde, Y.-A.: Physiology of nerve growth factor. Physiol. Rev., *60*:1284, 1980.

Thomas, P. K.: The connective tissue of peripheral nerve: an electron microscopic study. J. Anat., *97*:35, 1963.

Thomas, P. K.: The deposition of collagen in relation to Schwann cell basement membrane during peripheral nerve regeneration. J. Cell Biol., *23*:375, 1964.

Thomas, P. K., and Jones, D. G.: The cellular response to nerve injury. II. Regeneration of the perineurium after nerve section. J. Anat., *101*:45, 1967.

Thomas, P. K., Landon, D. N., and King, R. H. M.: Normal structure of the peripheral nerve. *In* Adams, J. H., Corcellis, J., and Duchen, L. W. (Eds.): Greenfield's Neuropathology. New York, John Wiley & Sons, 1984.

Thomas, P. K., and Ochoa, J.: Microscopic anatomy of peripheral nerve fibers. *In* Dyck, P. J., Thomas, P. K., Lambert, E. H., and Bunge, R. (Eds.): Peripheral Neuropathy. Philadelphia, W. B. Saunders Company, 1984, pp. 39–96.

Thomas, P. K., and Olsson, Y.: Microscopic anatomy and function of the connective tissue components of peripheral nerve. *In* Dyck, P. J., Thomas, P. K., Lambert, E. H., and Bunge, R. (Eds.): Peripheral Neuropathy. Philadelphia, W. B. Saunders Company, 1984, pp. 97–120.

Tinel, J.: The sign of "tingling" in lesions of the peripheral nerves. J. Presse Med., *23*:388, 1915. (Translated in Arch. Neurol., *24*:574, 1971.)

Torlov, I. M., and Epstein, V. H.: Nerve grafts. The importance of an adequate blood supply. J. Neurosurg., *2*:49, 1945.

Torvik, A., and Skjörten, F.: Electron microscopic observations on nerve cell regeneration and degeneration after axon lesions. I. Changes in the nerve cell cytoplasm. Acta Neuropathol. (Berl.), *17*:248, 1971.

Townsend, P. L. G., and Taylor, G. I.: Vascularized nerve grafts using composite arterialised neuro-venous systems. Br. J. Plast. Surg., *37*:1, 1984.

Tsukita, S., and Ishikawa, H.: The movement of membranous organelles in axons. Electron microscopic identification of anterogradely and retrogradely transported organelles. J. Cell Biol., *84*:513, 1980.

Tytell, M., Black, M. M., Garner, J. A., and Lasek, R. J.: Axonal transport: each major rate component reflects the movement of distinct macromolecular complexes. Science, *214*:179, 1981.

Ueyama, T.: The topography of root fibres within the sciatic nerve trunk of the dog. J. Anat., *127*:277, 1978.

Urbaniak, J. R.: Fascicular nerve suture. Clin. Orthop., *163*:57, 1982.

Van Beek, A., Glover, J. L., and Zook, E.: Primary versus delayed-primary neurorrhaphy in rat sciatic nerve. J. Surg. Res., *18*:335, 1975.

Van Beek, A. L., Hubble, B., Kinkead, L., Torros, S., and Suchy, H.: Clinical use of nerve stimulation and recording techniques. Plast. Reconstr. Surg., *71*:225, 1983.

Van Beek, A. L., Massac, E., Jr., and Smith, D. O.: The use of the signal averaging computer for evaluation of peripheral nerve problems. Clin. Plast. Surg., *13*:407, 1986.

Varon, S. S., and Adler, R.: Nerve growth factors and control of nerve growth. Curr. Top. Dev. Biol., *16*:207, 1980.

Varon, S. S., and Bunge, R. P.: Trophic mechanisms in the peripheral nervous system. Annu. Rev. Neurosci., *1*:327, 1978.

Waggener, J. D., Bunn, S. M., and Beggr, J.: The diffusion of ferritin within the peripheral nerve sheath: an electron microscopy study. J. Neuropathol. Exp. Neurol., *24*:430, 1965.

Waller, A.: Experiments on the section of glossopharyngeal nerves of the frog and observations of the alterations produced thereby in the structure of their primitive fibres. Philos. Trans. R. Soc. Lond. (Biol. Sci.), *140*:423, 1850.

Watson, W. E.: Observations on the nucleolar and total cell body nucleic acid of injured nerve cells. J. Physiol. (Lond.), *196*:655, 1968.

Webster, H. D.: Transient focal accumulation of axonal mitochondria during the early stage of wallerian degeneration. J. Cell Biol., *12*:361, 1962.

Webster, H. D., Martin, J. R., and O'Connell, M. F.: The relationships between interphase Schwann cells and axons before myelination: a quantitative electron microscope study. Dev. Biol., *32*:401, 1973.

Weddell, G.: Nerve endings in mammalian skin. Biol. Rev., *30*:159, 1955.

Weinberg, H. J., and Spencer, P. S.: The fate of Schwann cells isolated from axonal contact. J. Neurocytol., *7*:555, 1978.

Weiss, P.: Nerve patterns. The mechanics of nerve growth. Growth, *5*(Suppl.):163, 1941.

Weiss, P.: The technology of nerve regeneration: a review. Sutureless tubulation and related methods of nerve repair. J. Neurosurg., *1*:400, 1944a.

Weiss, P.: Sutureless reunion of severed nerves with elastic cuffs of tantalum. J. Neurosurg., *1*:219, 1944b.

Weiss, P., and Hoag, A.: Competitive reinnervation of rat muscles by their own and foreign nerves. J. Neurophysiol., *9*:413, 1946.

Weiss, P., and Taylor, A. C.: Histochemical analysis of nerve reunion in the cat after tubular splicing. Arch. Surg., *47*:419, 1943.

Weiss, P., and Taylor, A. C.: Further experimental evidence against "neurotropism" in nerve regeneration. J. Exp. Zool., *95*:233, 1944a.

Weiss, P., and Taylor, A. C.: Impairment of growth and

myelinization in regenerating nerve fibers subjected to constriction. Proc. Soc. Exp. Biol., *55*:77, 1944b.

Westgaard, R. H.: Influence of activity on the passive electrical properties of denervated soleus muscle fibres in the rat. J. Physiol. (Lond.), *251*:683, 1975.

Wilgis, E. F. S.: Nerve repair and grafting. *In* Green, D. P. (Ed.): Operative Hand Surgery. New York, Churchill Livingstone, 1982.

Williams, H. B.: The painful stump neuroma and its treatment. *In* Terzis, J. K. (Ed.): Microreconstruction of Nerve Injuries. Philadelphia, W. B. Saunders Company, 1987, pp. 161–171.

Williams, H. B., and Terzis, J. K.: Single fascicular recording: an intraoperative diagnostic tool for the management of peripheral nerve lesions. Plast. Reconstr. Surg., *57*:562, 1976.

Williams, L. R., Powell, H. C., Lundborg, G., and Varon, S.: Competence of nerve tissue as distal insert promoting nerve regeneration in a silicone chamber. Brain Res., *293*:201, 1984.

Williams, P. L., and Landon, D. N.: Paranodal apparatus of peripheral nerve fibres of mammals. Nature (Lond.), *198*:670, 1963.

Williams, P. L., and Landon, D. N.: The energy source of the nerve fiber. New Scientist, *21*:166, 1964.

Williams, P. L., and Wendell-Smith, C. P.: Some additional parametric variations between peripheral nerve fibre populations. J. Anat., *109*:505, 1971.

Wilson, D. L., and Stone, G. C.: Axoplasmic transport of proteins. Annu. Rev. Biophys. Bioeng., *8*:27, 1979.

Wilson, R. L.: Management of pain following peripheral nerve injuries. Orthop. Clin. North Am., *12*:343, 1981.

Winkleman, R. K.: Nerve Endings in Normal and Pathologic Skin. Springfield, IL, Charles C Thomas, 1960.

Wood, V. E., and Mudge, M. K.: Treatment of neuromas about a major amputation stump. J. Hand Surg., *12A*:302, 1987.

Woodhall, B.: Peripheral nerve injuries. II. Basic data from the Peripheral Nerve Registry concerning 7,050 nerve sutures and 67 nerve grafts. J. Neurosurg., *4*:146, 1947.

Wortis, H., Stein, M. H., and Jalliffe, N.: Fiber dissociation in peripheral neuropathy. Arch. Intern. Med., *69*:222, 1942.

Yahr, M. D., and Beebe, G. W.: Recovery of motor function. *In* Woodhall, B., and Beebe, G. W. (Eds.): Peripheral Nerve Regeneration. A Follow-up Study of 3656 World War II Injuries. Washington, U.S. Govt. Printing Office, 1956, VA Medical Monograph, Chap. 3.

Yamada, K. M., Spooner, B. S., and Wessells, N. K.: Ultrastructure and function of growth cones and axons of cultured nerve cells. J. Cell Biol., *49*:614, 1971.

Yates, A. J., Bouchard, J. P., and Wherrett, J. R.: Relation of axon membrane to myelin membrane in sciatic nerve during development: comparison of morphological and chemical parameters. Brain Res., *104*:261, 1976.

Young, L., Wray, R. C., and Weeks, P. M.: A randomized prospective comparison of fascicular and epineural digital nerve repairs. Plast. Reconstr. Surg., *68*:89, 1981.

Zachary, R. B., and Holmes, W.: Primary suture of nerves. Surg. Gynecol. Obstet., *82*:632, 1946.

Zelena, J.: Bidirectional movements of mitochondria along axons of an isolated nerve segment. Z. Zellforsch. Mikrosk. Anat., *92*:186, 1968.

Zenker, W., and Hohberg, E.: A-α-nerve fiber: number of neurotubules in the stem fiber and in the terminal branches. J. Neurocytol., *2*:143, 1973.

20

Ralph E. Holmes

Alloplastic Implants

In the history of man's efforts to reconstruct tissue loss and deformity, his attempts to use implant materials have probably paralleled those of autogenous tissues. Reliable clinical success in the use of implant materials did not emerge, however, until the twentieth century with the advent of biocompatible metals, followed by polymers and ceramics. During the past two decades there has been an acceleration of collaboration by materials scientists, biomaterials engineers, and clinical investigators resulting in an increased understanding of the requirements and potential of implant materials. The development of newer techniques to transfer autogenous tissues, such as myocutaneous flaps and free microvascular flaps, has not replaced the need for implant materials. For some procedures, such as increasing breast volume or chin projection, suitable autogenous tissue may be unavailable or implants may be more predictable. As the technology and understanding of alloplastic implants increase, it is likely that the spectrum of their use in plastic surgery will continue to increase.

Grafts, transplants or implants of biologic origin can be autogenous, allogenous, or xenogenous according to their source. "Transplanting" focuses on the movement of tissue from one site to another. "Implanting" refers to the recipient site placement of tissue, while "grafting" emphasizes the incorporation of tissue by recipient site healing processes. Traditionally, alloplastic materials have been called implants since they have not functioned as transplants or grafts. This thinking is likely to change as implants of synthetic origin come to play a more integral role in the reconstructive process. For example, an anterior trachea was experimentally recon-structured when a porous alloplast was *implanted* under the inferior end of the sternocleidomastoid muscle (Holmes, 1978). The implant became *grafted* to the muscle by the ingrowth of fibrovascular connective tissue. A mucosal lining was next placed against the vascularized implant opposite the muscle. At a third stage the implant was *transplanted* on a muscle pedicle to the trachea to provide structure and lining. Since all alloplastic materials must first be implanted, it should remain logical to call them implants.

Alloplastic implant materials are by definition biomaterials used to augment or replace a tissue, organ, or function of the body. Such materials must be biocompatible and must not elicit toxic, immunogenic, or carcinogenic reactions. Permanent implants must provide maintenance-free function in a physiologic environment over the patient's lifetime. Temporary implants must disintegrate gradually within a predictable time without the production of noncompatible, harmful disintegration products. Additionally there is a need for esthetic acceptability of the implant or the effect created by its implantation. These requirements reduce the material choices to a limited number that may be categorized as metals, polymers, and ceramics.

MECHANICAL TESTING

One of the most important properties of a material, whether it is used as a temporary skin cover, suture material, soft tissue substitute, or hard tissue replacement, is its ability to withstand the various mechanical forces placed upon it. These forces are *tension, compression, shear,* and *bending* (Fig. 20–1). In most clinical situations several forces are likely to act simultaneously, but for purposes of mechanical testing they are usually measured separately.

Stress-Strain Curve

Whenever one or more loads are placed on a material, it tends to deform in an amount related to the magnitude of the applied load. When the load is removed, the material tends to return to its original shape. For illustration, the pulling of a uniform cross sectional metal rod in tension along its axis will be considered (Frankel and Nordin, 1980).

When a load is applied to the rod in tension, the deformation or elongation of the rod can be measured and plotted on a load-deformation curve. From this curve the strength and stiffness of the structure can be determined. A hypothetical load-deformation curve is shown in Figure 20–2. When a load is applied within the elastic region of the curve (X-Y) and is then released, the structure returns to its original shape. If loading is continued beyond the yield point (Y) and into the nonelastic (plastic) region of the curve (Y-F) and is then released, the structure does not return to its original shape. The amount of permanent deformation of the structure that occurs if the structure is loaded to point D and then unloaded is represented by the distance between X and X′. If loading continues in the nonelastic region, the ultimate strength (U) and ultimate failure (F) points will be reached.

The load-deformation curve provides several measures of strength: (1) the ultimate strength of the structure, (2) the deformation it can sustain before failure, and (3) the

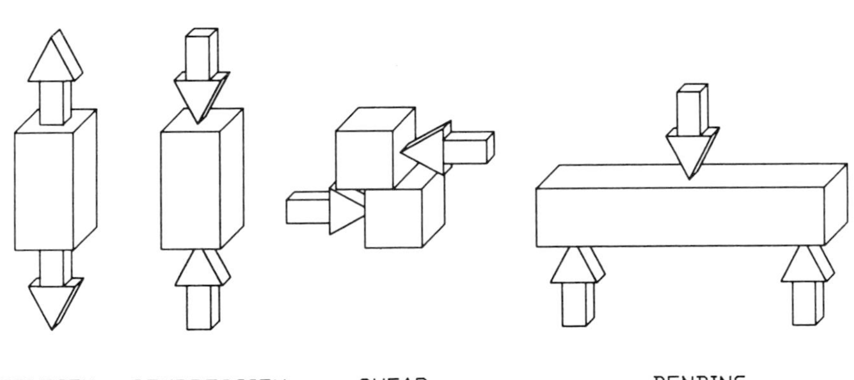

Figure 20–1. Types of force application in tests of implant mechanical properties.

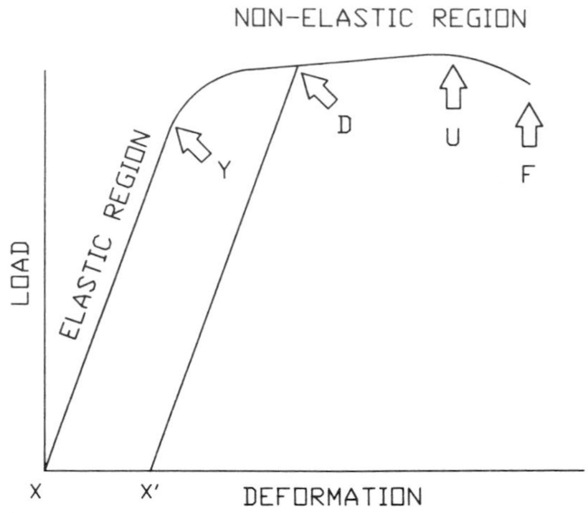

Figure 20–2. Load-deformation curve typical of ductile materials.

energy it can store before failure (area under the curve). In addition the stiffness of the structure, called the elastic modulus, is indicated by the slope of the curve in the elastic region.

To compare the mechanical properties of different materials it is necessary to express the applied force as load per unit area (stress) and the deformation as percentage lengthening or shortening (strain) of the test specimen. The stress-strain curve has an appearance similar to that of the load-deformation curve. Stress and strain values, however, are theoretically independent of the structural shape of the material and therefore reflect the material properties, rather than the structural properties, of an implant.

Materials are classified as brittle, ductile, or rubbery depending on the amount of deformation they undergo before and after failure (Van Vlack, 1975). Ceramic, a typical brittle material, deforms little before failure, as indicated by the absence of a plastic region on the stress-strain curve shown in Figure 20–3. Metals are typically ductile materials and may deform extensively before failure. A ductile material that is pieced together after fracture does not conform to its original shape, whereas a brittle material does. Polymers in some rubbery forms also undergo considerable deformation. Bone consists of a ceramic (hydroxyapatite) and a polymer (collagen) and thus exhibits intermediate properties.

The area under the stress-strain curve represents the amount of energy required to produce a failure. This quantity is called toughness. A material that can withstand high stresses and undergoes considerable plastic deformation is tougher than one that resists high stresses but has no capacity for deformation, or one that has a high capacity for deformation but can withstand only relatively low stresses.

Time Dependent Response

In the elastic region, metals and ceramics undergo all their deformation immediately upon application of a load, and the deformation remains constant as long as the load continues to be applied. However, polymers may continue to deform for some time after the application of a constant load (creep). Conversely, maintenance of a constant deformation of the polymer may require application of a decreasing load for some time (stress relaxation).

Fatigue

In some clinical situations loading of implant materials may be cyclic rather than static. Failure of an implant produced by a single load may also be produced by repeated application of a lower load. The interplay of load and repetition for all materials can be plotted as a fatigue curve (Figure 20–4). For some materials the fatigue curve is *asymptotic,* indicating that if the load is kept below a certain level the material remains intact

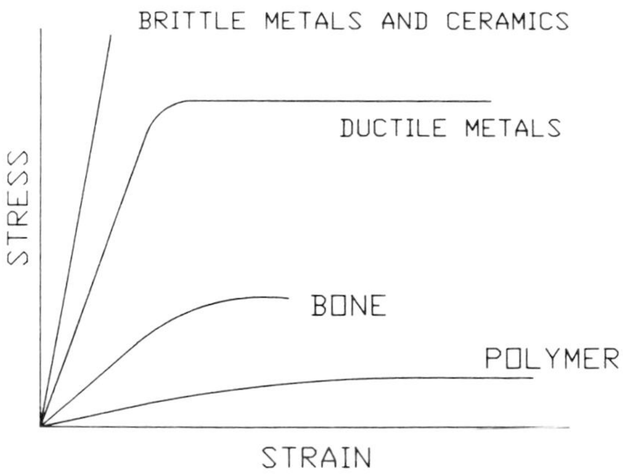

Figure 20–3. Stress-strain curves for four types of materials.

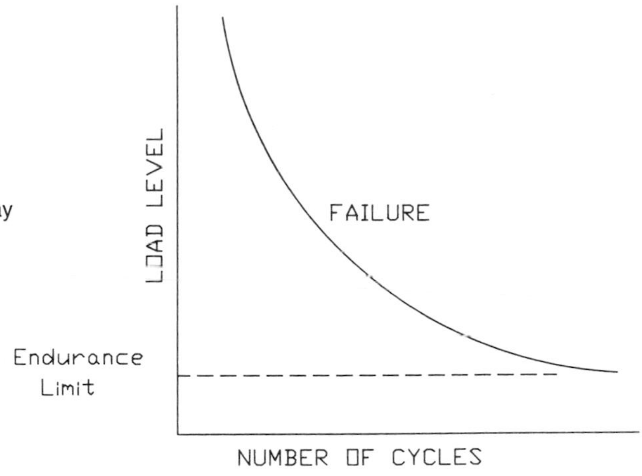

Figure 20–4. A fatigue curve representing the interplay of load levels, load repetitions, and specimen failure.

no matter how large the number of repetitions. This stress level is called the fatigue endurance limit. Metals often have endurance limits of about 50 per cent of their ultimate strength. Although many ceramics have low tensile properties, their fatigue endurance limits can be as high as 90 per cent of their ultimate strength.

It appears that fatigue normally begins on the surface of the implant in a region of tension, often at a surface imperfection or a region of stress concentration. Under the action of a tensile stress, a small crack begins at the imperfection and propagates during subsequent cyclic loading. Fatigue testing therefore involves evaluating stress levels and repetitions needed for crack initiation, and evaluating stress levels required for continued crack propagation.

Many inherent material factors influence the eventual fatigue life (Bapna, Lautenschlager, and Moser, 1975). Fine grain materials and implants with relatively few surface defects display greater fatigue resistance. The susceptibility of a material to corrosion or degradation by physiologic fluids may accelerate crack initiation or propagation. Ultimately the adequacy of an implant's mechanical properties can be determined only from the real life test of clinical use.

BIOLOGIC TESTING

The biologic testing of alloplastic materials includes the assessment of harmful and beneficial cellular and tissue responses by means of a variety of in vitro and in vivo tests. Attention is initially focused on toxicity testing, which may include testing for immunogenicity and carcinogenicity. If these effects are absent, the material is considered biocompatible and safe. The efficacy of an implant is then assessed using models appropriate to its use. For mammary implants, beneficial tissue responses include the formation of a noncontracted fibrous capsule. For bone implants, union and incorporation by bone ingrowth are desirable responses.

Toxicity

Most instances of implant toxicity are due to the release of substances to the biologic system (Hayes, 1982). The oxidation of metals, leaching of polymers, and biodegradation of ceramics cause release of potentially bioactive elements and molecules. The mechanical tests previously discussed can measure the changes in implant strength due to this release. However, only biologic tests can measure the changes in tissue response due to this release. While in vitro tests using tissue culture systems to identify cytotoxic effects are sensitive, they may be misleading if the release of bioactive substances is due to interaction between the biologic environment and the material. The most common tests therefore involve histologic observation after surgical implantation into laboratory animals.

Following the injury of surgical placement, a nonspecific inflammatory response occurs around all implants (Hurley, 1983). Any increase in the extent and duration of the acute and chronic inflammatory responses evoked by an implant indicates a degree of toxicity. Activated macrophages are observed at the surface of all implanted biomaterials. The macrophage population usually remains inconspicuous and by two weeks it is replaced by fibroblasts. In the presence of toxic substances a self-replicating population of macrophages may remain adjacent to the implant. In some instances giant cells are formed at sites of chronic inflammation by the fusion of newly arriving monocytes with aging macrophages (Chambers, 1978). No unique role for giant cells in chronic inflammation is evident, because their phagocytic function is less developed than that of macrophages and their ability to secrete enzymes is similar to that of macrophages. Nevertheless, the turnover of giant cells may become indolent in the presence of implant fragments resistant to degradation.

Immunogenicity

Another form of toxicity results from the interaction of implantable materials with the immune system (Merritt, 1984). The consequences of an immune reaction are varied, ranging from mild, fleeting symptoms to severe compromise of host or implant function. Substances must be foreign and of large molecular weight to be immunogenic. Most biomaterials are foreign and large. Thus, it is their chemistry and degradation by corrosion, wear, and dissolution that decides whether or not they will be immunogenic. Although the exact mechanism is unknown, it appears that many substances are first internalized by macrophages and then presented to the immune system for a subsequent response. The most common reaction associated with biomaterials is a cell-mediated sensitivity that involves T cells and does not involve antibody or B cells. Many of the symptoms can be accounted for by the soluble lymphokines released by T cells. Although the skin reaction of contact dermatitis remains local, the reaction to an implant may be systemic and not easily recognized.

Carcinogenicity

Observations of malignant tumors in association with alloplastic materials have been reported in both human and experimental animals. The question of whether there is a cause and effect relationship between implanted materials and tumor development in humans is still not resolved. However, continued clinical reports of tumor occurrence, coupled with demonstrated production of tumors by implanted materials in animals, have created concern that implanted biomaterials may induce malignant tumor formation in humans.

In experimental studies, tumors (principally sarcomas) have been produced by almost all solid materials, a phenomenon termed "solid-state carcinogenesis" (Bischoff and Bryson, 1964). From these studies, several major characteristics have been derived (Brand, Johnson, and Buoen, 1976). The composition of the material per se appears to be of little importance (unless it contains leachable carcinogens) because a wide variety of materials elicit a similar response. Maximal tumorigenesis is present when the material has a smooth, continuous surface. Perforations, weaves, or powders tend to reduce or abolish implant tumorigenicity. Solid-state tumor induction requires the implant to be of a minimal size below which tumors are not induced, and above which tumor-inducing activity increases with size. In the rat this critical size is 0.5 × 0.5 cm. The threshold size for humans is not known. Another characteristic is the requirement for the implant to remain in situ for a minimal period. Short-term contact appears to be ineffective. The minimal period in the rat is about six months; the tumors appear after a latency period of approximately 300 days. Comparable periods have not been established in humans, although it has been suggested that the latent period may be as long as 50 to 60 years in some cases (Brand and Brand, 1980). Currently, some authors believe that materials implanted in humans pose a significant risk for tumor induction given sufficient time. On the other hand, many contend that the solid-state mechanism of carcinogenesis does not operate in humans, and that the low incidence of reported material-associated tumors in humans is simply coincidental and not induced by the material.

Efficacy

After histologic testing has confirmed the safety of an implant material, there still remains the question: does it work? Unlike toxicity, efficacy is uniquely defined by the intended clinical application for each implant material. Will a dressing material remain occlusive and adherent and properly control evaporative loss? Will a mammary implant material remain soft and yet resist rupture? Will a bone implant undergo union and incorporation? If used in cranial reconstruction, will it provide adequate cranial protection? If used in contour defects, will it be dimensionally stable and impact resistant? Almost by definition, efficacy studies require observation and measurement after surgical implantation into animals. An implant intended for use as a bone graft substitute, for example, requires measurement of the amount of bone ingrowth.

Although the different biologic tests of implant efficacy are beyond the scope of this chapter, their interpretation by the clinician should be performed with care. In some instances the simple choice of animal may significantly alter this interpretation. Suture material performance, for example, may be studied in the rat. However, use of a rat model to measure the ability of an implant material to be incorporated by bone ingrowth yields overly optimistic and misleading results if translated to the clinical setting. This is due in part to species differences in bone morphology. Rats lack the secondary osteons predominant in humans.

Potentiation of Infection

The potential of an implant material to potentiate infection is an important property to be determined. The earliest biologic testing of this type was performed in human volunteers. After establishing the requirement of 10^6 *Staphylococcus pyogenes* to produce a pus-forming clinical infection, the addition of a braided silk suture was found to reduce the required bacteria to 100 organisms (Elek and Conen, 1957). Subsequent studies of the mechanisms of this potentiation have generally followed the work done on the effects of reactive biologic materials such as blood clot and necrotic tissue. Any reactivity contributed by an implant further activates local host defenses and triggers the release of tissue toxic inflammatory mediators such as lysosomal enzymes and oxygen-derived free radicals. This type of local tissue destruction establishes an environment adjacent to the alloplast that favors survival of bacteria and thus dramatically increases the likelihood of infection. The effects of implant reactivity on the complement system and the clotting cascade may also contribute to the tissue-destructive process (Dougherty and Simmons, 1982).

In addition to local tissue destruction, there are other infection-promoting consequences of implant materials. An interaction between the implant and host immune system may be significant. Contact between neutrophils and implant reduces the bactericidal capacity of the cells. Opsonization of *Staphylococcus aureus* also decreases markedly after implantation (Zimmerli, Waldvogel, and Vaudaux, 1982). If an implant material has not damaged host tissue or incapacitated white blood cells, it may still promote infection through the direct protection of bacteria, namely by bacterial adherence to the surface (Gristina and Costerton, 1984). Organisms, including *S. aureus, S. epidermidis, Streptococcus viridans,* and *Pseudomonas aeruginosa,* are capable of synthesizing a fibrous glycocalyx that allows them to adhere to and grow on implant surfaces (Marrie and Costerton, 1982). This might explain the temporal differences in the potentiation of infection by porous and dense implants. Following acute bacterial inoculation, the infection rate for porous implants (more surface for adherence) is greater than for dense implants. However, following late inoculation, after tissue ingrowth of the pores, the infection rate with dense materials (limited host access to organisms) is greater (Merritt, Shafer, and Brown, 1979). Less well studied are the recursive effects of the infectious process on implants. Since the solubility of hydroxyapatite increases with decreasing pH, the degradation of these implants may be potentiated by the presence of a transitory or chronic infection. Implant materials that do not potentiate infection are unlikely to be realized. It therefore behooves the surgeon to use the full knowledge of implant and wound biology to maximize the achievements of implant surgery.

METALS

All materials exist in one of three atomic forms: amorphous, mesomorphic, or crystalline. *Amorphous* materials (gases and liquids) possess atoms or molecules randomly distributed in space. *Mesomorphic* materials (some ceramics and polymers) are those in which the atoms or molecules have regular arrangements in some directions but not in others. The relatively weak intermolecular forces binding the molecules together contribute to the soft quality and lower mechanical properties of these materials as contrasted with those of crystalline materials. *Crystalline* materials (metals and some ceramics and polymers) are those in which the material is characterized by a three-dimensional orderly arrangement of atoms or molecules over large atomic distances. These materials tend to be strong, hard substances. The atomic order of each particular crystal can be conceptualized by the arrangement of spherical atoms into unique geometric positions known as lattice structures.

In order to obtain desirable mechanical and biophysical properties, combinations of metals (alloys) are often employed in implant materials. When combined by melting or solid-state diffusion, combinations of elements often form stoichiometric compounds, solid solutions and mixtures. In this alloying process the added atoms are accommodated within the parent lattice structure. In the case of steel the carbon atoms occupy interstitial sites between iron atoms, and form what is called an interstitial solid solution. If two metal atoms are roughly the same size, have the same bonding tendencies, and tend to crystallize in the same type of crystal structure, a substitutional solid solution may form. The crystal structure and solubility limits for a given alloy are strongly dependent on temperature. High temperatures followed by rapid cooling or quenching are commonly used to achieve the desired alloy composition.

Limited almost exclusively to skeletal applications, metals have been widely used for fracture plates, screws, cranial plates, mandible trays, and many joint replacement parts. The metals used in medical application are carefully alloyed to withstand the corrosive saline environment of the body. Since metals cannot repair or heal the damage caused by plastic deformation or fatigue, they must be both stronger and stiffer than the bone they support or replace. Typical mechanical properties for several metals used in medical implants are compared with bone in Table 20–1 (Keller and Lautenschlager, 1986).

The biologic responses to metals is similar to those for any implant material. Against the metal surface a layer of fibrous connective tissue forms, which can be quite thin in areas of close bone approximation. This general response can be modified by the ability of metals to corrode under attack by chloride ions (Williams, 1981). The biologic effect of corrosion, the electrochemical conversion of a metal to a metal compound, depends on the toxicity of the particular metal ions released (Meachim and Pedley, 1981). Fortunately, corrosion can be controlled by the formation of an oxide film. Both titanium and chromium naturally (passively) form a film and they are therefore used as alloys to increase corrosion resistance.

Stainless Steel

Stainless steel has been used as a standardized implant material since the 1920's (Williams and Roaf, 1973). The composition of stainless steel used for metallic implants is listed in Table 20–2 (ASTM, 1984). The most desirable composition of stainless steel would include a high concentration of nickel (Ni) to permit work hardening, a low concen-

Table 20–1. Mechanical Properties of Metallic Implant Materials and Bone

Material	Tensile Strength (MPa)	Compressive Strength (MPa)	Yield Point (MPa)	Elongation (%)	Elastic Modulus (GPa)
Stainless steel 316L					
Annealed	550	550	240	50	200
Cold-worked	965	965	790	20	200
Co-Cr (ASTM-F75)	700	700	500	10	240
Ti (ASTM-F67)	620	620	500	18	100
Ti-6Al-4V (ASTM-F135)	900	900	840	12	110
Tooth enamel	70	265	70	0	50
Cortical bone	140	130	130	1	18
Cancellous bone	1–2	4–8	–	–	0.2

Co = cobalt; Cr = chromium; Ti = titanium.

Table 20–2. Composition of Stainless Steel Alloy (Wrought, ASTM-F55)

Element	Weight %
Chromium	17–20
Nickel	12–17
Molybdenum	2–4
Carbon	0.03 max
Manganese	2.00 max
Phosphorus	0.03 max
Sulfur	0.03 max
Silicon	0.75 max
Nitrogen	0.10 max
Copper	0.50 max
Iron	Balance

tration of carbon (C) to prevent carbide formation, sufficient chromium (Cr) for corrosion resistance, and a small concentration of molybdenum (Mo) to resist pitting corrosion. Stainless steels are perhaps the easiest metal implant materials to fabricate. However, strict care is required for the manufacturing of quality implants. Although it is possible to cast these materials to shape, the impurity levels produced by this technique may lead to inferior corrosion and mechanical properties compared with forged and cold-worked implants.

The typical mechanical properties of the 316L stainless steel alloys used for implants are listed in Table 20–1. Fully annealed (softened) stainless steels exhibit a fairly high ultimate tensile strength, but the yield strength is low and the ductility is high. As a result, plastic deformation occurs readily with these materials. These alloys can be strengthened by cold working, which does not change the elastic modulus but does increase the yield and ultimate strengths.

Cobalt-Chromium Alloys

The Co-Cr alloys have played a significant role in the history of metallic implants. The early biologic acceptance demonstrated by Stellite (Co-Cr alloys with starlike microstructures) during the 1920's led to the introduction of Vitallium. When used in metal implant applications, Co-Cr alloys demonstrate an overall balance of corrosion resistance, fatigue resistance, and strength. The composition of cast Co-Cr alloys is shown in Table 20–3 (ASTM, 1984). The Co-Cr alloys used for implants have an approximate composition of 60 to 65 per cent Co and 25 to 30 per cent Cr. The alloys are essentially solid solutions of Cr in Co, with the addition of Mo to reduce grain size and Ni to toughen the material. The major disadvantage of the cast Co-Cr alloy system is that the materials harden rapidly, rendering the materials brittle and subject to premature fracture. The mechanical properties of a medical grade Co-Cr alloy are listed in Table 20–1. Depending on the annealing and cold-working treatments employed, a wide range of strength and ductility may be achieved.

Table 20–3. Composition of Co-Cr Alloy (Cast, ASTM-F90)

Element	Weight %
Chromium	27–30
Nickel	2.50 max
Molybdenum	5–7
Iron	0.75 max
Carbon	0.35 max
Manganese	1.00 max
Silicon	1.00 max
Cobalt	Balance

Titanium

Of the major metallic implant systems, titanium (Ti) and its alloys are the most recently introduced (Luckey and Kubli, 1983). Because of their combination of strength, light weight, corrosion resistance, and biocompatibility, Ti and its alloys have rapidly gained popularity. The compositions of Ti and its principal alloy used as implant materials are listed in Table 20–4 (ASTM, 1984). The Ti-6Al-4V alloy has a two-phase structure. By careful heat treatment, the size, shape, and distribution of the second-phase particles in the matrix can be controlled. The properties of the alloy may thereby be enhanced considerably compared with commercially pure Ti.

The fabrication and processing of Ti materials are more difficult than those of the

Table 20–4. Composition of Ti (ASTM-F67) and Ti-6Al-4V Alloy (ASTM-F136)

Element	Pure Ti (Weight %)	Ti-6Al-4V (Weight %)
Iron	0.5 max	0.25 max
Carbon	0.10 max	0.08 max
Oxygen	0.45 max	0.13 max
Aluminum	–	5.5–6.5
Vanadium	–	3.5–4.5
Titanium	Balance	Balance

stainless steel or Co-Cr alloys. In addition to its very high melting point, Ti is very reactive with the atmosphere. The environment must therefore be carefully controlled during fabrication. The mechanical properties of Ti and Ti-6Al-4V alloy are listed in Table 20–1. The mechanical properties of Ti are strongly dependent on the purity of the material and the degree and type of alloying. Increased oxygen content in Ti increases the tensile strength but at the expense of ductility. The heat treatments used to sinter spheres of Ti alloy onto solid alloy cores in order to produce porous implants for bone ingrowth also appear to affect adversely the fatigue life of these materials (Yue, Pilliar, and Weatherly, 1982).

Other Metals

Tantalum has considerable historical value as a potential metallic implant material because of its biologic acceptance, which stems from its relative chemical inertness and corrosion resistance. The major drawback to the use of tantalum as an implant material lies in its somewhat poor mechanical properties. The elastic modulus is relatively high, but the tensile strength is low. However, tantalum does appear to possess good fatigue properties (Plenk and associates, 1981).

A nickel-titanium (Ni-Ti) alloy (Nitinol) has been explored as a candidate implant material because of its unusual deformation characteristics (Bensmann, Baumgart, and Haasters, 1982). This alloy is said to have "memory" in that when deformed at room temperature and heated slightly, the alloy returns to its original shape. The temperature at which this transformation takes place is altered by alloying. Slight additions of iron and molybdenum enhance the mechanical properties and corrosion resistance of the alloy. Further research may result in its use as an implant with the ability to alter shape and forces in vivo.

POLYMERS

For the restoration of soft tissue deficiency, polymers provide the principal source of implant materials. As implant materials, polymers are available with a wide variety of mechanical and physical properties, are readily formed into desired shapes, and are relatively inert in their reactions with host tissue. Polymers derive their wide range of properties from a combination of their chemical composition and their structure (Leininger, 1972). The chemical composition of some polymers used as implants is listed in Table 20–5. The important role of chemical composition in the determination of polymer properties can be illustrated with polyethylene. Because of its hydrocarbon composition, it is relatively weak and easily extensible.

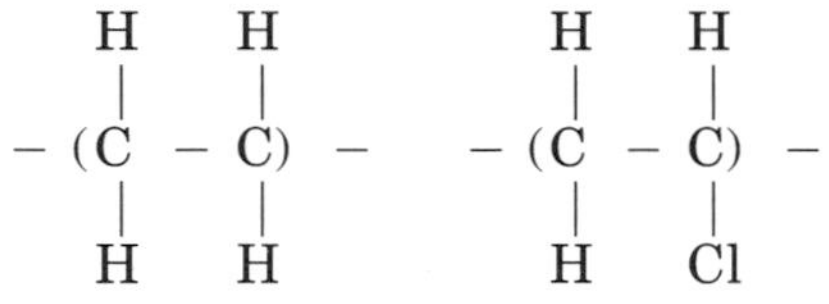

poly(ethylene) poly(vinylchloride)

If one hydrogen atom per ethylene unit is replaced by a chlorine atom, the tensile strength and modulus are more than doubled. Another effect of chemical composition is that of resistance to the physiologic environment. The presence of ester and amide links may permit enzymatic degradation if access is not limited by crystallinity of the polymer. The composition of polymers may include the addition of low molecular weight materials, known as plasticizers, if the polymer is too hard and rigid. In the case of polyvinylchloride, hydrocarbon esters are added to increase its flexibility. Because plasticizers are potentially leachable, these materials are restricted to implants of short-term use such as shunts and catheters. Fillers are rarely used in implant polymers except for silica to reinforce polydimethylsiloxane.

Polymers are structurally composed of long chains of repeating units that can reach molecular weights of hundreds of thousands of daltons (Leininger and Bigg, 1986). These chains may be linear, with or without branches, and may be crosslinked to adjacent chains. Polymers in the solid state can be either completely amorphous or semicrystalline. Crystallinity can vary from a low percentage, in low-tacticity polyvinylchloride, to over 90 per cent in a highly linear polyethylene. No polymer is completely crystalline, owing to the presence of lattice defect regions that contain unordered amorphous material. The high molecular weight that arises from the repetitive linking of the repeating units and the length of these units have a profound

Table 20–5. Composition of Polymers Used in Implants

Polymer	Repeating Unit
Poly(dimethylsiloxane)	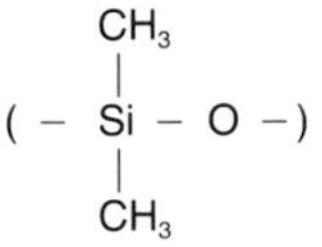
Poly(urethane)	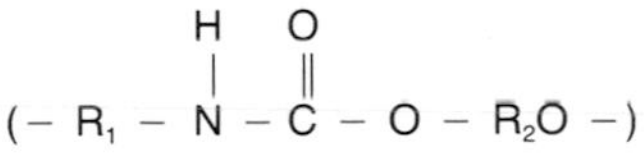
Poly(ethylene)	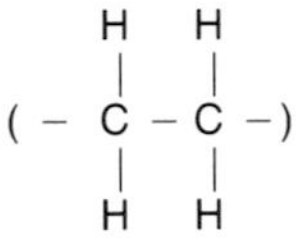
Poly(tetrafluoroethylene)	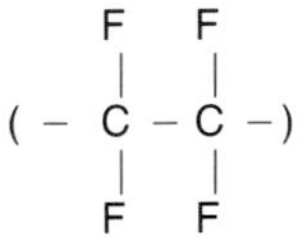
Poly(ethylene terephthalate)	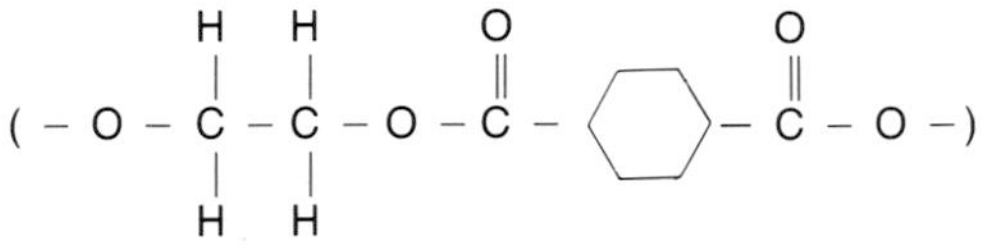
Poly(methylmethacrylate)	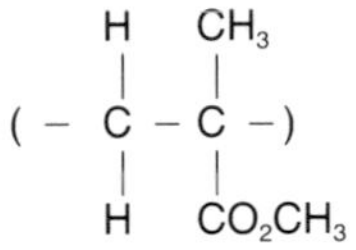
Poly(glycolide)	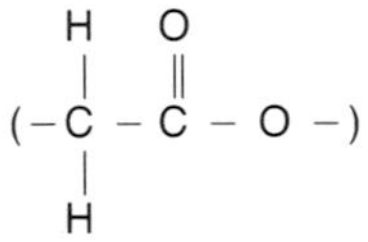
Poly(lactide)	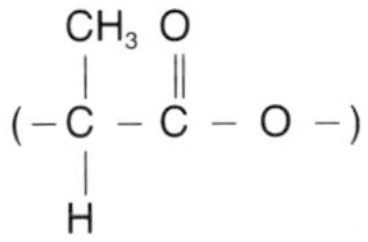
Poly(amide)	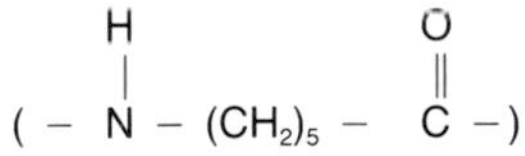

R_1 = diisocyanate: R_2 = polyether.

effect on the properties of a polymer. Using polyethylene again as an example, low molecular weight polymers exist as liquids, but as the length of the chains increase the liquids become more viscous, then waxy, and finally a plastic. The low interchain attraction between polymers can be increased by bringing the chains more closely together into a regular crystalline structure. This closer packing of the chains increases tensile strength and results in decreased solubility because reactive molecules can less easily penetrate the polymer and separate the chains. Further increases in material stiffness and stability can be achieved by the formation of crosslinks between the polymer chains.

In the liquid or melt state of a polymer, thermal energy is sufficiently high for long segments of each macromolecule to move in random brownian motion. As the melt is cooled, a temperature is reached at which all long-range segmental motions cease. This temperature, which is indicative of the abrupt cessation of large-scale polymer backbone rotation, is called the *glass transition temperature*. Below this temperature the modulus of a polymer increases several orders of magnitude, and it changes from a rubbery material to a glassy state. Polymers such as polydimethylsiloxane, with a glass transition temperature of −123°C, therefore exist in the rubbery or elastomeric state at room and body temperatures. Polymethylmethacrylate has a glass transition temperature of 105°C, thus accounting for its glassy state at physiologic temperatures.

The fabrication methods used for polymer implants generally depend on the presence of crosslinking (Billmeyer, 1971). Non-crosslinked polymers are thermoplastic and reversibly soften upon heating. For these polymers, processing is done while it is in the heat-softened state. By use of injection molding, the viscous polymer is forced by pressure into a closed mold, cooled, and ejected as the finished part. In some instances it is necessary to anneal the molded implant material to reduce residual stresses. Crosslinked polymers are thermosetting materials in which the polymer cures to an infusible, insoluble solid. By use of transfer molding, these polymers are heated in a chamber and forced into a mold before curing is complete. This process differs from injection molding in that the residence time in the heated mold must be long enough for curing to take place. Several polymers, notably methacrylates and silicones, may be cast as a curable liquid in a mold and allowed to thermoset at room temperature. The mechanical stresses imposed on polymer implants are small when used in soft tissue applications. As can be seen by comparison of their mechanical properties with those of human tissue (Yamada, 1970), the polymeric implants generally have higher strength than do the tissues (Table 20–6).

The biologic response to the polymer group of materials generally consists of a normal inflammatory response, deposition of collagen fibers, and finally maturation into a mature fibrous connective tissue that completely encapsulates the implant. The fibrous tissue reaches maturation in four to six weeks, and contains numerous discrete bundles of collagen and reticular fibers. The fibrous sheath is normally flexible and its inner surface is smooth and glistening. In some instances a constrictive fibrosis occurs, a biologic response that may require surgical correction. Wear of these polymers, with release of small particles, appears to evoke an inflammatory response. Liquid forms of polymers such as dimethylsiloxane and tetrafluoroethylene have been associated with inflammation and multinucleated giant cell reactions, and therefore are little used.

The Silicones or Poly(dimethylsiloxane)

This class of polymers has probably been more widely implanted than any other because of its soft tissue compatibility, easy formability, resistance to the physiologic environment, and wide range of mechanical properties. The silicones, or more precisely polydimethylsiloxane and related polymers, are the only noncarbon chain polymers used as implants (van Noort and Black, 1981). The dimethysiloxane unit can be polymerized into long chain molecules with average molecular weights in the millions. Although the methyl side groups predominate, occasionally a vinyl or phenyl group replaces the methyl group.

Table 20–6. Mechanical Properties of Polymeric Implant Materials and Soft Tissues

Material	Tensile Strength (MPa)	Elongation To Break (%)	Elastic Modulus (GPa)
Poly(dimethylsiloxane)	2–7	100–600	0.01
Poly(urethane)	1–69	10–1000	0.07–6.9
Poly(ethylene)	21–38	20–1000	0.4–1.2
Poly(tetrafluoroethylene)	10–20	200–400	0.4
Poly(ethylene terephthalate)	1–5	30–490	–
Poly(methylmethacrylate)	55–85	2–7	2.4–3.3
Skin	6–14	110–140	0.02–0.04
Fascia	12–14	14–17	0.3
Tendon	59–69	8–9	1.0
Elastic cartilage	3	30	0.015

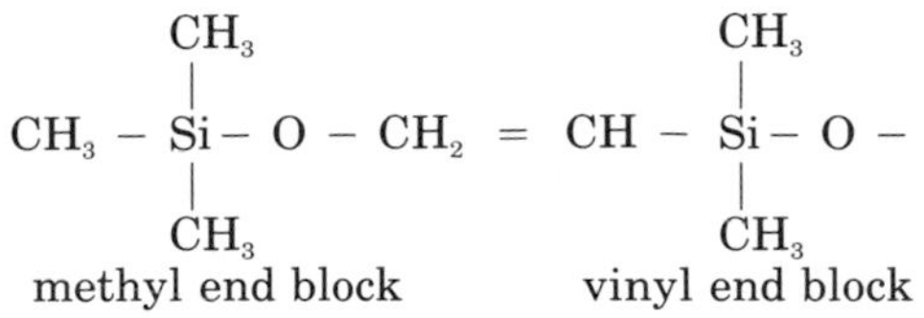

$$CH_3 - Si - O - CH_2 = CH - Si - O -$$

methyl end block   vinyl end block

The polymer chains are end-blocked with a methyl or a vinyl end block as shown above.

If the short chains of polymer are end-blocked, a silicone fluid results. With longer chain lengths, fluids of increased viscosity can be produced. To produce a gel or rubber (elastomer) requires the crosslinking of polymer chains. The polymer chains used in gels contain 50 to 500 dimethylsiloxane units, whereas elastomers require longer lengths with 500 to 2000 units.

Crosslinking or vulcanization is the process by which a polymer is turned into the three dimensional structure of a rubber with all its associated properties. This process consists of coupling the polymer chains together by primary chemical links at widely separated points, generally with several hundred monomer units separating each crosslink. In the case of heat-vulcanizing silicone rubber, the crosslinking is initiated by a benzoyl peroxide catalyst that breaks down upon heating to form free radicals. The strong dehydrogenating property of these radicals activates the methyl and vinyl groups, which subsequently crosslink as shown at the bottom of this page.

Other links such as trimethyl or propyl links may also be formed between chains. Because of the low intermolecular attraction in the silicone polymer, its tensile strength is extremely low (Braley, 1970). In order to have any practical use, a filler of fine silica with a particle size of about 30 microns is added before the vulcanization process. The amount of filler is usually in the range of 15 to 20 per cent by volume.

Silicone gels contain both crosslinked silicone and silicone fluid (Blais, 1983). Instead of the short dimethyl crosslinks used for elastomeric silicone, gels have long crosslinks consisting of many dimethylsiloxane units. The result is an open-mesh type of polymer network that is able to retain and occlude large amounts of silicone fluid. The elastic properties of the polymer network and the viscous properties of the polymer fluid account for the viscoelastic properties of the silicone gels.

The usual method of fabricating implants from silicone rubber is by transfer molding. Implants that require thin silicone envelopes, such as mammary and testicular implants, are typically fabricated by dipping and removing a mandrel, a method called solvent casting. A layer of silicone remains coated on the mandrel after solvent evaporation, and multiple dips can be used to increase the envelope thickness (Frisch, 1983). After vulcanization the silicone envelope is separated from the mandrel for use in further fabrication.

It is apparent from the different fabrication methods that a wide range of mechanical properties can be achieved. Tensile strengths can range from 2 to 10 MPa and extensibility from 100 to 600 per cent. One of the major limitations of the silicone rubbers is their poor resistance to tearing. After introducing a notch of 0.1 mm, the tensile strength of a silicone was reduced by 50 per cent, while a polyurethane, for example, showed only a 20 per cent reduction in tensile strength for the same size notch (van Noort and Black, 1981).

The biologic properties of silicone consist of the formation of a fibrous connective tissue capsule against the implant surface. In some instances this fibrous tissue undergoes contracture, a process that may be related to myofibroblast activity (Fig. 20–5).

Poly(urethane)

The urethane polymers include a wide variety of materials based on the urethane group (see Table 20–5) and having in common the same general classes of starting materials—diisocyanates and either polyesters or polyethers (Leininger and Bigg, 1986). The broad possibilities for the design and synthe-

$$CH_3 - \underset{|}{\overset{O}{Si}} - CH_2 + CH_2 - \underset{|}{\overset{O}{Si}} - CH_3 \longrightarrow CH_3 - \underset{|}{\overset{O}{Si}} - CH_2 = CH_2 - \underset{|}{\overset{O}{Si}} - CH_3$$

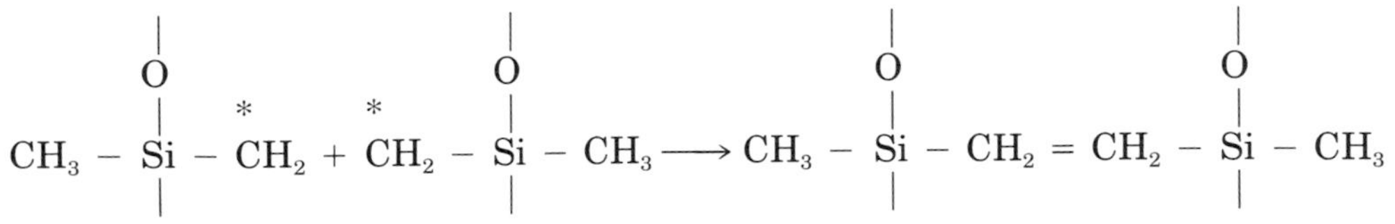

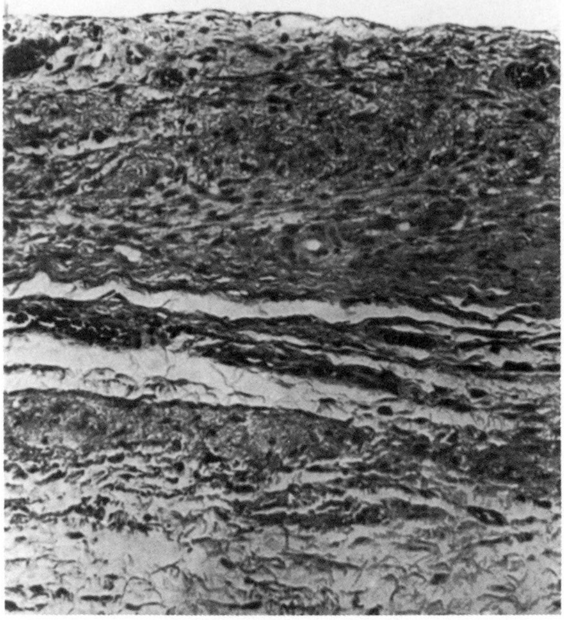

Figure 20–5. Mature fibrous connective tissue adjacent to a silicone implant. In situ the silicone was present against the upper surface of the connective tissue. ×125. (From Gayou, R.M.: A histological comparison of contracted and non-contracted capsules around silicone breast implants. Plast. Reconstr. Surg., *63*:700, 1979.)

sis of different polyurethanes with excellent mechanical and biologic properties contributed to their early appeal as implant materials. In the 1950's polyurethanes were implanted as foams and elastomers in a variety of applications. Unfortunately, most of these implants failed in the living system over long-term use because they were polyester polyurethanes (Lyman and associates, 1977). These materials were subsequently shown to possess poor hydrolytic stability and thus to be susceptible to degradation in the biologic environment. This problem has been overcome through the incorporation of hydrolytically stable polyether soft segments in most of the polyurethane implants used today, and polyurethanes now rank high among the list of acceptable implant materials.

The urethane polymers differ from the other polymer families in that each chain is composed of alternating hard (urethane) and soft (polyether) segments, which are respectively polar and nonpolar in nature (Boretos, 1981). This property causes the segmented copolymers to have a two-phase microstructure. The isocyanate (urethane) crystalline domains are dispersed in a macroglycol (polyether) amorphous matrix. The flexible amorphous segments provide elastic recovery properties to the polymer, and the hard crystalline segments act as reinforcing fillers that increase the modulus properties. The hard segments also provide intermolecular sites for secondary bindings. Although thermoplastic segmented polyurethanes are valuable in such medical items as extruded blood tubing, thermoset (crosslinked) polyurethanes are desirable for long-term surgical implants.

The most common prepolymer used for the urethane segment in implant materials is diphenylmethane diisocyanate (Lelah and Cooper, 1986). A polyether segment in common use is polytetramethylene oxide. Fabrication methods in use include both molding and solvent casting techniques. In some applications an open-cell foam is desired to allow connective tissue ingrowth and dispersion of the contractile forces of a fibrous capsule. Since CO_2 is generated in situ from the reaction of isocyanate with water, open-cell foams, with interconnecting pores between cells, can be made with expansion-free processes. Because of the large range of molecular weight and molar ratios possible for the segment copolymers, the polyurethane materials demonstrate the broadest range of mechanical properties (Table 20–6). The biologic properties of polyurethane include the normal sequence of repair leading to a mature fibrous capsule. The porosity of the material may result in an interconnected network of connective tissue ingrowth (Fig. 20–6).

Poly(ethylene)

The commercial polymerization of ethylene oxide gas was introduced in 1939 to produce what is now referred to as low density polyethylene (LDPE). The reaction takes place at pressures of 100 to 300 MPa and uses small amounts of peroxides to initiate the polymerization (Bloch and Hastings, 1972). These polymers consist of a large number of ethylene units linked together to form a highly branched chain macromolecule. Approximately 10 to 30 branches are present per 1000 carbon atoms. These branches limit the closeness of chain packing and hence account

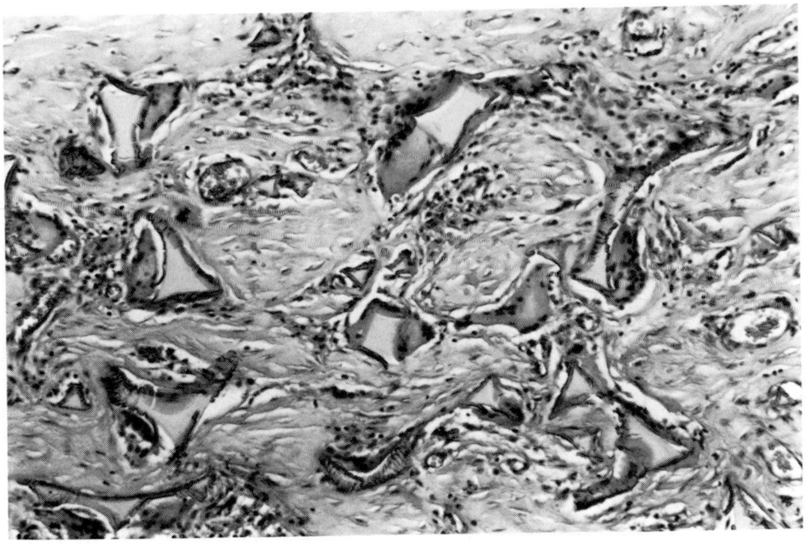

Figure 20–6. Porous polyester polyurethane (clear) with connective tissue ingrowth after three months. Foreign body cells are numerous and possibly related to hydrolytic degradation of this form of polyurethane. ×200. (From Smahel, J.: Tissue reactions to breast implants coated with polyurethane. Plast. Reconstr. Surg., *61*:80, 1978.)

for the lower density of LDPE. The chain branches also reduce crystallinity, increasing the ratio of amorphous material, and result in lower yield strength and lower stiffness.

Another type of polyethylene with different properties is made by low pressure polymerization at pressures less than 10 MPa. This polymer, referred to as high density polyethylene (HDPE), is a substantially linear molecule with few side chain branches. Consequently a higher density is attainable and both tensile strength and stiffness are improved. For non–weight-bearing applications, HDPE in solid and porous forms has overshadowed LDPE materials (Hastings, 1981). To attain the wear properties required by weight bearing, a polyethylene with molecular weights of approximately 4 million is polymerized by yet another process. This ultra high molecular weight polyethylene (UHMWPE) enjoys considerable popularity as a component in some total hip prostheses. The mechanical properties listed in Table 20–6 for polyethylene represent the HDPE form. When porous HDPE is placed against bone, it may become stabilized by the ingrowth of connective tissue and the close approximation of bone (Fig. 20–7). When mesh forms of HDPE are used to bridge cavity wall defects, fibrous tissue infiltration extends throughout the sheet. Because its higher melting point permits steam autoclaving, polypropylene

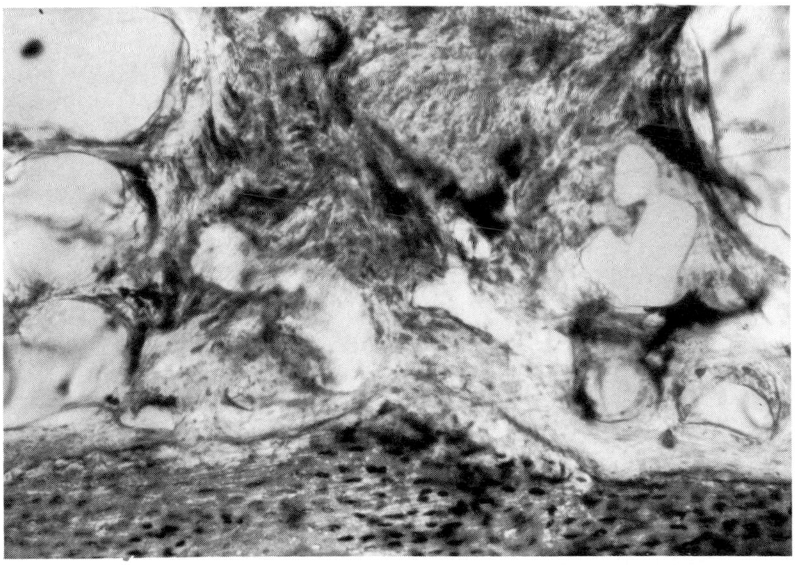

Figure 20–7. Porous high density polyethylene implant (clear) on top of a rat calvarial bone for 30 weeks demonstrates connective tissue ingrowth and close proximity of bone. ×10.

has replaced HDPE in the manufacture of surgical mesh. Polypropylene results from the substitution of one methyl group for a hydrogen atom in each polyethylene unit, and the biologic properties of the two materials are similar (DiBenedetto and Fleischer, 1983).

Poly(ethylene terephthalate)

The most common of the polyesters, polyethylene terephthalate (PET), is widely used in the texile garment industry. As an implant material, PET was early identified to be inert, biocompatible, flexible, resilient, and resistant to sterilization treatments (Guidoin and associates, 1977). As an implantable fabric, PET is used as a patch that permits tissue anchoring to a smooth substrate such as silicone. In addition, PET is the currently preferred polymer for the manufacture of medium and large caliber arterial prostheses.

The PET monomer is synthesized from two monomers under catalytic conditions (King and associates, 1981). One common technique makes use of ethylene glycol and terephthalic acid (see the bottom of this page).

Under a vacuum or an inert atmosphere, the polymerization proceeds until one of the reactants is totally depleted. The linear polymer chains used for forming fibers generally contain an average of 70 to 110 PET monomer units.

The PET polymer is converted to a filament by melt-spinning. This involves heating the polymer above its crystalline melting point and extruding it through small holes in a spinneret. After melt-spinning the continuous filaments are drawn or stretched between five and seven times their original length at an elevated temperature below the melting point. This drawing process rearranges the molecules and orients them more closely to the axis of the fiber. This also increases the crystallinity or compactness of the polymer, thereby improving the strength, dimensional stability, and fatigue resistance of the filaments. The PET fibers are used to produce the woven, knitted, and velour fabric configurations used in implant applications (Weselow and Snyder, 1983). The variety of fabric patterns accounts in part for the range of mechanical properties available in PET implants. Designs are selected to avoid bursting or aneurysm formation when used in the vascular system. Although it is desirable to maintain the compliance and flexibility of these fabrics, these properties are markedly reduced when encapsulation with new collagenous tissue occurs (Fig. 20–8).

Poly(tetrafluoroethylene)

The unusual chemical stability of the perfluorocarbon polymers, along with their unique nonadhesion and antifrictional properties, led to an interest in their potential as implant materials. This group of perfluorocarbon polymers—polymers containing only carbon, fluorine, and oxygen—includes several similarly biocompatible members, but only polytetrafluorethylene (PTFE) has received significant attention (Homsy, 1983). PTFE is a linear polymer prepared by aqueous polymerization processes that result in molecular weights ranging from 6 to 10 million. Crosslinks are not formed and the natural intermolecular attraction is weak. Consequently the bulk properties of these polymers include low tensile strength and flexural modulus. The intramolecular (interatomic) bond strengths reflect the strong carbon-carbon and carbon-fluorine covalent bonds (see Table 20–5). The strengths of these covalent bonds account for the inert, nonadhesive, and antifriction properties of PTFE.

Although PTFE exhibits a crystalline melting point, the melt viscosity is too high for fabrication by usual melt-molding technique (Homsy, 1981). Therefore, sintering (firing) procedures using PTFE powder are used to fabricate implants. Space between the fused polymer particles may be preserved to provide a porosity that permits tissue ingrowth. To

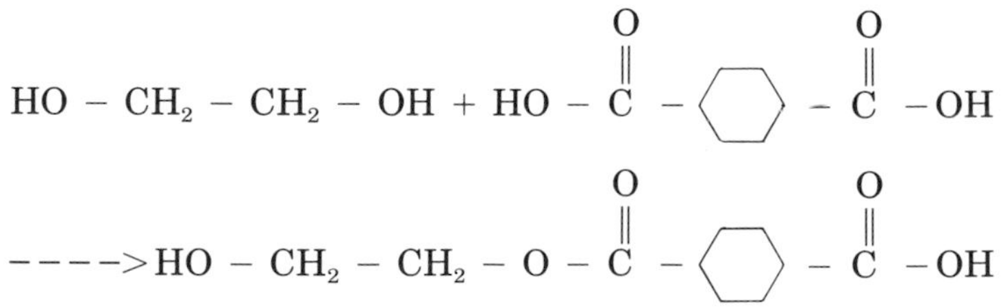

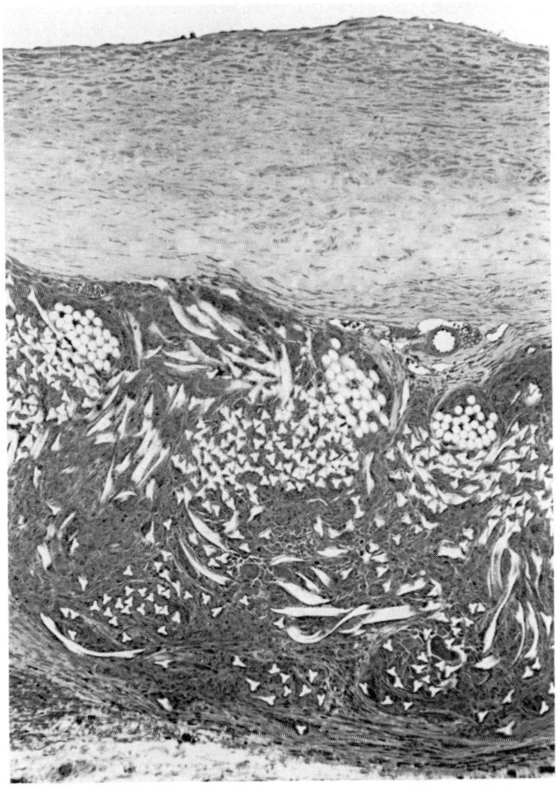

Figure 20–8. Section through polyethylene terephthalate vascular graft after one year. The interstices of the graft are packed with densely staining cells, distinguishing this region from the inner and outer capsules, which are composed of connective tissue. ×120. (From Burkel, W.E., and Kahn, R.H.: Biocompatibility of prosthetic grafts. *In* Stanley, J.C. (Ed.): Biologic and Synthetic Vascular Prostheses. New York, Grune & Stratton, 1982.).

modify the surface energy and therefore enhance the ability of cells to attach to its surface, PTFE powder has been composited with pyrolytic carbon fibers and aluminum oxides before sintering. The introduction of porosity into PTFE significantly reduces its strength, and a tensile strength of 1 MPa has been reported (Homsy and associates, 1972). When porous PTFE-carbon fiber implants are placed against bone, a fibrous tissue layer forms at the boundary, and stabilization consists of connective tissue ingrowth (Fig. 20–9).

Poly(methylmethacrylate)

Among the high molecular weight polymers developed during the first three decades of this century, polymethylmethacrylate (PMMA) was probably the first to find application as biomaterials. By the early 1940's it had been used for dentures, artificial teeth, inlays, crowns, and bridges, and also for artificial eyes, noses, and ears (Munson and Heron, 1941). Although external prostheses are not implants, it was in these applications that PMMA as a biomaterial was born.

When MMA monomer is combined in a chain reaction to form macromolecules (polymer), it acquires the desirable properties of transparency and relatively high strength and toughness. This polymerization is brought about by chemical activation of the monomer mediated

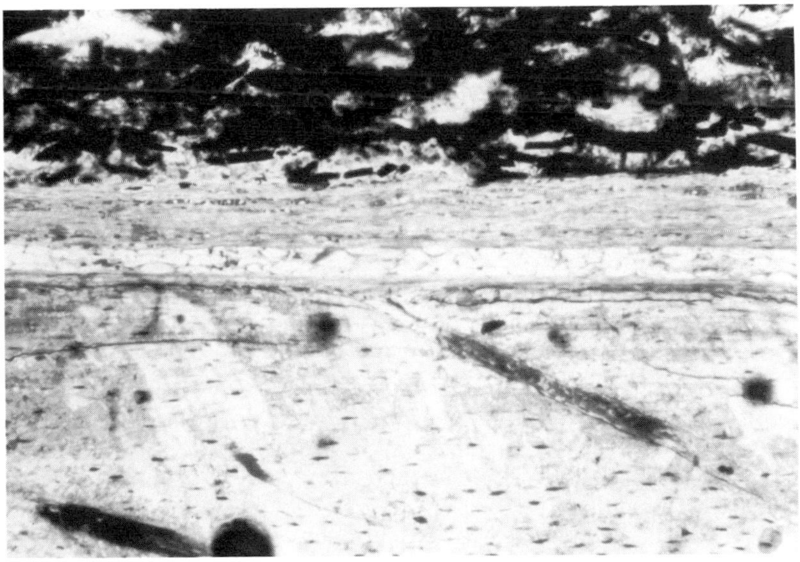

Figure 20–9. Polytetrafluoroethylene-carbon fiber implant on top of a rat calvarium after 30 weeks. In addition to connective tissue ingrowth, a characteristic fibrous layer between bone and implant is present. ×10.

by free radicals formed from the splitting of a benzoyl peroxide initiator (de Wijn and van Mullem, 1981). Heating is required to decompose benzoyl peroxide into its radical form. Thus, polymerization may be achieved by heating a mixture of MMA and benzoyl peroxide, giving the so-called heat-cured acrylic. The decomposition or splitting of the initiator at room temperatures can be achieved by the addition of a tertiary amine accelerator, resulting in polymerization of MMA without the addition of heat (cold-cured acrylic). Once initiated, the rate at which successive monomers are added to the chain is high, and up to several thousand monomer units can be linked together in a single polymer molecule in a few seconds.

Although this thermoplastic material can be fabricated using conventional mold techniques, the ability to shape it as an implant in situ represents the method of choice in many situations. The reaction mixture for cold-cured acrylic consists of a powder and a liquid. The powder consists of MMA polymer particles 10 to 30 microns in diameter to which the benzoyl peroxide initiator has been added. The liquid consists of MMA monomer in which the amine accelerator has been dissolved. After mixing together, the monomer polymerizes and binds together the preexisting polymer particles to form an easily moldable dough that cures in about ten minutes. When used as a load-distributing filler in the anchorage of hip prostheses, cold-cured PMMA (bone cement) has been shown to contribute to tissue damage (Linder, 1982). This is due in part to the exothermic reaction of polymerization, which can generate temperatures exceeding 70°C, and possibly also to the direct toxicity of the monomer. In other sites of application, these concerns are addressed by avoiding tissue contact with the monomer and minimizing tissue contact during the time of maximal exothermia. When used with proper care, PMMA demonstrates a high degree of tissue compatibility.

CERAMICS

Ceramics are the oldest man-made materials. Since ancient times, ceramic materials have found extended applications in products serving human health needs such as sewage pipe systems and sanitary ware. In restorative dentistry the classical silicate ceramics have been used widely. The systematic and detailed evaluation of ceramics as possible implant materials did not begin, however, until the 1960's, after metals and plastics had been in use for several decades (Hulbert, Klawitter, and Bowman, 1973). The purity and strength of different ceramics were significantly improved during this time. New and favorable material properties of some ceramics, such as high wear resistance and low friction, were also recognized. Furthermore, surprising features in biologic environments were discovered, ranging from an almost complete inertness for some materials to an active behavior that leads to bonding with the surrounding tissue or to degradation and conversion into bone.

From the huge number of ceramics available, only a few have been found suitable for implant purposes (Vincenzini, 1983). These include oxide ceramics, ceramics of calcium phosphate salts, some glass ceramics, and certain modifications of carbon. The fabrication of oxide and calcium phosphate ceramics usually involves the transformation of a shaped agglomeration of powder particles into a polycrystalline solid by solid-state reactions (mostly diffusion), which bond the particles together without melting (Wang, 1976). The powders are shaped by compaction and transformed by heat treatment at temperatures between 700° and 2000°C. This transformation process is called firing or sintering. The fabrication of glass ceramics may include liquid-phase sintering. The carbon ceramics require less generic methods for their fabrication.

As far as structure is concerned ceramics are dramatically different from metals and plastics (Heimke, 1986). Solid compounds are generally divided according to their bonding into two types: homopolar and heteropolar. In the homopolar bond, the valence electrons are shared with no close localization at one or the other of the atoms. In heteropolar compounds, the valence electrons are rather clearly bound to one or the other of the atoms, rendering them markedly ionic. In metals (homopolar) the valence electrons are freely moving and are not associated with the bond between any particular pairs of atoms. These freely moving electrons (the electron gas) are an essential feature controlling most basic properties of metals. In ceramics (heteropolar) the ionic nature of the bond is predominant. This implies that ceramics always contain more than one kind of atom, carbon being the only exception.

The typical properties of ceramic materials are closely related to the strong localization of electrical charges to the crystal lattice entities, the ions, and the necessity of maintaining electrical neutrality within the unit crystal. Because of the high binding forces in the ionic crystals, the deformation per unit force is relatively small. As a result, ceramics maintain their shape and dimension up to the breaking point, a property known as brittleness. The deformation available to be measured is often so little as to make measurements of tensile and bending strengths impractical, and compression strengths are more commonly reported. Also, because of their higher binding energies, ceramics may have higher ultimate strengths than metals, if dislocations, flaws, and microcracks can be avoided during fabrication. Unfortunately, microcracks are difficult to avoid in polycrystalline materials. In metals a defect or dislocation in the crystal lattice can be moved to an area of lower stress by the plasticity of its atoms. The ionic arrangements in ceramics reduce the mobility of any dislocation, leading to stress concentration around the microfracture and susceptibility to failure. The strength of ceramics is thus controlled by flaws present in the material (Soltesz and Richter, 1984).

The biologic properties of the ceramic materials range from nearly inert to bioactive. The dense alumina and carbon ceramics undergo a minimal alteration of the implant surface. A thin fibrous capsule only several cell layers in depth forms against the surface of these nearly inert materials. In many cases under load-bearing conditions the presence of a fibrous capsule eventually leads to loosening. Efforts to solve the problem of interfacial fixation of implants led to the development of surface-active biomaterials. While the calcium phosphate ceramics have a naturally active surface that bonds to bone, this property can be conferred upon ceramics called bioactive glass ceramics.

A novel feature of some ceramics is the ability to fabricate pores for tissue ingrowth and even subsequent replacement if the implant is resorbable. These pores, called macropores, must be 40 microns or greater for fibrous tissue ingrowth and 100 microns or greater for bone ingrowth (Hulbert and associates, 1972). If ingrowth is to be complete, the implant pores must be interconnected or the implant must rapidly resorb in front of the advancing ingrowth of tissue. Although this is not yet well understood, it appears that implant resorption is in part a function of its microporosity. Micropores are spaces left when powder particles are not completely joined together after sintering (Peelen and associates, 1977). Since particles have sizes on the order of microns, micropores have the same size. The mechanism of resorption of microporous materials presumably consists of extracellular fluid dissolution of necks between sintered particles and intracellular digestion of the isolated particles. Materials containing less than 5 per cent micropores are arbitrarily considered dense and have demonstrated minimal resorption. It should be noted that implant design may treat tissue ingrowth and degradation independently. It is possible for a material to be both dense and macroporous, or both microporous and macroporous.

Hydroxyapatite

Apatites consist of a large family of solids with a range of solid solutions due to the variety of ionic substitutions that are possible (Van Raemdonck, Ducheyne, and De Meester, 1984). Among the apatites, calcium hydroxyapatite ($Ca_{10}[PO4]_6[OH]_2$) has been of major interest because its crystals, the inorganic constituent of osseous and dental tissues, can be man-made. Synthetic hydroxyapatite is composed of 39.9 wt per cent Ca, 18.5 per cent P, and 3.4 per cent OH with a Ca:P ratio of 1.67. Biologic hydroxyapatite differs by the presence of small amounts of CO_3, Mg, and Na and trace amounts of F and Cl (Jaffe, 1972).

Hydroxyapatite is generally fabricated in an aqueous solution. Whenever a powder with a Ca:P ratio of 1.5 to 1.7 is sintered in a water-containing atmosphere at temperatures up to 1100° to 1300°C, an end product that is crystallographically apatitic is the result (de Groot, 1981). Transformation of carbonates into apatites has also been achieved by hydrothermal exchange reaction, leading to the use of invertebrate marine skeletons as implant precursors (White and associates, 1975). In the absence of water, hydroxyapatite can be fabricated by solid-state diffusion or precipitated from a melt.

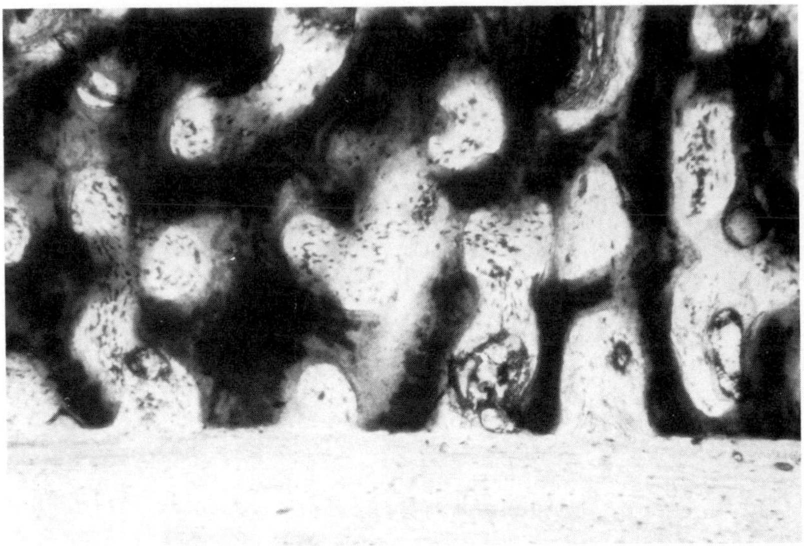

Figure 20–10. Microporous hydroxyapatite containing interconnected macropores after 30 weeks on top of rat calvarial bone. Note that the ingrowth of bone extends through the width of the implant. ×4.

All these manufacturing methods require careful control to maintain the purity of the hydroxyapatite material.

Depending on the preparation and sintering conditions and the presence of porosity, a wide range of mechanical properties is obtained. Dense hydroxyapatites demonstrate the highest compressive strengths with values around 400 MPa (Akao, Aoki, and Kato, 1981). Although hydroxyapatite implants, especially in their dense form, appear to be adequate in strength, the unavoidable presence of dislocations and microcracks limits their use to non–load-bearing applications. Load sharing, by bone ingrowth into porous forms of hydroxyapatite implants, represents a promising method of recruiting biologic assistance in the attainment of greater tensile strength (Holmes, 1979). To confer the benefits of bioactivity on traditional load-bearing materials, composites of hydroxyapatite and metals have been fabricated (Ducheyne and associates, 1980). The proclivity for bone ingrowth (Fig. 20–10) and bone bonding (Fig. 20–11) characterizes the biologic properties of hydroxyapatite ceramics.

Tricalcium Phosphate

Although the main mineral constituent of hard tissue is calcium hydroxyapatite, a variety of other calcium phosphates are present either in early development or in later

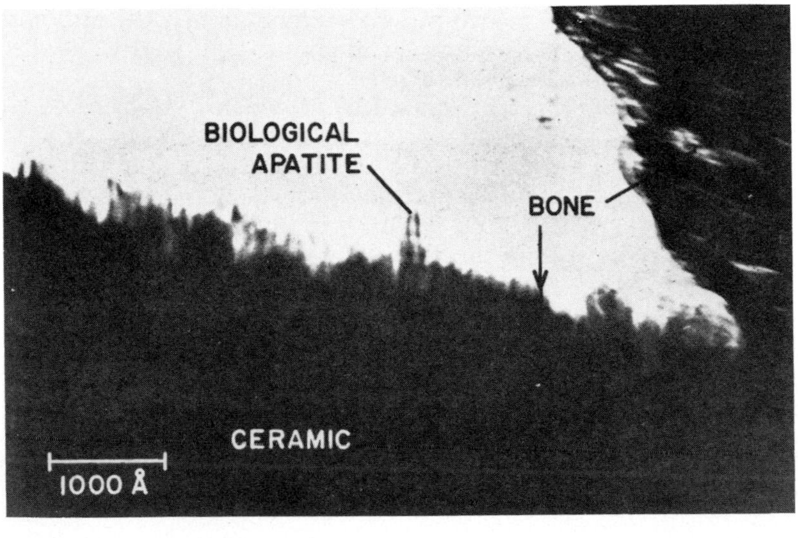

Figure 20–11. Transmission electron micrograph of bone-dense hydroxyapatite interface after six months in a canine femur. Ion beam micromilling demonstrates bonding of bone to the implant. ×50,000. (From Jarcho, M., Kay, J.F., Gumaer, K.I., Doremus, R.H., and Drobeck, H.P.: Tissue, cellular and subcellular events at a bone-ceramic hydroxylapatite interface. J. Bioeng., *1*:79, 1977. Reproduced with permission. Copyright 1977, Pergamon Journals, Ltd.)

stages of hard tissue maturation. Included in the early development is an amorphous calcium phosphate with a formula approaching $Ca_3(PO4)_2$. Research efforts to augment human bone have focused on this material.

Fully precipitated tricalcium phosphate is amorphous with an apatitic lattice containing defects. When compacted and fired under proper conditions, both dense and microporous materials have been produced (Cameron, MacNab, and Pilliar, 1977; Rootare and Craig, 1978). Most tricalcium phosphate materials have been fabricated with macropores. The most widely used technique consists of mixing the calcium phosphate powder with appropriately sized organic powders such as cellulose or naphthalene. These organic powders have a lower burning temperature than the sintering temperature. The evaporation of the organic materials leaves macropores that are preserved during sintering. The macropores substantially reduce the mechanical properties of the materials, and compressive strengths are typically 20,000 to 70,000 Pa.

The tricalcium phosphate materials are generally considered more resorbable. Macropores, and especially micropores, dramatically increase the specific surface area of these materials. Surface ions are relatively weakly held compared with the interior ions and are therefore more soluble. The chemical reactivity of solids also varies inversely with their crystalline perfection and crystal dimension. Thus, the greater number of dislocations and crystal defects in these materials may affect the diffusion and dissolution phenomena (Chuong, 1973). Because of this ability to resorb, wound healing may be prolonged until resorption is complete.

Glass

The most thoroughly studied of the bioactive glasses and glass ceramics is composed of 45 wt per cent SiO_2, 24.5 per cent CaO, 24.5 per cent Na_2O, and 6 per cent P_2O_5 (Hench and Clark, 1982). Liquid-phase melting and casting is used to produce the glasses with surface active silica, calcium, and phosphate groups. When exposed to physiologic solutions, a calcium-phosphate rich gel forms on the implant surface that appears to nucleate hydroxyapatite crystals and lead to chemical bonding with bone (Hench, 1981). Because of the relatively low intrinsic strength of this class of materials, they are generally used as composites or coatings on such materials as stainless steel, Vitallium, and dense alumina (Greenspan and Hench, 1976). The strength of the composite is then primarily dependent on the physical properties of the substrate, while the surface response to the biologic environment is controlled by the chemical activity of the coating (Fig. 20–12).

Oxide

Oxide ceramics are known by the metals from which they are formed. The crystal

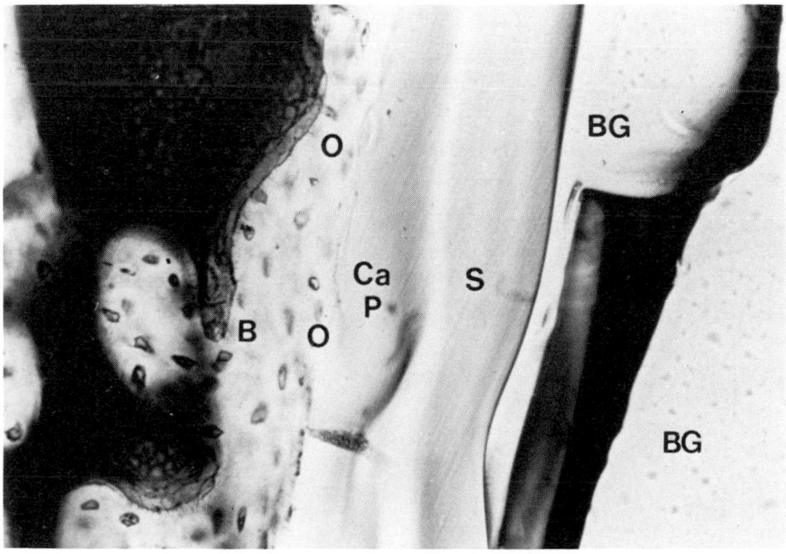

Figure 20–12. Transmitted light micrograph of a glass ceramic implant in a rat tibia after one month, showing bone bonded to the implant. BG = bulk implant; S = silica-rich layer; CaP = calcium phosphate–rich layer; O = osteocytes; B = bone. (From Hench, L.L., and Clark, A.E.: Adhesion to bone. *In* Williams, D.F. (Ed.): Biocompatibility of Orthopedic Implants. Vol. II. Boca Raton, CRC Press, 1982. Reprinted with permission. Copyright The Chemical Rubber Co., CRC Press, Inc.)

structures of these ceramics are determined by a closely packed arrangement of the oxygen ions, with the metal ions distributed in the interstices between the oxygen atoms (Heimke, 1986). The main representative of the oxide ceramics in medical implants is alumina (Al_2O_3). The main attraction of alumina is its corrosion resistance, low wear resistance, and coefficient of friction when used in joint applications (Griss and Heimke, 1981). The material is fabricated from highly purified Al_2O_3 by isostatic pressing and subsequent firing at 1500° to 1700°C. Compressive strengths of 500 MPa are readily achieved with these materials. Close contact may form between bone and the surface of these inert alumina materials, especially in the complete absence of motion (Fig. 20–13).

Carbon

The carbons used in implant materials represent offspring of nuclear development programs (Bokros, 1964). In the late 1950's the search for a durable, long-lived fuel for use in high temperature graphite nuclear reactors led to the discovery of a new family of carbon structures. Applications as implant materials followed the discovery that these carbons were strong, tough, and highly inert to tissues, including blood. All the carbons used in implants have a quasicrystalline turbostratic structure (Bokros, 1969). In the common graphite crystal a three-dimensional hexagonal lattice is formed by stacking layers of atoms in a parallel and regular sequence. In turbostratic structures the stacking is completely haphazard. The strong covalent bonding of atoms within layers is responsible for the high strength of these structures. The weak Van der Waals–type bonding between the randomly oriented layers is responsible for the large deformations that can be elastically absorbed by these materials.

The extremely high melting temperature of carbon makes it quite difficult to fabricate (Haubold, Shim, and Bokros, 1981). It is not possible to produce slabs of turbostratic carbon from which implants can be machined. Instead, it is necessary to form the material by the pyrolysis of hydrocarbons or by depositing carbon atoms in a vacuum. Compressive strengths range from 170 MPa for vitreous or glassy carbon to over 500 MPa for silicon-alloyed pyrolytic carbon. The elastic modulus or stiffness of carbon falls in the range of 21 to 26 GPa and closely approximates that of bone. This is relevant because materials joined with tissues of like stiffness carry loads with minimal concentration of stresses at the interface, and therefore have less propensity for loosening. These biomechanical properties are useful in the design of carbon dental implants and carbon finger joints (Hulbert and associates, 1975). In braided form, carbon fibers have been studied as scaffolds for the regeneration of tendons and ligaments (Wolter and associates, 1977). Carbon fiber has also been composited with polytetrafluoroethylene (Homsy, 1981) and polylactide (Parsons, Alexander, and Weiss, 1983) to serve as a scaffold for connective tissue ingrowth in reconstructive surgery (Fig. 20–14).

SUTURE MATERIALS

The oldest of the implant materials, sutures are referenced in ancient Egyptian writings

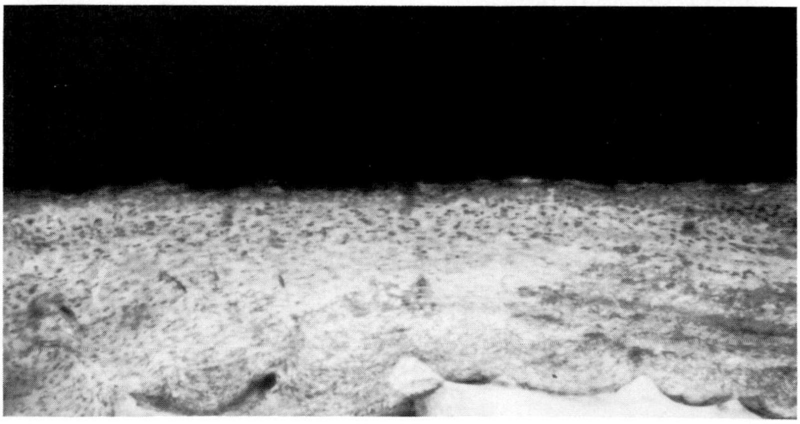

Figure 20–13. Dense alumina implant placed against a rat calvarial bone for 30 weeks appears in contact with the bone. Under higher magnification a thin layer of cells is present at the boundary. ×4.

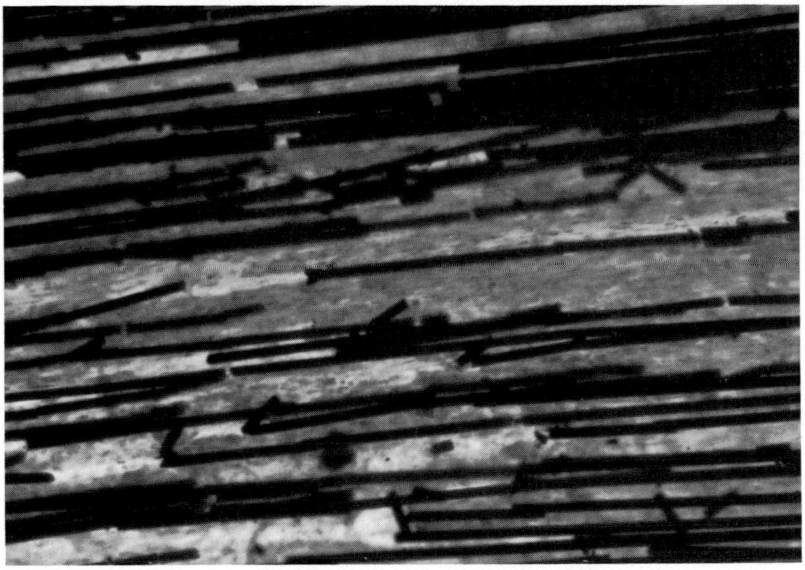

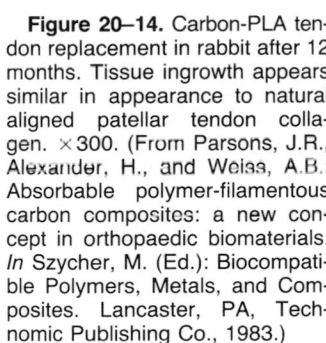

Figure 20–14. Carbon-PLA tendon replacement in rabbit after 12 months. Tissue ingrowth appears similar in appearance to natural aligned patellar tendon collagen. ×300. (From Parsons, J.R., Alexander, H., and Weiss, A.B.: Absorbable polymer-filamentous carbon composites: a new concept in orthopaedic biomaterials. *In* Szycher, M. (Ed.): Biocompatible Polymers, Metals, and Composites. Lancaster, PA, Technomic Publishing Co., 1983.)

(Majno, 1975). In 600 B.C. Suśrutaś' Samhita describes sutures made from ligaments, horsehair, leather, and vegetable fibers. The advances of polymer chemistry have led to synthetic sutures that are in many ways superior to the older natural polymeric materials. These natural and synthetic polymeric materials continue to be dominant, the only nonpolymeric suture material remaining in common use being stainless steel. The polymeric materials used in suture fabrication are conventionally classified as absorbable or nonabsorbable. Several of these materials are selected to represent the available diversity of mechanical and biologic properties (Table 20–7).

Protein

Catgut and regenerated collagen are resorbable materials of natural origin. Catgut is derived from the submucosa of sheep intestines and the serosa of beef intestines (Peacock, 1984). The jejunum and ileum of these animals are slit into longitudinal ribbons. The mucosa, muscularis, and other unwanted layers are removed by a combination of mechanical and chemical treatments. The cleaned ribbons are treated with a dilute solution of formaldehyde, which blocks hydroxyl and amino groups on the collagen polymer, thus increasing its strength and resistance to enzymatic attack in the body. Depending on the size of suture desired, a number of ribbons or strips are twisted together, dried under tension on frames, and polished to a uniform diameter. If more resistance to resorption is desired, an additional treatment with basic chromium salts is given.

Reconstituted collagen sutures are prepared by dissolving bovine deep flexor tendon in cyanoacetic acid. The collagen dispersion, a viscous gel, is then extruded through a

Table 20–7. Mechanical Properties of Polymeric Suture Materials

Material	Tensile Strength* (MPa)	Tensile Strength† (MPa)	Elongation To Break (%)	Elastic Modulus (GPa)
Catgut	310–380	110–210	15–35	2.4
Silk	370–570	240–290	9–31	8.4–12.9
Poly(glycolic acid)	760–920	310–590	18–25	7–14
Poly(glycolide-lactide)	570–910	300–400	18–25	7–14
Poly(ethylene terephthalate)	510–1060	300–390	8–42	1.2–6.5
Poly(amide) nylon 6	460–710	300–330	17–65	1.8–4.5
Poly(propylene)	410–460	280–320	24–62	2.2–6.9

*Straight pull breaking strength.
†Knot pull breaking strength.

spinneret into an acetone bath and formed into a ribbon. The ribbon is treated with formaldehyde, twisted, stretched, and dried in a manner similar to the way catgut is treated. The strengths of these collagen polymers typically drop to 25 per cent or less of their original values after 15 days in the body (Casey and Lewis, 1986). Complete absorption may require two to eight months. The mechanism by which collagen sutures degrade is one of lysozomal enzyme cleavage (Salthouse, Williams, and Willigan, 1969).

Silk is generally categorized as a nonresorbable protein material. However, it may gradually disappear and should be classed as a slowly absorbable suture material. A natural product of the silkworm cocoon, silk consists of 95 per cent proteins and 5 per cent wax, fats, and salts. In contrast to wool and other keratins, silk does not include sulfur-containing amino acid residues such as cystine, and is composed mainly of glycine, alanine, and serine residues with relatively small amounts of the more bulky side chains (Chu, 1983). To produce a cocoon for a future chrysalis, the silkworm secretes the protein substance through its spinneret, a small opening under its jaws. The liquid substance, called fibroin, polymerizes immediately upon exposure to the air. With a bending motion the filament is spun around the worm in the form of a figure of eight and is held together with sericin, a silk glue. At this point the cocoon is harvested and the chrysalis is suffocated. The sericin is softened by hot immersions, which allows unwinding of the filament in one continuous thread. The sericin coating is further removed from the natural silk, and the filaments are braided or twisted to form sutures. Silk sutures gradually lose all strength after two years in vivo (Casey and Lewis, 1986). Silk is also the most reactive of the suture materials, evoking a more extensive inflammatory response from polymorphonuclear cells, lymphocytes, and macrophages (Salthouse, 1983).

Polyester

Polymers with absorbable and nonabsorbable properties have been synthesized from polyester compounds. The search for synthetic biodegradable alternatives to collagen began with an attempt to synthesize a simplified collagen structure from the common amino acid residues glycine and proline. Polyglycine and polyproline have been synthesized, but they were not biodegradable. Aliphatic polyesters, however, were recognized to be particularly sensitive to hydrolysis. Advantage has been taken of the fact that aliphatic polyesters are hydrolytically unstable in the cases of polyglycolic acid (PGA) and polylactic acid (PLA).

PGA is synthesized by the ring-opening polymerization of glycolide at 220°C, using a tin catalyst (Gilding, 1981a) (see the bottom of this page).

The symmetry of the PGA leads to a highly crystalline polymer, and its normal crystallinity in suture fibers is 50 per cent. PGA fibers are prepared by melt-extrusion and drawing. PGA is the most hydrophilic of all the polyesters, and hydrolysis of the ester bond takes place preferentially in the amorphous phase of the material within two to three days after placement in vivo. The tensile strength is reduced to zero in 28 to 32 days, although mass loss does not begin until 21 days. Complete mass loss occurs over an 80 day period.

The next homologue in the series, PLA, may be prepared in the same manner as PGA, using lactide at 180° to 200°C (Gilding, 1981a) (see the top of p. 721).

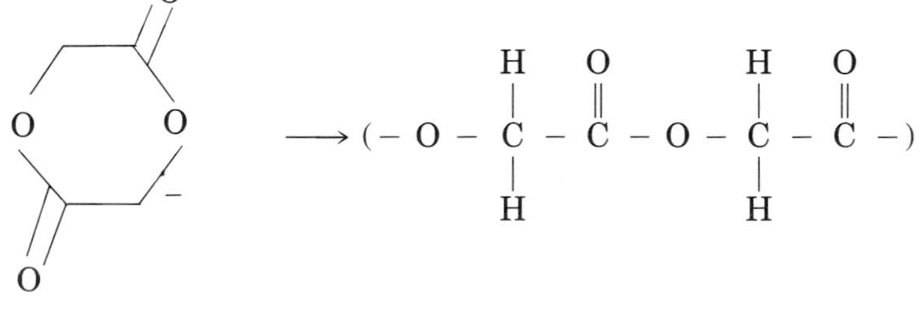

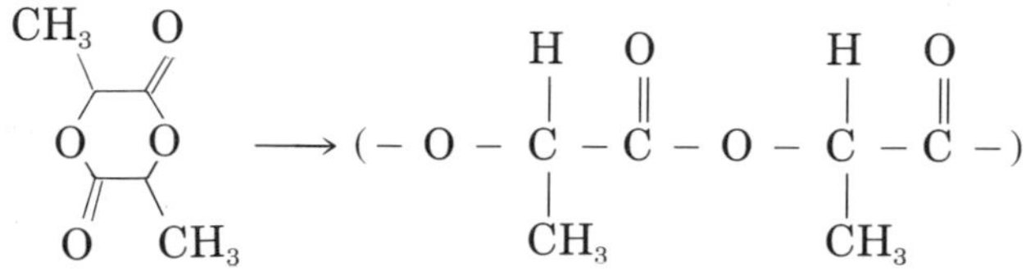

The pendant methyl group has two effects on biodegradation kinetics. First, it decreases the hydrophilicity and lowers the water uptake of the molecule to about 2 per cent. Second, it provides a significant steric hindrance to the hydrolysis reaction. As a result the rate of degradation is reduced dramatically and only a 10 per cent mass loss occurs over a six month implantation period. To achieve properties of both PGA and PLA polymers, a copolymer of glycolide (90 per cent) and lactide (10 per cent) is being used as a suture material.

The aromatic polyester polyethylene terephthalate (PET) has been discussed earlier. Because of the increased hydrophobicity of the aromatic moieties, the aromatic polyesters are less susceptible to hydrolysis (Gilding, 1981b). The increased crystallinity due to the increased symmetry of the chain, and the increased steric hindrance to hydrolytic attack associated with the shape of the aromatic moiety, confer additional stability on the polyester chain. All these factors led to PET being a valuable fiber in the fabrication of material for arteries, patches, and suture material when biodegradation is not desirable.

Polyamide and Polyolefin

Occupying a role of historical importance, the polyamide known generically as nylon was the first commercial polymer, made initially in the 1930's. Polyamides are polymers that have recurring amide groups as part of their molecular chains. The polyamides may be prepared by several different types of polymerization (Refojo, 1983). Opening of a lactam ring is used to form nylon 6, and reaction of a diamine with a dicarboxylic acid is used in forming nylon 66. A lactam of aminocaproic acid, caprolactam, undergoes a condensation polymerization when catalyzed at 240° to 280°C (see the bottom of this page).

The polyamide fibers are fabricated using melt-extrusion and drawing, as previously described (Casey and Lewis, 1986). Because some hydrolysis of the amide groups occurs over time, sutures made from these fibers lose strength in vivo, reaching a 25 per cent loss after two years.

Polypropylene, a member of the polyolefin group, has been previously discussed. A feature of its polymerization methods is control over the orientation of the monomer molecules as they join the chain. All the methyl groups may be made to lie on the same side (isotactic) or their placement may be alternated (syndiotactic) (see the top of p. 722).

Other arrangements are possible, including a random (atactic) form (Hastings, 1981). Of the different forms, isotactic polypropylene is the most regular (and hence most crystalline) structure because all its methyl groups are arranged along one side of the molecule. The

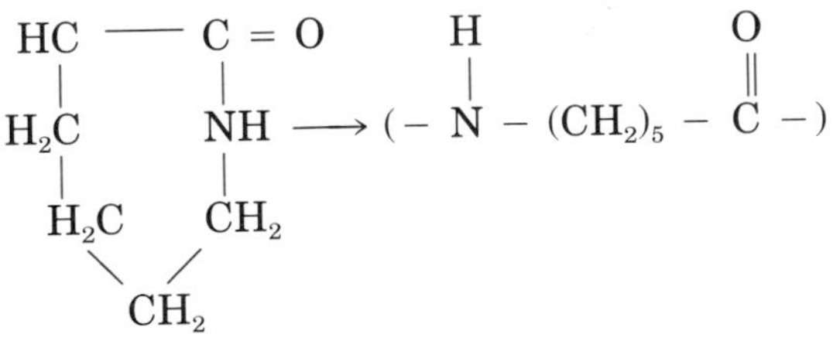

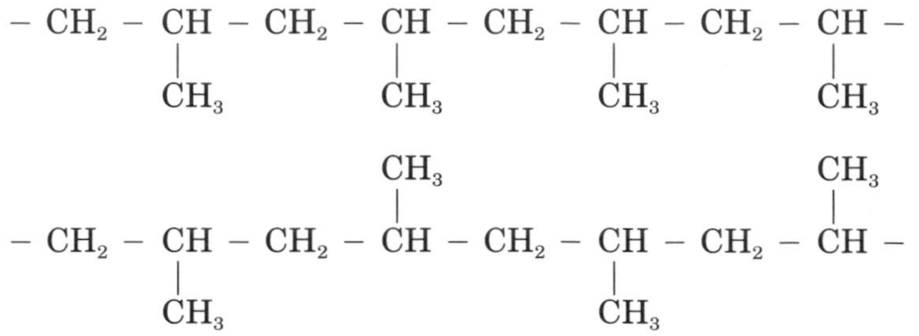

$$- CH_2 - CH - CH_2 - CH - CH_2 - CH - CH_2 - CH - \text{ Isotactic}$$

$$\qquad\quad |\qquad\qquad |\qquad\qquad |\qquad\qquad |$$

$$\qquad\quad CH_3\qquad\quad CH_3\qquad\quad CH_3\qquad\quad CH_3$$

$$\qquad\qquad\qquad\quad CH_3\qquad\qquad\qquad\qquad CH_3$$

$$\qquad\qquad\qquad\quad |\qquad\qquad\qquad\qquad |$$

$$- CH_2 - CH - CH_2 - CH - CH_2 - CH - CH_2 - CH - \text{ Syndiotactic}$$

$$\qquad\quad |\qquad\qquad\qquad\qquad\qquad |$$

$$\qquad\quad CH_3\qquad\qquad\qquad\qquad CH_3$$

effect of tacticity is also exerted through the degree of interchain hydrogen bonding that can be brought into play. This has been shown to be particularly important during the drawing and annealing process. Because of its molecular stereoregularity and the absence of any hydrolyzable linkage, polypropylene is neither weakened nor resorbed by the action of physiologic fluids or tissue enzymes (Casey and Lewis, 1986). These structural characteristics account for the finding that polypropylene is among the least histologically reactive of the suture materials (Fig. 20–15).

DRESSING MATERIALS

Dressing materials are not classically considered implant materials, since they are only temporarily applied to a wound surface until healing or skin grafting takes place. However, because of their contact with fluids, cells, and tissues, these materials must have many of the same properties as implant materials. Most of the materials used in synthetic wound dressings have previously been described in this chapter. While all dressings must adhere to the wound and keep it moist, they may basically deal with excess exudate either by absorbing it or by allowing vapor transport through the dressing. Absorption may include both fluid and macromolecular components of exudate, whereas vapor transport may be limited to fluid and may result in macromolecular concentration.

The first strategy for fluid management, absorption into the dressing, has utilized the properties of hydrogels. Hydrogels are polymeric chains with low crosslinking density, high chain flexibility, and high free volume that are capable of strong interactions with H_2O (Ratner, 1981). When a hydrogel polymer is placed in water, there is an osmotic driving force for the water to enter the water-

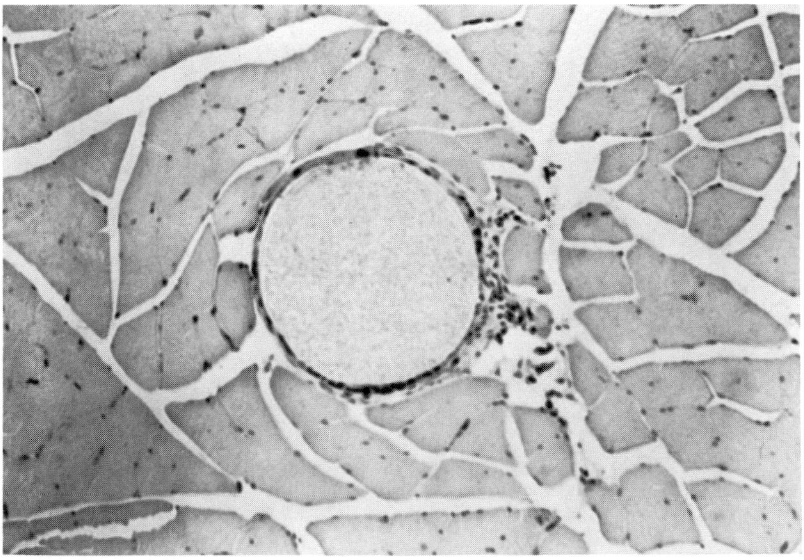

Figure 20–15. Polypropylene suture in rat gluteal muscle after 90 days. Only a thin collagen capsule surrounds the suture. ×110. (From Salthouse, T.N.: Tissue response to sutures. *In* Rubin, L. (Ed.): Biomaterials in Reconstructive Surgery. St. Louis, C.V. Mosby Company, 1983. Courtesy of Ethicon, Inc., Somerville, NJ 08876.)

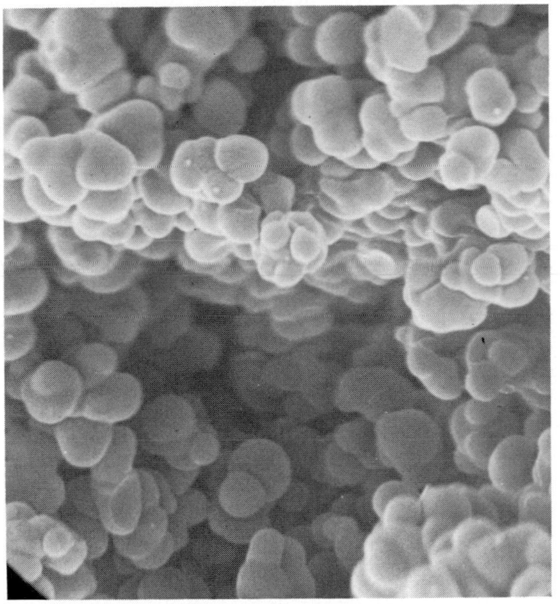

Figure 20–16. Scanning electron micrograph of PHEMA crosslinked hydrogel. The low crosslinking density, high chain flexibility, and high free volume of these polymeric chains permit them to expand and absorb a large amount of water. (From Ratner, B.D.: Biomedical applications of hydrogels: review and critical appraisal. *In* Williams, D.F. (Ed.): Biocompatibility of Clinical Implant Materials. Vol. II. Boca Raton, CRC Press, 1981. Reprinted with permission. Copyright The Chemical Rubber Co., CRC Press, Inc.)

free region within the polymer. Strong positive interactions between chemical structures on the polymer and the water (hydrogen bonding) further increase the driving force for swelling. As water enters and expands the hydrogel, the polymer chains become extended and exert a resistive force. When the osmotic force driving water into the system is balanced by the force exerted by the polymer chains in resisting expansion, the equilibrium degree of swelling has been achieved and no further water or fluid is absorbed. A representative of this class of materials is polyhydroxyethylmethacrylate (PHEMA) (Fig. 20–16). This polymer is usually obtained by free radical copolymerization of hydroxyethylmethacrylate with a difunctional monomer such as ethylenedimethacrylate (Migliaresi and associates, 1981). The resulting polymer has a glassy transition temperature of $-50°C$ and is therefore rubbery and soft at physiologic temperatures. Its equilibrium water content of 40 per cent accounts for the ability to absorb substantial amounts of fluid in a wound dressing. As with most hydrogels, PHEMA has a low mechanical strength and must be bonded to a film of mechanically stronger polymer such as silicone or polyurethane for practical use.

An example of use of transport for fluid management is a dressing made from silicone, nylon, and collagen. In this dressing a knitted nylon fabric is mechanically bonded to a thin silicone film and coated with collagen (Woodroof, 1984). The silicone membrane is 6 μm thick and the nylon fibers are 360 μm in diameter (Fig. 20–17). Thus, only a small portion of a nylon fiber is embedded in the silicone film, the remainder forming a mesh or series of loops for contact with the wound surface. The collagenous peptides, of porcine origin, are covalently bonded to both

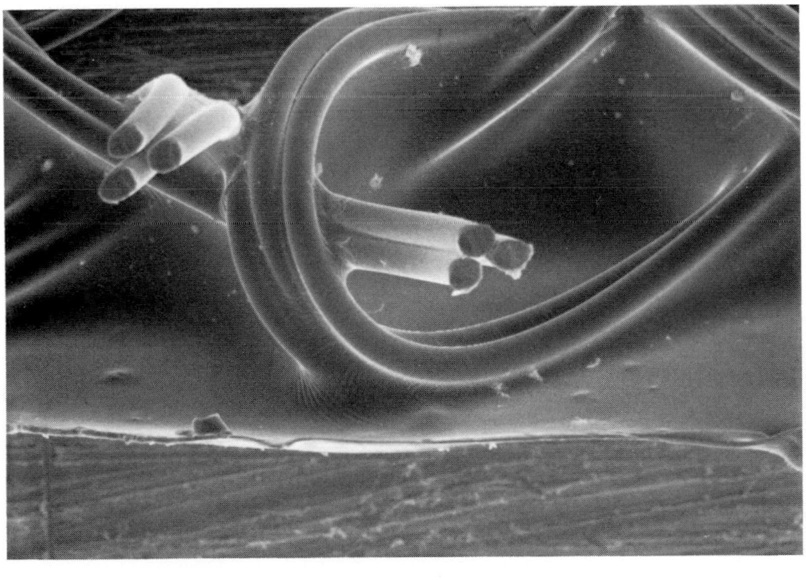

Figure 20–17. Scanning electron micrograph of a dressing composed of a nylon fabric–silicone rubber composite. (From Woodroof, A.E.: Biobrane, a biosynthetic skin prosthesis. *In* Wise, D.L. (Ed.): Burn Wound Coverings. Vol. II. Boca Raton, CRC Press, 1983. Reprinted with permission. Copyright The Chemical Rubber Co., CRC Press, Inc.)

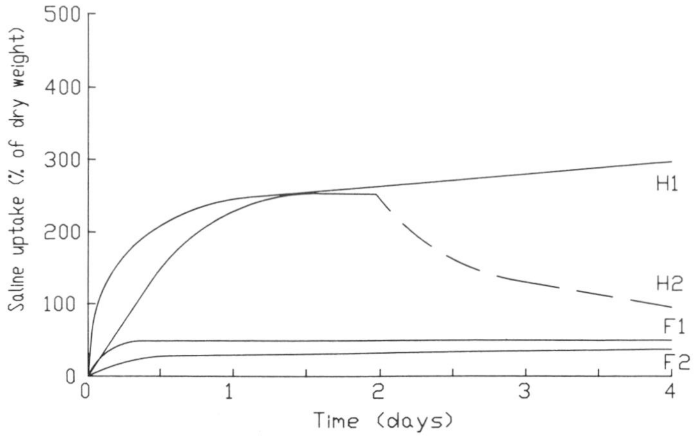

Figure 20–18. Moisture absorption of two hydrogel (H1, H2) and two film (F1, F2) dressings. Hydrogels manage excess exudate by absorbing it. After two days the hydrogel coating of H2 began to dissolve and enter the wound site. (From Cochran, J. H., Reed, A. M., and Schauer, M.A.: Physical characteristics of synthetic wound dressings: a comparison of physical properties and their clinical significance. In preparation.)

the silicone and nylon. The collagen coating maintains dressing adherence, the nylon mesh maintains surface moisture, and the permeable silicone film allows vapor transport of excess fluid. A less complex approach to vapor transport has been the simple use of a polyurethane film with either polyvinyl ether or polyacrylate-based, pressure-sensitive adhesive. The fluid absorption and fluid vapor transport of two hydrogel (occlusive) and two film (semiocclusive) dressings, plotted over time in Figures 20–18 and 20–19, clearly differentiate the two mechanisms by which they function (Cochran and Reed, 1988).

THE FUTURE

Over the past 50 years implants have changed from being rarely and seldom used to becoming safe and routinely used components of the surgical armamentarium. The development of a dialogue between materials and biologic scientists has resulted in recognition of the unique requirements of biomaterials. This fruitful collaboration has produced an array of permanent and resorbable substitute materials only dreamed of a generation ago. It would thus seem likely that the dreams of today's scientists represent the future of alloplastic implant materials. Few goals are as enticing to the plastic surgeon as that of regeneration, and materials scientists are increasingly directing their skills to help achieve this objective.

In the course of evolution the more advanced animals appear to have given up much of their spontaneous regenerative capacity in return for specialization. Complex organs such as the kidney and liver, when liquefied by bacterial infections, can be healed only with scar tissue. However, it is often observed that if only the parenchyma of these organs are destroyed, as in some viral infections, the remaining intact stroma enables a remarkable degree of regeneration to take place. Guided regeneration through

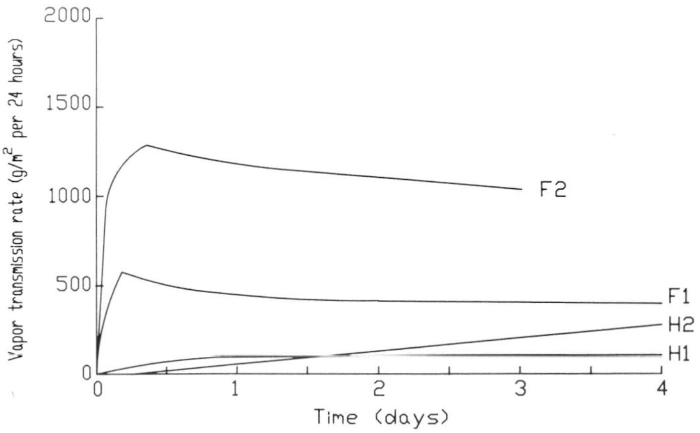

Figure 20–19. Moisture vapor transmission rates for two hydrogel (H1, H2) and two film (F1, F2) dressings. Films manage excess exudate by means of their gaseous transport properties. After three days the water dish ran dry under film F2 owing to its high permeability. (From Cochran, J.H., Reed, A.M., and Schauer, M.A.: Physical characteristics of synthetic wound dressings: a comparison of physical properties and their clinical significance. In preparation.)

the use of surgically implanted lattice materials that serve as synthetic stroma would represent an incremental step toward the goal of regeneration. Several areas of implant investigation illustrate the rapidly evolving reality of this progress.

The stromal component of bone is the interstitial hard tissue within which the haversian systems, or osteons, are located. Nourished by haversian canals and canaliculi, populated by osteocytes within lacunae, and demarcated from osseous stromal support by cement lines, osteons are the parenchymal component of bone (Fig. 20–20). When cortical bone is used as a graft material, it is the osteons that are evacuated to leave a stroma into which parenchymal regeneration is guided (Fig. 20–21). An idealized cortical graft material would thus contain channels of osteonic diameter and channel wall fenestrations for interosteonic vascular communication (Fig. 20–22). Implant lattices, made of hydroxyapatite for its bioactive properties, have demonstrated a high degree of bone ingrowth in both cortical (Fig. 20–23) and cancellous (Fig. 20–24) configurations (Holmes, Bucholz, and Mooney, 1986, 1987). The prospect appears bright that future lattices will have more of the mechanical properties of stromal bone, will be seeded with osteoprogenitor cells, and will be impregnated with osteoinductive factors to allow further control of the regenerative process.

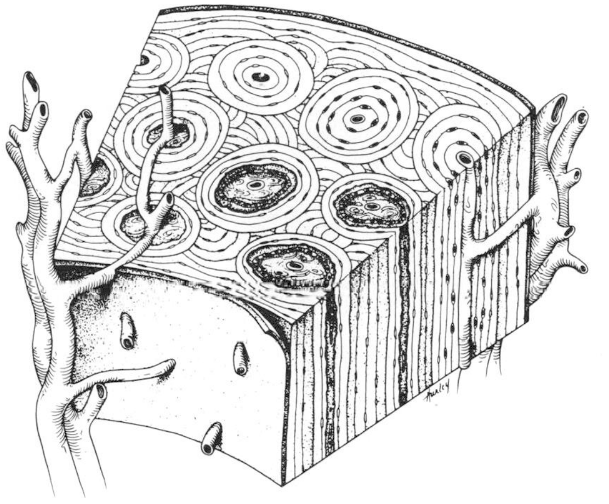

Figure 20–21. After grafting the devitalized osteons *(upper left)* are evacuated *(lower left)*. Osteoblastic apposition of new bone *(lower right)* results in regeneration of the osteons *(upper right)*.

The stromal component of skin is the dermal framework of collagen fibers within which the parenchymal components of fibroblasts, vessels, nerves, and skin appendages are located and upon which an epithelial barrier resides. After skin is grafted, regeneration is guided by the residual collagenous lattice and conduits of the dermis. Substan-

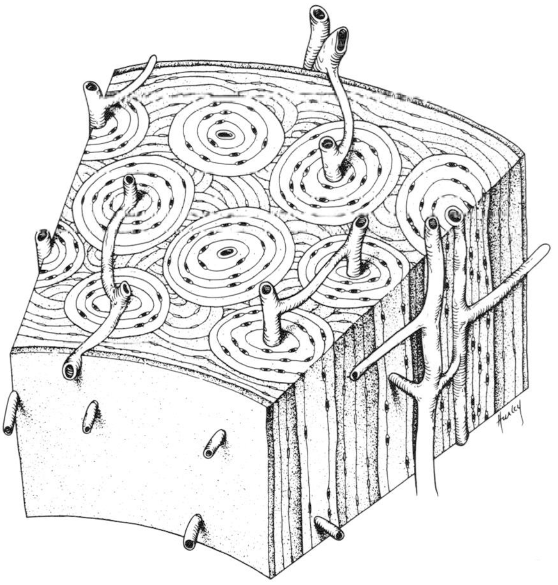

Figure 20–20. Osteons represent the living parenchymal component of bone and are sustained by a vascular network that interconnects through the stromal or interstitial supporting bone.

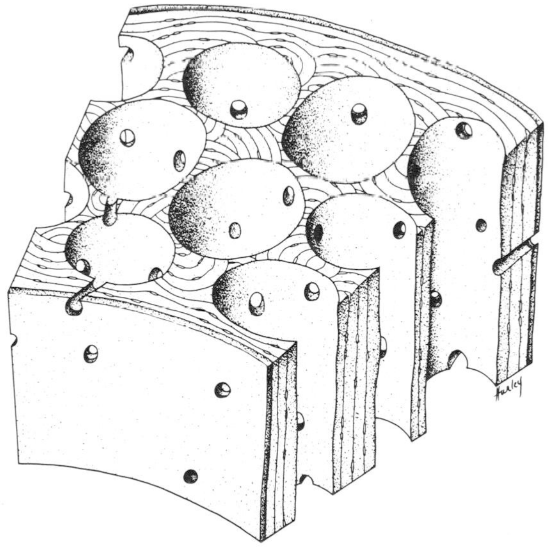

Figure 20–22. The requirements of a stromal framework for bone regeneration include the presence of channels of osteonic diameter and channel wall fenestrations for the interosteonic vascular network.

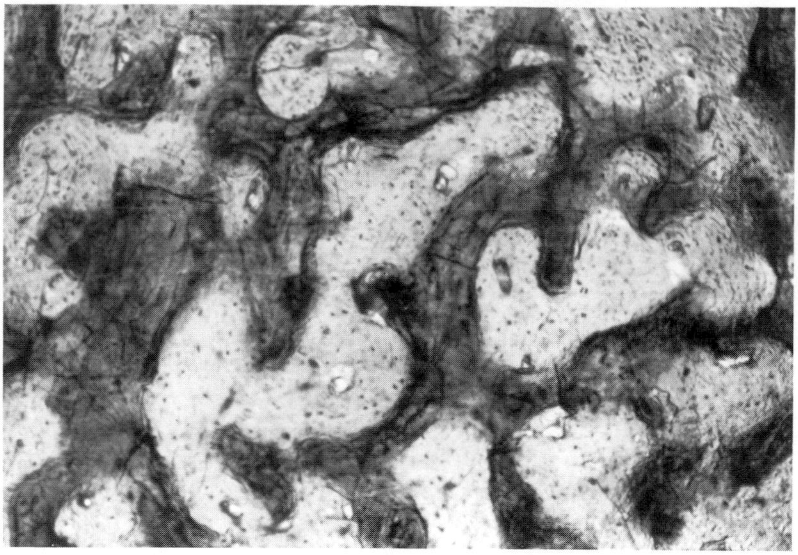

Figure 20–23. A macroporous hydroxyapatite implant with average pore diameters of 600 μm and pore interconnections of 260 μm demonstrates regeneration of trabeculae after six months in a canine tibial metaphysis. (From Holmes, R.E., Bucholz, R.W., and Mooney, V.: Porous hydroxyapatite as a bone graft substitute in metaphyseal defects: a histometric study. J. Bone Joint Surg., *68A*:904, 1986.)

tial replacement of fibroblastic, endothelial, and axonal elements occurs, usually without interruption of the passive diffusion of nutrients to the overlying epidermis. To achieve this success with biomaterials engineering, a bilayer membrane has been developed (Yannas and associates, 1984). The upper layer is a conventional silicone elastomer; the bottom layer is a highly porous, covalently cross-linked network of purified bovine collagen and glycosaminoglycans (GAG). The bottom layer acts as a lattice to guide and support the regeneration of neodermal tissue. The upper layer is eventually removed and replaced with a layer of epidermal cells. The ability of a neodermis to replace the synthetic dermal stroma and support the epidermal graft has been histologically demonstrated (Burke and associates, 1981). Recently, a one-stage approach has been demonstrated (Boyce, Christianson, and Hansbrough, 1988; Boyce and Hansbrough, 1988). Acellular sheets of collagen-GAG membranes stored in the dry state (Fig. 20–25) are rehydrated shortly before use. Human basal keratinocytes in log phase growth are then inoculated onto the dermal membrane and further incubated to epidermal confluence (Fig. 20–26). After one-stage transfer of the composite graft, fibrovascular ingrowth into the syn-

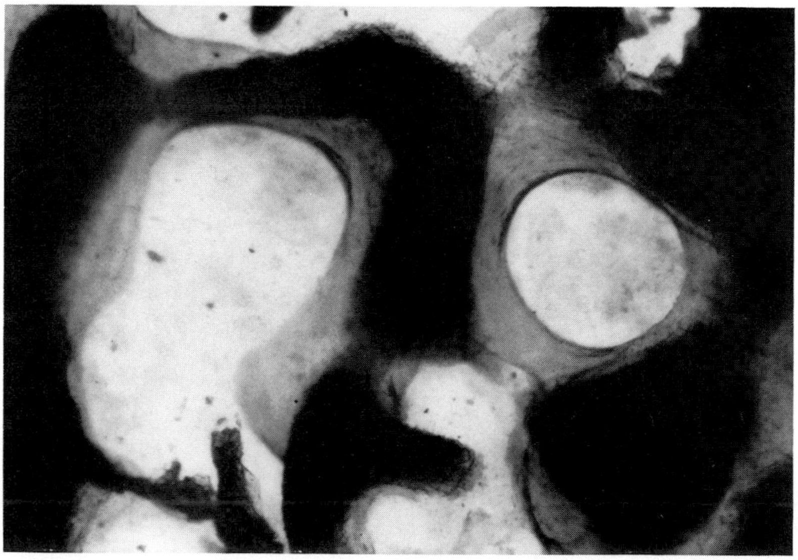

Figure 20–24. A macroporous hydroxyapatite implant with average pore diameters of 230 μm and pore interconnections of 190 μm demonstrates regeneration of osteons after 12 months in a canine radial diaphysis. (From Holmes, R.E., Bucholz, R. W., and Mooney, V.: Porous hydroxyapatite as a bone graft substitute in diaphyseal defects: a histometric study. J. Orthop. Res., *5*:114, 1987.)

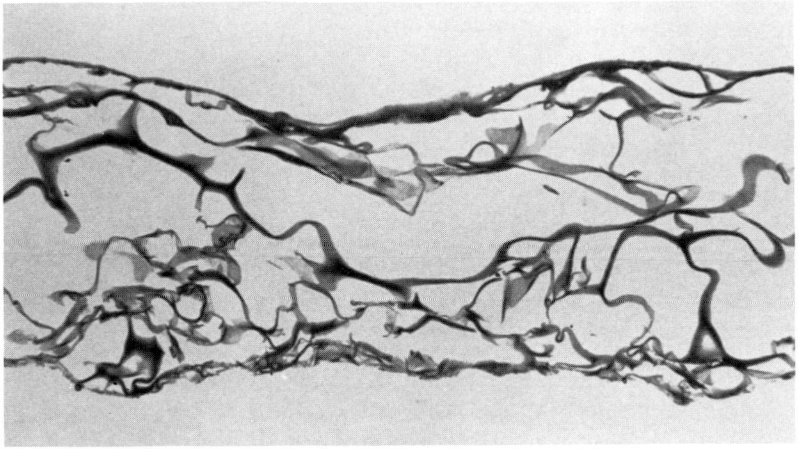

Figure 20–25. Photomicrograph of synthetic dermal membrane composed of collagen and glycosaminoglycan. (From Boyce, S.T., and Hansbrough, J.F.: Biological attachment, growth and differentiation of cultured human epidermal keratinocytes on a graftable collagen and chondroitin-6-sulfate substrate. Surgery, *103*:421, 1988.)

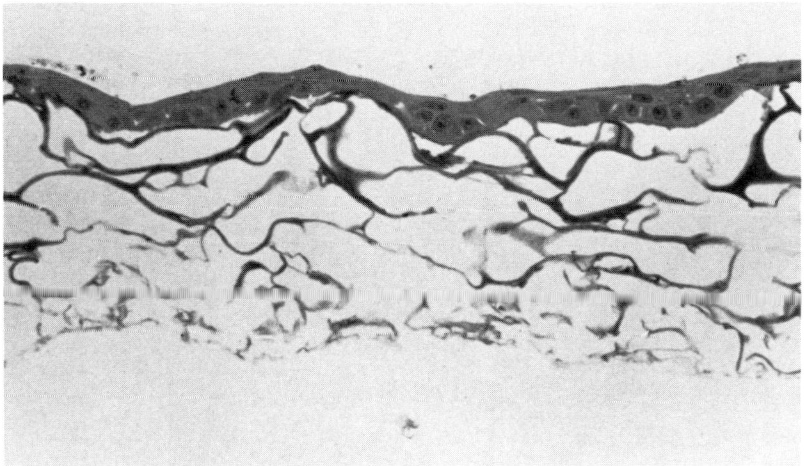

Figure 20–26. Cultured human keratinocytes have been inoculated onto the surface of a synthetic dermal membrane and cultured to confluence. (From Boyce, S.T., and Hansbrough, J.F.: Biological attachment, growth and differentiation of cultured human epidermal keratinocytes on a graftable collagen and chondroitin-6-sulfate substrate. Surgery, *103*:421, 1988.)

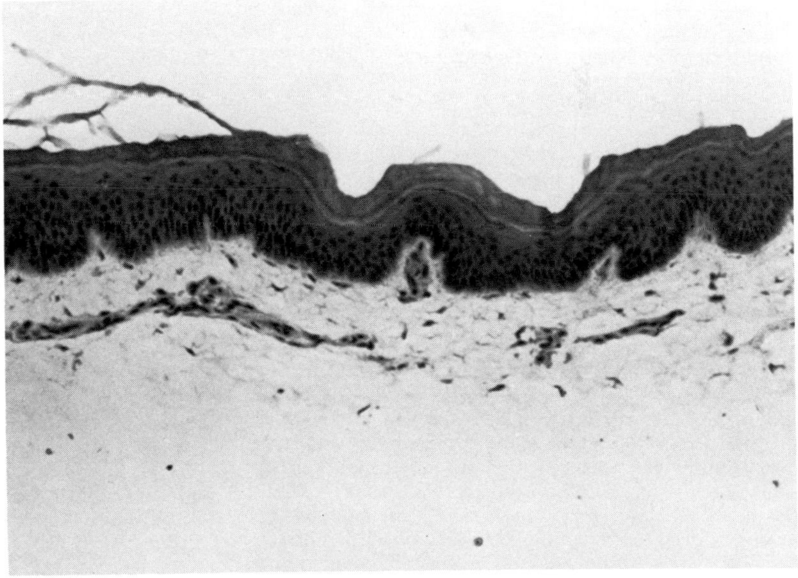

Figure 20–27. Dermal regeneration within the synthetic collagen-GAG framework provides support for the cultured epidermal cell layer after a one-stage grafting procedure. (From Boyce, S.T., and Hansbrough, J.F.: Biological attachment, growth and differentiation of cultured human epidermal keratinocytes on a graftable collagen and chondroitin-6-sulfate substrate. Surgery *103*:421, 1988.)

thetic dermal lattice yields a regenerated dermis supporting an epidermal lining (Fig. 20–27). It seems only a matter of time until seeding with other cell types, and impregnation of the implant with epidermal growth factor, fibroblast growth factor, angiogenic factor, and other factors still being studied, will allow further control over the regenerative process. The imaginative application of materials science to the regeneration of nerves, vessels, and tendons, coupled with the new discoveries of molecular engineering, promises similar advances in surgical management. It appears certain that in the future the use of implant materials will not only continue to parallel, but will increasingly merge with, the use of natural tissues.

REFERENCES

Akao, M., Aoki, H., and Kato, K.: Mechanical properties of sintered hydroxyapatite for prosthetic application. J. Mater. Sci., *16*:809, 1981.

ASTM: Annual Standards Book, Vol. 13.01, Medical Materials and Devices. Philadelphia, American Society for Testing and Materials, 1984.

Bapna, M. S., Lautenschlager, E. P., and Moser, J. B.: The influences of electrical potential and surface finish on the fatigue life of surgical implant materials. J. Biomed. Mater. Res., *9*:611, 1975.

Bensmann, G., Baumgart, F., and Haasters, J.: Application of memory alloy Ni-Ti as an implant material. Trans. Soc. Biomater., *4*:90, 1982.

Billmeyer, F. W.: Textbook of Polymer Science, 2nd Ed. New York, John Wiley & Sons, 1971.

Bischoff, F., and Bryson, G.: Carcinogenesis through solid state surfaces. Progr. Exp. Tumor. Res., *5*:85, 1964.

Blais, P.: Silicone breast implant: technological and physicochemical aspects. *In* Rubin, L. R. (Ed.): Biomaterials in Reconstructive Surgery. St. Louis, C. V. Mosby Company, 1983.

Bloch, B., and Hastings, G. W.: Plastics Materials in Surgery. 2nd Ed. Springfield, IL., Charles C Thomas, 1972.

Bokros, J. C.: Random pyrolytic carbon. Nature (Lond.), *202*:1004, 1964.

Bokros, J. C.: Deposition, structure and properties of pyrolytic carbon. *In* Walker, P. L. (Ed.): Chemistry and Physics of Carbon. Vol. 5. New York, Marcel Dekker, 1969.

Boretos, J. W.: The chemistry and biocompatibility of specific polyurethane systems for medical use. *In* Williams, D. F. (Ed.): Biocompatibility of Clinical Implant Materials. Vol. II. Boca Raton, CRC Press, 1981.

Boyce, S. T., Christianson, D. J., and Hansbrough, J. F.: Structure of a collagen-GAG dermal skin substitute optimized for cultured human epidermal keratinocytes. J. Biomed. Mater. Res., *22*:939, 1988.

Boyce, S. T., and Hansbrough, J. F.: Biological attachment, growth and differentiation of culture human epidermal keratinocytes on a graftable collagen and chondroitin-6-sulfate substrate. Surgery, *103*:421, 1988.

Braley, S.: The chemistry and properties of medical grade silicone rubber. J. Macromol. Sci. Chem., *23*:529, 1970.

Brand, K. G., and Brand, I.: Risk assessment of carcinogenesis at implantation sites. Plast. Reconstr. Surg., *66*:591, 1980.

Brand, K. G., Johnson, K. H., and Buoen, L. C.: Foreign body tumorigenesis. CRC Crit. Rev. Toxicol., *4*:353, 1976.

Burke, J. F., Yannas, I. V., Quinby, W. C., Bondoe, C. C., and Jung, W. K.: Successful use of a physiologically acceptable artificial skin in the treatment of extensive burn injury. Ann. Surg., *194*:413, 1981.

Cameron, H. U., MacNab, I., and Pilliar, R. M.: Evaluation of biodegradable ceramic. J. Biomed. Mater. Res., *11*:179, 1977.

Casey, D. J., and Lewis, O. G.: Absorbable and nonabsorbable sutures. *In* von Recum, A. F. (Ed.): Handbook of Biomaterials Evaluation. New York, Macmillan Publishing Company, 1986.

Chambers, T. J.: Multinucleate giant cells. J. Pathol., *126*:125, 1978.

Chu, C. C.: Survey of clinically important wound closure biomaterials. *In* Szycher, M. (Ed.): Biocompatible Polymers, Metals, and Composites. Lancaster, PA, Technomic Publishing Company, 1983.

Chuong, R.: Experimental study of surface and lattice effect on the solubility of hydroxyapatite. J. Dent. Res., *52*:911, 1973.

Cochran, J. H., Jr., and Reed, A.: Synthetic biomaterials for soft tissue. *In* Marsh, J. L. (Ed.): Current Therapy in Plastic and Reconstructive Surgery. Toronto & Philadelphia, B. C. Decker, 1989.

de Groot, K.: Degradable ceramics. *In* Williams, D. F. (Ed.): Biocompatibility of Clinical Implant Materials. Vol. I. Boca Raton, CRC Press, 1981.

de Wijn, F. R., and van Mullem, P. J.: Biocompatibility of acrylic implants. *In* Williams, D. F. (Ed.): Biocompatibility of Clinical Implant Materials. Vol. II. Boca Raton, CRC Press, 1981.

DiBenedetto, A., and Fleischer, A.: Biological properties of surgical mesh. *In* Rubin, L. R. (Ed.): Biomaterials in Reconstructive Surgery. St. Louis, C. V. Mosby Company, 1983.

Dougherty, S. H., and Simmons, R. L.: Infections in bionic man: the pathology of infections in prosthetic devices. Part I. Curr. Probl. Surg., *19*:221, 1982.

Ducheyne, P., Hench, L. L., Kagan, A., Martens, M., and Mulier, J. C.: Effect of hydroxyapatite impregnation on skeletal bonding of porous coated implants. J. Biomed. Mater. Res., *14*:225, 1980.

Elek, S. D., and Conen, P. E.: The virulence of *Staphylococcus pyogenes* for man: a study of the problems of wound infection. Br. J. Exp. Pathol., *38*:573, 1957.

Frankel, V. H., and Nordin, M. (Eds.): Basic Biomechanics of the Skeletal System. Philadelphia, Lea & Febiger, 1980.

Frisch, E. E.: Technology of silicones in biomedical applications. *In* Rubin, L. R. (Ed.): Biomaterials in Reconstructive Surgery. St. Louis, C. V. Mosby Company, 1983.

Gilding, D. K.: Biodegradable polymers. *In* Williams, D. F. (Ed.): Biocompatibility of Clinical Implant Materials. Vol. II. Boca Raton, CRC Press, 1981a.

Gilding, D. K.: Degradation of polymers: mechanisms and implications for biomedical applications. *In* Williams, D. F. (Ed.): Fundamental Aspects of Biocompatibility. Vol. I. Boca Raton, CRC Press, 1981b.

Greenspan, D. C., and Hench, L. L.: Chemical and mechanical behavior of bioglass coated alumina. J. Biomed. Mater. Res., *10*:503, 1976.

Griss, P., and Heimke, G.: Biocompatibility of high density alumina and its applications in orthopedic surgery. *In* Williams, D. F. (Ed.): Biocompatibility of Clinical Implant Materials. Vol. I. Boca Raton, CRC Press, 1981.

Gristina, A. G., and Costerton, J. W.: Bacterial adherence to biomaterials: the clinical significance of its role in sepsis. Trans. Soc. Biomater., *7*:175, 1984.

Guidoin, R., Gosselin, C., Domurado, D., Marcois, M., Levaillant, P. A., et al.: Dacron as arterial prosthetic material: nature, properties, brands, fate and perspectives. Biomater. Med. Dev. Artif. Organs, *5*:177, 1977.

Hastings, G. W.: Biocompatibility of polyethylenes and polypropylene. *In* Williams, D. F. (Ed.): Biocompatibility of Clinical Implant Materials. Vol. II. Boca Raton, CRC Press, 1981.

Haubold, A. D., Shim, H. S., and Bokros, J. C.: Carbon in medical devices. *In* Williams, D. F. (Ed.): Biocompatibility of Clinical Implant Materials. Vol. II. Boca Raton, CRC Press, 1981.

Hayes, A. W.: Principles and Methods of Toxicology. New York, Raven Press, 1982.

Heimke, G.: Ceramics. *In* von Recum, A. F. (Ed.): Handbook of Biomaterials Evaluation. New York, Macmillan Publishing Company, 1986.

Hench, L. L.: Stability of ceramics in the physiological environment. *In* Williams, D. F. (Ed.): Fundamental Aspects of Biocompatibility. Vol. I. Boca Raton, CRC Press, 1981.

Hench, L. L., and Clark, A. E.: Adhesion to bone. *In* Williams, D. F. (Ed.): Biocompatibility of Orthopedic Implants. Vol. II. Boca Raton, CRC Press, 1982.

Holmes, R. E.: Tracheal reconstruction with a porous hydroxyapatite implant. Unpublished data, 1978.

Holmes, R. E.: Bone regeneration within a coralline hydroxyapatite implant. Plast. Reconstr. Surg., *63*:626, 1979.

Holmes, R. E., Bucholz, R. W., and Mooney, V.: Porous hydroxyapatite as a bone graft substitute in metaphyseal defects: a histometric study. J. Bone Joint Surg., *68A*:904, 1986.

Holmes, R. E., Bucholz, R. W., and Mooney, V.: Porous hydroxyapatite as a bone graft substitute in diaphyseal defects: a histometric study. J. Orthop. Res., *5*:114, 1987.

Homsy, C. A.: Biocompatibility of perfluorinated polymers and composites of these polymers. *In* Williams, D. F.: Biocompatibility of Clinical Implant Materials. Vol. II. Boca Raton, CRC Press, 1981.

Homsy, C. A.: Proplast: chemical and biological considerations. *In* Rubin, L. R. (Ed.): Biomaterials in Reconstructive Surgery. St. Louis, C. V. Mosby Company, 1983.

Homsy, C. A., Cain, T. E., Kessler, F. B., Anderson, M. S., and King, J. W.: Porous implant systems for prosthesis stabilization. Clin. Orthop., *89*:220, 1972.

Hulbert, S. F., Cooke, F. W., Klawitter, J. J., Leonard, R. B., Sauer, B. W., et al.: Attachment of prostheses to the musculo-skeletal system by tissue ingrowth and mechanical interlocking. J. Biomed. Mater. Res., 7:1, 1972.

Hulbert, S. F., Kent, J. N., Bokros, J. C., Shim, H. S., and Reed, O. M.: Design and evaluation of LTI-Si carbon endosteal implants. Oral Implant., *6*:79, 1975.

Hulbert, S. F., Klawitter, J. J., and Bowman, L. S.: History of ceramic orthopaedic implants. Mater. Res. Bull., *7*:1239, 1973.

Hurley, J. V.: Acute Inflammation. 2nd Ed. Edinburgh, Churchill Livingstone, 1983.

Jaffe, H. L.: Metabolic, Degenerative and Inflammatory Diseases of Bones and Joints. Philadelphia, Lea & Febiger, 1972, p. 125.

Keller, J. C., and Lautenschlager, E. P.: Metals and alloys. *In* von Recum, A. F. (Ed.): Handbook of Biomaterials Evaluation. New York, Macmillan Publishing Company, 1986.

King, M., Blais, P., Guidoin, R., Prowse, E., Marcois, M., et al.: Polyethylene terephthalate vascular prostheses—material and fabric construction aspects. *In* Williams, D. F. (Ed.): Biocompatibility of Clinical Implant Materials. Vol. II. Boca Raton, CRC Press, 1981.

Leininger, R. I.: Polymers as surgical implants. CRC Crit. Rev. Bioeng., *1*:333, 1972.

Leininger, R. I., and Bigg, D. M.: Polymers. *In* von Recum, A. F. (Ed.): Handbook of Biomaterials Evaluation. New York, Macmillan Publishing Company, 1986.

Lelah, M. D., and Cooper, S. L.: Polyurethanes in Medicine. Boca Raton, CRC Press, 1986.

Linder, L.: The tissue response to bone cement. *In* Williams, D. F. (Ed.): Biocompatibility of Orthopedic Implants. Vol. II. Boca Raton, CRC Press, 1982.

Luckey, H. A., and Kubli, F. (Eds.): Titanium Alloys in Surgical Implants, ASTM Special Technical Publication 796. Philadelphia, American Society for Testing and Materials, 1983.

Lyman, D. J., Seare, W. J., Albo, D., Bergman, S., Lamb, J., et al.: Polyurethane elastomers in surgery. Int. J. Polym. Mater., *5*:211, 1977.

Majno, G.: The Healing Hand: Man and Wound in the Ancient World. Cambridge, MA, Harvard University Press, 1975.

Marrie, T. J., and Costerton, J. W.: Glycocalyx enclosed mode of growth of bacteria on a variety of prostheses. Abst. 359, 22nd Interscience Conference on Antimicrobial Agents and Chemotherapy, 1982.

Meachim, G., and Pedley, R. B.: The tissue response at implant sites. *In* Williams, D. F. (Ed.): Fundamental Aspects of Biocompatibility. Vol. I. Boca Raton, CRC Press, 1981.

Merritt, K.: Role of medical materials, both in implant and surface applications in immune response and in resistance to infection. Biomaterials, *5*:47, 1984.

Merritt, K., Shafer, J. W., and Brown, S. A.: Implant site infection rates with porous and dense materials. J. Biomed. Mater. Res., *13*:101, 1979.

Migliaresi, C., Nicodemo, L., Nicolais, L., and Passerini, P.: Physical characterization of microporous poly (2-hydroxyethyl methacrylate) gels. J. Biomed. Mater. Res., *15*:307, 1981.

Munson, F. T., and Heron, D. F.: Facial reconstruction with acrylic resin. Am. J. Surg., *53*:291, 1941.

Parsons, J. R., Alexander, H., and Weiss, A. B.: Absorbable polymer–filamentous carbon composites: a new concept in orthopaedic biomaterials. *In* Szycher, M. (Ed.): Biocompatible Polymers, Metals, and Composites. Lancaster, PA, Technomic Publishing Company, 1983.

Peacock, E. E.: Wound Repair. 3rd Ed. Philadelphia, W. B. Saunders Company, 1984.

Peelen, J. G. J., Rejda, B. V., Vermeiden, J. P. W., and de Groot, K.: Sintered tricalcium phosphate as bioceramic. Sci. Ceram., *9*:226, 1977.

Plenk, H., Pfluger, G., Schider, G., Bohler, N., and Grundschober, F.: Tantalum and niobium implants for high stress conditions. Trans. Soc. Biomater., *4*:40, 1981.

Ratner, B. D.: Biomedical applications of hydrogels: review and critical appraisal. *In* Williams, D. F. (Ed.): Biocompatibility of Clinical Implant Materials. Vol. II. Boca Raton, CRC Press, 1981.

Refojo, M. F.: Polymers in ophthalmology. *In* Rubin, L. R. (Ed.): Biomaterials in Reconstructive Surgery. St. Louis, C. V. Mosby Company, 1983.

Rootare, H. M., and Craig, R. G.: Characterization of hydroxyapatite powders and compacts at room temperature and after sintering at 1200 degrees C. J. Oral Rehab., *5*:293, 1978.

Salthouse, T. N.: Tissue response to sutures. *In* Rubin, L. R. (Ed.): Biomaterials in Reconstructive Surgery. St. Louis, C. V. Mosby Company, 1983.

Salthouse, T. N., Williams, J. A., and Willigan, D. A.: Relationship of cellular enzyme activity to catgut and collagen suture absorption. Surg. Gynecol. Obstet., *129*:691, 1969.

Soltesz, U., and Richter, H.: Mechanical behavior of selected ceramics. *In* Ducheyne, P., and Hastings, G. W. (Eds.): Metal and Ceramic Biomaterials. Vol. II. Boca Raton, CRC Press, 1984.

van Noort, R., and Black, M. M.: Silicone rubbers for medical applications. *In* Williams, D. F. (Ed.): Biocompatibility of Clinical Implant Materials. Vol. II. Boca Raton, CRC Press, 1981.

Van Raemdonck, W., Ducheyne, P., and De Meester, P.: Calcium phosphate ceramics. *In* Ducheyne, P., and Hastings, G. W. (Eds.): Metal and Ceramic Biomaterials. Vol. II. Boca Raton, CRC Press, 1984.

Van Vlack, L. H.: Elements of Materials Science and Engineering. 3rd Ed. Reading, MA, Addison-Wesley, 1975.

Vincenzini, P. (Ed.): Ceramics in Surgery. Amsterdam, Elsevier, 1983.

Wang, F. F. Y. (Ed.): Treatise on Materials Science and Technology. Vol. 9. Ceramic Fabrication Processes. New York, Academic Press, 1976.

Weselow, A., and Snyder, R. W.: Textiles. *In* Rubin, L. R. (Ed.): Biomaterials in Reconstructive Surgery. St. Louis, C. V. Mosby Company, 1983.

White, E. W., Weber, J. N., Roy, D. M., Owen, E. L., Chiroff, R. T., and White, R. A.: Replamineform porous biomaterials for hard tissue implant applications. J. Biomed. Mater. Res., *6*:23, 1975.

Williams, D. F.: Electrochemical aspects of corrosion in the physiological environment. *In* Williams, D. F. (Ed.): Fundamental Aspects of Biocompatibility. Vol. I. Boca Raton, CRC Press, 1981.

Williams, D. F., and Roaf, R.: Implants in Surgery. London, W. B. Saunders, 1973.

Wolter, D., Kitzer, E., Heldin, G., and Coldewey, J.: Ligament replacement in the knee joint with carbon fibers coated with pyrolytic carbon. Trans. Soc. Biomat., *1*:126, 1977.

Woodroof, E. A.: Biobrane, a biosynthetic skin prosthesis. *In* Wise, D. L. (Ed.): Burn Wound Coverings. Vol. II. Boca Raton, CRC Press, 1984.

Yamada, H.: Strength of Biological Materials. Baltimore, Williams & Wilkins Company, 1970.

Yannas, I. V., Burke, J. F., Warpehoski, M., Stasikelis, P., Skrabut, E. M., et al.: Prompt, long-term functional replacement of skin. *In* Wise, D. L. (Ed.): Burn Wound Coverings. Vol. II. Boca Raton, CRC Press, 1984.

Yue, S., Pilliar, R. M., and Weatherly, G.: Heat treatments to improve the fatigue resistance of porous coated Ti-6Al-4V implants. Trans. Soc. Biomater., *5*:93, 1982.

Zimmerli, W., Waldvogel, F. A., and Vaudaux, P.: Pathogenesis of foreign body infection: description and characteristics of an animal model. J. Infect. Dis., *146*:487, 1982.

Additional Reading

Boretos, J. W.: Concise Guide to Biomedical Polymers: Their Design, Fabrication and Moulding. Springfield, IL, Charles C Thomas, 1973.

Boretos, J. W., and Eden, M. (Eds.): Contemporary Biomaterials: Material and Host Response, Clinical Applications, New Technology and Legal Aspects. Park Ridge, NJ, Noyes Publications, 1984.

Bruck, S. D.: Properties of Biomaterials in the Physiological Environment. Boca Raton, CRC Press, 1980.

Christel, P., Meunier, A., and Lee, A. J. C. (Eds.): Biological and Biomechanical Performance of Biomaterials. Amsterdam, Elsevier, 1986.

Cooper, S. L., and Peppas, N. A. (Eds.): Biomaterials: Interfacial Phenomena and Applications. Washington, DC, American Chemical Society, 1982.

de Groot, K. (Ed.): Bioceramics of Calcium Phosphate. Boca Raton, CRC Press, 1983.

Ducheyne, P., and Hastings, G. W. (Eds.): Functional Behavior of Orthopedic Biomaterials. Vols. I and II. Boca Raton, CRC Press, 1984a.

Ducheyne, P., and Hastings, G. W. (Eds.): Metal and Ceramic Biomaterials. Vols. I and II. Boca Raton, CRC Press, 1984b.

Ducheyne, P., Van der Perr, G., and Aubert, A. E. (Eds.): Biomaterials and Biomechanics. Amsterdam, Elsevier, 1984.

Gebelein, C. G., and Carralier, C. E. (Eds.): Bioactive Polymeric Systems: An Overview. New York, Plenum Press, 1985.

Goldberg, E. P., and Nakajima, A. (Eds.): Biomedical Polymers. New York, Academic Press, 1980.

Gregor, H. P. (Ed.): Biomedical Applications of Polymers. New York, Plenum Press, 1975.

Hastings, G. W., and Ducheyne, P. (Eds.): Macromolecular Biomaterials. Boca Raton, CRC Press, 1984a.

Hastings, G. W., and Ducheyne, P. (Eds.): Natural and Living Biomaterials. Boca Raton, CRC Press, 1984b.

Kronenthal, R. L., Oser, Z., and Martin, E. (Eds.): Polymers in Medicine and Surgery. New York, Plenum Press, 1977.

Lee, A. J. C., Albrektsson, T., and Branemark, P. E. (Eds.): Clinical Applications of Biomaterials. Chichester, John Wiley & Sons, 1982.

Lelah, M. D., and Cooper, S. L.: Polyurethanes in Medicine. Boca Raton, CRC Press, 1986.

Park, J. B.: Biomaterials: An Introduction. New York, Plenum Press, 1979.

Planck, H., Egbers, G., and Eyre, I. (Eds.): Polyurethanes in Biomedical Engineering. Amsterdam, Elsevier, 1984.

Rubin, L. R. (Ed.): Biomaterials in Reconstructive Surgery. St. Louis, C. V. Mosby Company, 1983.

Smith, D. C., and Williams, D. F. (Eds.): Biocompatibility of Dental Implant Materials. Vols. I to IV. Boca Raton, CRC Press, 1982.
Szycher, M. (Ed.): Biocompatible Polymers, Metals, and Composites. Lancaster, PA, Technomic Publishing Company, 1983.
Vincenzini, P. (Ed.): Ceramics in Surgery. Amsterdam, Elsevier, 1983.
von Recum, A. F. (Ed.): Handbook of Biomaterials Evaluation: Scientific, Technical, and Clinical Testing of Implant Materials. New York, Macmillan Publishing Company, 1986.
Williams, D. F. (Ed.): Biocompatibility of Clinical Implant Materials. Vols. I and II. Boca Raton, CRC Press, 1981a.
Williams, D. F. (Ed.): Fundamental Aspects of Biocompatibility. Vols. I and II. Boca Raton, CRC Press, 1981b.
Williams, D. F. (Ed.): Systemic Aspects of Biocompatibility. Vols. I and II. Boca Raton, CRC Press, 1981c.
Williams, D. F. (Ed.): Biocompatibility of Orthopedic Implants. Vols. I and II. Boca Raton, CRC Press, 1982.
Williams, D. F. (Ed.): Biocompatibility of Tissue Analogs. Vols. I and II. Boca Raton, CRC Press, 1985.
Winter, G. D., Leray, J. L., and de Groot, K. (Eds.): Evaluation of Biomaterials. New York, John Wiley & Sons, 1980.
Wise, D. L. (Ed.): Burn Wound Coverings. Vols. I and II. Boca Raton, CRC Press, 1984.

21

I. Kelman Cohen
Erle E. Peacock, Jr.

Keloids and Hypertrophic Scars

ETIOLOGIES OF ABNORMAL SCAR FORMATION

BIOCHEMICAL OBSERVATIONS

DIAGNOSIS

TREATMENT MODALITIES
- Pharmacologic
- Mechanical
- Radiation
- Surgical

The biochemical processes of wound repair normally culminate in fine-line scars as the only evidence of dermal injury. In certain individuals, however, the repair process may go awry and wounds may heal with large, raised collagenous scars known as keloids or hypertrophic scars. Both lesions have the annoying clinical symptoms of itching, tenderness, and pain. Although both types of lesions are characterized by excessive collagen deposition (Blackburn and Cosman, 1966; Cohen, Diegelmann and Keiser, 1976), the causes remain obscure. The clinical course and physical appearance define keloid and hypertrophic scar as separate entities. Keloids (Fig. 21–1) frequently persist at the site of injury, often recur after excision, and always overgrow the boundaries of the original wound (Peacock, Madden, and Trier, 1970). In contrast, hypertrophic scars, although often red and raised, remain within the confines of the original wound and tend to regress over an extended period (Fig. 21–2). However, hypertrophic scars frequently recur after excision and closure.

The complications of these abnormal scar formations are often severe and their clinical management is frustrating. Both surgeon and patient must accept the reality that neither pharmacologic intervention nor technical skill will ensure prevention or cure. Potential control of abnormal scar formation is thus of paramount interest to the plastic surgeon.

This chapter reviews some of the proposed etiologies and biochemical findings regarding keloids and hypertrophic scars. It also explores the biochemical rationale for treating abnormal scars by surgical, mechanical, hormonal, pharmacologic, or radiation modalities.

ETIOLOGIES OF ABNORMAL SCAR FORMATION

For unknown reasons, keloid and hypertrophic scar formation is unique to man. Attempts to develop animal models for abnormal scar formation have always proved unsuccessful. Despite numerous studies, there is no valid theory or explanation to indicate which factor(s) initiate keloid or hypertrophic scar formation.

For example, although the increased incidence of keloids and hypertrophic scars in dark-skinned races has been documented in several studies (Bloom, 1956; Crockett, 1964; Koonin, 1964; Oluwassanmi, 1974), the lesions are found in all races and populations. Proposed causes of abnormal scar formation have included foreign body reaction (Mowlem, 1951), bacterial infection (Brenizer, 1915), or the possibility that degraded or

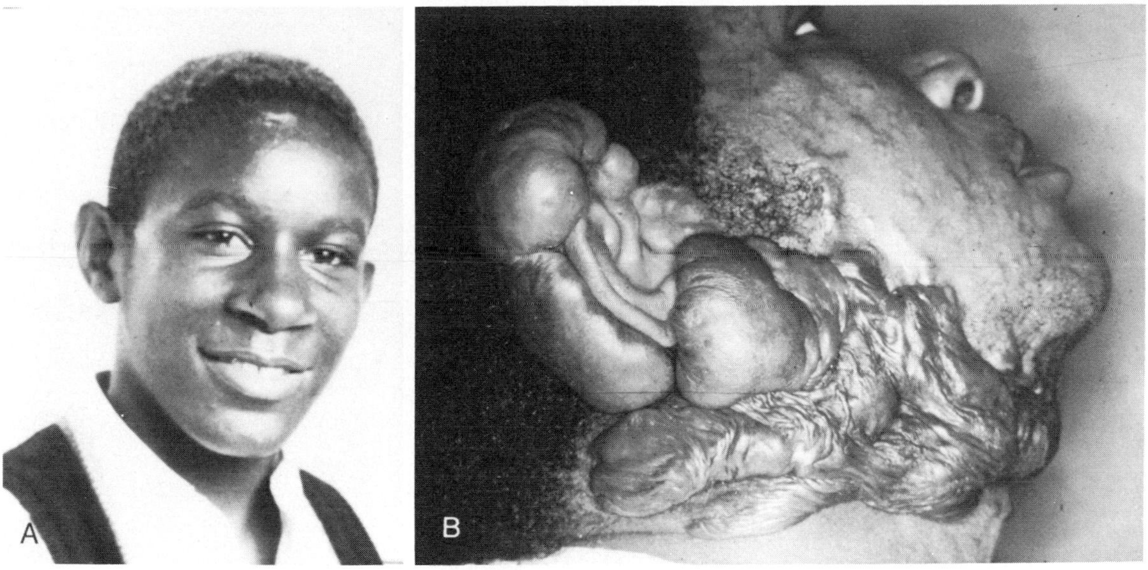

Figure 21–1. Keloid development. *A,* Patient at age 16 before keloid formation. *B,* The same patient at age 32 after shaving cuts initiated the development of keloids.

denatured collagen serves as a catalyst for scar hyperplasia (Keiser and associates, 1963). None of these theories is supported by reproducible data. The genetic patterns of patients with keloids have not been elucidated clearly. HLA types seem to be unrelated (Cohen and associates, 1979) in studies from the authors' laboratory, in contrast to the work of others (Laurentaci and Dioguardi, 1977). However, family members are commonly afflicted (Fig. 21–3).

The role of the immune system in abnormal scar formation is unclear. Initial studies that showed increased IgG in keloid tissue compared with normal dermis Table 21–1 and other preliminary studies (Chytilova, Kul-

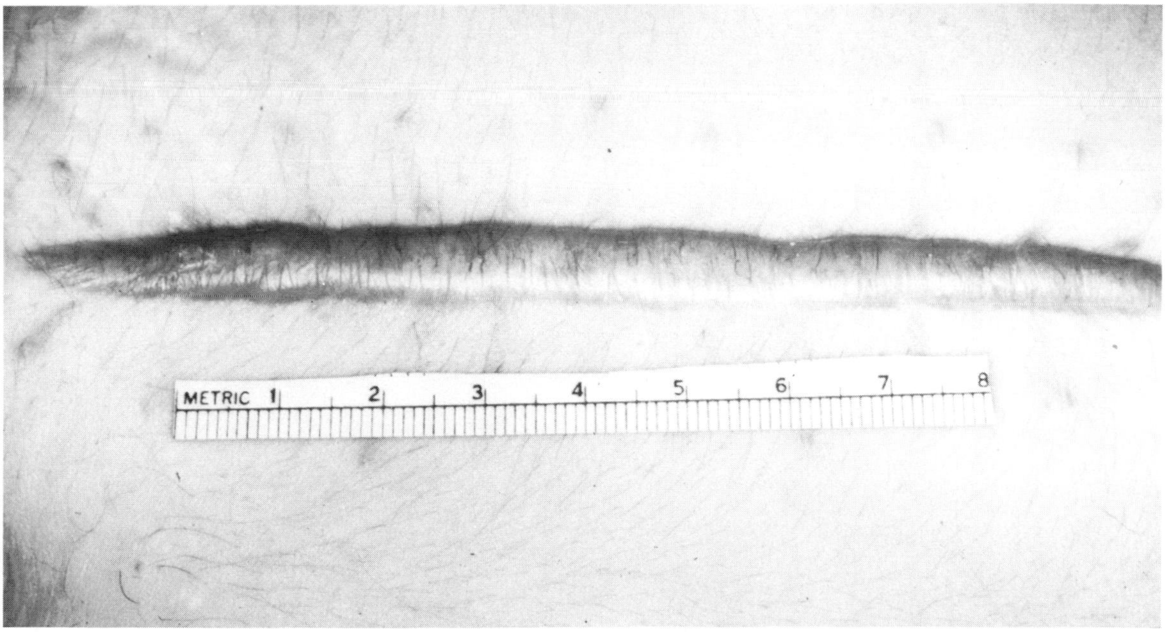

Figure 21–2. Hypertrophic scar. Although red and raised, the scar remains within the limits of the original wound, and in time the hypertrophic scar often regresses.

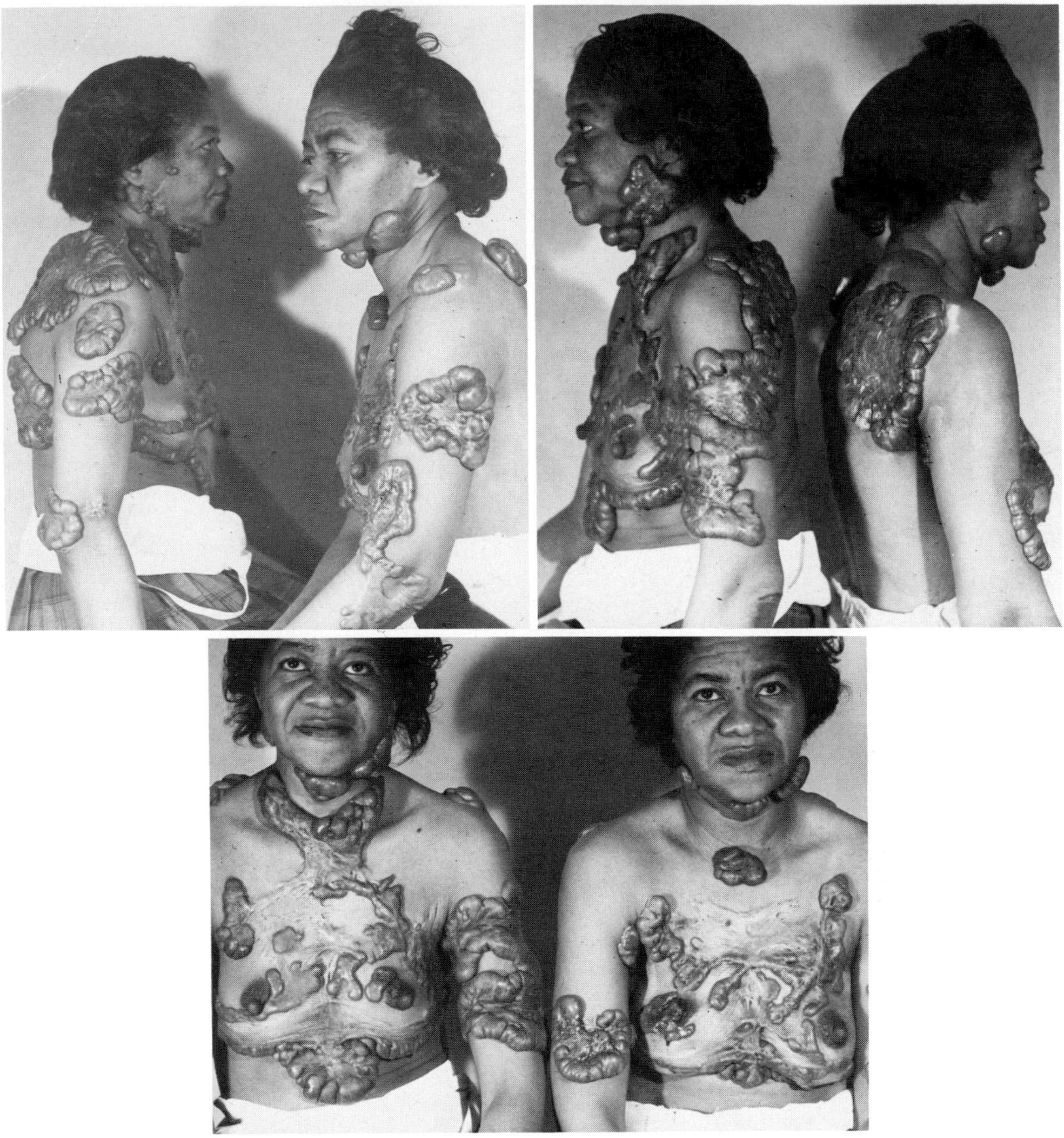

Figure 21–3. Severe keloid formation in identical twins. Note the similar locations of the keloids in each despite different initiating traumas. Their mother and maternal grandmother also had keloids.

Table 21–1. Saline-Extractable Tissue IgG

Specimens	No. of Patients	Mg IgG / *Mg Protein*	Mg IgG / *Mg Dry Wt*
Normal dermis	14	0.46 ± 0.11	8.4 ± 2.2
Normal scar	15	0.61 ± 0.13	13.23 ± 2.71
Keloid	16	1.05 ± 0.16*	18.72 ± 2.37*

Results are expressed as mean ± SEM.

*p value equal to or less than 0.05 compared with normal dermis and scar (Wilcoxon two sample test).

Reprinted in part from Cohen, I. K., McCoy, B. J., Mohanakumar, T., and Diegelmann, R. F.: Immunoglobulin, complement, and histocompatibility antigen studies in keloid patients. Plast. Reconstr. Surg., *63*:689, 1979.

hanek, and Horn, 1959; Oluwassanmi, Lucas, and Chvapil, 1976; Hazrati and Hoomad, 1977; Janssen de Limpens and Cormane, 1982) suggested immune system involvement in keloid pathogenesis. However, subsequent detailed studies of other immunologic parameters, such as serum IgG, and C1q complement component, immune lymphocyte characterization, and specific tissue immunoglobulins, failed to demonstrate cellular, systemic, or local immunologic factor(s) in keloid formers associated with abnormal scar etiology (Cohen and associates, 1979; Kischer and associates, 1983). In addition, there appears to be no correlation between histocompatibility antigens (HLA typing) and keloid formation (Cohen and associates, 1979), as occurs in some immune-associated disease states (Katz, 1977). Moreover, no known circulating stimulatory factor, immune or otherwise, that could account for excessive collagen production in keloids, has been documented (McCoy and Cohen, 1981). However, it may be possible that wounding results in the production of some sort of material that the body recognizes as foreign and may even be antigenic; hence, a chronic inflammatory reaction could result in excessive collagen production characteristic of keloids.

Other possible causes of keloid formation include thyroid hormone alterations, ingrown hairs, and melanocyte stimulating hormones and are discussed in a comprehensive review of the subject by Crikelair, Ju, and Cosman (1977). Again, none of the hypotheses has ever been validated.

Kischer, Thies, and Chvapil (1982) compared the microvasculature of hypertrophic scars and keloids with that of normal dermis and normal scar. They observed increased occlusion of the microvessels by endothelial cell proliferation in abnormal scars when compared with normal dermis (Fig. 21–4). These authors suggested that perivascular myofibroblast contraction may contribute significantly to increased microvascular occlusion—and resulting hypoxia—in hypertrophic scars and keloids. Myofibroblasts have been found in both keloids (James, Besanceney, and Odom, 1980) and hypertrophic scars (Baur, Barratt, and Linares, 1978), although their role in abnormal scar formation is obscure. If hypoxia is a major factor contributing to excessive collagen deposition in abnormal scars, the findings noted above may explain how hypoxia is established and how it persists in abnormal wounds. The hypothesis that hypoxia may significantly influence abnormal scar formation is reasonable, since Hunt and associates (1978) demonstrated the modulating effects of hypoxia on collagen production. Kischer, Shetlar, and Chvapil (1982) hypothesized that normal endothelial cell proliferation, probably stimulated by fibrin and thrombin during early wound repair, is prolonged or exaggerated in abnormal scar formation. They suggested that subsequent microvascular occlusion, owing to epithelial hyperplasia and myofibroblast contraction, may stimulate excessive collagen production in keloids and hypertrophic scars. The theory needs further study, yet appears plausible in view of the histologic and biochemical findings. Preliminary fibroblast tissue culture studies in the authors' laboratory suggest that hypoxia may select a homogeneous fibroblast population that produces collagen at a rate significantly greater than that of a heterogeneous fibroblast population.

BIOCHEMICAL OBSERVATIONS

Biochemical data gathered over the past decade indicate that multiple factors are involved in scar formation, and have put investigators and clinicians on the brink of unraveling the cause of abnormal scars. Early biochemical studies of keloids and hypertrophic scars focused on quantitating enzyme levels and the degree of cellularity in the lesions. Various glycogenic-related enzymes such as lactic dehydrogenase were found to be increased in keloid compared with normal skin (Hoopes, Su, and Im, 1971; Kemble and Brown, 1976). The collagen-related enzyme prolyl hydroxylase was also reported to be elevated in keloid compared with normal skin

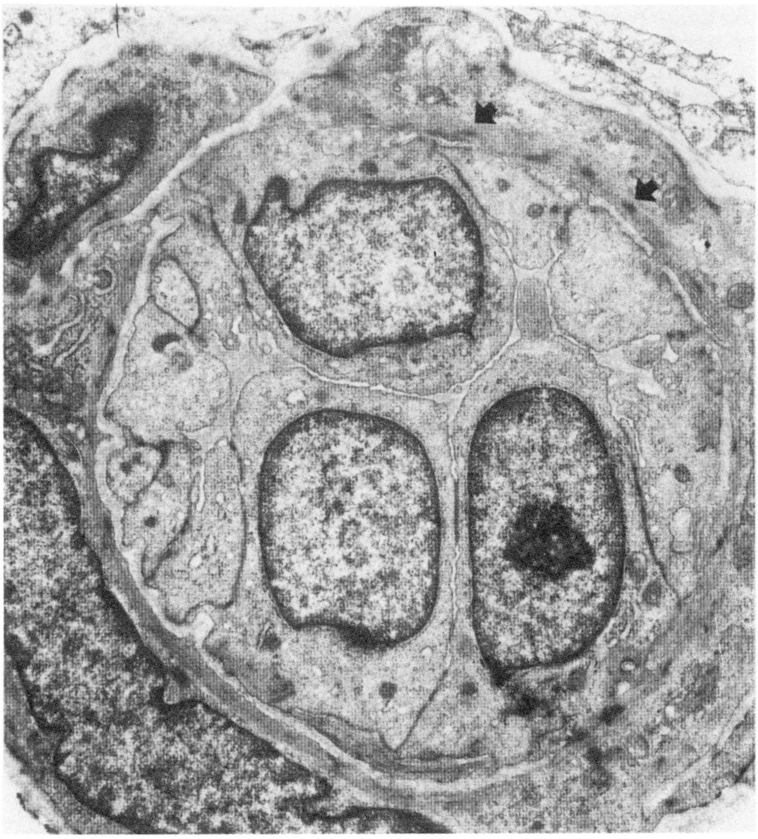

Figure 21–4. Cross section of a microvessel from a hypertrophic scar. Profiles of at least 12 endothelial cells are present. A satellite cell is present with an inner rim of microfilaments and cytoplasmic densities *(arrows).* Note also the high position of interendothelial tight junctions (× 10,200). (From Kischer, C. W., Thies, A. C., and Chvapil, M.: Perivascular myofibroblasts and microvascular occlusion in hypertrophic scars and keloids. Hum. Pathol., *13*:819, 1982.)

(Cohen, Keiser, and Sjoerdsma, 1971). Prolyl hydroxylase is required for the hydroxylation of proline during collagen biosynthesis, and this finding suggested that collagen overproduction was the characteristic abnormality in keloid lesions.

It is possible that the biochemical defect responsible for abnormal scar formation is expressed early in the course of wound repair and cannot be detected by the time abnormal lesions are fully developed. Unfortunately, there are no studies on early formation of keloids to test such a hypothesis. Collagen production is elevated in keloid biopsies (Cohen and Keiser, 1973; Cohen, Diegelmann, and Keiser, 1976) and in cultured fibroblasts derived from keloids (Diegelmann, Cohen, and McCoy; 1979; McCoy, Galdun, and Cohen, 1982). Moreover, increased collagen production by cultured fibroblasts derived from keloids persists throughout their in vitro life span (McCoy, Galdun, and Cohen, 1982). It appears, therefore, that once keloid fibroblasts responsible for keloids overcome entropy, they do not revert to normal even after being removed from the lesions and placed in culture. No significant differences in DNA content or cellularity were observed in keloid compared with normal dermis, although this matter is still debated (Blackburn and Cosman, 1966; Hoopes, Su and Im, 1971; Diegelmann, Cohen, and McCoy, 1979). These data suggest that each fibroblast within a keloid is producing excessive collagen, as opposed to an increased number of fibroblasts each producing a normal amount of collagen.

One of the authors (IKC) is currently attempting to explain why excessive collagen production occurs and persists in abnormal scars as well as in the fibroblasts derived from these lesions. As mentioned, it may be that excessive collagen-producing fibroblasts are *selected by the wound environment* and that this selection results in excessive collagen production and deposition by fibroblasts in the lesions. This hypothesis is supported by several studies. First, Hunt and associates (1978) reported that increased hypoxia is noted in early animal wounds and that hypoxia stimulates macrophages, in turn, to stimulate fibroblast collagen production. There is reason to believe that keloids are hypoxic, because microvascular occlusion (Kischer, Shetlar, and Chvapil, 1982; Kischer, Thies, and Chvapil, 1982) is frequent and some portions of keloids are relatively avascular (Linares and associates, 1972). Moreover, increased lactate (Hoopes, Su, and Im, 1971), increased histamine (Hakanson and associates, 1969; Cohen and associates, 1972; Kischer, Buncc, and Shetlar, 1978) and decreased pH (unpublished observation) are characteristics of abnormal scars that conceivably could create a "stressed" environment selecting fibroblasts that are high collagen producers.

The hypoxia-selectivity hypothesis is substantiated by several reports demonstrating that heterogenous populations of fibroblasts with particular biochemical characteristics can be isolated from normal tissue (Martin and associates, 1974; Bordin, Page, and Narayanan, 1984). Perhaps certain kinds of fibroblasts predominate in abnormal wounds and either (1) fail to respond to regulatory signals ending increased collagen production during early wound healing or (2) are selected and proliferate more abundantly in the "stressed" environment of the early wound the possible "stress" factors mentioned above. There is evidence that keloid-derived fibroblasts, which can be isolated in vitro, are a selected subset of normal dermal fibroblasts that occur more abundantly in abnormal scars. For example, fibroblasts grown out of keloid tissue produce increased extracellular matrix components in vitro (Diegelmann, Cohen, and McCoy, 1979; McCoy, Galdun, and Cohen, 1982; Kischer and Hendrix, 1983), and demonstrate a differential response to hydrocortisone (Russell, Russell, and Trupin, 1982) and histamine (Russell, Russell, and Trupin, 1977; Topol, Lewis, and Benveniste, 1981) compared with normal fibroblasts. Recent studies by Russell and associates (1988) have shown that keloid-derived fibroblasts have reduced growth factor requirements. Such studies indicate that the "type" of fibroblast in abnormal scars is different from fibroblasts in normal dermis. However, such "abnormal" cells are morphologically identical to normal fibroblasts and grow at the same rate (Diegelmann, Cohen, and McCoy, 1979). Further studies are necessary to verify the intriguing hypothesis that abnormal scars result from a population of normal cells in the dermis that have gone awry or are preferentially selected during wound healing. Such in vitro findings are important because they may eventually lead to an improved understanding of the regulatory stimuli that "turn on" and "turn off" the events of normal wound repair in man.

It is important to consider the possibility that keloids and hypertrophic scars may result not only from increased collagen production but also from decreased collagen degradation. There is biochemical evidence for an increased level of α_2-macroglobulin, a collagenase inhibitor, in keloid lesions (Diegelmann, Bryant, and Cohen, 1977). Although the collagenase found in keloids appears to be similar to that of normal dermis (Milsom and Craig, 1973; McCoy and Cohen, 1982), increased collagenase inhibitors may contribute to a lack of collagen degradation and, therefore, increased collagen deposition within abnormal scars.

The question of collagen type abnormalities in abnormal scars is raised frequently. After injury to normal skin, the ratio of Type III to Type I collagen increases and then subsides to a normal value of about 17 to 20 per cent of total collagen as wound healing progresses (Bailey and associates, 1975a,b; Gay and associates, 1978). It is known that Type III collagen is increased in granulation tissue (Hayakawa and associates, 1979) and in hypertrophic scars (Bailey and associates, 1975a; Craig, Schofield, and Jackson, 1975), but Type III collagen appears to occur in a normal amount in keloids. Uitto and associates (1985) reported that keloid fibroblasts overproduce Type I collagen while Type III collagen expression remains unchanged. This finding also suggests that keloid is dissimilar to an early wound. This is surprising because other parameters such as elevated water content (Cohen, Diegelmann, and Keiser, 1976), increased soluble collagen (Cohen, Diegelmann, and Keiser, 1976), and increased histamine (Cohen and associates, 1972) indicate that mature keloids resemble early wounds. It is possible that abnormal collagen types have not been found because of limitations of typing methodology. More sophisticated typing methods may identify abnormal ratios and types of collagen in abnormal scars.

There has never been a clear histologic differentiation between keloids and hypertrophic scars. Blackburn and Cosman (1966) differentiated keloids from hypertrophic scars on the basis that keloids appeared to contain bundles of collagen with focal proliferation or nodules and increased quantities of mucopolysaccharides. Kischer, Shetlar, and Chvapil (1982) reviewed the literature on histology of abnormal scars and reported that collagen in *both* keloids and hypertrophic scars is organized into discrete nodules, frequently (but not always) obliterating the rete pegs in the papillary dermis of the lesions. Whereas collagen in normal dermis is arranged in discrete fascicles, separated by considerable interstitial space, the collagen nodules in keloids and in hypertrophic scars appear avascular and unidirectional, and are aligned in a "highly stressed" configuration. The origin and significance of characteristic collagen nodules in abnormal scars are unknown at the present time. It is interesting that myofibroblasts have been found in keloids and hypertrophic scars, but their role in abnormal scar formation remains obscure. The relationship between the histology and pathophysiology of these lesions remains an enigma.

Although the biochemical and histologic puzzles of abnormal scar formation are slowly being solved, questions still remain regarding the clinical findings in abnormal scars. For example, why do certain individuals seem more likely to produce keloids and hypertrophic scars? Why do certain areas of the body seem to form abnormal scars more often than others? Why do abnormal scars form after one type of injury but not after another in the same individual?

DIAGNOSIS

Before a keloid or hypertrophic scar is treated, a theoretical diagnosis distinguishing one from the other should be formed. Hypertrophic scar appears to be a self-limiting type of overhealing following injury. With time, the raised, red hypertrophic scar becomes flat and pale. The true keloid, however, extends beyond the confines of the original wound and does not regress (see Figs. 21–1 to 21–3). Aside from clinical diagnosis by careful observation, there is no absolute way to distinguish with certainty a keloid from a true hypertrophic scar. Dermatofibrosarcoma protuberans or other malignant fibromatous lesions can appear clinically quite similar to keloid (Manalan, Cohen, and Theogaraj, 1974) and should be ruled out. If there is doubt that the lesion may be neither a keloid nor a hypertrophic scar, biopsy is mandatory.

TREATMENT MODALITIES

Several forms of treatment have been utilized for keloids and hypertrophic scars, with varying degrees of success. At an early stage, the surgeon should ascertain whether the patient's objective is to eradicate the esthetic and/or functional deformity, to prevent recurrence by surgery and adjuvant pharmacologic therapy or whether the objective is merely to ameliorate the physical discomfort and itching. If eradication is the objective, patients must be warned that recurrence not only is likely but may be more severe than the original lesion. Many lesions are not esthetically displeasing to the patient, and there is no need for operative intervention in these cases. If symptoms of burning and itching are the major problem, control may be possible with intralesional injection of triamcinolone and/or systemic antihistamines (Cohen and associates, 1972). Diphenhydramine hydrochloride (Benadryl), 50 mg by mouth at bedtime, may be effective. The efficacy of H_2 blockers has not been tested. Unfortunately, keloids frequently recur after excision even when surgery is supplemented with other forms of therapy such as intralesional corticosteroids. Excision is beneficial only when used in conjunction with pharmacologic treatment to prevent the inevitable recurrence of keloids after excision alone. Conversely, it is improbable that pharmacologic therapy alone can eradicate large keloids, although corticosteroids used by themselves may alleviate some discomfort such as burning and itching, and often may reduce the size of the lesion.

Pharmacologic

Pharmacologic treatment of lesions characterized by excessive collagen production has been historically directed toward either decreasing protein production (specifically, collagen production) or enhancing collagen turnover by rendering the collagen molecule more soluble or more susceptible to enzymatic degradation. Steroids affect the former, and lathyrogens such as β-aminopropionitrile (BAPN) and penicillamine are agents used to accomplish the latter.

Steroids have been shown to decrease the size of keloids in a number of clinical studies (Ketchum and associates, 1966; Ketchum, Cohen, and Masters, 1974) and decrease collagen synthesis in in vitro studies specifically performed on keloid and normal dermal fibroblasts (McCoy, Diegelmann, and Cohen, 1980). Surprisingly, collagen production as measured by prolyl hydroxylase (Cohen and Keiser, 1973) was not decreased in lesions previously treated with triamcinolone. Nevertheless, triamcinolone acetonide is the steroid of choice for intralesional treatment of keloids. Moderately insoluble intralesional triamcinolone acetonide has been claimed to be effective in reducing the size of keloids and hypertrophic scars (Fig. 21–5). It has also been suggested that keloid resorption after steroid treatment may, in part, be due to steroid enhancement of collagenase activity (Ketchum, Robinson, and Masters, 1967; Houck and Sharma, 1968). There are data to suggest that corticosteroids not only inhibit protein synthesis but also enhance collagenase activity (McCoy, Diegelmann, and Cohen, 1980).

Triamcinolone acetonide is best used in a concentration of 40 mg per ml; smaller concentrations are ineffective. Local infiltration of the lesion with a Wyeth metal syringe containing a needle that is part of the syringe barrel itself and is not detached by high pressure injection is recommended. The bevel of the needle should be directed down during injection and, when possible, injection should be into the upper dermis, because there seems to be wider dispersion of the drug by means of this technique. The metal syringe also protects the surgeon's hand from injury during injection. Local anesthesia is not necessary and only adds to the patient's discomfort because of the additional injections necessary. Dermojet does not appear to be useful in keloid therapy, and there are no data suggesting that Dermojet injections are better than direct injections.

Injections are usually staged six to eight weeks apart. In hypertrophic scars and smaller keloids, caution should be exercised because overtreatment may result in the development of telangiectasias and severe tissue atrophy, which may create additional significant deformity. Similarly, depigmentation in dark-skinned patients may cause patient dissatisfaction. Pregnancy or planned pregnancy are contraindications to treatment since corticosteroids may induce birth defects.

Colchicine is a pharmacologic agent that has had limited use in treating abnormal scars. This agent is able to inactivate microtubules within collagen-producing fibroblasts so that collagen cannot be secreted from the cells. (Diegelmann and Peterkofsky, 1972; Ehrlich, Grisilis, and Hunt, 1977). Colchicine may also enhance collagenase activity (Harris and Krane, 1971; Labandter, 1978). Unfortunately, it appears that the effective dose of colchicine lies close to its toxic dose, and therefore this agent and other drugs with a similar mode of action have limited clinical application in the treatment of abnormal scars when used by themselves. In fact, there are no animal or human data to substantiate the efficacy of systemic colchicine in the treat-

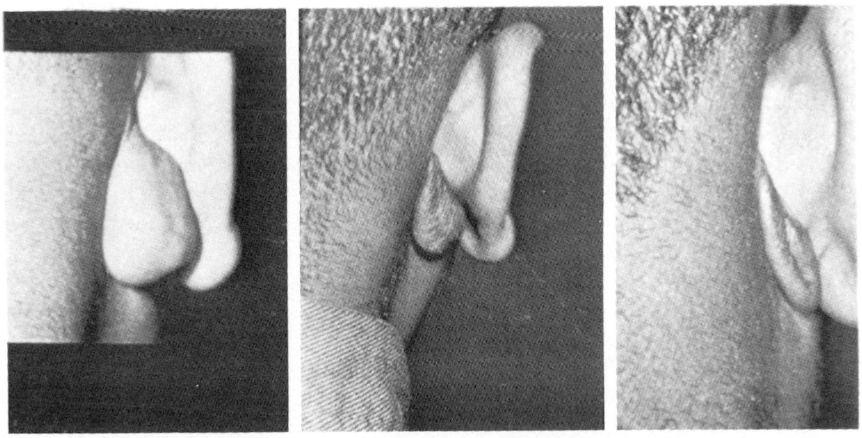

Figure 21–5. Keloid behind the ear of a 17 year old patient. It regressed after four monthly intralesional injections of triamcinolone acetonide. (From Ketchum, L. D., Smith, J., Robinson, D. W., and Masters, F. W.: The treatment of hypertrophic scar, keloid, and scar contracture by triamcinolone acetonide. Plast. Reconstr. Surg., *38*:209, 1966.)

ment of these conditions. One of the authors (EEP) has reported preliminary data to suggest that colchicine, in combination with other agents, may decrease collagen deposition in animal wounds as well as in human beings (Peacock, Madden, and Trier, 1970; Labandter, 1978). It seems likely, therefore, that the clinical use of colchicine in the treatment of abnormal scars will probably be in conjunction with other agents.

Beta-aminopropionitrile (BAPN) is a lathyrogenic agent that is receiving renewed clinical interest as a scar-controlling drug. First investigations in 1966 (Peacock and Madden) demonstrated the ability of BAPN to act clinically as a collagen crosslinking inhibitor. The integrity of the collagen molecule depends, to a large extent, on crosslinking and fibril formation of the molecule in the extra cellular space. Agents such as BAPN and D-penicillamine prevent collagen crosslinking and thereby render the molecule more susceptible to enzymatic degradation (Peacock, Madden, and Trier, 1970; Labandter, 1978). Subsequent use of BAPN in preventing tendon adhesions (Craver, Madden, and Peacock, 1968), joint stiffness in immobilized limbs (Furlow and Peacock, 1965), and esophageal stricture (Davis, Madden, and Peacock, 1972) has proved its potential usefulness in preventing fibrosis, but not without undesirable side effects that appear to be by-products of its metabolism. It is believed now that if metabolism of the agent can be blocked (by monoamine oxidase inhibitors such as pargyline) (Arem, Rasmussen, and Peacock, 1977), the lathyrogenic properties of BAPN can be maximized while the toxic effects are minimized. At present, long-term use of systemic BAPN is clearly not the answer to the control of abnormal scar because of its generalized effects on body collagen. Another agent, D-penicillamine, inhibits collagen crosslinking at different sites from those affected by BAPN; the combined use of two such agents may prove more efficacious than either alone. For lesions such as keloid and hypertrophic scar, systemic toxicity of BAPN could be avoided completely by development of an efficient topical delivery system. The basal turnover rate of collagen in unwounded tissue is extremely slow, and BAPN does not alter collagen that has already been crosslinked. BAPN only *prevents* newly synthesized collagen from being crosslinked in a mature insoluble form. Therefore, to use topical BAPN for treatment of keloids, excision of the lesion is required before the drug is administered. Perhaps, if esthetic surgical procedures are performed on known keloid formers, topical BAPN or topical D-penicillamine *may* be effective in preventing keloid formation in the new incisions. Although at this time the clinical use of these topical agents can be classified only as investigative, their widespread use may be anticipated within the next decade.

Other efforts to control or prevent abnormal scar formation pharmacologically include the use of iron chelators such as α,α'-dipyridyl or *o*-phenanthroline (Brada, Chvapil, and Bulba, 1972). These agents interfere with hydroxyproline formation and therefore render the collagen molecule more susceptible to degradation. The direct effects of iron-chelating agents on specific collagen metabolism in vivo have not been fully determined and the agents may have undesirable toxic, nonspecific iron-chelating properties. The use of proline or lysine analogues such as 3,4-dehydro-L-proline, *cis*-4-fluoro-L-proline, and *cis*-4-hydroxy-L-proline to create underhydroxylated collagen has also been attempted (Rosenbloom and Prockop, 1971; Bora, Lane, and Prockop, 1972). The efficacy of these agents appears to depend on the available in vivo amino acid pools of proline and lysine as well as on other factors that significantly curtail the effectiveness of analogues in treating fibrosis. This type of biochemical approach to wound healing control was an excellent concept, but similar to other treatment modalities, has not proved practical clinically because of associated drug toxicity.

Mechanical

Mechanical pressure has been reported to inhibit hypertrophic scar formation (Shoemaker, 1901). Dunoff and Burke (1978) hypothesized that mechanical pressure altered the glycosaminoglycan (GAG) content and blood vessel permeability of healing wounds and thus subsequently curtailed scar formation by altering normal collagen-GAG interaction during wound healing. Others suggested that mechanical pressure increases tissue collagenase activity, which in turn prevents excessive collagen deposition (Kischer, Shetlar, and Shetlar, 1975; Larson and associates, 1976; Brent, 1978); this notion has not been substantiated. Nevertheless, pressure therapy is used widely to control abnormal scar formation after burn injury, for example, even though the mechanisms by which mechanical pressure works are unknown. The procedure involves prolonged application of pressure wraps (four to 12 months for burn scars) (Larson and associates, 1976); in the case of keloids, a pressure earring may be applied (Brent, 1978) to prevent their recurrence. Problems have been encountered, however, in that when the pressure is removed for any length of time, hypertrophic scarring may occur. Sasaki (1988) attempted to treat sternal keloids by tissue expansion followed by tension-free wound closure. His unpublished data clearly demonstrate, however, that keloids still recur in the presence of tension-free closure after skin expansion.

Radiation

The use of ionizing radiation as a means of treating keloids was first attempted in the early 1900's (DeBeurman and Gougerot, 1906) and thereafter with questionable success (Stark, 1963; Spector, 1969). Radiation nonselectively destroys collagen-producing fibroblasts in the lesions as well as in surrounding connective tissue and cells—a significant drawback to its use. Even when combined with surgery and chemotherapy, radiation does not appear to provide an effective, preventive modality for abnormal scar or keloid formation. Although there are no known reports of radiation-induced carcinoma following treatment of abnormal scars with radiation, caution is always recommended because of this possibility.

Surgical

Manipulation of the type of suture material and experiments with different suture techniques have been proposed as methods of obviating possible abnormal scar formation. There are no data to suggest that the type of suture material or surgical closure technique is in any way involved in the etiology of abnormal scar. However, tension and lines of relaxed skin tension (see Chap. 1) may be related to hypertrophic scar formation (Flint, 1976). Experienced surgeons recognize that preauricular rhytidectomy closure with tension often results in hypertrophic scarring. Wound closure in the lines of relaxed skin tension (i.e., the transverse forehead) usually produces fine-line scars, whereas perpendicular forehead scars tend to be hypertrophic. W- or Z-plasty (see Chap. 1) correction of hypertrophic scars must be done with great caution to avoid the greater deformity of a hypertrophic W or Z (Flint, 1976). Some authors have suggested that a rim of keloid, allegedly to splint the wound, should remain at the time of excision (Peacock, Madden, and Trier, 1970). There are no data to support this concept. Similarly, there is the clinical impression (personal observation) of reduced incidence of recurrent earlobe keloid if the entire epithelial tract resulting from the original ear-piercing event is removed. However, there are no statistical data to confirm this clinical impression. Perhaps it is not too speculative to conceive of a pharmacologic suture capable of controlling collagen deposition or the inflammatory process in the healing wounds after closure.

MECHANICAL FACTORS OF SURGICAL WOUND CLOSURE AFFECTING SCAR APPEARANCE

Amount of Scar Tissue. The amount of scar tissue or collagen deposited in a wound has remained out of the control of the surgeon. Perhaps, avoiding the use of large foreign body sutures, applying pressure, and preventing hematoma may alter the ultimate appearance of scar. Many authors believe that the fibroplastic response is greater in children and during pregnancy. Elderly people often have less inflammatory response and less scar tissue than the young.

Lines of Minimal Tension (Langer's Lines). In 1861 Langer observed the directional spreading of puncture wounds in cadavers, which, in general, correspond to the lines of minimal tension in the skin (see Chap. 1). In general, these lines are perpendicular to the underlying muscle. It has been argued that scars parallel to the muscle pull (in Langer's lines) resolve earlier and remain finer and more delicate than those where muscular activity results in tension on the skin. Although this clinical observation and hypothesis are often valid, there are many cases in which fine-line scars occur with skin tension and hypertrophic scars may occur in tension-free closure. Tension probably represents only one of many multifactorial elements affecting the resultant scar.

To avoid tension on skin closure and to place incisions parallel to the lines of minimal tension, or as close to parallel as possible, surgeons often perform Z- or W-plasties (see Chap. 1). Although these mechanical maneuvers may indeed result in esthetically improved scars, one must remember that hypertrophic or wide scars may also occur with these procedures. *There are no mechanical alterations of skin that will control keloid recurrence.* Z-plasty correction of a keloid almost always results in another keloid.

A Z-plasty can be used to relax areas of skin tension and provide a greater range of motion when additional skin is available adjacent to the area of tension. The aphorism of Sir Harold Gillies over 30 years ago remains valid that one can rob Peter to pay Paul when Peter can afford to pay the price. Thus, a large Z-plasty can relieve an axillary contracture (Fig. 21–6) without the use of a skin graft. The Z-plasty principles of Davis and Kitlowski espoused in 1939 are as sound today as they were then (Fig. 21–7).

Shape of a Scar. A semicircular scar may become puffy and raised, and is called a "trapdoor" scar (Fig. 21–8). There is no validity to the hypothesis that the trapdoor deformity is secondary to lymphatic or venous obstruction. Rather, as the curvilinear scar contracts, there is an almost pursestring-type effect (scar contraction), which raises the level of the tissue within the semicircle, resulting in the trapdoor effect (Fig. 21–9, 21–10).

Skin Suture Marks. Any mark left by a suture (Fig. 21–11) is the result of mechanical trauma from the suture material and manifests the same histologic features as those of an incisional scar (Gillman and Penn, 1956; Ordman and Gillman, 1966). Gillies' advice (1943) remains as meaningful today as it was then. "How tight to tie is a matter of experience and lies between that adequate to bring the edges closely opposed and that that cuts through by causing tissue necrosis. Err on the loose side. Stitch marks are indisputable evidence of a stitch that has caused a local pressure necrosis and its accompanying infection" (Fig. 21–12).

Avoidance of suture marks may be ascribed to a number of techniques. For example, as early as 1949 Webster stated that "buried sutures take the burden of tension from the skin sutures and allow the early removal of the latter so that they leave no scars. Constriction of the skin by sutures causes necrosis, and necrosis means scarring and deformity. The more loosely the skin stures can be tied, in conformance with good approximation of the cut surface, and the earlier they can

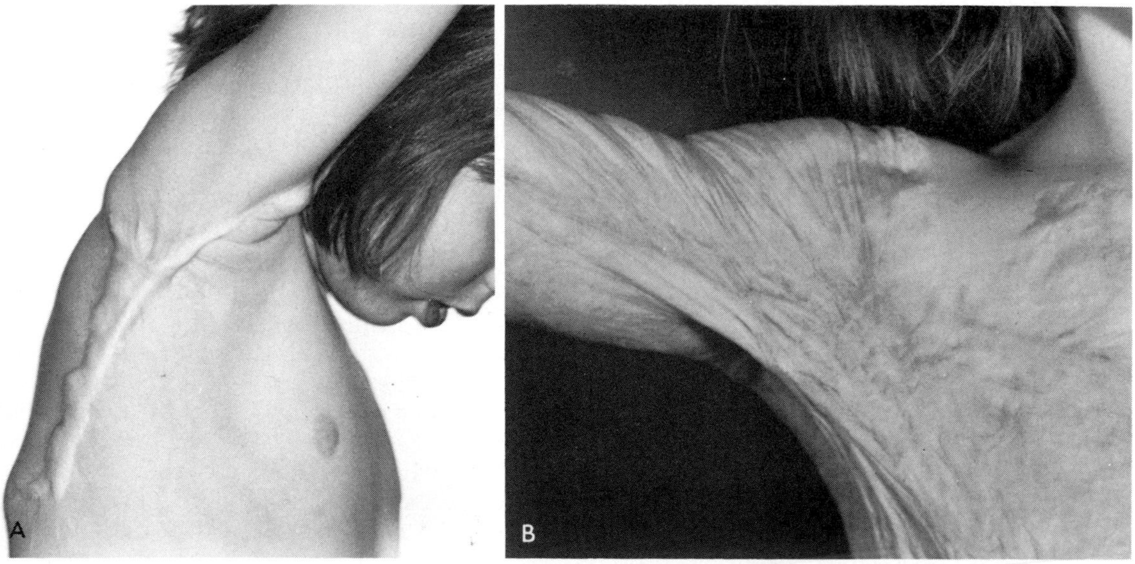

Figure 21–6. Contracture and hypertrophy of an incision crossing the axillary flexion crease *(A)* and an elevated contracture band without hypertrophy *(B)* of a burn scar involving the anterior axillary line.

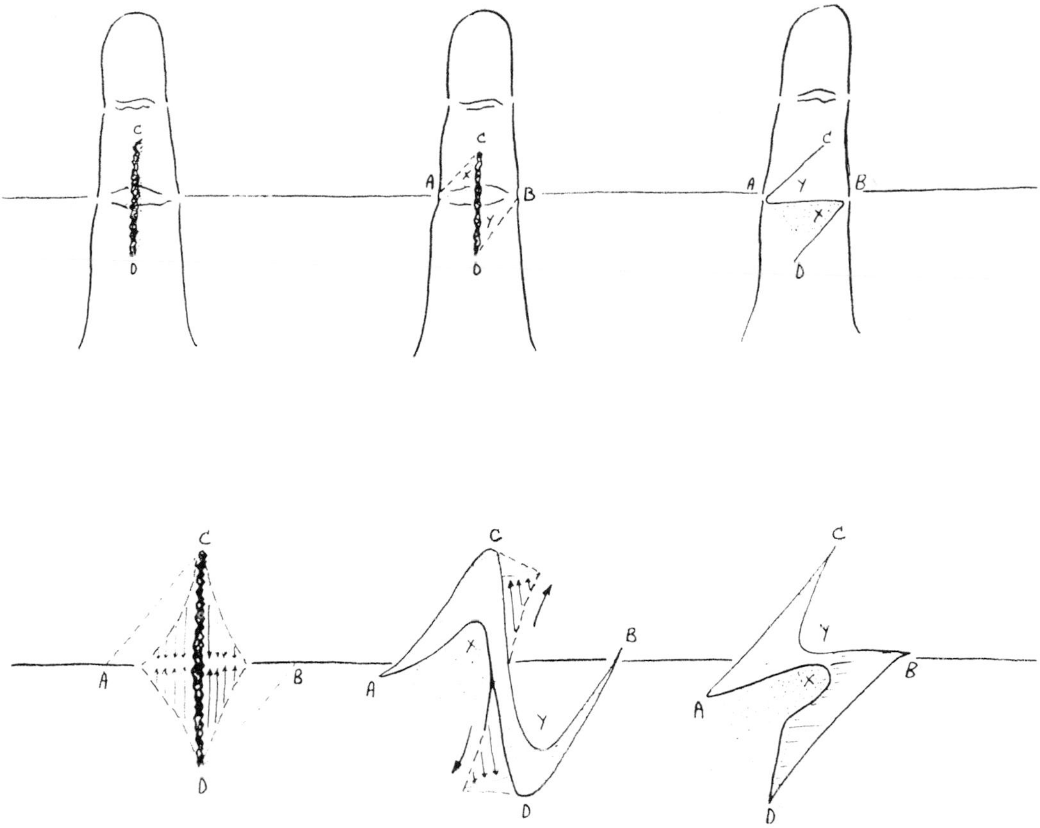

Figure 21–7. Correction of a crossjoint scar by Z-plasty. CD is converted to CA–AB–BD. As soon as the incisions AC and DB are made, the triangular flaps X and Y tend to transpose themselves to the desired position because of the inherent contraction forces in the scar.

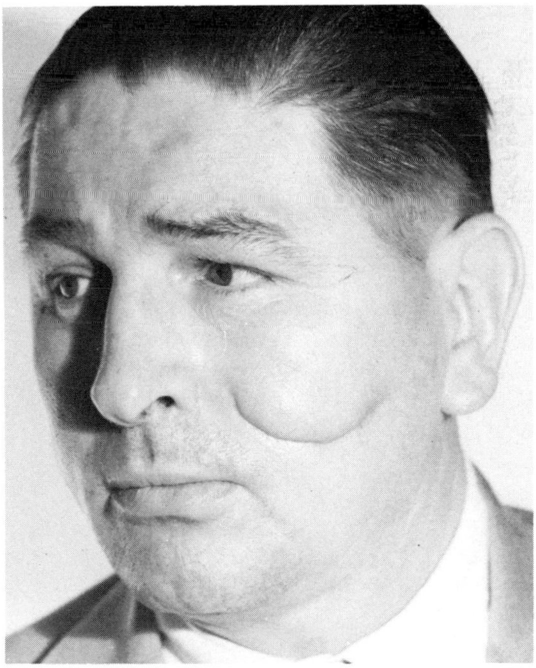

Figure 21–8. Trapdoor scar of the cheek.

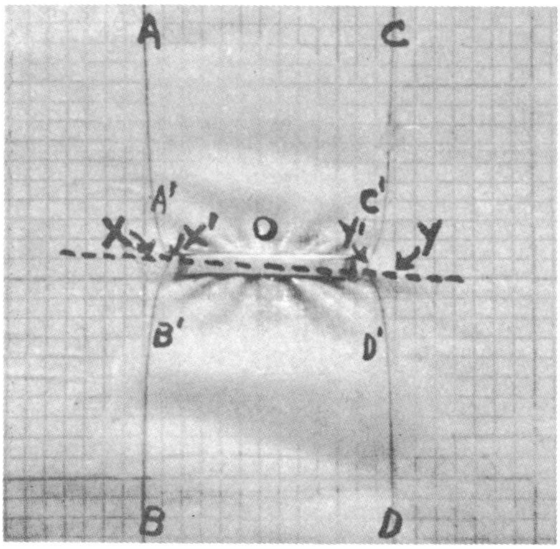

Figure 21–9. Experimental study of scar contraction. A rubber band is glued under tension onto an elastic membrane. Contraction of the rubber band pulls straight lines AXB to A′X′B′ and CYD to C′Y′D′. Note also the wrinkles above and below the rubber band X′OY′. The forces of contractions can be graphically represented by triangle A′X′B′ and triangle C′Y′D′ (JU, 195′).

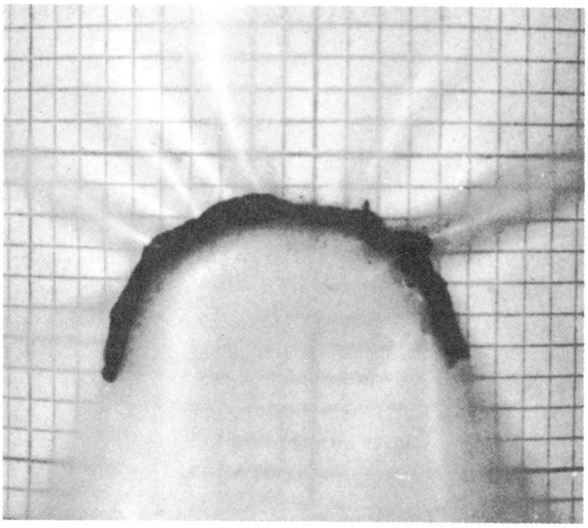

Figure 21–10. Experimental production of the trapdoor effect. A semicircular rubber band under tension is glued onto the elastic membrane. The membrane within the semicircle becomes raised and puffy (JU, 1951).

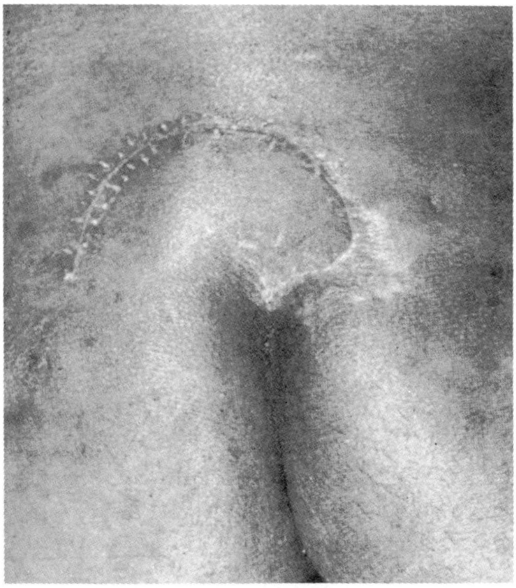

Figure 21–11. Excision of a sacral pressure sore and closure of the defect by a rotation flap. Note the suture marks in the left half of the incision.

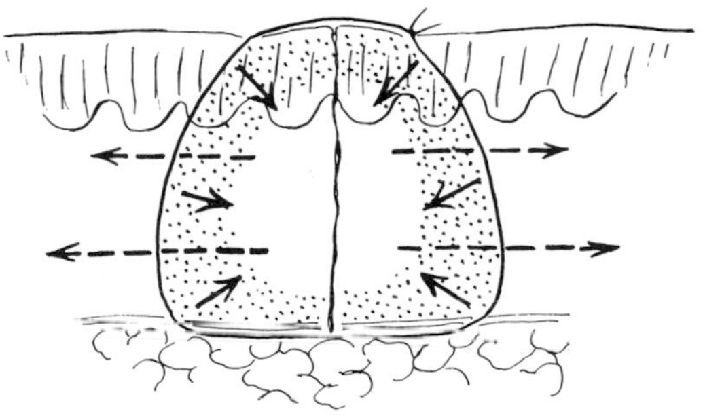

Figure 21–12. If the suture is tied too tightly, the intrinsic tension is toward the center, and ischemia and necrosis occur in the encompassed tissue *(stippled area).* If extrinsic tension tends to distract the wound edges, the force is away from the center, but the adversely affected tissue area is the same.

be removed, the smaller will be the permanent mark on the skin."

Without reviewing historical observations, it is clear that closure with subcuticular sutures alone avoids most risks of suture marks. Skin tape closures with or without dermal sutures may be indicated. Although sutures through the entire skin may be appropriate, they should be removed as early as possible to prevent epithelial tracking and skin necrosis. The astute technician is also aware that the trauma caused as the back end of the needle passes through skin may also cause sufficient damage to leave a permanent skin mark.

Location of a Scar. Some areas of the body heal with less noticeable scars than others. Incisions in the eyelids usually leave fine, almost invisible, scars, as do those in the forehead, the palms and soles, the penis and scrotum, and all mucous membranes generally. However, over the distal portion of the nose, scars become depressed. Scars about the chin, sternal area, shoulders, and upper back tend to spread, as do incisions on the lower extremities. This all too frequently happens despite proper attention to surgical precepts. Certain conditions such as acne and lymphedema also predispose to unsightly scars.

REFERENCES

Arem, A. J., Rasmussen, D., and Peacock, E. E., Jr.: Monoamine oxidase inhibition during the control of scar formation. Surg. Forum, *28*:528, 1977.

Bailey, A. J., Bazin, S., Sims, T. J., Le Lous, M., Nicoletis, C., and Delaunay, A.: Characterization of the collagen of human hypertrophic and normal scars. Biochim. Biophys. Acta, *405*:412, 1975a.

Bailey, A. J., Sims, T. J., Le Lous, M., and Bazin, S.: Collagen polymorphism in experimental granulation tissue. Biochem. Biophys. Res. Commun., *66*:1160, 1975b.

Baur, P. S., Barratt, G., and Linares, H. A.: Wound contractions, scar contractures and myofibroblasts: a clinical case study. J. Trauma, *18*:8, 1978.

Blackburn, W. R., and Cosman, B.: Histologic basis of keloid and hypertrophic scar differentiation. Arch. Pathol., *82*:65, 1966.

Bloom, D.: Heredity of keloids. Review of the literature and a report of a family with multiple keloids in five generations. N. Y. State J. Med., *56*:511, 1956.

Bora, F. W., Jr., Lane, M. M., and Prockop, D. J.: Inhibitors of collagen biosynthesis as a means of controlling scar formation in tendon injury. J. Bone Joint Surg., *54A*:1501, 1972.

Bordin, S., Page, R. C., and Narayanan, A. S.: Heterogeneity of normal human diploid fibroblasts: isolation and characterization of one phenotype. Science, *223*:171, 1984.

Brada, Z., Chvapil, M., and Bulba, S.: Influence of 1,10-phenanthroline on pathologic changes in liver of ethionine fed rats. Life Sci., *11*:2277, 1972.

Brenizer, A. G.: Keloid formation in the Negro. Ann. Surg., *61*:83, 1915.

Brent, B.: The role of pressure therapy in management of earlobe keloids: preliminary report of a controlled study. Ann. Plast. Surg., *1*:579, 1978.

Chvapil, M., and Hurych, J.: Control of collagen biosynthesis. *In* Hall, D. A. (Ed.): International Review of Connective Tissue Research. Vol. 4. New York, Academic Press, 1968, p. 67.

Chytilova, H., Kulhanek, V., and Horn, V.: Experimental production of keloids after immunization with autologous skin. Acta Chir. Plast. (Praha), *1*:70, 1959.

Cohen, I. K., Beaven, M. A., Horakova, Z., and Keiser, H. R.: Histamine and collagen synthesis in keloid and hypertrophic scar. Surg. Forum, *23*:509, 1972.

Cohen, I. K., Diegelmann, R. F., and Keiser, H. R.: Collagen metabolism in keloid and hypertrophic scar. *In* Longacre, J. J. (Ed.): The Ultrastructure of Collagen. Springfield, IL, Charles C Thomas, 1976, pp. 199–212.

Cohen, I. K., and Keiser, H. R.: Collagen synthesis in keloid and hypertrophic scar following intralesional use of triamcinolone. Surg. Forum, *24*:521, 1973.

Cohen, I. K., Keiser, H. R., and Sjoerdsma, A.: Collagen synthesis in human keloid and hypertrophic scar. Surg. Forum, *22*:488, 1971.

Cohen, I. K., McCoy, B. J., Mohanakumar, T., and Diegelmann, R. F.: Immunoglobulin, complement, and histocompatibility antigen studies in keloid patients. Plast. Reconstr. Surg., *63*:689, 1979.

Craig, R. D. P., Schofield, J. D., and Jackson, D. S.: Collagen biosynthesis in normal and hypertrophic scars and keloid as a function of the duration of the scar. Br. J. Surg., *62*:741, 1975.

Craver, J. M., Madden, J. W., and Peacock, E. E., Jr.: Biological control of physical properties of tendon adhesions: effect of beta-aminopropionitrile in chickens. Ann. Surg., *167*:697, 1968.

Crikelair, G. F., Ju, D. M. C., and Cosman, B.: Scars and keloids. *In* Converse, J. M. (Ed.): Reconstructive Plastic Surgery. 2nd Ed., Philadelphia, W. B. Saunders Company, 1977, p. 413.

Crockett, D. J.: Regional keloid susceptibility. Br. J. Plast. Surg., *17*:245, 1964.

Davis, J. S., and Kitlowski, E. A.: The theory and

practical use of the Z-incision for the relief of scar contractures. Ann. Surg., *109*:1001, 1939.

Davis, W. M., Madden, J. W., and Peacock, E. E., Jr.: A new approach to the control of esophageal stenosis. Ann. Surg., *176*:469, 1972.

DeBeurman, C., and Gougerot, H.: Cheloides des muguescises. Ann. Dermatol. Syphil., *7*:151, 1906.

Diegelmann, R. F., Bryant, C. P., and Cohen, I. K.: Tissue alpha-globulins in keloid formation. Plast. Reconstr. Surg., *59*:418, 1977.

Diegelmann, R. F., Cohen, I. K., and McCoy, B. J.: Growth kinetics and collagen synthesis of normal skin, normal scar, and keloid fibroblasts in vitro. J. Cell Physiol., *98*:341, 1979.

Diegelmann, R. F., and Peterkofsky, B.: Inhibition of collagen secretion from bone and cultured fibroblasts by microtubular disruptive drugs. Proc. Natl. Acad. Sci. U.S.A., *69*:892, 1972.

Dunoff, R. B., and Burke, J. F.: Abnormality of hypertrophic scar blood vessels. J. Surg. Res., *25*:251, 1978.

Ehrlich, H. P., Grisilis, G., and Hunt, T.: Evidence for the involvement of microtubules in wound contraction. Am. J. Surg., *133*:706, 1977.

Flint, M. H.: The biological basis of Langer's lines. *In* Longacre, J. J. (Ed.): The Ultrastructure of Collagen. Springfield, IL, Charles C Thomas, 1976, pp. 132–140.

Furlow, L. T., Jr., and Peacock, E. E., Jr.: Effect of beta-amino propionitrile on the prevention and treatment of joint stiffness in rats. Surg. Forum, *16*:457, 1965.

Gay, S., Viljanto, J., Rackellio, J., and Penttinen, R. P.: Collagen types in early phases of wound healing in children. Acta Chir. Scand., *144*:205, 1978.

Gillies, H.: Technique of good suturing. Clin. J., *72*:223, 1943.

Gillman, T., and Penn, J.: Studies on the repair of cutaneous wounds. M. Proc. Johannesburg (Suppl.), *2*:1, 121, 150, 1956.

Griffith, B. H.: The treatment of keloids with triamcinolone acetonide. Plast. Reconstr. Surg., *38*:202, 1966.

Hakanson, R., Owman, C., Sjoberg, N. O., and Sporrong, B.: Direct histochemical demonstration of histamine in cutaneous mast cells: urticaria pigmentosa and keloids. Experientia, *25*:854, 1969.

Harris, E. D., Jr., and Krane, S. M.: Effects of colchicine on collagenase in cultures of rheumatoid synovium. Arthritis Rheum., *14*:669, 1971.

Hayakawa, T., Hashimoto, Y., Myokei, Y., Aoyama, H., and Izawa, Y.: Changes in type of collagen during the development of human post-burn hypertrophic scars. Clin. Chem. Acta, *93*:119, 1979.

Hazrati, E., and Hoomad, A.: The keloidal diathesis, a resistant state to malignancies. Plast. Reconstr. Surg., *59*:555, 1977.

Hoopes, J. E., Su, C. T., and Im, M. J. C.: Enzyme activities in hypertrophic scars and keloids. Plast. Reconstr. Surg., *47*:132, 1971.

Houck, J. C., and Sharma, U. K.: Induction of collagenolytic and proteolytic activities in rat and human fibroblasts by anti-inflammatory drugs. Science, *161*:1361, 1968.

Hunt, T. K., Conolly, W. B., Aronson, S. B., and Goldstein, P.: Anaerobic metabolism and wound healing: an hypothesis for the initiation and cessation of collagen synthesis in wounds. Am. J. Surg., *135*:328, 1978.

James, W. D., Besanceney, C. D., and Odom, R. B.: The ultrastructure of a keloid. J. Am. Acad. Dermatol., *3*:50, 1980.

Janssen de Limpens, A. M. P., and Cormane, R. H.: Studies on the immunologic aspects of keloids and hypertrophic scars. Arch. Dermatol. Res., *274*:259, 1982.

Ju, D. M. C.: The physical basis of scar contracture. Plast. Reconstr. Surg., *7*:343, 1951.

Katz, S. I.: Histocompatibility antigens and disease. Arch. Dermatol., *113*:1716, 1977.

Keiser, H., Leroy, E. C., Udenfriend, S., and Sjoerdsma, A.: Collagen-like protein in human plasma. Science, *142*:1678, 1963.

Kemble, J. V. H., and Brown, R. F. R.: Enzyme activity in human scars, hypertrophic scars and keloids. Br. J. Dermatol., *94*:301, 1976.

Ketchum, L. D., Cohen, I. K., and Masters, F. W.: Hypertrophic scars and keloids. A collective review. Plast. Reconstr. Surg., *53*:140, 1974.

Ketchum, L. D., Robinson, D. W., and Masters, F. W.: Degradation of mature collagen: a laboratory study. Plast. Reconstr. Surg., *40*:89, 1967.

Ketchum, L. D., Smith, J., Robinson, D. W., and Masters, F. W.: The treatment of hypertrophic scar, keloid, and scar contracture by triamcinolone acetonide. Plast. Reconstr. Surg., *38*:209, 1966.

Kischer, C. W., Bunce, H., III, and Shetlar, M. R.: Mast cell analyses in hypertrophic scars, hypertrophic scars treated with pressure, and mature scars. J. Invest. Dermatol., *70*:355, 1978.

Kischer, C. W., and Hendrix, M. J.: Fibronectin in hypertrophic scars and keloids. Cell Tissue Res., *231*:29, 1983.

Kischer, C. W., Shetlar, M. R., and Chvapil, M.: Hypertrophic scars and keloids: a review and new concept concerning their origin. Scan. Electron Microsc., *4*:1699, 1982.

Kischer, C. W., Shetlar, M. R., and Shetlar, C. L.: Alteration of hypertrophic scars induced by mechanical pressure. Arch. Dermatol., *111*:60, 1975.

Kischer, C. W., Shetlar, M. R., Shetlar, C. L., and Chvapil, M.: Immunoglobulins in hypertrophic scars and keloids. Plast. Reconstr. Surg., *71*:821, 1983.

Kischer, C. W., Thies, A. C., and Chvapil, M.: Perivascular myofibroblasts and microvascular occlusion in hypertrophic scars and keloids. Hum. Pathol., *13*:819, 1982.

Koonin, A. J.: The aetiology of keloids: a review of the literature and a new hypothesis. S. Afr. Med. J., *38*:913, 1964.

Labandter, H.: Potentiation of colchicine-induced collagenolysis. Surg. Forum, *29*:592, 1978.

Langer, C.: Zur Anatomie und Physiologie der Haut. Sitzungsb. Acad. Wissensch., *45*:223, 1861.

Larson, D. L., Willis, B., Linares, H., Shetlar, M. R., and Kischer, C. W.: *In* Longacre, J. J. (Ed.): The Ultrastructure of Collagen. Springfield, IL, Charles C Thomas, 1976, p. 269.

Laurentaci, G., and Dioguardi, D.: HLA antigens in keloids and hypertrophic scars. Arch. Dermatol., *113*:1729, 1977.

Linares, H. A., Kischer, C. W., Dobrkovsky, M., and Larson, D. L.: The histiotypic organization of the hypertrophic scar in humans. J. Invest. Dermatol., *59*:323, 1972.

Manalan, S. S., Cohen, I. K., and Theogaraj, S. D.: Dermatofibrosarcoma protuberans or keloid—a warning. Case report. Plast. Reconstr. Surg., *54*:96, 1974.

Martin, G. M., Sprague, C. A., Norwood, T. H., and Pendergrass, W. R.: Clonal selection, attenuation and differentiation in an *in vitro* model of hyperplasia. Am. J. Pathol., *74*:137, 1974.

McCoy, B. J., and Cohen, I. K.: Effects of various sera

on growth kinetics and collagen synthesis by keloid and normal dermal fibroblasts. Plast. Reconstr. Surg., *67*:505, 1981.

McCoy, B. J., and Cohen, I. K.: Collgenase in keloid biopsies and fibroblasts. Connect. Tissue Res., *9*:181, 1982.

McCoy, B. J., Diegelmann, R. F., and Cohen, I. K.: In vitro inhibition of cell growth, collagen synthesis, and prolyl hydroxylase activity by triamcinolone acetonide. Proc. Soc. Exp. Biol. Med., *163*:216, 1980.

McCoy, B. J., Galdun, J., and Cohen, I. K.: Effects of density and cellular aging on collagen synthesis and growth kinetics in keloid and normal skin fibroblasts. In Vitro, *18*:79, 1982.

Milsom, J. P., and Craig, R. D. P.: Collagen degradation in cultured keloid and hypertrophic scar tissue. Br. J. Dermatol., *89*:635, 1973.

Mowlem, R.: Hypertrophic scars. Br. J. Plast. Surg., *4*:113, 1951.

Oluwasanmi, J. O.: Keloids in the African. Clin. Plast. Surg., *1*:179, 1974.

Oluwasanmi, J. O., Lucas, D. O., and Chvapil, M.: Effect of a concurrent immune response on the collagen synthesis around implanted Ivalon sponges. Plast. Reconstr. Surg., *58*:601, 1976.

Ordman, L. J., and Gillman, T.: Studies in the healing of cutaneous wounds. II. The healing of epidermal, appendageal, and dermal injuries inflicted by suture needles and by the suture material in the skin of pigs. Arch. Surg., *93*:883, 1966.

Peacock, E. E., Jr., and Madden, J. W.: Some studies on the effect of α-aminopropionitrile on collagen in healing wounds. Surgery, *60*:7, 1966.

Peacock, E. E., Jr., Madden, J. W., and Trier, W. C.: Biologic basis for the treatment of keloids and hypertrophic scars. South. Med. J., *63*:755, 1970.

Rosenbloom, J., and Prockop, D. J.: Incorporation of *cis*-hydroxyproline into protocollagen and collagen. J. Biol. Chem., *246*:1549, 1971.

Russell, J. D., Russell, S. B., and Trupin, K. M.: The effect of histamine on the growth of cultured fibroblasts isolated from normal and keloid tissue. J. Cell Physiol., *93*:389, 1977.

Russell, J. D., Russell, S. B., and Trupin, K. M.: Fibroblast heterogeneity in glucocorticoid regulation of collagen metabolism: genetic or epigenetic? In Vitro, *18*:557, 1982.

Russell, S. B., Trupin, K. M., Rodriguez-Eaton, S., Russell, J. D., and Trupin, J. S.: Reduced growth factor requirement of keloid-derived fibroblasts may account for tumor growth. Proc. Natl. Acad. Sci. U.S.A., *85*:587, 1988.

Sasaki, G.: Personal communication, 1988.

Shoemaker, J. V.: A Practical Treatise on Diseases of the Skin. 4th Ed. New York, D. Appleton Company, 1901.

Spector, W. G.: Inflammation in repair and regeneration. *In* Dunphy, J. E., and Van Winkle, H. W., Jr. (Eds.): Repair and Regeneration; The Scientific Basis for Surgical Practice. New York, McGraw-Hill Book Company, 1969, p. 8.

Stark, R.: Plastic Surgery. New York, Harper & Row, 1963.

Topol, B. M., Lewis, V. L., Jr., and Benveniste, K.: The use of antihistamine to retard the growth of fibroblasts derived from human skin, scar, and keloid. Plast. Reconstr. Surg., *68*:227, 1981.

Uitto, J., Perejda, A. J., Abergel, R. P., Chu, M.-L, and Ramirez, F.: Altered steady-state ratio of type I/III procollagen mRNAs correlates with selectively increased type I procollagen biosynthesis in cultured keloid fibroblasts. Proc. Natl. Acad. Sci. U.S.A., *82*:5935, 1985.

Webster, J. P.: Plastic surgery: general principles. *In* Christopher, F. (Ed.): Textbook of Surgery. 5th Ed. Philadelphia, W. B. Saunders Company, 1949, p. 1403.

22

Thomas J. Baker
James M. Stuzin

Chemical Peeling and Dermabrasion

A direct surgical approach is of limited usefulness for treating problems isolated to the dermis and epidermis. Multiple fine facial rhytides, an uneven area of skin pigmentation or hyperpigmentation, and acne scarring are conditions in which standard surgical techniques have limited application. These problems are better approached through other treatment modalities: chemical peeling and dermabrasion.

Chemical peeling and dermabrasion involve the controlled removal of the epidermis and superficial areas of dermis, thereby smoothing surface irregularities and altering areas of discoloration. While both modalities have been used in the past to treat similar clinical problems, trial and error have given the clinician a better understanding of which is better suited to the various pathologic conditions; they should no longer be used interchangeably.

CHEMICAL PEELING

Chemical peeling is a process in which chemicals are applied to the skin in order to obtain alteration in the gross and microscopic anatomy of the dermis and epidermis. The application of certain chemical mixtures produces a controlled, predictable chemical injury to the skin. After healing, chemical peeling results in a smoother, firmer skin, which appears more youthful and less lined. Chemical peeling is most commonly used to remove fine facial wrinkles, to treat irregular hyperpigmentation of facial skin, and to ablate other minor skin blemishes (Baker and Gordon, 1986).

Historical Background

Although there is no recorded evidence, it is likely that prehistoric people recognized and used abrasives, oils, and simple drugs as a beautification treatment for aging skin. The oldest record of cosmetic treatment by physicians is the Ebers papyrus circa 1560 B.C., (Ebbell, 1937), which outlines methods for removing wrinkles, dyeing hair and eyebrows, and correcting squints, along with other procedures for beautifying the body. Early chemosurgery probably took the form of certain types of acid treatment. Exfoliation of the skin was accomplished by the direct application of poultices made from mineral and plant substances. Sulfur, mustard, and limestone are known to have been used (Baker and Gordon, 1987).

During the early part of the twentieth century, chemical face peeling was periodically used by lay operators, although MacKee and Karp (1952) are reported to have used liquefied phenol for the treatment of acne scars as early as 1903. Early references in the medical literature are sparse, but an article published by Bames (1927) gave some background in the clinical observations made after the use of chemical peeling.

During the late 1940's and early 1950's, the treatment was given considerable publicity by the news media. Claims were made that the "Fountain of Youth" had been found at last, and miraculous results were illustrated in "before" and "after" pictures in advertisements by "lay" clinics. Throughout this period, despite the resolution of facial wrinkles, there remained a good deal of skepticism among the medical community. Most physicians concluded that the cases illustrated represented a hoax and that the photographs shown were touched up.

Despite the lack of medical acceptance, some physicians continued to investigate the use of chemical exfoliation. Urkov (1946) described his method of superficial exfoliation using a mixture of resorcinol and salicylic acid for light peeling; he preferred liquid phenol for acne scars and wrinkles. Another report by Sulzberger (1961) described treating acne scars with similar chemical agents.

As peeling became more commonplace, results observed by physicians of patients being treated in "lay" clinics stimulated a greater interest in the scientific investigation and evaluation of chemical peeling. The "secret" formulas of the lay operators were difficult to obtain, and discussions with them produced only a superficial understanding regarding the use of their formula. Over a period of years information was gradually gathered from both lay operators and their patients.

Brown, Kaplan, and Brown (1960a) are credited with introducing chemical peeling in the plastic surgery literature, although Gillies, without publishing his technique, is reported to have used pure carbolic acid many years previously in a painting and taping technique for the correction of "slight laxity of the lid" (Gillies and Millard, 1957; Batstone and Millard, 1968). Following the report of Brown, Kaplan, and Brown (1960a), numerous studies were published in both the plastic surgery and dermatology literature, demonstrating the clinical effectiveness of the procedure and the histopathologic changes accompanying chemical peeling (Baker, 1961, 1962; Baker and Gordon, 1963; Baker, Gordon, and Seckinger, 1966; Baker and associates, 1974; Litton, 1962, 1966; Litton, Fournier, and Capinpin, 1973; Combes, Sperber, and Reisch, 1960; Ayres, 1960, 1962, 1964; Sperber, 1963, 1965; Spira, Gerow, and Hardy, 1974).

The acceptance of chemical peeling by plastic surgeons has been gradual, although over time its safety, effectiveness, and longevity have been substantiated, and its use in the plastic surgery community is now widespread (Litton and Trinidad, 1981). From a secret treatment performed by lay operators, chemical peeling has become a safe, medically supervised technique that is widely used as an adjunct in treating certain dermatologic conditions.

Histology of Sun-Damaged and Aging Skin

Patients seeking chemical peel are generally middle-aged women who have had excessive sun exposure and have suffered structural skin damage, in addition to the normal aging process. Degenerative changes occur in both the dermis and epidermis (Kligman, 1969). The histologic changes that occur in aging parallel those that arise from actinic damage, the difference being perhaps more quantitative than qualitative. More accelerated and severe changes are seen after chronic sun exposure (Montagna and Carlisle, 1979).

Elastosis is the hallmark of sun-damaged skin (Fig. 22–1). It represents a degenerative process whereby dermal collagen is replaced by a thickened, tangled, dense mass of altered elastic fibers. Routine H and E (hematoxylin and eosin) stains of actinic skin reveal a basophilic degeneration of collagen and elastic fibers (Rudolph and Woodward, 1981). Mowry staining shows an increase in ground substance in the form of acid mucopolysac-

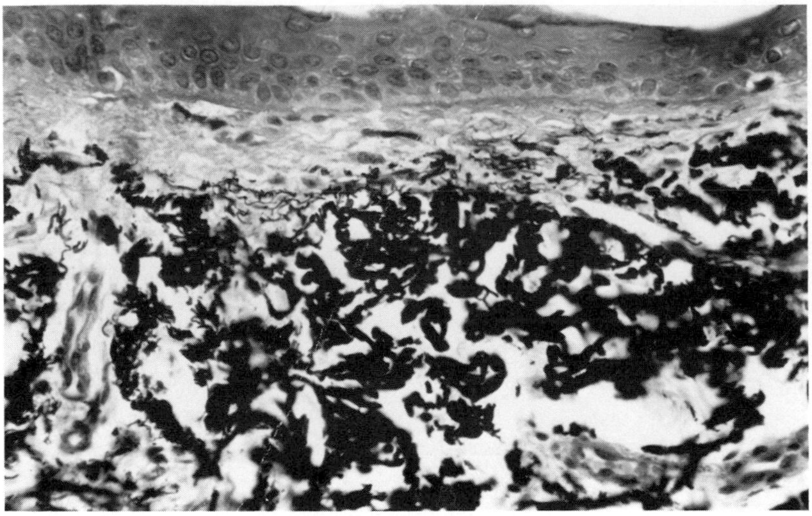

Figure 22–1. Histology of sun-damaged facial skin. The epidermal cells are in disarray, showing variability in size and staining properties. Beneath the flat epidermis, there is a thin, clear band of collagen ("grenz zone"), an ongoing attempt to repair dermal damage. The deep dermis is composed of thickened, tangled, abnormal elastic fibers (solar elastosis). (Luna stain, × 406.) (From Kligman, A. M., Baker, T. J., and Gordon, H. L.: Long-term histologic follow up of phenol face peels. Plast. Reconstr. Surg., *75*:652, 1985.

charides present within the dermis (Kligman, Baker, and Gordon, 1985). Elastic tissue stains reveal that the dermis appears to be replaced by a solid mass of damaged elastic fibers, which in undamaged skin comprise less than 5 per cent of the dry weight of the dermis. As the elastosis deepens, the collagen disappears proportionately. Thus, the fibrous network that normally provides dermis with its viscoelastic properties is degraded and the skin shows little resistance to stretching. Other findings in sun-damaged skin include a sparsity of vessels, which are irregularly placed and variably dilated. Large, thin-walled veins account for the telangiectasia of photo-damaged skin. A chronic inflammation signifying chronic injury is reflected in the patchy perivascular infiltration of lymphocytes, histiocytes, and mast cells observed histologically in these specimens (Fig. 22–1).

A thin subepidermal band of fine collagen seems to be exempt from the above degenerative changes. This eosinophilic band of collagen, without elastin being present, is termed the "grenz zone" and represents the region where new collagen is generated continuously by hyperplastic fibroblasts in an attempt to repair the ravages of ultraviolet light. This region of the papillary dermis, immediately below the basal layer of the epidermis, is largely responsible for the regenerative changes seen after chemical peeling (Stegman, 1982; Kligman, Baker, and Gordon, 1985).

The epidermis in sun-damaged skin appears disorderly, and is variably thickened

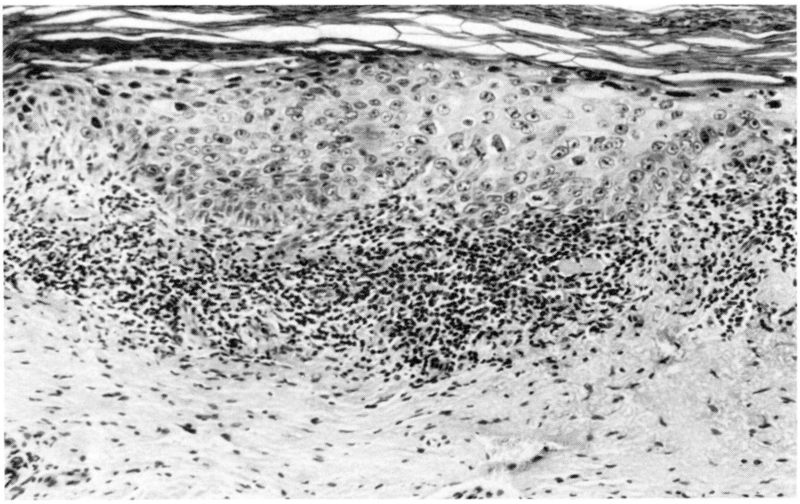

Figure 22–2. Early, subclinical actinic keratosis. The epidermis shows atypical cells and cytologic variability, and there is a dense subepidermal lymphocytic infiltrate. (H & E stain, × 160.) (From Kligman, A. M., Baker, T. J., and Gordon, H. L.: Long-term histologic follow up of phenol face peels. Plast. Reconstr. Surg., *75*:652, 1985.)

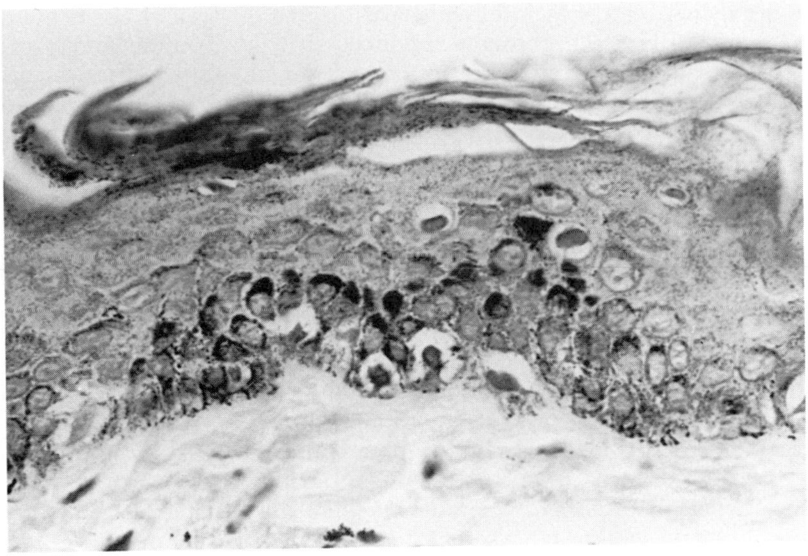

Figure 22–3. Uneven distribution of melanin granules in the epidermis. Some cells are engorged with melanin, while others contain little pigment. In the center are three large adjacent melanocytes, probably nonfunctional. The blotchiness of sun-damaged skin is largely attributed to irregular pigment distribution. (Fontana stain, × 650.) (From Kligman, A. M., Baker, T. J., and Gordon, H. L.: Long-term histologic follow up of phenol face peels. Plast. Reconstr. Surg., *75*:652, 1985.)

and composed of cells varying in size, shape, and staining properties. These cells are small with pyknotic nuclei, and exhibit cellular disarray with loss of vertical polarity. The basement membrane is thickened, ragged, and often blurred (Fig. 22–2).

Melanocytes within the epidermis are increased in number, hypertrophic, and unevenly distributed. The quantity of melanin granules within the keratinocytes is extremely variable; some cells are engorged with pigment, while others appear virtually empty. The uneven distribution of melanin explains the blotchiness of photo-damaged skin (Fig. 22–3).

In response to ultraviolet (UV) light, freckle-like, deeply pigmented macules are commonly produced, termed "solar lentigo" (or senile lentigo). These represent a downgrowth of pigment-laden cells produced by hyperplastic melanocytes (Fig. 22–4).

Histologic Changes After Chemical Peeling

The application of phenol produces a controlled chemical injury. The depth of penetration into the dermis is between 0.3 and 0.6 mm, extending into the papillary dermis (Ayres, 1960; Litton, 1962; Spira and associates, 1970; Stegman, 1982). The histologic

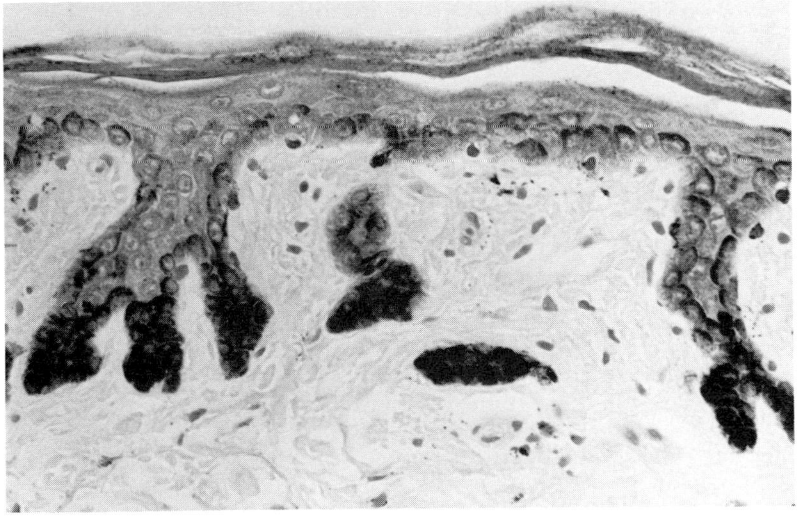

Figure 22–4. Solar lentigo represented by branching downgrowths of epidermis containing large amounts of pigment, secreted by numerous melanocytes clustered at the tips of the rete pegs. (Fontana stain, × 406.) (From Kligman, A. M., Baker, T. J., and Gordon, H. L.: Long-term histologic follow up of phenol face peels. Plast. Reconstr. Surg., *75*:652, 1985.)

and clinical changes following peeling are a direct result of the changes produced in the superficial dermis and epidermis: the removal of the damaged elastotic skin and the reconstruction of this layer with neocollagen after wound healing. As with other partial-thickness injury to the skin, the healing seen after chemical peeling proceeds from the epithelial appendages (Campbell, 1977; Kligman, Baker, and Gordon, 1985).

Biopsies obtained 48 hours after phenol peeling demonstrate a keratocoagulation necrosis of the epidermis, extending through the papillary dermis, surrounded by a marked inflammatory reaction (Litton, 1962). Epidermal regeneration begins at 48 hours and is usually completed within seven days. Dermal regeneration lags behind epidermal healing, and biopsies taken two weeks after treatment show only a partial reconstitution of the dermis; attempts at reformation of the rete pegs, dermal thickening, fibroblastic proliferation, and deposition of new collagen are also observed (Spira and associates, 1970). By three months the most striking change apparent in dermal anatomy is the alteration of the upper dermal collagen from a wavy, disorganized form to a rigid, compact shape, replacing the disorganized collagen seen in elastosis (Baker, 1962; Brown, Kaplan, and Brown, 1960a; Ayres, 1962; Stegman, 1982).

Over the years the authors have published the constant histologic changes seen in human skin after chemical peeling (Baker, Gordon, and Seckinger, 1966; Baker and Gordon, 1971; Baker and associates, 1974). These findings are:

1. Homogenization of the dermal collagen architecture.
2. Marked diminution of the quantity of melanin granules within the basal layer of the epidermis.
3. An increase in the amount of elastic staining tissue within the dermis.

The clinical conclusions based on the consistency of these histologic findings are as follows:

1. The microscopic changes induced by chemical peeling with phenol are permanent or nearly so.
2. The skin changes that occur after chemical peeling can be accurately predicted.
3. The histologic changes and alterations in dermal anatomy are responsible for the clinical reaction to peeling.

The etiology of the improved appearance of skin following regeneration of dermal collagen has been the subject of controversy (Baker and asociates, 1974; Bhangoo, 1974; Spira and associates, 1970; Spira, 1980). The best way to study the long-term effects of peeling is to examine the border zone of adjacent peeled and unpeeled skin in the same patient, so that adjoining specimens can be directly compared. Since most patients are reluctant to have their faces biopsied, specimens have been obtained after face lifting of patients who had been peeled earlier (Fig. 22–5) (Baker and associates, 1974; Kligman, Baker, and Gordon, 1985). The contrasts in changes between peeled and unpeeled skin are readily apparent and are most obvious within the first few months after treatment, although distinct differences remain even as long as 20 years later. The aging process continues, but the histologic changes produced by peeling are permanent and their clinical appearance is long-lasting.

Dermis. Even under low power magnification, the changes within the dermis after peeling are profound and contrast with the histologic appearance of the adjacent un-

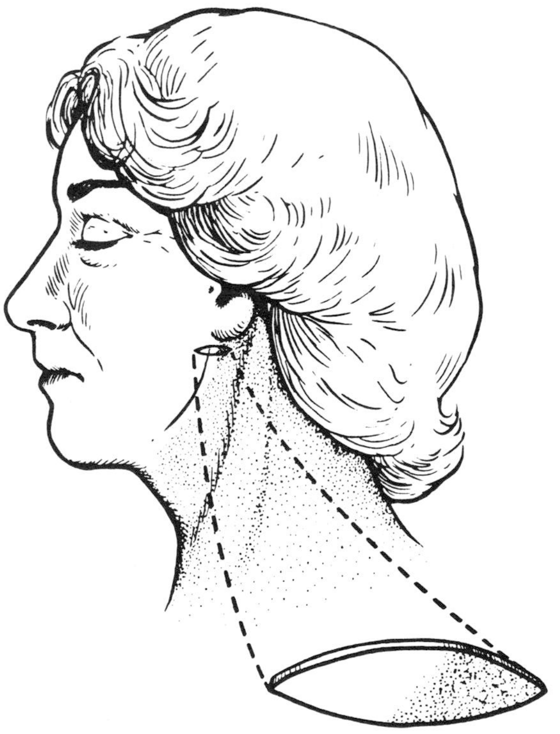

Figure 22–5. Study model to examine histologically the border zone between peeled and unpeeled skin in patients undergoing face lifting following a phenol peel of the face. (From Baker, T. J., and Gordon, H. L.: Surgical Rejuvenation Of The Aging Face. St. Louis, MO, C.V. Mosby Company, 1986.)

peeled skin. A new, wide band of dermis, measuring 0.2 to 0.3 mm in width, is found directly beneath the epidermis and is sharply defined from the tangled mass of elastotic fibers representing the old, unpeeled dermis. The newly formed matrix consists of compact and parallel bundles of collagen arranged horizontally. A fairly dense network of fine elastic fibers course through this zone, often disposed in a parallel pattern conforming to the configuration of the collagen fibers. Even in specimens obtained as long as 20 years after peeling, these elastic fibers remain fine and numerous (Fig. 22–6).

Mowry staining shows a considerable diminution in the presence of ground substance within this dermal band, as compared with adjacent unpeeled skin (Kligman, Baker, and Gordon, 1985). Small blood vessels in the reconstructed zone appear normal and are not surrounded by lymphocytic infiltrates. Inflammatory signs of chronic actinic damage are not present. Telangiectatic vessels are found only within the deep dermis, which is beyond the reach of the peeling solution (Fig. 22–7).

Epidermis. The epidermis is no longer in disarray after peeling; the cells stain evenly and are of uniform shape, and there is a return of vertical polarity. Lentiginous downgrowths are rarely seen.

Although peeled skin tends to be hypopig-

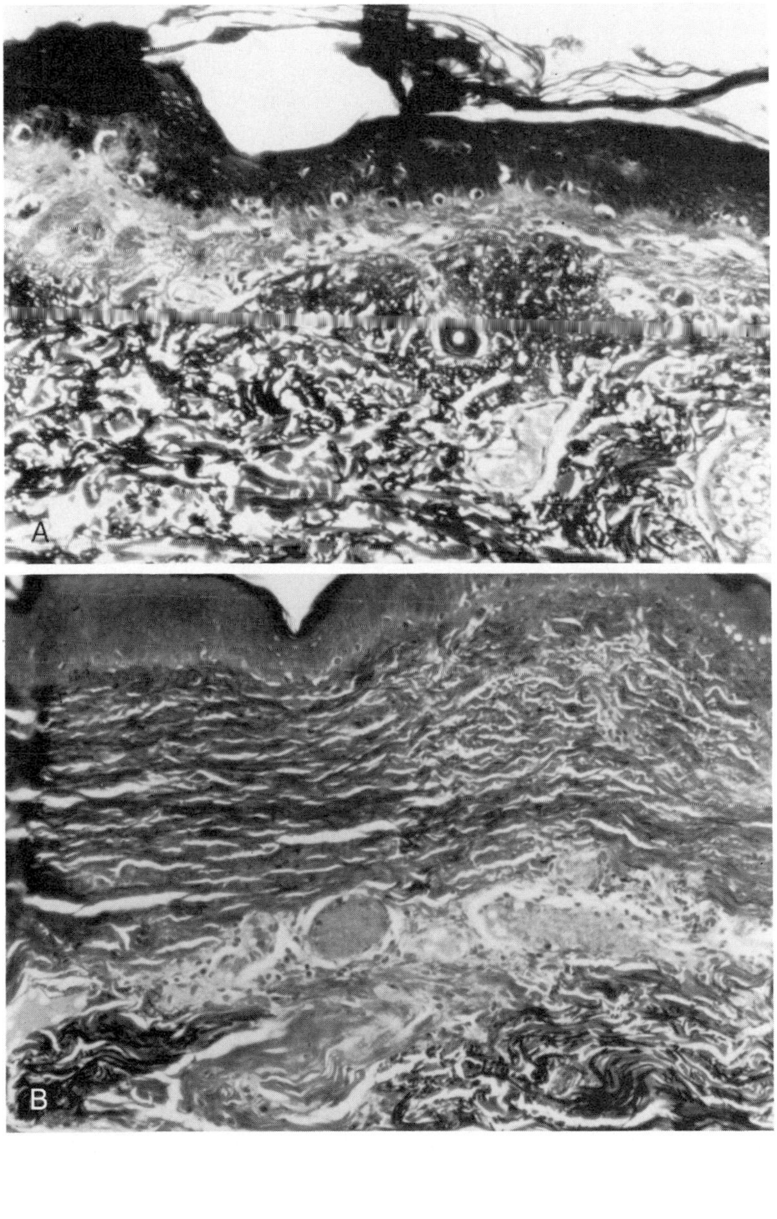

Figure 22–6. *A,* Unpeeled specimen showing eosinophilic "grenz zone" and marked dermal elastosis below. *B,* Same patient 12 years after peeling showing a wide band of new, fine, parallel collagen bundles. (From Kligman, A. M., Baker, T. J., and Gordon, H. L.: Long-term histologic follow up of phenol face peels. Plast. Reconstr. Surg., *75*:652, 1985.)

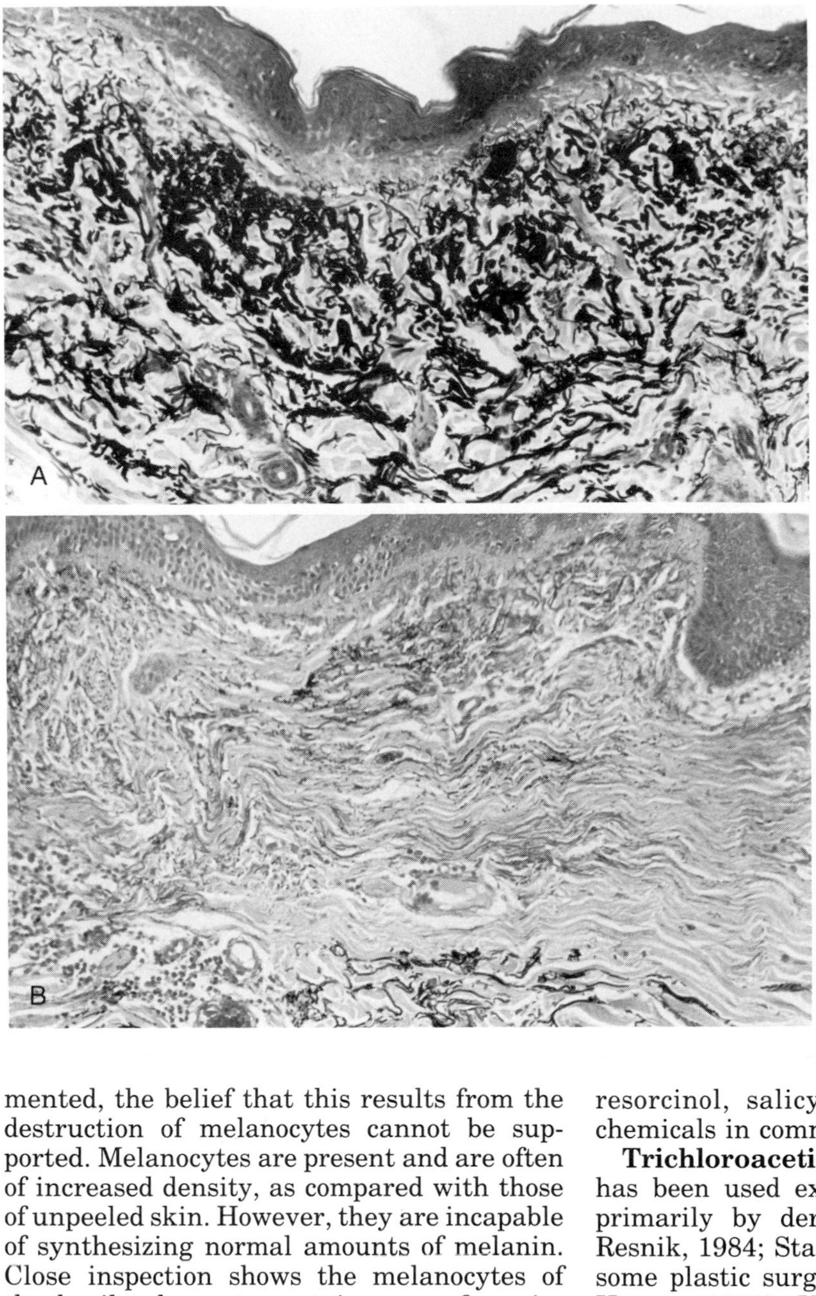

Figure 22–7. *A,* Unpeeled specimen illustrating intense elastosis. (Luna stain, × 160.) *B,* Same patient 14 years after peeling, showing a wide band of horizontally arranged collagen bundles that intertwine with fine elastic fibers. (Luna stain, × 96.) (From Kligman, A. M., Baker, T. J., and Gordon, H. L.: Long-term histologic follow up of phenol face peels. Plast. Reconstr. Surg., *75*:652, 1985.)

mented, the belief that this results from the destruction of melanocytes cannot be supported. Melanocytes are present and are often of increased density, as compared with those of unpeeled skin. However, they are incapable of synthesizing normal amounts of melanin. Close inspection shows the melanocytes of the basilar layer to contain many fine pigment granules, and this pigment is evenly dispersed with no tendency to form local accumulation of pigment or lentigos. Microscopic actinic keratoses are not observed in peeled skin (Fig. 22–8) (Kligman, Baker, and Gordon, 1985).

Chemical Agents and Toxicology

Numerous agents have been used over the years in peeling skin. Trichloroacetic acid, resorcinol, salicylic acid, and phenol are chemicals in common use today.

Trichloroacetic Acid. Trichloroacetic acid has been used extensively for many years, primarily by dermatologists (Ayres, 1962; Resnik, 1984; Stagnone, 1987), as well as by some plastic surgeons (Wolfort, Dalton, and Hoopes, 1972). Unlike phenol, its strength can be varied. A 10 to 25 per cent solution is used for light peeling, 35 to 50 per cent for intermediate peeling, and 50 to 75 per cent for deep peeling (Stagnone, 1987). There is also a greater safety of action with trichloroacetic acid, as its systemic toxicity is less than that of phenol (Ayres, 1962; Campbell, 1977; Stagnone, 1987).

Light peeling, using 15 to 25 per cent trichloroacetic acid, is performed in several sessions. The chemical is applied for one to two minutes, then neutralized either with benzalkonium chloride or by thorough washing with water. Generally, with light peeling, there is mild skin erythema for two to three days and light exfoliation of skin at three to five days. The peeling is equivalent to a mild sunburn and can be repeated one week later.

Intermediate peeling is performed in a similar fashion, using 35 to 50 per cent trichloroacetic acid without taping. Erythema and desquamation are greater with intermediate concentrations of trichloroacetic acid, and healing is usually seen in one week. Proponents of intermediate peeling state that pigmentary changes are much less than those seen after deep peeling with phenol or stronger concentrations of trichloroacetic acid. Intermediate peeling can be repeated several weeks later if clinically necessary.

Fifty to 75 per cent trichloroacetic acid with taping produces a deep chemical peel, the results of which are stated to be the equivalent to peeling with phenol, without the risks of the systemic toxicity of phenol (Ayres, 1962; Wolfort, Dalton, and Hoopes, 1972; Resnik, 1984; Stagnone, 1987).

Although the authors have little experience with trichloroacetic acid, their initial experience produced unpredictable results with tendencies to hyperplastic scarring at high concentrations. Others have described similar problems with trichloroacetic acid (Aronsohn, 1972; Litton, 1966). More important, in the patient with severe sun damage and deep rhytides, the effects of trichloroacetic acid peeling are not as profound as those seen with phenol. Histologic studies show that 60

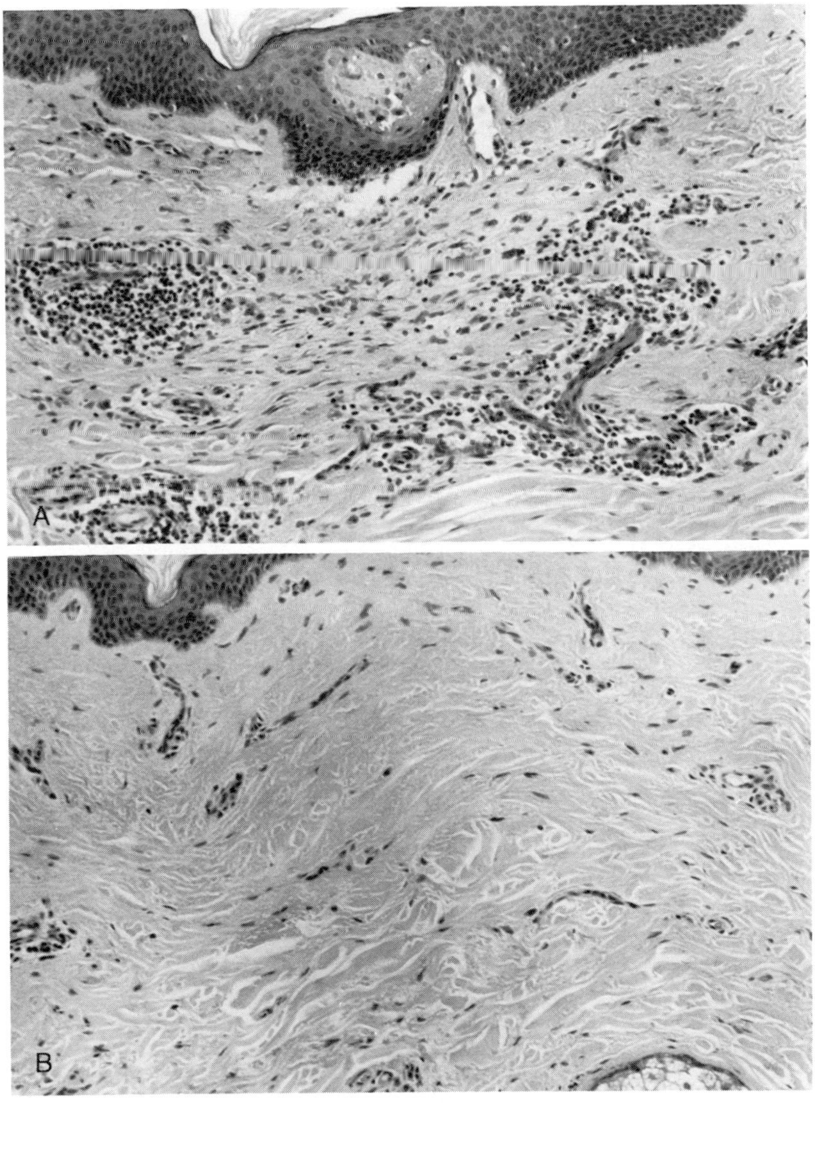

Figure 22–8. *A,* Unpeeled specimen showing perivenular lymphocytic infiltrate, practically always present in sun-damaged skin. *B,* Specimen from the same individual 18 years after peeling. There is no sign of inflammation. The population of dermal mesenchymal cells, including fibroblasts, is seemingly normal. (Luna stain, × 153.) (From Kligman, A. M., Baker, T. J., and Gordon, H. L.: Long-term histologic follow up of phenol face peels. Plast. Reconstr. Surg., *75*:652, 1985.)

per cent trichloroacetic acid, used with and without taping, has only half the degree of penetration into the dermis, and half the amount of neocollagen formation within the "grenz zone," compared with that seen with the use of phenol (Stegman, 1980, 1982). In these studies, 25 per cent trichloroacetic acid barely penetrated beyond the epidermis.

Trichloroacetic acid should be reserved for light peeling, i.e., to correct epidermal abnormalities such as mild actinic damage or superficial pigmentary changes from chloasma or melasma that do not respond to bleaching creams. In the authors' experience, the improved skin fullness and rubor seen with trichloroacetic acid are often short-lived, largely reflecting transient edema. Deeper rhytides, severely sun-damaged skin, and deep pigmentary problems lend themselves to more efficacious treatment with phenol, which produces a deeper penetration into the dermis, a greater degree of resultant formation of neocollagen, and a longer-lasting effect, compared with trichloroacetic acid.

Resorcinol. Resorcinol is another substance used in chemical peeling. The Combes formula uses resorcinol, salicylic acid, and lactic acid in equal amounts in an alcohol base. It is used widely in lay clinics and beauty salons. Treatments are given weekly and more coats of solution are applied in subsequent treatments. The depth of peeling is controlled by the number of coats of solution and the results are reported to be similar to those from light peeling with trichloroacetic acid (Stagnone, 1987). The authors have no experience with the use of resorcinol peeling.

Phenol. Phenol is a keratocoagulant, originally used in carbolic acid as a disinfectant. It has been mixed with other substances in various combinations to enhance its effectiveness. Combes, Sperber, and Reisch (1960) combined salicylic acid, citric acid, and glycerine with phenol. Litton (1962) recommended a 50 per cent phenol solution combined with glycerine, distilled water, and croton oil. Brown, Kaplan, and Brown (1960a) utilized phenol in a 60 to 95 per cent solution with cresol, olive oil, and distilled water added.

The formula used for years by the authors was obtained after careful search of the literature, discussion with lay users of phenol, animal experimentation, and finally clinical use. The safety and efficaciousness have been demonstrated over time. The formula consists of a 50 per cent phenol solution in a saponified suspension as follows:

3 ml U.S.P. phenol (C_6H_5OH)
2 ml tap water
8 drops liquid soap (Septisol)
3 drops croton oil (from the seed of *Croton tiglium*)

In determining the optimal concentration to use, it became apparent, when varying the concentration of phenol, that phenol peeling produces an "all or none" response. Unlike trichloroacetic acid, low concentrations of phenol do not produce a light peel, and higher concentrations of phenol do not produce a more profound, deeper peel. In fact, the opposite appears true. When one uses high concentrations of phenol, a more rapid and complete coagulation of the keratin in the epidermis occurs and the coagulant layer produces a barrier to further penetration of the acid, lessening its effect on the dermis (Brown, Kaplan, and Brown, 1960a; Spira and associates, 1970). Spira and associates (1970) noted little histologic difference when using 50, 75, and 100 per cent phenol solution; raising the concentration of phenol increased the risk of toxicity without producing improved clinical results. Similar results were noted by Stegman (1982), who showed in his histologic studies that 100 per cent phenol produced 35 to 50 per cent less penetration than a 50 per cent phenol solution.

The liquid soap used by the authors is Septisol, but any liquid soap suffices. The soap acts as a wetting agent to reduce surface tension, and helps to emulsify the mixture.

Croton oil is extracted from the seeds of *Croton tiglium* and is an additional irritant that speeds the destruction of the epidermis, enhancing the penetrating action of the mixture. Croton oil can be difficult to obtain, as it is an archaic medicine; if it is not available, the peeling can be done without it. Spira and associates (1970) noted no difference in histologic specimens peeled with and without the use of croton oil.

The action of phenol can be prolonged and deepened by the use of a vapor barrier such as occlusive tape, which acts to confine the active ingredients to the region of application, to promote maceration, and to enhance phenol penetration (Rees, 1980). Various histologic studies have demonstrated the enhanced effect of occlusive taping after phenol peeling and this phenomenon has been confirmed clinically (Spira and associates, 1970; Stegman, 1982; Baker, Gordon and Seckinger, 1966; Litton, 1962; Brown, Kaplan, and Brown, 1960a).

Systemic absorption of phenol through the skin is seen after chemical peeling. Phenol is detoxified in the liver and eliminated in the urine. A toxic dose produces injury to both liver and kidney and can depress the respiratory centers and the myocardium. Litton (1962) observed blood levels of 0.68 mg per 100 ml one hour after application of 3 ml of a 50 per cent phenol solution, 0.19 mg per 100 ml two hours after application, and 0.10 mg per 100 ml four hours after exposure. Since blood levels of 25 mg per 100 ml after phenol ingestion have been associated with survival, it appears that careful application of small volumes of phenol poses little risk of producing phenol toxicity (Deichmann and Witherup, 1944; Litton, 1966; Mosienko and Baker, 1978). On the other hand, it should be remembered that Brown, Kaplan, and Brown (1960a) noted two deaths from phenol by lay operators after the application of the chemical to extensive areas of the body over a short time. Lotter (1979) reported one death in her series of 408 patients undergoing chemical peeling.

Truppman and Ellenby (1979) studied the apparent systemic effects of full face phenol peeling and noted a high incidence of significant cardiac arrhythmias when 50 per cent of the face was treated in less than 30 minutes. *When the same area was treated over 60 minutes or more, arrhythmias did not occur.* Presumably, higher levels of phenol absorption produce myocardial irritability, with arrhythmias ranging from atrial tachycardia to premature ventricular contractions to ventricular tachycardia. The authors recommend cardiac monitoring of all patients undergoing peeling, and resuscitation equipment should be available. Rather than applying the mixture to the whole face over a short time, the clinician should apply the phenol regionally to small areas, spaced over long time intervals. This maneuver serves to prevent rapid absorption and arrhythmia complications. Similar findings and recommendations were noted by Gross (1984), who reported primarily atrial arrhythmias with rapid phenol absorption, as well as by Litton and Trinidad (1981), who noted that 13 per cent of plastic surgeons performing chemical peeling had noticed some type of cardiac complication or arrhythmia.

Indications

Proper patient selection is the most important aspect of obtaining satisfactory results following treatment. In the beginning, the authors used phenol peeling to treat many conditions, until by trial and error it was gradually discovered what the chemical peel was best suited for. For example, little benefit was seen after chemical peeling for the treatment of acne scarring. Chemical peeling also did not improve the appearance of capillary hemangioma and telangiectasia. It has little effect in reducing the hyperpigmentation seen in some split-thickness skin grafts.

Two clinical conditions have responded well to chemical peeling. It is effective for someone whose skin is finely wrinkled, the so-called weather-beaten look. It is also helpful for the individual with blotchy skin pigmentation caused by pregnancy, chloasma, birth control pills, chronic solar exposure, and various dermititides.

Patients with fair complexions are better candidates than those with olive-toned skin. Darker complexioned individuals tend to show an obvious line of dermarcation between the treated and untreated areas after the bleaching produced by chemical peeling. Caution should also be exercised in peeling black and Oriental patients. In general, regional peeling can be performed in fair-complexioned patients, while olive complexions usually require full face peeling to minimize the contrasting hypopigmentation observed in peeled skin. Thick and oily skin seems to respond less favorably to peeling and has a greater tendency to develop areas of spotty hyperpigmentation.

Red-haired, freckle-faced patients with fine wrinkles around the eyes and mouth are poor candidates for peeling because they usually show an obvious line of demarcation. While the peeling removes the wrinkles, it also bleaches the pale freckles present in these patients and makes it difficult to blend the peeled and unpeeled skin. There is no satisfactory method to "feather" the line of demarcation and make it less obvious in these patients.

Males, with few exceptions, are not good candidates, because the use of covering cosmetics is not appropriate and because the thick male skin in most instances does not respond as well as the thinner skin of females (Mosienko and Baker, 1978; Baker and Gordon, 1987).

Chemical peeling should not be used to treat rhytides or pigmentation of the neck, thorax, or extremities. Attempts at peeling these areas have occasionally resulted in hypertrophic scarring and may relate to the paucity of skin appendages, as compared with facial skin (Rees, 1980). Because of the large areas to be treated, there is also the danger of systemic phenol toxicity.

Spot peeling can be performed on individual lentigos on the dorsum of the hands and fingers, and the judicious application of pure phenol directly on these pigmented lesions predictably eliminates these common signs of aging.

In summary, the conditions that can be treated with chemical peeling are listed in descending order of responsiveness:

1. Fine facial wrinkles: excellent response (Figs. 22–9, 22–10).
2. Spotty hyperpigmentation: excellent response for hyperpigmentation localized to the face. The technique is also useful in removing individual lentigos of the hands and fingers (Figs. 22–11, 22–12).
3. Precancerous lesions following radiation (solar) exposure. While fluorouracil (5-FU) has largely replaced chemical peeling in treating these, this is an added benefit in patients with sun-damaged skin and actinic keratoses undergoing peeling for facial wrinkles (Spira and associates, 1971). Chemical peeling has also been used with good results to treat dermal changes after radiation therapy in patients with juvenile acne.
4. Superficial acne scarring. This condition is usually more effectively treated by dermabrasion and the treatment should be reserved for patients whose acne scars are *very* superficial.

Chemical peeling is not indicated to treat port wine stains, telangiectasias, hypertrophic scars, and scars resulting from burns. Little benefit is seen in these conditions after chemical peeling.

Preoperative Evaluation

Most patients who come for consultation have some kind of surgical face lifting procedure in mind to improve the appearance of

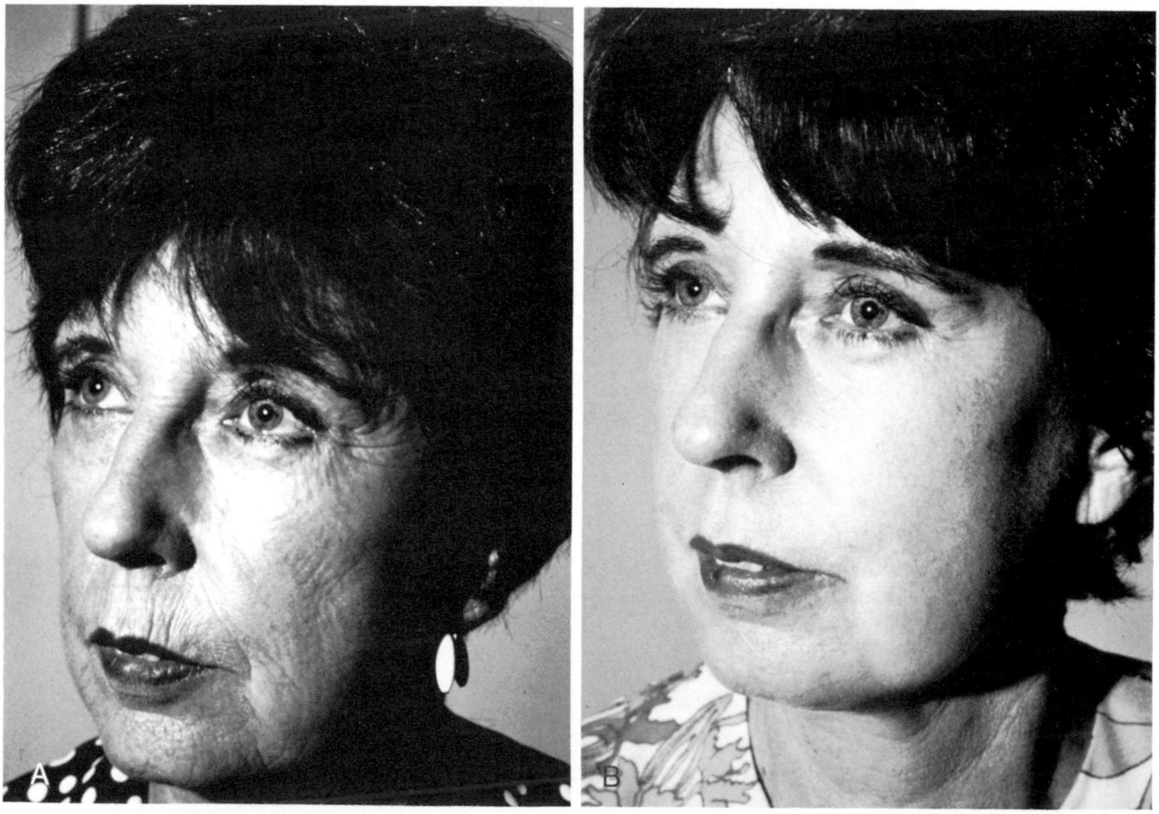

Figure 22–9. *A,* A 48 year old woman with severely sun-damaged skin. There is deep wrinkling in all areas, causing the skin to appear prematurely aged. *B,* One year after a full face peel. No surgery has been performed. (From Baker, T. J., and Gordon, H. L.: Surgical Rejuvenation Of The Aging Face. St. Louis, MO, C.V. Mosby Company, 1986.)

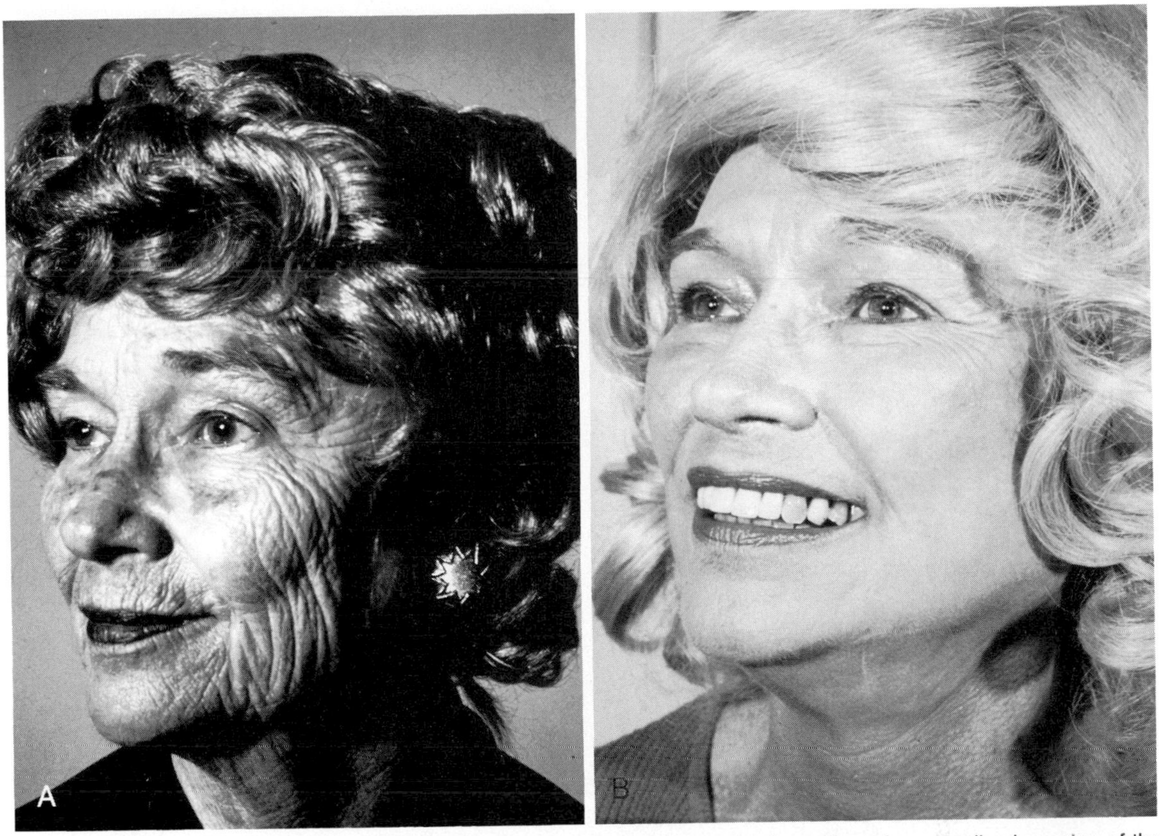

Figure 22–10. A 67 year old woman with the common stigmata of the aging face. There is generalized sagging of the skin and subcutaneous tissues of the face and neck. Note the abundance of fine wrinkling, as well as blotchy hyperpigmentation. A surgical face lift and blepharoplasty were performed and three months later a chemical peel was done. *B,* The patient's appearance six months after the combined peeling and surgery. (From Baker, T. J., and Gordon, H. L.: Surgical Rejuvenation Of The Aging Face. St. Louis, MO, C.V. Mosby Company, 1986.)

their face. The most common public misconception is that surgical face lifting removes all facial wrinkles, an obvious limitation of rhytidectomy. Thorough discussion of the expected benefits of peeling as opposed to rhytidectomy must be explained to the patient before a chemical peel is undertaken. If the patient is likely to benefit from both procedures, it is preferable to perform the face lift first and follow with the chemical peeling three months later (Baker, 1962; Baker and Gordon, 1963, 1987; Litton, Fournier, and Capinpin, 1973). *Under no circumstances should chemical peeling be performed on undermined skin at the time of rhytidectomy. This is an invitation to the catastrophic possibility of full-thickness skin loss.* Eyelid peeling and blepharoplasty should *never* be performed at the same time.

Regional perioral peeling in properly selected candidates is a useful adjunct to rhytidectomy and can be performed simultaneously without complications (Baker and Gordon, 1979).

The entire procedure and postoperative course following chemical peeling should be explained in detail to the patient preoperatively. This should include information about the indications for peeling and the anticipated results; the need to rest the voice for 48 hours (after full face peeling) and to go on a clear liquid diet with a straw for the same period; the transient 48-hour visual impairment secondary to eyelid edema; the eschar formation, desquamation, and discomfort to be expected; the ointment application required; and details of local hygiene. The reddish appearance of the skin after peeling should be emphasized and the length of time required for the healing process to be completed is also discussed, including the need to avoid the sun for several months (Mosienko and Baker, 1978). Since the skin is dryer after peeling, the patient should be instructed

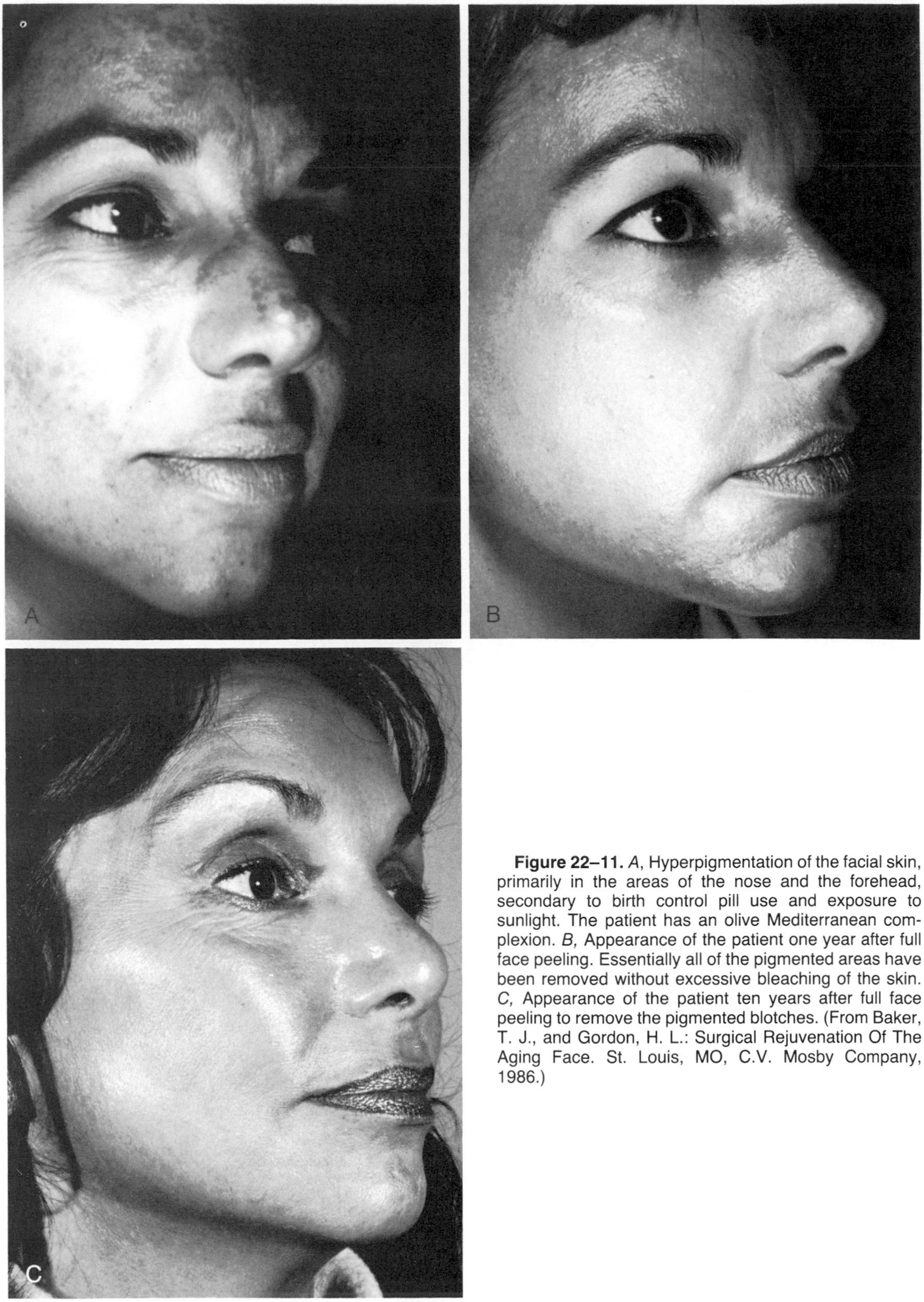

Figure 22–11. *A*, Hyperpigmentation of the facial skin, primarily in the areas of the nose and the forehead, secondary to birth control pill use and exposure to sunlight. The patient has an olive Mediterranean complexion. *B,* Appearance of the patient one year after full face peeling. Essentially all of the pigmented areas have been removed without excessive bleaching of the skin. *C,* Appearance of the patient ten years after full face peeling to remove the pigmented blotches. (From Baker, T. J., and Gordon, H. L.: Surgical Rejuvenation Of The Aging Face. St. Louis, MO, C.V. Mosby Company, 1986.)

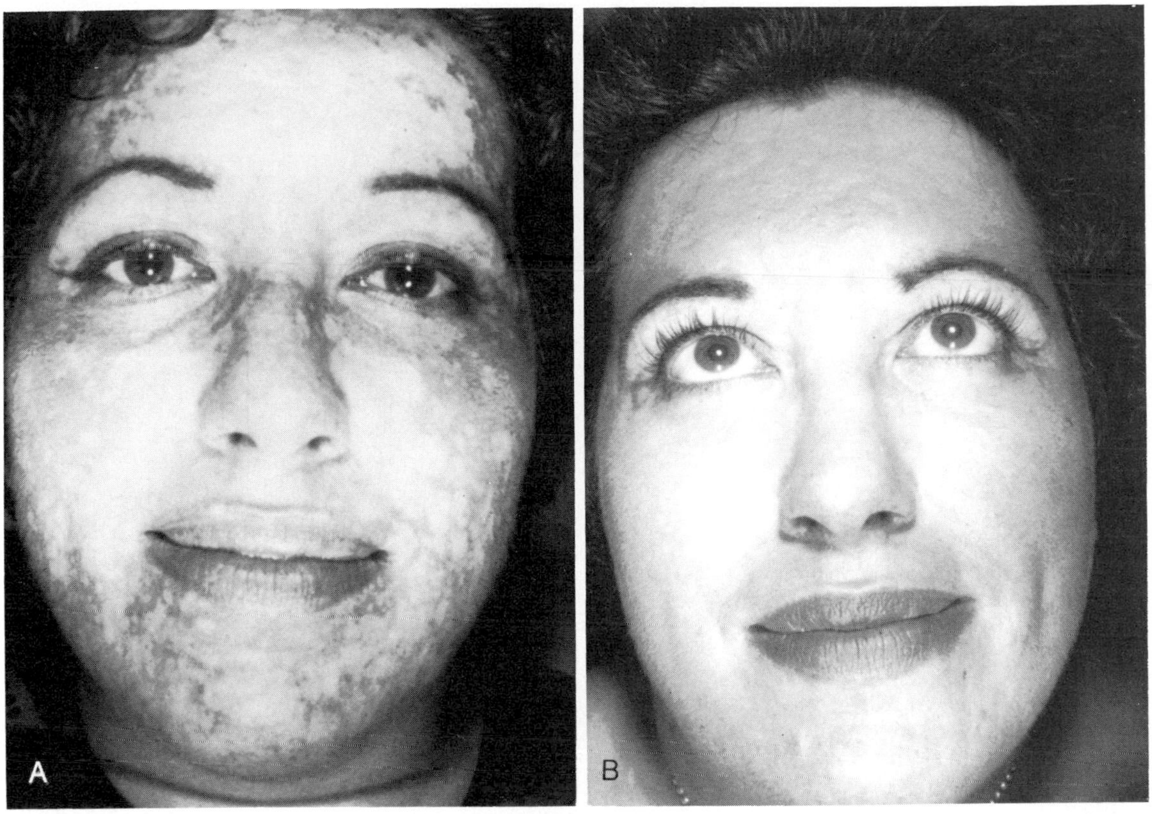

Figure 22–12. *A*, A 28 year old woman who had a generalized allergic drug reaction of the facial skin and developed hyperpigmentation. *B*, Appearance of the patient seven months after full face peeling to remove the areas of hyperpigmentation. (From Baker, T. J., and Gordon, H. L.: Surgical Rejuvenation Of The Aging Face. St. Louis, MO, C.V. Mosby Company, 1986.)

in the use of moisturizers and daily lubrication. It is imperative to maintain photographic records of patients to use as a basis for comparison at the conclusion of the treatment.

Technique: Full Face Peeling

Chemical peeling should be performed in a hospital or an ambulatory surgical facility. Full face peeling requires sedation before and during the procedure. An intravenous catheter should be in place and the patient should be monitored with electrocardiographic and pulse/oximetry equipment. Because of the anticipated eyelid edema for two to three days after full face peeling, experienced personnel must be available if the procedure is performed on an outpatient basis. For regional perioral or spot peeling of the face, the need for sedation, monitoring, and postoperative care is minimized. The night before the procedure, the patient thoroughly washes her face to remove all traces of make-up, and this is repeated the next morning. Upon arrival at the hospital or clinic, the patient is premedicated, the authors' preference being oral diazepam. Before the application, intravenous meperidine (50 mg) is effective in alleviating the discomfort of the peel, and this can be supplemented as needed. Local anesthestic agents are not used.

The skin is again cleansed with liquid soap and water, thoroughly dried, and washed with diethyl ether to remove all surface oils that might interfere with the peeling.

The chemical mixture for peeling is freshly prepared before each case. The ingredients do not readily mix and need to be stirred vigorously before each application (Fig. 22–13).

The peeling mixture is applied to the face with a cotton-tipped applicator. The mixture is applied evenly and uniformly over the entire area and into each wrinkle. The skin becomes pearly white on contact with the

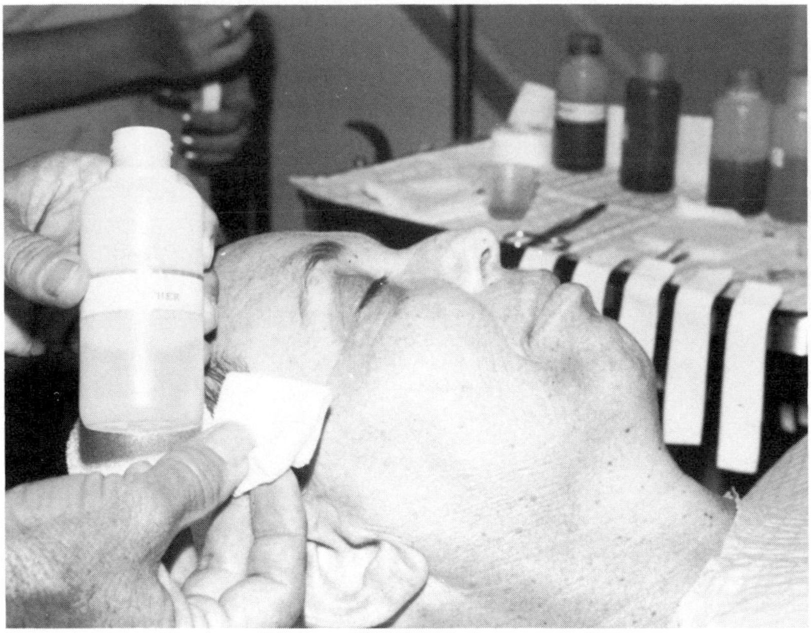

Figure 22–13. The sedated patient has her face cleaned with diethyl ether to remove superficial skin oils. The phenol mixture has been freshly made and is on the tray in the background. (From Baker, T. J., and Gordon, H. L.: Surgical Rejuvenation Of The Aging Face. St. Louis, MO, C.V. Mosby Company, 1986.)

chemicals, and the patient experiences a mild burning sensation, which gradually subsides as the local anesthetic property of phenol takes effect. The application is carried slightly into the hairline to minimize the line of demarcation where the peeling stops. The peeling process does not affect the hair follicles and therefore does not cause alopecia. The applicator is semimoist rather than saturated to prevent the solution from dripping onto areas where it is not desired. Any site that the solution touches will be affected. Lightly rolling the applicator onto a piece of gauze absorbs the excess liquid and helps to avoid this problem (Fig. 22–14).

The phenol is applied slowly to lessen patient discomfort and minimize the possibility of rapid phenol absorption. The solution is

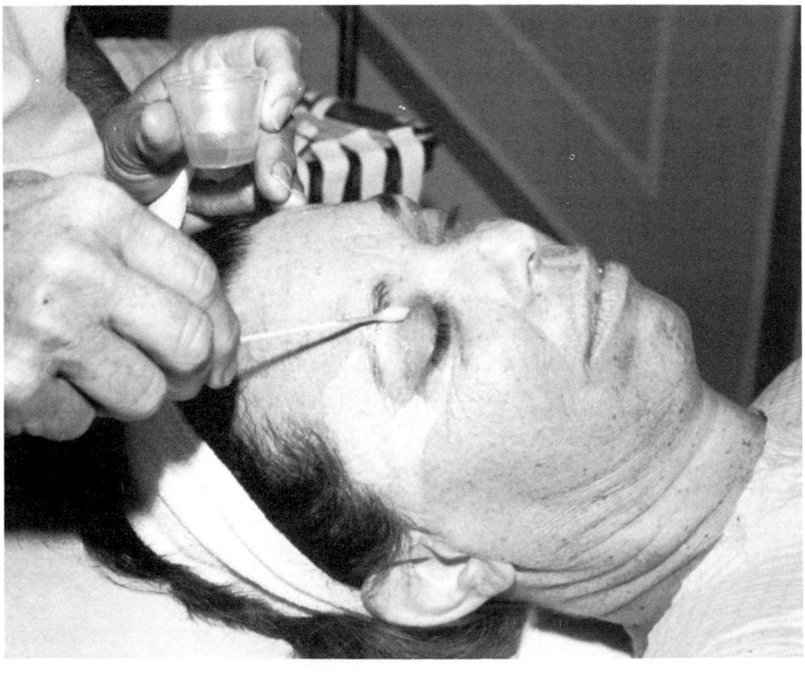

Figure 22–14. The phenol mixture is applied to the facial skin with a cotton-tipped applicator. Note that the skin immediately turns a distinctive grayish-white color. The patient experiences a burning sensation. (From Baker, T. J., and Gordon, H. L.: Surgical Rejuvenation Of The Aging Face. St. Louis, MO, C.V. Mosby Company, 1986.)

applied to the forehead first. The painting is carried close to and into the eyebrows. If the upper eyelids are to be treated, the applicator must be almost dry to prevent the phenol coming into contact with the cornea and conjunctiva. The mixture is applied to the skin between the brow and the upper tarsal fold, but the skin overlying the tarsal plate is left untreated. Peeling in this region leads to enormous eyelid edema, which can be slow to resolve. The upper lid skin can be taped, but no tape is applied directly over the eyebrows.

After the first area is treated, it is covered with an occlusive dressing, usually waterproof tape, and 20 to 30 minutes elapse before proceeding to the next area. The malar region and cheeks, including the lower eyelids, are then treated. When chemical peeling of the lower eyelids is performed, the skin is moistened to within 2 mm of the ciliary margin. An assistant holds the upper eyelids open to prevent blinking until each of the lower lids has been treated, blotted, and allowed to air dry. A supply of water to irrigate the eye in case of mishap is an important safeguard. With this method, the possibility of corneal injury is minimized.

The mixture is regionally applied to the entire face as far inferiorly as a line 2 to 3 cm below the inferior margin of the mandible. If a natural skin crease is present in the upper neck, this forms a logical area to terminate the peel. If there is no obvious crease, the mixture should extend onto the neck only far enough to camouflage the treated area as well as possible. Around the mouth, care should be taken to apply the chemicals at least to the vermilion border and preferably slightly into it. Application along the vermilion removes the vertical wrinkles of the upper lip, especially the smaller ones that radiate from the vermilion border. The earlobes are commonly wrinkled, and can be treated if it is deemed desirable to remove the fine wrinkles in the lobes themselves.

Application of the Waterproof Mask. After the skin has been completely covered with the chemical mixture, a mask of waterproof adhesive tape is applied directly to the skin (Fig. 22–15). The eyes, eyebrows, nostrils, and mouth are all that is left exposed after taping. Short pieces of tape are easier to apply than long ones and seem to conform to the curves of the face better. When the tape is first applied, it may not adhere well, but as the body heat warms the adhesive and early edema occurs, adherence of the tape improves. The short strips should not be applied tightly: if they are improperly applied, the skin beneath can become folded or pleated and the skin in the depth of the fold will not be in contact with the tape. This produces

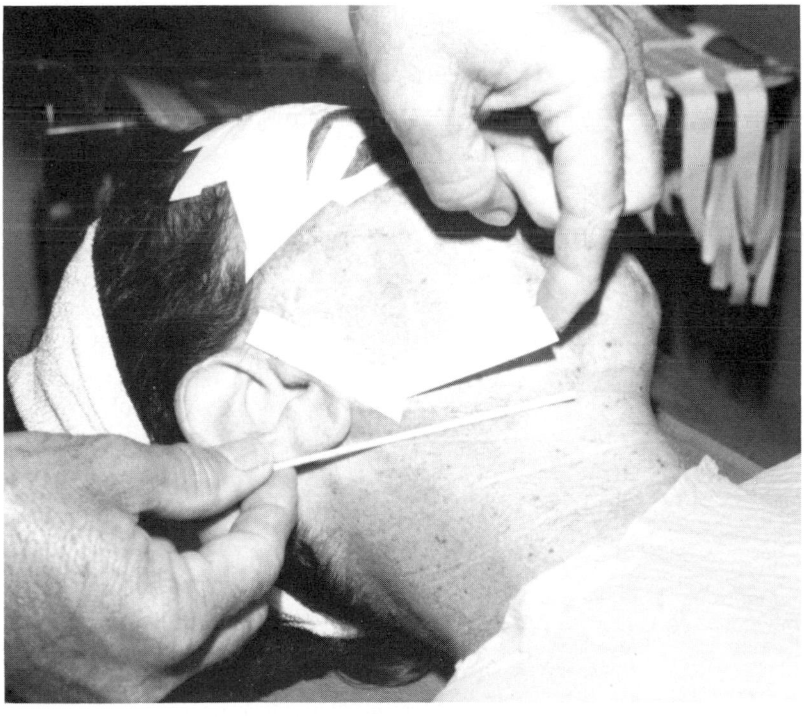

Figure 22–15. Each of the areas (forehead, cheeks, and perioral area) is individually painted with the phenol mixture and immediately covered with waterproof adhesive tape before proceeding to the next area. (From Baker, T. J., and Gordon, H. L.: Surgical Rejuvenation Of The Aging Face. St. Louis, MO, C.V. Mosby Company, 1986.)

streaking and unevenness in the final texture and color of the skin.

After the area to be treated is covered with strips of ½-inch tape, a second layer is placed over the first, using strips of 1-inch tape. The second layer reinforces the mask and ensures that all areas are covered (Fig. 22–16).

It has long been the authors' impression that occlusive taping maintains the concentration of phenol at the skin surface and produces a more complete and longer-lasting peel. The effectiveness of taping has been confirmed clinically by others (Brown, Kaplan, and Brown, 1960a; Litton, 1962) and by histologic studies (Spira and associates, 1970; Stegman, 1982). If a lesser result is desired, peeling without taping may be used.

The disadvantages of taping include patient discomfort and inability to evaluate what is going on beneath the mask. Mask removal is uncomfortable. Drying of the skin after application of thymol iodide at the time of tape removal is unpleasant, and separation of the crusts from the face after desquamation and healing is at times painful.

A new method of occlusive dressing that abandons taping is currently being evaluated. For patients with fine wrinkles that are not too deep, and in all peels performed for pigmentation problems, Vaseline (petroleum jelly) is immediately applied thickly over the peeled areas to serve as a lubricant and occlusive dressing (Stuzin, Baker, and Gordon, 1988). Wound lubrication is continued throughout the early postoperative period with A & D ointment or an antibiotic ointment. Gentle washing of the peeled areas is begun on the second day after peeling. This routine is continued until wound healing is complete (five to seven days), at which time facial lubrication with a lighter moisturizer is begun.

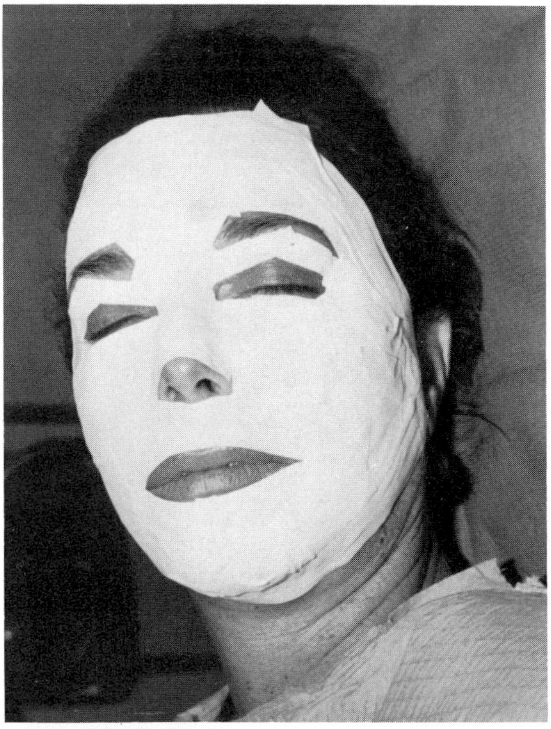

Figure 22–16. All of the treated skin has been covered with waterproof adhesive tape. (From Baker, T. J., and Gordon, H. L.: Surgical Rejuvenation Of The Aging Face. St. Louis, MO, C.V. Mosby Company, 1986.)

As the authors have gained experience using Vaseline as the occlusive dressing, they have become impressed with its efficaciousness in producing results similar to those following occlusive taping. Patients are more comfortable, as the skin is constantly kept moist after peeling, and eschar formation with crust separation is prevented. The use of Vaseline obviates the need for tape mask removal, and the treating physician can observe the peeled areas at all times. We now use a Vaseline occlusive dressing for all regional peels and in all peels performed for facial hyperpigmentation (Fig. 22–17). We reserve tape occlusion for the deeply lined face that appears "weather-beaten" and has sustained significant actinic damage.

Regional Peeling

There are instances in which only an isolated area of the face needs to be treated, most commonly the upper lip alone or the entire perioral region. The same formula as in full face peeling is utilized in regional peeling, and care is taken to apply the mixture slightly onto the vermilion border and to include not only the nasolabial folds but also an area extending 2 to 3 mm beyond. If the peel stops at the nasolabial fold, it will merely accentuate the line rather than partially eliminate it.

Regional perioral peeling is excellent treatment for the fine upper lip wrinkles and the lines radiating from the vermilion into which lipstick tends to run. Deep lines beneath the lower lip, especially those below the commissure of the mouth and paralleling the mentalis muscle, are perhaps the most difficult

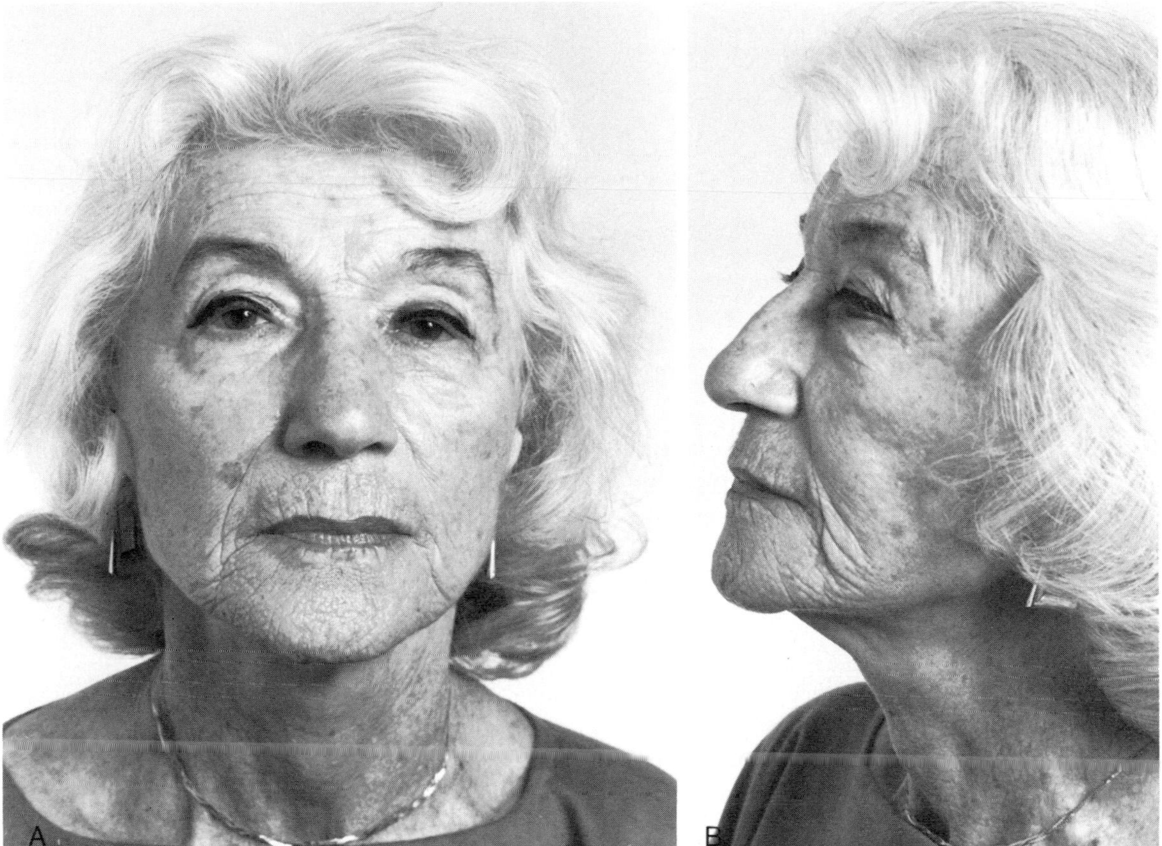

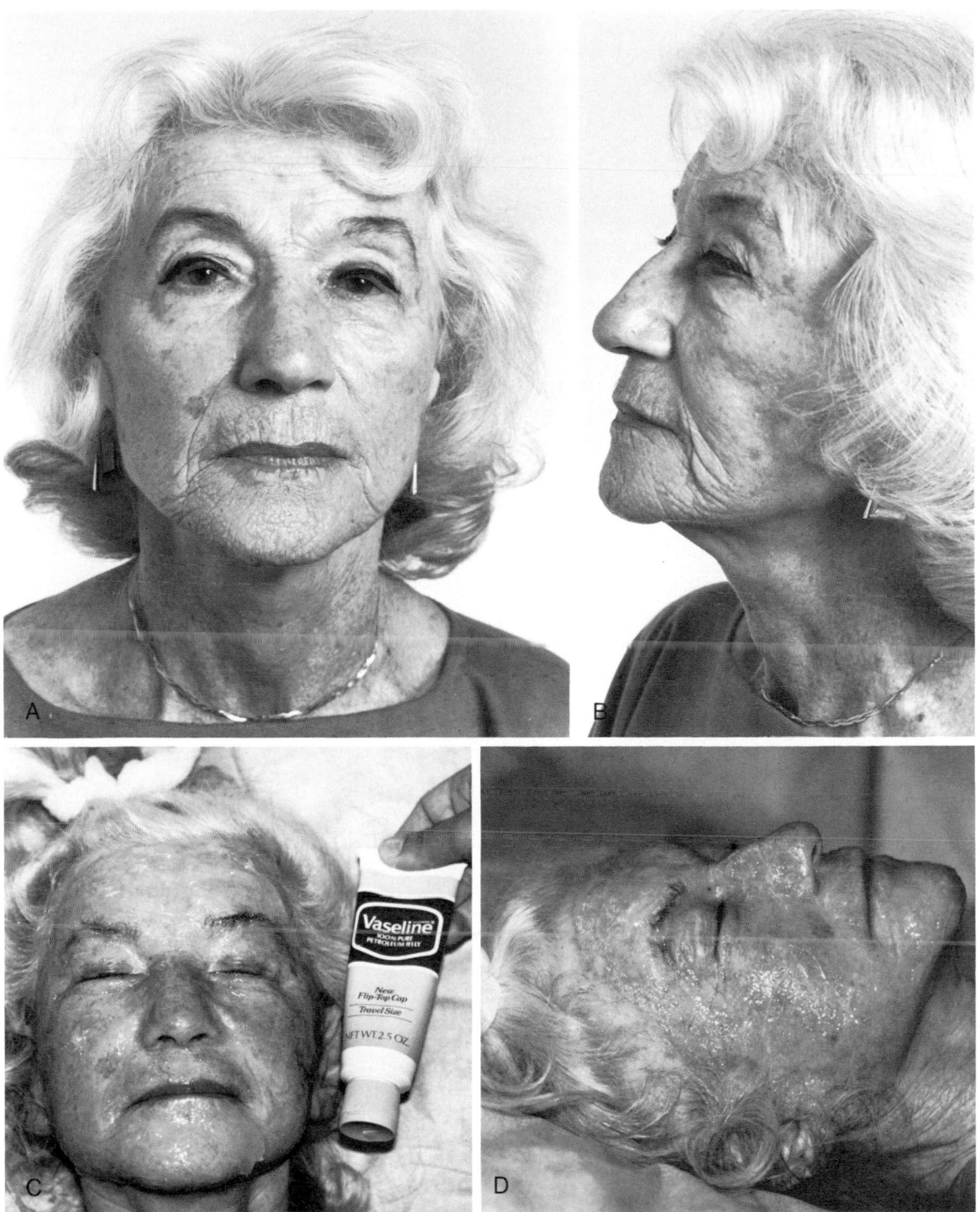

Figure 22–17. *A, B,* Appearance before chemical peeling. *C, D,* Chemical peeling was done in conjunction with a Vaseline occlusive dressing.

Illustration continued on following page

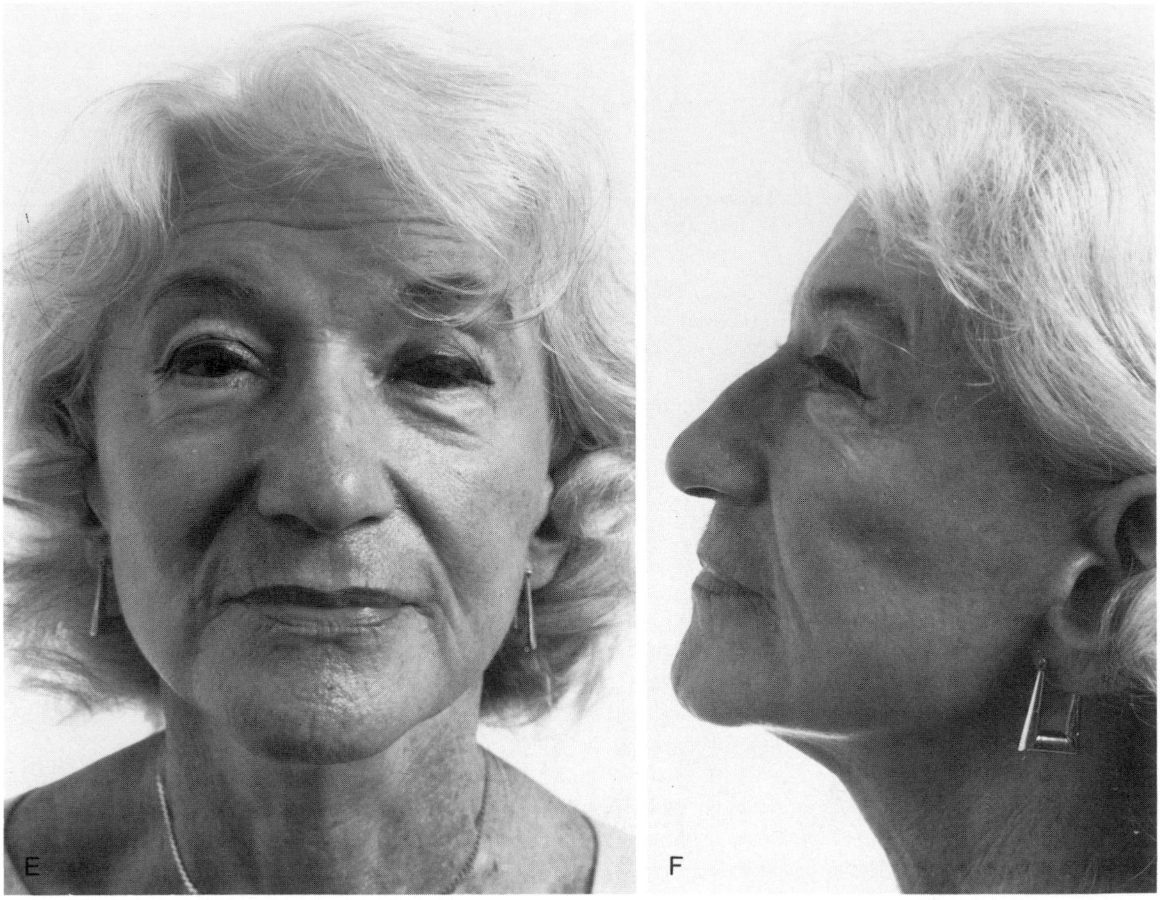

Figure 22–17 *Continued E, F,* Postoperative appearance. (From Stuzin, J. M., Baker, T. J., and Gordon, H. L.: Chemical peel—a change in routine. Accepted for publication, Plast. Reconstr. Surg., 1988.)

lines in the face to eliminate, and only modest improvement is seen in this region after peeling (Fig. 22–18).

Regional perioral peeling can be done on an outpatient basis, often as an isolated procedure without sedation or monitoring. It also can be combined safely with rhytidectomy (Baker and Gordon, 1963, 1979). The glabellar region or periorbital areas can also be regionally peeled and the postoperative care is similar to that after full face peeling.

Postoperative Care

Within one to two minutes after the phenol mixture is applied, the initial burning sensation subsides because of the local anesthetic action of the phenol. Approximately 20 to 30 minutes after the tape mask is applied, the burning sensation returns, this time to a greater degree and for a longer period. Analgesia is helpful in keeping the patient comfortable during this time, and narcotics are usually necessary. Facial edema reaches a maximum during the first six to 12 hours after treatment. The eyelids often swell shut and the patient may not be able to open her eyes for about 48 hours.

The patient is instructed in voice rest to ensure that the tape remains adherent to the skin, and there should be a minimum of chewing. Liquids are encouraged and taken with the use of a straw. The head of the bed is elevated and the patient is allowed out of bed with assistance.

Most of the burning sensation subsides after the first 12 to 24 hours and so does the necessity for medication. Patients can ambulate during the second 24 hours, their mobility limited only by their ability to see between the edematous lids.

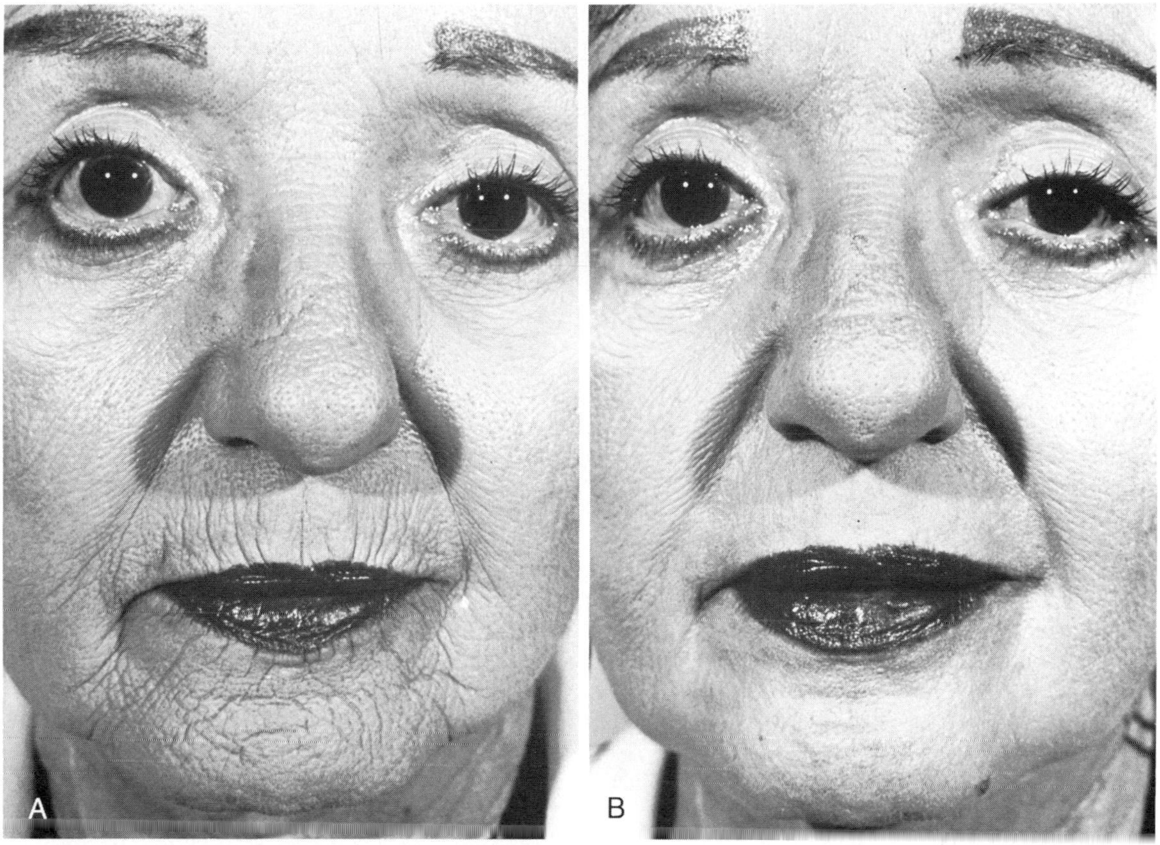

Figure 22–18. *A,* A 62 year old woman with generalized wrinkling and sagging of the facial skin. The most severe wrinkling is in the perioral area. The general complexion is fair and without freckles. *B,* The patient is shown one year after chemical peeling of only the perioral area. No surgery has been performed. (From Baker, T. J., and Gordon, H. L.: Surgical Rejuvenation Of The Aging Face. St. Louis, MO, C.V. Mosby Company, 1986.)

If a mask is used, it is removed after 48 hours. The removal may be somewhat painful and may require medication. At 48 hours, many areas of taping begin to separate spontaneously. The tape mask is split in several places to facilitate removal. A superficial layer of epithelium, adherent to the undersurface of the dressing, is usually removed with the tape. The appearance of the newly uncovered skin can be alarming to the uninitiated, resembling a uniform second degree burn. The skin is edematous and moist. It is covered with a thin layer of loose necrotic epithelium and coagulated exudate. Any loose material or crusts can be lightly washed away at this time (Fig. 22–19).

After the mask has been completely removed, the skin is covered with thymol iodide powder, for its drying and bacteriostatic effects. A large cotton ball twisted around the end of an applicator stick can be used as a powder puff (Fig. 22–20).

The powdered surface is left open and allowed to dry for 24 hours. A thin, yellow-brown crust forms. Twenty-four hours after mask removal the face is covered, powder and all, with A & D ointment to soften and loosen the crusts. The face is washed with warm water and ointment applied several times daily until crust separation occurs, usually one week after peeling.

After crust separation the skin appears erythematous, but the edema usually subsides rapidly. The patient is instructed to continue washing several times daily and to lubricate the skin between washings with a moisturizer. Pain is not common during this period, but itching can be a problem. Ice water compresses are useful in controlling this symptom, but rarely sedatives or topical steroids may prove necessary.

The patient can begin to use cosmetics over the treated areas at the end of two weeks if healing is proceeding in a normal fashion.

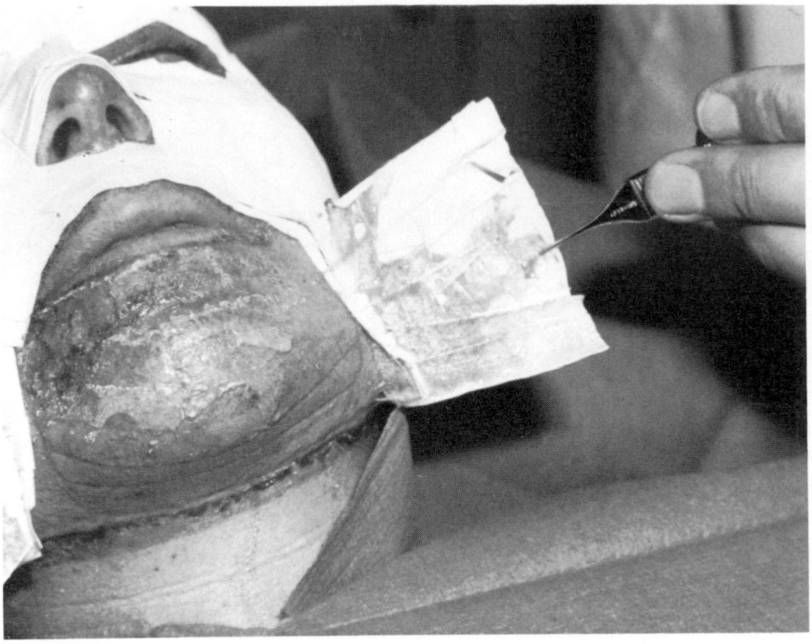

Figure 22–19. The tape mask is split in several places to facilitate removal. There is necrotic epithelial debris adherent to the underside of the tape. (From Baker, T. J., and Gordon, H. L.: Surgical Rejuvenation Of The Aging Face. St. Louis, MO, C.V. Mosby Company, 1986.)

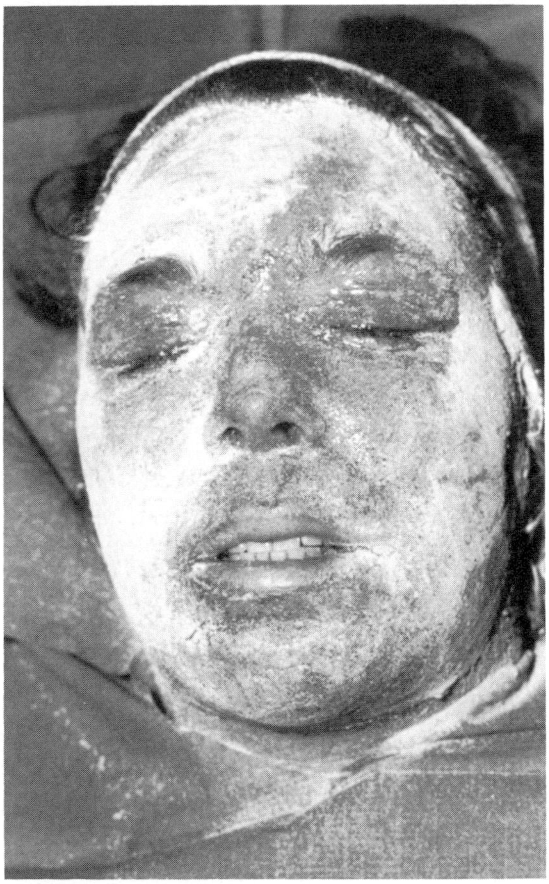

Figure 22–20. The face has been dusted with thymol iodide powder immediately after removal of the tape. (From Baker, T. J., and Gordon, H. L.: Surgical Rejuvenation Of The Aging Face. St. Louis, MO, C.V. Mosby Company, 1986.)

The erythematous color usually persists for 10 to 12 weeks, but in rare cases may last up to six months.

Since chemical peeling removes a significant amount of pigment from the basal layer of the epidermis, the process eventually lightens the skin and reduces natural protection against the sun. Patients who undergo peeling should be warned to avoid direct or reflected sunlight for extended periods until healing is complete. This precaution is especially important in the postoperative period when the skin remains erythematous and has not faded in color. Most cases of blotchy pigmentation following chemical peel arise in patients who have disregarded the advice to avoid solar exposure.

Specific recommendations with reference to the sun should include the following:

1. Peeled skin will never tan normally and precautions for lifetime use of sunscreens need to be followed.
2. Patients should avoid direct sunlight for three to six months, especially during the middle of the day. If they must be in the sun, they should wear a wide-brimmed hat and apply sunscreens.
3. Reflected sunlight should be avoided. This is a particular problem when driving automobiles. Make-up bases with sunscreen and sunscreens with high sun protection factors must be worn at all times.

Problems with blotchy hyperpigmentation are virtually eliminated in patients who rigidly avoid the sun and protect their skin after chemical peeling.

Complications

Skin Depigmentation. Hypopigmentation or bleaching of the skin is almost unavoidable except in fair-skinned individuals. Patients with dark complexions show more bleaching than those with light complexions, and red-haired, freckled individuals exhibit a pronounced bleaching effect. Many of the problems seen because of a poor blending between treated and untreated skin can be avoided by proper patient selection.

The peel should be stopped at a point just beneath the jawline to conceal the line of demarcation as much as possible. Some patients have little or no contour definition at the jawline because of an obtuse cervicomental angle, and these individuals should be forewarned preoperatively that the line may be conspicuous. It is helpful to stop the occlusive taping just short of the point of application of the mixture in an attempt to "feather" the peeled area into the untreated skin of the neck.

Milia. Milia are occasionally seen after peeling although less frequently than after dermabrasion. They usually are seen in the first six to eight weeks after treatment, and may be few in number or quite numerous and confluent. Milia often regress spontaneously, but if they are persistent the patient can use a soft complexion brush on the skin several times daily. Persistent milia can be surgically opened and drained in the office.

Erythema. Prolonged erythema occasionally persists beyond 10 to 12 weeks after peeling. The authors have observed patients in whom the skin was significantly red for up to six months, but in no case did the erythema persist permanently. Spira, Gerow, and Hardy (1974) recommended the use of topical steroids for this problem, but reassurance and patience are probably the best form of therapy.

Hypertrophic Scarring. Scarring is the rarest but most catastrophic complication after peeling. Most problems occur around the mouth, mostly as a transverse band of hypertrophic scar on both the upper or lower lips adjacent to the vermilion border. This is most commonly seen when perioral peeling is combined with rhytidectomy, and may relate to excessive edema in this region when the peeling is performed along with surgical face lifting. Currently, it is our opinion that occlusive taping should rarely be used when combining perioral peeling and rhytidectomy; Vaseline occlusive dressings are perhaps safer in this circumstance.

The worst scars are observed along the anterior neck and have been associated with flexion contractures requiring surgical release (Fig. 22–21). Peeling of this area should be avoided, not only because of possible poor healing in this region, but also because of the development of a noticeable line of demarcation if the peel is carried into the supraclavicular region.

The treatment of hypertrophic scars includes massage, steroid injection, and finally surgical revision. Fortunately, most small scars respond to conservative treatment, but only after a long and trying course for both patient and doctor (Fig. 22–22).

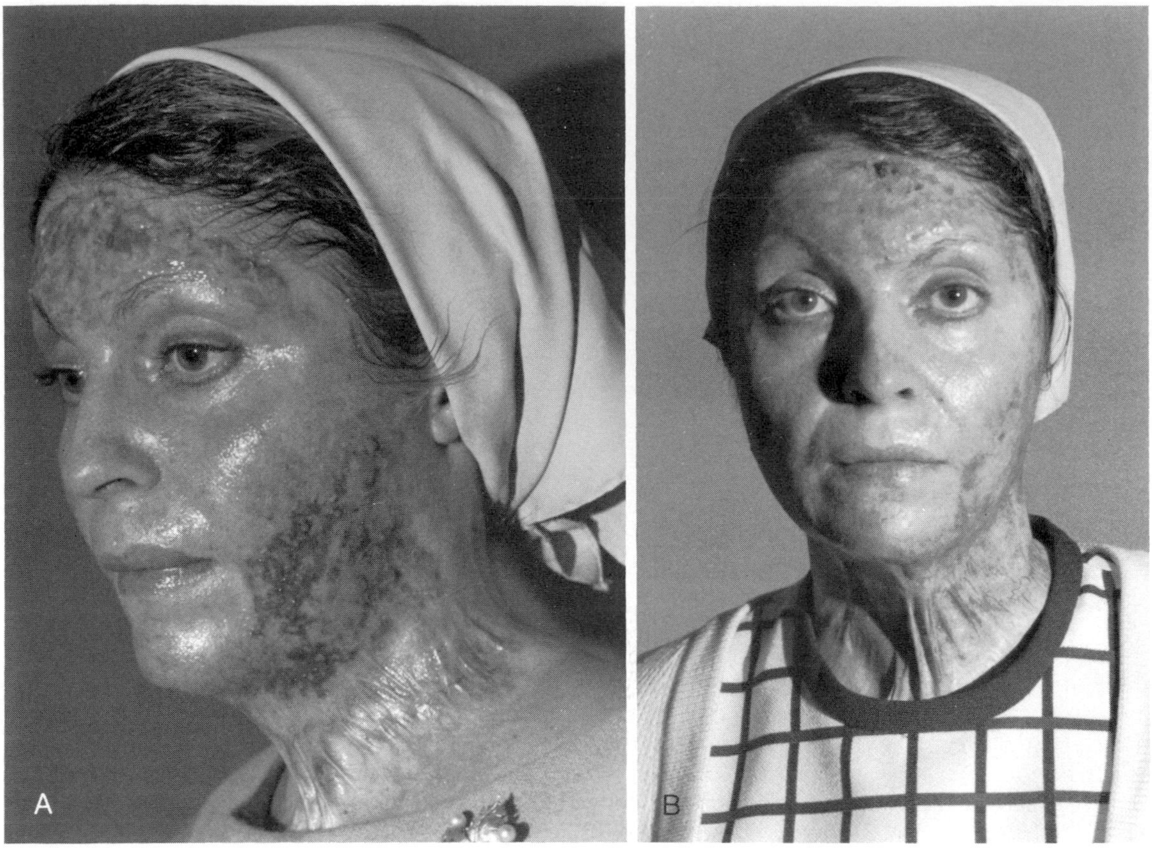

Figure 22–21. *A,* A 38 year old woman who had chemical peeling of the face and neck performed four weeks earlier in a lay clinic. Deep second and scattered third degree burns resulted. Contractions are seen developing in the neck. *B,* After seven weeks the burn scar contractures are well developed and the areas of deep burns are reepithelizing. (From Baker, T. J., and Gordon, H. L.: Surgical Rejuvenation Of The Aging Face. St. Louis, MO, C.V. Mosby Company, 1986.)

Ectropion of the Lower Eyelid. Ectropion of the lower eyelid has been seen in patients who have undergone blepharoplasty before peeling. Unrecognized incipient senile ectropion predisposes to this problem. The authors hesitate to perform full face peeling on a patient who has undergone a previous lower lid blepharoplasty, and in cases in which the lower lids are peeled an occlusive dressing is not used.

Blotchy Hyperpigmentation. Blotchy hyperpigmentation is most often seen in dark-skinned individuals who have a degree of skin blotchiness before treatment. Early exposure to sunlight is a common etiologic factor, and avoidance of and protection from the sun help to prevent this problem. The use of Valium (diazepam) and birth control pills has also been implicated in the development of hyperpigmentation changes after peeling (Ferreira, 1978, 1980).

In treating this condition, one should use bleaching creams such as 4 per cent hydroquinone, which is usually required for several months. If hyperpigmentation persists for longer than one year, repeeling of the entire face without using a tape mask is generally effective.

Alteration of Existing Skin Conditions. Alteration of previously existing skin conditions is common after peeling and this should be explained to the patient before treatment.

Existing nevi are not removed with peeling and actually appear darker after treatment.

Patients with multiple spider telangiectasias often find these areas more noticeable after peeling and they should be advised of this possibility. The dilated blood vessels are usually deep within the dermis and are not removed by peeling.

As in dermabrasion, pores appear larger after chemical peeling. Some patients request chemical peeling to treat enlarged pores and have the mistaken idea that chemical peeling reduces pore size. The opposite is true.

Rarely, it may be necessary for a patient

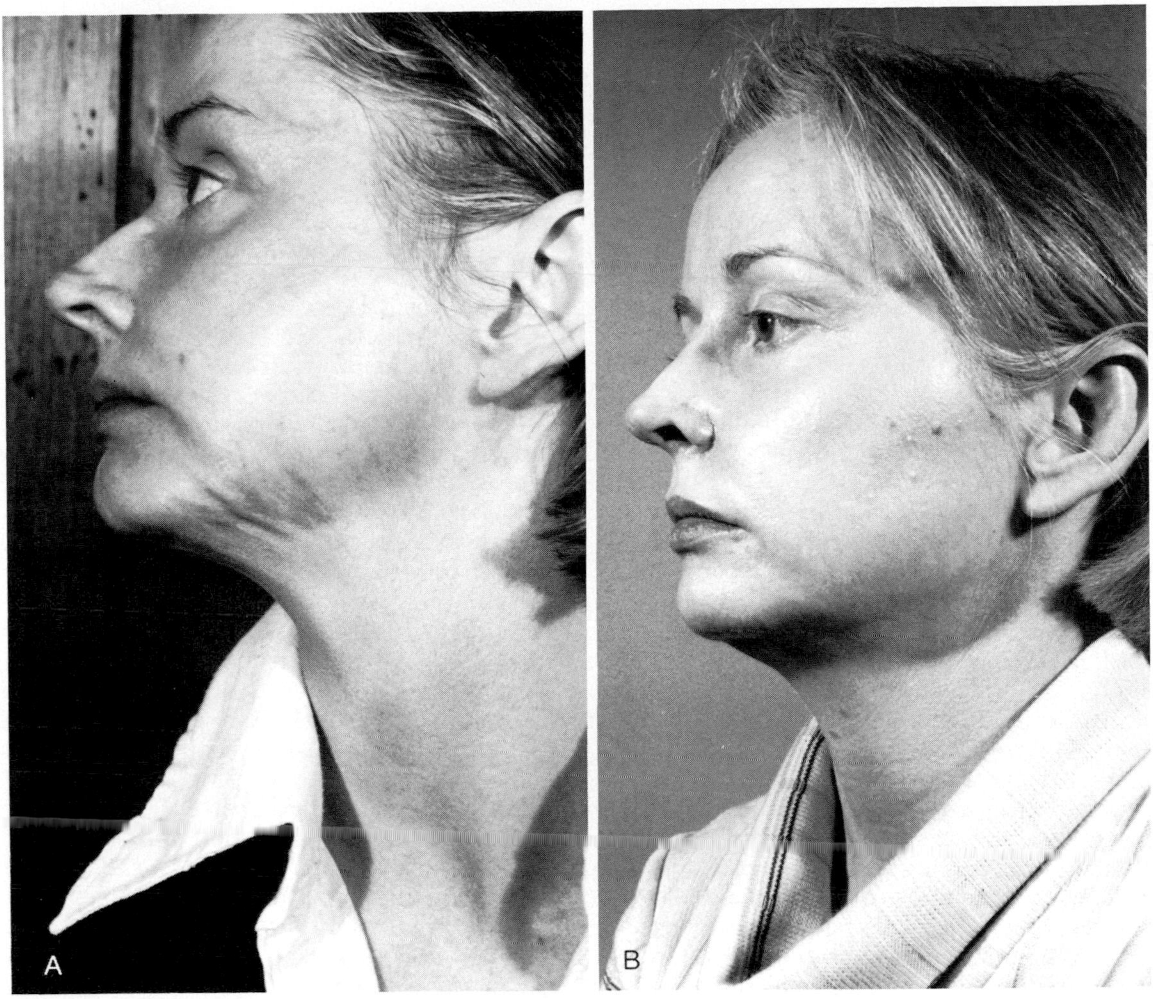

Figure 22–22. *A,* Hypertrophic scar formation in the submental area after a full face peeling. *B,* Appearance of the patient six years after peeling. Improvement is apparent in the areas of scar hypertrophy. Treatment consisted of topical steroids given over a period of several months during the first year. (From Baker, T. J., and Gordon, H. L.: Surgical Rejuvenation Of The Aging Face. St. Louis, MO, C.V. Mosby Company, 1986.)

to undergo a second chemical peeling. This is usually performed because of the development of blotchy hyperpigmentation after peeling, although occasionally it is necessary to treat recalcitrant facial rhytides. Eight to 12 months should elapse before repeeling and occlusive taping should never be used after the second peeling. The results of repeating the chemical peeling have been uniformly satisfactory and the treatment does not appear to increase the prevalence of hypertrophic scarring.

DERMABRASION

Dermabrasion is an abrasive process to remove the epidermis and superficial dermis, resulting in a smoothing of contour irregularities. It is also beneficial in the removal of superficial skin pigmentation. It is most commonly employed to ameliorate facial wrinkling, acne scarring, traumatic scars, scars resulting from smallpox or varicella, and superficial lentigos, and to treat dermal tattoos. Dermabrasion is also employed in dermal overgrafting techniques which are useful in increasing the thickness and improving the color of transplanted skin grafts.

Historical Background

The modern use of surgical planing was pioneered by Kromayer (1905) who reported the use of rasps and rotating wheels in the treatment of acne scars, keratoses, and hyperpigmentation. Kromayer (1905, 1914, 1930) termed this technique "scarless surgery" and over time it evolved from the use of hand-powered instruments to dental burs driven by electric motors. An astute observer, Kromayer noted that the healing seen after dermabrasion was from the epithelium of deep adnexal structures and that, if surgical planing was not carried below the papillary layer of the dermis, uneventful healing without hypertrophic scarring would follow.

Dermabrasion was not widely practiced after the initial reports by Kromayer. General acceptance of the technique began after World War II, following reports by Iverson (1947, 1953), who noticed favorable results in treating traumatic tattoo injuries by manual abrasion with sandpaper. McEvitt (1950) described a similar technique for the treatment of acne scarring.

The 1950's witnessed renewed interest in dermabrasion including a refinement in technique. Motor-driven cylinders and a variety of abrasive materials replaced manual abrasion. Kurtin (1953) described his procedure that used a rapidly revolving wire brush after application of ethyl chloride spray for anesthesia and hardening of the skin surface. Diamond-impregnated burs also became popular for the fine and easily controllable depth of abrasion produced. As the technical aspects of abrasion improved, the results became more predictable (Small, 1956; Burks, 1956, 1959; Burks, Marascalco, and Clark, 1963; Pegum and associates, 1959).

More recent modifications of technique include the introduction of high speed cutting tools, a variety of abrasive burs, and the use of Freon as a skin refrigerant in place of ethyl chloride (Stolar, 1984; Orentreich and Dunn, 1984; Alt, 1987). Nonetheless, the basic principles of mechanical abrasion or planing of the skin have remained unchanged. What has been learned over the years, largely by trial and error, are the clinical conditions that can be effectively treated with dermabrasion and the degree of improvement to be expected. With an understanding of its limitations as well as its efficacy, dermabrasion has become a widely practiced technique to treat a host of dermatologic conditions.

Healing of Abraded Areas

The success of surgical abrasion is dependent on the ability of the skin to reconstitute a new epidermal layer from the deep-lying dermal appendages. For this reason, favorable healing is seen in regions of the skin that have the largest number of adnexal structures and where the skin is thickest. Conversely, thin skin and skin with a paucity of sebaceous glands and hair follicles (eyelids, lower anterior neck, and medial surface of the arms) tend to exhibit delayed healing and hypertrophic scarring after dermabrasion. The face, with the exception of the eyelids, consists of thick skin, well endowed with epithelial adnexa, and heals rapidly after surgical planing. The back, despite its thickness, is often deficient in adnexa and may exhibit unsatisfactory healing in some individuals. The lower neck and suprasternal and sternal regions similarly respond poorly to dermabrasion.

Healing of abraded areas is comparable with that seen in the donor sites of split-thickness skin grafts. As in skin graft donor sites, the more superficial the abrasion, the faster is the subsequent healing and the less the tendency to heal with scarring. To be effective, planing must extend below the level of the epidermis into varying depths of the dermis. Judgment and experience dictate the appropriate level of abrasion that will produce the desired clinical result, although the planing should rarely be carried deeper than the base of the papillary dermis.

Immediately after dermabrasion, the serum from the wound forms a coagulum across the abraded surface entrapping necrotic cells and other surface debris. If allowed to dry, an eschar develops along the wound surface. Beneath this, an intense epithelial proliferation of adnexal elements is observed and is most marked 3 to 4 days after treatment (Eisen, Holyoke, and Lobitz, 1955; Luikart, Ayres, and Wilson, 1959; Odland and Ross, 1968; Hill, 1980). Between the third and fifth postoperative days, a thin layer of epidermis, lacking rete pegs, has regenerated and there is evidence of re-formed hair follicles and sebaceous glands. This histologic finding correlates with the loosening of surface crusts and the presence of thin, shiny red skin beneath the eschar. Epidermal regeneration is completed within seven days and always precedes dermal regeneration. With time, the epidermis gradually thickens and differentiates to assume its normal architecture.

Immediately after wounding of the skin, fibroblasts begin to migrate into the abraded area. Dermal regeneration parallels the fibroblastic proliferation. Early evidence of dermal reconstitution is noted at five days and continues for up to one year (Hill, 1980). In the first two weeks after abrasion, a considerable amount of collagen is synthesized, forming a horizontal striated pattern in the subepidermal layer similar to what is seen after chemical peeling (see Fig. 22–6) (Luikart, Ayres, and Wilson, 1959; Behin, Feuerstein, and Marovitz, 1977; Stegman, 1980, 1982). The development of a neocollagen layer represents an attempt by the dermis, which has not been removed by the abrasion but has sustained a direct traumatic injury, to heal itself. The newly regenerated dermal layer contributes to the smoothness and tightening of the skin that is commonly observed after dermabrasion. An additional factor in the tighter appearance of skin following abrasion is the inter-island contraction phenomenon (Converse and Robb-Smith, 1944). This phenomenon is a progressive approximation of new islands of epithelium in the contracting, healing dermal wound. Inter-island contraction is responsible for a reduction in the surface area of the dermal wound, and accounts for a tendency to constrict and collapse the deep pits of acne scars after dermabrasion (Campbell, 1977).

Late biopsy of an abraded area shows that the basic architecture of the skin is unchanged (Baker and Gordon, 1971.) The epidermis is of normal thickness, and in an average patient a normal amount of pigmentation is present within the basal layer. The adnexal structures appear and function normally. The vascularity is normal. Regeneration of the removed dermis is limited, being replaced by the forces of scar formation and contracture.

Compared with chemical peeling, the histologic changes after dermabrasion are more moderate. Dermabrasion does not produce a homogenization of the dermal collagen architecture. There is much less effect in the quantity of pigment present within the basal layer of the epidermis, and there is not the increase in the elastic fibers noted within the dermis after healing. Neocollagen regeneration in the dermis is smaller and less profound than that seen after chemical peeling (Behin, Feuerstein, and Marovitz, 1977). The major change seen after dermabrasion is a permanent removal of dermis, which does not regenerate to its original thickness (Baker and Gordon, 1971; Sawhney, Subbaraju, and Chakravarti, 1969). Mechanical dermis removal directly lessens and smooths contour irregularities along the skin surface. The presence of neocollagen within the regenerated dermis and the presence of inter-island contraction are secondary contributors to the overall salutary effects produced by dermabrasion.

Indications

Acne. The most common use of dermabrasion today is for the treatment of acne scarring. An abrasion extending to a moderate depth, approaching the base of an acne pit, commonly yields a significant improvement in facial appearance. Dermabrasion acts essentially as a camouflage procedure and, while not removing a scar, makes it less obvious by lessening the distinction between the pock mark and the surrounding skin. The shadow cast by the acne pit becomes less apparent after treatment. When deep lesions are present, a second or even a third dermabrasion may be necessary, although there is a smaller percentage of improvement following each procedure. Results of dermabrasion for acne scars tend to be better than those seen after chemical peeling, and dermabrasion or dermaplaning has essentially replaced peeling in the treatment of all but the most superficial of acne scars (Fig. 22–23).

Scars. Traumatic or surgical scars often respond favorably to dermabrasion. Both elevated and depressed scars can be improved by surgical planing, which produces a leveling in contour between the scar and the surrounding tissue and diminishes the shadow cast by contour irregularities. Elevated scars are directly dermabraded, whereas depressed scars are best treated by planing down adjacent skin. When dealing with scars wider than 5 mm, trapdoor injuries, and scars that run against relaxed skin tension lines, consideration should be given to other forms of scar revision such as direct excision, Z-plasty, or W-plasty (Figs. 22–24 to 22–26). The residual of certain viral infections can result in significant facial scarring, especially after infection with smallpox, varicella, and herpes zoster. Significant improvement has been noted in the appearance of these lesions after dermabrasion (Maneksha, 1960; Roenigk, 1977).

Hypertrophic burn scars lack adnexal components for regeneration and respond poorly to direct dermabrasion. On the other hand,

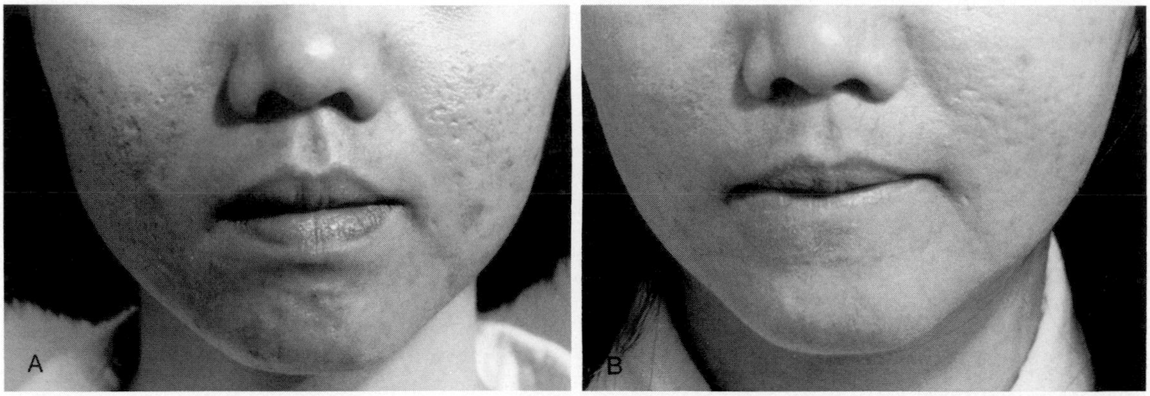

Figure 22–23. Treatment of acne facial scars by dermaplaning. *A*, Preoperative view. *B*, Postoperative view. (Courtesy of Dr. Melvin Spira.)

dermabrasion followed by overgrafting has proved somewhat useful in the revision of hypertrophic burn scars in selected patients (Hynes, 1957; Webster, Peterson, and Stein, 1958; Rees and Casson, 1966). Dermal overgrafting involves the planing of the epidermis of a previously placed split-thickness skin graft followed by the reapplication of another skin graft directly to the abraded dermal surface. Overgrafting has also been shown to be useful in treating unstable depressed scars and chronic radiodermatitis, and in tattoo removal (Hynes, 1957; Rees and Casson, 1966; Krant and Arons, 1977).

Tattoos. Amateur and traumatic tattoos are often improved by dermabrasion. The more superficial the presence of pigment within the dermis, the greater is the improvement after treatment (Fig. 22–27). Occasionally, the removal of the superficial dermis exposes more deeply situated particles, which can be removed directly or curretted. Professional tattooing places the pigment deep within the dermis, and these lesions are usually beyond the reach of dermabrasion. Direct excision, skin grafting, salabrasion (see Chap. 73), or laser removal (see Chap. 75) are more effective in the treatment of professional tattoos (Rosenberg, 1952; Strakosch, 1953; McDowell, 1974; Clabaugh, 1975; Reid and Muller, 1980).

Pigmentation. Pigmented nevi commonly recur after dermabrasion unless the pigment is confined to the basal layer of the epidermis. Similarly, blotchy hyperpigmentation, as seen in chloasma and melasma, can be improved by dermabrasion, although the bleaching effects following surgical planing are much less than those seen with chemical peeling, and the results tend to be less dramatic and less permanent.

Keratotic Lesions. Senile or seborrheic keratoses can be safely and quickly removed following dermabrasion with excellent results (Pickrell and associates, 1962). These lesions similarly can be treated by electrodesiccation and curettage with equally good results, as is the authors' preference. The use of dermabrasion as a prophylactic or therapeutic measure for treatment of actinic keratoses has been advocated by many (Burks, 1959; Epstein, 1987), although fluorouracil (5-FU) is easier, less traumatic, and generally preferable to treat premalignant lesions.

Wrinkles. Solar elastosis and fine facial rhytides show improvement following dermabrasion, although the effects are less marked than those after chemical peeling. For the patient with leathery, weathered skin requiring full facial treatment, chemical peeling is more efficacious and longer lasting. The limitations of abrasion of rhytides of the eyelids have previously been noted.

Dermabrasion is efficacious in removing the rhytides present in the upper lip as well as the lines adjacent to the vermilion along both the upper and lower lips. It also effectively removes fine glabellar wrinkles. Rhytides in these areas tend to be narrow and superficially located within the dermis, and for these reasons respond favorably to dermabrasion. Although the effect is not as dramatic as chemical peeling nor quite as long lasting, the results are often gratifying.

While the authors have advocated chemical peeling for the treatment of perioral rhytides,

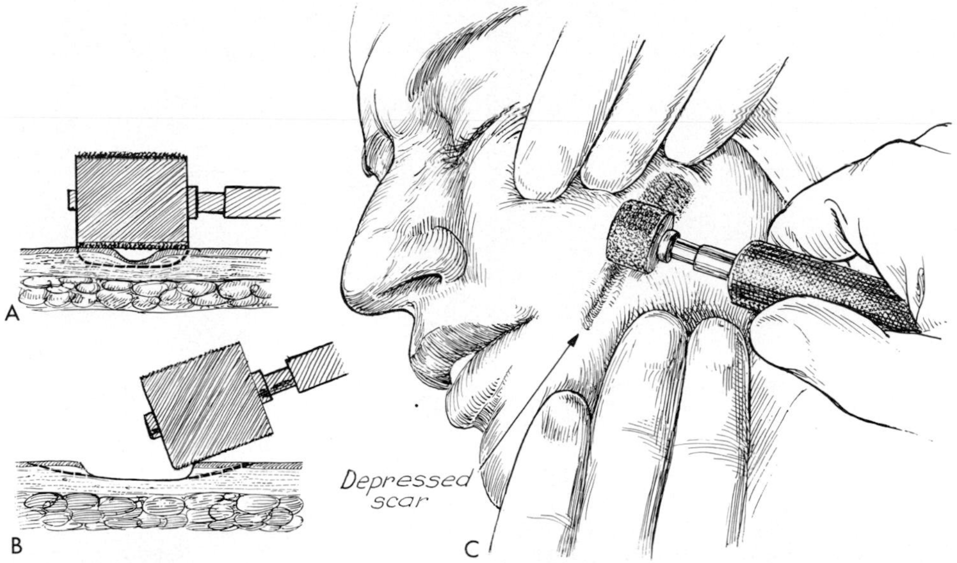

Figure 22–24. Dermabrasion of a depressed scar. *A,* Position of the head parallel to the scar. *B,* Beveling of edges. *C,* Direction of dermabrasion.

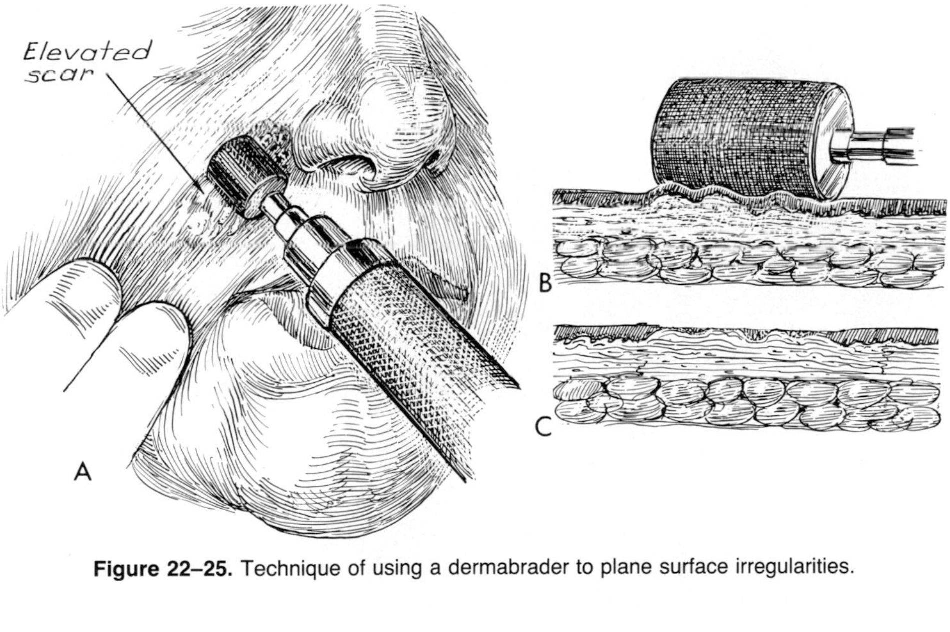

Figure 22–25. Technique of using a dermabrader to plane surface irregularities.

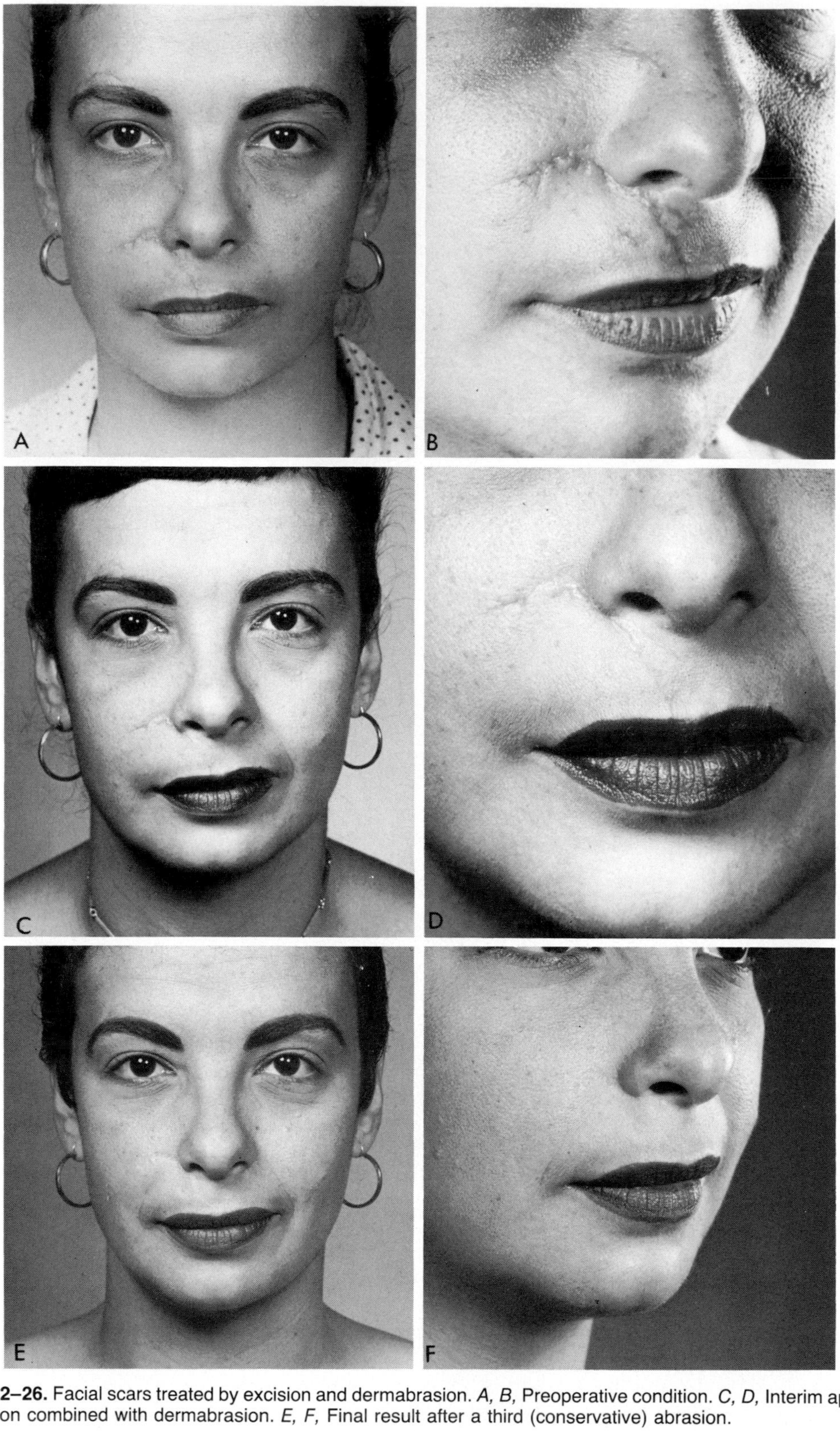

Figure 22–26. Facial scars treated by excision and dermabrasion. *A, B,* Preoperative condition. *C, D,* Interim appearance after excision combined with dermabrasion. *E, F,* Final result after a third (conservative) abrasion.

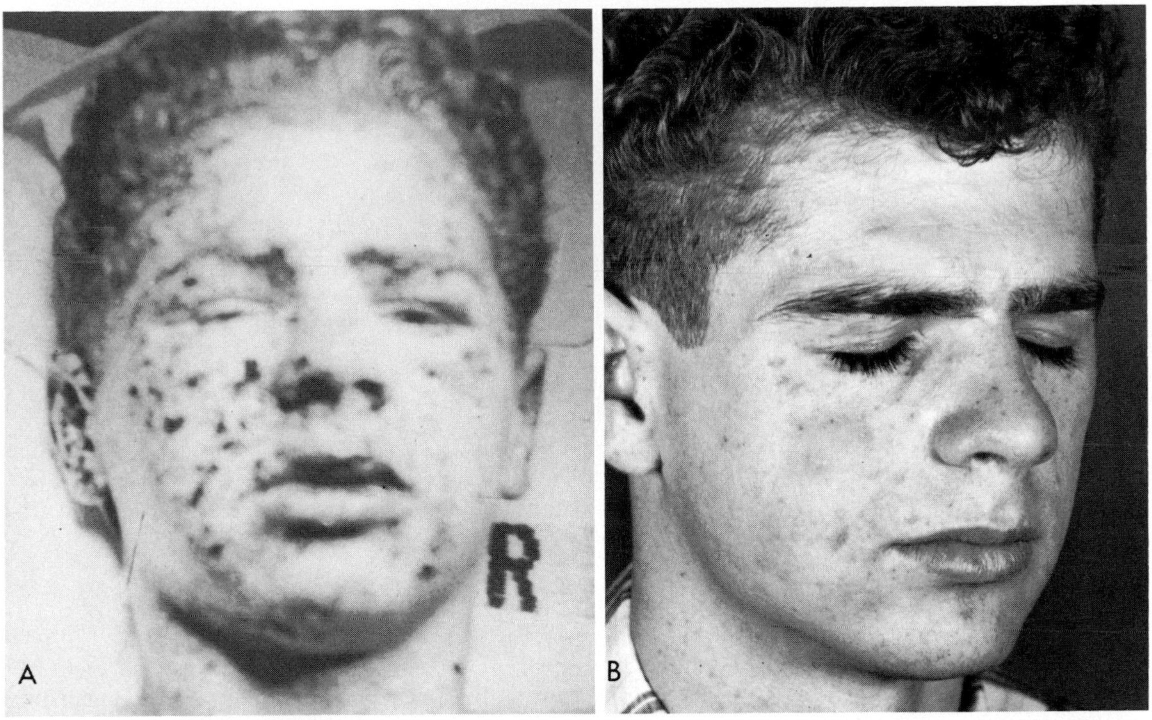

Figure 22–27. *A,* Widespread post-traumatic (gunpowder explosion) tattooing of the face treated by scrubbing, abrading, and curettement. *B,* Appearance after an additional abrasion treatment. Note that some marks are likely to be permanent because of the deep deposition of the pigment. Further excision combined with abrasion is indicated.

alone or accompanying surgical face lifting (Baker and Gordon, 1979), they have recently begun to use dermabrasion to a greater extent in treating these problems. The main advantage of dermabrasion is that as the depth of treatment is more controllable and presumably lighter than chemical peeling, patients tend to heal faster and with less discomfort than those undergoing peeling. The period of erythema following abrasion is shorter. For the dark-complexioned individual, the bleaching effect of dermabrasion is less and the contrasting color changes between the treated and untreated skin are minimized. At this time, perioral peeling is reserved for light-complexioned individuals who present with significant perioral wrinkles. Dermabrasion is especially indicated for the deep lines of the lower lip lying below the oral commissure and paralleling the mentalis muscle (Fig. 22–28).

Miscellaneous Conditions. Syringomas, trichoepitheliomas, adenoma sebaceum, and neurofibromatosis have all been reported to respond favorably to dermabrasion (Alt, 1987). Dermabrasion has also been shown to be a useful adjunct in the treatment of rhinophyma (Ortiz-Monasterio, Lopez-Mas, and Araico, 1974).

Limitations

Like chemical peeling, dermabrasion has its limitations. While almost all acne scars or pitting are improved after dermabrasion, it is a rare case of acne scarring in which a superior result is achieved and the acne scars rendered imperceptible. The deep "icepick" type of acne scars are especially recalcitrant to treatment and may require a direct surgical approach in conjunction with dermabrasion (Iverson, 1953; McAndrew, 1959; Orentreich and Dunn, 1984).

The often cited quote "fifty per cent improvement or better" (Alt, 1987) is a subjective evaluation that is another way of stating that the condition is improved, but scarring remains. The limitations of the procedure must be emphasized to the patient preoperatively, and the need for a second treatment six to 12 months later discussed when evaluating acne scars.

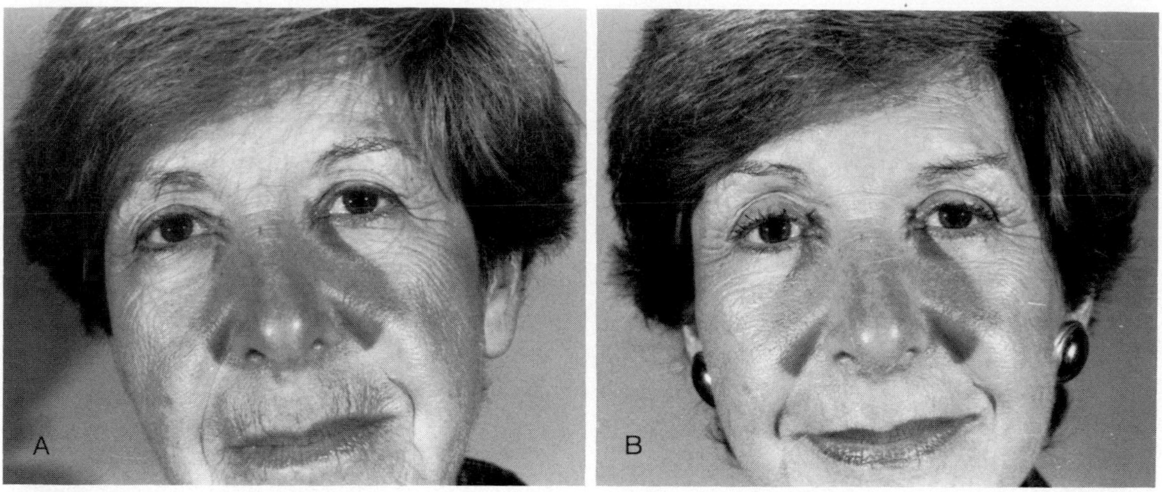

Figure 22–28. Typical improvement seen in perioral rhytides following dermabrasion. The patient also underwent a face lift at the time of the dermabrasion. *A,* Preoperative appearance. *B,* Postoperative appearance.

Technique

All patients undergoing dermabrasion are best treated in a hospital operating room or ambulatory surgical facility, which allows proper sedation and monitoring. Anesthesia can be either local or general. Local infiltration anesthesia combined with regional blocks are often used with satisfactory results. Refrigerants tend to be cumbersome and provide less than ideal anesthesia during the procedure. The authors see no advantage in freezing the skin rather than using local anesthetics (Campbell, 1977; Abadir and Abadir, 1980), and have noted no improvement in the results when the dermabrasion is performed on frozen skin. This experience contrasts with varying reports in the dermatology literature noting that freezing the skin and placing it in a semisolid state are important factors in obtaining satisfactory results with the procedure (Orentreich and Dunn, 1984; Alt, 1987).

Dermabrasion is usually performed with a motor-driven instrument attached to either wire brushes, cylinders of sandpaper, or stainless steel burs. The authors' preference is to use a relatively low speed, motor-driven hand piece (12,000 to 15,000 rpm) with various-sized diamond-tipped fraises. The diamond-impregnated burs produce a fine, easily controllable depth of abrasion and, when driven at relatively low speeds, yield a superficial to medium depth of surgical planing. The control provided with this equipment has essentially eliminated postoperative hypertrophic scarring. A 5 mm wheel-shaped bur is useful for abrading around the vermilion border. On the flat surface of the upper lip or cheeks, a larger, cylindrical bur is usually preferable (Fig. 22–29).

Before infiltration with local anesthesia, the depth of the pock marks or pits should be marked with surgical ink and the extent of the dermabrasion outlined. The abrader is moved slowly with even pressure across the skin surface, removing the epidermis and superficial dermis down to the desired level. The abrading drum should parallel the surface of the skin (see Figs. 22–24 and Fig. 22–25), the sanding process consisting of light brushing strokes that run at right angles to the plane of rotation of the instrument. In performing the abrasion, it is important to use even pressure and to let the machine do the work of abrading the skin. The hand piece is kept moving, rather than remaining stationary over an abraded area. This maneuver minimizes the possibility of deep planing secondary to a combination of pressure, heat, and friction. Frequent inspection of the skin surface, with the appearance of fine punctate bleeding and removal of the previously placed surgical ink, offers guidelines to the proper depth of abrasion (Fig. 22–30).

Placing the skin on stretch is useful for obtaining a proper tension against which to dermabrade, and it helps to produce a smooth, even planing. Intraoral packs can also be placed to provide a hard surface on which to

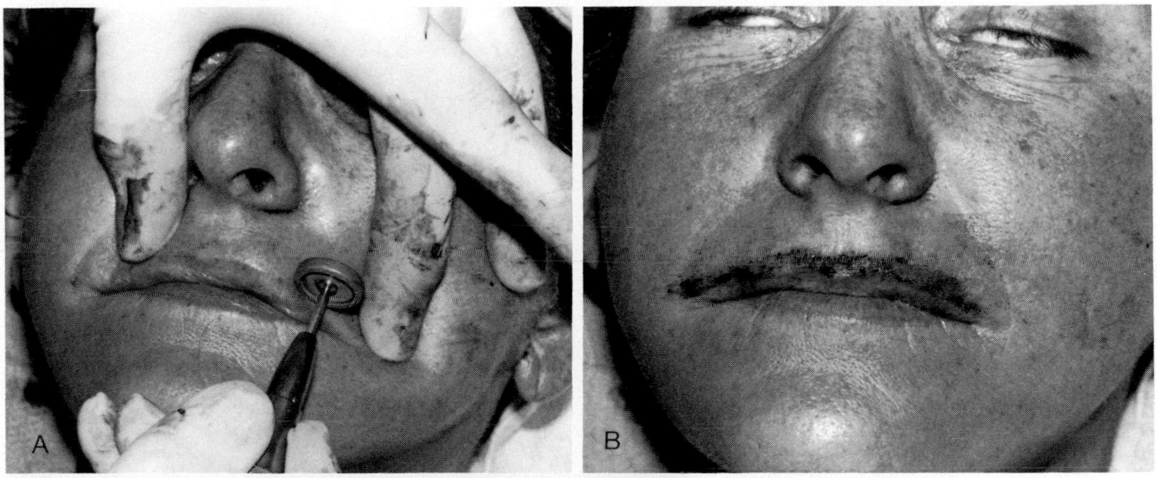

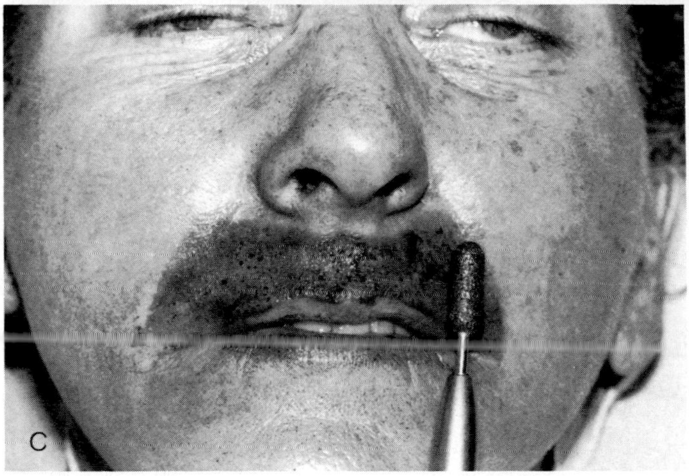

Figure 22–29. *A,* A 5 mm wheel-shaped bur is used along the vermilion border carrying the abrasion into the vermilion itself. *B,* Appearance of the lip after dermabrasion of the vermilion border. *C,* The remainder of the upper lip is abraded with a cylindrical fraise, abrading to the base of the nose and just beyond the nasolabial fold. Fine punctate bleeding delineates the proper depth of the abrasion.

work. Lighter pressure is advisable when abrading bony prominences, to control the depth of abrasion.

The depth of the abrasion should be confined to a superficial or, at most, intermediate thickness of dermis. The proper level is apparent from the multiple fine bleeding points seen as the abrasion is carried into the vessels that lie within the dermal papillae. While the object of treatment is to remove and blend surface irregularities, it can be risky to abrade adjacent skin aggressively in treating deeply situated scars. It is preferable to re-abrade in one or two additional sessions rather than attempt complete obliteration of scar irregularities, risking hypertrophic scarring.

As the planing is carried to the periphery, the edges of the abrasion should be "feathered" into the surrounding skin, performing a superficial abrasion along the treatment margins. A fine bur, lighter pressure, and fewer strokes along the periphery all produce a more superficial abrasion. In this manner, the dermabrasion is blended into the surrounding area (see Fig. 22–24), and this maneuver lessens the line of demarcation between treated and untreated skin.

Postoperative Care

After abrasion, the area is irrigated with normal saline. If necessary, hemostasis is obtained with gauze sponges soaked in 1:50,000 epinephrine solution, topically applied.

Dressings are to be avoided, as is the use of air blowing or otherwise allowing the abraded area to become desiccated. If gauze is allowed to remain in contact with the skin or the abraded area, an eschar or crust will form along the wound surface as the gauze rigidly adheres to the skin. Gauze dressings

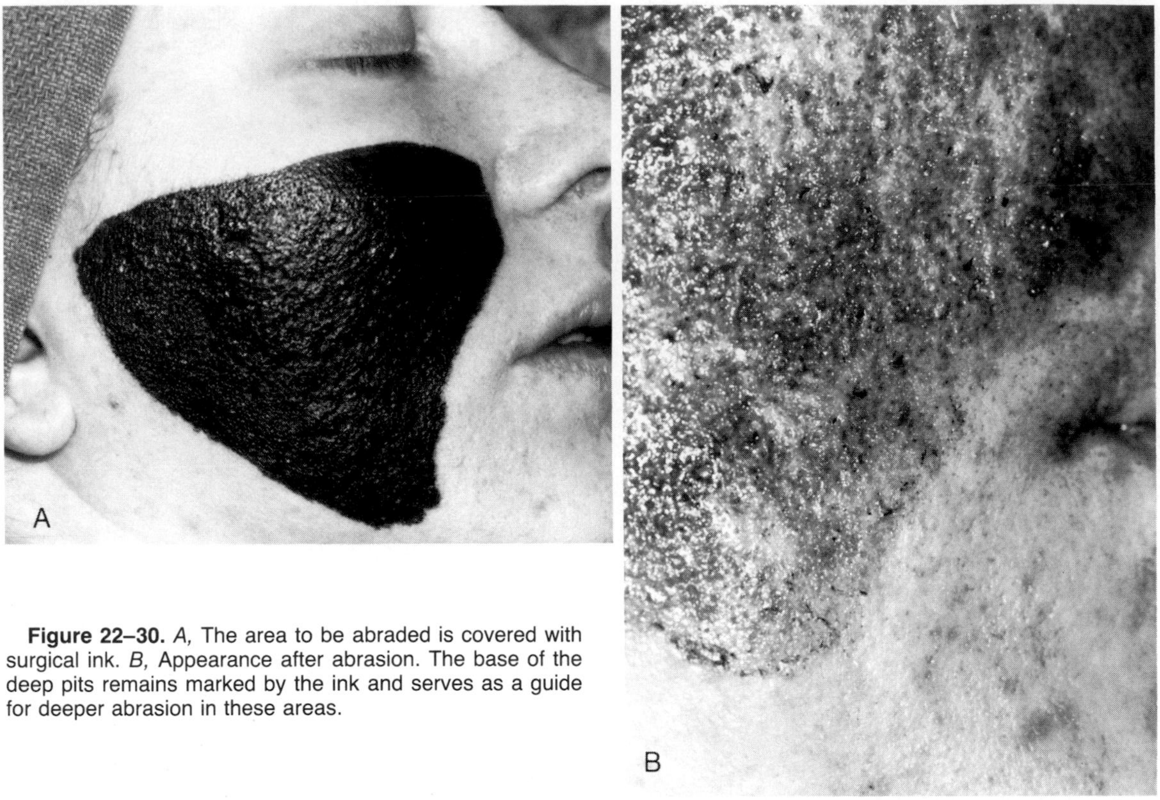

Figure 22–30. *A,* The area to be abraded is covered with surgical ink. *B,* Appearance after abrasion. The base of the deep pits remains marked by the ink and serves as a guide for deeper abrasion in these areas.

increase patient discomfort and delay the healing time until eschar separation is complete. It is preferable to apply a topical antibiotic ointment directly to the abraded area following treatment and to keep the face lubricated with A & D ointment until wound healing is complete. The patient may wash the face with clear water a day after surgery and is instructed to keep the abraded area moist with ointment until reepithelization is complete, usually in five to seven days.

The appearance of the healing surface parallels that of chemical peeling, although erythema of the skin tends to resolve more quickly. In ten days the patient can wear cosmetics and largely cover the erythema present within the abraded area. Moisturizers are necessary until the skin returns to its normal appearance, to prevent dryness and cracking. Avoidance of sunlight and the use of sunblocks and coverage make-up base are critical to protect the skin from pigmentary changes during the period of wound healing.

Complications

With proper patient selection and technique, complications are few after dermabrasion. The most common problem relates to patient dissatisfaction from incomplete resolution of deep pock marks secondary to acne scarring. Repeat dermabrasion of these areas often produces an improvement over the initial result.

Milia. All patients undergoing dermabrasion should be warned that milia may occur, and they are seen in approximately 50 per cent of the patients, usually two to four weeks after planing. Milia usually disappear spontaneously within a few weeks following the use of local hygiene and abrasive soap, although occasionally they may require individual incision and expression of their contents.

Erythema of the Skin. All patients have skin erythema after dermabrasion. This commonly disappears within four to eight weeks but occasionally lasts up to 12 weeks. Erythema can be effectively covered with facial cosmetics.

Hyperpigmentation of the Abraded Area. This has been noted in many patients and is seen more frequently than in those undergoing chemical peeling. The use of sunscreens and heavy covering make-up base are important in avoiding this troublesome problem. If the condition is persistent, bleaching cream with 4 per cent hydroquinone produces improvement in some patients. Secondary abrasion six months later, followed by meticulous sun avoidance, usually takes care of the remaining area of hyperpigmentation.

In most patients, there is a gradual lightening of the skin after dermabrasion, although this is easily concealed with make-up. The significant bleaching effect seen with phenol peeling is not as pronounced after surgical planing.

Hypertrophic Scarring. Scarring follows if the dermabrasion is carried deeply or if the patient develops a secondary infection postoperatively. Dermabrasion in unfavorable anatomic areas, such as the base of the neck, can produce similar problems even if the abrasion is superficial. Conservatism in abrasion and repeat dermabrasion are the best ways to avoid this complication.

Dermabrasion With Chemical Peeling

A combination of dermabrasion with chemical peeling has received attention (Horton and Sadove, 1987), although the concept was introduced by Dupont and associates (1972) and later by Stagnone (1977), who applied dermabrasion after initially treating facial skin with a 50 per cent trichloroacetic acid solution.

The indications for this combined procedure are the same as for chemical peeling, primarily the treatment of facial rhytides. The proposed advantage is that the results are alleged to be more profound and longer lasting from the combination of the two techniques (Horton and Sadove, 1987). Although used in full face treatments, the combination of chemical peeling and abrasion has most commonly been performed for regional problems: perioral, glabella, and "crow's feet" rhytides. The peeling solution is applied first. After it dries to a pearly white color, it is dermabraded down to a fine, superficially bleeding surface. The patient is not taped postoperatively but rather managed with ointment, eliminating the problem of crusting and eschar formation.

The results of this technique are satisfactory and complications are few. Histologic studies show that the changes following the combination technique are similar to those after chemical peeling alone.

The authors have used the combination of chemical peeling and dermabrasion for several years and have found the results indistinguishable from those seen after chemical peeling alone. It appears that the peeling produces the desired results, and the addition of dermabrasion is an unnecessary step (Baker and Gordon, 1987). Moreover, in inexperienced hands there is the risk that deeply abrading peeled skin may lead to hypertrophic scarring.

"Chemabrasion" should be limited to those patients who present with both acne scarring and facial rhytides. In these difficult situations, total face peeling is preferred, followed by dermabrasion along the areas of the acne scarring.

INJECTABLE COLLAGEN

Injectable collagen is a product that has been developed over the last 12 years and is composed of purified bovine dermal collagen emulsified in buffered saline and 0.3 per cent lidocaine base. It is used to fill in contour depressions of facial skin, to improve fine facial rhytides, and to augment depressed acne scars.

Injectable collagen is synthesized from calf hide and is composed mainly of Type I collagen (95 per cent) together with a small amount of Type III (5 per cent). Selective proteolytic hydrolysis of the collagen molecule allows for a reduction in the low antigenic potential of this material. In this process, the nonhelical portion of the mammalian collagen molecule, which accounts for most of the antigenicity, is removed leaving the monotonously repetitious and tightly bound triple helix, which is only weakly antigenic (Knapp, Kaplan, and Daniels, 1977; Knapp, Luck, and Daniels, 1977).

Injectable collagen is marketed in three forms: Zyderm I, Zyderm II, and Zyplast. Zyderm I contains 35 mg per ml of collagen. Approximately 25 to 30 per cent of the total injected volume is collagen, the remainder being saline base. As the saline is absorbed over two to three weeks, the initial correction of contour is diminished, necessitating overcorrection and multiple treatments. Zyderm II, introduced in 1983, contains 65 mg per ml of collagen, and because of the higher concentration of collagen requires less overcorrection. Zyplast collagen, introduced in 1985, is a glutaraldehyde crosslinked Zyderm collagen that appears to be degraded more slowly than Zyderm, producing longer-lasting results (Kligman and Armstrong, 1986).

Histopathology of Collagen Injection

It was originally believed that following Zyderm collagen injection, the implant would be invaded by host tissue cells, develop a vascular supply, and become histologically blended with the host connective tissue (Knapp, Kaplan, and Daniels, 1977; Knapp, Luck, and Daniels, 1977). Follow-up studies have failed to confirm this and there is no evidence of Zyderm collagen becoming incorporated into normal host tissue (Kligman and Armstrong, 1986). Biopsies at varying intervals reveal that the implant remains clearly distinguishable from surrounding host dermis and appears as an amorphous mass surrounded by host dermal collagen. If there is no allergic or foreign body reaction, very few fibroblasts are noted growing into the implant, and there is no vascular ingrowth. Bovine collagen appears as an inert implant in the dermis and does not appear to stimulate new native collagen production (Stegman, 1987a). In patients exhibiting clinical reaction at the implant site, foreign body granulomas with infiltration of giant cells, lymphocytes, histocytes, and plasma cells characterize a delayed hypersensitivity reaction to the collagen (Swanson and associates, 1983; Labow and Silvers, 1985).

Loss of clinical improvement after initial implantation of Zyderm collagen is seen beginning at six months after injection (Rapaport, Salit, and Rivkin, 1984; Pharriss, 1984; Robinson and Hanke, 1985). The ultimate fate of injected collagen is undetermined at this time. Degradation of the collagen remains a distinct possibility (Robinson and Hanke, 1985). On the other hand, Stegman (1987b) postulates that over time there is a migration of the implant deeper into the skin, causing the collagen eventually to be extruded from the dermis into the underlying subcutaneous tissue. In this location, the implant no longer exerts an upward pressure on the dermis to correct scars and rhytides. All authors agree that retreatment is usually required within six to 24 months after collagen injection (Collagen Corporation, see references).

Indications

Injectable collagen has been used primarily to correct facial rhytides resulting from aging and actinic damage. It is also recommended to correct depressed scarring secondary to acne, trauma, viral infections, and iatrogenic sequelae (Stegman and Tromovitch, 1980; Courtiss, 1982; Bailin and Bailin, 1982; Kaplan, Falces, and Tolleth, 1983; Webster, Kattner, and Smith, 1984).

Fine facial rhytides, especially perioral wrinkles, rhytides along the nasolabial folds, and those in the glabellar region can respond favorably to collagen injection. Forehead lines, creases in the chin, and "crow's feet" exhibit a less dramatic result after treatment (Stegman, 1987a). Proper patient selection is important for satisfactory results from injectable collagen.

It is alleged that the vertical glabellar lines respond the most favorably to treatment and exhibit the longest-lasting degree of correction (Robinson and Hanke, 1985). Zyderm injected directly into the dermis is the preferred material for this region.

Perioral rhytides of the upper lip can be treated with Zyderm injected directly into the individual crease. Care is required, since overcorrection in the vermilion and periorbital areas is slow to resolve because of the thin dermis and hyperextensibility at these sites (Kaplan, Falces, and Tolleth, 1983). Conservatism in implanting small amounts of collagen over several treatment sessions often provides adequate, if only temporary, relief of the rhytides. In the authors' opinion, a more complete and more long-lasting solution to perioral wrinkles is seen following dermabrasion or chemical peeling.

Deep nasolabial folds are best treated with Zyplast injected subdermally along the nasolabial groove. This elevates the depressed area between lips and cheeks, and softens the appearance of a deep line often present in this area. Subsequently, if a persistent superficial crease remains, Zyderm injected directly into the dermis usually obliterates the remaining rhytide in this location.

Injectable collagen may be of some help in the treatment of depressed scars resulting from acne. The collagen is injected at the base of the pock mark to elevate it and make it less obvious when contrasted with the surrounding skin. Each acne scar must be individually injected, usually with Zyderm. Soft, distensible scars with relatively smooth margins respond more favorably than heavy, indurated lesions with a large amount of surrounding fibrosis. Icepick scars show little or no improvement with collagen.

Injectable collagen has also been used to provide contour restoration of depressed scars after trauma or surgery. Zyplast is the preferred agent to treat these scars and can provide a restoration of subcutaneous tissue that is often lacking in these lesions. The agent is injected directly into the subcutaneous layer beneath the scar to bring it to the level of the surrounding skin.

Technique

Zyderm imparts the best correction if it is injected directly within the dermis at the time of treatment (Tromovitch, Stegman, and Glogau, 1984). Subcutaneous injection may correct depressed deformities temporarily, but it is short-lived. To treat fine facial rhytides, collagen is injected directly into the dermis underlying the skin crease. Overcorrection is necessary to compensate for the absorption of saline and lidocaine present within the suspension. The end point of injection is usually a white blanching, with the skin appearing slightly thickened and brawny, and the wrinkle becoming slightly elevated from the surrounding tissue. Zyplast should be placed subcutaneously, immediately beneath the dermis. If placed within the dermis, it appears as an irregular and obvious mass and does not blend in as well as injected Zyderm. Once injected, the Zyplast bolus can be repositioned within the subcutaneous plane by massaging and pinching the fluid into the desired shape, producing a more even contour in this area.

There is less bruising and pain with Zyplast injection, although much more material is required to achieve contour correction after a subcutaneous injection. Small amounts of Zyderm usually alleviate fine facial rhytides, and the longevity of this injection is six to eight months in most reports. Zyplast appears to hold its correction for 12 to 18 months (Stegman, 1987b).

Complications

Complications after collagen injection are small and usually relate to its synthesis from a bovine source. The main drawbacks of collagen injection have been its short duration and limited effectiveness. After six months clinical resolution is quite common and often repeat treatment is required. The cost of the material, which is substantial, and the need for serial injections must be completely explained to the patient before treatment with injectable collagen is undertaken.

Approximately 3 per cent of patients are allergic to injectable collagen, and all patients should be skin tested before undergoing treatment. The screening skin test detects both humoral and cell-mediated immune responses. It is read at 72 hours and again at four weeks. Two-thirds of all patients react by 72 hours and the remaining allergic patients show a cutaneous reaction by the end of the four week period. A positive skin test demonstrates a surrounding zone of induration, swelling, erythema, and pruritus in response to the collagen. Any erythema or induration that persists for more than six hours after skin testing, or appears 24 hours after implantation, is considered a positive skin test. The allergies presumably relate to dietary exposure to beef, and skin testing is indispensable to discover patients with allergy to bovine collagen.

Patients who show negative skin test results can rarely exhibit allergic reactions at the treatment site after reinjection. Delayed hypersensitivity as well as the development of anti–bovine collagen antibodies have been documented in these patients (Castrow and Krull, 1983; Cooperman and Michaeli, 1984). Treatment site reactions appear similar to those in a positive skin test, are erythematous and indurated, and require several months before resolution of the symptoms and disappearance of the lesions. A positive skin test on the arm is much easier for most patients to experience than a positive treatment site reaction on the face, and constant reassurance and patience are necessary in dealing with this distressing development. Treatment site reactions of erythema and transient swelling have been noted following alcohol ingestion, sinusitis, or exposure to sunlight (Swanson and associates, 1983). Localized areas of infarction, presumably secondary to injection in underlying blood vessels, have also been seen.

Systemic symptoms such as arthralgia, arthritis, fever, and urticaria rarely occur after injection with bovine collagen and are a manifestation of immune response. These reactions, which are usually self-limiting, are treated symptomatically. Fears of introducing autoimmune cross reactivity to human collagen have been raised (Cohen, Peacock, and Chvapil, 1984), but have not been substantiated by numerous clinical trials. Overall, the systemic immunogenicity of bovine collagen appears low (Cooperman and Michaeli, 1984; Siegle and associates, 1984; Stegman, 1987b).

Personal Note on Collagen. At the time of writing, the authors no longer use injectable collagen. Although it is efficacious in treating localized rhytides and scar depressions, we have become frustrated by short-lasting results and the cost of the material.

REFERENCES

Abadir, D. M., and Abadir, A. R.: Dermabrasion under regional anesthesia without refrigeration of the skin. J. Dermatol. Surg. Oncol., *6*:119, 1980.

Alt, T. H.: Therapeutic facial dermabrasion. *In* Epstein, E. (Ed.): Skin Surgery. 6th Ed. Philadelphia, W. B. Saunders Company, 1987, p. 327.

Aronsohn, R. B.: Complications of chemosurgery. Eye Ear Nose Throat Mon., *51*:19, 1972.

Ayres, S.: Dermal changes following application of chemical cauterants to aging skin (superficial chemosurgery). Arch. Dermatol., *82*:578, 1960.

Ayres, S.: Superficial chemosurgery in treating aging skin. Arch. Dermatol., *85*:385, 1962.

Ayres, S.: Superficial chemosurgery: its current status and relationship to dermabrasion. Arch. Dermatol., *89*:395, 1964.

Bailin, P. L., and Bailin, M. D.: Correction of depressed scars following Mohs' surgery: the role of collagen implantation. J. Dermatol. Surg. Oncol., *8*:845, 1982.

Baker, T. J.: The ablation of rhytides by chemical means: a preliminary report. J. Fla. Med. Assoc., *47*:451, 1961.

Baker, T. J.: Chemical face peeling and rhytidectomy. A combined approach for face rejuvenation Plast. Reconstr. Surg., *29*:199, 1962.

Baker, T. J., and Gordon, H. L.: Chemical face peeling, an adjunct to surgical face lifting. South. Med. J., *56*:412, 1963.

Baker, T. J., and Gordon, H. L.: Chemical face peeling and dermabrasion. Surg. Clin. North Am., *51*:387, 1971.

Baker, T. J., and Gordon, H. L.: Chemical peeling as a practical method of removing rhytides of the upper lip. Ann. Plast. Surg., *2*:209, 1979.

Baker, T. J., and Gordon, H. L.: Chemical face peel. *In* Goldwyn, R. M. (Ed.): The Unfavorable Result in Plastic Surgery. 2nd Ed. Boston, Little, Brown & Company, 1984, p. 633.

Baker, T. J., and Gordon, H. L.: Chemical face peeling. *In* Surgical Rejuvenation of the Aging Face. St. Louis, MO, C. V. Mosby Company, 1986, p. 37.

Baker, T. J., and Gordon, H. L.: Chemical peel with phenol. *In* Epstein, E. (Ed.): Skin Surgery. 6th Ed. Philadelphia, W. B. Saunders Company, 1987, p. 423.

Baker, T. J., Gordon, H. L., Mosienko, P., and Seckinger, D. L.: Long-term histological study of skin after chemical face peeling. Plast. Reconstr. Surg., *53*:522, 1974.

Baker, T. J., Gordon, H. L., and Seckinger, D. L.: A second look at chemical face peeling. Plast. Reconstr. Surg., *37*:487, 1966.

Baker, T. J., Horton, C. E., and Sadove, R. C.: Discussion. Refinements in combined chemical peel and simultaneous abrasion of the face. Ann. Plast. Surg., *19*:510, 1987.

Bames, H. O.: Truth and fallacies of face peeling and face lifting. Med. J. Rec., *126*:86, 1927.

Batstone, J. H., and Millard, D. R., Jr.: An endorsement of facial chemo-surgery. Br. J. Plast. Surg., *21*:193, 1968.

Behin, F., Feuerstein, S. S., and Marovitz, W.: Comparative histological study of mini pig skin after chemical peel and dermabrasion. Arch. Otolaryngol., *103*:271, 1977.

Bhangoo, K. S.: Letter: Histological changes following chemical face peeling. Plast. Reconstr. Surg., *54*:599, 1974.

Brown, A. M., Kaplan, L. M., and Brown, M. E.: Phenol-induced histological skin changes: hazards, techniques, and uses. Br. J. Plast. Surg., *13*:158, 1960a.

Brown, A. M., Kaplan, L. M., and Brown, M. E.: Cutaneous alterations induced by phenol: a histologic bioassay. Int. Surg., *34*:602, 1960b.

Burks, J. W.: Wire brush planing—an office procedure. Postgrad. Med., *20*:652, 1956.

Burks, J. W.: Prophylactic planing of the aged patient for cancer of the skin. J. La. Med. Soc., *111*:169, 1959.

Burks, J. W., Marascalco, J., and Clark, W. H., Jr.: Half-face planing of precancerous skin after five years. Arch. Dermatol., *88*:572, 1963.

Campbell, R. M.: Surgical and chemical planing of the skin. *In* Converse, J. M. (Ed.): Reconstructive Plastic Surgery. 2nd Ed. Philadelphia, W. B. Saunders Company, 1977, p. 442.

Castrow, F. F., 2nd, and Krull, E. A.: Injectable collagen implant—update. J. Am. Acad. Dermatol., *9*:889, 1983.

Clabaugh, W. A.: Tattoo removal by superficial dermabrasion. Five year experience. Plast. Reconstr. Surg., *55*:401, 1975.

Cohen, I. K., Peacock, E. E., and Chvapil, M.: Zyderm (letter). Plast. Reconstr. Surg., *73*:857, 1984.

Collagen Corporation, Palo Alto, CA: Package insert with injectable collagen (Zyderm).

Combes, F. C., Sperber, P. A., and Reisch, M.: Dermal defects: treatment by a chemical agent. N.Y. Physicians & Am. Med., *55*:36, 1960.

Converse, J. M., and Robb-Smith, A. H. T.: The healing of surface cutaneous wounds: its analogy with the healing of superficial burns. Ann. Surg., *120*:873, 1944.

Cooperman, L., and Michaeli, D.: The immunogenicity of injectable collagen. I. A one year prospective study. J. Am. Acad. Dermatol., *10*:638, 1984.

Courtiss, E. H.: Cosmetic defects and collagen injection. J. Am. Acad. Dermatol., *247*:3360, 1982.

Deichmann, W., and Witherup, S.: Phenol studies. VI. The acute and comparative toxicity of phenol and *o*-, *m*-, and *p*-cresols for experimental animals. J. Pharmacol. Exp. Ther., *80*:233, 1944.

Dupont, C., Ciaburro, H., Prevost, Y., and Cloutier, G.: Phenol skin tightening for better dermabrasion. Plast. Reconstr. Surg., *50*:588, 1972.

Ebbell, B. (Translator): The Papyrus Ebers: The Greatest Egyptian Medical Document. Copenhagen, Levin & Munksgaard, 1937.

Eisen, A. Z., Holyoke, J. B., and Lobitz, W. C.: Responses of superficial portion of human pilosebaceous apparatus to control injury. J. Invest. Dermatol., *25*:145, 1955.

Epstein, E.: Dermabrasion for therapeutic purposes. *In* Epstein, E. (Ed.): Skin Surgery. 6th Ed. Philadelphia, W. B. Saunders Company, 1987, p. 344.

Ferreira, J. A.: Dermabrasion of the skin: prevention and/or treatment of hyperpigmentation. Aesthetic Plast. Surg., *1*:381, 1978.

Ferreira, J. A.: The role of diazepam in skin hyperpigmentation. Aesthetic Plast. Surg., *4*:343, 1980.

Gillies, H. D., and Millard, D. R.: The Principles and Art of Plastic Surgery. Boston, Little, Brown & Company, 1957, p. 493.

Gross, B. G.: Cardiac arrhythmias during phenol face peeling. Plast. Reconstr. Surg., *73*:590, 1984.

Hill, T. G.: Cutaneous wound healing following dermabrasion. J. Dermatol. Surg. Oncol., *6*:487, 1980.

Horton, C. E., and Sadove, R. C.: Refinements in combined chemical peel and simultaneous abrasion of the face. Ann. Plast. Surg., *19*:504, 1987.

Hynes, W.: The treatment of scars by shaving and skin graft. Br. J. Plast. Surg., *10*:1, 1957.

Iverson, P. C.: Surgical removal of traumatic tattoos of the face. Plast. Reconstr. Surg., *2*:427, 1947.

Iverson, P. C.: Further developments in the treatment of skin lesions by surgical abrasion. Plast. Reconstr. Surg., *12*:27, 1953.

Kaplan, E. N., Falces, E., and Tolleth, H.: Clinical utilization of injectable collagen. Ann. Plast. Surg., *10*:437, 1983.

Kligman, A. M.: Early destructive effects of sunlight on human skin. J.A.M.A., *210*:2377, 1969.

Kligman, A. M., and Armstrong, R. C.: Histologic response to intradermal Zyderm and Zyplast (glutaraldehyde cross-linked) collagen in humans. J. Dermatol. Surg. Oncol., *12*:351, 1986.

Kligman, A. M., Baker, T. J., and Gordon, H. L.: Long-term histologic follow-up of phenol face peels. Plast. Reconstr. Surg., *75*:652, 1985.

Knapp, T. R., Kaplan, E. N., and Daniels, J. R.: Injectable collagen for soft tissue augmentation. Plast. Reconstr. Surg., *60*:398, 1977.

Knapp, T. R., Luck, E., and Daniels, J. R.: Behavior of solubilized collagen as a bioimplant. J. Surg. Res., *23*:96, 1977.

Krant, S. M., and Arons, M. S.: Dermabrasion debridement of the deep dermal burn. Plast. Reconstr. Surg., *60*:68, 1977.

Kromayer, E.: Rotationsinstrumente: ein neues technisches Verfahren in der dermatologischen Kleinchirugie. Chir. Dermatol. Ztschr., Berlin, *12*:26, 1905.

Kromayer, E.: Repetitorium der Haut und Geschlechtskrankheiten für Studierende und Aerzte. Jena, Gustav Fischer, 1914, p. 24.

Kromayer, E.: The Cosmetic Treatment of Skin Complaints (English translation of 2nd German [1929] Edition). New York, Oxford University Press, 1930, p. 9.

Kurtin, A.: Corrective surgical planing of skin: new technique for treatment of acne scars and other skin defects. Arch. Dermatol. Syph., *68*:389, 1953.

Labow, T. A., and Silvers, D. N.: Late reactions at Zyderm skin test sites. Cutis, *35*:154, 1985.

Litton, C.: Chemical face lifting. Plast. Reconstr. Surg., *29*:371, 1962.

Litton, C.: Follow-up study of chemosurgery. South. Med. J., *50*:1007, 1966.

Litton, C., Fournier, P., and Capinpin, A.: A survey of chemical peeling of the face. Plast. Reconstr. Surg., *51*:645, 1973.

Litton, C., and Trinidad, G.: Complications of chemical face peeling as evaluated by a questionnaire. Plast. Reconstr. Surg., *67*:738, 1981.

Lotter, A.: Human pigment factors relative to chemical face peeling. Ann. Plast. Surg., *3*:231, 1979.

Luikart, R., Ayres, S., and Wilson, J. W.: Surgical skin planing. N.Y. State J. Med., *59*:3413, 1959.

MacKee, G. M., and Karp, F. L.: The treatment of post-acne scars with phenol. Br. J. Dermatol., *64*:456, 1952.

Maneksha, R. J.: Dermabrasion therapy for scars. Experience of 150 cases of smallpox scars. Plast. Reconstr. Surg., *25*:615, 1960.

McAndrew, J. J.: Removal of linear scars. A. M. A. Arch. Dermatol., *80*:227, 1959.

McDowell, F.: Editorial: Tattoo erasing. Plast. Reconstr. Surg., *53*:580, 1974.

McEvitt, W. G.: Treatment of acne pits by abrasion with sandpaper. J.A.M.A., *142*:647, 1950.

Montagna, W., and Carlisle, K.: Structural changes in aging human skin. J. Invest. Dermatol., *73*:47, 1979.

Mosienko, P., and Baker, T. J.: Chemical peel. Clin. Plast. Surg., *5*:79, 1978.

Odland, G., and Ross, R.: Human wound repair. I. Epidermal regeneration. J. Cell Biol., *39*:135, 1968.

Orentreich, N., and Dunn, N. P.: Dermabrasion. *In* Goldwyn, R. M. (Ed.): The Unfavorable Result in Plastic Surgery. 2nd Ed. Boston, Little, Brown & Company, 1984, p. 919.

Ortiz-Monasterio, F., Lopez-Mas, J., and Araico, J.: Rhinoplasty in the thick-skinned nose. Br. J. Plast. Surg., *27*:19, 1974.

Pegum, J. S., Ridley, C. M., Russell, B., Thorne, B., and Morrison, S. L.: Dermabrasion: an appraisal. Br. J. Dermatol., *71*:371, 1959.

Pharriss, B. B.: Zyderm (letter). Plast. Reconstr. Surg., *74*:849, 1984.

Pickrell, K., Matton, G., Huger, W., and Pound, E.: Dermabrasion of extensive keratotic lesions of the forehead and scalp. Plast. Reconstr. Surg., *30*:32, 1962.

Rapaport, M. J., Solit, R., and Rivkin, L.: Collagen injections for aging skin lines (wrinkles). J. Am. Acad. Dermatol., *11*:250, 1984.

Rees, T. D.: Chemabrasion and dermabrasion. *In* Rees, T. D. (Ed.): Aesthetic Plastic Surgery. Philadelphia, W. B. Saunders Company, 1980, p. 749.

Rees, T. D., and Casson, P.: Indications for cutaneous dermal overgrafting. Plast. Reconstr. Surg., *38*:522, 1966.

Reid, R., and Muller, S.: Tattoo removal by CO_2 laser dermabrasion. Plast. Reconstr. Surg., *65*:717, 1980.

Resnik, S. S.: Chemical peeling with trichloroacetic acid. J. Dermatol. Surg. Oncol., *10*:549, 1984.

Robinson, J. K., and Hanke, C. W.: Injectable collagen implant: histopathologic identification and longevity of correction. J. Dermatol. Surg. Oncol., *11*:124, 1985.

Roenigk, H. H., Jr.: Dermabrasion for miscellaneous cutaneous lesions (exclusive of scarring from acne). J. Dermatol. Surg. Oncol., *3*:322, 1977.

Rosenberg, W. A.: Accidental tattooing of the face treated by abrasion with sandpaper. A.M.A. Arch. Dermatol. Syph. *65*:466, 1952.

Rudolph, R., and Woodward, M.: Ultrastructure of elastosis in facial rhytidectomy skin. Plast. Reconstr. Surg., *67*:295, 1981.

Sawhney, C. P., Subbaraju, G. V., and Chakravarti, R. N.: Healing of donor sites of split skin grafts. An experimental study in pigs. Br. J. Plast. Surg., *22*:359, 1969.

Ship, A. G., and Weiss, P. R.: Pigmentation after dermabrasion: an avoidable complication. Plast. Reconstr. Surg., *75*:528, 1985.

Siegle, R. J., McCoy, J. P., Jr., Schade, W., and Swanson, N. A.: Intradermal implantation of bovine collagen. Humoral immune responses associated with clinical reactions. Arch. Dermatol., *120*:183, 1984.

Small, A. A.: Kurtin's surgical planing procedure: a review of experience with special reference to post-acne scarring. Can. Med. Assoc. J., *75*:279, 1956.

Sperber, P. A.: Chemexfoliation: a new term in cosmetic therapy. J. Am. Geriatr. Soc., *11*:58, 1963.

Sperber, P. A.: Chemexfoliation for aging skin and acne scarring. Arch. Otolaryng., *81*:278, 1965.

Spira, M.: Notes on chemical peeling. Ann. Plast. Surg., *5*:416, 1980.

Spira, M., Dahl, G., Freeman, R., Gerow, F. J., and Hardy, S. B.: Chemosurgery—a histological study. Plast. Reconstr. Surg., *45*:247, 1970.

Spira, M., Freeman, R. F., Arfai, P., Gerow, F. J., and Hardy, S. B.: A comparison of chemical peeling, dermabrasion and 5-fluorouracil in cancer prophylaxis. J. Surg. Oncol., *3*:367, 1971.

Spira, M. R., Gerow, F. J., and Hardy, S. B.: Complications of chemical face peeling. Plast. Reconstr. Surg., *54*:397, 1974.

Stagnone, J. J.: Chemabrasion, a combined technique of chemical-peeling and dermabrasion. J. Dermatol. Surg. Oncol., *3*:217, 1977.

Stagnone, J. J.: Chemical peeling and chemabrasion. *In* Epstein, E. (Ed.): Skin Surgery. 6th Ed. Philadelphia, W. B. Saunders Company, 1987, p. 412.

Stegman, S. J.: A study of dermabrasion and chemical peels in an animal model. J. Dermatol. Surg. Oncol., *6*:490, 1980.

Stegman, S. J.: A comparative histologic study of the effects of three peeling agents and dermabrasion on normal and sundamaged skin. Aesthetic Plast. Surg., *6*:123, 1982.

Stegman, S. J.: Zyderm collagen. *In* Epstein, E. (Ed.): Skin Surgery. 6th Ed. Philadelphia, W. B. Saunders Company, 1987a, p. 357.

Stegman, S. J.: Injectable collagen (letter). Plast. Reconstr. Surg., *80*:866, 1987b.

Stegman, S. J., and Tromovitch, T. A.: Implantation of collagen for depressed scars. J. Dermatol. Surg. Oncol., *6*:450, 1980.

Stolar, R.: Abrasive planing with high-speed cutting tools (30,000 to 85,000 rpm). Dermatol. Clin., *2*:285, 1984.

Strakosch, E. A.: Sandpaper-abrasion treatment of tattoos. A.M.A. Arch. Dermatol. Syphl., *67*:53, 1953.

Stuzin, J. M., Baker, T. J., and Gordon, H. L.: Chemical peel—a change in routine. Accepted for publication, Plast. Reconst. Surg.

Sulzberger, M. B.: Dermatology: Diagnosis and Treatment. 2nd Ed. Chicago, Year Book Medical Publishers, 1961.

Swanson, N. A., Stoner, J. G., Siegle, R. J., and Solomon, A. R.: Treatment site reactions to Zyderm collagen implantation. J. Dermatol. Surg. Oncol., *9*:377, 1983.

Tromovitch, T. A., Stegman, S. J., and Glogau, R. G.: Zyderm collagen: implantation techniques. J. Am. Acad. Dermatol., *10*:273, 1984.

Truppman, E. S., and Ellenby, J. D.: Major electrocardiographic changes during chemical face peeling. Plast. Reconstr. Surg., *63*:44, 1979.

Urkov, J. C.: Surface defects of skin treated by controlled exfoliation. Ill. Med. J., *89*:75, 1946.

Webster, G. V., Peterson, R. A., and Stein, H.: Dermal overgrafting of the leg. J. Bone Joint Surg., *40A*:796, 1958.

Webster, R. C., Kattner, M. D., and Smith, R. C.: Injectable collagen for augmentation of facial areas. Arch. Otolaryngol., *110*:652, 1984.

Wolfort, F. G., Dalton, W. E., and Hoopes, J. E.: Chemical peel with trichloroacetic acid. Br. J. Plast. Surg., *25*:333, 1972.

23

Roger E. Salisbury

Thermal Burns

HISTORY OF TREATMENT

In considering the history of the treatment of burn injuries, one might quote Adam MacDougall, who in 1819 stated that "it would equally exceed the bounds of convenience and utility to particularize all the remedies that have been recommended in the treatment of accidents of this kind."

The writings on this subject (Table 23–1) reflect the fact that burn care evolved slowly as a rational treatment process. Pack and Davis (1930) described the treatments of the ancients such as the salve of Paracelsus containing the fat of old wild hogs, wasted angle worms, moss "from the skull of a person hung." Paulus Aeginata advocated light herbs mixed with vinegar to prevent blisters, and bull's gall dissolved with water. Pigeons' dung, burned and mixed with oil, was also recommended. The British, at the Battle of Crecy in 1346, were the first to use gunpowder, and this development gave rise to many medical problems including those associated with the treatment of burns. The stimulus of the war experience initiated new and experimental types of treatment. In 1596, Clowes wrote a treatise on gunpowder burns. He did not differentiate the depth of burns but rather described multiple types of treatment on different parts of the body. He suggested oily dressings containing many drugs, did not open the blisters, and was an advocate of bleeding. Fabricius Hildanus (1610), who wrote *De Combustionibus,* was the first to classify burns into three categories, and also showed pictorially the early successful surgical release of hand contractures. Paré (1634) clearly described the differences between second and third degree burns, early excision of the burn wound, and those burns that frequently developed contractures. "One must be careful if burns affect the palpebres or the legs or the fingers or the throat or the axilla or the joint of the knee or of the arm for these joints should not stick together."

Richard Wiseman in 1676 wrote several "chirurgical treatises" and discussed splinting to avoid contractures. He advised refrigerants or calefactive medicaments. Edward Kentish (1797) described pressure dressings as a relief for pain, and in his essay on burns promised to "rescue the healing art from empiricism and to reduce it to established laws." The use of ice and ice water for analgesia and the prevention of edema was explained by H. Earle in his essay "The Means of Lessening The Effects of Fire on the Human Body" in 1799. Controversies over the best method to treat the burn wound persist to the present day. Dressings remained pop-

Table 23–1. Burn Treatment History

Neanderthal Man	Extracts of plants
Smith papyrus (1500 B.C., Egyptians)	Gum and goat's milk mixed with mother's milk
	Strips soaked in oil
Chinese (600–500 B.C.)	Extracts of tea leaves
Hippocrates (430 B.C.)	Swine's semen, resin, and bitumen
	Oak bark solutions
Celsus (ancient Rome)	Honey and bran
Galen (ancient Rome)	Vinegar or wine
Rhases (9th century)	Cold water
Paré (1517–1596)	Excision and ointments
David Cleghorn (1792)	Vinegar and chalk poultice
Edward Kentish (1797)	Pressure dressings
Syme (1827)	Wool dressings
Lisfranc (1835)	Calcium chloride dressings
Passavant (1858)	Saline baths
Tomasalis (1897)	Salt water injections

ular until Wallace in 1949 advocated exposure treatment for burns of the face, buttock, and perineum.

Dupuytren (1832), the brilliant French surgeon, made multiple contributions to burn research, including the documentation of the degree of injury to depth and the description of the phases of the postburn course—irritation, inflammation, suppuration, and exhaustion. In 1823 the Edinburgh Medical Journal published two papers on postmortem findings in two burn deaths. One patient had a gastric ulcer and another gastric congestion. Multiple lecturers at this time were describing perforation of the stomach following burn death, and there was increased interest in studying both the pathology and treatment of thermal injuries. Cotton dressings over burns were first discussed in a Glasgow medical journal in 1828. Readers were told how to apply dressings and were cautioned against changing them more than once daily.

Sir George Ballingall in 1833 gave one of the best descriptions of death from burn sepsis: "sinking in a hectic state, exhausted by a profuse discharge of matter from an extensive separating surface." James Sim (1799–1870) advocated pressure dressings for burns. In a landmark decision in 1848, the managers of the Royal Infirmary in Edinburgh designated one building for all burn cases, and this became known as the Burn Hospital. In 1875 Joseph Lister recommended boric acid and carbolic acid for burn wounds in order to kill bacteria. In 1881 Tappeiner of Munich studied autopsies of burn deaths and recognized the concentration of blood, increased hemoglobin concentration, and decreased blood and water volume. In spite of a speech by Robert Hornby in 1833 to the Royal Medical Society in which he recognized burn shock as similar to that seen with acute peritonitis, and in which he argued against bleeding and purging, these practices persisted through the latter part of the nineteenth century. The appreciation by Tappeiner of burn pathology, however, was a significant event. In 1905 Sneve noted the importance of intravenous saline for resuscitation, and wrote an article in the Journal of the American Medical Association advocating early skin grafting.

The understanding of burn pathology took a great leap forward when Underhill (1930) studied a group of patients burned in a theatre fire in 1921. He analyzed the content of blister fluid and determined that burn shock was due to fluid loss, not toxins (a popular theory of that time). The Cocoanut Grove fire in Boston in 1942 resulted in extensive studies by Cope and Moore on the diagnosis and treatment of burn shock. Formulas gradually evolved to calculate fluid losses; Evans in 1952 used burn skin surface area and weight as the principal variables. The Brooke formula was a modification of the Evans formula and utilized salt, colloid, and water. Moyer and associates (1965) recommended only Ringer's lactate solution, yielding alert, oriented patients even when the body surface area burn was large. Baxter (1978) modified the latter recommendation with the Parkland formula. With these advances in the understanding of burn shock and vigorous fluid resuscitation, a dramatic improvement in early survival occurred.

The pattern of triage of burn patients changed dramatically in the 1960's. The U.S. Army Research Unit was initially guided by Pulaski and Artz, who stressed patient care, as well as clinical and laboratory burn related research. Critically injured patients, civilian and military, were referred to the Center, and the concept of the multidisciplinary burn team evolved. In 1962 the Shriners fraternal organization in the United States began development of three burn centers affiliated with universities and dedicated specifically to the care of burned children.

These centers served as role models that have completely altered burn care around the world. Their superb survivival statistics made others realize that patients with large burns were not automatically doomed but had a chance of survival if cared for in a specialized center. Laboratory and clinical research in burn injury ultimately improved other areas of trauma care. It became obvious that the burn patient with multisystem involvement was the perfect trauma model. The universality of the burn problems provided a reason for better international cooperation and exchange of ideas. In 1960 the first International Congress on Research in Burns was held in Washington, DC. At the second meeting in 1963, the International Society for Burn Injuries was founded, and it has been conducting meetings every four years. The American Burn Association was founded in 1968. The Society's membership was unique in that it consisted of all the members of the burn team, including nonphysicians (dietitians, physical and occupational therapists, nurses, and psychologists).

EPIDEMIOLOGY

Previous attempts to document the incidence of burn injury, the morbidity and mortality rates, and the costs have been hampered by lack of scientific technique by the investigators and the multifactorial variability associated with the subject. Subsequent studies have attempted to bring objectivity and numerical analysis, but the results must be interpreted carefully. For example, Wheeler and associates (1983), studying the effects of burn severity and institutional differences on the cost of care, found that expenditures per patient could be eight times higher in a burn center than in a general hospital. It is noteworthy, however, that patients in centers are often much more severely injured than those sent to general hospitals. Therefore, one should consider other factors such as the size and depth of the burn, the presence of inhalation injury, and the age of the patient before comparing costs.

Expenses increase rapidly as the burn depth increases, even with small total body surface injuries. The location of care for the small burn was found to be important. The cost per day of treating a small burn in a specialized facility was more than twice the daily costs in a general care facility. However, many of the services utilized in the specialized care facility are not available in the general care facility, and their use causes the increased cost. It is indeed true that many patients treated in burn centers do not have sufficiently serious injuries to justify this highly technical facility, with all its ancillary personnel and costs. Treating the smaller burn in the nonburn facility saves money. The problem, however, faced by many burn centers is what is known as the "social admission." Specifically, many small burns occur in the elderly who cannot care for themselves and thus require inpatient treatment that ordinarily might be provided on an outpatient basis for a younger patient. In addition, the efforts to mobilize and care for such a patient would involve many members of the burn team who might not be utilized for the younger patient. Lastly, the increased attention, and thus costs, that are mobilized for the older patient and are not available in a general hospital might be the deciding factor in returning such a patient to his home rather than to a nursing home. Studies remain to be done to demonstrate that both quality and quantity of life are enhanced by treating these patients at burn centers and that the extra cost is justified.

In studying the epidemiology of minor burn injuries, Edlich and associates (1982) reported interesting data. In analyzing burns that required only emergency room or outpatient attention, it became obvious that cause and frequency of injury differed according to age, race, and sex. For example, for nonwhites the risk was greater than for whites; men seemed to be more prone than women to be injured; and individuals' risk increased as their income decreased. The highest incidence was in young adults (ages 20–29) and those under 1 year old. Scalding was the most important cause of minor burns. Women seemed most at risk from grease and hot surfaces, whereas men sustained flame, chemical, and flash injuries most frequently. There was also a seasonal incidence, highest in July and lowest in February.

The epidemiology of burns in children continues to be a subject for special attention because of the problems of child abuse. Children most at risk have been found to be males and the very young. There is often only a single parent in a poor household. Frequently there is a history of burn injury and of psychosocial disorders in the family. Most commonly, neither the child nor the parents admit to abuse. The incidence of acute burn admissions in these children varies from 1.7 to 8 per cent in burn units across the United States. The burden of proof rests with the attending physicians that child abuse or neglect has or has not been the cause of the injury. Although it is almost impossible to make the diagnosis in the emergency room, it is suggested by the history and physical examination. The burns may have a symmetric stocking distribution over the lower extremities, or there may be symmetric burns of the hands or buttocks suggesting immersion. The presence of unexplained scars on other parts of the body, which may have been caused by previous cigarette burns, is also highly suggestive of child abuse.

Although protocols differ in burn centers around the country, reports suggest a steady increase in survival rates and a decrease in hospitalization time. Feller, Tholen, and Cornell (1980) noted through a national burn information exchange that, in an evaluation of the results from 37,000 patients from 120 burn facilities, there was at least a 25 per cent reduction in hospital stay in every age group since the 1971 study. Curreri and associates (1980) reviewed a personal series of 937 patients and noted that in the LA_{50} (burn size in which 50 per cent of patients survive) had improved in the 0 to 14 year age group to 62 per cent and in those over 40 years of age to 38 per cent. The techniques used for determining treatment results in a center are important and, as Wachtel (1982) noted, may not be transposable from one center to another. In his burn center he noted that the important prognostic variables included admission white blood cell count, serum osmolality, involvement of a flammable liquid, preexisting mental disorders, or the presence of cardiovascular or gastrointestinal diseases. The LA_{50} for a total area burn was 58.1 per cent and for a total area third degree burn was 40.9 per cent, a decided improvement over the results of 20 years earlier. Caldwell (1983) used statistical methods to predict morbidity and mortality, especially multiple regression analysis. Using a probit analysis for predicting probability of mortality, he compared his survival results at the University of Arkansas with the National Burn Information Exchange and found a significant improvement in the survival of children, young adults to age 34, and the elderly (ages 60–74). The advantage of a multiple regression analysis as a statistical tool is that it can explain complex multivariable relationships. In reviewing 806 adult and pediatric burn admissions, Caldwell found that for the pediatric patient the percentage of total body burn best correlated with the length of hospital stay. Likewise the percentage of full-thickness burn was also an extremely important prognostic factor. For adults, the percentage of full-thickness burn best correlated with the length of hospital stay. For predicting mortality, the important variables included age, percentage full-thickness burn, percentage total body burn, incidence and severity of inhalation injury, and etiology (e.g., flame burn of clothing, chemical, etc.). Although the results and the statistical tools used may differ from center to center, this scientific approach will gradually lead to more uniform treatment protocols. As the emphasis shifts from subjective clinical impressions to objective data, certain treatment modalities will be found to be superior to others and will gain broad-based approval.

PATHOLOGY

Many factors influence the extent of burn injury on exposure to heat. Some tissues such as nerves and vessels are much more sensitive than is bone, for example. Thickness of the skin (location or part of the body) and buffering materials, such as hair or clothing, may affect the extent of the burn. The time/temperature relationship is crucial to an understanding of thermal destruction. Even a low temperature (below 44°C) will result in tissue death if the duration of exposure is prolonged. Between 44° and 51°C the rate of cell destruction doubles with each degree rise in temperature. At above 70°C the tissue destruction is instantaneous.

Partial-thickness (*second degree*) burns may be superficial or deep. The superficial second degree is blistered or appears pink, and has intact epithelium and dermal appendages. The regeneration is complete within 10 to 14 days. The deep second degree burn often appears white, but is soft and resilient. The entire epithelium and dermal papillae are destroyed but some hair follicles and sweat glands survive, from which epithelialization occurs. Healing may take three to four weeks and skin quality is frequently poor, resulting in hypertrophic scar formation.

Full-thickness (*third degree*) burns are brown and dry, and have thrombosed vessels. The eschar is unyielding and hard. The entire epithelium and dermis are destroyed and any spontaneous healing that occurs is due to wound contraction. The source of the burn is often a clue to the depth of injury. Brief exposure to flame, scald, or flash results most often in burns of partial thickness. Prolonged exposure to flame, immersion, and high voltage electrical injuries result in full-thickness burns (*third degree*).

On a microscopic level, burn injury is followed by an increased capillary permeability that ends at 24 to 36 hours. The increased permeability is even observed in uninjured tissue in patients with large total body burns, resulting in generalized edema. A free leakage of plasma proteins into the extravascular space leads to decreased oncotic intravascular pressure and increased colloid pressure in the extravascular space.

Changes in the blood include red blood cell destruction, usually less than 10 per cent of the total red blood cell mass unless prolonged exposure has occurred. The red blood cells also have a reduced life span (Baxter, 1970). Some type of detrimental plasma factor is present because, when the red cells are injected into a normal person, they survive a normal length of time. Blood viscosity increases in proportion to the increase in the hematocrit.

RESUSCITATION

Considering that more than 50 per cent of all burn deaths occur within the first five days after injury, it is obvious that there is still a lack of understanding of the pathophysiology of burn shock and inhalation injury. The burn injury results in loss of capillary integrity and the outpouring of a plasma-rich fluid into the interstitium. If a large burn is untreated, hypovolemic shock and death result. The likelihood of fatal burn shock occurring is obviously related to the extent and depth of total body burn. For a greater than 25 per cent total body surface burn, edema results not only in the burned tissue, but also in unburned skin and organs. There is a generalized increase in capillary permeability because of mediators such as histamine, serotonin, kinins, and prostaglandins (all elevated in burned tissue). Edema increases for approximately 36 hours post burn because of the increased hydrostatic effect of the tissue pressure. Vasoconstriction and hemoconcentration result. Nicotinic acid and heparin are not effective in reducing permeability and decreasing intravenous fluid needs. Fluid loss has been documented as being most severe during the eight hours immediately post injury. Therefore, most resuscitation formulas suggest giving one-half of the 24 hour fluid requirements in the first eight hours after a burn.

To prevent shock, the most important questions one must answer are: who needs intravenous resuscitation and how should this be managed? A general rule of thumb would be that a child with less than a 10 per cent partial-thickness burn or an adult with less than a 15 per cent partial-thickness burn does not require intravenous resuscitation. However, a child with a 10 per cent burn that has a deep second degree or third degree component or an adult with a less than 20 per cent burn, but mostly third degree, might well need intravenous support. Reliance on a fixed formula number as an absolute is an invitation to disaster. For example, an elderly patient who has had previous myocardial disease and is taking digoxin and diuretics may be in a tenuous balance, which can be upset easily by a 10 per cent full-thickness contact burn. Likewise, an infant with a 6 per cent total body burn who refuses oral resuscitation and vomits may well be a candidate for severe complications. Therefore, each case must be individualized. In hospitalized patients, as the total body burn approaches 10 per cent in a child or 20 per cent in an adult, monitoring must be stringent if intravenous fluid is not given. For the child or adult with a marginal burn, it is always safe to insert an intravenous line and give parenteral fluids until one is certain that the patient will tolerate oral resuscitation. Twenty-four hours of intravenous fluids and monitoring of urine output are not fraught with complications; a more cavalier approach can lead to serious problems.

A review of the formula chart (Table 23–2) suggests that many different approaches to resuscitation have been tried. Opinions differ over whether to give colloid, what concentration of salt is appropriate, and so forth. The fact that so many patients have been resus-

Table 23–2. Resuscitation Formulas

	Brooke	Modified Brooke	Parkland	Monafo	Evans
Day 1					
Colloid	0.5 ml/kg/% burn	None	None	None	1 ml/kg/% burn
Crystalloid	Lactated Ringer's solution, 1.5 ml/kg/% burn	Lactated Ringer's solution, 2 ml/kg/% burn (adult), 3 ml/kg/% burn (child)	Lactated Ringer's solution, 4 ml/kg/% burn	250 mEq Na, 150 mEq lactate, 100 mEq Cl, titrate to urine flow	Lactated Ringer's solution, 1 ml/kg/% burn
5% D/W	2000 ml/m^2	None	None	"Liberal" free water by mouth	2000 ml/m^2
Urine	30–50 ml/hr (adult)	30–50 ml/hr (adult) 1 ml/kg/hr (child)	50–70 ml/hr (adult)	30–50 ml/hr (adult)	30–50 ml/hr (adult)
Rate	½ total in first 8 hr, ¼ total in next 8 hr, ¼ total in next 8 hr	Same as Brooke	½ total in first 8 hr, ¼ total in next 8 hr, ¼ total in next 8 hr	Infuse constantly	½ total in first 8 hr, ¼ total in next 8 hr, ¼ total in next 8 hr
Calculation of volume	Same as Evans	Same as Parkland	Use total burn area for all sizes of burn	Titrate to urine production, not burn	Use burn area up to a total of 50% TBSA; above 50% TBSA burn, calculate as 50% burn
Day 2					
Colloid	0.25 ml/kg/% burn	0.3–0.5 ml/kg/% burn	700–2000 ml (adult) as required to maintain urine	–	0.5 ml/kg/% burn
Crystalloid	Lactated Ringer's solution 0.5 ml/kg/% burn	None	None	–	Lactated Ringer's solution, 0.5 ml/kg/% burn
5% D/W	1500–2000 ml	Sufficient to maintain urine	Sufficient to maintain urine	–	1500–2000 ml

citated successfully with different fluid formulas attests to the built-in flexibility and tenacity of the human body. For example, the original Brooke formula successfully resuscitated many young adults but was deficient in dealing with infants or the elderly. An examination of the formula reveals that it is a hypotonic approach to resuscitation from burn shock. Giving a large amount of free water only increases the volume of total fluid that is being given to the patient, and this will result in more edema. Administration of colloid in the first 24 hours has been rejected by most clinicians because the colloid is transferred into the interstitium and does not remain in the vascular tree any more efficiently than does sodium. Thus, colloid replacement is a very expensive form of resuscitation. The use of free water replacement therapy in infants has led to a significant incidence of hyponatremia and the possibility of seizures during the first 72 hours. The widespread use of the Baxter (1978) formula has caused many to believe that it gives more fluid than is necessary in the first 24 hours and could create problems, particularly in the elderly or the very young burn patient.

Hypertonic saline has been advocated because of the possibility of giving less total volume, with a resulting decrease in edema and the need for escharotomy. Some studies, however, suggest that volume restoration is at the expense of intracellular water and may cause an even greater depression of plasma volume and cardiac output, with resulting cellular dehydration. If the serum sodium level reaches 165 mEq or more, urine output will decrease and resuscitation must then be done with a more dilute fluid. Cellular function may be impaired when intracellular fluid loss exceeds 15 per cent.

The use of dextran for fluid resuscitation has been popular in Europe, where it is administered up to 150,000 molecular weight with 5 per cent D/W (dextrose and water) and blood. The patients potentially have an increased bleeding tendency, which has not been a clinical problem. However, dextran interferes with blood typing, and therefore blood samples should be obtained and sent for typing before this type of treatment is begun.

The modified Brooke formula (2 ml/kg Ringer's lactate per percentage burn in adults and 3 ml/kg per percentage burn in children) has been a popular form of resuscitation and is obviously a direct descendant of the technique of Moyer, Margraf, and Monafo (1965) using lactated Ringer's solution. The patient is given intravenous lactated Ringer's solution, one-half the total volume in the first eight hours, the remainder being divided over the remaining 16 hours. The patient is given nothing by mouth, and if there is an ileus, a nasogastric tube is inserted.

A formula does not deal with every possible variable, and monitoring of the resuscitation effort is very important. Some of the usual parameters for monitoring a patient in shock are not extremely helpful for someone who has had a serious burn injury. For example, it may be difficult to record the blood pressure, not only because of peripheral vasoconstriction but also because of extremity edema. In circumferentially burned extremities, it is difficult to take an accurate blood pressure reading even when the Doppler is used. If there are other complicating injuries, an arterial line should be inserted for accurate pressure measurement. If a noninvasive technique is deemed suitable, the Doppler flow meter is infinitely more sensitive than the stethoscope. A central venous pressure (CVP) line and a Swan-Ganz monitor to measure capillary wedge pressure are useful in patients with a history of cardiac disease, those who do not respond initially to resuscitation, those with a complicating inhalation injury, or those with severe antecedent systemic diseases that result in marginal preburn volume status. Only a small percentage of patients actually require this type of monitoring technique, and one should not administer intravenous fluids to attain a mythical CVP or Swan-Ganz numerical value. During insertion, one must also consider possible injury to the cardiac valves or pulmonary vessels.

Anxiety and restlessness may well be indicative of hypoxia and hypovolemia, and are best treated by oxygen and intravenous fluid administration. Electrocardiographic monitoring is useful after electrical injury or in patients with antecedent cardiopulmonary disease.

The most effective hourly monitor for intravenous resuscitation remains urine output. During the first 24 hours after injury, a urine ouput of 30 ml per hour in an adult or 1 ml/kg. per hour in a child indicates adequate renal perfusion, and thus internal organ flow. During the second 24 hours, fluid regimens once again differ, but it is possible to use several different techniques for satisfactory resuscitation. First, because there is no further capillary leakage, colloid may be useful in restoring plasma volume to normal. Empirically, 0.50 ml/kg per percentage burn, administered slowly over the second 24 hour period, is utilized by many centers. The colloid may be supplemented with D5/W or, if urine output precipitously drops, half-strength saline may be added, as the patient may still have a continued need for salt (depending on how resuscitation was performed during the first 24 hours). For children it is best to continue intravenous fluid administration with D5/0.45 PSS (5% dextrose and half normal saline) rather than D5/W alone, in order to prevent the development of sudden hyponatremia.

Blood cell loss in the first 24 hours may be 0.50 to 1 per cent of the total red cell blood mass for each 1 per cent of full-thickness burn. Blood should be given during the first 24 hours only to those patients with an antecedent anemia or to patients with severe associated injuries, as the blood viscosity is already elevated because of the hypovolemia associated with plasma loss. Since these patients usually have increased peripheral resistance and poor flow, administration of blood merely accentuates the circulatory problem. For patients with a hematocrit of less than 40, blood replacement is begun on the third day. Allowing anemia to persist results in continued poor peripheral flow and deprives the wound of the oxygen needed for wound healing. The patient is frequently hypermetabolic from the injury, with an increased cardiac output to satisfy his oxygen needs. Maintenance of anemia only further stresses a hyperdynamic heart.

After 48 hours, the patient should be reevaluated for the possibility of nasogastric feedings. If there is still an ileus, all fluids should continue to be given intravenously. If bowel sounds are audible, sips of fluids by mouth or nasogastric tube can be initiated, but most of the patient's fluid requirements on the third day should be given intravenously, in order to allow the bowel to regain its tone and activity. On the third day, intravenous salt solution is not indicated. Instead, D5/W, approximately 1 ml/kg per percentage burn (for replacement of evaporative water losses plus the remainder of the patient's maintenance fluids), is administered. Blood and/or colloid supplements should be given as needed.

The complications of resuscitation are multiple, and some are almost impossible to treat. For example, an infant or adult who has had delayed resuscitation may not respond to normal or increased fluid resuscitation. The child has a noncorrectable metabolic acidosis, and reconstitution of plasma volume may be followed by cerebral edema, convulsions, and death. Delayed resuscitation in the aged can lead to irreversible myocardial problems that do not respond to either fluid load or inotropic agents. Significantly, in a normal patient the cardiovascular output peaks at 50 to 100 per cent above normal when plasma volume is reconstituted on the second day, and stabilizes at about two times normal. The increased cardiac output is attributed to the magnitude of the injury, and it returns to normal when the wounds are covered. It can be exacerbated by anemia, inadequate nutrition, and infection. The unsuccessful resuscitation may be characterized initially by several hours of satisfactory urine output and reasonable cardiac function followed by a precipitous drop from which the patient does not recover. Another type of unsuccessful resuscitation occurs in which the patient has a low cardiac output from the beginning of resuscitation and simply never responds. Prophylactic use of digitalis is not indicated in patients because they already have higher than normal cardiac activity. The continued and rapid sodium shifts during the first 72 hours may result in an unacceptably high incidence of arrhythmias when digitalis is given. Although a myocardial depressant factor has been postulated by Baxter (1978) and others, it has not been universally accepted. Echocardiographic studies in large burns failed to document abnormal left ventricular function, and the left ventricular ejection fraction was normal (Dorethy and associates, 1977).

Other resuscitative complications include hypernatremia and hyponatremia. Hypernatremia may be due to inadequate replacement of evaporative water losses. The estimated loss in milliliters per hour equals 25 (plus the percentage body surface burned) $\times$ the total body surface in square meters. An approximate estimation of this formula would be 1 ml/kg per percentage burn over 24 hours. Body weight, serum osmolality, and urine and serum sodium levels should also be monitored. A common cause of underreplacement of evaporative water losses is discontinuation of intravenous support on day 3 and the attempt to force the patient to take all his liquid requirements by mouth or by nasogastric tube.

Hyponatremia may result when silver nitrate is the topical agent of choice, when the Brooke formula is used in children, or when one uses biologic dressings without appreciating that there should be a decrease in fluid needs as a result of diminished evaporative loss.

Hyperkalemia may occur owing to tissue and red blood cell destruction, and potassium should not be given in the first 48 hours after injury. Hypokalemia is the more common complication and is attributed to increased urinary potassium losses. Topical Sulfamylon (mafenide acetate) and silver nitrate may increase potassium loss.

If laboratory tests reveal a marked aberration in serum electrolyte values, one should never treat the patient until a repeat set of studies has been performed for confirmation purposes. The patient must be evaluated by using all parameters of resuscitation. For example, hyponatremia may be due to overestimation of water requirements. Weighing the patient may provide a clue by demonstrating that he should be water restricted rather than given more salt. Administering more salt in the face of increased circulating antidiuretic hormone (ADH), which is present for the first five or six days post injury, merely leads to additional water retention. Urine sodium normally should be 50 to 125 mEq/liter per day. Less than 20 mEq of sodium per liter of urine signals an explained plasma deficit and reflects a volume deficit, not a lack of salt.

In the elderly burn patient, one must be aware of limited cardiac reserve and the possibility of pulmonary edema in someone with an already impaired heart. Therefore, these patients should be monitored closely with a Swan-Ganz catheter. At the first signs of failure, they should be treated with cardiac inotropic agents and fluid administration, limited as much as possible to maintain a normal urine output. Diuretics are rarely helpful as they usually exacerbate systemic hypovolemia. This type of patient is the ideal candidate for resuscitation with hypertonic saline, in order to decrease the total volume of fluid administration.

Prolonged hypovolemia after a delayed resuscitation may result in renal failure, but this is a rare event. If it is obvious that the patient is in renal failure and does not respond to a trial of fluid challenge, mannitol, or furosemide administration, the rate of intravenous fluid administration must be reduced and only evaporative water losses should be replaced. Peritoneal dialysis will be of limited value because of the catabolic state, especially if the patient has an abdominal wall burn. A nephrology consultation to consider hemodialysis should be obtained immediately, without waiting until the patient is in extremis.

INHALATION INJURY: DIAGNOSIS AND TREATMENT

Of the 12,000 annual deaths attributed to burns, approximately 50 to 60 per cent involve inhalation injury as a contributing factor. The injury may manifest itself early or late. The early complication of carbon monoxide intoxication occurs because the affinity of carbon monoxide for hemoglobin is approximately 210 times that of oxygen. A carbon monoxide concentration of only 0.1 per cent room air (21 per cent oxygen) may cause a 50 per cent reduction in the oxygen-carrying capacity of the blood. The resulting tissue hypoxia is caused by a shift in the dissociation curve for oxyhemoglobin, leading to an increased affinity for hemoglobin by oxygen and a decreased release of oxygen to the tissues. The diagnosis of carbon monoxide intoxication is suspected when the patient complains of headache, fatigue, or nausea (carbon monoxide content less than 30 per cent). When the carbon monoxide content is greater than 40 per cent, the patient may complain of visual impairment, have difficulty in walking, exhibit personality changes, and present with a cherry-red facies. When the concentration is greater than 50 per cent there may be profound evidence of central nervous system damage, with paresis and loss of consciousness. Arterial blood specimens may reveal low oxyhemoglobin saturation with a normal PaO_2. Lactic acidosis may be common, while the $PaCO_2$ may be low, normal, or elevated.

There may be injury to the airway as a result of the hot air, which causes laryngeal spasm and edema. The smoke may contain soot and other particulate matter that carries toxic materials such as sulfur dioxide (SO_2) and nitrogen dioxide (NO_2). There may also be smoke poisoning due to the presence of noxious gases such as hydrochloric acid, sulfuric acid, and hydrogen cyanide. The temporal sequence from this insult may be bronchiolar edema, atelectasis, pseudomembranous tracheobronchitis, intra-alveolar hemorrhage, and eventually alveolar pulmonary edema and/or bacterial pneumonia.

The diagnosis of smoke inhalation injury is made by history, physical examination, and laboratory determinations. The history of a burn in a closed space is highly suggestive. The patient who is found unconscious in a house fire or a burning building is a leading candidate for smoke inhalation injury. On physical examination the patient may have burns of the head and neck, but this finding is only suggestive and not diagnostic. The findings of soot in the mouth, burned nasal hairs (vibrissae), or intraoral burns are suggestive of inhalation. Auscultation and examination of the chest that reveal dyspnea, stridor, coughing, and a subjective difficulty in breathing should raise the suspicion of inhalation injury. Direct laryngoscopy and fiberoptic bronchoscopy remain accurate techniques to document upper and lower airway inhalation injury with an over 95 per cent diagnostic accuracy rate. Fiberoptic bronchoscopy can be performed at the bedside by a skilled examiner, with no significant complication rate. The xenon scan has also been reasonably accurate in diagnosing inhalation injury, but necessitates removing the patient from the burn center. There is an incidence of false-positive results in patients who are heavy smokers and have antecedent pulmonary disease. Trapping of the radioactive xenon in the injured pulmonary tree, however, identifies the area of injury rapidly.

Treatment of inhalation injury depends on the mechanism. For carbon monoxide intoxication, administration of 100 per cent oxygen is the obvious treatment and the only question is how it should be delivered. The half-life of carbon monoxide in the hemoglobin molecule is approximately four hours on room air but only one half-hour when 100 per cent oxygen is breathed. Oxygen administered by face mask is often ineffective in a patient who is in pain or uncooperative. Endotracheal intubation is usually reserved for moderate or severe cases, but is completely appropriate in an uncooperative patient. Mucolytic agents, high humidity oxygen, frequent suctioning, and bronchodilators are helpful therapeutic adjuncts.

The indications for intubation (Fig. 23–1) for upper airway injury include progressive

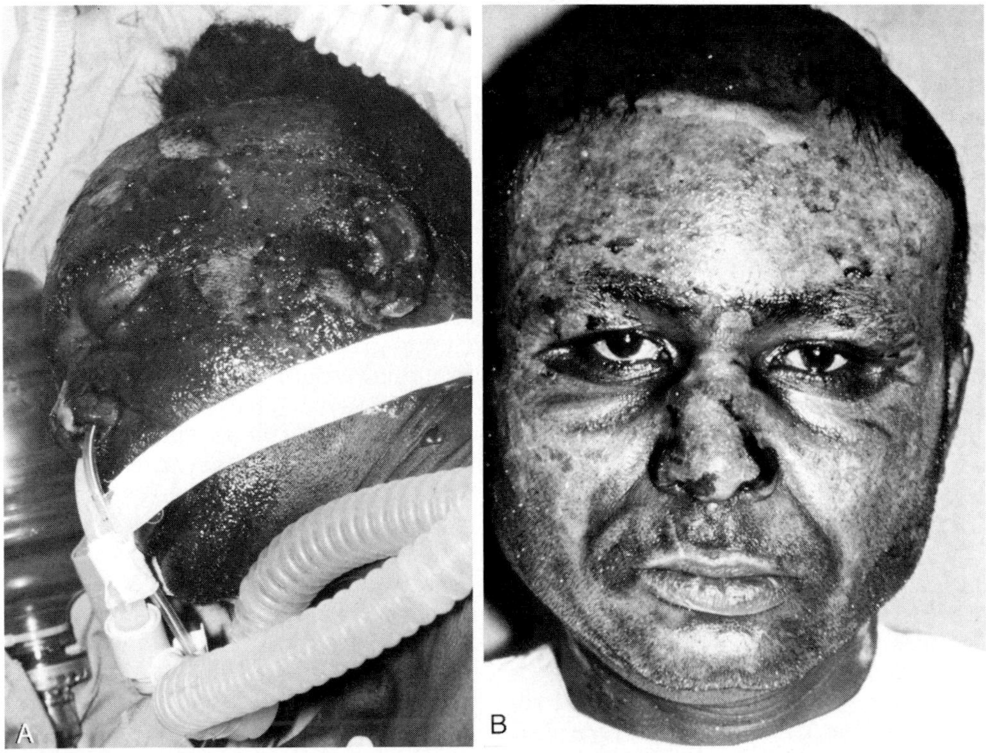

Figure 23–1. When possible, intubation is always preferable to tracheostomy. *A,* Three days post burn injury, the edema is resolving. *B,* By one week post burn injury, the endotracheal tube has been removed.

stridor, hoarseness, a subjective feeling of inability to breathe, and deteriorating blood gas values. It is imperative that the treating physician realize that the inhalation injury, if supraglottic in location, is a progressive phenomenon. If time is wasted in deciding whether or not to intubate the patient, it may be impossible to do so and an emergency trachcostomy will be required. Closure of the airway may be abrupt, resulting in sudden respiratory arrest, or the airway may be so narrowed, especially in a child, that it is impossible for even the most skilled anesthesiologist to intubate the patient. It is extremely common for the supraglottic edema to resolve in 72 to 96 hours post injury and for the patient to be extubated without any further difficulty.

For a lower airway injury, the indications for intubation and ventilation, as set forth by Trunkey (1978), are as follows:

1. Parenchymal lung failure.
2. Infiltrates on chest radiograph.
3. Tachypnea greater than 35/min.
4. $(A-a)DO_2$ greater than 300 torr.
5. Compliance less than 30 ml per cm of water.
6. Shunt fraction of 15 per cent or greater.

When there is any suggestion of carbon monoxide poisoning, administration of 100 per cent oxygen by tube for several hours is indicated, as this markedly increases the dissociation of the carbon monoxide from the hemoglobin. For the patient who fails to respond to 100 per cent oxygen therapy, hyperbaric oxygenation has been reported to be helpful in some situations. The use of PEEP (positive end expiratory pressure) ensures adequate oxygenation, and it is also wise to insert a Swan-Ganz catheter to monitor pulmonary capillary wedge pressure, cardiac output, and mixed venous oxygen content. Intravenous resuscitation must be performed judiciously and fluids restricted to a minimum to avoid overhydration of the compromised lungs. With the abnormal capillary permeability resulting from the inhalation injury, excess intravenous fluid administration leads only to additional sequestration of extravascular fluid in the lungs.

The use of steroids is mentioned only to be condemned. There is no evidence, either experimentally or clinically, that steroids provide any benefit for inhalation injuries. In fact, they have been associated with an increased incidence of infection in a controlled study. Likewise, prophylactic antibiotic therapy does not prevent infection and merely gives rise to the emergence of resistant organisms. It is, however, worthwhile to obtain serial cultures, and treat pneumonitis if it occurs with appropriate antibiotics.

BURN METABOLISM

A hyperdynamic state and increased cardiac output following thermal injury persist for many weeks and may be elevated to two to four times normal. The metabolic sequelae of the injury cease when wound healing has occurred. Much of the increased blood flow is directed to the wound, as reported by Aulick and Wilmore (1977). Total limb blood flow was measured by venous occlusion plethysmography, and the high levels of flow also tended to increase wound temperature.

The basal metabolic rate and temperature tend to remain elevated after thermal injury even in the absence of infection. Regardless of dietary protein intake, the catabolism of protein is greater than normal and may lead to loss of skeletal mass, decreased host resistance, and impaired wound healing. There is a distinct relationship between the size of the burn and the degree of hypermetabolism observed after injury. Part of the elevated VO_2 (oxygen consumption) is due to evaporative heat loss from the wound. Placing the patient in a warm environment and covering the wounds, however, do not eliminate hypermetabolism. It was thought that patients with uncontrolled evaporative water loss became cold and that therefore a hypermetabolic state resulted. Wilmore and associates (1974a) showed that this theory was not true and that, although warming the environment can decrease heat production, it does not return the basal metabolic rate (BMR) to normal. They concluded that an internal reset of the "thermostat" caused increased metabolic activity, the direct effect of beta stimulation from elevated catecholamines. There is not, however, complete acceptance of these results. For example, Arturson and associates (1969) treated patients with infrared heat lamps and could decrease the elevated BMR.

It is believed that the central nervous system is important in mounting a response to stress, as a brain-dead patient is unable to become hypermetabolic. The response of the hypothalamus and pituitary to afferent stimuli results in adjustments in thermoregulation and metabolism. Studies of burn patients fail to disclose a hyperthyroid state. There is an increased level of human growth hormone (HGH) in the acute and recovering phase of burn injury, while thyroxine (T_4) and triiodothyronine (T_3) levels are reduced and thyrotropin (TSH) remains normal (Wilmore and associates, 1974a, b).

After the balance of energy expenditure is understood, it is possible with a combination of oral and enteral feedings to prevent the patient from "parasitizing" himself nutritionally. The total body glucose stores are limited, yet glucose remains the primary fuel for wound healing. Hepatic glucose production is related to the size of the injury, and may be two times normal in patients with severe burns. Body protein stores are broken down to amino acids in the liver and converted to glucose in the absence of adequate alimentation. While the body temporarily keeps "the ship afloat" by this technique, starvation, sepsis, and death ultimately result. Wolfe and Burke (1979) reported that glucose production is constantly elevated in burn patients owing to increased glycogen, cortisol, and catecholamine production. A glucose infusion, however, is effective in protein sparing and in decreasing glucose production via protein breakdown.

A significant amount of energy is derived from the oxidation of free fatty acids, which are also elevated. An infusion of Intralipid may provide caloric support but is not protein sparing. Nitrogen excretion is always increased in the burn patient, regardless of the diet, owing to a decreased rate of protein synthesis and/or an increased rate of breakdown. Low serum albumin is attributed to redistribution rather than to decreased protein production. While Wilmore and associates (1974b) reported that a supranormal diet did not decrease the BMR, Wolfe and Burke (1979) found that increased intake resulted in an increased VO_2.

In summary, the hypermetabolic response is due to an alteration of the neural-humoral control mechanism. Some type of internal reset of the central nervous system regulatory mechanism occurs, leading to an increase in core temperature, sympathetic activity, and levels of plasma catecholamines, all of which participate in heat production and mobilization of substrate. Without appropriate nutritional support, severe catabolism characterizes the postburn period. An increased rate of glucose production, increased protein breakdown, decreased level of insulin production, and an increased catabolism occur at a level the patient can tolerate only for a short time. More than 10 per cent of weight loss leads to an inhibition of wound healing and a depressed immunologic response to injury. More than 30 per cent weight loss results in death. The loss of respiratory muscle mass eventually causes decreased ventilation and increased susceptibility to pulmonary infections. At the cellular level, there is evidence of the "sick cell." The cellular sodium pump fails, leading to an increase in intracellular sodium. Active transport of sodium becomes inhibited in both the red blood cell and the muscle cells.

Aggressive caloric support may be combined with many modalities. As emphasized by Wilmore and associates (1971), one can reduce pain with the judicious use of narcotics, increase the temperature in the room to diminish cold stimuli, and give sedatives to reduce anxiety. All these ancillary measures decrease catecholamine output and thus decrease caloric demand.

In determining the caloric needs of the patient, one can use the formula postulated by Curreri and Luterman (1978) (Table 23–3). There is a difference of opinion, however. The formula of 25 kcal/kg body weight plus 40 kcal per percentage burn works satisfactorily in adults. Children's requirements are higher: 40 to 60 kcal/kg body weight. The calorie:nitrogen ratio should be approximately 150:1.

Hyperalimentation should be initiated as soon as the patient is able to tolerate a diet. It is unusual for a patient with a total body burn of greater than 30 per cent surface area to be able to take all his calories by mouth, and the insertion of a small feeding tube is mandatory to maintain nitrogen balance. Although results differ from patient to patient, one should start with a complete liquid diet and slowly advance according to patient tolerance. Elemental diets are not routinely used; they are hyperosmolar and one has to limit volume and concentration, or significant diarrhea can occur. Any of the complete liquid diets (Tables 23–4 and 23–5) are satisfactory and should slowly be increased in volume and concentration as tolerated.

For larger total body burns it may be impossible to achieve all the desired volume and caloric support by the enteral route. Thus, peripheral and central intravenous support

Table 23–3. Protocols For Calculating Calorie and Protein Needs

Author	Age	Percentage of Burn	Calories	Protein
Wilmore	Adult	Any	Use normograms to calculate BMR, % change in BMR, energy requirements	Adjust nitrogen/total calorie to 1:150
Wilmore	All	≥ 30	2000–2200 kcal/m²/day	15 gm nitrogen/m²[a]
Muir	Adult	Less than 20	35 kcal/kg	1.5 gm/kg
		20–30	40 kcal/kg	2.0 gm/kg
		30–40	50 kcal/kg	3.0 gm/kg
		40–50	60 kcal/kg	4.0 gm/kg
Davies	Adult	Up to 50[b]	(20 kcal × body wt in kg) + (70 kcal × % burn)	(1 gm × body wt in kg) + (3 gm × % burn)
Davies	Child[c]	Up to 50[b]	(60 kcal × body wt in kg) + (35 kcal × % burn)	3 gm × body wt in kg) + (1 gm × % burn)
Curreri	Adult	Any	(25 × body wt in kg) + (40 × % burn)	Not calculated

BMR = basal metabolic rate. [a]1 gm nitrogen = 6.25 gm protein. [b]>50% surface injuries are calculated as a 50% injury. [c]Up to 12 yrs of age.

will be necessary. Central venous lines must be inserted with care and some trepidation. Unlike the general trauma patient, the skin of the burn patient is covered with organisms, and the potential for suppurative thrombophlebitis and sepsis is increased. The central venous line should be removed and rotated every three days. As with other trauma patients, the concentration of carbohydrate in the infusion must be slowly increased according to patient tolerance. Blood and urine glucose should be checked frequently because, if the patient is not tolerating the glucose, it will act as a diuretic and cause dehydration. Intractable hyperglycemia is one of the earliest signs of sepsis, and hyperalimentation should be suspected immediately while the source of the offending organism is sought and intravenous antibiotic administration is begun.

Although feedings usually are not begun for three or four days after a large burn injury (until it is certain that the ileus has ended), several new research approaches offer promise. McArdle and associates (1984) have reported that the small intestine retains its mobility or peristalsis immediately after burn injury. They have passed a small nasal feeding tube into the duodenum and immediately begun elemental diet feedings by bypassing the stomach. Their elemental diet consisted of 7 per cent amino acids, 25 per cent glucose, with electrolytes and vitamins. All patients achieved positive nitrogen balance in ten days and tolerated the diet. The patients did not show evidence of hyperglycemia. There was no persistent neutrophilia, and serum proteins remained within normal range. These patients had burns within a 40 to 70 per cent range of total body surface. With the feeding of an elemental diet instead of complex carbohydrates, fats, and proteins, the demand for increased circulation in an already hypovolemic patient was obviated. Since the stomach was bypassed, there was no fear of gastric dilatation and aspiration. This work seems promising and additional investigation is warranted.

The accurate assessment of nutritional adequacy is critical. Monitoring of daily weight changes is important and anthropometric measurement, such as the triceps skin fold thickness or midarm muscle circumference in patients with unburned extremities, can be valuable. There is no one satisfactory parameter for studying nutritional adequacy because there are so many possible misinterpretations. For example, serum albumin may be a good indicator of visceral protein activity, but it can also be reduced as a result of overhydration or the presence of edema or cirrhosis. Serum transferrin, if reduced, has been linked to an increased incidence of bacteremia. A reduced value may also be observed in liver disease, fluid overload, or iron overload. Nitrogen balance may be measured by taking a 24 hour urine specimen, so long as there are no inadvertent discards of specimens or omissions to make the result appear falsely normal. Skin tests may be of value in assessing the nutritional status and also in predicting mortality, but anergy may exist for other reasons such as infection, shock, trauma, or the age of the patients. Thus, a

Table 23–4. Composition of Several Commercially Available Enteral Formulas

Per 1000 Calories Formula	Protein (gm)	kcal/ml	Carbohydrate (gm)	Fat (gm)	Potassium (mEq)	Sodium (mEq)	kcal/N	Lactose (gm)	Osmolality (mOsm/kg)
Intact Protein									
Carnation Instant Breakfast	55.2	1.1	124.1	27.6	63.3	37.0	113:1	84	–
Protein Isolates									
Ensure Plus[a]	36.6	1.5	133.2	35.5	32.4	30.7	117:1	0	600
Magnacal[b]	35.0	2.0	125.0	40.0	16.0	21.7	178:1	0	520
Isocal[c]	32.5	1.0	125.0	42.0	32.1	21.7	192:1	0	300
Osmolite[a]	35.0	1.1	136.8	36.3	21.7	23.5	178:1	0	300
Sustacal[c]	60.3	1.0	137.8	32.0	52.7	40.2	104:1	0	625
Precision Isotonic[d]	30.0	1.0	150.0	31.3	25.6	34.8	208:1	0	300
Travasorb MCT[e]	49.2	2.0	122.8	33.0	44.6	15.2	127:1	0	475
Hydralized Protein, Amino Acids									
HN Vivonex[f]	43.3	1.0	211.0	0.9	18.0	33.5	150:1	0	312
Vi-Pep[g]	25.0	1.0	175.0	25.0	21.8	32.6	250:1	0	520
Vital[a]	41.7	1.0	185.0	10.3	29.8	16.7	150:1	0	450
Supplements, Nutrient Modules									
Citrotein[d]	60.5	0.7	184.2	2.6	28.8	45.8	103:1	0	496
Pro-Mix (2T)[h]	90.0	40	1.0	*	5.0	0.7	37:1	<0.09	–
Polycose (1T)[a]	0.0	32	8.0	0.0	0.02	0.38	–	0	–
Hi-Protein Gelatin (5 oz)[d]	15.0	0.9	18.0	0.0	4.9	11.9	54:1	0	757
Sustacal Pudding (5 oz)[c]	6.8	1.9	32.0	9.5	7.4	5.2	220:1	9.7	–

All values taken from manufacturers' information. [a]Ross Laboratories. [b]Organon. [c]Mead Johnson. [d]Doyle Pharmaceutical Company. [e]Travenol Laboratories. [f]Norwich Easton Pharmaceuticals. [g]Cutter Laboratories. [h]Brunswick Laboratories.

Table 23–5. Supplemental Feedings

Diet Supplement	Protein (gm)	Carbohydrate	Fat (gm)	Calories/ml	Na (mEq)*	K (mEq)*	Total Calories	Ingredients
Chocolate milk shake	65	270	60	1.9	43	80	1900	Skim milk powder, 100 gm Dextrose, 100 gm Vanilla ice cream, 300 gm Chocolate syrup, 50 ml Whole milk,* q.s. 1000 ml
Lemonade	0	250	0	1	8	9	1000	Corn syrup, 160 gm Lemon juice, 180 ml Sugar, 110 gm Water,* q.s. 1000 ml
Low sodium supplement	45	180	45	1.3	1	45	1300	Lonalac,† 150 gm Chocolate syrup (low sodium), 120 ml Sugar, 65 gm Vanilla, 30 ml Water,* q.s. 1000 ml
Eggnog	55	90	50	1	30	34	1000	Eggs, 4 Sugar, 50 gm Vanilla, 10 ml Whole milk,* q.s., 1000 ml

*Milk or water to make the total feeding equal to 1000 ml.
†Mead Johnson.

profile of all these studies may be necessary to provide an idea of the adequacy of nutritional status.

IMMUNOLOGY

Patients who sustain thermal injury may already have impaired immune function for reasons other than the burn. For example, immune function is decreased in the very young, the very old, patients with diabetes, and those with poor nutrition who have suppressed humoral and cell mediated immunity. Patients on drugs (tetracycline, chloramphenicol, streptomycin, gentamicin, or kanamycin) may have suppression of cell mediated immune response. Mafenide and sulfadiazine can inhibit chemotaxis by the polymorphonuclear leukocytes. Anesthesia can alter immune function even in normal patients, as B cell and T cell mitogenic capabilities are inhibited by inhalation agents such as halothane, ether, and nitrous oxide. Phenobarbital decreases the production of antibody by the spleen cells of rats and mice.

Many investigators have documented general and specific immunologic changes following thermal injury. Alexander and associates (1966, 1967, 1968, 1970; Alexander and Wixson, 1970) found an increased rate of phagocytosis and decreased intracellular killing of bacteria in the burned patient. Abnormalities of the neutrophil bacteria cell index frequently preceded the onset of sepsis; conversely, neutrophil function became normal after skin coverage. These authors also reported a decrease of opsonins in the serum of patients with severe burns. The reticuloendothelial system was found by Rittenbury and Hanback (1967) to have a decreased clearance of colloidal carbon before death in burned dogs. Dressler and Scornick (1974) showed that burned animals with infected wounds had a decreased resistance to aerosol challenges of *Pseudomonas* compared with those without infected wounds. Multiple studies have demonstrated defects in the humoral immune system following thermal injury. Arturson and associates (1969) reported a decrease in all serum immunoglobulins two days after burn injury that returned to normal after several weeks. Immunoglobulin M concentration was the most depressed. In burned children, immunoglobulin G and N depression persisted for at least 60 days. Serum complement is also decreased after burns.

Cell mediated immunity is severely limited after burn injury. There is increased survival of skin grafts before rejection and a decreased skin reactivity to antigens. Ninnemann, Fisher, and Frank (1978) reported that allograft survival was directly related to the immunosuppressive activity of a patient's serum. There was decreased phytohemagglutinin responsiveness of the lymphocytes. The lymphocytes had altered reactivity to mitogens. There was an increase in spontaneous DNA synthesis by lymphocytes in the burned patient, suggesting a strong antigenic challenge either from bacteria in the wound or the burned skin.

WOUND MANAGEMENT

The management of the burn wound has undergone remarkable changes in the past 20 years, resulting in an increased incidence in patient survival. Bacterial proliferation causing burn wound sepsis and disseminated infection was the rule rather than the exception in patients with large thermal injuries. Since the middle of the 1960's, the burn physician has multiple agents to choose in controlling bacterial growth in the burn wound, and different modalities of treatment are available to achieve a healed wound.

Small second or third degree burns may be treated on an outpatient basis, and therapy should consist of cleaning the wounds with a mild soap and debriding ruptured bullae or blisters. Intact blisters that do not impede motion need not be ruptured. The wound should be covered by a sterile dressing, which may consist of impregnated gauze, a bulky gauze dressing to absorb drainage, and a splint if the hand and wrist are involved. If these dressings are changed three times a week, second degree burns heal promptly and the eschar gradually separates from the small third degree wounds. The use of Silvadene (silver sulfadiazine) or Sulfamylon (mafenide acetate) for burns in outpatients is a classic case of "overkill." These agents were designed for large and deep total body burns in which infection is a major concern. Their use for outpatient care is needlessly expensive and may give rise to the emergence of resistant organisms.

For the inpatient treatment of burns there are three commonly used modalities of treatment:

1. Enzymes.
2. Topical chemotherapeutic agents.
3. Primary eschar excision and skin grafting.

The use of enzymes is an attractive therapeutic alternative in that it requires no surgical skill to remove the eschar, does not incite bleeding, causes rapid dissolution of the necrotic tissue, and would seem to decrease hospitalization time. Unfortunately, use of the enzymes presently available does not make it possible to cover a 70 per cent full-thickness burn with the enzymatic agent and eradicate the eschar within 24 hours. Various studies (Law and MacMillan, 1973; Krizek, Robson, and Groskin, 1974) with the preparations currently available have revealed a significant chance of sepsis if the agent is applied over too large an area of the body surface without concurrent use of a topical chemotherapeutic agent. Thus, the enzymes have been found most efficacious for deep second degree burns of the hands or intermediate second degree burns covering less than 20 per cent of the total body surface area. If an enzyme is applied with moistened saline dressings within a few hours of injury and if the dressings are changed several times in the first 24 hours, the eschar is definitely softened and can be merely scraped off with the handle of a scalpel. In many instances of deep second degree burn, the wound is then ready for overgrafting if necessary, with a reasonable chance that the skin graft will take. For patients with large areas of third degree burn, the wound is not always ready for grafting and there is residual necrotic collagen, which must be removed before any skin grafting can be done. The wound often appears boggy and is of questionable viability. For circumferential burns of the upper or lower extremity, the application of an enzyme has been found useful in softening the eschar and decreasing the need for mechanical escharotomy. Instead, the "chemical escharotomy" property of the enzyme has been sufficient to prevent severe constriction of the extremity. The use of this technique by the uninitiated must be viewed with some caution, because it may increase the need for fluid administration during the first 24 hours post burn. The enzyme should be used for no more than 24 hours, and if the wound is not to be mechanically debrided and grafted at that time, Silvadene should be applied liberally to the remaining burn wound.

The use of topical chemotherapeutic agents evolved in the 1960's with the widespread use of 0.5 per cent silver nitrate, Sulfamylon, and Silvadene (Table 23–6). Each drug has its advantages and disadvantages. Some drugs are definitely second line therapeutic weapons, while others are frankly dangerous. For example, gentamicin cream has an unacceptable incidence of ototoxicity and nephrotoxicity, and a rapid rate of emergence of resistant organisms. Betadine (povidone-iodine) has been used more commonly in

Table 23–6. Topical Chemotherapeutic Agents

	Silvadene (silver sulfadiazine)	Sulfamylon (mafenide acetate)	Silver Nitrate
Advantages	Painless Wound visible Easy to use Motion maintained	Penetrates eschar Wound visible Easy to use No resistance Motion maintained	No hypersensitivity Painless No resistance
Disadvantages	Neutropenia	Pain Carbonic anhydrase inhibitor Pulmonary?	Poor penetration Hyponatremia Discolors burn wound

Europe, but is not as effective as other agents in laboratory and clinical trials. The preparation has not been found as efficacious against all organisms in the burn wound as Silvadene or Sulfamylon. The issue of iodine absorption still remains unsettled, and incidences of toxicity have been reported (Pietsch and Meakins, 1976).

Silver nitrate (0.5 per cent) remains an effective form of treatment of the burn wound in patients with fresh injuries. The 0.5 per cent silver nitrate is applied to the wound in wet, bulky dressings that must be changed several times daily and frequently wetted in order to maintain the activity of the silver nitrate at the wound surface. The 0.5 per cent silver nitrate solution is nontoxic and no instances of the emergence of resistant organisms have been reported. There are, however, several problems with this agent. First, the activity of the 0.5 per cent silver nitrate at the wound surface can act as a leech of sodium and render the patient hyponatremic. Therefore, blood electrolytes must be serially monitored. The agent is not satisfactory in small children because, when they become hyponatremic, they tend to have convulsions. The agent is not effective in patients who have neglected burn wounds or who have been transferred several days after injury with a wound that is not under bacteriologic control. Silver nitrate does not penetrate the eschar as effectively as Silvadene and Sulfamylon, and burn wound sepsis may result. The agent acts at the wound surface to suppress bacteria, but does not reach the bacteria in the depths of the burn wound, which proliferate and cause burn wound sepsis.

Sulfamylon has become a second line drug in the last ten years. It was tested extensively during the Vietnam war and found to be most useful in penetrating the burn eschar and in suppressing bacterial proliferation. As with all agents, the wound is not sterilized, but bacterial growth is suppressed sufficiently to avoid burn wound sepsis. Sulfamylon is easily applied and dressings may or may not be used. This drug simplifies nursing care, in contrast to silver nitrate, which stains everything with which it comes into contact.

Although Sulfamylon is well accepted by nursing staff, it causes certain problems for the patient. First, it is painful, and patients complain of extreme burning when it is applied. Second, and most important, it is a carbonic anhydrase inhibitor and may cause an increased burden on injured lungs in the elimination of hydrogen ion. Patients can develop a respiratory alkalosis, exhaling CO_2 in an attempt to maintain a pH of 7.4 because of the activity of the carbonic anhydrase inhibitor. For patients with an inhalation injury or pneumonia, this physiologic response may produce an unacceptable pulmonary burden. Furthermore, patients who have large burns treated with Sulfamylon can develop an abnormally high incidence of pulmonary problems in the first four days post injury. For these reasons, the drug is not commonly used as the first choice in patients with large burns. It is indicated for electrical injuries as it penetrates the wound better than Silvadene to maintain bacteriologic control. Sulfamylon is also the agent of choice in a patient who has a neglected wound or one that has become infected.

Silvadene remains the drug of first choice in most burn centers in the United States. It has a broad spectrum of activity, has a low incidence of development of resistant organisms, is relatively pain free, is easily applied, and is efficacious against a broad spectrum of organisms. It may be used with an open technique or applied on dressings and changed once or twice daily. There is a small incidence of hypersensitivity reaction to this drug, resulting in neutropenia. Jarrett, Ellerbe, and Demling (1978), however, did not find any change in the mortality rate in those patients who developed leukopenia. One can either continue or suspend treatment with this agent, but the neutrophil count eventually returns to normal.

When the burn wound is treated with topical agents, intermediate and deep second degree burns may heal without the complication of burn wound sepsis. Before the development of effective topical chemotherapy, deep second degree burns commonly converted to full-thickness skin loss because of unchecked bacterial proliferation. If a nonexcision protocol is used, the common treatment is to apply Silvadene or the topical agent of choice once or twice daily to the burn wounds. The patient's wounds can be cleaned daily by the bedside or in the shower. Necrotic debris can be removed as it separates from the underlying viable tissue. There is no advantage in attempting to remove the burn eschar prematurely, since a new, quasi-eschar merely forms in its place. With a regimen of daily dressing changes and wound inspection, judicious debridement, intermediate and deep second degree burns gradually heal over a period of two to four weeks. Full-thickness injury becomes obvious as the eschar separates, leaving a granulating wound.

After the bulk of the eschar has separated, mechanical means are employed to remove the remnants of adherent necrotic debris. These may consist of excising pieces of adherent collagen during the dressing changes. The patient is given ketamine anesthesia and the eschar is removed with a scalpel, wire brush, or curette. Wet to dry dressing changes are then made with coarse mesh gauze.

Quantitative biopsies are taken of the wound to determine if skin grafting is feasible. It has been clearly shown that, if quantitative biopsies reveal greater than 10^5 organisms per gram of tissue in the wound, the chances for skin graft vascularization are minimal, whereas if the wound counts are fewer than 10^5 organisms, there is an excellent chance for skin graft take (Krizek, Robson, and Klio, 1967). A qualitative analysis of the wound should also be done to determine the presence or absence of *Streptococcus*. The presence of *Streptococcus* in any concentration is an indication to postpone surgery, as skin grafts are exquisitely sensitive to the ravages of this organism.

Biologic Dressings

The use of biologic and synthetic dressings has been another major advance in wound care. As Table 23–7 indicates, biologic dressings perform many beneficial functions in wound care.

The serial application of a biologic dressing to a wound can gradually decrease the bacterial counts and prepare the wound for skin grafting. When a biologic dressing adheres to a granulating or excised wound, it is a clear indication that the recipient bed is ready for skin autografting. Covering the wounds with biologic dressings decreases wound pain, so that the patient can more readily perform therapy exercises and take part in his own rehabilitation. Since biologic dressings also serve to decrease evaporative water and protein losses, the physician must restrict fluid administration to avoid pulmonary edema. For patients with intermediate or deep second degree burns, the serial application of biologic dressings appears to hasten wound healing by providing a protective milieu in which epithelial proliferation can occur.

The standard by which all biologic dressings are judged is, of course, the *human skin allograft*. The techniques for collection and preservation of skin allograft have advanced markedly in the last 20 years. An allograft stored only in a refrigerator at 4°C has a limited half-life but, when it is fresh frozen under controlled conditions, it can be used for as long as six months after procurement. Unfortunately, the procurement and freezing of skin allograft are expensive and the constant demand exceeds the availability. Caution must be used in selecting donors as it is possible to transmit infectious diseases such as hepatitis. Thus, the continuing demand has given rise to a search for other dressings.

Amnion is an effective biologic covering for the wound. It is inexpensive, may be obtained in any delivery room by a skilled technician,

Table 23–7. Role of Biologic Dressings in Wound Care

1. To decrease bacterial count
2. To decrease evaporative water and protein loss
3. To diminish pain
4. To prevent desiccation of vital structures
5. To protect the wounds until skin grafting
6. As a test to determine if wounds are ready to accept a skin graft

and is most effective when covered with an occlusive dressing.

Porcine xenograft, commercially available, has been especially helpful in centers that cannot afford or do not have skin banking facilities. Because of differences in production, different types of available skin (fresh, frozen, lyophilized) and variable quality of production, the results of clinical research have been contradictory. For example, while it is agreed that skin xenograft does not adhere to the wound as well as an allograft, there is disagreement as to whether xenograft is as efficacious as allograft in clearing the bacterial population from the wound (Salisbury, Carnes, and McCarthy, 1980).

Attempts continue to produce synthetic wound covers, but none at this time have replaced biologic dressings. Hydron (an amalgam of polyethylene glycol-400 and polyhydroxyethyl methacrylate) was tried as a spray-on dressing but it was found that it did not adhere properly, did not always seal the wound, and allowed subgraft fluid collection with bacterial proliferation.

The use of collagen has been attempted in multiple forms, but as a unilaminate dressing it does not decrease evaporative water loss and has problems with adherence and conformability to an uneven surface. At present, Biobrane, a bilaminate membrane consisting of an outer layer of silicone bonded to a flexible nylon with a "dermal" layer of Type 1 porcine collagen, is the most promising of the synthetic dressings. It controls evaporative water loss, is elastic, and conforms to wound surfaces. The bacteriologic control of the wound has been quite satisfactory in clean wounds. This dressing has been found useful not only on donor sites but also on freshly excised wounds and open-mesh grafts.

Burke and associates (1981) have developed a bilaminate membrane consisting of a Silastic epidermis and a bovine collagen dermis. This dressing, when applied to the wound, develops vascularization of the neodermis and acts as a template for the formation of a new dermis. When donor sites are available in the patient with a large burn, the Silastic epidermis can be removed and skin grafts applied to the neodermis. This concept is exciting in that large wounds can be safely covered, a neodermis can be created from the template of the dressing, and thin grafts can be applied if available. Long-term follow-up is lacking and there is so far no confirmation of these results from other centers.

Tissue culture of epidermal cells has continued to be an area of clinical and laboratory evaluation. It has been demonstrated that suspensions of human epidermal cells can be grown on collagen film into a structure that appears similar to a normal multilayered epidermis. O'Connor and associates (1981) have shown that epidermal cells can be grown into sheets in culture discs and subsequently applied to full-thickness burn wounds. Biopsies of this skin six months later demonstrated that all epidermal layers were present. This remains a fruitful area for laboratory investigation as it is obvious that, if sheets of skin can be grown from only a few cells, even the largest total body surface burns can be salvaged.

Excision of Burn Eschar

Excision of the burn wound has received a great deal of attention as a way of reducing hospitalization time and possibly increasing patient survival. Candidates for excision of burn eschar are patients with deep second degree or third degree burns who can tolerate anesthesia. Small, deep second degree or third degree burns can be excised and grafted and patients released from the hospital much earlier than with nonsurgical intervention. Patients with large total body burns and questionable chances of survival are also excellent candidates, because early excision of the wound and skin grafting reduce the physiologic effect of total size of body burn, and thus enhance the chances of survival (Fig. 23–2). Excision is not a benign procedure, however, and should be undertaken only by an experienced team with the full support of a blood bank.

Second degree burns that are intermediate or deep may be *tangentially* excised with the Braithwaite knife or the dermatome, but this maneuver should be performed over a limited area; bleeding can be extensive and is invariably underestimated by the inexperienced surgeon. Hemostasis is achieved by elevation of an extremity, when possible, applications of thrombin-soaked sponges, and judicious use of electrocautery. When the extremities are involved, the application of tourniquets diminishes blood loss.

Unless tourniquets are used for extremity excisions, it is wise to limit excision to 15 per cent of a total body surface burn because of difficulties with the control of bleeding, pro-

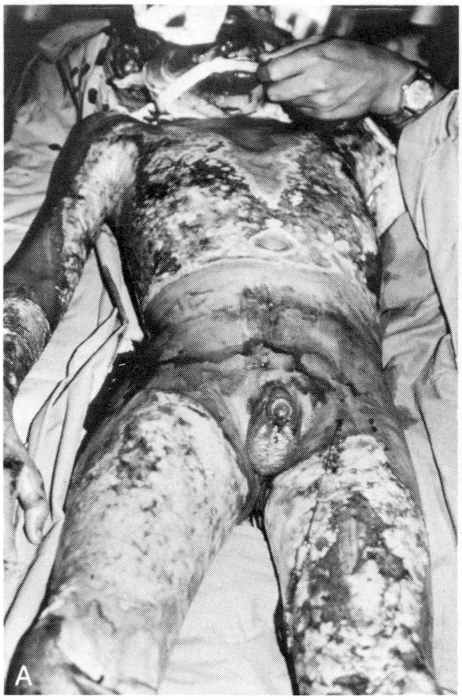

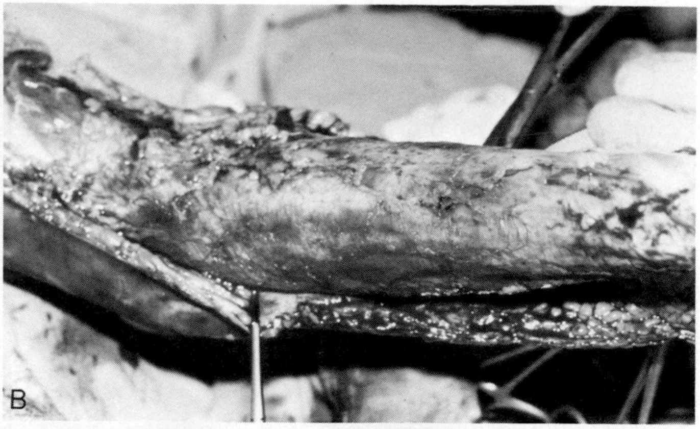

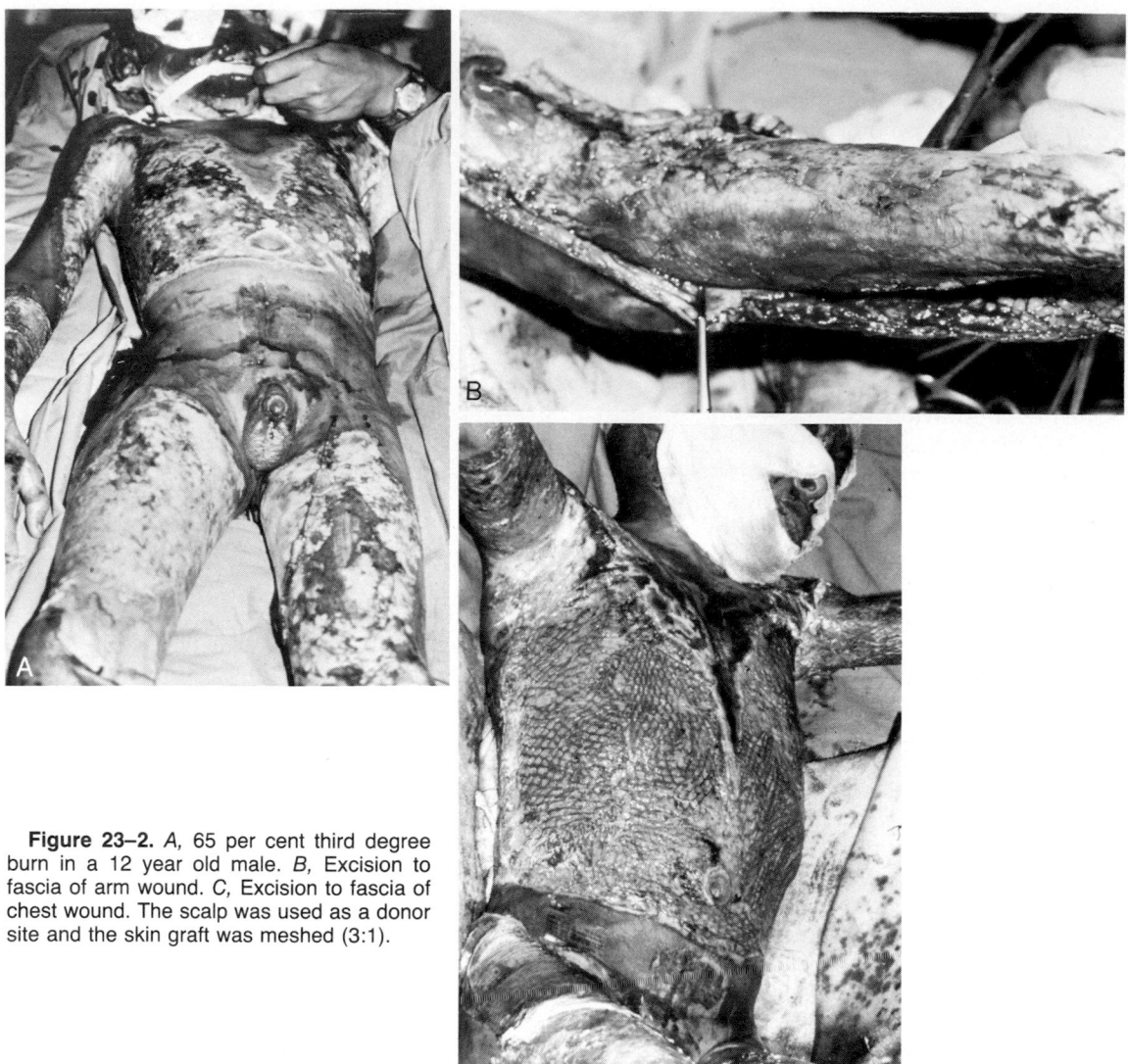

Figure 23–2. *A,* 65 per cent third degree burn in a 12 year old male. *B,* Excision to fascia of arm wound. *C,* Excision to fascia of chest wound. The scalp was used as a donor site and the skin graft was meshed (3:1).

longed operative time, and the dangers of hypothermia and hypovolemia. In a life-threatening burn that requires surgery, excision to fascia is indicated even though it is cosmetically less desirable. Blood loss is easier to control; the surgery can be performed more rapidly; and skin grafts are well vascularized on fascia. It is imperative that the patient be transfused to a normal hematocrit before the operation begins, otherwise hypotension may ensue as anesthesia is commenced. Several large intravenous lines should be inserted so that one is available for constant blood administration, which is started before the first incision is made. Another intravenous route can be used for medications and for giving patients their normal fluid requirements, independent of whatever intraoperative blood losses there may be. For patients with life-threatening injury, careful monitoring in the operating room includes the recording of hourly urine output and of arterial blood gas values, and accurate estimation of the blood loss. Prophylactic antibiotics are given before surgery and for 72 hours thereafter, because of the risk of bacteremia resulting from incisions through heavily contaminated tissue. Patients are returned to the operating room every five to seven days for serial excision of the eschar.

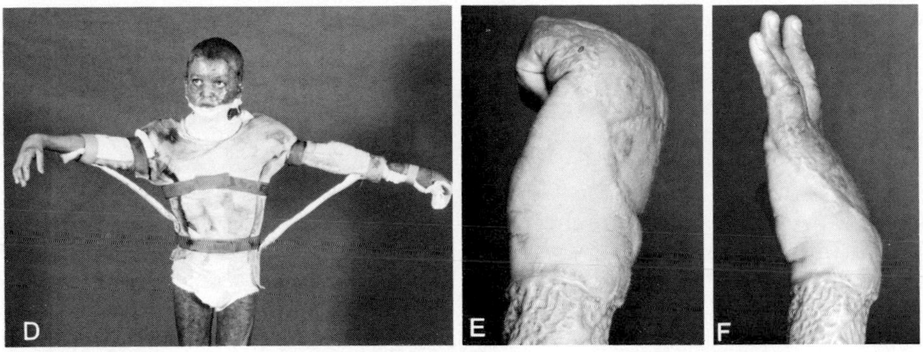

Figure 23–2 *Continued D, E, F,* Two months post burn, the patient is wearing splints and shows no evidence of flexion contractures.

If donor sites are not available for skin grafting, biologic dressings are applied to the wound and grafting is done when these are available. The important goal is to remove the eschar as quickly as possible and to reduce the size of the total body burn to one more compatible with life.

COMPLICATIONS

It is unquestionably easier to prevent complications following thermal injury than to treat them. In the immunosuppressed burn patient with multiple system problems, any complication may be fatal. With the introduction of effective topical chemotherapeutic agents and more aggressive surgical excision, *burn wound sepsis* has become less common. The clinical signs of burn wound sepsis include:

1. Sudden color change in the wound to black, dark brown, or red-violet (Fig. 23–3).
2. Hemorrrhage of the subeschar fat.
3. Seeming conversion of partial- to full-thickness injury or sudden breakdown of healed second degree burn to a new eschar.
4. Premature eschar separation.
5. Appearance of purple or black eruptions in unburned skin.
6. Sudden development of hypotension, ileus, and hypothermia.

Rapid confirmation of the clinical diagnosis can be confirmed by a frozen section biopsy of the burn wound to show any hemorrhage in the unburned tissue, small vessel thrombosis, vasculitis, bacteria in unburned tissue, or proliferation of organisms in the subeschar space.

The treatment for this life-threatening complication is to perform an excision of the burn wound that is obviously affected, change the topical agent, and give intravenous antibiotics. A mere change in topical chemotherapeutic agent will not solve the problem, however, as the quantity of organisms be-

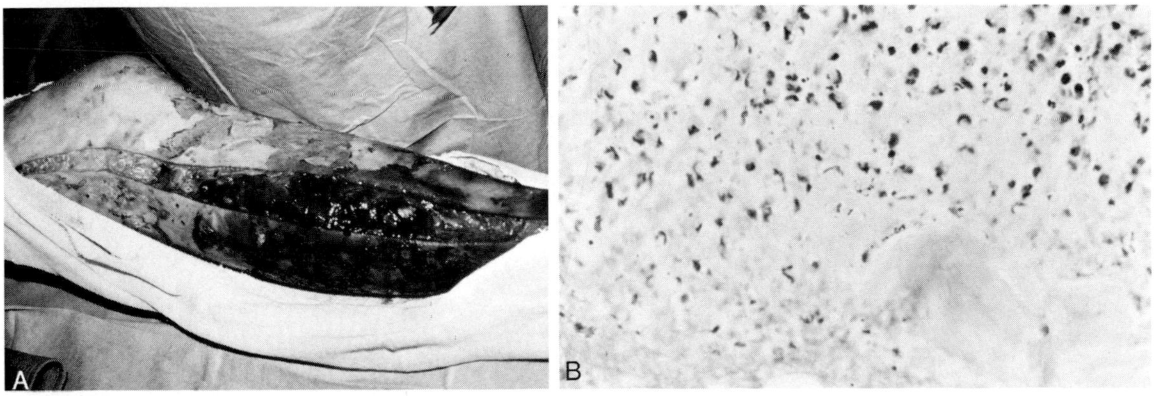

Figure 23–3. *A,* Burn wound sepsis diagnosed by a change in color of the eschar. Note the nonviable muscle where the eschar has been incised. *B,* Gram stain smear (400 ×) showing negative rods.

neath the eschar and the rapidity of the progression of the disease are too great. Application of the new topical agent should follow the entire excision of the affected burn wound. Subeschar infusion of an appropriate antibiotic has been found to be effective as an adjunct in some cases. The patient's wound cultures for the previous week are checked. One or two antibiotics, to which the organisms are sensitive, are selected and injected by syringe locally into the subeschar space of the entire burn wound. Occasionally, in individuals too ill to be taken to the operating room, this step is effective in conjunction with a change in the topical chemotherapeutic agent. It is most reasonable to carry out the subeschar infusion shortly before taking the patient to the operating room for excision of the wound in conjunction with a change in the topical chemotherapeutic agent.

When operative examination of the burn wound sepsis reveals spread of disease beneath the fascia, extirpation of the large muscle groups in the area must be performed. For example, if the burn wound sepsis begins in an extremity, the patient's family must understand that amputation to the more proximal joint above the site of infection may be necessary. Resection of the abdominal or chest wall is occasionally necessary as a last attempt at salvage.

Pulmonary complications remain the most common cause of sepsis, especially airborne pneumonia. The pneumonia may begin as bronchiolitis secondary to bacterial involvement of the tracheobronchial tree. Many patients have had an inhalation injury requiring intubation that predisposes to this problem, as does the presence of a tracheostomy or antecedent aspiration. Any or all of these problems in a patient with a large total body burn seem to increase the frequency of this septic complication.

Hematogenous pneumonia may account for only one-third of pulmonary infections, but carries an extremely high mortality rate because the "cannonball" lesions apparent on chest radiograph reflect an embolism from a distant source of sepsis that may well be occult. The patient must be examined closely for other sources of infection such as perirectal abscess, prostatitis, suppurative thrombophlebitis, burn wound sepsis, or even a perforated viscus. The initiating cause of sepsis must be eradicated and a vigorous pulmonary regimen instituted, including intravenous antibiotics, tracheobronchial suctioning, and ventilatory support if necessary.

Suppurative thrombophlebitis (Fig. 23–4) is a treatable and curable form of sepsis as long as the diagnosis is made early. Preventive therapy dictates that no intravenous line should be in the same site longer than 72 hours, as it is simply a foreign body that places the patient at risk. The diagnosis is suggested by the sudden development of gram-positive or -negative sepsis with clinical deterioration and positive blood cultures. A systematic examination must be performed in any site in which the patient had cannulation of a vessel. Often there are no clinical signs such as cellulitis, lymphangitis, edema, or increased heat of the intact skin. One must systematically open the sites of the previously cannulated veins and examine the point of entrance. The patient may have frank pus exuding from the vein or simply thrombosis. Open dissection of the vein must be performed

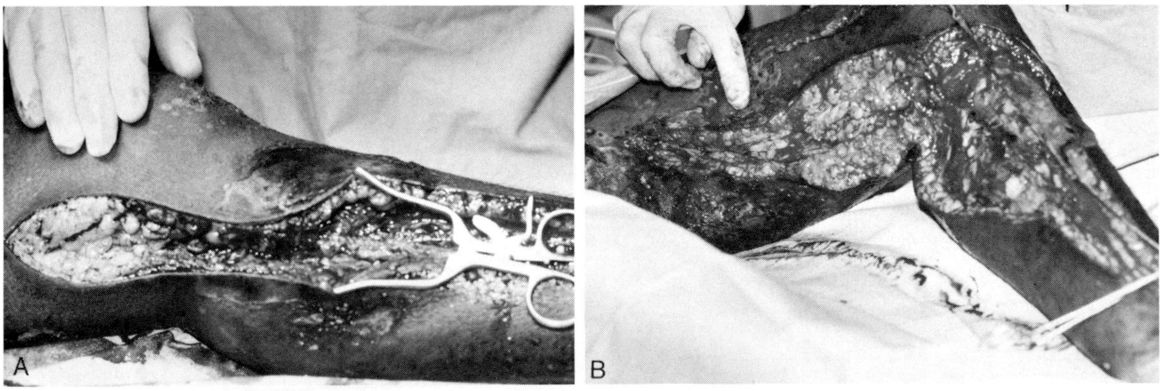

Figure 23–4. *A,* Suppurative thrombophlebitis involving a long segment of the saphenous vein. Treated by excision of the vein and all of the suspicious overlying tissue. *B,* Appearance following treatment.

in a proximal direction until normal vein is encountered. The entire vein is excised, the wound being left open and covered with a topical agent. The wound may be loosely approximated with Steri-strips or a few sutures 72 hours later.

Gastrointestinal complications appear to be less frequent since an improved understanding of the pathophysiology of ulcer disease has developed, better nutritional support provided, and more effective wound care achieved. Patients who suddenly show clinical signs of sepsis and abdominal distention with ileus must be considered as having developed a perforated viscus. Examination is often difficult because there may be a burn of the abdominal wall. Ultrasonographic examination is indispensable in making this diagnosis.

Curling's ulcer, which formerly had an incidence of approximately 12 per cent in all burn patients, has become an infrequent complication even in patients with large burns. Gastroduodenoscopy studies by Czaja, McAlhany, and Pruitt (1975) revealed that one could document gastric lesions as early as five hours after burn injury. Such patients could be followed serially with gastroduodenoscopy and it was observed that the ischemic areas could progress to frank ulcerations.

Prevention has been effective in reducing the incidence of ulceration. Serial specimens of the gastric aspirate are monitored and, when the pH becomes acidic, administration of antacids via a nasogastric tube is effective in maintaining the pH in the alkaline range. Prophylactic administration of antacids is continued when the patient begins oral feedings, and cimetidine and H_2 blockers have likewise been effective. The goal of antacid therapy is to maintain the pH of gastric fluid at greater than seven; antacids should be given two hours after meals, at bedtime, and in the late afternoon. Frequent feedings with a high caloric substrate over 24 hours have made the nutritionally depleted patient a rarity. Better nutrition and more effective wound care have decreased the incidence of infection. In the past, gastrointestinal bleeding was often the first sign of a septic patient, and neither medical nor surgical therapy was effective once this complication occurred.

Superior mesenteric artery syndrome is another gastrointestinal complication that has decreased in frequency with the increased emphasis on improved nutrition. In the past it was seen in 1 per cent of patients at the Institute of Surgical Research of the Brooke Army Medical Center. The mean weight loss sustained was approximately 25 per cent in these patients, who presented clinically with abdominal distention and projectile vomiting after eating. Radiographs revealed a characteristic dilatation of the proximal duodenum and obstruction of the small bowel at the level of the mesenteric vessels. Retrograde peristalsis could be seen on fluoroscopy. Treatment includes passage of a long nasogastric tube past the site of obstruction for improved feeding, placing the patient on his side during and after oral intake in an attempt to allow passage of gastrointestinal contents, and vigorous intravenous nutritional support. After the patient has regained normal body weight, the problem should be resolved. If these measures are not successful, a duodenojejunostomy for feeding purposes may be required.

Common *orthopedic complications* include osteomyelitis, heterotopic ossification, and nonhealing of fractures. Osteomyelitis may occur as a result of burns sufficiently deep to injure the bone (Fig. 23–5) and may result in nonviability. Organisms proliferate in the

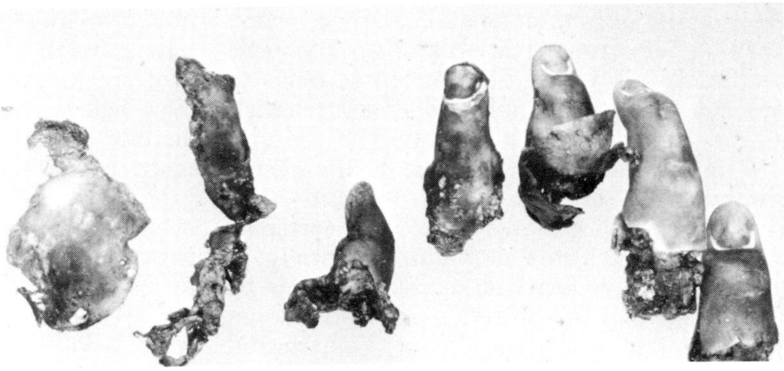

Figure 23–5. Burned bone necessitating multiple finger amputations.

exposed necrotic osseous tissue, and treatment must be directed toward extirpation of the necrotic bone. This condition is unlike the osteomyelitis seen as a result of infection at the site of an unhealed fracture. In this instance, the bone itself is rendered necrotic because of the thermal injury, and bacterial proliferation is purely a secondary phenomenon.

Unhealed fractures can occur for multiple reasons, including depressed wound healing in a cachectic patient with a large burn, but most frequently they are due to inadequate immobilization. For patients who sustain a fracture in an unburned extremity, casting is a reasonable alternative. This treatment obviously cannot be given in a patient who has a cutaneous burn, as unchecked bacterial proliferation would result. In the patient who has a burned extremity with an underlying unstable fracture, the burn wound should be excised, and open reduction and internal fixation of the fracture performed. Otherwise, mobilization and movement of the ends of the fractured bone will result in a hematoma. If the patient has a transitory bacteremia from manipulation of the burn wound, the hematoma may become infected, and osteomyelitis and sepsis may result. Unfortunately, the treatment for this life-threatening complication is amputation of the injured extremity plus vigorous systemic intravenous therapeutic support.

Heterotopic ossification continues to be a puzzle, its etiology being poorly understood and the appropriate treatment uncertain. Early, overvigorous therapy in areas of deep injury of the extremities is thought to be a possible, but never proved, etiologic factor. The treatment remains surgical in severely symptomatic patients. It is believed that serial radioactive technetium scans should be taken until it is obvious that active bone deposition at the site of ossification has ceased, and only then should extirpative surgery be performed. The area of symptomatic ossification is excised, care being taken to avoid damage to normal vital structures such as the ulnar nerve at the elbow.

A major complication of the healing burn wound is *hypertrophic scar formation*. Although there are many different theories as to the cause of this problem, one study in children revealed that no correlation could be found between the patient's age and the development of wound problems (Velasco and associates, 1978). As suspected, blacks develop more hypertrophic scar than do whites. A most significant variable noted was the time required for a burn wound to heal. If it healed in 14 to 21 days, approximately one-third of the sites became hypertrophic, but if it healed after 21 days, 78 per cent of the burn sites developed hypertrophic scars (Velasco and associates, 1978). In the past it was noted that some wounds required as long as four or five weeks to heal, but poor quality skin that was easily damaged by pressure or the mildest trauma remained hyperemic and developed hypertrophic scar. Thus, when possible, it is reasonable to excise tangentially the eschar and skin graft wounds that will take longer than two weeks to heal. If this treatment is not possible, wounds that take longer to heal should be treated prophylactically with pressure dressings rather than wait for hypertrophic scars to appear. The use of silicone gel has been helpful in controlling the appearance of burn scars, especially in concave areas such as the axilla, neck, face, and clavicle and other areas over which a pressure garment is ineffective. The exact mode of action of this elastomer or silicone gel is unknown, but it has been noted that, if it is used properly, hypertrophic scars lose their erythematous appearance and become smoother and less edematous. Contractures also resolve. Studies by scanning and transmission electron microscopy indicate a reduction in collagen cohesiveness and an increased number of vestibular fibroblasts (Larson and associates, 1979). The clinical use of compression garments, silicone gel, and judicious splinting should decrease the need for surgical release of scar contractures.

BURN REHABILITATION

The issues of burn rehabilitation are probably the most provocative of any aspect of burn care in the remainder of the twentieth century. More burns are being salvaged than ever before, but the social mechanisms for dealing with the recovered patients are far more primitive than the care rendered in intensive care units. Specifically, there is not even an accepted definition of what constitutes adequate rehabilitation after burn injury.

A recent survey by the American Burn Association Committee on Organization and

Table 23–8. Time Commitment of Psychologic Care Personnel

	Mean No. of Treatment Hours per Week (Year)			
	Group 1	***Group 2***	***Group 3***	***Group 4***
Psychologic Personnel	(58 adm)*	(101 adm)*	(150 adm)*	(259 adm)*
Psychiatrist	5.0 (260)	1.7 (88)	2.8 (146)	4.1 (213)
Psychologist	0	0	1.3 (68)	5.6 (291)
Registered nurse, BSN or MSN	0	0.2 (10)	1.0 (52)	0.6 (31)
Clergy	1.5 (78)	0.3 (16)	1.8	0
Social worker or MSW	0	0	0.2 (10)	0
Total†	9.0 (468)	1.7 (88)	8.0 (416)	9.8 (510)

*Mean number of acute burn admissions.
†Independently calculated mean total number of hours per group (not sum of column data).

Delivery of Burn Care found some disturbing contradictions in care. They agreed that every discharged patient deserves a team effort that involves a reconstructive plastic surgeon, a physical and occupational therapist with access to a cosmetologist, a psychiatrist or psychologist, and a vocational rehabilitation counselor. After a review of the personnel available in larger and smaller units, it was obvious that the number of admissions did not in any way predetermine that the staff would be larger. For example, it was noted that 50 per cent of the largest facilities had a full-time social worker, but only 15 to 22 per cent of the smaller units (under 200 patients per year) provided full-time social work coverage. The choice of half-time or full-time staff was not based on the number of admissions but on poorly defined administrative decision. Only one-fifth of the burn care facilities used psychiatrists or psychologists on even a part-time basis, even though it is well documented that a very high incidence of postburn patients suffer psychologic problems (totally unrelated to the size of the burn). The largest facilities with the greatest number of admissions did not differ from the smallest units in terms of their commitment to psychiatric help for the patient. While there always seems to be provision for a surgeon to repair a wound contracture, only 50 per cent of the facilities surveyed offered vocational rehabilitation counseling. The most disturbing finding of the survey was the extreme variation in the number of care hours rendered per week by rehabilitation specialists in the various facilities.

This finding raises the question: what constitutes reasonable and effective care? Is it possible that one unit, which gives three times as much psychologic care to the postburn patient as another, can be rendering the same quality of care? Table 23–8 indicates that centers that are admitting four times as many patients as the smaller units are not necessarily making a greater time commitment to the patients. At present, there is not even a generally accepted definition of burn rehabilitation or any mechanism for assessing what is adequate care, or what are the minimal number and types of rehabilitation personnel that burn units should have. The American Burn Association has formed a committee to study these problems.

Reconstruction of burn deformities is discussed in Chapters 21 (keloids and hypertrophic scars), 32 (forehead and scalp), 34 (eyelid), 37 (nose), 38 (lips and cheeks), 39 (cervical region), 40 (auricle), 41 (face), and 132 (hands).

REFERENCES

Alexander, J. W., Fisher, M. W., and MacMillan, B. G.: Immunological determinants of *Pseudomonas* infections in man accompanying severe burn injury. J. Trauma, *10*:565, 1970.

Alexander, J. W., Hegg, M., and Altemeier, W. A.: Neutrophil function in selected surgical disorders. Ann. Surg., *168*:447, 1968.

Alexander, J. W., and Moncrief, J. A.: Alterations of the immune response following severe thermal injury. Arch. Surg., *93*:75, 1966.

Alexander, J. W., and Moncrief, J. A.: Immunologic phenomenona in burn injuries. J.A.M.A., *199*:257, 1967.

Alexander, J. W., and Wixson, D.: Neutrophil dysfunction and sepsis in burn injury. Surg. Gynecol. Obstet., *130*:431, 1970.

Arturson, G. S.: Transport and demand of oxygen in severe burns. J. Trauma, *17*:179, 1977.

Arturson, G. S., Hogman, C. F., Johansson, S. G., and Killander, J.: Changes in immunoglobulin levels in severely burned patients. Lancet, *1*:546, 1969.

Artz, C. P., Moncrief, J. A., and Pruitt, B. A., Jr.: Burns: A Team Approach. Philadelphia, W. B. Saunders Company, 1979.

Aulick, L. H., and Wilmore, D. W.: Influence of the burn wound on peripheral circulation in thermally injured patients. Am. J. Physiol., *237*:901, 1977.

Ballingall, Sir G.: Outlines of Military Surgery. Edinburgh & London, A. Balfour, 1833.

Baxter, C. R.: Problems and complications of burn shock resuscitation. Surg. Clin. North Am., *58*:1313, 1978.

Berry, C. C., Wachtel, T. L., and Frank, H. A.: An analysis of factors which predict mortality in hospitalized burn patients. Burns Incl. Therm. Inj., *9*:38, 1982.

Bjornson, A. B., Altemeier, W. A., and Bjornson, W. S.: Changes in humoral components of host defense following burn trauma. Ann. Surg., *186*:88, 1977.

Bowser, B. H., Caldwell, F. T., Baker, J. A., and Walls, R. C.: Statistical methods to predict morbidity and mortality: self assessment techniques for burn units. Burns Incl. Therm. Inj., *9*:318, 1983.

Brown, W. L., Bowler, E. G., Mason, A. D., Jr., and Pruitt, B. A., Jr.: Protein metabolism in burned rats. Am. J. Physiol., *231*:476, 1976.

Burke, J. F., Yannas, I. V., Quinby, W. C., Jr., Bondoc, C. C., and Jung, W. K.: Successful use of a physiologically acceptable artificial skin in the treatment of extensive burn injury. Ann. Surg., *194*:413, 1981.

Caldwell, F. T.: Statistical methods to predict morbidity and mortality. Burns Incl. Therm. Inj., *9*:319, 1983.

Clowes, W.: A Profitable and Necessary Book of Observations for All Those Burnt with the Flame of Gunpowder. London, E. Bollisant, 1596.

Cockshott, W. P.: The history of the treatment of burns. Surg. Gynecol. Obstet., *102*:116, 1956.

Curreri, P. W., and Luterman, A.: Nutritional support of the burned patient. Surg. Clin. North Am., *58*:1151, 1978.

Curreri, P. W., Luterman, A., Braun, D. W., Jr., and Shires, G. T.: Burn injury: analysis of survival and hospitalization time for 937 patients. Ann. Surg., *192*:472, 1980.

Czaja, A. J., McAlhany, J. C., and Pruitt, B. A., Jr.: Acute duodenitis and duodenal ulceration after burns. Clinical and pathological characteristics. J.A.M.A., *232*:621, 1975.

Daniels, J. C., Cobb, E. K., Lynch, J. B., Lewis, S. R., and Larson, D. L.: Altered nucleic acid synthesis in lymphocytes from patients with thermal burns. Surg. Gynecol. Obstet., *130*:783, 1970.

Daniels, J. C., Sakai, H., Cobb, E. K., Lewis, S. R., and Larson, D. L.: Evaluation of lymphocyte reactivity studies in patients with thermal burns. J. Trauma, *11*:595, 1971.

Deitch, E. A., Wheelahan, T. M., Rose, M. P., Clothier, J., and Cotter, J.: Hypertrophic burn scars: analysis of variables. J. Trauma, *23*:895, 1983.

Dorethy, J. F.: The efficacy of colloid crystalloid resuscitation fluid in the earlier reestablishment of an adequate hemodynamic state in postburn shock. Fifth International Congress on Burn Injuries, Stockholm, Sweden, June 20, 1978.

Dorethy, J. F., Welch, G. W., Treat, R. C., Mason, A. D., Jr., and Pruitt, B. A., Jr.: Sequential hemodynamic alterations in severe thermal injury in the military population—colloid-crystalloid vs. crystalloid fluid resuscitation. Annual Research Progress Report. U.S. Army Institute of Surgical Research, 120–139, 1977.

Dressler, D. P., Barbee, W. K., and Sprenger, R.: The effect of Hydron burn wound dressing on burned rat and rabbit ear wound healing. J. Trauma, *20*:1024, 1980.

Dressler, D. P., and Skornick, W. P.: Alveolar macrophage in the burned rat. J. Trauma, *14*:1036, 1974.

Dupuytren, G.: Leçons orales de clinique chirurgicale. Vol. I, 1832, p. 459.

Earle, J.: Means of Lessening the Effect of Fire on the Human Body. London, C. Clark, 1799.

Edlich, R. F., Glasheen, W., Attinger, E. O., Anne, A., Haynes, B., and Hiebert, J. T.: Epidemiology of serious burn injuries. Surg. Gynecol. Obstet., *154*:505, 1982.

Fein, A., Leff, A., and Hopewell, P. C.: Pathophysiology and management of the complications resulting from fire and the inhaled products of combustion: review of the literature. Crit. Care Med., *8*:94, 1980.

Feller, I., Tholen, D., and Cornell, R. G.: Improvements in burn care, 1965 to 1979. J.A.M.A., *244*:2074, 1980.

Glasheen, W. P., Attinger, E. O., Anne, A., Boyd, D. R., Ruffin, W., et al.: Epidemiology of minor burn injuries. Burns Incl. Therm. Inj., *8*:423, 1982.

Hanback, C. D., and Rittenbury, M. S.: Response of the reticuloendothelial system in thermal injury. Surg. Forum, *16*:46, 1965.

Heimbach, D. M., Afromowitz, M. A., Engrav, L. H., Marvin, J. A., and Perry, B.: Burn depth estimation—man or machine. J. Trauma, *24*:373, 1984.

Hildanus, Fabricius: De Combustionibus. Frankfort, 1610.

Imlach, H.: Dissertation, Royal Medical Society. Edinburgh, (M.S.), 1835.

Jarrett, F., Ellerbe, S., and Demling, R.: Acute leukopenia during topical burn therapy with silver sulfadiazine. Am. J. Surg., *135*:818, 1978.

Kentish, E.: Essay on Burns. London, 1797.

Krizek, T. J., Robson, M. C., and Groskin, M. G.: Experimental burn wound sepsis—evaluation of enzymatic debridement. J. Surg. Res., *17*:219, 1974.

Krizek, T. J., Robson, M. C., and Klio, E.: Bacterial growth and skin graft survival. Surg. Forum, *18*:518, 1967.

Kumar, P.: Child abuse by thermal injury—a retrospective study. Burns Inc. Therm. Inj., *10*:344, 1984.

Larson, D., Huang, T., Lumares, H., Dobrbeovsky, M., Baur, P., and Parks, D.: Prevention and treatment of scar contracture. *In* Artz, C. P., Moncrief, J. A., and Pruitt, B. A., Jr. (Eds.): Burns: A Team Approach. Philadelphia, W. B. Saunders Company, 1979, p. 466.

Law, E. J., and MacMillan, B. G.: Excision of acute burns with immediate meshed autografting. Presentation, American Burn Association, Dallas, TX, 1973.

Levine, N. S., Lindberg, R. A., Salisbury, R. E., Mason, A. D., Jr., and Pruitt, B. A., Jr.: Comparison of coarse mesh gauze with biologic dressings on granulating wounds. Am. J. Surg., *131*:727, 1976.

Levine, N. S., Salisbury, R. E., and Mason, A. D., Jr.: The effect of early surgical excision and homografting on survival of burned rats and of intraperitoneally-infected burned rats. Plast. Reconstr. Surg., *56*:423. 1975.

Libber, S. M., and Stayton, D. J.: Childhood burns reconsidered: the child, the family, and the burn injury. J. Trauma, *24*:245, 1984.

Lister, J.: A Contribution to the Germ Theory of Putrefaction and Other Fermentative Changes, and to the Natural History of Torulae and Bacteria. Edinburgh, Neill & Company, 1875.

MacDougall, A.: Probationary Essay on Burns. Edinburgh, 1818.

Malick, M. H., and Carr, J. A.: Flexible elastomer molds in burn scar control. Am. J. Occup. Ther., *34*:603, 1980.

May, R. S.: Burn rehabilitation in the United States. J. Burn Care Rehab., *5*:69, 1984.

McArdle, A. H., Palmason, C., Brown, R. A., and Williams, H. B.: Early enteral feeding of patients with major burns: prevention of catabolism. Ann. Plast. Surg., *13*:396, 1984.

Miller, C. L., and Trunkey, D. D.: Thermal injury: defects in immune response induction. J. Surg. Res., *22*:621, 1977.

Moyer, C.: An assessment of the therapy of burns. Ann. Surg., *137*:628, 1953.

Moyer, C. A., Margraf, H. W., and Monafo, W. W., Jr.: Burn shock and extravascular sodium deficiency—treatment with Ringer's solution with lactate. Arch. Surg., *90*:799, 1965.

Moylan, J. A.: Inhalation injury. J. Trauma, *21*:720, 1981.

Muir, I. F. K.: The treatment of electrical burns. Br. J. Plast. Surg., *10*:292, 1958.

Muir, I. F. K.: Red cell destruction in burns, with particular reference to the shock period. Br. J. Plast. Surg., *14*:273, 1961.

Ninnemann, J. L., Fisher, J. C., and Frank, H. A.: Prolonged survival of human skin allografts following thermal injury. Transplantation, *25*:69, 1978.

O'Connor, N. E., Mulliken, J. B., Banks-Schlegel, S., et al.: Grafting of burns with cultured epithelium prepared from autologous epidermal cells. Lancet, *1*:75, 1981.

Pack, G. T., and Davis, A. H.: Burns: Types, Pathology, and Management. Philadelphia, J. B. Lippincott Company, 1930.

Paré, A.: The Workes of that Famous Chirurgion, Ambrose Parey. Translated out of the Latin and compared with the French by T. Johnson. London, T. Cotes & R. Young, 1634.

Perkins, K., Davey, R. B., and Wallis, K. A.: Silicone gel: a new treatment for burn scars and contractures. Burns Incl. Therm. Inj., *9*:201, 1983.

Pietsch, J., and Meakins, J. L.: Complications of povidine-iodine absorption in topically treated burn patients. Lancet, *1*:280, 1976.

Polk, H. C., Jr.: Prolongation of xenograft survival in patients with *Pseudomonas* sepsis: a clarification. Surg. Forum, *19*:514, 1968.

Pruitt, B. A., and Levine, N. S.: Characteristics and uses of biologic dressings and skin substitutes. Arch. Surg., *119*:312, 1984.

Rittenbury, M. S., and Hanback, L. D.: Phagocytic depression in thermal injuries. J. Trauma, *7*:523, 1967.

Robson, M. C., and Krizel, T. J.: Predicting skin graft survival. J. Trauma, *13*:213, 1973.

Robson, M. C., Krizel, T. J., Koss, N., and Samburg, J. L.: Amniotic membranes as a temporary wound dressing. Surg. Gynecol. Obstet., *136*:904, 1973.

Salisbury, R. E., Carnes, R., and McCarthy, L. R.: Comparison of the bacterial clearing effects of different biologic dressings on granulating wounds following thermal injury. Plast. Reconstr. Surg., *66*:596, 1980.

Shedd, D. P.: Historical landmarks in the treatment of burns. Surgery, *43*:1024, 1958.

Sneve, H.: The treatment of burns and skin grafting. J.A.M.A., *45*:1, 1905.

Tappeiner: Ueber Veränderungen des Blutes und der Muskeln nach ausgedehnten Hautverbrennungen. Centralbl. Med. Wiss. (Berlin), *19*:385, 401, 1881.

Trunkey, D. D.: Inhalation injury. Surg. Clin. North Am., *58*:1133, 1978.

Underhill, F. P.: The significance of anhydremia in extensive superficial burns. J.A.M.A., *95*:852, 1930.

Vander Elst, E.: Historical aspects of the treatment of burns. *In* Lorthioir, J. (Ed.): Physiopathology and Treatment of Burns. Brussels, Presses Academiques Européennes, 1964, pp. 1–23.

Velasco, M. G., Mutch, D., Surkes, N., and Williams, H. B.: Compression treatment of hypertrophic scars in burned children. Can. J. Surg., *21*:450, 1978.

Wachtel, T.: An analysis of factors which predict mortality in hospitalized burn patients. Burns, *9*:38, 1982.

Wallace, A. B.: Treatment of burns. Ann. R. Coll. Surg., *5*:283, 1949.

Wheeler, J. R., Van Harrison, R., Wolfe, R. A., and Payne, B. C.: The effects of burn severity and institutional differences on the costs of care. Med. Care, *21*:1192, 1983.

Wilmore, D. W., Curreri, P. W., Spitzer, K. W., Spitzer, M. E., and Pruitt, B. A., Jr.: Supranormal dietary intake in thermally injured hypermetabolic patients. Surg. Gynecol. Obstet., *132*:881, 1971.

Wilmore, D. W., Long, J. M., Mason, A. D., Jr., and Pruitt, B. A., Jr.: Catecholamines: mediators of the hypermetabolic response to thermal injury. Ann. Surg., *180*:653, 1974a.

Wilmore, D. W., Moylan, J. A., Breslow, B., Mason, A. D., Jr., and Pruitt, B. A., Jr.: Human growth hormone and high caloric feeding. Surg. Gynecol. Obstet., *183*:875, 1974b.

Wilmore, D. W., Orcutt, T. W., Mason, A. D., Jr., and Pruitt, B. A., Jr.: Alterations in hypothalamic function following thermal injury. J. Trauma, *15*:697, 1975.

Wiseman, R.: Severall Chirurgical Treatises. London, R. Royston, 1676.

Wolfe, R. R., and Burke, J. F.: Effect of caloric intake on hypermetabolic response to burn injury. Circ. Shock, *6*:170A, 1979.

Yannas, I. V., Burke, J. F., Orgill, D. P., and Skrabut, E. M.: Wound tissue can utilize a polymeric template to synthesize a functional extension of skin. Science, *215*:174, 1982.

24

Edward A. Luce

Electrical Injuries

HISTORY

The commercial use of electrical power began in the mid-nineteenth century, and serious injuries and fatalities were soon to follow. The first recorded fatality occurred in 1879 (Jex-Blake, 1913), a stage hand in Lyons, France. In his Goulstonian Lecture, Jex-Blake said that "the first use of electricity was employed in lighting the operatic stage in Paris (at the first performance of Meyerbeer's *La Prophète*) in 1849 and in lighthouses off the English coast in the 1850's. A stage carpenter was killed in Lyon in 1879 with an alternating current of 250 volts from a Siemens dynamo. The victim became insensible and died within twenty minutes; no artificial respirations were given." Jex-Blake (1913) estimated that in 1901 to 1910, 183 deaths occurred in England. He continued: "as regards the USA, where electricity is so extensively used, I have not been able to find any statistical records. One must remember that in America life is held very cheap and that safeguards and protective legislation tend to be regarded as undue restrictions upon industry and commerce."

Today, approximately 1000 to 1200 fatalities occur annually in the United States, 20 to 25 per cent from lightning (Campbell, Campbell, and Fletcher, 1969). Electrical burns account for 3 to 4 per cent of admissions to burn units (DiVincenti, Moncrief, and Pruitt, 1969).

PATHOPHYSIOLOGY

The principal determinant of tissue damage is voltage. Ohm's law states that the intensity of the current (amperage) is directly proportional to the potential (voltage) and inverse to the resistance, $I = V/R$. More pertinent is Joule's law, stating that the heat generated is directly proportional to the resistance and to the square of the voltage, or heat $= 0.24$ $(\text{voltage})^2 \times$ resistance. The two critical components in both equations are *tension* and *resistance*. Besides the magnitude of voltage, the duration and surface area of contact is important. The resistance is determined by the nature of the conductor, length, and cross section. In the limited situation, the factor that affects conduction is the nature of the tissue, i.e., nerves and blood vessels are good conductors, dry skin and bone are poor. The poor conduction or, more appropriately, the high resistance to the passage of current effectively transfers electrical energy to thermal energy, consistent with Joule's law. It must be recalled that the heat generated varies proportionately to resistance, but to the *square* of the voltage. An analogous equation is the relationship of tissue destruction produced by the passage of a missile, $K = MV^2$; velocity is the principal determinant.

Most commonly, exposure to 1000 volts or greater is considered a high tension electrical burn.

In the past, the passage of current through the body was thought to occur preferentially through tissues of low resistivity such as nerves and blood vessels. Experimental studies (Hunt and associates, 1976; Sances and associates, 1981) have demonstrated that the internal milieu acts as a single uniform resistance. This resistance is a function of volume or cross sectional diameter. For example, an extremity has a higher current density and higher production (Joule effect) than the trunk. This clarification of the pathophysiology of electricity and electrical injury has direct clinical application.

The type of current, direct or alternating, is important at low voltage levels. Slow alternating current can induce tetanic muscle spasm so that the victim cannot release a grip on the current source. Cardiac arrhythmias are more readily induced with alternating current, and fatalities can occur easily with household current of 110 volts if skin resistance is low. Virtually all electrical injuries occur with alternating current.

Most classifications of types of electrical burns list three: thermal, arc, and direct electrical injury (Esses and Peters, 1981). The distinction is probably artificial, and a useful division of high tension injuries is into flash and "true" high tension electrical burns (Luce and Gottlieb, 1984).

INITIAL ASSESSMENT AND RESUSCITATION

The initial assessment of the electrically injured patient should consider associated injuries. A careful history taking from witnesses may reveal an associated fall that could be responsible for fractures or visceral injury.

Case Discussion. A 19 year old male was assisting his father in painting a barn when he grasped a high tension wire. He was seen in the Emergency Room, and plastic surgery consultation was obtained for the upper and lower extremity burns. The patient was tachycardiac and initial hematocrit was 30 per cent, unexpectedly low for the magnitude of the burn. Diagnostic peritoneal lavage was positive and subsequent exploratory laparotomy revealed a ruptured spleen. In the confusion and concern over the electrical burn, the father had forgotten the history of a fall from the ladder at the time of injury, and was not questioned.

Careful questioning about the circumstances surrounding the injury is important. The voltage in the line source, as well as the environmental conditions, should be ascertained, if possible. The patient should be examined with particular attention directed toward entry and exit sites of the current passage. The skin of the flexion creases of the extremities are examined for evidence of "arc" burns, a finding that may indicate extensive destruction of underlying tissue. An entry or exit site may be present in the scalp, concealed by hair.

Initial therapeutic steps are the same in electrical burns as in thermal burns (see Chap. 23). Inhalation injury is rarely an associated condition, and intervention to maintain the airway is infrequently necessary. A notable exception is direct electrical burn to the neck when, because of the injury and associated edema, the upper airway can become compromised. Nasotracheal intubation should be performed prophylactically soon after admission in such instances.

Early electrocardiographic abnormalities are present in approximately one-third of electrical burn patients, but are usually transient and not clinically significant (Luce and Gottlieb, 1984; Housinger and associates, 1985). Operative intervention should not be deferred because of ECG abnormalities in an otherwise hemodynamically stable patient.

Prompt fluid resuscitation of the electrical burn patient is the keystone to the prevention of acute renal failure. Although the body surface area burn is often small, the fluid requirements are much greater than in a comparable thermal burn. Standard resuscitation formulas based on body weight and percentage body surface area burned are not applicable to high tension electrical burns (Artz, 1974). The incidence of acute renal failure has been from 1.5 to 7.5 per cent of large series (Baxter, 1970; Solem, Fischer, and Strate, 1977; Rouse and Dimick, 1978; Wilkinson and Wood, 1978) with a comparable increase in mortality rate. The combination of hypovolemia and the circulating pigment load of myoglobin and hemoglobin pose a distinct threat of pigment precipitation in the renal tubules. To minimize this risk, the use of mannitol to increase renal perfusion

Table 24–1. Fluid Requirements in "True" versus Flash Electrical Burns

	"True"	Flash
Percentage BSA burn	18.8	16.0
Fluid in first 24 hours (ml)	11,610.0 (n = 18)*	4100.0 (n = 12)*

*n = Numbers of patients used for calculation of fluid requirements.

and sodium bicarbonate to achieve urine alkalinity has been an integral part of the resuscitation program for electrical burns (DiVincenti, Moncrief, and Pruitt, 1969; Baxter, 1970; Artz, 1974; Hunt, Sato, and Baxter, 1980). The resuscitation protocol of the author consists of vigorous infusion of Ringer's lactate without either bicarbonate or mannitol. Urine pH has been consistently neutral or alkaline in resuscitated patients. A high volume of fluids is administered until the urine clears of gross pigment. The decision about the volume of administered fluids is based on the appearance of the urine, not necessarily the output, although the restoration of high urine output usually has been heralded by the clearance of pigment. To achieve this goal in a series of true high tension burns required approximately 7 ml/kg of fluids per percentage body surface area burned within the first 24 hours (Luce and Gottlieb, 1984) (Table 24–1).

Patients aged 45 years or older who have also sustained large body surface area involvement and a mixture of thermal and electrical burns may require Swan-Ganz catheterization of the pulmonary artery for more accurate determination of cardiac function during the resuscitation period.

WOUND MANAGEMENT

The clinical differentiation of flash or thermal burns from "true" high tension electrical burns is usually possible. Flash burns are typically mixed full- and partial-thickness burns without characteristic entry or exit wounds. "True" high tension electrical burns are sharply demarcated, full thickness, and leathery in appearance and on palpation. The determination hinges on the presence of tissue destruction deeper than the skin and subcutaneous tissue.

Topical antibiotic cream coverage for the thermal component is usually Silvadene, but Sulfamylon is an excellent choice for the full-thickness current contact points.

The appropriate management of the electrical burn wound has engendered considerable discussion and controversy. A dichotomy of opinion is evident in early investigative work between (1) those who subscribed to the concept that high tension electricity inflicts an injury with unique characteristics, intrinsic and separate from that of thermal burns (Jellinek, 1936) and (2) those who attributed the pathologic condition of electrical lesions to the heat of resistance generated by the passage of the current (Jaffé, 1928). The former school of thought gave rise to the concept of progressive or de novo necrosis that occurred after injury, possibly secondary to delayed vascular damage and occlusion from the current. As described above, experimental studies (Hunt and associates, 1976; Sances and associates, 1981; Laberge, Ballard, and Daniel, 1984) have not demonstrated evidence of delayed or progressive vascular occlusion and have established electrical injury as essentially a burn. However, the concept of progressive necrosis, particularly myonecrosis, persists in many discussions of electrical burns (Butler and Gant, 1977; Solem, Fischer, and Strate, 1977; Rouse and Dimick, 1978; Sullivan, Scott, and Boswick, 1981). The argument is not of academic interest alone since two divergent philosophies of wound management have emerged. One school of opinion has advocated conservative, cautious debridement and late wound closure. According to this philosophy, early coverage risks infection due to incomplete excision of necrotic muscle. Others propose early excision and repair. The point is crucial, particularly with regard to the extremities, since the sequelae of scar contracture, stiff joints, and limitation of function are incurred by delayed or prolonged closure of extremity wounds (Luce and Griffen, 1978).

Electrical injury should appropriately be considered a burn, as for practical purposes the extent of necrosis is complete at the time of injury. Patients with high tension injuries should be taken to the operating room within the first few hours after injury for wound exploration and debridement. Debridement consists of escharectomy and aggressive excision of devitalized muscle, as judged by color and lack of contractility. Contractile response to the stimulus of electrocautery has been a valuable guide to viability. Ancillary measures such as technetium muscle scans (Hunt and associates, 1979) and frozen section microscopy (Quinby and associates, 1978) have been used, but have not become standard therapy because of significant logistic problems. Experience is probably the best diagnostic tool. Most areas of muscle necrosis correspond closely to the area of skin burns in the trunk. Additional areas of deep tissue necrosis can be detected in the periosseous tissues in the extremities, as well as beneath the skip or arc burns at flexion creases.

Debrided wounds are covered with biologic dressings of porcine skin or allografts. Patients are returned to the operating room 24 to 48 hours later for a second wound exploration and debridement. If necessary, amputation should be performed at this procedure. If additional debridements are warranted, some consideration should be given to the vascular supply of the muscle or muscles involved. Debridement may devascularize retained muscle (Laberge, Ballard, and Daniel, 1984). In the lower extremity, on occasion, the author has debrided from origin to insertion of a muscle or compartment to avoid this complication.

Dressing changes of large, open, debrided electrical burn wounds are extremely painful. Rapid wound closure is advantageous to reduce pain, reverse the catabolic state, minimize contracture, and hasten rehabilitation (Luce, 1982). Until wound closure is obtained, maximal nutritional support and active physical therapy participation is critical. Pain with dressing changes can be addressed with patient-controlled analgesia, a useful technique for electrical burns but less so for thermal burns.

Scalp and Skull

The head is not infrequently a contact or entry point in high tension burns. The method of management is dependent on the depth of injury. The anatomic lesion has been described as saucer shaped (Stuckey, 1963) when viewed in cross section. The most superficial burn of the lateral margins extends to the deepest point, the cranium, at the center (Fig. 24–1). With loss of pericranium and exposure or involvement of the underlying bone, the approach in the past has been conservative. The calvarium was left exposed for an indeterminate time, usually months, and eventually nonviable bone was sloughed or removed as a sequestrum. The defect was closed with a split-thickness skin graft or flap. Delay while sequestration is awaited can be complicated by the occurrence of epidural abscess and meningitis (Kragh and Erich, 1961; DiVincenti, Moncrief, and Pruitt, 1979; Skoog, 1970). The outer table can be removed to expose a viable diploic cavity, if performed sufficiently early in the postinjury period. With the subsequent development of granulation tissue, the defect can be covered with split-thickness skin grafts (Fig. 24–2). The intermediate and long-term results of this technique may not be

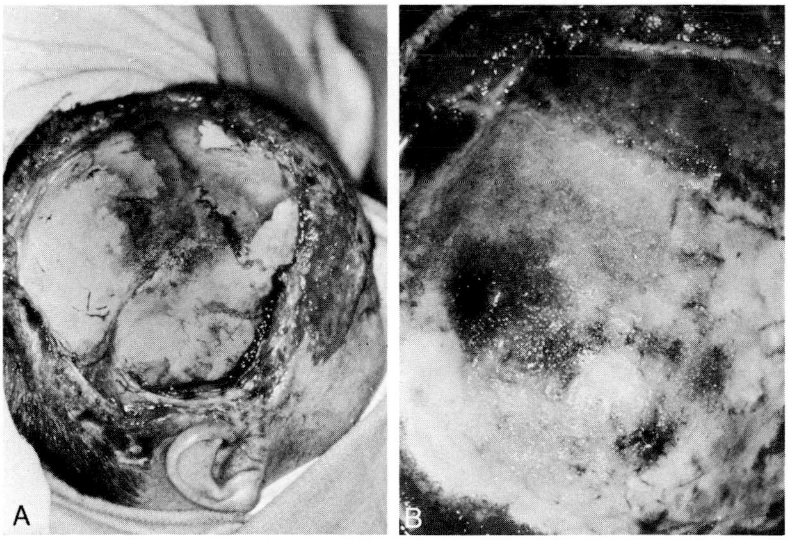

Figure 24–1. *A,* High tension electrical injury of the scalp and skull. The soft tissue destruction is greater than that of bone. The periphery of the bony exposure is white with viable-appearing bone. *B,* Close-up view of the central area of bone exposure, which appears necrotic.

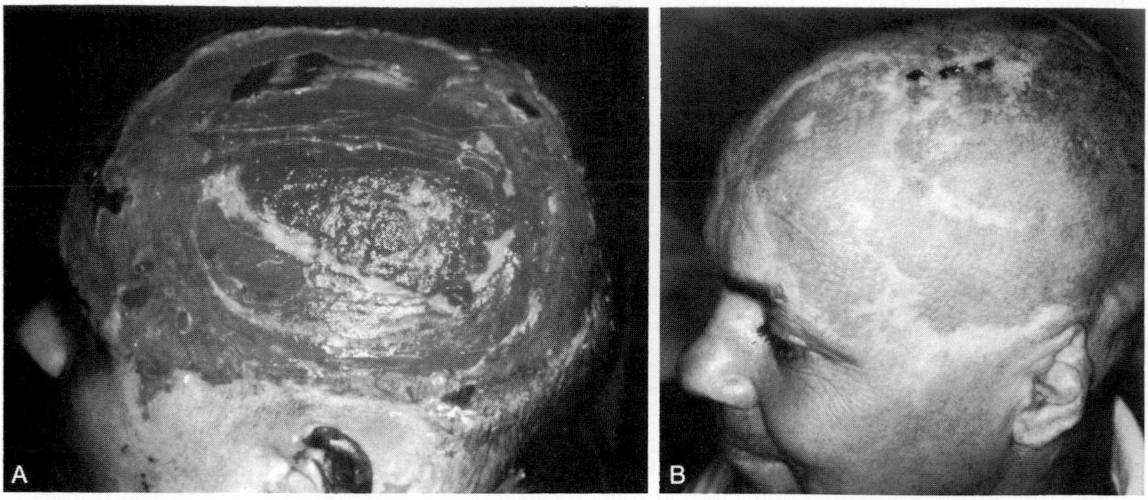

Figure 24–2. *A,* Large area of exposed bone secondary to contact point with 20,000 volts, after decortication and development of granulation tissue. *B,* Healed wound after application of a split-thickness skin graft.

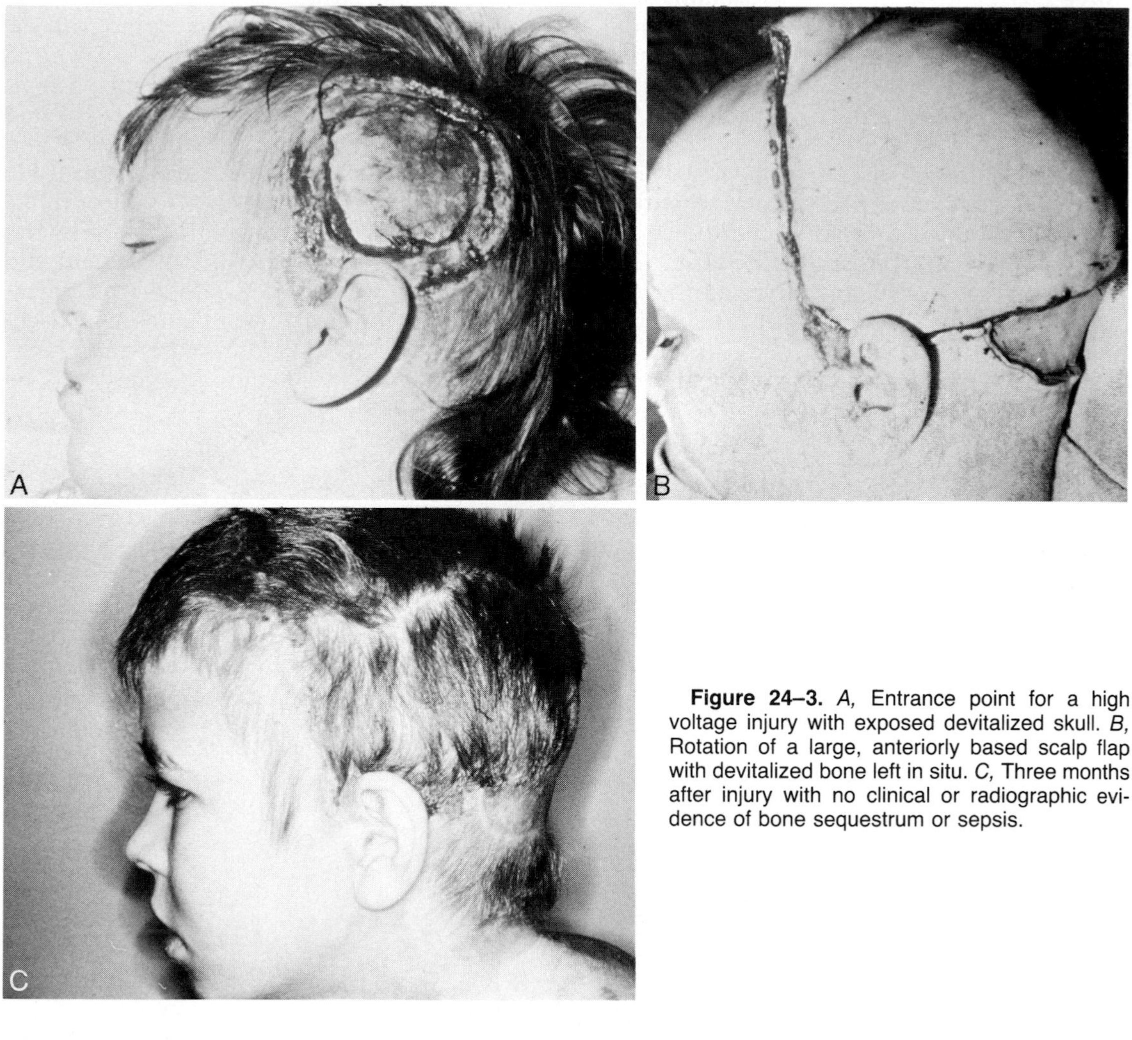

Figure 24–3. *A,* Entrance point for a high voltage injury with exposed devitalized skull. *B,* Rotation of a large, anteriorly based scalp flap with devitalized bone left in situ. *C,* Three months after injury with no clinical or radiographic evidence of bone sequestrum or sepsis.

acceptable (Curtin and associates, 1963; Caffee, 1980). The sequelae of ulceration and fibrosis may eventually require flap coverage. If the bony injury is full thickness, the diploic cavity is destroyed. Excision of the full-thickness bone in this situation is feasible, and closure is accomplished with skin grafts on the dura. Early excision of full-thickness bone invites the complications of hemorrhage, cerebrospinal (CSF) leak, and meningitis (Robinson, Masters, and Forrest, 1965).

An alternative approach is early excision of the eschar and flap coverage of the exposed bone with adjacent uninjured scalp without regard for the degree of bone devitalization (Luce and Hoopes, 1974) (Fig. 24–3). The devitalized bone is regarded as an in situ bone graft, which is covered by well-vascularized soft tissue. This concept regards electrically injured bone as salvageable if the cycle of desiccation, colonization, and sequestration can be interrupted. Crucial to the outcome is early debridement and coverage before the bone becomes sufficiently colonized to become osteomyelitic (Silverberg and associates, 1986). If the defect is so large that the remaining uninjured scalp is inadequate for coverage, free microvascular transfer of distant tissue, preferably omentum, is warranted (Caffee, 1980; Silverberg and associates, 1986). Recipient vessels should be sought beyond the immediate zone of injury.

In the author's experience, the delayed onset of central nervous system complications, including mixed neurologic lesions, paraplegia, and quadriplegia, has occurred in patients with high tension skull injury.

Trunk and Perineum

The primary concern in truncal electrical burns is injury to the enclosed viscera. The author has treated two patients with contact points of the anterior chest wall who developed a lesion of the underlying lung similar to pulmonary contusion. The radiographic picture was that of focal atelectasis and edema of the involved lung field. Both patients recovered quickly with ventilatory support and PEEP (positive end expiratory pressure).

Abdominal visceral damage from high tension electrical burns has been uncommon, but is attended by a high fatality rate (Almgard, Liljedahl, and Nylen, 1965; Newsome, 1972; Yang, Tsai, and Noordhoff, 1985). The clue is a contact point on the anterior abdominal wall. Intestinal injury and perforation have also been described in fatal low voltage electrocution (Williams and Karl, 1981). Full-thickness loss of the abdominal wall and intestinal injury may be obvious at the time of presentation by prolapse of the perforated intestinal loops through the wound (Fig. 24–4). The injury may be less obvious, for example, if the current passes through the abdominal wall and injures intestine immediately adjacent to the entry site. Perforation may not occur for several days while the integrity of the intestinal wall deteriorates, and fatalities can be attributable to the delay in diagnosis. Appropriate management of high tension contact burns of the abdomen consists of immediate wound exploration and debridement (Fig. 24–5). The eschar, subcu-

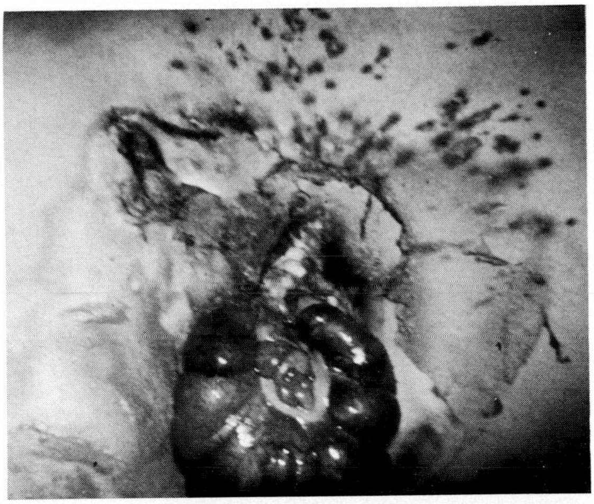

Figure 24–4. High tension injury of the abdomen with spontaneous evisceration of necrotic colon.

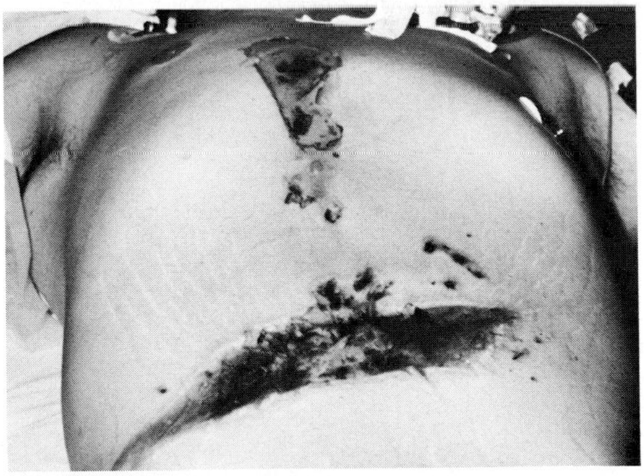

Figure 24–5. Contact points of the anterior chest wall and abdomen. Appropriate management requires operative escharotomy and exploration of the wound.

taneous fat, fascia, and muscle are progressively debrided until viable tissue is encountered. If debridement proceeds to an injured peritoneum, formal exploratory laparotomy is indicated, since the loop of injured intestine may be in an entirely different quadrant of the abdomen. If laparotomy is necessary, primary closure of the excised wound by advancement or rotation of a myocutaneous flap is prudent.

Perineal wounds are managed by early debridement and excision, urinary diversion, if indicated, and early wound closure. Full-thickness loss of the scrotum is treated in a manner similar to that for an avulsive injury. Shaft penile burns are excised as a unit and replaced with thick split-thickness skin grafts (Fig. 24–6).

Extremities

Electrical burns of the extremities are the most frequent site of injury. A common pattern is entrance of the current in the upper extremity and exit through the lower extremity (Figs. 24–7 and 24–8). When the injury is secondary to high tension current, the upper

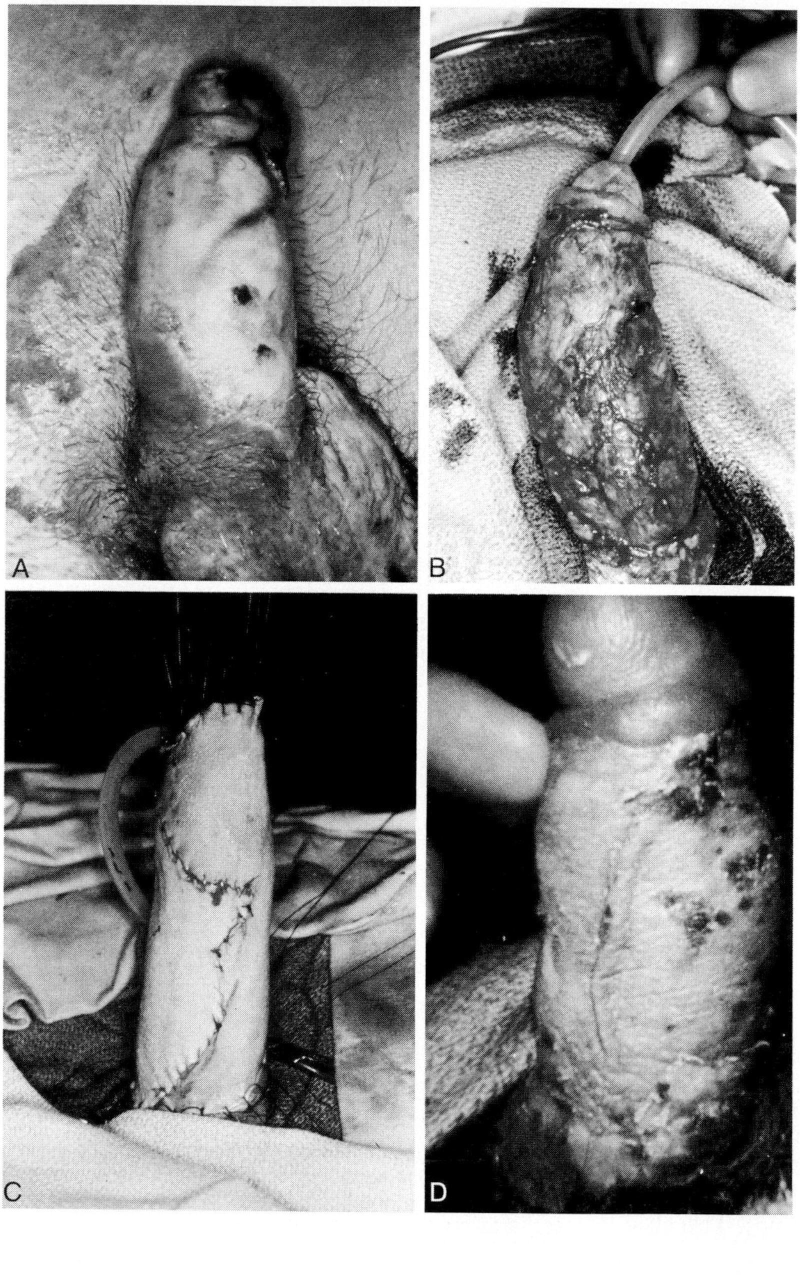

Figure 24–6. *A,* Full-thickness loss of penile shaft skin from contact injury. *B,* Primary excision of eschar from base of shaft to corona. *C,* Application of a split-thickness skin graft. Note the interdigitation of the suture line to avoid straight line contracture. *D,* Appearance one month postoperatively.

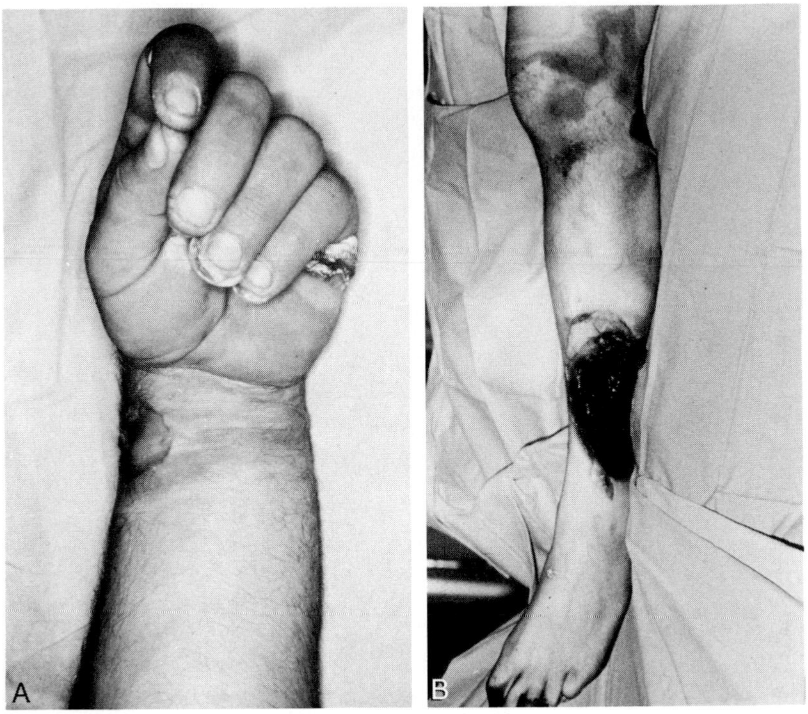

Figure 24–7. *A,* Entrance injury of 14,000 volts in the palm. *B,* Exit point in the left lower extremity. Although an obvious exit wound existed at the midcalf level, the entire extremity from the distal thigh is nonviable.

extremity or a portion thereof is often lost (Robson, Murphy, and Heggers, 1984).

Patients are typically employed as linemen or injured in an industrial accident. The erection of television and Citizens' Band radio home transmitter antennae have been responsible for some of the patient population. In the author's series of patients, the range of exposure was 3000 to 70,000 volts (mean of 30,800) (Luce and Gottlieb, 1984). The eventual outcome is usually dictated in large part by the status of the extremity on presentation. If the extremity is ischemic without a pulse, anesthetic, and maintained in a flexed and contracted position, either amputation or salvage of a functionless part is a distressingly frequent result, despite aggressive decompression and debridement (Fig. 24–9). These results have stimulated a consideration of the pathophysiologic process in high tension electrical injury of the upper extremity.

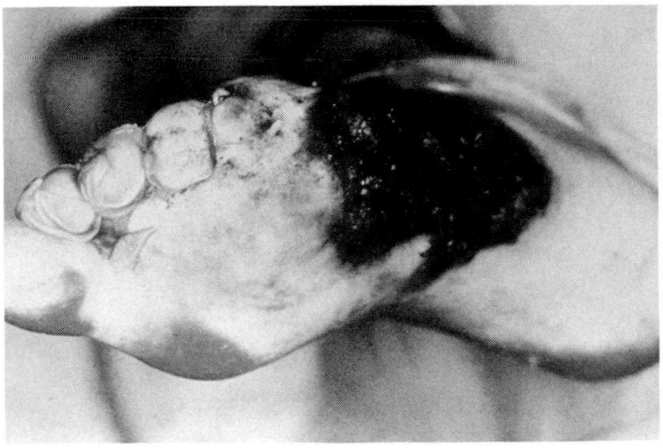

Figure 24–8. Exit wound on the lateral aspect of the foot.

Virtually all patients have been injured by grasping the line source or ground (exit). In doing so, they have sustained a significant cutaneous burn of the volar wrist in association with a palmar burn (Fig. 24–10). The mechanism may be a tetanic contraction of the digits, the wrist, and possibly the elbow and shoulder. The current is induced to travel the shortest distance, a straight line, and it arcs across the flexion creases of wrist, elbow, and shoulder (Fig. 24–11). If this concept is correct, the sharply demarcated burns seen in these areas represent both entrance and exit wounds as the current arcs. Arcing current ionizes air particles and can raise temperature into the 2500° to 3000°F range. Exploration of the wrist burn has revealed a coagulative necrosis of the underlying structures. Tremendous thermal damage is inflicted on muscle bellies, tendons, nerves, and (most significantly) both radial and ulnar arteries. Pulsatile flow has been traced from

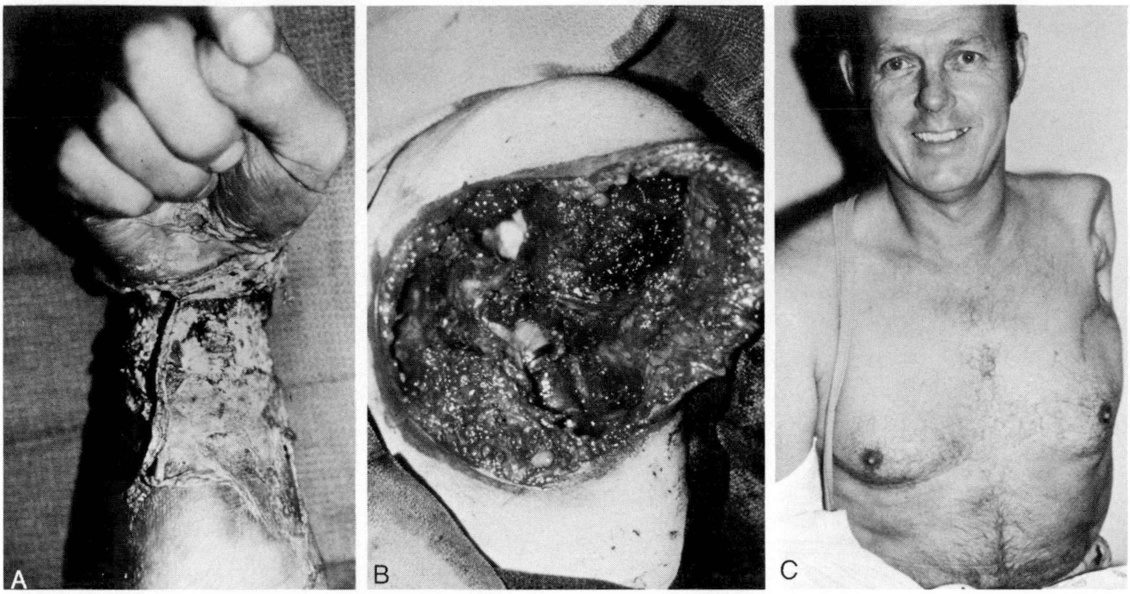

Figure 24–9. *A,* Contact point in the hand and forearm. Additional areas of injury were present at the antecubital fossa and axilla. *B,* The wound in the same patient after glenohumeral disarticulation and debridement of the chest wall musculature. *C,* The wound healed primarily. The patient was fitted with an upper extremity disarticulation prosthesis.

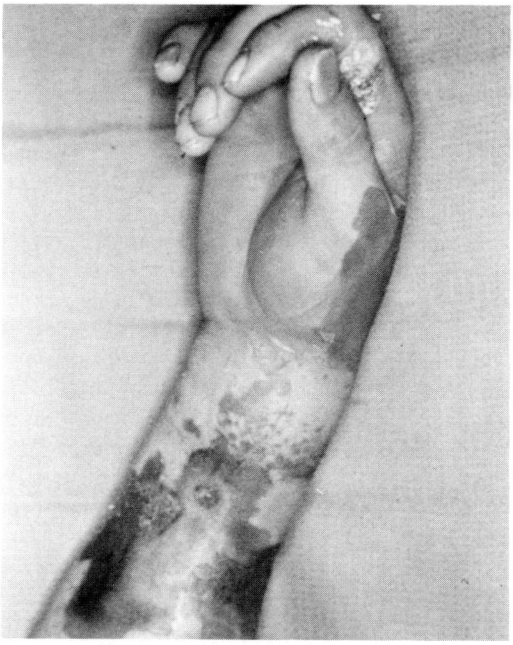

Figure 24–10. Injury sustained during erection of a Citizens' Band antenna. The palmar wound is minor but an extensive arc injury has been inflicted on the distal forearm.

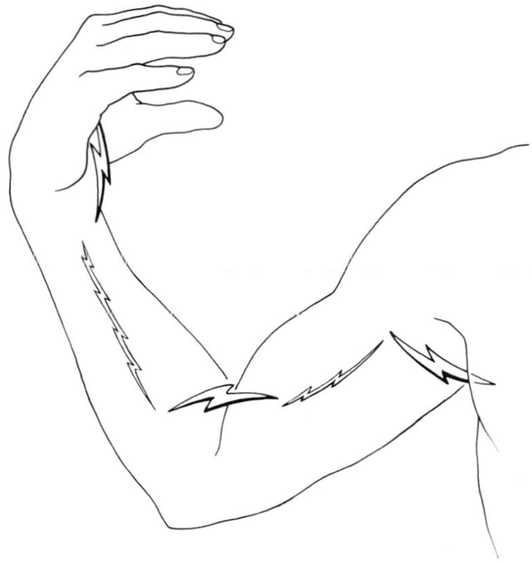

Figure 24–11. The passage of current through the upper extremity in a high tension injury. The contact point is in the palm. The current arcs at the wrist, travels up the forearm, arcs at the antecubital fossa, courses the upper arm, and possibly arcs at a third point at the axilla.

proximal to distal to the level of the severe wrist burn (Fig. 24–12). Precisely at that point the vessels were without flow, and nearly indistinguishable as discrete structures.

Further passage of the current in a more proximal direction may create additional skip areas of burn at the flexion creases of the antecubital fossa and axilla (Fig. 24–13). These innocuous appearing burns often conceal considerable deep tissue necrosis (Fig. 24–14).

Additional areas of concealed necrosis, some more proximal than the principal cutaneous burn, are the periosseous muscle groups. Presumably since bone is a poor conductor, the increased heat of resistance damages immediately adjacent tissue. Likewise, these areas of myonecrosis may be occult and unsuspected (Fig. 24–15).

If the concept of regarding electrical injury as a thermal burn is valid, the hypothesis of zones of differing degrees of tissue damage is also valid (Robson, Murphy, and Heggers, 1984). As discussed above, tissue necrosis is most extensive at the zone or zones of current concentration. Necrosis may be less uniform and more patchy in occurrence in the more proximal and peripheral area or zone.

Discussion of the differing views of the pathophysiology of electrical injury, *progressive or de novo myonecrosis versus the concept of electrical injury as a thermal burn,* is particularly pertinent in the management of high tension electrical injury of the extremities. From this controversy, two divergent therapeutic philosophies have emerged. One school of thought advocates conservative, wait-and-see therapy and cautious periodic debridement. Inadequate excision is the rule and early coverage is placed at risk, according to this philosophy. The other school proposes early excision and repair, avoiding the problems of scar contracture, stiff joints, and lim-

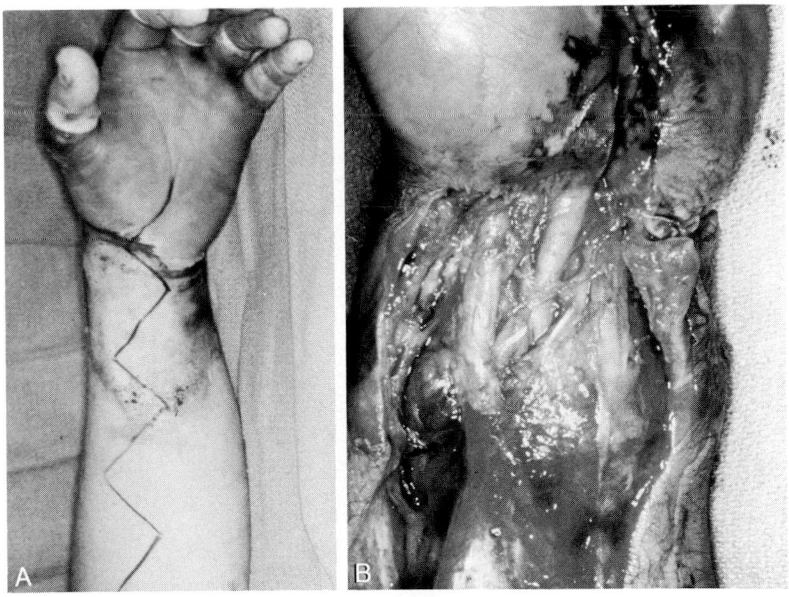

Figure 24–12. *A,* High tension injury of the upper extremity. The forearm has been prepared for a decompressive fasciotomy. *B,* The same patient after fasciotomy and exploration. Considerable thermal damage has been inflicted on the wrist structures with a sharp demarcation point proximally.

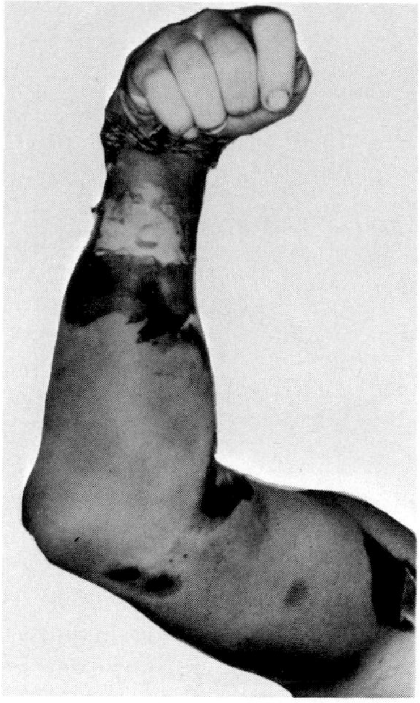

Figure 24–13. Nonviable extremity distal to the elbow with arcing points at the wrist, antecubital fossa, and axilla.

itation of function due to prolonged or delayed closure of extremity wounds.

Necrosis is not uniform or predictable. The three mechanisms of flexion crease arcing, periosseous tissue damage, and patchy necrosis at the periphery of the central zone may have been interpreted in the past as progressive necrosis (Figs. 24–16 and 24–17). Necrotic or questionable muscle retained at the time of early debridement provides the nidus for additional tissue loss. Contamination and desiccation initiate the cycle of compromised viability and diminished resistance followed by infection, hypoxia, and further compromise of the circulatory status that results in manifest necrosis. Adjacent muscle, although viable but adversely affected by this process, may perpetuate the cycle.

Only early, aggressive, and complete debridement of devitalized skin and muscle can prevent the cycle and provide the setting for definitive coverage. In patients with high

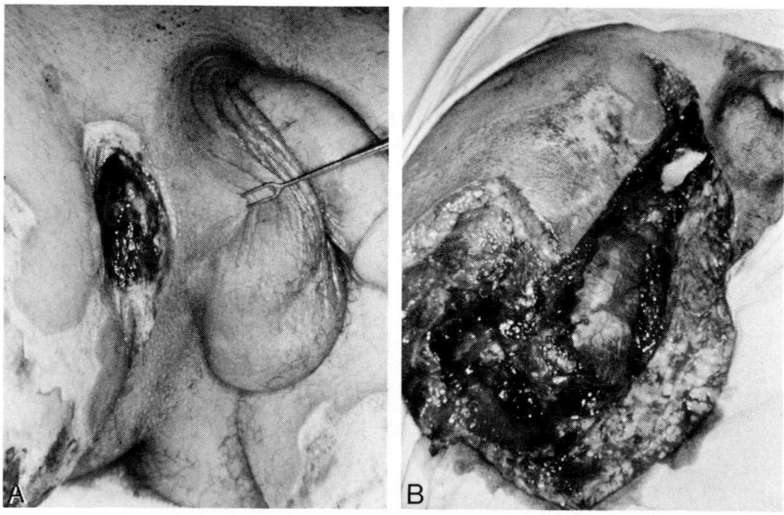

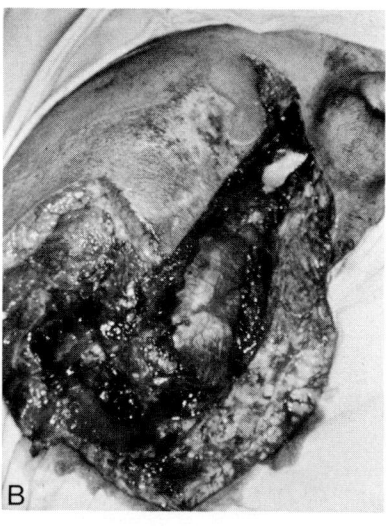

Figure 24–14. *A,* Arc injury of the groin. *B,* Appearance after a high above-knee amputation, wound exploration, and debridement of the groin. The cutaneous component of the arc burn concealed a deep destructive wound of the underlying structures.

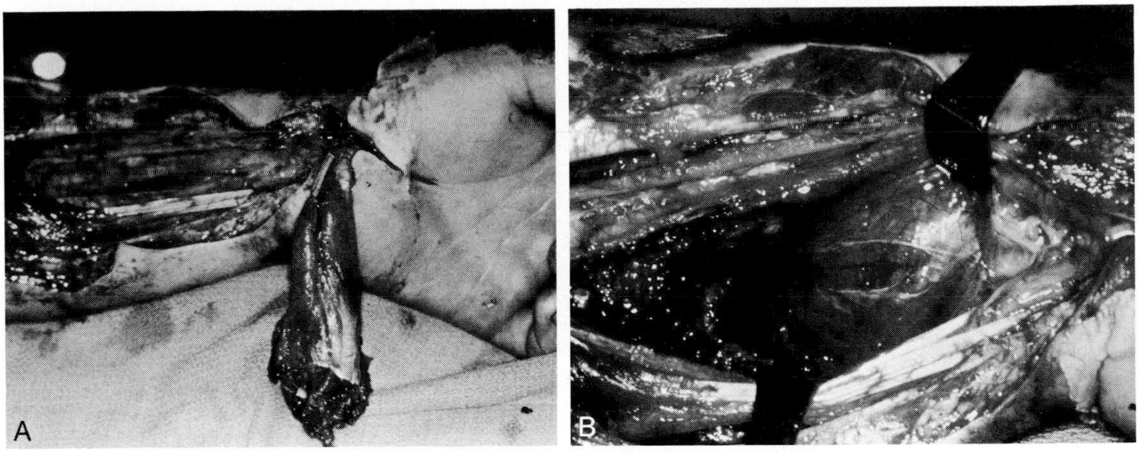

Figure 24–15. *A,* Fasciotomy, wound exploration, and debridement of necrotic muscle of a portion of the flexor compartment, including the flexor sublimis and carpi radialis. The flexor profundi are viable. *B,* Beneath the viable layer of the muscle and tendon is a nonviable pronator quadratus, presumably resulting from the heat of resistance generated by the radius and ulna.

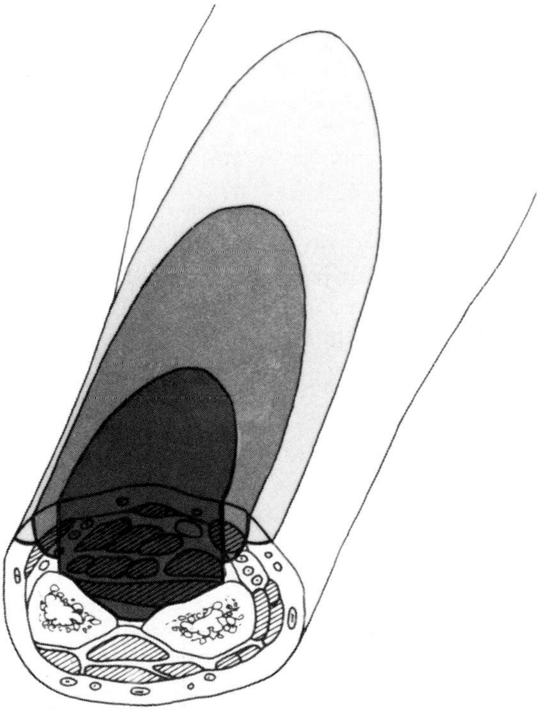

Figure 24–16. The zones of injury in an electrical burn. In three dimensions the deepest injury occurred at the wrist with thermal destruction of skin, subcutaneous fat, and underlying muscles and nerves. More proximal to the arc injury is full-thickness skin loss but sparing of the underlying structures. The most proximal and peripheral zone consists of only partial-thickness skin loss.

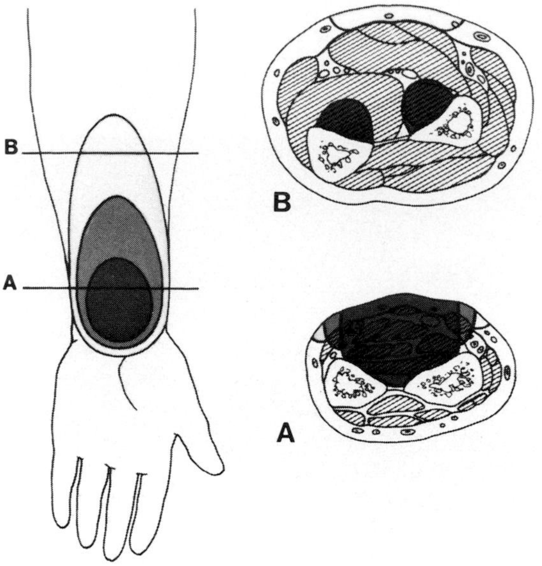

Figure 24–17. Cross sectional representation through the forearm. *A* Represents the most distal point seen in Figure 24–16. *B,* The proximal cross sectional area demonstrates hidden areas of periosseous myonecrosis under a skin burn that appears more superficial than in *A*.

tension injury, fasciotomy, wound exploration, and debridement should be accomplished within the first few hours after injury. Debridement consists of escharectomy and aggressive excision of devitalized muscle, as judged by color and lack of contractility to stimulation. Bleeding is often from larger vessels and does not represent true nutrient flow. Particular attention should be directed toward the skip areas of flexion creases and adequate exposure of the periosseous muscle groups. The use of ancillary measures of technetium muscle scans or frozen section microscopy has not gained widespread application. Mummified or irretrievable extremities should be amputated at the initial surgical procedure.

Patients are returned to the operating room 24 to 48 hours later for a second wound exploration and debridement. At this juncture, the periphery of the zone of injury should be carefully inspected for areas of patchy necrosis. Wounds may need to be extended for adequate exposure. Nerves and tendons are a notable exception to this conceptual approach and should be preserved even if they appear devitalized. Direct thermal damage at the wrist combined with contamination and desiccation, particularly in open fasciotomy wounds, can lead to necrosis and loss of nerves and tendons.

Definitive coverage is provided as rapidly as feasible. The goals of pain relief, enhancement of nutrition, deterrence of sepsis, and rehabilitation of the extremity to provide early motion and salvage of nerve and tendons, are promoted by early coverage. Early coverage can be obtained only by aggressive and complete debridement. Coverage has been provided by split-thickness skin grafts in the lower extremity and groin or abdominal flaps in the upper extremity. Split-thickness skin grafts have been used on occasion in the upper extremity (Fig. 24–18), but they do not provide the stable coverage often required. The use of free flaps for definitive coverage of upper extremity electrical injury wounds has been attempted with some success (Grotting and Walkinshaw, 1985; Silverberg and associates, 1986). Microvascular free tissue transfer is an attractive option for coverage of bone, tendon, and nerve without the limitations of more conventional flaps. The concern that the recipient vessels have sustained an occult injury that contraindicates free tissue transfer is not justified, and this technique deserves much wider application in the management of patients with electrical burns.

COMPLICATIONS

Complications of electrical injury include sequelae common to electrical and thermal burns alike, as well as problems unique to electrical burns.

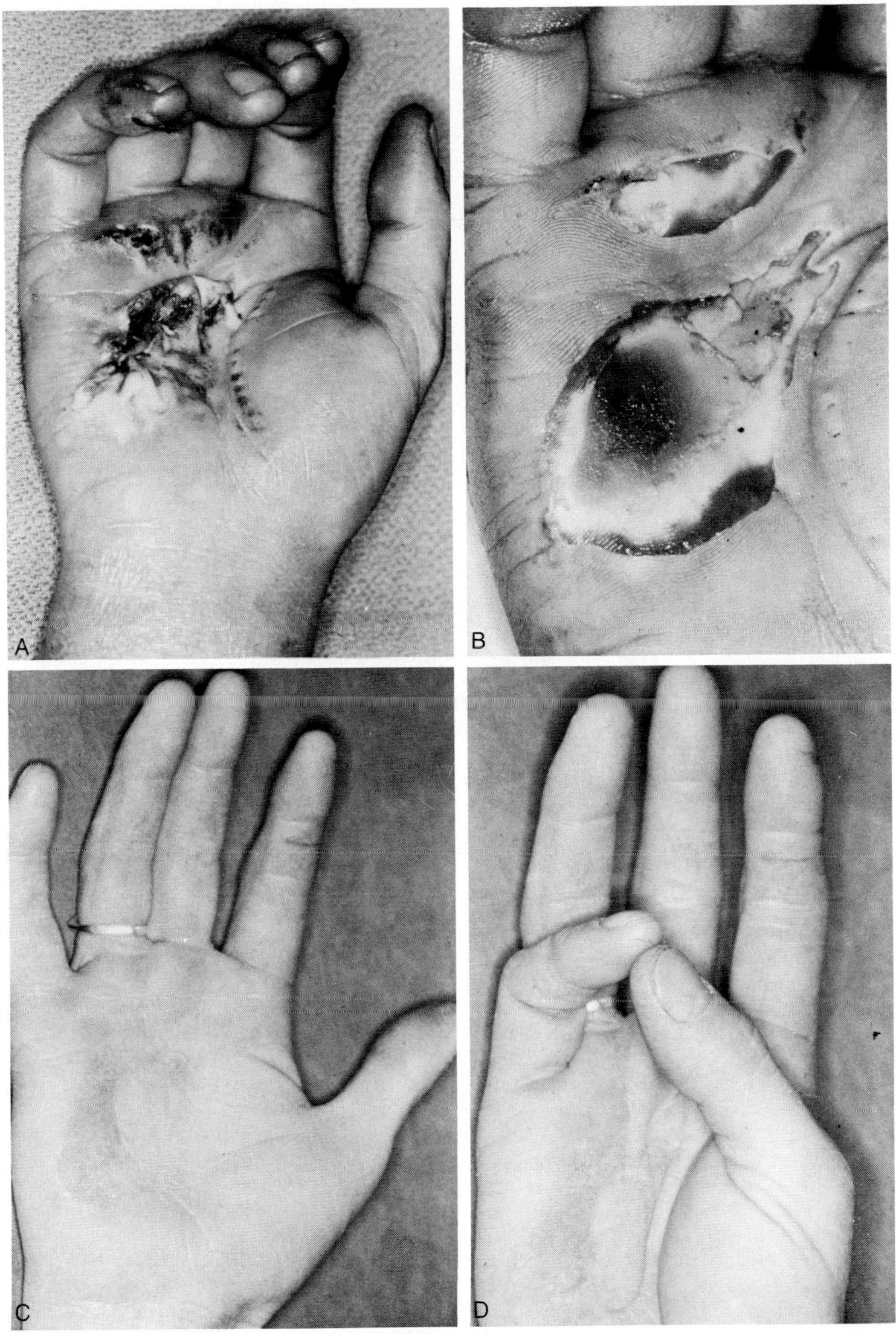

Figure 24–18. *A, B,* High tension contact injury of the palm. *C, D,* Normal function after excision and primary split-thickness skin grafting.

Central Nervous System

Patients who sustain an entrance or exit wound of the scalp and skull seem at most risk for central nervous system (CNS) complications. The most devastating is the delayed onset of paraplegia or quadriplegia. Amply described in the literature, the onset is described as occurring weeks or months after the injury (Levine and associates, 1975; Christensen and associates, 1980). The three cases in the author's experience all arose within three weeks after the injury. One quadriplegic and one paraplegic patient had a presentation that the consulting neurologist believed was consistent with vascular occlusion or a spinal artery syndrome. One patient had a mixed sensory-motor deficit of different levels that actually improved gradually over a period of weeks. All three patients had high tension entrance sites in the scalp and skull.

Other nervous system sequelae include nonfocal neurologic signs and symptoms. Patients may develop problems with gait and balance, speech, memory, personality changes, or seizures. The author managed two patients with contact injury of the neck who experienced delayed onset of difficulty with gait and balance. Both patients demonstrated nonspecific neurologic conditions in the lower extremities and did not show improvement on long-term follow-up.

Cataracts

The traditional impression was that cataract occurrence was limited to patients who sustained injuries with entrance sites in the head. However, a report of a series of cataracts in major electrical injuries indicates that only half the patients sustained head and neck injuries (Saffle, Crandall, and Warden, 1985). The first clinical presentation is a complaint of decreased visual acuity one to 12 months post injury, although onset can be as late as 30 months after the injury. More often than not, the occurrence is bilateral. The true incidence is not known, but probably ranges from 6 to 10 per cent of all high tension injuries. The magnitude of voltage must play a role, since up to 50 per cent of survivors of lightning injury suffer some type of eye damage (Castren and Kytila, 1964). However, cataracts have been described in cases of exposure to as little as 220 volts. Because of the subtle nature of the problem against the background of more obvious and dramatic injury elsewhere, one must specifically question and examine the patient to determine the possibility of cataracts developing.

Gastrointestinal

Electrical burn patients are subject to the same acute and subacute complications of the gastrointestinal tract that occur in thermal injury (see Chap. 23). These include stress ulceration and bleeding, acalculous cholecystitis, and perhaps pancreatitis (Pruitt, 1974).

The occurrence of direct intestinal injury and perforation has been previously described. Long-term follow-up of patients who have recovered from high tension electrical injury has revealed an unusually high incidence of gastrointestinal complaints and problems. Baxter (1970) reported that three-fourths of the patients in his series had some dysfunction of the gastrointestinal tract and a significant incidence of gallstones 12 to 18 months post injury. Since these patients are often young males, gastrointestinal complaints may be overlooked or regarded as functional in origin.

Skeletal

The principal late skeletal complications have consisted of heterotopic bone formation and bone cysts in the extremity amputation stumps, as well as periarticular ectopic calcification. Ectopic calcification about the joints, particularly the elbows, is a well-recognized complication in burns, both thermal and electrical. There is evidence that one causative factor may be iatrogenic, namely, vigorous or forced passive mobilization of joints in the postinjury period.

Heterotopic bone formation and bone cysts in the amputation stumps have occurred in most of the author's patients with high tension injury of the extremity. Both have been a source of difficulty. Bone cysts have become secondarily inflamed and have culminated in sinus tracts. The tracts and cysts have been managed with curettement, packing, and secondary closure and the results were satisfactory. Heterotopic bone formation has produced areas of skin erosion, difficulty with amputee prostheses, and limitation of motion (Clark, Naso, and Ditunno, 1980). Management has consisted of conservative excision where indicated and reinstitution of general range of motion.

RESULTS

Traditionally, exposure to 1000 volts or more is considered a high tension injury. Actually, high tension electrical injuries can usually be further subdivided, on the basis of circumstances and type and distribution of injury, into *flash* and *"true"* high tension burns. The former typically are mixed full- and partial-thickness burns without characteristic entry and/or exit wounds. The voltage in "true" high tension injury is usually considerably greater than 1000 volts. The subdivision of patients in this manner is important clinically, since virtually all amputations and flap procedures are limited to the "true" subgroup. The duration of hospital stay is nearly twice as long in the "true" subgroup (45.7 days) as in the flash subgroup (23.1 days). The incidence of acute renal failure in the series of electrical burns has been 1.5 to 7.5 per cent, and the overall mortality rate from renal failure and sepsis, including clostridial myonecrosis, has been 3 to 14 per cent (Luce and Gottlieb, 1984). With prompt, vigorous resuscitation and early, aggressive debridement, renal failure and death should not occur.

REFERENCES

Almgard, L., Liljedahl, S., and Nylen, B.: Electrical burns of the abdomen. Acta Chir. Scand., *130*:550, 1965.

Artz, C. P.: Changing concepts of electrical injury. Am. J. Surg., *128*:600, 1974.

Baxter, C. R.: Present concepts in the management of major electrical injury. Surg. Clin. North Am., *50*:1401, 1970.

Butler, E. D., and Gant, T. D.: Electrical injuries with special reference to the upper extremities. Am. J. Surg., *134*:95, 1977.

Caffee, H.: Scalp and skull reconstruction after electrical burn. J. Trauma, *20*:87, 1980.

Campbell, J. R., Campbell, T. J., and Fletcher, W. S.: Severe electrical burns. Am. Surg., *35*:779, 1969.

Castren, J. A., and Kytila, J.: Eye symptoms caused by lightning. Acta Ophthalmol., *42*:139, 1964.

Christensen, J. A., Sherman, R. T., Balis, G. A., and Wuamett, J. D.: Delayed neurologic injury secondary to high-voltage current, with recovery. J. Trauma, *20*:166, 1980.

Clark, G. S., Naso, F., and Ditunno, J. F., Jr.: Marked bone spur formation in a burn amputee patient. Arch. Phys. Med. Rehabil., *61*:189, 1980.

Curtin, J. W., Latham, W. D., Greely, P. W., et al.: Catastrophic loss of the scalp and contiguous structures. Plast. Reconstr. Surg., *32*:1, 1963.

DiVincenti, F. C., Moncrief, J. A., and Pruitt, B. A., Jr.: Electrical injuries: a review of sixty-five cases. J. Trauma, *9*:497, 1969.

Esses, S. I., and Peters, W. J.: Electrical burns; pathophysiology and complications. Can. J. Surg., *24*:11, 1981.

Grotting, J., and Walkinshaw, M.: The early use of free flaps in burns. Ann. Plast. Surg., *15*:127, 1985.

Housinger, T. A., Green, L., Shahangian, S., et al.: A prospective study of myocardial damage in electrical injuries. J. Trauma, *25*:122, 1985.

Hunt, J., Lewis, S., Parkey, R., and Baxter, C.: The use of technetium[99m] stannous pyrophosphate scintigraphy to identify muscle damage in acute electrical burns. J. Trauma, *19*:409, 1979.

Hunt, J. L., Mason, A. D., Jr., Masterson, T. S., and Pruitt, B. A., Jr.: Pathophysiology of acute electrical injuries. J. Trauma, *16*:335, 1976.

Hunt, J. L., Sato, R. M., and Baxter, C. R.: Acute electrical burns: current diagnostic and therapeutic approaches to management. Arch. Surg., *115*:434, 1980.

Jaffé, R. H.: Electropathology. Arch. Pathol., *5*:837, 1928.

Jellinek, S.: Causation, pathology, and therapeutics of electrical injuries. Edinburgh Med. J., *43*:587, 1936.

Jex-Blake, A. J.: Death by electric currents and by lightning. Br. Med. J., *1*:425, 1913.

Kragh, L. V., and Erich, J. B.: Treatment of severe electric injuries. Am. J. Surg., *101*:419, 1961.

Laberge, L. C., Ballard, P. A., and Daniel, R. K.: Experimental electrical burns: low voltage. Ann. Plast. Surg., *13*:185, 1984.

Levine, N. S., Atkins, A., McKeel, D. W., Jr., et al.: Spinal cord injury following electrical accidents: case reports. J. Trauma, *15*:459, 1975.

Luce, E. A.: Rehabilitation following electrical injury. Ann. Plast. Surg., *8*:442, 1982.

Luce, E. A., Dowden, W. L., Su, C. T., and Hoopes, J. E.: High tension electrical injury of the upper extremity. Surg. Gynecol. Obstet., *147*:38, 1978.

Luce, E. A., and Gottlieb, S. E.: "True" high-tension electrical injuries. Ann. Plast. Surg., *12*:321, 1984.

Luce, E. A., and Griffen, W. O.: Shotgun injuries of the upper extremity. J. Trauma, *18*:487, 1978.

Luce, E. A., and Hoopes, J. E.: Electrical burn of the scalp and skull. Plast. Reconst. Surg., *54*:359, 1974.

Newsome, T. W.: Visceral injuries: an unusual complication of an electrical burn. Arch. Surg., *105*:494, 1972.

Pruitt, B. A., Jr.: Complications of thermal injury. Clin. Plast. Surg., *1*:667, 1974.

Quinby, W. C., Burke, J. F., Trelstad, R. L., and Caulfield, J.: The use of microscopy as a guide to primary excision of high-tension electrical burns. J. Trauma, *18*:423, 1978.

Robinson, D. W., Masters, F. W., and Forrest, W. J.: Electrical burns: a review and analysis of thirty-three cases. Surgery, *57*:385, 1965.

Robson, M. C., Murphy, R. C., and Heggers, J. P.: A new explanation for the progressive tissue loss. Plast. Reconst. Surg., *73*:431, 1984.

Rouse, R. G., and Dimick, A. R.: Treatment of electrical injury compared to burn injury: a review of pathophysiology in comparison of patient management protocols. J. Trauma, *18*:43, 1978.

Saffle, J. R., Crandall, A., and Warden, G. D.: Cataracts: a long-term complication of electrical injury. J. Trauma, *25*:17, 1985.

Sances, A., Jr., Myklebust, J. B., Larson, S. J., et al.: Experimental electrical injury studies. J. Trauma, *21*:589, 1981.

Silverberg, B., Banis, J. C., Jr., Verdi, G. D., and Acland, R. D.: Microvascular reconstruction after electrical and deep thermal injury. J. Trauma, *26*:128, 1986.

Skoog, T.: Electrical injuries. J. Trauma, *10*:816, 1970.

Solem, L., Fischer, R. P., and Strate, R. G.: The natural history of electrical injury. J. Trauma, *17*:487, 1977.

Stuckey, J. G.: The surgical management of massive electrical burns of the scalp. Plast. Reconst. Surg., *32*:538, 1963.

Sullivan, W. G., Scott, F. A., and Boswick, J. A., Jr.: Rehabilitation following electrical injury to the upper extremity. Ann. Plast. Surg., *7*:347, 1981.

Wilkinson, C., and Wood, M.: High-voltage electrical injury. Am. J. Surg., *136*:693, 1978.

Williams, D. B., and Karl, R. C.: Intestinal injury associated with low-voltage electrocution. J. Trauma, *21*:246, 1981.

Yang, J. Y., Tsai, Y. C., and Noordhoff, M. S.: Electrical burn with visceral injury. Burns, *11*:207, 1985.

25

Stephan Ariyan
Thomas J. Krizek

Radiation Effects: Biologic and Surgical Considerations

On a cold, wintry evening in Bavaria in January, 1896, Rudolph Albert von Kölliker, an 80 year old biologist, stood before a strange machine, placed his hand on the glass part of the machine, and waited as Wilhelm Konrad Roentgen (1845–1923) pressed the electric switch. A red light appeared and a photographic plate was exposed. A few minutes later the picture was developed and showed clearly the bones of von Kölliker's hand against the soft tissue background. When this was reported the next day in the press, the world learned of a "new kind of ray." Because its characteristics were unknown, it was labeled "X"—x-ray.*

Roentgen's discovery (1895) actually occurred several months earlier when he observed a greenish glow near a Crookes tube that had the ability to penetrate solid matter and expose photographic plates. The discovery ushered in the era of modern medicine, provided a diagnostic tool without which some specialties could not exist, and offered a therapeutic modality that has cured disease and alleviated the suffering of untold thousands. However, like many other potent agents, its use may be attended by accidental injury or serious side effects. The first cases of acute radiation dermatitis were reported within a year (Daniel, 1896). Soon thereafter, the effect of chronic exposure to small doses of radiation was noted as skin cancer on the hand of a technician who had been demonstrating this new "x-ray" for four years (Frieben, 1902).

The discovery of additional injuries identified over the years has lead to a high degree of protection for, and awareness on the part of, those likely to be chronically exposed. There remain several circumstances in which the effects of radiation require or influence the care provided by reconstructive surgeons: (1) patients accidentally exposed to high doses of radiation from either industrial accidents or war; (2) patients who require surgery after planned preoperative therapeutic radiation or after radiation therapy failure; (3) patients who develop radiation injury either shortly after or many years after therapeutic radiation.

ETIOLOGY

In contrast to other forms of radiation such as visible light or infrared, the effects of radiation therapy are due to "ionizing radiation." This means simply that photons are

*The origins of "X," the 24th letter of the English alphabet, are unknown before its appearance in the Greek alphabet. In mathematics, the symbol X has long been used to represent the unknown quantity.

delivered that have sufficiently high energy to ionize and disrupt chemical bonds. Photons are small packages of energy, of which there are several types.

Alpha Particles. These particles are relatively large, are positively charged, and are, in fact, helium nuclei. Because of their relatively large mass, they are stopped by 2 to 9 cm of air. None can pass through a thin sheet of paper. Radium and radioactive isotopes, when injected or taken orally, will emit alpha particles into surrounding tissues.

Beta Particles. These are negatively charged particles with very small masses traveling at very high speeds. They are actually electrons. With their high speeds, they may penetrate up to 1 cm of tissue but are easily stopped by thin sheets of metal. They are therapeutically useful in thin and superficial layers of tissue and are used, for example, in the electron beam therapy of mycosis fungoides.

Gamma Rays. These are uncharged photons of energy traveling at the speed of light. They have the ability to penetrate to deep layers of tissue and have a therapeutic value. They are a product of the natural decay of radioactive material, e.g., radium and cobalt-60.

Roentgen or X-rays. These are identical in basic properties with gamma rays, but are produced artificially by the bombardment of electrons onto a tungsten target, from which the x-rays are emitted. For practical purposes, gamma rays and x-rays are the same.

Orthovoltage. Orthovoltage refers to the range of radiation particles whose energy is less than 1 million volts, generated by machines delivering energy in the range of 80,000 to 400,000 volts, or 80 to 400 kilo electron volts (kev).

Supervoltage. Supervoltage describes the range of particles or radiation whose energy exceeds 1 million volts. These are generated by particle accelerators such as the betatron, cyclotron, or linear accelerator. The usual therapeutic range is between 4 and 8 million electron volts (Mev). The recently introduced Sagittaire units deliver energy in excess of 22 million electron volts (Mev).

Brachytherapy. Brachytherapy is the application of radioactive material directly adjacent to or into the tumor that is being treated. While the oldest treatment by this means is by radium, newer methods include the application of seeds or strands incorporating isotopes of iridium-192, iodine-125, cesium-137, or gold-198. The advantage of brachytherapy is that it delivers higher doses directly to the tumor and less to the surrounding tissues because of its lesser penetration (or greater fall-off), which is at the rate of the square of the distance from the radioactive source.

Rad. The rad is the most common unit of measurement in therapeutic radiation. It does not represent the energy that leaves the machine but rather the energy absorbed from the ionizing particles per unit mass of irradiated tissue. This is calculated from the known energy source, the distance to the tissue, and the types of tissue irradiated. One rad represents 100 ergs absorbed per gram of tissue irradiated. This concept of volume of tissue is most important. It is, for example, meaningless to say that a patient who has received 6000 rads to his tongue, 4000 rads to his neck, and 4000 rads to his chest has received 14,000 rads. It is like saying that a five-room house has a temperature of 350°F because the temperature of each room is 70°F. The volume of tissue must be identified.

BIOLOGIC EFFECTS

The total effect of radiation on tissues is not thoroughly understood. Ionizing radiation damages biologic material in a unique way, unlike mechanical, thermal, or chemical injury, and it is probably a confusing misnomer to label it a "burn." The effects at the molecular level are both random and an "all or none" phenomenon. The resultant damage to a cell is determined by the relative importance of the destroyed molecule to the function of the cell. In the dose ranges employed clinically (1000 to 10,000 rads), the biologically significant damage is that which occurs to DNA. Most of this damage can be repaired, and enzymatic processes may continue. However, genetic information is lost, and the cell loses its ability to divide indefinitely and produce a clone.

The clinical significance of this is clear. At doses 100 to 1000 times the usual therapeutic dose, rapid dissolution of cells occurs, and there are early gross and microscopic alterations in tissue. In the therapeutic range, there are no such clinical or microscopic changes until that time at which the injured cells attempt to divide, often many weeks later. In rapidly dividing cell populations, such as lymphocytes or intestinal mucosal cells, the effects may be manifest within hours or days. In populations of cells such as neurons or striated muscle that do not normally reproduce, even though the radiation may have destroyed the same genetic information in the DNA, the effect is never clinically or microscopically observed since the cell usually does not replicate. These tissues are therefore said to be "radioresistant."

However, it is emphasized that these "kills" are random events that hit normal cells as well as tumor cells. If we conceive of a room (a tumor) full of red balloons (tumor cells) and blue balloons (normal cells), and place ourselves in one corner with a bushel basket full of darts (rads), we have an appropriate analogy. As we stand blindfolded throwing darts (rads), we will begin breaking balloons. In the beginning we will break many red balloons (tumor cells), and after 1000 darts (rads) we will have broken 90 per cent of them, and some blue balloons (normal cells) as well. After another 1000 darts (rads) we will have destroyed another 90 per cent of what remains. Therefore, success is based solely on random chance. If the room (tumor size) is small, the red balloons (tumor cells) few, and the darts (rads) many, we will frequently succeed. Conversely, if the room is large, we will be only partially successful.

The ability of tissue to repair itself after radiation injury is related entirely to the population of surviving cells. The biology of tumors is such that the tumor cells are turning over more slowly and are less numerous than the surrounding normal tissue. Since they are more numerous and have a rapid turnover rate, the surrounding normal cells are able to repopulate the area and allow healing to occur, even though some of their population has been destroyed in the same random fashion as tumor cells. If this were not the case, all therapeutic radiation of tumors would result in a residual open wound as the tumor disappeared.

Diagnosis

A complete description of the problem or injury related to radiation requires documentation of a number of factors. The evaluation should include (1) a description of the area or region that has been exposed to radiation; (2) an assessment of the total dose that has been absorbed by the tissue; (3) the duration of the exposure to the radiation (hours, days, weeks); and (4) a description of the source of the radiation.

For example, when a patient who has received therapeutic radiation to a tongue neoplasm is being evaluated, an appropriate description would be that the patient received "6000 rads to his oral cavity and upper neck, in 30 treatments over a 40 day period, using a 6 Mev linear accelerator, ending three months ago."

Systemic Effects

In contrast to radiation administered to local areas of the body, intense whole body radiation, as in those who were exposed to the atomic bombs, results in "radiation sickness." The latter may be separated into three phases—prodromal, latent, and main.

Prodromal Phase. This phase is characterized by gastrointestinal symptoms of anorexia, nausea, vomiting, and diarrhea. The dose necessary to cause the symptoms varies among individuals but is in the range of 50 rads total body dosage.

Latent Phase. This is the time necessary for the depletion of cells irreparably damaged by the radiation. It is only after this interval that the sustained disturbances are manifest. The rapidity with which the cells are depleted depends on the dose and the tissues involved, and this period may last hours to weeks.

Main Phase. This phase of the syndrome begins as the effects of the depletion of the cells during the latent phase become clinically manifest. The degree depends on the number of immature cells remaining to preserve or restore function. However, severe radiation damage to the brain or cardiovascular systems (20,000 rads) may result in death within minutes to hours. In the absence of such damage, death in severe injuries usually results from irreparable bone marrow or intestinal injury. It is estimated that 2000 rads to the whole body results in fatal enteritis within two weeks (Upton, 1968). Damage to the other tissues is usually of secondary importance in such severe radiation injuries.

Local Effects

The local effects of radiation injury may be grouped for purposes of discussion into three major categories: acute, subacute, and chronic radiation injury.

Acute Radiation Injury. Acute radiation injury is usually the result of accidental injury, such as in industry, and most often involves orthovoltage radiation. Exposure to a high dose of radiation in a short time (for example, 5000 to 10,000 rads in one day) produces injury of the skin and local tissues that resembles thermal burns in appearance but differs from burns by evolving more slowly and deeply. These changes were well described in a treatise by Warren (1943). The basal cells, which must divide regularly to maintain the epidermis, are damaged and show mitotic derangement immediately. In response to this injury, a transitory erythema may develop within minutes and may recur in cyclic waves. The recurrent nature of the erythema is not well understood.

The erythema is soon accompanied by edema, itching, and pain. These findings are followed by "dry desquamation" (scaling and flaking), "wet desquamation" (blistering and weeping), and sloughing and ulceration of the skin. There may be ischemic necrosis of the underlying tissue, as well as progressive, diffuse, obliterative endarteritis (Knowlton and associates, 1949; Upton, 1968). The chronic vasculitis causes pain of an unrelenting nature. The most serious sequelae to the vasculitis are progressive tissue ischemia, secondary infection, and necrosis.

Subacute Radiation Injury. This may result from the administration of repeated doses of lower intensity radiation over a longer period. There is also an erythema of the skin with associated edema. Mucous membranes may become inflamed. There is usually no ulceration or necrosis, and the edema and erythema subside over several weeks. After several months, the skin and subcutaneous tissue become thickened and harden into a "woody induration"; the skin subsequently develops a darker pigmentation. These changes are usually seen in the therapeutic ranges of radiation therapy, particularly when it has been delivered by orthovoltage machines.

Several authors have performed histologic studies of vessels within irradiated fields. Sams (1965) and Watson (1979) have described thickening of the walls of these vessels, increased deposition of collagen, and fragmentation of the elastic lamina. Guelinckx and associates (1984) not only reported thickening of the vessel walls, but also demonstrated dehiscence of the endothelial cells by scanning electron microscopy; furthermore, their studies illustrated microthrombi and fibrin depositions in irradiated vessels. These studies show that, although the radiated tissues are abundant in the number of vessels present in these tissues, the vessel walls have fibrosis and do not permit adequate diffusion of nutrients, antibiotics, and antibodies.

Chronic Radiation Injury. Chronic radiation damage results from repeated exposures to low dose radiation, often over an extended period. It has historically occurred as an occupational hazard among x-ray technicians and dentists. It can also be observed many years later in those who received therapeutic radiation, often tragically, for benign disease. The chronic changes may progress to the most serious of sequelae, namely malignant transformation of skin, soft tissue, or bone.

The histologic changes that occur through these phases are the same as those for acute and subacute radiation injury, but vary in the time of evolution and the intensity with the type of injury (Allen, 1954). Changes in the epidermis include early swelling of the prickle cell layer, edema of the basal cell layer, and increased melanin production. Large nuclei first appear, followed by development of hyperkeratosis, acanthosis, and finally atrophy of the epidermis. The effects on the dermis are even more profound. In the acute phase there is edema and vesiculation of the upper dermis, which may lead to separation of the epidermis or subsequent dense scarring. There is progressive atrophy of the hair follicles, sebaceous glands, and eccrine glands. Loss of elastic fibers and severe fibrosis may also be observed.

The most profound changes, and those of greatest concern to the surgeon, are the alterations in vascularity. An initial vasodilatation is followed by fibrinoid necrosis of the vessel walls and thromboses. The end result is an obliterative endarteritis with chronic ischemia. The vascular changes pose the greatest challenge to the reconstructive surgeon.

The effects of surgery are permanent ... the effects of radiation are permanent, continuous, and progressive.

ANONYMOUS

Infections

Over the years, the clinical experience of surgery within irradiated tissue has demonstrated a high incidence of wound infections. This is particularly true in the head and neck area because the oral cavity is an abundant reservoir of virulent bacteria, with counts in the range of 10^7 to 10^8 organisms per ml (Richardson and Jones, 1958). The infections observed after surgery in the head and neck area are rarely a result of bacterial invasion from the outside, but rather a disruption in the balance between the local bacterial flora and the host defense mechanisms. The incidence of wound infections following composite resections of intraoral tumors combined with neck dissections has been reported to be as high as 60 to 65 per cent (Ketcham and associates, 1969; Kerth, Sisson, and Becker, 1973).

A study investigating the effects of surgery within previously irradiated tissue demonstrated that irradiated tissue could not tolerate bacterial contamination as well as normal tissue (Ariyan and associates, 1980). In this study of 144 rats wounded at various intervals after a single dose of 1050 rads (the biologic equivalent of 4000 rads in divided doses) or 1800 rads (biologic equivalent of 6000 rads in divided doses), there was satisfactory wound healing without evidence of infection in 80 to 100 per cent of each of the groups (Fig. 25–1). However, a larger number of animals whose wounds were contaminated with 10^4 *Staphylococcus aureus* demonstrated infection rates as high as 67 per cent (Fig. 25–2). The incidence of infections in this study rose significantly with the increasing dose of radiation and with the increasing interval from radiation to wounding.

Many factors contributed to this finding, but the most important one was believed to be the alteration in vascularity caused by the radiation. In an effort to determine whether antibiotics could diffuse effectively into the radiated tissues, a study was conducted on the effects of systemic treatment with gentamicin of the rats wounded and contaminated with the same investigative model (Cruz and associates, 1984). While the tissue levels of antibiotics were found to be equal in both the irradiated and nonirradiated skin at five weeks after radiation, these levels were found to decrease to 70 per cent of control levels at 10 weeks, and to 40 per cent of control levels at 15 weeks.

Therefore, in the event of a wound infection within a heavily irradiated tissue site, the resultant wound must be treated topically, because systemic antibiotics do not diffuse into the infected radiated bed. The wound should be debrided surgically and opened for proper drainage. Under most circumstances the wound should be treated by topical application of antibacterials that are known to penetrate tissue and eschar, such as silver sulfadiazine (Silvadene) cream, to obtain lo-

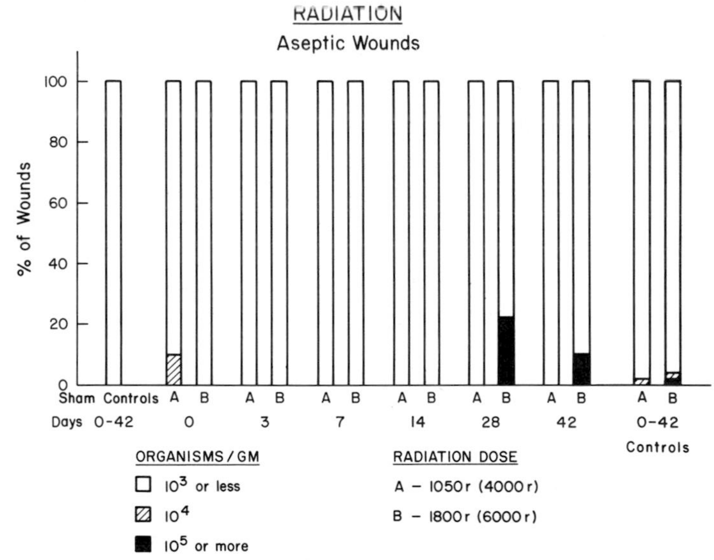

Figure 25–1. Bacterial counts of aseptic wounds made at various intervals after radiation therapy to the skin of rats. (From Ariyan, S., et al.: Plast. Reconstr. Surg., *65*:328, 1980.)

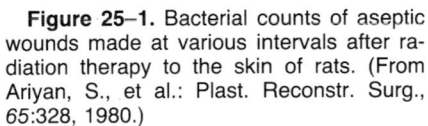

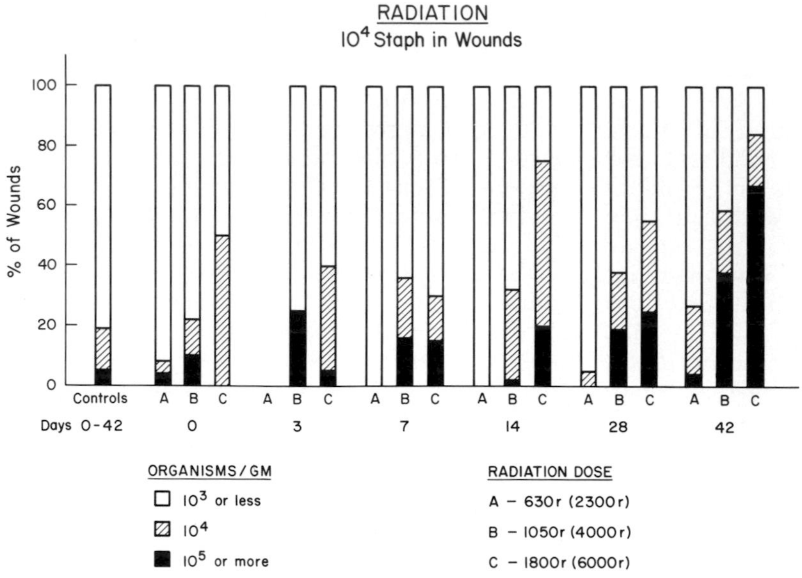

Figure 25–2. Distribution of bacterial counts of wounds contaminated with 10^4 *S. aureus* at various intervals after radiation therapy to the skin of rats. (From Ariyan, S., et al.: Plast. Reconstr. Surg., *65*:328, 1980.)

cal control of the bacterial contamination. Once the bacterial counts of the wound are reduced to levels below 10^5 organisms per gram of tissue, the wounds are ready for surgical coverage. If there is a satisfactory vascular bed at that time, a skin graft may be sufficient, otherwise the wounds require coverage by well-vascularized muscle flaps.

Malignant Transformation

Ionizing radiation not only cures cancer but also may cause it. The conditions that set the stage for malignant transformation may be chronic inflammation, chronic exposure to radiation, or a combination of these. Laboratory studies in animals have suggested a cocarcinogenic effect of inflammation and radiation. Radiation administered to wounds chronically infected with bacteria (Lacassagne and Vinzent, 1929a,b) or chronically inflamed by sterile foreign bodies (Lacassagne, 1933; Burrows and Clarkson, 1943) has led to the development of sarcomas, whereas none developed in control animals exposed to radiation alone.

Chronic or repeated exposure to radiation has also been shown to have a carcinogenic effect on tissues. This phenomenon was demonstrated by Hoffman (1925), Martland, Conlon, and Knef (1925), and Martland (1931) in radium watch dial painters who were exposed to repeated bombardment by alpha particles. The dial painters swallowed the radium in the fluorescent paint when they pointed the brush tips on their tongues. The radium was absorbed and deposited in bones and emitted radioactive alpha particles continuously. High levels of radiation located in the paranasal sinuses apparently disposed to malignancy in the mucous membranes of the sinuses (Fig. 25–3) (Warren, 1970). Warren also felt that this type of carcinogenesis, resulting from the chronic inhalation of radioactive gas in the air, was the cause of the bronchogenic carcinomas seen in the uranium miners of Colorado and the pitchblende miners of Europe (Ludewig and Lorenser, 1924). In addition, it has been noted that individuals receiving repeated small doses of radiation over long periods, such as physicians, dentists, radiologists, and technicians, have a higher incidence of skin cancer (Teloh, Mason, and Wheelock, 1950; Hueper, 1954) as well as leukemia (Ulrich, 1946; Warren, 1956; March, 1961).

Acute or short-term exposure may also be associated with malignant transformation of the tissue within the irradiated field. Through the joint efforts of the Atomic Bomb Casualty Commission of the United States and the Japanese National Institute of Health, extensive studies, conducted over 25 years, of the Japanese survivors of the atomic bombs have led to the conclusion that there is a greater incidence of leukemia and thyroid carcinoma among the people exposed to radiation (Brill, Tomonaga, and Heyssel, 1962; Socolow and associates, 1963; Zeldis, Jablon,

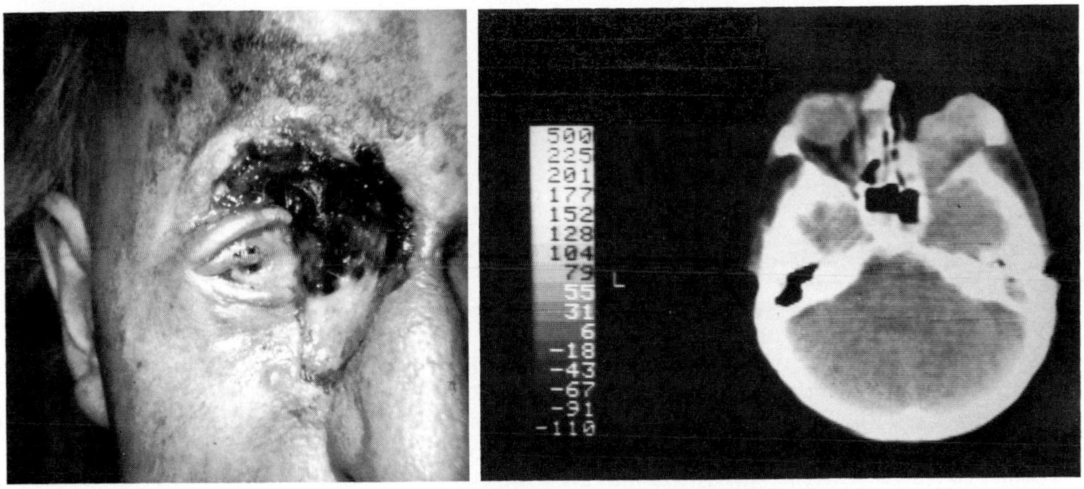

Figure 25–3. *Left,* A former radium watch dial painter who had developed epidermoid carcinoma in the ethmoid sinuses had been treated unsuccessfully with radiation therapy. Breakdown of tissue and secondary infection of the persistent periorbital cancer resulted. *Right,* A CT scan shows the extent of the tumor and periorbital tissue invasion. (From Ariyan, S., and Krizek, T.J.: Reconstruction after resection of head and neck cancer. Ciné Clinics, Clinical Congress of the American College of Surgeons, Dallas,1977.)

and Ishida, 1964; Miller, 1969). Nevertheless, there is still discussion regarding the atomic bomb survivors, because the bombs dropped at the two Japanese cities were not the same. Owing to differences in bomb structures, the Nagasaki bomb released gamma rays, while the Hiroshima bomb released both gamma rays and neutrons; neutrons produce greater damage per unit tissue than gamma rays, and indeed the incidence of cancers per dose of exposure was found to be higher from the Hiroshima bomb (Finch, 1979).

Radiation therapy from orthovoltage x-ray machines was used in the 1920's to treat children with enlarged thymus, tonsils, and adenoids. Simpson and Hempelmann (1957) studied these children and found an association between thyroid carcinoma and the radiation treatment of thymic enlargement. Well-controlled reviews (Pifer and associates, 1963; Toyooka and associates, 1963) of 2800 children treated with x-rays for thymic enlargement between 1926 and 1957 in an upstate New York county revealed a significantly higher frequency of thyroid carcinoma and leukemia than in untreated siblings or in the general population of children in the same area. In longer follow-up studies, several authors (Hempelmann and associates, 1975; Favus and associates, 1976; Shore and associates, 1980) found that both benign and malignant nodules developed among the irradiated patients, but only a few benign adenomas and no malignancies among the nonirradiated siblings.

Finally, clinical surveys of cohort studies have demonstrated a higher incidence of salivary gland tumors among the Japanese atomic bomb survivors (Takeichi and associates, 1983). This relationship between radiation and salivary gland tumors has been further elaborated by the demonstration of the latter developing among patients treated with radiation to the head and neck during childhood (Schneider and associates, 1977; Katz and Preston-Martin, 1984).

The potential for malignant transformation of soft tissue and bone in an area of radiation injury is of particular concern. Although the skin and soft tissue may be surgically replaced in the event of malignant transformation, it may be hazardous if the danger of subsequent development of osteogenic sarcoma in the underlying irradiated bone is high. A review of the 129 cases of osteogenic sarcoma following radiation reported in the literature indicates that the chances of malignant transformation must be very small (Krizek and Ariyan, 1973). Among these cases, 20 followed radium ingestion (radium dial painters), 35 followed radiation for chronic inflammation (co-carcinogenic effect), and 74 followed treatment of benign or malignant neoplasm. However, as Kilgore and

Abbott (1938) have emphasized, a diagnosis of malignant transformation must not be considered unless histologic evidence of nonmalignancy has been obtained before radiation. In fact, Cahan and associates (1948) have listed several criteria that should be operative before one considers radiation to be responsible for malignant transformation (Table 25–1). It is clear from this list that all but 20 of the reported 129 cases of osteogenic sarcoma did *not* meet the criteria.

Osteogenic sarcoma is among the least common forms of cancer, with an incidence in the normal population of one per 100,000 (Hatfield and Schulz, 1970; Warren, 1970). In fact, Warren (1970) emphasized that this rate had been decreasing over the previous 20 years, at a time when radiation fallout had been increasing. Burch (1960) and Newcombe (1957) attempted to extrapolate the incidence of carcinogenesis but were unsuccessful because the data were too scanty. Compared with the millions of people exposed to or treated by radiation who have survived a long latent period, the incidence must be small, if it is indeed any higher than the incidence of such sarcomas in the population at large.

Osteoradionecrosis

Since first described in 1926 by Ewing, osteoradionecrosis ("radiation osteitis") has been a dilemma for both radiotherapist and surgeon. Ewing believed that the changes observed in bone, particularly in the mandible and pelvis, were related to vascular damage, rendering the bones more susceptible to infection and trauma. Several reviews indicate that this problem has been in no way resolved by newer treatment techniques and modalities for delivering radiation (Bragg and associates, 1970; Kim and associates, 1974), and an incidence of mandibular osteoradionecrosis as high as 10 to 30 per cent has been reported for head and neck cancer patients treated by radiation (Rankow and Weissman, 1971). Although the influence of infection and trauma are probably operative, the changes in vascularity appear to be of paramount importance.

Table 25–1. Cahan's Criteria for Malignant Transformation

1. There should be histologic evidence that no malignancy was present before the radiation
2. The malignancy must occur within the field exposed to radiation
3. There should be a reasonable latent period (generally more than ten years)
4. The malignant change should be confirmed histologically

In addition to the dose of radiation, other factors influencing the development of mandibular radionecrosis include the size of the tumor treated, the proximity of the tumor to bone, the state of oral hygiene, and the number of dental extractions. Exposure of the bone to the oral cavity during or after radiation therapy is a common prelude to radionecrosis (Fig. 25–4). When dental extractions are accomplished and healing is proceeding before radiation, and when oral hygiene is meticulously maintained during radiation, the chances of radionecrosis are dramatically reduced. The most important surgical contribution to the prevention of osteoradionecrosis is adequate soft tissue coverage over the affected bone.

PRINCIPLES OF TREATMENT

There are several distinct circumstances in which the surgeon is called upon to treat the effects produced by radiation. The approach varies, depending on the nature of the problem, the anatomic site of involvement, and the phase of the injury (acute, subacute, or chronic). The most common categories of clinical problems are outlined below, and several illustrative cases are presented:

1. Acute radiation injury.
2. Planned surgery after therapeutic radiation.
3. Radiation ulcers.
4. Malignant transformation.

Acute Radiation Injury

Acute radiation injury is most often due to an industrial accident and usually involves the extremities, particularly the hands. The diagnosis is critical. To establish a diagnosis, the amount of radiation to the total body and to the involved local tissues should be known. The assistance of a radiation therapist and a radiation physicist is mandatory. The circumstances of the injury are reconstructed, the time of exposure estimated, and dosimetry studies carried out (often with water phantoms). Data usually indicate the amount of radiation absorbed per volume of tissue. For

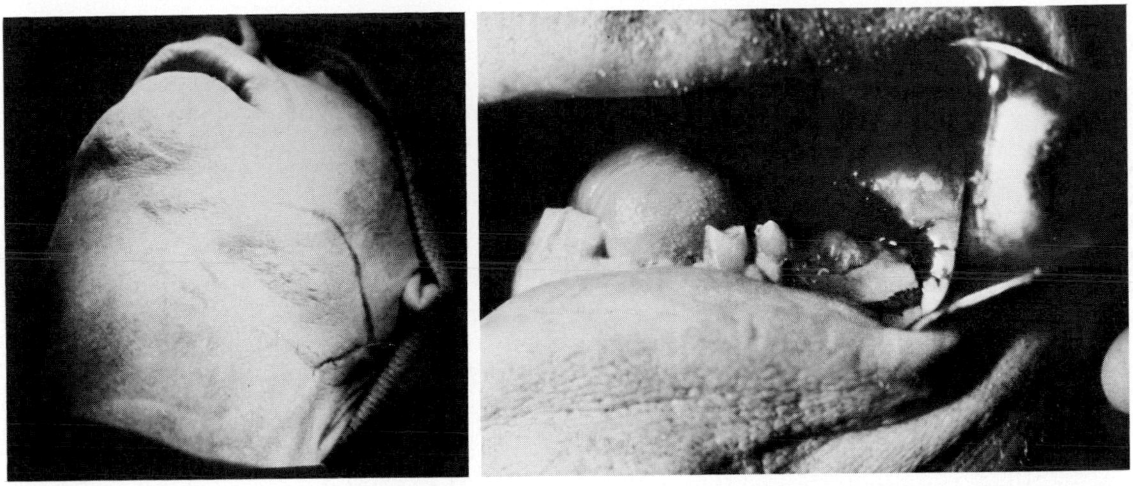

Figure 25–4. Osteoradionecrosis of the jaw with breakdown of the overlying skin *(left)* is invariably associated with an intraoral breakdown of mucosal lining and exposure of the bone *(right)* to the intraoral flora of virulent bacteria.

example, in the cases subsequently illustrated, such studies provided information about surface dose and exposure of underlying soft tissue and bone. The management of total body radiation is nonsurgical and beyond the scope of this chapter.

The initial approach is conservative. The local effects of radiation are progressive, and the extent of injury may not be readily apparent during the early phase. The outstanding clinical finding is pain, to such a degree that hospitalization is mandatory. Large doses of narcotics and sedatives are required, and narcotic addiction is a not uncommon sequela of the injury. Local skin care with bland ointments and steroid creams may provide some relief.

Since these injuries often involve the hands, the traditional principles of managing the acute injured hand should not be ignored simply because the injury is from radiation. Splinting is often necessary to maintain position: the metacarpophalangeal joints in full flexion and interphalangeal joints in extension, with the wrist above the neutral position. Splinting maintains position, but it is motion that preserves function; hydrotherapy and range of motion exercises are mandatory, even in the face of severe pain.

The conservative approach may be all that is required, and Brown, McDowell, and Fryer (1949a,b) and Brown and Fryer (1956, 1957, 1965) have reported large series of patients so managed. However, in more severe injuries, skin breakdown begins in the first few weeks post injury. Open wounds, secondary infection, and ischemia potentially set in motion recurrent cycles of ulcer formation, infection, and necrosis, leading finally to gangrene. Lanzl, Rozenfeld, and Tarlov (1967) have predicted the inevitability of this cycle and progression and have advised early amputation. Infection appears to be the key factor in triggering the cycle: an ischemic wound, infected often with *Pseudomonas aeruginosa*, not unlike that seen in thermal burns. The ischemic wound, isolated from the bloodstream (and from systemically administered antibiotics), should be treated like a burn with appropriate *topical* antibacterials.

No surgery is indicated until the wound passes into the subacute phase, characterized by the disappearance of much of the erythema and edema. At such time, wide excision of the involved tissue should be accomplished. Even the margins and the bed, admittedly, will also have been exposed to radiation. Since there is some evidence that this tissue, although viable and still vascular, has a diminished resistance to infection, systemic antibiotics may be helpful before, during, and for 48 hours after surgery.

The sine qua non of successful management is adequate soft tissue coverage. Except in the most exceptional circumstances, in which tendons, bone, or joints are actually exposed, the use of split-thickness skin grafts is still the treatment of choice. Since bleeding from these wounds may be troublesome and difficult to control, a delayed grafting technique may be employed, unless one is very confident of hemostasis. The open wound is covered with a biologic dressing (allograft or xenograft), and the patient is returned to the operating room in 24 to 48 hours for the definitive application of skin grafts. The grafts should be of medium thickness and without "pie-crusting"; mesh grafts have no place in the treatment of radiation lesions because the wound bed in the interstices may desiccate if not covered with tissue and will not support the migration of epithelial cells across the small defects. Postoperative care is similar to that for a thermal burn, and in the case of the hand, motion should be started by the fifth postoperative day. The most remarkable feature of the treatment is the immediate, dramatic relief of pain that the patient experiences after the removal of the injured tissue and coverage with skin.

The patient deserves a conscientious follow-up. Although the incidence of osteogenic sarcoma is small, routine radiologic examination of the part is indicated. The early radiographic changes occasionally seen in the bones may be due to disuse atrophy, not to osteoradionecrosis, and may totally revert to a normal appearance after adequate resurfacing.

Case 1: Acute Radiation Injury of the Hand (19,500 Rads). A 43 year old male was exposed to 19,500 rads (dominant right hand) over several hours from a faulty industrial 110-kev fluoroscope. This dosage of exposure was calculated from water phantom studies at the industrial machine through the assistance of radiophysicists. He initially complained of "dermatitis," with itching and erythema over the dorsum of his index and middle fingers, symptoms that occurred within a few hours. There were further signs of radiation injury, with pain and breakdown of the skin over the subsequent ten days.

Before the surgical consultation, the patient had been treated by immobilization of the hand. The hand was treated with topical antibiotics, which resulted in healing of the weeping wounds, only to be followed by local skin breakdown (Fig. 25–5). At the time of surgical consultation three months after injury, he had essentially no range of motion in the index finger and little motion in the middle finger. A biopsy showed ulceration and fibrinoid necrosis with vascular dilatation and arteriolar thickening (Fig. 25–6), findings usually seen in radionecrosis.

The patient was initially treated with analgesics and whirlpool therapy, accompanied by active and passive range of motion exercises. The hand was placed in a dynamic splint, with improvement of the range of motion. Two weeks after this therapy began, excision of the skin over the dorsum of the index and middle fingers and about half of the dorsum of the hand was accomplished. Active bleeding was observed in the wound bed, which was covered with a medium-sized split-thickness skin graft.

Motion was again instituted with physical therapy after surgery, and the patient returned to work two months following surgery. At the end of one year, he had full range of motion.

The radiographic appearance of the hand before surgery (Fig. 25–7) revealed demineralization and cystic degeneration, particularly adjacent to the interphalangeal joints. The findings were interpreted as being typical of osteoradionecrosis. Four months later, after motion had been restored and the wounds were healed, the radiographs were interpreted as being normal.

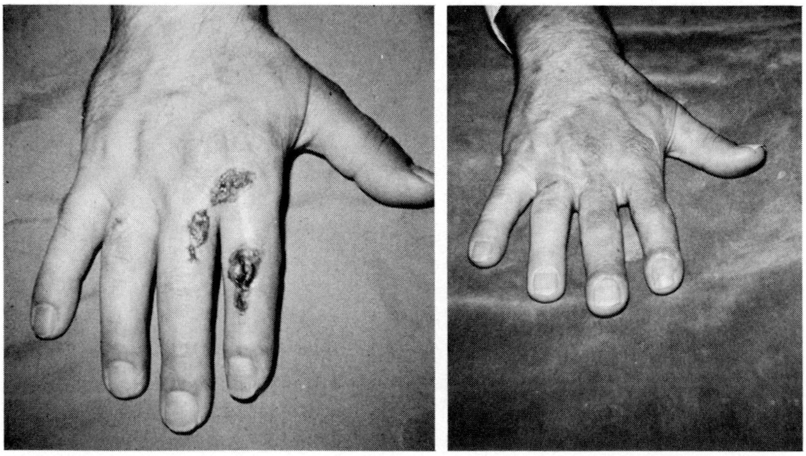

Figure 25–5. *Left,* A massive radiation injury from industrial exposure of the hand to 19,500 rads over a few hours. *Right,* Fifteen year follow-up after surgical debridement of the wound, and coverage with split-thickness skin grafts. There is no evidence of malignant transformation.

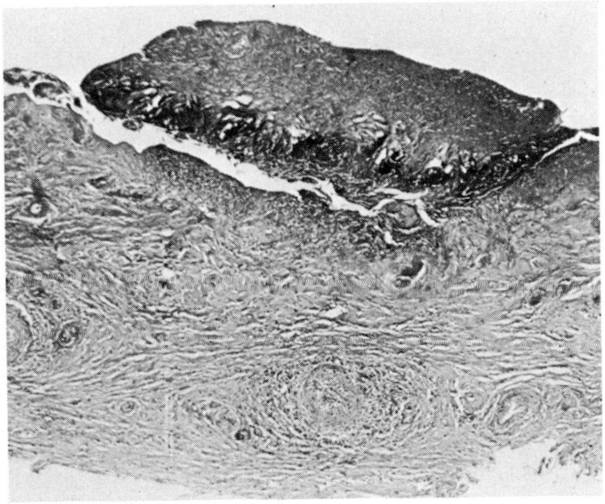

Figure 25–6. Histologic appearance of radiation injury with fibrinoid necrosis, vascular dilatation, and arteriolar thickening (see Fig. 25–5).

The patient was at work 15 years after injury with a functional hand. Occasional arthritic-type pain is relieved with salicylates, and the radiographs remain normal.

Case 2: Acute Radiation Injury of the Hand (250,000 Rads). A second patient, involved with the same faulty machine as in Case 1, was a 45 year old female who was exposed to 250,000 rads to both hands over a period of less than three hours. Additional calculations showed that a dose of 25,000 rads had been absorbed by the bone. She was initially treated in the same manner as the other patient before her transfer for surgical care, three months after the injuries. She had constant and excruciating pain and dry erythematous dermatitis over the dorsum of both index fingers and the tip of the left thumb (Fig. 25–8).

The patient was treated with active and passive range of motion exercises in a whirlpool. The involved skin was excised down to the extensor mechanism over the dorsum of the right index and middle fingers; part of the dorsum of the hand was also resected. Since the tendons were exposed and the blood supply of the bed did not appear satisfactory, the wound was covered with a deltopectoral

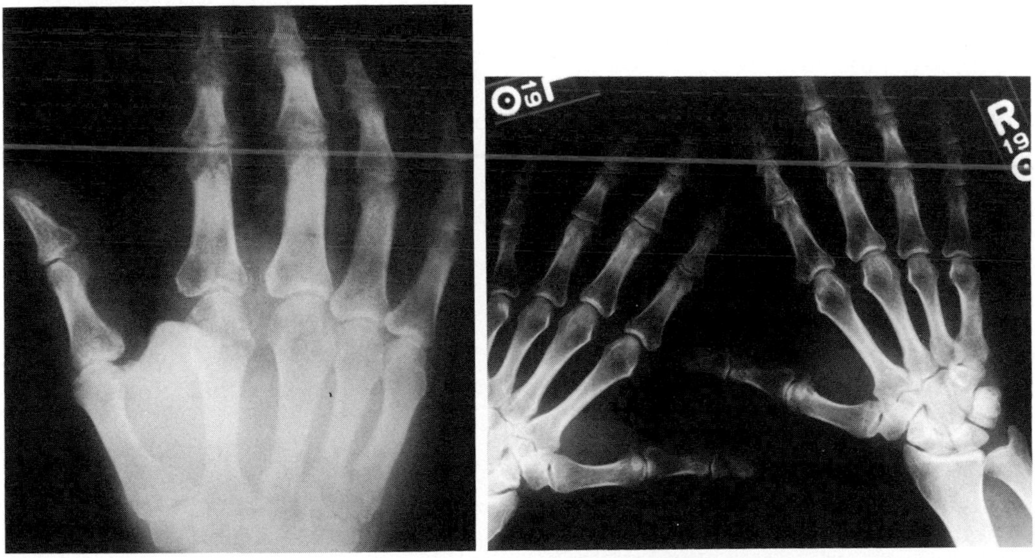

Figure 25–7. Preoperative radiograph of the hand *(left)* reveals demineralization, which was interpreted as evidence of osteoradionecrosis (see Fig. 25–5). Postoperative follow-up x-rays of the hand after motion and function were restored *(right)* revealed normally calcified bones.

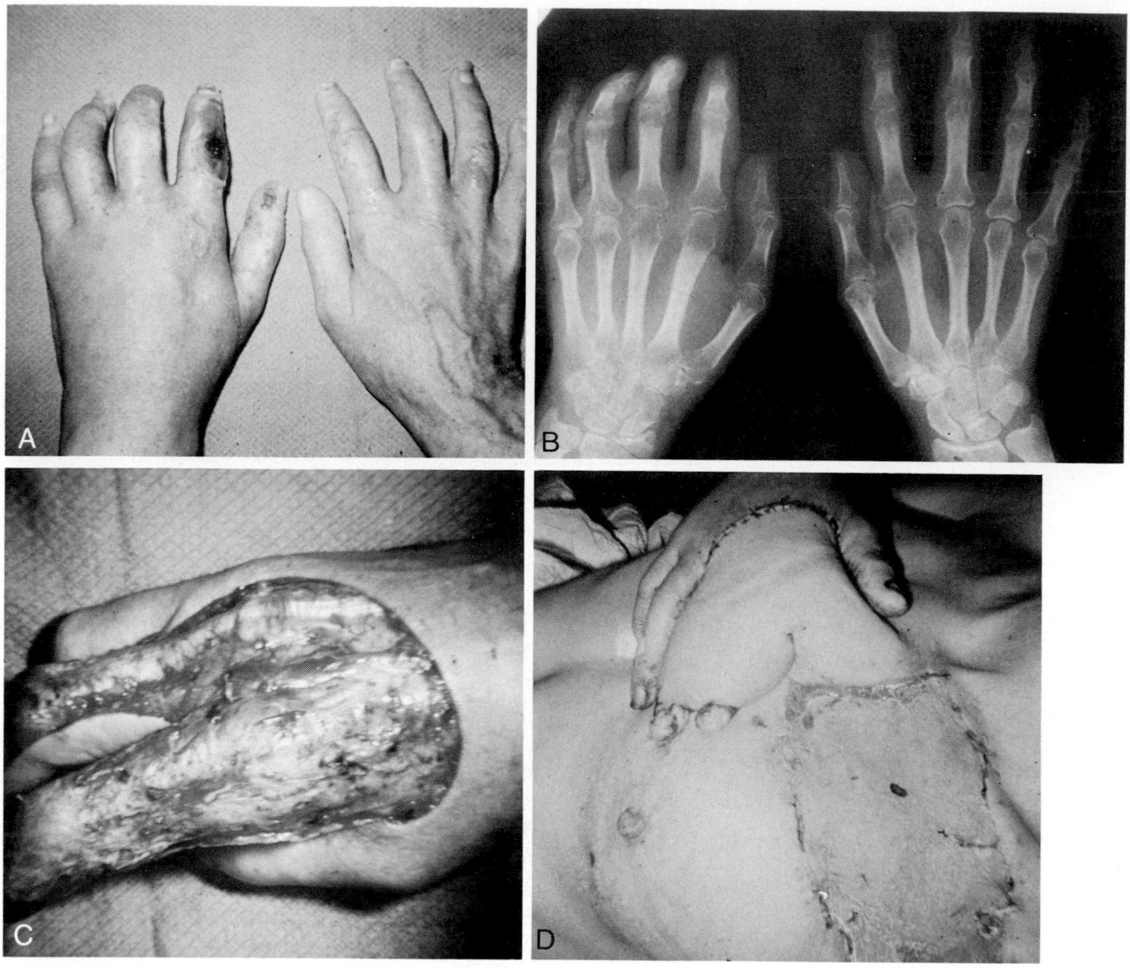

Figure 25–8. *A,* Massive radiation injury of both hands three months after exposure to 250,000 rads. *B,* X-rays demonstrating demineralization of the bones. *C,* Appearance following excision of the damaged skin. *D,* Because of exposure of tendons and poor bleeding from the wound bed, the defect was covered with a cutaneous flap.

flap. Following excision of the ischemic tissue and covering of the wound, there was immediate and complete relief of pain.

Six weeks later, with return of functional range of motion to the right hand, the left hand was surgically treated. Since the ulceration of the left index finger involved not only the cutaneous surface but also the extensor tendon mechanism and the joint, a ray amputation was performed. In addition, the skin was removed over the thumb, first web space, and dorsum of the hand. The wound was covered with a deltopectoral flap from the contralateral side.

After division, the flaps of both hands were revised and subsequently defatted. There was gradual increase in the ranges of motion in both hands. Postoperative x-rays showed no evidence of inflammatory or necrotic changes of the bone. An arteriogram performed just before surgery had demonstrated marked diminution of flow to the digital arteries, and the presence of precapillary arteriovenous shunts (Fig. 25–9). One year later, however, a repeat arteriogram showed revascularization and satisfactory blood flow throughout the hand.

Surgery After Radiation Therapy

Therapeutic radiation followed by definitive surgery is a common approach to the management of head and neck cancer in many centers. The rationale is predicated on the reasoning that surgical failures in head and neck cancer are related to an inability to provide adequate margins of resection, while

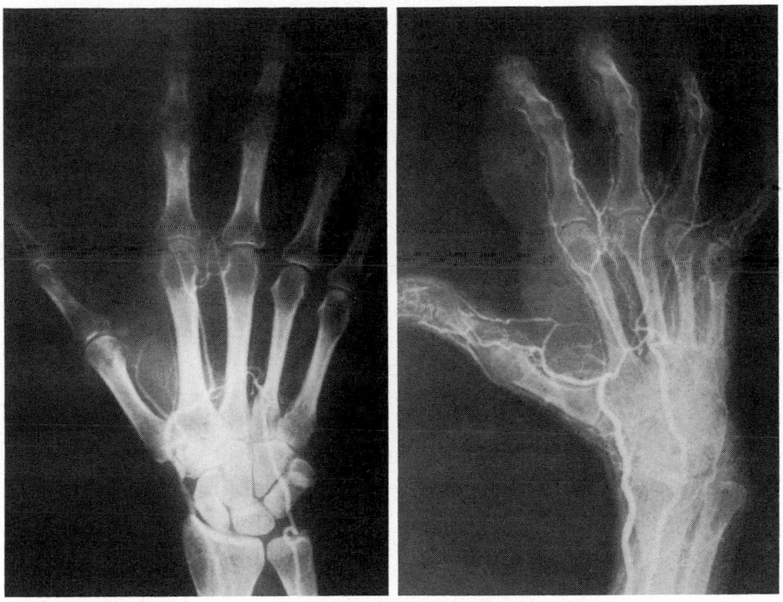

Figure 25–9. Arteriogram of the right hand of the patient in Fig. 25–8. The preoperative study *(left)* shows vasculitis and poor circulatory flow. The arteriogram at one year after resurfacing with a flap *(right)* shows normal vasculature.

radiation therapy fails because of an inability to control the large volume of tumor located centrally.

An understanding of radiation biology and radiation effects provides the basis for the surgical approach in these circumstances. Several principles are involved:

1. Radiation therapy may reduce bulk and render it technically feasible to remove "inoperable" cancers; it does not make them more curable.

2. The volume of tissue that must be removed for cure is exactly the same after radiation therapy as it was before treatment.

3. The rate of disappearance, or lack of shrinkage in tumor size, has nothing to do with the tumor's "response" to radiation.

4. The surgical approach to head and neck cancer must be altered when operating in radiated fields.

As discussed earlier in the chapter, the treatment of tumors with radiation therapy is analogous to throwing darts in a room full of balloons. At the beginning many balloons burst with few darts, but as there are less balloons remaining, few balloons will burst with many darts. Therefore, if the room (tumor size) is small, the balloons (cells) few, and the darts (rads) many, we always succeed. Conversely, if the room is large, we are only partially successful. The same is true of tumors. By random chance, each 1000 rads kills about 90 per cent of cells, and 4000 rads achieves 99.9 per cent success. However, as in the room, the *volume* in which the cells are contained does not change, and the cells may well be anywhere in that volume. For that reason, if the tumor was too large to operate on for cure before treatment, it probably remains so.

Likewise, the appearance of the tumor means little. If it is rapidly dividing, it may disappear quickly, and if 90 per cent of the tumor cells are killed following each 1000 rads, it may disappear completely. The more anaplastic a tumor is, the more rapidly it divides (disappears). However, no squamous cell cancer is ever cured with much less than 6000 rads. If it is dividing slowly, it may remain unchanged throughout the entire course of treatment, even though it may be cured.

If one makes the decision to employ radiation therapy, it should be recognized that curability by surgery and the operation required for this should be determined *before* radiation therapy. Evaluation during therapy is deceptive because the rate of tumor disappearance is deceptive. Finally, the surgical approach must be altered because of changes in the tissues.

As the evolution of the radiation effect is developing as outlined above, the acute, edematous phase is the least favorable time for surgery. At this time, bleeding is extensive and the tissues are prone to infection. Like any acutely inflamed tissue, meaningful fibroplasia does not occur until the inflammation subsides. In addition, the chronic phase of radiation injury is one of ischemia and dense fibroplasia, another period unfavorable for surgery. Timing is therefore critical, and the surgery should be performed after the acute inflammation subsides but before the time of dense fibroplasia and ischemia (and also before the tumor begins to recover and grow again). An adequate rule of thumb is to wait a week for each week during which therapy was administered.

The principles of surgery that are altered by radiation therapy include the following:

1. The use of primary closure in the mouth or in the hypopharynx should be restricted to those situations in which there is no tension on the suture line.

2. Flap tissue (local, cutaneous, myocutaneous) should be used whenever the defect does not allow closure without tension, or when there is exposed bone (Fig. 25–10).

3. Skin grafts should be employed only in areas that are not mobile (e.g., maxillary defects, cheek).

4. Neck dissection should be made through incisions that do not require a closure along the carotid artery.

5. Radiated tissue has diminished resistance to infection, and systemic antibiotics may be helpful even though the dose delivered may be significantly less in the radiated tissue.

6. Immediate bone grafts in irradiated beds are rarely successful.

It should again be noted that preoperative radiation does not yet have valid statistical confirmation as a therapeutic plan superior to other approaches.

Radiation Ulcers

Radiation ulcers are usually associated with previous therapeutic radiation rather than with accidental injury. Their distribution, therefore, is related to the areas where tumors are most commonly treated with therapeutic radiation, e.g., the oral cavity, neck, chest wall, anterior axillary fold, sacral region, and inguinal region.

The pathophysiology is not dissimilar to that of acute radiation injury and involves local ulceration, secondary infection, and finally necrosis. The symptoms and signs are similar to those of other ulcers but are characterized by the inordinate amount of pain that accompanies the ischemia. The margins of such ulcers, although viable, are usually severely compromised and often cannot be employed as part of the reconstruction.

The principles of therapy are as above: local wound care, control of infection with topical antibacterial agents, resection of the ulcer bed and margins of the wound (usually, resection of much of the original field of radiation is indicated), and finally adequate soft tissue coverage. In the oral cavity, particularly in the presence of osteoradionecrosis of the mandible, resection of the ulcer and necrotic bone allows sufficient collapse of adjacent tissue so that primary closure can be effected. On occasion, when the underlying

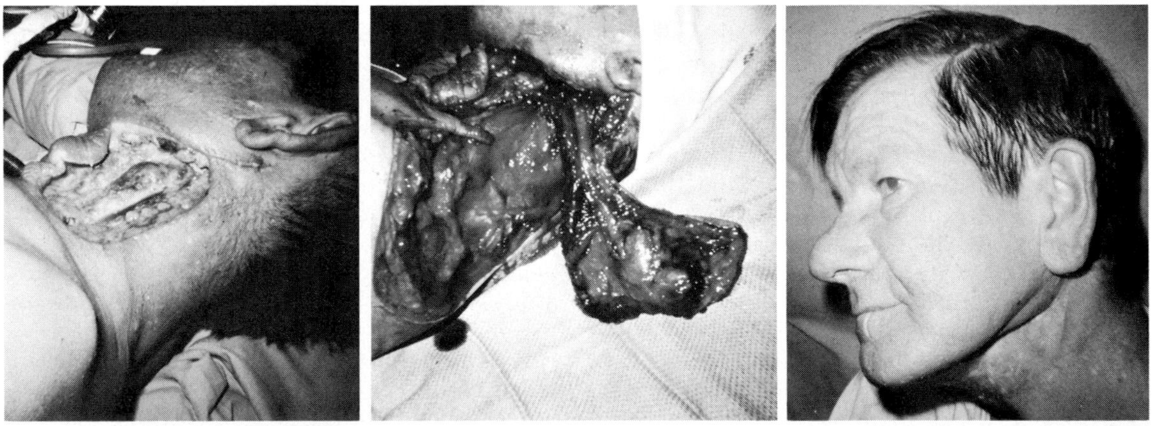

Figure 25–10. *Left,* Breakdown of tissue after resection of a tumor of the piriform sinus after a course of preoperative radiation therapy. There had been an infection with exposure of the mandible and carotid artery. *Center,* After topical treatment with antibacterial creams, the wound was debrided and the exposed mandible and carotid artery were covered with a trapezius myocutaneous flap. *Right,* The wound healed without further complications. (From Ariyan, S.: Clin. Plast. Surg., *6*:523, 1979.)

tissue bed is suitable, a split-thickness skin graft suffices. However, the principal indications for flap coverage as outlined by Robinson (1975) are appropriate:

1. For coverage of exposed, or potentially exposed, vital structures—large vessels, nerves, tendons, bones, cartilage, peritoneum, pleura, or dura.
2. To provide a moving or gliding surface for tendons and joints.
3. As a cover through which future reconstructive procedures can be accomplished.
4. For filling out contours, or for filling in cavities.
5. To allow more motion in kinetic areas—neck, joints, chest wall.

Case 3: Radiation Ulcer—Sacral Region (Split-Thickness Skin Graft). An example of this type of injury is seen in a 50 year old female with a history of an adenocarcinoma of the uterus that was treated by hysterectomy. After surgery, she had radium implant and external beam radiation of 4000 rads via double-opposing ports measuring 15 × 12 cm. An erythematous reaction in the gluteal crease subsequently resulted in early breakdown of the skin over the area. The area was hyperpigmented 18 months later, with a central ulcer that would not heal (Fig. 25–11).

The entire area was excised beyond the margins of pigmentation and beyond the area of vasculitis and ischemia. The excision was extended down to the sacral fascia, and there appeared to be healthy skin at the margins of resection. The wound was packed with saline-soaked gauze until adequate granula-

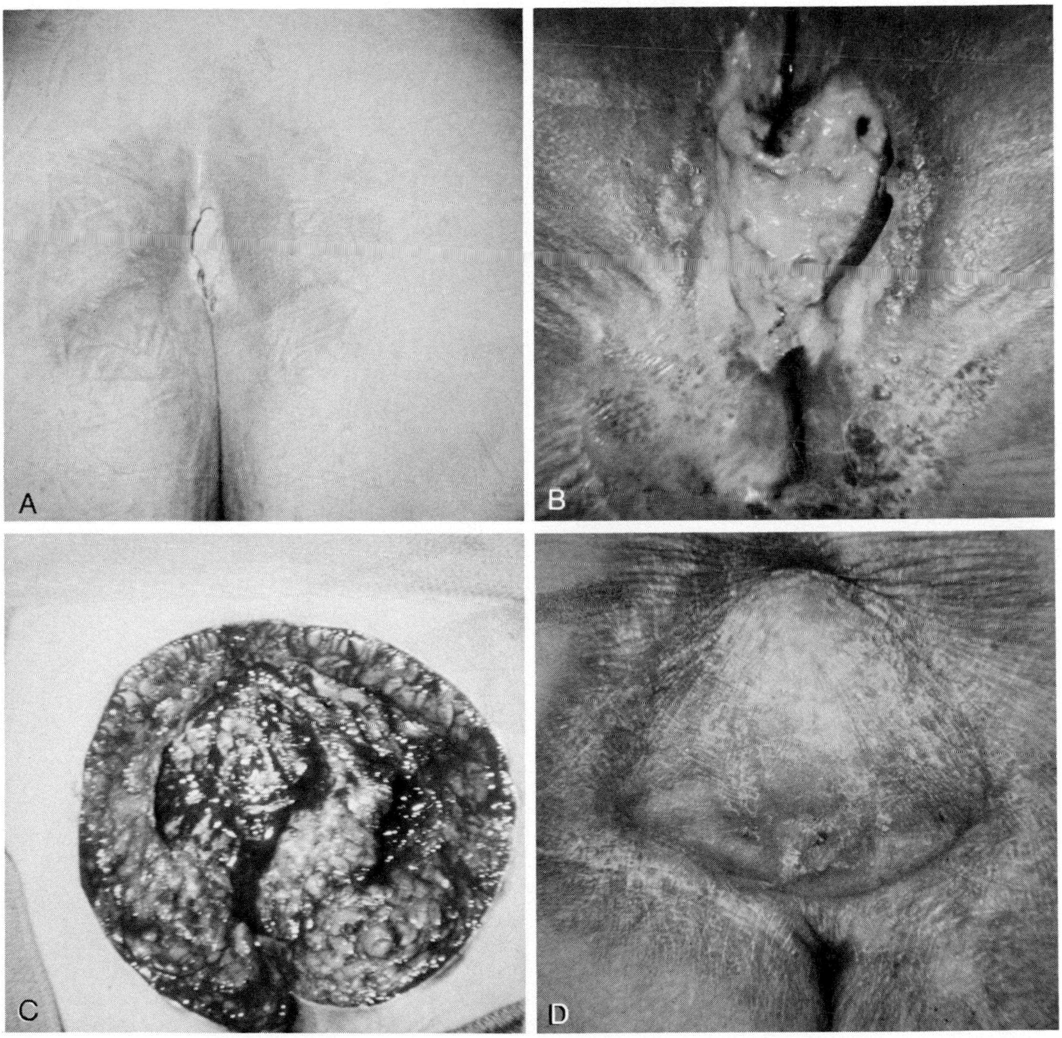

Figure 25–11. *A,* Hyperpigmentation and central ulceration *(B)* of an area of skin following radiation therapy. *C,* All ischemic tissue within the ports of radiation was excised. *D,* The area was covered with skin grafts.

tion tissue filled the bed, and a split-thickness skin graft was applied to the wound. The patient was pain free and the area remained healed two years later at the time of last follow-up.

Case 4: Radiation Ulcer—Sacral Region (Rotation Flap). A 55 year old male had received preoperative radiation for an adenocarcinoma of the rectum. Several weeks after an abdominoperineal resection, the perineal wound broke down and failed to heal (Fig. 25–12). The ulcer measured 2 × 3 cm across and was 5 to 6 cm deep. There was an additional problem in that there had already been disruption of the suture line and the wound was deep. After excision of the lesion, the resulting large cavity needed to be filled with well-vascularized tissue. This was accomplished by the transposition of gluteus maximus muscle flaps; cutaneous coverage was then achieved by the rotation of a large buttock flap. Since the tissues of the flap were outside the portals of radiation, they had a healthy blood supply and healed readily. The patient remained pain free with healed wounds until his death 18 months later from metastatic disease.

Malignant Transformation

It is well documented that low dose chronic exposure or even therapeutic radiation may result in malignant degeneration of the skin

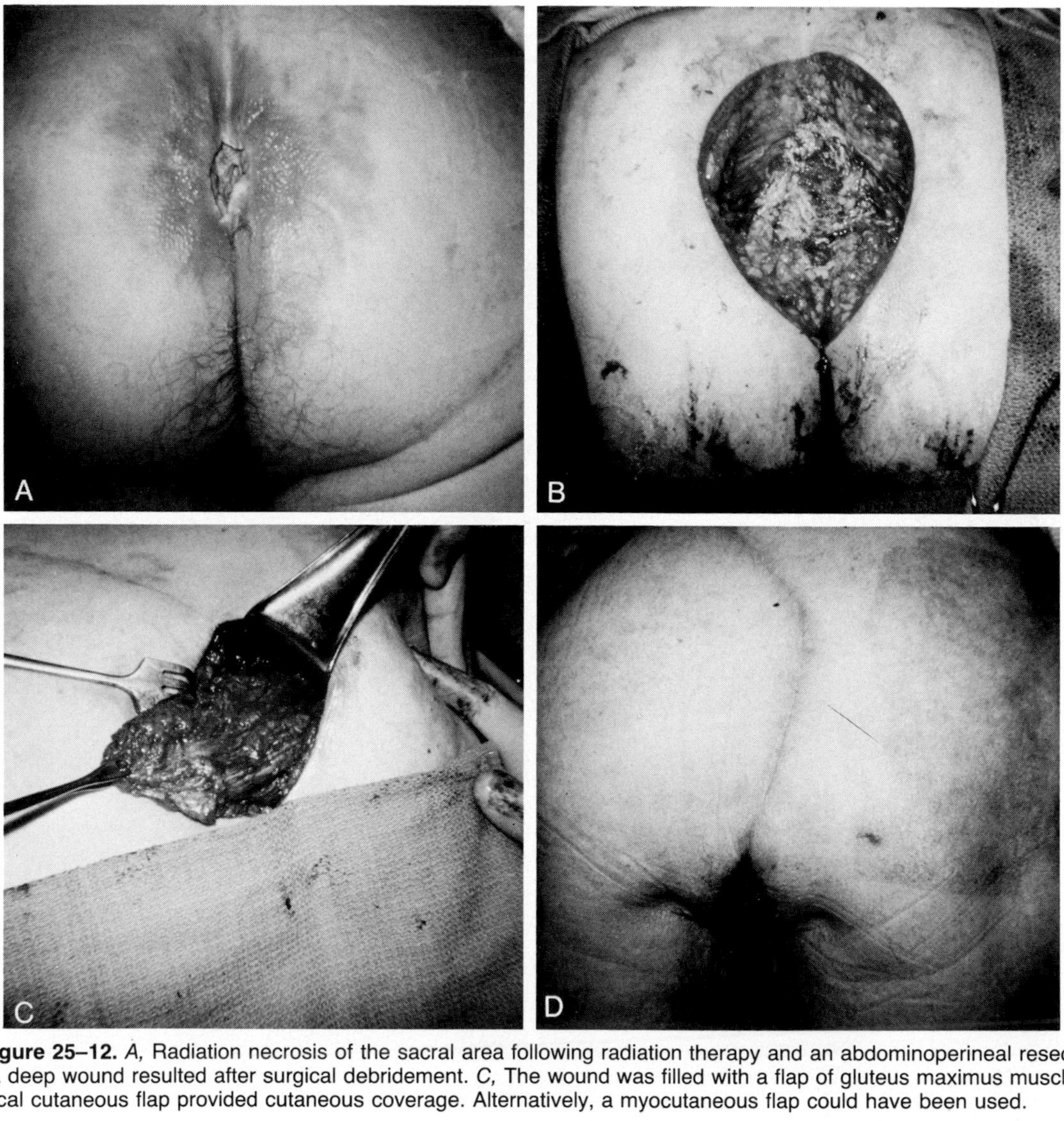

Figure 25–12. *A,* Radiation necrosis of the sacral area following radiation therapy and an abdominoperineal resection. *B,* A deep wound resulted after surgical debridement. *C,* The wound was filled with a flap of gluteus maximus muscle. *D,* A local cutaneous flap provided cutaneous coverage. Alternatively, a myocutaneous flap could have been used.

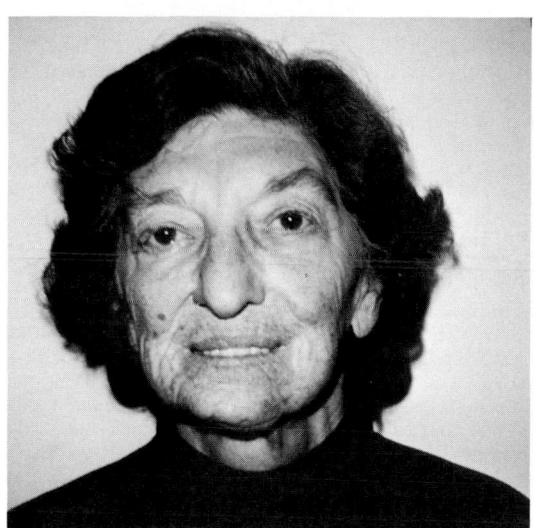

Figure 25–13. A patient who had been treated 50 years previously with repeated small doses of radiation for acne has developed a number of basal cell carcinomas and has a squamous cell carcinoma of the right cheek.

after an interval of many years. The involved sites are related to the reason for exposure, either occupational (hands) or therapeutic (acne or hirsutism of the face and upper neck) (Fig. 25–13). Carcinoma of the thyroid has also followed radiation to the thymus.

The pathophysiology appears to be the same as that for other similar injury-induced malignancies, such as burn scar carcinoma (Marjolin's ulcer). The chronic radiation changes render the tissue ischemic and susceptible to injury with easy breakdown; any subsequent reparative process is difficult or lacking. As the tissue progresses through the stages of atrophy, pseudoepitheliomatous hyperplasia, and finally carcinoma, the accessibility of the lesion allows for early diagnosis and early treatment. Since many of the lesions are superficial, topical chemotherapy may be effective. Ulcerated lesions, however, require excision and closure. A postirradiated site with multiple cancers and a wide area of breakdown is, although infrequent, among the most challenging of reconstructive problems, often requiring resurfacing of large areas of the face. Split-thickness skin graft coverage is usually effective, if not an esthetic triumph.

Deeply invasive malignancy should be treated in a manner similar to the therapy for other squamous cell carcinomas. Since the resected area is comparable with that seen in radiation ulcers, a similar approach and decision regarding graft coverage are appropriate.

REFERENCES

Allen, A. C.: The Skin, A Clinicopathologic Treatise. St. Louis, MO, C. V. Mosby Company, 1954.

Ariyan, S., Marfuggi, R. A., Harder, G., and Goodie, M. M.: An experimental model to determine the effects of adjuvant therapy on the incidence of postoperative wound infection. I. Evaluating preoperative radiation therapy. Plast. Reconstr. Surg., *65*:328, 1980.

Bragg, D. G., Shidnia, H., Chu, F. C., and Higinbotham, N. L.: The clinical and radiographic aspects of radiation osteitis. Radiology, *97*:103, 1970.

Brill, A. B., Tomonaga, M., and Heyssel, R. M.: Leukemia in man following exposure to ionizing radiation. A summary of the findings in Hiroshima and Nagasaki, and a comparison with human experience. Ann. Intern. Med., *56*:590, 1962.

Brown, J. B., and Fryer, M. P.: Report of surgical repair in the first group of atomic radiation injuries. Surg. Gynecol. Obstet., *103*:1, 1956.

Brown, J. B., and Fryer, M. P.: Reconstruction of electrical injuries, including cranial losses. With preliminary report of cathode-ray burns. Ann. Surg., *146*:342, 1957.

Brown, J. B., and Fryer, M. P.: High energy electron injury from accelerator machine. Radiation burns of chest wall and neck. 17-year follow-up of atomic burns. Ann. Surg., *162*:426, 1965.

Brown, J. B., McDowell, F., and Fryer, M. P.: Radiation burns, including vocational and atomic exposures. Treatment and surgical prevention of chronic lesions. Ann. Surg., *130*:593, 1949a.

Brown, J. B., McDowell, F., and Fryer, M. P.: Surgical treatment of radiation burns. Surg. Gynecol. Obstet., *88*:609, 1949b.

Burch, P. R. J.: Radiation carcinogenesis: a new hypothesis. Nature, *185*:135, 1960.

Burrows, H., and Clarkson, J. R.: The role of inflammation in the induction of cancer by x-rays. Br. J. Radiol., *16*:381, 1943.

Cahan, W. G., Woodard, H. Q., Higinbotham, N. L., Stewart, F. W., and Coley, B. L.: Sarcoma arising in irradiated bone. Cancer, *1*:3, 1948.

Cruz, N. I., Ariyan, S., Minitor, P., and Andriole, V. T.: An experimental model to determine the level of antibiotics in irradiated tissues. Plast. Reconstr. Surg., *73*:811, 1984.

Daniel, J.: The x-rays. New Science, *3*:562, 1896.

Ewing, J.: Radiation osteitis. Acta Radiol., *6*:399, 1926.

Favus, M. J., Schneider, A. B., Stachura, M. E., et al.: Thyroid cancer occurring as a late consequence of head and neck irradiation. Evaluation of 1056 patients. N. Engl. J. Med., *294*:1019, 1976.

Finch, S. C.: The study of atomic bomb survivors in Japan. Am. J. Med., *66*:899, 1979.

Frieben, E. A.: Cancroid des rechten Handrückens nach langdauernder Einwirkung von Roentgenstrahlen. Forstchr. Roentgenstr., *6*:106, 1902.

Guelinckx, P. J., Boeckx, W. D., Fossion, E., and Gruwez, J. A.: Scanning electron microscopy of irradiated recipient blood vessels in head and neck free flaps. Plast. Reconstr. Surg., *74*:217, 1984.

Hatfield, P. M., and Schulz, M. D.: Postirradiation sarcoma. Including five cases after x-ray therapy of breast carcinoma. Radiology, *96*:593, 1970.

Hempelmann, L. H., Hall, W. J., Phillips, M., Cooper, R. A., and Ames, W. R.: Neoplasm in persons treated with x-ray in infancy: fourth survey in 20 years. J. Natl. Cancer Inst., *55*:519, 1975.

Hoffman, F. L.: Radium (mesothorium) necrosis. J.A.M.A., *85*:961, 1925.

Hueper, W. C.: Recent developments in environmental cancer. Arch. Pathol., *58*:475, 1954.

Katz, A. D., and Preston-Martin, S.: Salivary gland tumors and previous radiotherapy to the head or neck. Report of a clinical series. Am. J. Surg., *147*:345, 1984.

Kerth, J. D., Sisson, G. A., and Becker, G. D.: Radical neck dissection in carcinoma of the head and neck. Surg. Clin. North Am., *53*:179, 1973.

Ketcham, A. S., Hoye, R. C., Chretien, P. B., and Brace, K. C.: Irradiation twenty-four hours preoperatively. Am. J. Surg., *118*:691, 1969.

Kilgore, A. R., and Abbott, L. C.: Sarcoma following benign bone lesions. West. J. Surg., *46*:348, 1938.

Kim, J. H., Chu, F. C., Pope, R. A., Woodard, H. Q., Bragg, D. B., and Shidnia, H.: Proceedings: time dose factors in radiation induced osteitis. Am. J. Roentgenol., *120*:684, 1974.

Knowlton, N. P., Leifer, E., Hogness, J. R., Hempelmann, L. H., Blaney, L. F., et al.: Beta-ray burns of human skin. J.A.M.A., *141*:239, 1949.

Krizek, T. J., and Ariyan, S.: Severe acute radiation injuries of the hands. Report of two cases. Plast. Reconstr. Surg., *51*:14, 1973.

Lacassagne, A.: Conditions dans lesquelles ont été obtenus, chez le lapin, des cancers par action des rayons X sur des foyers inflammatoires. C. R. Soc. Biol., *112*:562, 1933.

Lacassagne, A., and Vinzent, R.: Action des rayons X sur un foyer infectieux local, provoqué chez le lapin par l'injection de *Streptobacillus caviae*. C. R. Soc. Biol., *100*:247, 1929a.

Lacassagne, A., and Vinzent, R.: Sarcomes provoqués chez des lapins par l'irradiation d'abscès à *Streptobacillus caviae*. C. R. Soc. Biol., *100*:249, 1929b.

Lanzl, L. H., Rozenfeld, M. L., and Tarlov, A. R.: Injury due to accidental high-dose exposure to 10 MeV electrons. Health Phys., *13*:241, 1967.

Ludewig, P., and Lorenser, E.: Untersuchungen der Grubenluft in den Schneeberger Gruben auf den Gehalt an Radiumemanation. Strahlentherapie, *17*:428, 1924.

March, H. C.: Leukemia in radiologists, ten years later. With review of the pertinent evidence for radiation leukemia. Am. J. Med. Sci., *242*:137, 1961.

Martland, H. S.: The occurrence of malignancy in radioactive persons. A general review of data gathered in the study of the radium dial painters with special reference to the occurrence of osteogenic sarcoma and the interrelationship of certain blood diseases. Am. J. Cancer, *15*:2435, 1931.

Martland, H. S., Conlon, P., and Knef, J. P.: Some unrecognized dangers in the use and handling of radioactive substances: with special reference to the storage of insoluble products of radium and mesothorium in the reticulo-endothelial system. J.A.M.A., *85*:1769, 1925.

Miller, R. W.: Delayed radiation effects in atomic-bomb survivors. Major observations by the Atomic Bomb Casualty Commission are evaluated. Science, *166*:569, 1969.

Newcombe, H. B.: Magnitude of biological hazard from strontium-90. Science, *126*:549, 1957.

Pifer, J. W., Toyooka, E. T., Murray, R. W., Ames, W. R., and Hempelmann, L. H.: Neoplasms in children treated with x-rays for thymic enlargement. J. Natl. Cancer Inst., *31*:1333, 1963.

Rankow, R. M., and Weissman, B.: Osteoradionecrosis of the mandible. Ann. Otol. Rhinol. Laryngol., *80*:603, 1971.

Richardson, R. L., and Jones, M.: A bacteriologic census of human saliva. J. Dent. Res., *37*:697, 1958.

Robinson, D. W.: Surgical problems in the excision and repair of radiated tissue. Plast. Reconstr. Surg., *55*:41, 1975.

Sams, A.: Histologic changes in the larger blood vessels of the hind limb of the mouse after x-radiation. Int. J. Radiat. Biol., *9*:165, 1965.

Schneider, A. B., Favus, M. J., Stachura, M. E., Arnold, M. J., and Frohman, L. A.: Salivary gland neoplasms as a late consequence of head and neck irradiation. Ann. Intern. Med., *87*:160, 1977.

Shore, R. E., Woodard, E. D., Pasternack, B. S., and Hempelmann, L. H.: Radiation and host factors in human thyroid tumors following thymus irradiation. Health Phys., *38*:451, 1980.

Simpson, C. L., and Hempelmann, L. H.: The association of tumors and roentgen-ray treatment of the thorax in infancy. Cancer, *10*:42. 1957.

Socolow, E. L., Hashizume, A., Nerishi, S., and Niitani, R.: Thyroid carcinoma in man after exposure to ionizing radiation. A summary of the findings in Hiroshima and Nagasaki. N. Engl. J. Med., *268*:406, 1963.

Takeichi, N., Hirose, F., Yamamoto, H., Ezaki, H., and Fujikura, T.: Salivary gland tumors in atomic bomb survivors, Hiroshima, Japan. II. Pathologic study and supplementary epidemiologic observations. Cancer, *52*:377, 1983.

Teloh, H. A., Mason, M. L., and Wheelock, M. C.: A histopathologic study of radiation injuries of the skin. Surg. Gynecol. Obstet., *90*:335, 1950.

Toyooka, E. T., Pifer, J. W., Crump, S. L., Dutton, A. M., and Hempelmann, L. H.: Neoplasms in children treated with x-rays for thymic enlargement. II. Tumor incidence as a function of radiation factors. J. Natl. Cancer Inst., *31*:1357, 1963.

Ulrich, H.: Incidence of leukemia in radiologists. N. Engl. J. Med., *234*:45, 1946.

Upton, A. C.: Effects of radiation on man. Annu. Rev. Nucl. Sci., *18*:495, 1968.

Warren, S.: Effects of radiation on normal tissues. XIII. Effects on the skin. Arch. Pathol., *35*:304, 1943.

Warren, S.: Longevity and causes of death from irradiation in physicians. J.A.M.A., *162*:464, 1956.

Warren, S.: Radiation carcinogenesis. Bull. N.Y. Acad. Med., *46*:131, 1970.

Watson, J. S.: Experimental microvascular anastomoses in radiated vessels. Plast. Reconstr. Surg., *563*:529, 1979.

Zeldis, L. J., Jablon, S., and Ishida, M.: Current status of ABCC-NIH studies of carcinogenesis in Hiroshima and Nagasaki. Ann. N.Y. Acad. Sci., *114*:225, 1964.

26

Martin C. Robson
David J. Smith, Jr.

Cold Injuries

Human exposure to cold results in injury due to heat loss. Depending on the amount of unprotected or inadequately protected exposure, the injury can be localized, generalized, or both. Localized cold injury is categorized by its pathogenesis as frostbite, and generalized injury is discussed as systemic hypothermia. Although historically many syndromes secondary to cold exposure and heat loss were identified by their clinical presentations, it is preferable to present them as localized (frostbite) or generalized (systemic hypothermia).

The confusion in the literature concerning various treatment models is the result of multiple clinical descriptions of the local injury, suggesting different etiologies and a different sequence of cellular and chemical changes. The determination of the pathogenesis of localized injury as singular enabled prospective trials to be performed to demonstrate the inefficacy of many suggested remedies. Since the subclassifications simply represent different clinical descriptions of the same disease process, this chapter is devoted to discussing either local or generalized cold injuries.

Regardless of whether localized or generalized, the development of a cold injury does not depend only on the depth of the ambient temperature and the duration of exposure. Several other contributory conditions, or "predisposing factors," have been identified. One of the most significant is the wind velocity, which, combined with temperature, constitutes the wind-chill index. Although the time-temperature factor is basic to the severity of the cold injury, it may be modified by the wind-chill index (Fig. 26–1). Knowledge of this index is important to an understanding of how cold injuries occur when the absolute temperature is not low enough to cause tissue damage. Air itself is a poor thermal conductor, yet cold air is not nearly so dangerous a freezing factor as the combination of wind and cold. The chilling effect of a temperature of +20°F combined with a 45 mile/hr wind is identical to that of a −40°F temperature coupled with a 2 mile breeze (Washburn, 1962).

The humidity or wetness also predisposes to cold injury. Increased environmental humidity or localized moisture has been documented to increase the severity of tissue damage, again by increasing heat transfer. Small leaks in boots allowing small amounts of water to enter have been associated with localized injury on an otherwise protected foot (Boswick, 1976).

The degree of inadequacy of protective clothing varies with environmental conditions and may contribute to insufficient con-

INDEX OF WIND-CHILL FACTOR

Wind	Degrees Fahrenheit Dry-Bulb Temperature													
	35	30	25	20	15	10	5	0	−5	−10	−15	−20	−25	−30
	Equivalent Degrees													
Calm	35	30	25	20	15	10	5	0	−5	−10	−15	−20	−25	−30
			COLD								BITTER COLD			
5 mph	33	27	21	16	12	7	1	−6	−11	−15	−20	−26	−31	−35
10 mph	21	16	9	2	−2	−9	−15	−22	−27	−31	−38	−45	−52	−58
			VERY COLD											
15 mph	16	11	1	−6	−11	−18	−25	−33	−40	−45	−51	−60	−65	−70
20 mph	12	3	−4	−9	−17	−24	−32	−40	−46	−52	−60	−68	−76	−81
											EXTREME COLD			
25 mph	7	0	−7	−15	−22	−29	−37	−45	−52	−58	−67	−75	−83	−89
30 mph	5	−2	−11	−18	−26	−33	−41	−49	−56	−63	−70	−78	−87	−94
35 mph	3	−4	−13	−20	−27	−35	−43	−52	−60	−67	−72	−83	−90	−98
40 mph	1	−4	−15	−22	−29	−36	−45	−54	−62	−69	−76	−87	−94	−101

Figure 26–1. The combination of temperature and wind velocity results in a lower effective temperature for the exposed tissue.

servation of body heat. Tight-fitting clothing may produce areas of constriction that can hinder blood circulation and lessen the extent of heat-retaining air insulation. Wet clothing transmits heat from the body into the environment, because water is a thermal conductor (Knize, 1977). Clothing that allows transmission of moisture away from the body is important. In addition, an outer layer to protect from the wind decreases heat loss. This wind resistant layer must still have the same transmission capabilities. Clothes that decrease the amount of surface area are effective. Therefore, mittens are more protective than gloves since they prevent the air from circulating between the fingers. It is known that 80 per cent of the total body heat loss can occur through the exposed head and neck areas. These areas require coverage to prevent this loss. Foot covering can be a significant problem. The presence of deep snow is deceiving. It has been documented that when the air temperature is 0°F, the temperature beneath a foot of snow is −14°F (Washburn, 1962). Feet need to be dressed for the temperature where they are resting, not for the temperature around the person's head.

Clinical studies during World War II (Whayne and DeBakey, 1958) and the Korean conflict (Orr and Fainer, 1952) showed a high correlation between fatigue and apathy and the incidence of cold injury. Cold injuries occurred with high frequency among soldiers in retreat. Under such conditions or under starvation, men were often indifferent to their personal hygiene and to the condition of their clothing (Kinmouth, Rob, and Simeone, 1962).

Overexertion increases heat loss. Huge quantities of body heat can be lost through the lungs by panting, and perspiration causes further chilling (Washburn, 1962). Both panting and sweating require excess energy, a factor that adds to the fatigue factor.

Among civilians, the most common factor contributing to cold injury has been impairment of judgment due to excessive alcohol consumption. Intoxicated patients and others whose consciousness, judgment, or self-protective instincts are depressed by psychosis or drug abuse often expose themselves to dangerous environmental hazards. In the Denver series, alcohol intake or mental instability led directly to cold injury in 50 per cent of the patients (Knize and associates, 1969). Once the injury had occurred, however, alcoholic intake probably did not significantly alter the clinical outcome. In addition, alcohol results in vasodilatation and an increased blood flow to the body surface. The increased heat loss causes chilling of the blood. This has two detrimental effects: (1) it lowers the tissue temperature, making it more prone to freezing; and (2) the chilled blood can return to the heart and lungs and lower the total body temperature.

Because impaired local circulation is a primary cause of frostbite, an effort should be made to avoid anything that may adversely affect circulation. Cigarette smoking has been documented to cause vasoconstriction, decreased flow, and tissue loss in flaps (Lawrence and associates, 1984). It should be avoided during cold exposure and during the recovery period following cold injury. Any other drugs known to have vasoactive properties may also predispose to frostbite. Finally, disease states that have altered tissue perfusions (e.g., atherosclerosis, arteritis) are factors to be considered.

On the basis of clinical observations, an individual who has experienced a previous cold injury must be placed in a high risk category during subsequent exposure (Mills and Whaley, 1964; Whayne and DeBakey, 1958). For reasons not yet determined, a cold injury in some way sensitizes a person, with the result that subsequent cold exposure, even of a lesser degree, produces tissue damage more rapidly (Knize, 1977). Military studies have shown that long periods of physical immobility contribute to the extent of cold injury. Motion is necessary for the production of body heat and efficient circulation, especially with respect to endangered limbs.

While civilian clinical studies are inadequate for statistical evaluation of etiopathogenesis factors such as race and previous climatic environmental background, they suggest that dark-skinned soldiers under the same combat conditions are more susceptible to cold injury (Knize, 1977). Similarly, individuals from regions of warmer climates within the United States tend to be more susceptible (Whayne and DeBakey, 1958).

FROSTBITE: LOCALIZED COLD INJURY

History

Although Hippocrates described some of the symptoms and sequelae of frostbite injury, it is doubtful whether cold injuries were prevalent in ancient Greece.The first investigations on the effect of cold injury were in England in 1805 (Zingg, 1967). However, the first authoritative account of mass casualties was the description by Baron de Larrey, Surgeon-in-Chief of Napoleon's army during the invasion of Russia in 1812 (Larrey, 1814). During World War II frostbite was a major cause of morbidity among ground troops. From August, 1942 to January, 1944, there were more casualties from frostbite among the Eighth Air Force than from enemy gunfire (Lewis, 1952). With increased awareness of the importance of prevention of heat loss and rapid rewarming, casualties in the Korean war decreased, although long-term sequelae were frequent (Blair, Schatzki, and Orr, 1957).

Localized injuries secondary to cold have classically been defined by their clinical presentation. This has resulted in two systems of classification: one based on the acute physical findings observed after cold exposure and subsequent rewarming, and the other noting the physical findings but adding the environmental conditions under which the injury occurred. In the first system, which is still most commonly used, injuries are classified according to "degree of injury." *First degree* injury is characterized by a white or yellowish, firm plaque in the area of injury (Knize, 1977). Erythema and edema may also be present. Tissue necrosis or loss usually does not occur. However, lingering causalgia pain frequently develops, indicating that some element of nerve damage has been produced. *Second degree* frostbite consists of superficial blisters containing clear or milky fluid (Fig. 26–2). Erythema and edema frequently sur-

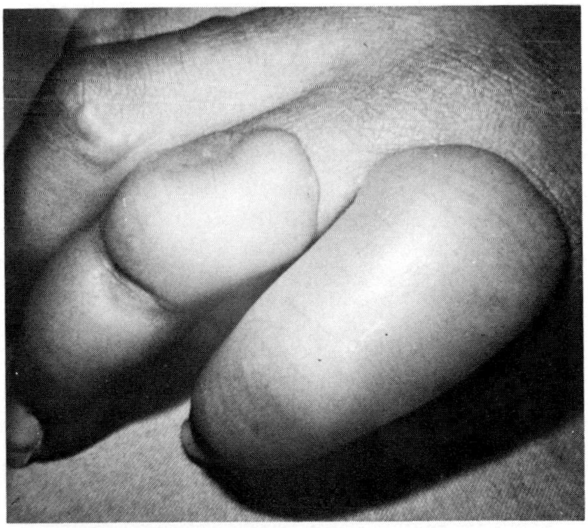

Figure 26–2. Second degree frostbite of the fingers. Note the clear or milky fluid-filled blisters.

round the blisters. These injuries usually heal spontaneously without deeper tissue necrosis unless the initial level of injury was sufficiently deep to progress to tissue loss. Injury to the blister may result in desiccation and tissue necrosis. *Third degree* frostbite consists of deeper blisters containing red or purple fluid or areas of darkly discolored skin without blisters. The prognosis for these injuries has been guarded, with tissue necrosis common. If only partial-thickness loss occurs, it is more commonly associated with areas of blister formation, while deeply discolored areas usually represent a full-thickness injury. *Fourth degree* frostbite consists of deep cyanosis of the injured part without vesicle formation or local edema. In these injuries, gangrene is often evident within hours of injury.

The other system correlates the physical findings with the environmental conditions at the time of injury. *Chilblain* is a skin condition resulting from chronic intermittent exposure to the environmental conditions of high humidity and low ambient temperature without the development of tissue freezing. It is characterized by discomfort in the involved limbs. The symptoms usually resolve spontaneously without tissue loss. *Trench foot* (immersion foot) develops slowly over a period of hours or days, without actual tissue freezing, and is due to the exposure of wet feet to a temperature range of 32° to 50°F (1° to 10°C) (White and Scoville, 1945; Knize, 1977). The extremity initially becomes anesthetic, pain being experienced only with motion or weight bearing. Immediately after exposure the skin appears erythematous, but it eventually appears pale and markedly swollen. As the lesion progresses, blisters filled with serous or serosanguineous fluid appear. Tissue loss is difficult to determine, but most frequently there is spontaneous healing beneath the nonviable tissue cover.

Frostbite occurs rapidly after exposure to temperatures at freezing levels or below. Clinically, this temperature has been shown to be 20°F (−6.5°C) or below for a duration of one hour or more (Knize and associates, 1969). The skin becomes blanched and a stinging sensation is noted. The part eventually becomes numb and a sensation of clumsiness is often reported. After rewarming, these injuries are indistinguishable from trench foot, although the prognosis for tissue survival is better for the trench foot injury.

Probably the most violent and rapid cases of frostbite were those reported by U.S. bomber crews during World War II. Most of these occurred at altitudes of 25,000 to 35,000 feet in temperatures of −25° to 45°F (Washburn, 1962). When attacked, the only manner in which "waist gunners" of the aircraft could operate their machine guns was to open "waist ports" through which to fire their guns. In order to ensure better dexterity, these gunners often discarded their gloves. Terrible cases of frostbite resulted from these brief exposures, which fulfilled all the criteria for acute injury: fear; exhaustion (German attacks were planned at the end of long flights); hypoxia; inadequate nourishment; and tight gripping of a frigid, solid object. These conditions, resulting in high altitude frostbite injuries, will probably never be repeated. The frigid temperature of outer space does not affect crews directly, since humans cannot exist outside a pressurized cabin at heights much above 40,000 feet, except briefly during free-fall parachute descents. At altitudes above 63,000 feet, humans cannot exist without a pressurized suit, for above this altitude human blood boils at body temperatures (Washburn, 1962).

Pathophysiology

Human skin may be injured by cold in two ways: by direct cellular injury or by indirect cellular effects resulting from microvascular changes leading to thrombosis and ischemia. Some of the recognized and documented changes from direct cellular injury include: (1) development of extracellular ice formation, (2) development of intracellular ice formation, (3) cell dehydration with cell shrinkage, (4) abnormal concentration of electrolytes within the cell, (5) thermal shock, and (6) denaturation of lipid-protein complexes (Zacarian, 1985).

When cells are subjected to a slow rate of cooling, ice crystals develop between the cells in their interspaces. On the other hand, rapid cooling produces intracellular ice crystals, which are more lethal to the cell and less favorable to cell survival. The rate of freezing in a clinical cold injury is not sufficiently fast to produce intracellular crystals (Merryman, 1970). The extracellular ice that forms is nevertheless not innocuous, because it causes the withdrawal of water across the cell membrane, contributing to cell dehydration. Mazur (1963, 1965) proposed the following sequence of injury: modification of protein structure by high electrolyte concentration, alteration of membrane lipids, alteration of cellular pH, and imbalance of chemical activity. This phenomenon subsequently permits the rapid and toxic increase of electrolytes within the cell, leading to partial shrinkage and collapse of its vital cell membrane. Moran (1929) originally proposed this theory of cellular dehydration, and it was subsequently supported by Merryman's study of "ice crystal nucleation" (Merryman, 1956). These events are incompatible with cell viability.

The entire volume or content of water within a given cell is not totally freezable. The small amount of unfrozen water, referred to as "bound water," constitutes as much as 8 to 10 per cent of the water content and is held tightly in the protein complex within the cell. No matter how rapid or profound the hypothermia, this bound water remains in liquid state. At temperatures below −20°C, approximately 90 per cent of the available water is frozen (Zacarian, 1985). Thus, the mechanical theory of ice crystals actually disrupting the cell is attractive but has little supporting evidence.

The phenomenon of sudden and profound temperature change in the biologic system is referred to as thermal shock (Greenfield, Shepherd, and Whelan, 1951). This precipitous chilling has been theorized to be incompatible to maintain homeostasis of a living system, and therefore incompatible with life. The severity of this phenomenon is open to debate. Another poorly understood concept is the manner in which subzero temperatures produce denaturation of lipid-protein complexes. Lovelock (1954, 1957) interpreted the detachment of lipids and lipid proteins from cell membranes as a consequence of the solvent action of the toxic electrolyte concentration within the cell. There is no direct evidence to confirm that enzyme activity is altered during freezing, but DNA synthesis is inhibited (Johnson and Daniels, 1974). On the other hand, Shikama and Yamazaki (1961) reported ox liver catalase activity changes and Markert (1963) suggested structural alteration of lactic acid dehydrogenase after freezing and thawing. Stowell and associates (1965) have described nuclear changes in the cell and the cytoplasmic structures, primarily mitochondria, endoplasmic reticulum, and Golgi bodies.

Indirect cellular damage is secondary to progressive microvascular insult and is more severe than the direct cellular type. This finding is emphasized by a study showing that skin tissue subjected to a standard freezing and thawing injury in vivo that consistently produced necrosis survived as a full-thickness skin graft transplanted to an uninjured recipient site (Weatherly-White, Sjostrom, and Paton, 1964). Conversely, uninjured full-thickness skin did not survive when transferred to a recipient area pretreated with the same freezing injury. Thus, the direct skin injury appears reversible and the progressive nature of injury is most likely due to microvascular changes.

Approximately 62 per cent of the capillary circulation ceases in the temperature range +11° to +3°C, while 35 to 40 per cent of blood flow ceases in the arterioles and venules (Rinfret, 1962). Capillary patency initially appears normal in post-thawed tissue, but blood flow subsequently declines in three to five minutes. Three phenomena are noticed after thawing: (1) the momentary and initial vasoconstriction of the arterioles and venules; (2) the resumption of circulation and blood flow, and (3) a simultaneous and continued shower of emboli coursing through the microvessels (Zacarian, 1985). Within minutes vasodilatation is noted, which continues and progresses to its peak 45 minutes after the freeze thaw insult. In any case, tissue injury secondary to vascular stasis leads to hypoxia and subsequent tissue necrosis.

Considerable evidence points to the primary damage of the cold injury being changes of the vascular endothelium. At 72 hours after freeze and rethawing, there is a loss of vascular endothelium in the capillary walls with significant fibrin deposition. The endothelium may be totally destroyed and the fibrin may saturate the arteriole walls (Zacarian, 1985). Rabb and associates (1974) used electron microscopy to demonstrate the effects of freezing and the early damage sustained by the endothelium of the capillaries of the hamster cheek pouch following subjection to subzero temperatures. They observed ultrastructural derangement of the endothelial cells after the thaw period and this progressed after one hour of observation. Zacarian, Stone, and Clater (1970) further confirmed this immediate injury by demonstrating fluid extravasation from vessels almost immediately after thawing. As in other trauma, the endothelial cells of the vascular walls began to swell and protrude inward into the lumen and then finally underwent lysis.

Cold injury appears to be greatest upon the venules, owing in part to their slower circulation. Arterioles, whose rate of flow is almost twice that of the venules, are less damaged by freezing and develop stasis later than the venules. Capillaries manifest the least direct effects of cold injury, but their flow is quickly arrested because of their position between the arterioles and venules. Generalized stasis and cessation of flow were noted at the point of freezing within 20 minutes. Platelet thrombi were followed by white thrombi (blood cells and fibrin) as blood flow progressively slowed. Sludging and stasis resulted in final thrombosis. Kulka (1956, 1964) also supported these observations. After cold insult to living tissue, he found local vascular thromboses advancing from the capillary levels to larger vessels and resulting in ischemic death of progressively larger areas. Viable cells were observed histologically in cold-injured tissues for as long as eight days or until occlusion of the local vessels occurred. These findings emphasize that a major role is played by vascular insufficiency and that the direct injury to cellular structures and mechanisms may be reversible.

Bellman and Adams-Ray (1956) studied the microvasculature of the cold injury with microangiography. Although spasm of the arterioles and venules did exist, it was not sufficiently marked to explain the decreased flow of progressive microvascular collapse. These authors postulated that the defects seen in the angiograms were caused by local factors and might also be due to thrombi. Because the changes observed in cold injury may be similar to those seen in other inflammatory states, Robson and Heggers (1981), postulated that the progressive ischemia seen in frostbite might be due to the same inflammatory mediators responsible for progressive dermal ischemia in the burn wound. They evaluated blister fluids from cases of hand frostbite, and found levels of PGE_2, $PGF_{2\alpha}$, and thromboxane B_2 (TXB_2) (Table 26–1). The vasoconstricting, platelet aggregating, and leukocyte sticking prostanoids ($PGF_{2\alpha}$ and TXB_2) were markedly elevated. These authors postulated that the massive edema described by Merryman (1956, 1960, 1970) following cold injury was either due to leakage of proteins caused by release of these prostaglandins and thromboxanes, or secondarily due to white blood cell agglutination in the capillaries and increased hydrostatic pressure.

Table 26–1. Prostanoid Derivative Levels in Blister Fluid Aspirated from Ten Patients with Frostbite*

PGE_2	PGF_{2a}	TXB_2
<0.10	1.4	3.36
<0.10	<0.5	6.04
0.19	<0.5	0.40
0.24	10.1	2.95
0.27	4.7	4.56
0.40	<0.5	0.81
0.47	19.3	2.60
0.49	15.1	1.65
0.59	66.9	3.91
2.54	11.6	1.22

*Note the high levels of the vasoconstricting prostanoid PGF_{2a} and TXB_2. The values are expressed in ng per ml. (From Robson, M. C., and Heggers, J. P.: Evaluation of hand frostbite blister fluid as a clue to pathogenesis. J. Hand Surg., *6*:43, 1981.)

Raine and associates (1980) used the frostbite rabbit ear model to test the hypothesis that the progressive ischemia was secondary to release of inflammatory mediators. They demonstrated increased survival when the arachidonic acid cascade was blocked at all levels. The most marked tissue salvage resulted when specific thromboxane inhibitors were used. This has since been shown to be effective in the clinical situation and is discussed below.

Treatment

Treatment is directed at the specific pathophysiologic effects of the cold injury and thus is aimed at either blocking the direct cellular damage, preventing the progressive microvascular thrombosis and tissue loss, or correcting the residual defect. There is little role for emergency or prehospital management of patients with frostbite. Certainly most of the treatment regimens previously advocated have no role and are, indeed, contraindicated. Snow or ice should not be applied since these only worsen the injury. Partial slow warming by blankets is also injurious. Blisters should not be disrupted in any way before hospitalization.

Although the transport of patients to an appropriate care facility previously might have involved a delay of several hours, severe winter conditions and an appreciation by the public of the importance of the wind-chill index have served to increase the awareness of such injuries in urban emergency departments. An appropriate history should be obtained and during transport all exposed parts, particularly the extremities, should be elevated and kept elevated until arrival at the treating facility. Upon arrival, constricting or wet clothing should be removed from the injured parts. Since the injured areas are insensate, care should be taken to avoid further trauma. Smoking is prohibited. It is critically important to avoid refreezing after the part has been thawed. Mills, Whaley, and Fish (1961) stated that in such cases, when "freeze-thaw-freeze" cycles occur, the cumulative insult to tissue is considerably more severe. Direct cellular damage is treated by thawing rapidly with immersion in water warmed to between 104° and 108°F (40° and 42°C) (Knize, 1977). This is the single, unanimously agreed treatment for frostbite of all degrees. The narrow temperature range should be observed closely, because rewarming at lower temperatures is less beneficial for tissue survival (Fuhrman and Crismon, 1947); rewarming at higher temperatures may produce a burn injury and thus compound the injury (Mills, Whaley, and Fish, 1961). If the core body temperature is low, measures for the resuscitation of patients with systemic hypothermia should be undertaken, as described later in the chapter.

Pain experienced with thawing is usually severe, and a parenteral analgesic such as morphine is recommended if not contraindicated. The frozen extremities should remain in the water bath until the skin becomes erythematous at the most distal parts of the frostbite injury. Usually this takes less than 30 minutes. Active motion of the part during rewarming is helpful. The tissue will become soft to palpation, but care must be exercised not to massage the area, since this may introduce further injury. All nonfreezing cold injuries should be rewarmed to normal body temperatures. The physical appearance of the thawed tissue may provide a prognostic indication. Rapid return of skin warmth and sensation with the presence of an erythematous color is a favorable sign. The persistence of cold, anesthetic, and pale skin is unfavorable.

This type of rapid rewarming therapy reverses the ice crystal formation in the tissue. However, it does nothing for the progressive phase of the injury. Therefore, additional treatment is necessary to prevent progressive dermal ischemia and tissue loss. This consists of topical and systemic agents to minimize the production of thromboxane by the injured cells.

McCauley and associates (1983), designed a protocol, based on the pathophysiology of progressive dermal ischemia, which has been therapeutically successful. Following rapid rewarming, the clear or white blisters are debrided, because they have been shown to contain thromboxane. The deeper hemorrhagic blisters are aspirated of fluid, but not debrided. The remainder of the protocol incliudes the administration of tetanus prophylaxis, intravenous or intramuscular narcotics as needed, systemic aspirin, parenteral penicillin during the edema phase, topical treatment with an antithromboxane agent, and elevation of the injured part.

This protocol has proved useful and effective (Fig. 26–3). It is used in all but the most minor localized cold injuries. All but the most minor frostbite cases should also be admitted to the hospital. The most superficial injuries can occasionally be sent home after rapid rewarming. Even these injuries should be admitted if, after rewarming, a warm environment cannot be ensured for the patient. The patient should not be discharged from an emergency department into subfreezing weather. If a warm car is waiting, the patient is allowed to leave only after proper clothing has been obtained (e.g., stocking cap, wool mittens, wool socks, and so forth).

Most frostbite injuries require admission to the hospital, after which the complete protocol is carried out. The white blisters or clear blisters that represent the more superficial injury are debrided to prevent further contact of $PGF_{2\alpha}$ or thromboxane with the already damaged underlying tissues. Unlike the clear blisters, the hemorrhagic blisters represent structural damage to the subdermal plexus. It is appropriate to aspirate the thromboxane from these blisters, but to debride them would allow desiccation of the deep dermis and conversion to a full-thickness injury. Therefore, these blisters are left intact. A specific thromboxane inhibitor is then placed on the wounds to further prevent formation of this vasoconstricting mediator. Tetanus prophylaxis is given if indicated by the history. Tetanus was a common historical complication; thousands of Napoleon's soldiers in the Russian campaign died of this complication (Campbell, 1964). However, a 1985 report documented tetanus in a frostbite injury (Didlake and

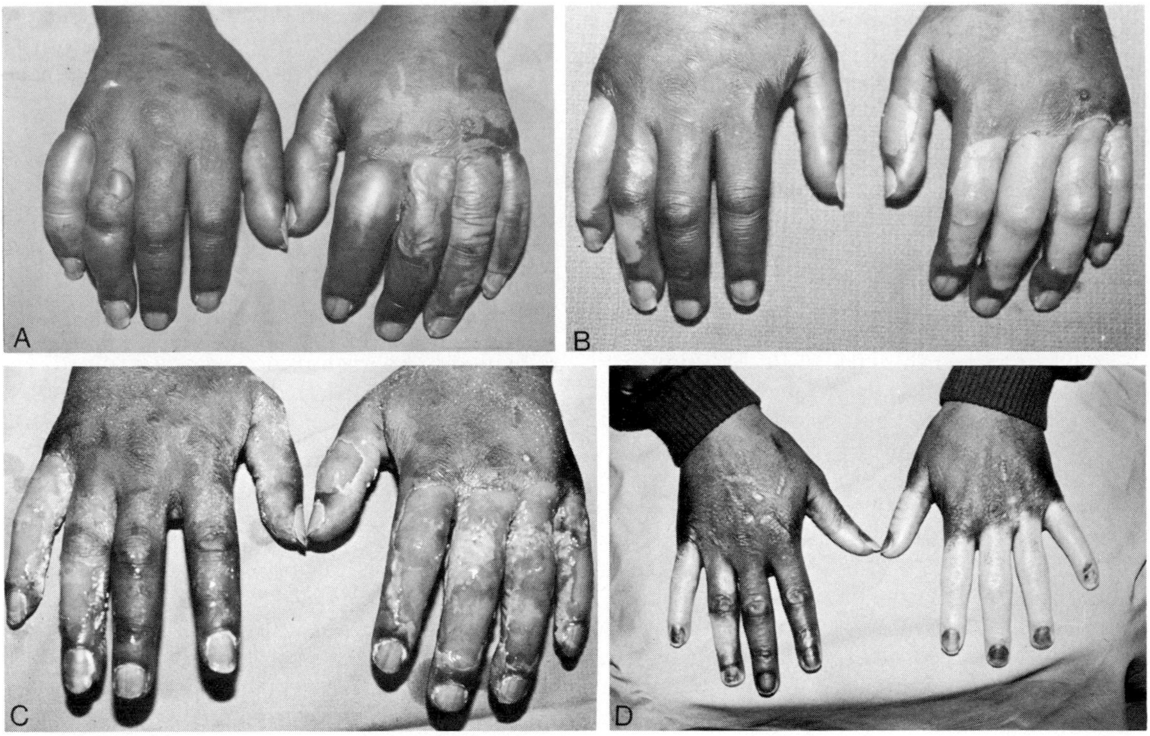

Figure 26–3. Patient treated with frostbite protocol. *A,* Appearance of hands on admission, demonstrating second degree frostbite. *B,* Appearance immediately following debridement. *C,* Following treatment with systemic antiprostaglandin and topical antithromboxane agent. *D,* Following healing. Note the areas of depigmented skin. (From McCauley, R. L., Hing, D. N., Robson, M. C., and Heggers, J. P.: Frostbite injuries: a rational approach based on the pathophysiology. J. Trauma, *23*:143, 1983. © by Williams & Wilkins, 1983.)

Kukora, 1985). Aspirin is given in this protocol as a means of systemically blocking further production of $PGF_{2\alpha}$ and thromboxane. It can be given in small doses to achieve the desired effects. Elevation is necessary as an attempt to minimize the edema; efforts to prevent edema formation by measures other than elevation have been successful. Since edema is known to inactivate the normal streptococcicidal properties of the skin, parenteral penicillin is given while the patient is in the edematous phase of the injury, to prevent streptococcal invasion.

Since frostbite generally involves injuries to the upper or lower extremities, appropriate physical therapy and occupational therapy are recommended. Daily hydrotherapy for active and passive range of motion has proved extremely valuable in the preservation of function.

Other therapeutic modalities have been tried in the attempt to prevent progressive thrombosis and tissue loss. Most of these were attempted before the pathophysiology of the injury with the inflammatory mediators had been elucidated. However, these therapeutic attempts deserve some comment. It has been noted that vessels, shortly after thawing, are dilated and filled with clumps of erythrocytes. These clumps can easily be dislodged by gentle manipulation, and therefore do not represent true thrombosis. Although the mechanism that leads to this erythrocyte clumping is not completely understood, it may reflect the presence of a cold induced increase in blood viscosity. This possibility suggests the use of low molecular weight dextran in the early treatment of cold injury. Although no controlled clinical trial of low molecular weight dextran has been reported, there has been experimental evidence to suggest its usefulness. It has been demonstrated that the use of 1 gm/kg per day of low molecular weight dextran protects against tissue loss in the rabbit ear model (Weatherly-White, Sjostrom, and Paton, 1964). This recommendation has led some to suggest giving 1 liter of 6 per cent dextran intravenously to patients on the day of injury, followed by 500 ml on each of the next five days (Robson, Krizek, and Wray, 1979).

Although true thrombi are not present in the dilated, erythrocyte filled vessels immediately after thawing, they do form over the next few days. This observation has led to the suggestion that heparin may be of use to treat frostbite. Lange and Loewe (1946) demonstrated its usefulness in experimental frostbite. Subsequent workers, however, have been unable to substantitate these findings and there is no current evidence that heparin alters the natural history of frostbite (Schumacker and associates, 1947).

Intra-arterial reserpine has also been shown experimentally to be of use in frostbite. Porter and associates (1976) reported its use in five patients, three of whom were treated within two weeks of their injuries. Angiography was performed both before and after injection. The reserpine appeared to be effective in relieving the vasospasm. However, the treatment had no effect on the progression of the cutaneous gangrene. Another study using reserpine compared slow rewarming combined with intravenous dextran, intra-arterial tolazoline, intra-arterial reserpine, and various combinations of these drugs (Snider and Porter, 1975). All the drug treatments were superior to simple slow rewarming. However, and most important, rapid rewarming was as effective as any of these drug therapies. Therefore, it appears that reserpine is possibly effective when patients present late and cannot be rapidly rewarmed immediately after injury. However, none of the anticoagulant or vasodilatation regimens has proved useful in controlled clinical trials.

Early surgical intervention has no role in the acute care of frostbite injuries unless there is ischemia from a constricting eschar or a subeschar infection that cannot be controlled by topical antimicrobials. Decompressing escharotomy incisions are rarely necessary to improve the distal circulation. If such escharotomies are necessary to decompress the digits and facilitate joint motion, incisions along the transaxial line are best employed. It is important that the incisions avoid injury to the underlying structures. If uncontrolled infection is present early, escharectomy may be necessary. However, this is rare with the use of penetrating antibacterials such as mafenide acetate.

Several reports from Europe and those after World War II supported the use of sympathetic block and sympathectomy (Robson, Krizek, and Wray, 1979). However, controversy continues about their role. If an influence of the sympathetic nervous system is involved, it seems reasonable that early sympathectomy would be beneficial. However, experimental evidence indicates that sympathectomy performed within the first few hours of injury increases edema formation and accelerates the pathologic process of tissue destruction (Golding and associates, 1963; Weatherly-White, Sjostrom, and Paton, 1964). On the other hand, in experimental injuries, sympathectomy performed 24 to 48 hours after thawing seems to hasten resolution of edema and decrease tissue loss (Golding and associates, 1963). It does seem significant that the precise role of sympathectomy remains poorly defined more than 45 years after Ducuing and associates (1940) reported the results of sympathetic nerve interruption in some 300 patients. This is due to both a lack of clinical means to evaluate the results and a lack of agreement on the rationale for the use of sympathectomy in frostbite injuries.

Surgical intervention is more properly reserved for later in the treatment of frostbite. Today this is most frequently seen if the frostbite is very severe or if treatment has been delayed. Otherwise the therapeutic measures outlined above should be sufficient to prevent progressive injury and gangrene. If gangrene ensues, amputation or debridement with resurfacing may be necessary, but should be done only after the area has been well demarcated. Aggressive early debridement or attempted salvage may jeopardize recovering tissue and add to the amount of tissue loss. Reconstructive procedures have no place before amputation or resurfacing with a skin graft.

Late Sequelae

Until 1957, little was recorded about the long-term sequelae of frostbite injuries. At that time, Blair, Schatzki and Orr (1957) studied 100 veterans of the Korean conflict followed for at least four years after their injuries. They reported the following chronic symptoms, in order of decreasing frequency: excessive sweating, pain, coldness, numbness, abnormal skin color, and joint stiffness. In addition, abnormalities of the nails, including ridging and inward curving of the edges, were observed. In general, the degree of long-term disability was related to the severity of the original injury, and the symptoms were more prominent in cold than in warm weather. The latter finding could be attributed to the fact that the ability of vessels to react to stress is diminished. In the study of Simeone (1960), previously injured blood vessels did not constrict as effectively as normal vessels when exposed to cold, and did not dilate as effectively when vasoconstriction was blocked.

It is likely that hyperhidrosis is both a cause and a result of cold injury. Hyperhidrosis suggests the presence of an abnormal sympathetic nervous system induced by cold injury and, in fact is abolished by sympathetic denervation. Sensitivity to cold and the predisposition to recurrent cold injury are, in some ways, analogous to the consideration of hyperhidrosis. Blanching and pain upon subsequent cold exposure may be troublesome or so dramatic as to suggest a diagnosis of Raynaud's phenomenon. Almost without exception, a painful, shiny, cyanotic, sweaty limb becomes a warm, dry, and useful extremity with sympathetic interruption. However, it seems unwarranted to conclude that this is necessarily a manifestation of an abnormality in the sympathetic nervous system, since hyperhidrosis and cold sensitivity are just as likely to precede the injury (Blair, Schatzki, and Orr, 1957).

The late abnormalities of change in skin color, including depigmentation in blacks and an appearance resembling erythrocyanosis in Caucasians, are most likely the result of ischemia (Blair, Schatzki, and Orr, 1957). Similarly, the abnormality of the nails is comparable with that observed with ischemia, regardless of the cause. Neither of these sequelae usually requires treatment.

Late symptoms of joint stiffness and pain on motion are relatively common, and undoubtedly are related to the underlying scars and to mechanical problems occasioned by the variety of amputations required. However, Blair, Schatzki, and Orr (1957) noted "punched out" defects in the subchondral bone of the involved limbs. These localized areas of bone resorption generally appear within five to ten months after injury and may heal spontaneously. Vascular occlusion was thought the most likely cause of the lesions. These bone changes, in close proximity to joint surfaces, may help to explain the joint symptoms.

The effects of frostbite on premature closure of the epiphyses in the growing hand has been reemphasized (Wenzl, Burke, and Bianco, 1967). The extent of premature closure was correlated with the severity of the frostbite, but it was also noted in partial-thickness injuries. In the digits, premature closure was more frequent from a distal to proximal direction (DIP > PIP > MP). The thumb was less often involved. In only 2 per cent did partial epiphyseal closure cause an angular deformity.

One of the characteristic features of frostbite is the surprising salvage possible in an apparently badly injured extremity. Amputation therefore should be performed with caution and deferred as long as possible. The line of demarcation may not be decided definitively for weeks or months after injury. As long as secondary sepsis does not intervene, patience often rewards the patient and the surgeon with the maximal surviving length of the limb.

SYSTEMIC HYPOTHERMIA: GENERALIZED COLD INJURY

Hypothermia becomes significant only when environmental exposures cause body temperature to fall below 35°C (95°F). Such exposures are relatively common and often fatal, most likely because they are unrecognized. Many diseases predispose to or abet the development of hypothermia: erythroderma, Paget's disease, malnutrition, central or peripheral thermoregulatory failure, poisoning, diabetes mellitus, and anemia (Pratt, 1980).

The temperature of the vital organs, as distinguished from the temperature of the extremities, is known as the *core temperature*. The vital organs, the contents of the skull, thorax, and abdomen, constitute the core of the body, and the extremities and surface of the body make up the shell. The temperature of the hypothalamus is the true core temperature (Pratt, 1980). When the core temperature drops below 35°C (95°F), an individual is considered to be in a hypothermic state.

Diagnosis can be made quickly, easily, and accurately by using a low temperature (subnormal) thermometer, placed either in the rectum or in freshly voided or catheterized urine.

History

As early as 1880 a Russian called Laptschinsky first proposed the use of rapid rewarming in "hot water" as a treatment for systemic hypothermia (Alexander, 1945, 1946). The infamous German experiments during World War II, as reported by Alexander (1945, 1946), clearly demonstrated the effectiveness of warm water baths to resuscitate those with hypothermia. Reports in the nonmedical literature have chronicled episodes in wars or disasters such as the sinking of the Titanic (Zingg, 1967). Pugh (1966) reported several deaths due to hypothermia in young hikers in Great Britain. Rapid bath rewarming was promoted for accidental hypothermia (Golden, 1973; Mills, 1976). In 1973, research scientists in Great Britain estimated that 10 per cent of the elderly population had suffered from chronic hypothermia (Irvine, 1973).

The reported incidence of hypothermia has increased as physicians and the public have become more aware of its possibility. Fuel shortages, increased age of the general population, exposure to cold environment, increased participation in winter sports and other outdoor activities, and immersion in cold water are factors that increase the incidence of hypothermia. In any of these situations or activities, protective clothing and body thermal regulatory mechanisms fail to retain body heat adequately.

Not unlike localized cold injury, systemic hypothermia may be divided into three categories: chronic, subacute, and acute. *Chronic hypothermia* results from exposure to a cold environment for extended periods. Elderly people attempting to conserve fuel and children under the age of 1 year are prime candidates. The metabolism of the elderly is slower and they cannot maintain a normal temperature when subjected to an environment below 18°C (64°F) (Pratt, 1980). These patients present as cold, slow-moving individuals who are often semiconscious. The face may be swollen and pink, the pulse slow and weak, the blood pressure low, and the cardiac rhythm irregular. The elderly hypothermia patient rarely shivers. The symptoms are such that a physician may believe the patient is having or has had a stroke, has Parkinson's disease, or has cardiac complications.

Subacute hypothermia occurs in patients suffering from cold exposure: for example, someone who has spent a winter night outdoors after a fall while inebriated or when involved in a skiing accident, with a core temperature below 33°C (91.4°F). The condition is seen in a very cold patient who may or may not be shivering, may or may not be conscious, and may have any or all of the following: low blood pressure, slurred speech, shallow breathing, cardiac arrhythmia, focal weakness, dilated pupils, ataxic gate, and sensory loss (Pratt, 1980). Because of the varied symptomatology associated with hypothermia, patients under treatment for other conditions, who also have been exposed to cold, should be evaluated for the presence of an abnormally low core temperature.

Acute hypothermia is a term generally reserved for cases of immersion in cold water, below 21°C (70°F) (Pratt, 1980). Although humans can become hypothermic when exposed to a water temperature of 21°C, acute hypothermia is usually seen after exposure to water below 10°C (50°F). The resultant quick cooling of the body does not allow time for development of the dramatic electrolyte imbalance present in chronic and subacute hypothermia. These victims become quickly immobilized and have reduced respiratory and metabolic rates, temporarily increased urine output, and a low level of consciousness.

As the exterior of the body cools, vasoconstriction reduces blood flow to the limbs. This life-saving mechanism of the body renders the limbs useless after a short time. Such vasoconstriction is a part of the mammalian diving reflex, which slows many body functions when cold water or air makes contact with the bridge of the nose (Pratt, 1980). It is one reason that near-drowning victims may be revived after long immersion with no permanent brain damage.

As body temperature falls, the victim becomes unconscious, physiologic activity slows, and cellular metabolism is greatly reduced. Because of reduced cardiac output, in addition to reduced pulmonary and renal function, the patient may be pronounced dead, when in reality he has severe but reversible bradycardia. The body size, fat content, time of cold exposure, and type of protective clothing are all factors that influence the rate of cooling. For this reason, the length of time during which a person may be immersed and still survive varies.

Table 26–2. Physiologic Responses to Decreasing Body Temperature*

Temperature and Zones	Level of Consciousness	Voluntary Movements	Muscle Tone	Reflexes	Electrical Activity: Cardiac	Electrical Activity: Brain	Hemodynamics	Renal Function	Respiration and Metabolism
Safe									
37°–35° C 98.6°–95.0° F	Normal		Shivering	Vessel constriction	Amplitude of ECG falls as temperature decreases		Heart rate rises, blood pressure rises, cardiac output increases	Increased renal function	Both increase
34°–33° C 93.2°–91.4° F	Normal, some amnesia	Ataxic gait; pain readily appreciated		Hoffmann's sign; ankle clonus present				Urine flow increases 1.002–1.006 specific gravity	
Transitional									
33°–32° C 91.4°–89.6° F	Some dysarthria		Aggressive shivering	Maximum shivering					Both decrease, respiration shallow
32°–31° C 89.6°–87.8° F				Exaggerated tendon reflex	Pathognomonic "J" wave associated with QRS complex		Cardiac output 30% below normal		
31°–30° C 87.8°–86.0° F	Stuporous; may recognize relations and friends	Slow movements and delayed reactions	Shivering	Less hyperactive, more lethargic as temperature drops			Heart rate decreases, prolonged systole		
30°–29° C 86.0°–84.2°F			Shivering ceases	Hoffmann's sign; ankle clonus absent		Appearance of large amplitude slow delta wave		Renal blood flow decreased by 50%, urine output decreased	

Danger									
29°–28° C 84.2°–82.4° F	Simple questions can be answered	Little voluntary motion except eye tracking	Spontaneous or provoked myoclonus and facial spasm start	Abdominal reflex sluggish		Appearance of theta activity followed by disorganized high voltage activity		Urine output 1–3 ml/min	Production of CO_2 severely reduced
28°–27° C 82.4°–80.6° F	Only grunts and groans	Limbs move to noxious stimuli		Pupil responds to light only slightly; equal and normal	Arterial dysrhythmias		Arterial blood pressure normal		Basal metabolic rate falls 50%; apnea present
27°–26° C 80.6°–78.8° F	Fails to speak	Movement replaced with rigor		Pupil miotic response to light, plantar response disappears, gag reflex lost, deep tendon reflex lost	Ventricular fibrillation or standstill		Decreased cardiac output, blood pressure drops severely		
26°–24° C 78.8°–75.2° F	Unconsciousness	None		Corneal reflex disappears					
24°–23°C 75.2°–73.4°F									
20°–15°C 68.0°–59.0° F						Paroxysmal spike activity present			

*As depicted by Pratt, R. S.: Hypothermia: the chill that need not kill. Bull. Am. Coll. Surg., *65*:28, 1980.

Pathophysiology

The first and earliest physiologic changes associated with hypothermia consist of peripheral vasoconstriction. The result is an increase in cardiac activity, blood volume in the core, renal output, and respiratory and metabolic rates. As the low temperature persists and decreases, depression of cerebral, renal, cardiac, respiratory, and metabolic functions follows until they virtually cease.

After the initial increase in respiratory rate and tidal volume, respiration is inexorably decreased as core temperature falls (Pratt, 1980). The heart initially attempts to compensate for the loss of body heat by increasing the cardiac rate, stroke volume, and blood pressure. As the core temperature decreases, cardiac rate, stroke volume, and blood pressure decrease. "J" waves, which are typical of hypothermia, appear on an electrocardiogram at 89.6° to 87.8°F (Pratt, 1980).

Hypovolemia is the immediate result of hypothermia as fluid from the vascular component moves into the extracellular compartment, expands the extracellular fluid volume, and produces generalized edema. The hemoglobin concentration increases briefly during this time, but then falls steadily during the remaining period as a result of hemodilution association with the redistribution of extracellular fluid to the vascular compartments (Pratt, 1980). White blood cell counts fall in direct relation to the reduction of body temperature. The differential count in the response to infection remains unimpaired. Platelet counts fall during hypothermia, but are quickly restored during rewarming. Coagulation is impaired during hypothermia, but this deficiency disappears on rewarming.

Cold diuresis results from the increased renal perfusion that occurs when vasoconstriction shunts blood from the shell to the core. The rise in cardiac output and in blood pressure increases the perfusion, but as the core temperature falls further and cardiac output is lowered, renal filtration also decreases (Pratt, 1980).

Three phases or zones of progressive hypothermia are clinically recognized: (1) at the rectal temperature of 33° to 37°C (91.4° to 98.6°F), thermal regulatory mechanisms act against continued chilling by promoting shivering, increasing the pulse rate and blood pressure, and constricting the skin capillaries (Table 26–2); (2) at 29° to 33°C (84.2° to 91.4°F), the general body tissue metabolic rate is depressed, while the pulse rate, blood pressure, and respiratory rate progressively decrease as body temperature falls; and (3) below 29°C or 84.2°F, cardiac arrhythmias frequently occur. Finally, when the core temperature is lower than 24°C (75°F), temperature regulatory centers cease to function, and heat is lost as from an inanimate object (Hervey, 1973; Pratt, 1980).

The symptoms of mild hypothermia are subtle: they may appear in association with other symptoms or mimic a completely different illness. Cardiac arrhythmia is suggestive of heart failure; low levels of consciousness may indicate head trauma; a stumbling gait may lead one to suspect central nervous system disorders. All these symptoms may be the result of hypothermia alone. Lack of shivering should not preclude consideration of a diagnosis of hypothermia, because many people, especially the elderly, do not shiver even when their temperature has dropped below 32°C (89.0° to 84.2°F).

At 35° to 33°C (95° to 91.4°F), the patient is usually alert, cooperative, and well oriented (Pratt, 1980) (Table 26–2). As the core temperature falls below 34° to 33°C (93.2° to 91.4°F), the patient becomes drowsy, has increasing difficulty in understanding and responding, and has great difficulty in speaking. Amnesia usually occurs when the temperature falls below 32°C (89.6°F), although conscious responses may occur at this level. At 34° to 32°C (93.2° to 89.6°F), dysarthria is a striking sign. At 31° to 30°C (87.8° to 86.0°F), the patient is stuporous but can be aroused to answer simple questions, although speech has deteriorated. At 29° to 28°C (84.2° to 82.4°F), the patient can still answer questions, but usually only after long delay. At 27° to 26°C (80.6° to 78.8°F), only groaning responses are made, and below 26° (78.8°F), consciousness is usually lost.

The skin of a hypothermic victim has a cadaveric pallor and patchy mottling over dependent areas. Edema in the subcutaneous tissue causes turgor and puffiness of the face. Bradycardia is often present. The gastrointestinal tract is less active, and bowel sounds and peristalsis are commonly absent. Polyuria is present but is replaced by oliguria, which is seen late in the more acute stage.

Treatment

Immediately upon admission to the emergency department, the core temperature of any patient suspected of being hypothermic is obtained. A laboratory thermometer or thermocouple probe reading to 20°C (68°F) is used, since the routine clinical thermometer is not calibrated below 34°C (93.2°F). All patients with a rectal temperature below 34°C (93.2°F) are entered into the hypothermia treatment protocol and the resuscitation team is notified (Frank and Robson, 1980). The airway is secured, as needed, and any cold or wet clothing is cut away with a minimum of disturbance to the patient. The leads of a portable electrocardiographic monitor with defibrillator unit are applied, and urinary and central venous pressure catheters are inserted. Baseline arterial blood gases and serum electrolyte levels are obtained and any acidosis or arrhythmias are treated. A rapid physical examination is performed to determine any associated injury or disease. Family, friends, and police or paramedics who deliver the patient are occasionally able to provide useful information.

Within 15 minutes, the patient is transferred to an area for rapid rewarming. This is most often and conveniently in a hospital burn center that has a Hubbard tank available for patient immersion (Fig. 26–4). The tank should be filled at the time when the resuscitation team was notified by the emergency department. The water should be at 40°C (104° to 105°F). The ECG leads and wires are left attached to the patient and continue to function. The platform supporting the patient in the water is left attached to a mechanical hoist in case the patient needs rapid removal.

Arterial blood gases, corrected for patient temperature, are measured at 15 minute intervals, and sodium bicarbonate is given as necessary to treat the acidosis. Balanced electrolyte sodium is given rapidly to maintain a urinary output between 30 and 50 ml per hour. Blood pressure and pulse are monitored, and serve as additional aids for the adequacy of the fluid and temperature resuscitation. Central venous pressure is usually low and is monitored only to protect against a rapid increase if overhydration or pulmonary edema develop. A Swan-Ganz catheter gives more information but has not been needed in reported series; the added time required for insertion does not seem to justify its routine use (Frank and Robson, 1980; Zachary and associates, 1982). Cardiac arrhythmias are treated as needed, but are usually self-correcting as the temperature begins to rise. When the core temperature reaches 37°C (98.6°F), which may take between one and three hours, the patient is removed from the warming tank, placed in an intensive care unit, and monitored for the next 24 to 48 hours. Associated injuries and medical problems are treated as necessary. Frequently, when the initial laboratory results are obtainable, the blood glucose may be low. This

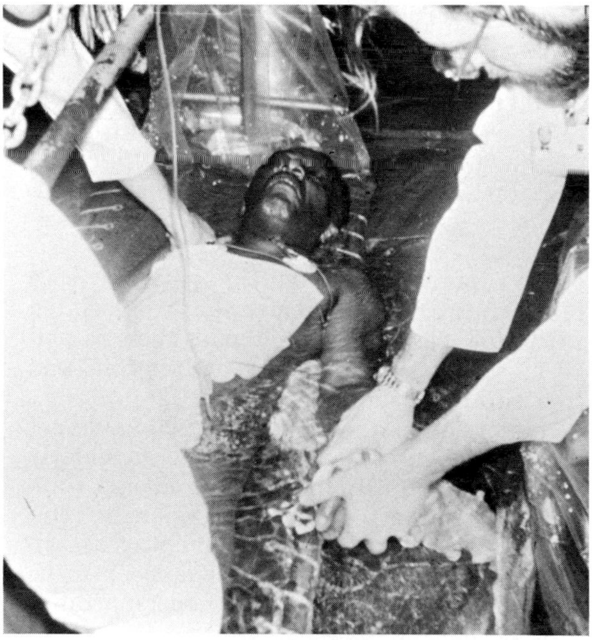

Figure 26–4. Example of a patient in a Hubbard tank undergoing rapid immersion rewarming according to the hypothermia protocol.

can be corrected with rapid intravenous administration of 50 per cent glucose.

Controversy exists with regard to the optimal core rewarming techniques. Weyman and associates (1974) found that in the presence of an underlying disease, the mortality rate was 75 per cent. On the other hand, Frank and Robson (1980) and Zachary and associates (1982) reported a mortality rate of less than 4 per cent with rapid immersion rewarming.

Concern about external rewarming centers on two issues: (1) the "afterdrop" phenomenon and (2) vascular collapse secondary to hypovolemia. None of the patients in the two series reported by the author (Frank and Robson, 1980; Zachary and associates, 1982) experienced any clinically apparent afterdrop. The mechanism of the afterdrop has been postulated to be the result of shunting of cold blood to the core, with a paradoxical drop in core temperature following peripheral vasodilatation with external rewarming. Cardiac arrhythmias have been described as a consequence of this phenomenon. In a study performed on volunteers, afterdrop was shortest in patients treated with trunk immersion, probably because immersion rapidly reheats the core as well as the external surface, as shown by rectal and esophageal thermometers (Zachary and associates, 1982). No patients in the two reported series developed ventricular fibrillation during resuscitation, suggesting that there is little clinical correlation with temperature afterdrop. All patients underwent central venous pressure monitoring as a guide for fluid replacement. Resuscitation with balanced salt solution, titrated for urine output, was used to avoid the relative hypovolemia associated with rewarming and vasodilatation. Dopamine was introduced for inotropic support when needed, but only after satisfactory volume replacement had been achieved.

By rapidly correcting the patient's core temperature, the problems usually associated with slow rewarming methods, such as acidosis and hypoxemia, were minimized and treated appropriately.

Immersion rewarming proved effective not only in young patients but also in elderly victims with multiple medical problems. Rapidly rewarming patients to physiologic temperatures facilitates the treatment of associated medical problems, which appear to be the major cause of morbidity and mortality in hypothermic patients.

For opponents of rapid rewarming by immersion, internal rewarming has been suggested. Theoretically, rewarming "internally" should eliminate the problem of peripheral vasodilatation. Internal rewarming has been attempted in a variety of ways, including thoracotomy and direct warming of the mediastinum with heated physiologic solution (Linton and Ledingham, 1966) and peritoneal dialysis with warm solutions (Grossheim, 1973). Other methods attempted have been extracorporeal circulation systems, incorporating a heat exchanger with either hemodialysis equipment (Davies, Millar, and Miller, 1967) or cardiopulmonary bypass equipment (Towne and associates, 1972) and centripetal carotid infusion (Rogers and Hillman, 1970). Inhalation of heated gases administered with anesthesiology equipment has also been used (Henderson and Pettigrew, 1971). The advantage of the latter technique is that it can be carried out with portable equipment, and theoretically can be initiated before the patient is transferred to a hospital facility, while at the same time providing oxygen. Respiratory assistance with oxygen is important during rewarming. Stewart and Hillman (1972) concluded that the most critical defect in the hypothermic patient is hypoxemia from respiratory depression, and correction of this state should be begun at the earliest possible time. It has been reported that once the blood has been oxygenated, the rewarming rate can proceed as fast as is convenient (Hillman, 1971). Therefore, if warm oxygen is started before hospitalization, it should be possible to carry out rapid rewarming as soon as the diagnosis is made.

Late Sequelae

Zingg (1967) has documented late complications after successful rewarming of hypothermic patients. He reported the possibility of subsequent renal failure and death several days after normal body temperature had been reached. He stated that bronchopneumonia was the contributing factor to these late deaths in some individuals, but in others the cause of death was unknown. In the two series reviewed by the author (Frank and Robson, 1980; Zachary and associates, 1982), these observations were not made. Patients who survive the rapid immersion rewarming did amazingly well. The occasional late death was secondary to the associated medical conditions that contributed to the hypothermia. Certainly, in many of these patients, septic conditions are the inciting cause of the hypothermia, and need to be diagnosed and treated accordingly. Tuberculosis has often been present. However, if the associated medical conditions are successfully treated, there are remarkably few sequelae secondary to the hypothermic state. The central nervous system appears to function quite well despite prolonged periods of apparent death at the time of initial presentation (Zingg, 1967).

COMBINED FROSTBITE AND SYSTEMIC HYPOTHERMIA

A final word is needed about the few patients who present with both localized (frostbite) and generalized (systemic hypothermia) cold injuries. If the primary treatment techniques recommended in this chapter are used for each of the injuries, there is no specific problem when they occur in combination. Rapid rewarming is the first treatment for the local cold injury, and if it is also used for generalized systemic hypothermia, the patient receives treatment for both conditions simultaneously. Following a rapid rewarming, the systemic hypothermic patient is placed in an intensive care unit, and the frostbite protocol can be used for local injuries. The associated medical conditions may prohibit as vigorous a physical and occupational therapy protocol as might be carried out without these conditions; otherwise, the treatment regimen should be the same. If the associated conditions require strict bed rest in the intensive care unit, bedside physical therapy is necessary to maintain range of motion of the locally injured part.

REFERENCES

Alexander, L.: The treatment of shock from prolonged exposure to cold, especially in water. Item No. 24, File No. XXVI-37 (Combined intelligence objectives Subcommittee, U. S. Army, July 1945), also Report No. 250, Office of the Publication Board, Department of Commerce, Washington, DC, 1946.

Bellman, S., and Adams-Ray, J.: Vascular reactions after experimental cold injury. Angiology, 7:339, 1956.

Blair, J. R., Schatzki, R., and Orr, K. D.: Sequelae to cold injury in one hundred patients: follow-up study four years after occurrence of cold injury. J.A.M.A., *163*:1203, 1957.

Boswick, J. A., Jr.: Cold injuries. *In* Salisbury, R. E., and Pruitt, B. A. (Eds.): Burns of the Upper Extremity. Philadelphia, W. B. Saunders Company, 1976, p. 96.

Campbell, R.: General outcooling and local frostbite. *In* Viereck, E. (Ed.): Proceedings Symposia on Arctic Biology and Medicine. IV. Frostbite. Fort Wainwright, Alaska, Arctic Aeromedical Laboratory, 1964, p. 254.

Davies, D. M., Millar, E. J., and Miller, I. A.: Accidental hypothermia treated by extracorporeal blood-warming. Lancet, *1*:1036, 1967.

Didlake, R. H., and Kukora, J. S.: Tetanus following frostbite injury. Contemporary Orthopaedics, 10:69, 1985.

Ducuing, J., D'Harcourt, J., Folch, A., and Bofill, J.: Les troubles trophiques des produits par de froid sec en pathologie de guerre. J. Chir., *55*:385, 1940.

Frank, D. H., and Robson, M. C.: Accidental hypothermia treated without mortality. Surg. Gynecol. Obstet., 151:379, 1980.

Fuhrman, F. A., and Crismon, J. M.: Studies on gangrene following cold injury. VII. Treatment of cold injury by immediate rapid warming. J. Clin. Invest., *26*:476, 1947.

Golden, F. S.: Proceedings: Recognition and treatment of immersion hypothermia. Proc. R. Soc. Med., *66*:1058, 1973.

Golding, M. R., De Jong, P., Sawyer, P. N., et al.: Protection from early and late sequelae of frostbite by regional sympathectomy: mechanism of "cold sensitivity" following frostbite. Surgery, *53*:303, 1963.

Greenfield, A. D. M., Shepherd, J. T., and Whelan, R. F.: Cold vasoconstriction and vasodilatation. Ir. J. Med. Sci., *309*:415, 1951.

Grossheim, R. L.: Hypothermia and frostbite treated with peritoneal dialysis. Alaska Med., *15*:53, 1973.

Henderson, M. A., and Pettigrew, R. T.: Induction of controlled hyperthermia in treatment of cancer. Lancet, *1*:1275, 1971.

Hervey, G. R.: Physiological changes encountered in hypothermia. Proc. R. Soc. Med., *66*:1053, 1973.

Hillman, H.: Treatment after exposure to cold. Lancet, *2*:1257, 1971.

Irvine, R. E.: Hypothermia. Modern Geriatrics, *3*:464, 1973.

Johnson, B. E., and Daniels, F., Jr.: Enzyme studies in experimental cryosurgery of the skin. Cryobiology, *11*:222, 1974.

Kinmouth, J. B., Rob, C. G., and Simeone, F. B.: The cryopathies. *In* Vascular Surgery. London, E. Arnold, 1962, pp. 164–182.

Knize, D. M.: Cold injury. *In* Converse, J. M. (Ed.): Reconstructive Plastic Surgery. Vol. 1. Philadelphia, W. B. Saunders Company, 1977, p. 516.

Knize, D. M., Weatherly-White, R. C., Paton, B. C., and Owens, J. C.: Prognostic factors in the management of frostbite. J. Trauma, *9*:749, 1969.

Kulka, J. P.: Histopathologic studies in frostbitten rabbits. *In* Ferrer, M. I. (Ed.): Cold Injury. New York, Josiah Macy, Jr., Foundation, 1956, p. 97.

Kulka, J. P.: Microcirculatory impairment as a factor in inflammatory tissue damage. Ann. N.Y. Acad. Sci., *116*:1018, 1964.

Lange, K., and Loewe, L.: Subcutaneous heparin in the pitkin menstruum for the treatment of experimental human frostbite. Surg. Gynecol. Obstet., 82:256, 1946.

Larrey, D. J.: Memoirs of Military Surgery. Vol. II. Baltimore, Joseph Cushing, 1814, pp. 156–164.

Lawrence, W. T., Murphy, R. C., Robson, M. C., and Heggers, J. P.: The detrimental effect of cigarette

smoking on flap survival: an experimental study in the rat. Br. J. Plast. Surg., *37*:216, 1984.
Lewis, R. B.: The Wellcome Prize Essay for 1951. Local cold injury—frostbite. Military Surgeon, *110*:25, 1952.
Linton, A. L., and Ledingham, I. M.: Severe hypothermia with barbiturate intoxication. Lancet, *1*:24, 1966.
Lovelock, J. E.: Physical instability and thermal shock in red blood cells. Nature, *173*:659, 1954.
Lovelock, J. E.: The denaturation of lipid-protein complexes as a cause of damage by freezing. Proc. R. Soc. Biol., *147*:427, 1957.
Markert, C. L.: Lactate dehydrogenase isozymes: dissociation and recombination of subunits. Science, *140*:1329, 1963.
Mazur, P.: Studies on rapidly frozen suspensions of yeast cells by differential thermal analysis and conductometry. Biophys. J., *3*:323, 1963.
Mazur, P.: Causes of injury in frozen and thawed cells. Fed. Proc., *24*:(Suppl. 15):5–175, 1965.
McCauley, R. L., Hing, D. N., Robson, M. C., and Heggers, J. P.: Frostbite injuries: a rational approach based on the pathophysiology. J. Trauma, *23*:143, 1983.
Merryman, H. T.: Mechanisms of freezing in living cells and tissues. Science, *124*:515, 1956.
Merryman, H. T.: General principles of freezing and freezing injury in cellular materials. Ann. N.Y. Acad. Sci., *85*:503, 1960.
Merryman, H. T.: The exceeding of a minimum tolerable cell volume in hypertonic suspension as a cause of freezing injury. *In* Walstenhome, G., and O'Connor, M. (Eds.): The Frozen Cell. London, Churchill, 1970, p. 51.
Mills, W. J.: Out in the cold. Emerg. Med., *8*:134, 1976.
Mills, W. J., and Whaley, R.: Frostbite: a method of management. *In* Viereck, E. G. (Ed.): Proceedings Symposia on Arctic Biology and Medicine. IV. Frostbite. Fort Wainwright, Alaska, Arctic Aeromedical Laboratory, 1964, p. 127.
Mills, W. J., Whaley, R., and Fish, W.: Frostbite: experience with rapid rewarming and ultrasonic therapy. Alaska Med., *3*:28, 1961.
Moran, T.: Critical temperature of freezing living muscle. Proc. R. Soc. Biol., *105*:177, 1929.
Orr, K. D., and Fainer, D. C.: Cold injuries in Korea during the winter of 1950–1951. Medicine, *31*:177, 1952.
Porter, J. M., Wesche, D. H., Rosch, J., and Baur, G. M.: Intra-arterial sympathetic blockade in the treatment of clinical frostbite. Am. J. Surg., *132*:625, 1976.
Pratt, R. S.: Hypothermia: the chill that need not kill. Bull. Am. Coll. Surg., *65*:28, 1980.
Pugh, L. G.: Accidental hypothermia in walkers, climbers, and campers: report to the Medical Commission on Accident Prevention. Br. Med. J., *1*:123, 1966.
Rabb, J. M., Renaud, M. L., Brandt, P. A., and Witt, C. W.: Effect of freezing and thawing on the microcirculation and capillary endothelium of the hamster cheek pouch. Cryobiology, *11*:508, 1974.
Raine, T. J., London, M. D., Goluch, L., Heggers, J. P., and Robson, M. C.: Antiprostaglandins and antithromboxanes for treatment of frostbite. Surg. Forum, *31*:557, 1980.
Rinfret, A. P.: Cryobiology. *In* Vavice, R. W. (Ed.): Cryogenic Technology. New York, John Wiley & Sons, 1962, pp. 528, 577.
Robson, M. C., and Heggers, J. P.: Evaluation of hand frostbite blister fluid as a clue to pathogenesis. J. Hand Surg., *6*:43, 1981.
Robson, M. C., Krizek, T. J., and Wray, R. C., Jr.: Care of the thermally injured patient. *In* Zuidema, G. D., Rutherford, R. B., and Ballinger, W. F., II (Eds.): The Management of Trauma. 3rd Ed. Philadelphia, W. B. Saunders Company, 1979, p. 666.
Rogers, P., and Hillman, H.: Increased recovery of anaesthetized hypothermic rats induced by intracarotid infusion. Nature (Lond.), *228*:1314, 1970.
Schumacker, H. B., White, B. H., Wrenn, E. L., Cordell, A. R., and Sanford, T. F.: Studies in experimental frostbite—I. The effect of heparin in preventing gangrene. Surgery, *22*:900, 1947.
Shikama, K., and Yamazaki, I.: Denaturation of catalase by freezing and thawing. Nature (Lond.), *190*:83, 1961.
Simeone, F. A.: Surgical volumes of the history of the United States Army Medical Department in World War II. Cold injury. Arch. Surg., 80:396, 1960.
Snider, R. L., and Porter, J. M.: Treatment of experimental frostbite with intra-arterial sympathetic blocking drugs. Surgery, *77*:557, 1975.
Stewart, T., and Hillman, H.: Treatment after exposure to cold. Lancet, *1*:140, 1972.
Stowell, R. E., Young, D. E., Arnold, E. A., and Trump, B. F.: Structural, chemical, physical, and functional alterations in mammalian nucleus following different conditions of freezing, storage and thawing. Fed. Proc., *24*(Suppl. 15):S-115, 1965.
Towne, W. D., Geiss, W. P., Yanes, H. O., and Rahimtoola, S. H.: Intractable ventricular fibrillation associated with profound accidental hypothermia—successful treatment with partial cardiopulmonary bypass. N. Engl. J. Med., *287*:1135, 1972.
Washburn, B.: Frostbite. N. Engl. J. Med., *266*:974, 1962.
Weatherly-White, R. C. A., Sjostrom, B., and Paton, B. C.: Experimental studies in cold injury. J. Surg. Res., *4*:17, 1964.
Wenzl, J. E., Burke, E. C., and Bianco, A. J., Jr.: Epiphyseal destruction from frostbite of the hands. Am. J. Dis. Child., *114*:668, 1967.
Weyman, A. E., Greenbaum, D. M., and Grace, W. J.: Accidental hypothermia in an alcoholic population. Am. J. Med., *56*:13, 1974.
Whayne, T. F., and DeBakey, M. F.: Cold Injury, Ground Type. Washington, U.S. Government Printing Office, 1958.
White, J. C., and Scoville, W. B.: Trench foot and immersion foot. N. Engl. J. Med., *232*:415, 1945.
Zacarian, S. A.: Cryogenics: the cryolesion and the pathogenesis of cryoneerosis. *In* Zacarian, S. A. (Ed.): Cryosurgery for Skin and Cutaneous Disorders. St. Louis, MO, C. V. Mosby Company, 1985.
Zacarian, S. A., Stone, D., and Clater, M.: Effects of cryogenic temperatures in the microcirculation in the golden hamster cheek pouch. Cryobiology, *7*:27, 1970.
Zachary, L., Kucan, J. O., Robson, M. C., and Frank, D. H.: Accidental hypothermia treated with rapid rewarming by immersion. Ann. Plast. Surg., *9*:238, 1982.
Zingg, W.: The management of accidental hypothermia. Can. Med. Assoc. J., *96*:214, 1967.

Index

Note: Page numbers in *italics* refer to illustrations; page number followed by *t* refer to tables.